MAGNETIC RESONANCE
OF THE SPINE

MAGNETIC RESONANCE OF THE SPINE

Dieter R. Enzmann, M.D.
Professor (Neuroradiology)
Director of MRI
Department of Diagnostic Radiology and Nuclear Medicine
Division of Diagnostic Radiology
Stanford University School of Medicine
Stanford, California

Robert L. DeLaPaz, M.D.
Assistant Professor of Radiology
Neuroradiology
Department of Diagnostic Radiology and Nuclear Medicine
Division of Diagnostic Radiology
Stanford University School of Medicine
Stanford, California

Jeremy B. Rubin, M.D.
Co-director
Magnetic Resonance Imaging
Department of Diagnostic Imaging
The Good Samaritan Hospital of Santa Clara Valley
San Jose, California

With 1645 illustrations

The C.V. Mosby Company
St. Louis Baltimore Philadelphia Toronto 1990

Mosby

Editor: George Stamathis
Developmental editor: Maureen Slaten
Project manager: Carol Sullivan Wiseman
Production editor: Florence Achenbach
Designer: Rey Umali

Printed in the United States of America

The C.V. Mosby Company
11830 Westline Industrial Drive, St. Louis, Missouri 63146

Library of Congress Cataloging in Publication Data

Enzmann, Dieter R.
Magentic resonance of the spine/Dieter R. Enzmann, Robert L. DeLaPaz, Jeremy B. Rubin.
p. cm.
ISBN 0-8016-2787-7
1. Spine—Magentic resonance imaging. 2. Spine—Diseases—Diagnoses. I. DeLaPaz, Robert L. II. Rubin, Jeremy B. III. Title.
[DNLM: 1. Magnetic Resonance Imaging. 2. Spinal Diseases—diagnosis. 3. Spine—anatomy & histology. WE 725 E61m]
RD768.E59 1990
617.3′7507548—dc20
DNLM/DLC
for Library of Congress

89-12785
CIP

GW/MV/MV 9 8 7 6 5 4 3 2 1

Preface

As many of the readers of this book will be aware, MR can be a challenging imaging technique to master. This is especially true for MR of the spine. As it has evolved, MR has done for the spine what x-ray CT initially did for the brain; it has opened up extraordinary new opportunities for investigating spine and spinal cord diseases never before available. Although many excellent texts already exist dealing with MR of the central nervous system, a more detailed text dedicated to the spine now seems appropriate. A book always risks obsolescence, especially in a fast moving field such as MR. The timing of this book, however, has been fortunate in that there has been some stabilization of the pulse sequences used in spine imaging. This book also illustrates the value of procrastination—by employing this age-old behavior we were able to incorporate the use of MR contrast media, GdDTPA, into the book.

How should one use this book? Although it is assumed that the reader has some knowledge of basic MR terminology and physics, this book deals with both the technical aspects of scanning and individual disease processes. Clinical background is provided especially in those instances where knowledge of the clinical history is important in choosing the appropriate scanning technique. Although specific protocols are suggested (in Chapter 2) it is more important to understand the rationale behind them. This will help the reader to understand *why* a particular protocol is used; this will facilitate incorporating new developments in spine imaging into one's scanning repertoire. There is no intention in this book to prescribe the "right" way to perform MR scans since that concept doesn't exist given the wide variety of techniques and machines available. Rather, we have tried to stress comparison of different techniques while providing a rationale for advantages and disadvantages of each. From our own experiences, we have obviously developed some biases with regard to scanning sequences, but we have tried to keep our preferences within tolerable limits. Much of what is recommended in this book is most directly applicable to high field systems (1.0-1.5 Tesla). For midfield and lower field systems specific scanning parameters may not apply directly, although the basic principles and findings will still hold.

This book is purposefully heavily illustrated. The legends for the illustrations are used to make points that may not be stressed in the text to avoid redundancy. Figure illustrations, therefore, are an important feature of this book. We have spent considerable effort to optimize the illustrations since we do feel an MR picture is worth maybe not a thousand words but at least several sentences.

Both the technical and interpretative aspects of spine imaging represent a challenge and we think this book can help individuals meet this challenge.

Contents

1

Basic Principles of CSF Flow

Jeremy B. Rubin

Magnetic resonance (MR) imaging is exquisitely sensitive to proton motion.* Spinal cerebral spinal fluid (CSF) undergoes an oscillatory motion that increases or decreases signal intensity and causes errors in the spatial localization of the signal.[45-48] These motion artifacts degrade the quality of images by reducing image contrast and by increasing image noise.[45-48]

Understanding how CSF motion influences the appearance of spine images is vital to the diagnostician because it avoids potential false negative and false positive errors in interpretation.[45] False negative errors occur when CSF motion artifacts reduce image contrast and obscure pathologic lesions that are in close proximity to moving CSF.[45] False positive errors occur when CSF motion artifacts simulate pathologic conditions in the CSF (intradural-extramedullary lesions), at the CSF-dura interface (extradural lesions), or in the spinal cord (intramedullary lesions).[45] An appreciation of the physical basis for CSF motion artifacts permits a rational approach to optimizing spine image quality[18,47,48] and facilitates the implementation of methods that can be used to measure CSF motion directly.* Furthermore, the absence of normal CSF motion may be an important clue to the presence of an abnormality at that location or elsewhere in the spine.[45]

This chapter describes the appearance of CSF motion artifacts on both spin echo (SE) and short-repetition time (TR) variable flip angle/gradient echo spine images and their effects on image contrast. The physical basis for these artifacts, as well as methods available to eliminate them, will be discussed. The conclusion describes how CSF motion may be imaged directly. CSF flow images generated using this approach illustrate a variety of pathologic conditions in later chapters.

PHYSIOLOGY OF CSF MOTION

A review of some aspects of CSF physiology and motion can help to understand how MR artifacts are caused by moving CSF. CSF production and circulation in humans has been extensively studied.[13] Approximately 500 cc of CSF is produced per day (0.35 cc/min), predominantly in the choroid plexus of the lateral ventricles. During the course of several hours, CSF circulates through the ventricular system and subarachnoid space to be absorbed by the arachnoid villi of the dural sinuses. This slow

*References 2, 6, 7, 23, 25, 54, 56.

*References 4, 9, 15, 21, 52, 53.

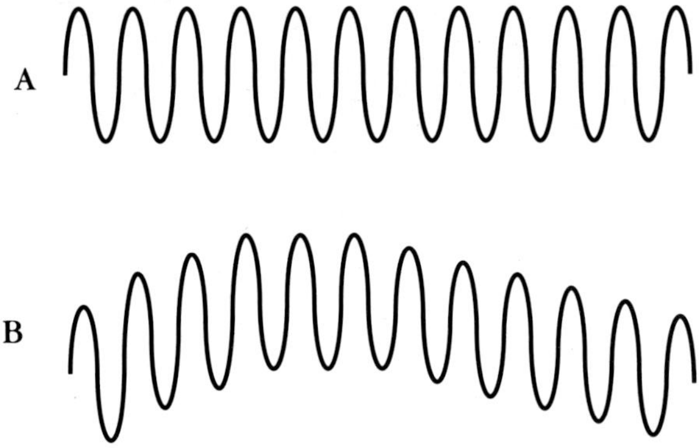

FIGURE 1-1. **A,** Cardiac and **B,** combined cardiac and respiratory CSF motion. Each curve represents a plot of CSF position within subarachnoid space vs. time. Cardiac CSF motion occurs secondary to cerebral perfusion, which causes CSF to oscillate at heart rate. Respiratory CSF motion occurs secondary to respiration-dependent transmitted venous pressures, causing CSF to oscillate at respiratory rate. Under resting conditions, respiratory component of CSF motion is usually small compared to cardiac component of CSF motion. (From Rubin JB, Enzmann DR. CSF flow effects during MRI of the central nervous system. In: Magnetic resonance annual 1988. New York: Raven Press, 1988. With permission.)

circulation of CSF has relatively little influence on MR because its velocity is very low compared to the time required for MR imaging.[46]

Of greater significance to MR is the *oscillatory* CSF motion, which is commonly observed on myelography.[14,24,33] This complex motion is related to both cardiac and respiratory cycles[1] (Figure 1-1). The cardiac-dependent CSF motion is synchronous with the cardiac cycle and occurs secondary to cerebral perfusion, which displaces CSF from the ventricular system and cranial subarachnoid space into the spinal subarachnoid space. The respiratory-dependent CSF motion is synchronous with the respiratory cycle and occurs secondary to variations in venous pressure that are transmitted to CSF by the lumbar epidural venous plexus and dural sinuses. In most individuals the cardiac mechanism is responsible for the majority of CSF motion. Respiratory CSF motion is usually not very prominent during resting conditions and is superimposed on cardiac CSF motion. However, respiratory CSF motion may be increased by cough, Valsalva maneuver, hyperventilation, or venous hypertension.

In the spinal subarachnoid space, a caudal displacement of CSF occurs synchronously with cerebral perfusion, whereas the reciprocal cranial motion occurs during cerebral venous drainage.[14] CSF pulsation amplitude is greatest within the cervical spine (3 to 30 mm, mean 9.6 mm), intermediate within the thoracic spine, and lowest within the lumbar spine (0 to 7 mm, mean 1.7 mm).[14,33] Preferential CSF motion may be observed within characteristic spinal subarachnoid locations because normal anatomic structures, including nerve roots and arachnoid septations, may act as hydraulic baffles to focally dampen or redirect CSF motion.[45]

CSF motion occurs during both cardiac systole and diastole. The distinction between CSF systole and CSF diastole is that spinal CSF motion is caudal in systole and cranial in diastole and that the average CSF velocity is slightly greater in systole than in diastole. In principle, CSF is stationary at each extreme of its oscillatory excursion; however, this is so brief that it may be considered perpetually moving. In the past, manometric and myelographic methods were the only means available to study CSF motion. With the advent of MR, CSF motion may be evaluated with flow sensitive pulse sequences, which are described later.

CSF MOTION ARTIFACTS ON CLINICAL IMAGES

This section examines the appearance of CSF motion artifacts on both SE and short-TR variable flip angle/gradient echo images. The effects of these artifacts on spine image contrast are discussed later.

Spin Echo Imaging

Physiologic CSF motion on conventional SE images influences both CSF signal intensity and spatial localization of the signal.[45,46] In this chapter, a reduction in CSF signal intensity relative to stationary CSF is referred to as signal-loss, an increase in CSF signal intensity relative to stationary CSF is referred to as signal-gain, and spatially mismapped CSF signal intensity is referred to as ghosts. The appearance of these motion artifacts is often complicated because several of them usually occur simultaneously.[46,47,48] Some motion artifacts may be dominant and hide others that are less prominent.[46,48] As discussed

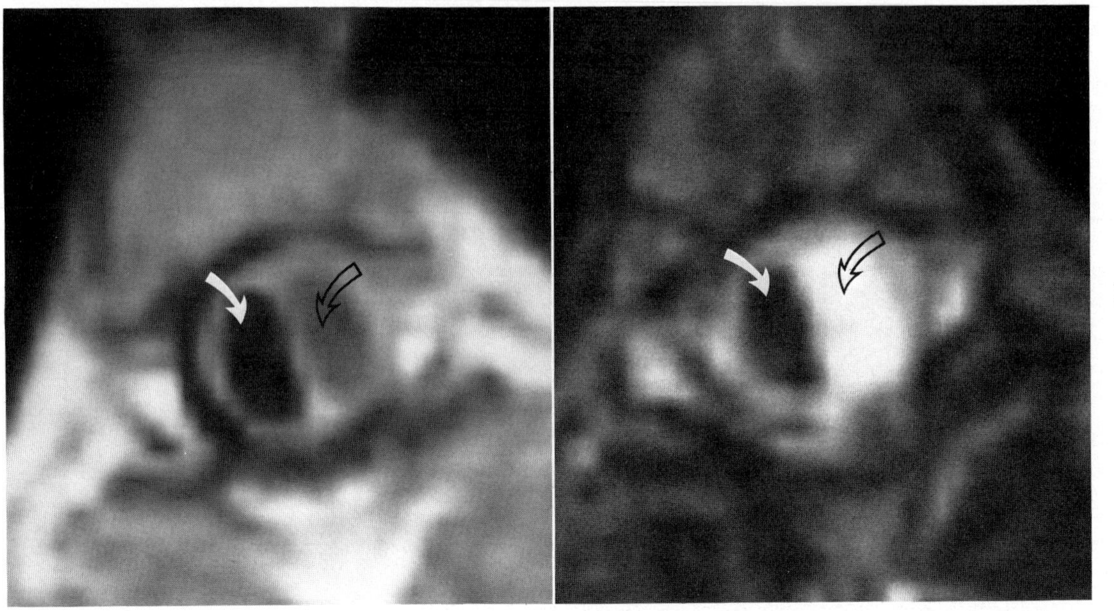

FIGURE 1-2. Signal-loss on SE images. Axial cervical spine images **A,** T1W SE 800/20 and **B,** T2W SE 2000/80 in patient with syrinx. Two compartments are present within the syrinx, one containing pulsatile CSF *(solid arrow)* and the other containing stationary CSF *(open arrow)*. On T2W image, stationary CSF is hyperintense to spinal cord as expected, whereas oscillatory CSF exhibits signal-loss. Signal-loss is prominent on T2W image and less prominent on T1W image.

later in this chapter, there are methods that may be used to minimize the detrimental effects of CSF motion on spine image quality. These methods, known as motion compensation techniques, are available on commercial imagers and are being increasingly used for spine imaging.* However, a familiarity with CSF motion artifacts is important to avoid errors in interpretation because motion compensation techniques are not always used and they occasionally are not effective in eliminating CSF motion artifacts.

Signal-loss

Signal-loss on SE images is recognized as decreased signal intensity of moving CSF compared to stationary CSF. Signal-loss may be observed on T1-weighted (T1W), proton density-weighted (PDW), and T2-weighted (T2W) spine images[45] (Figure 1-2). Signal-loss is commonly observed on long-TR pulse sequences (balanced or T2W) where it is easy to recognize because stationary CSF is relatively high signal intensity. It is usually more difficult to appreciate on T1W images because CSF is already relatively low signal intensity secondary to its long T1 relaxation time. As shown later in this chapter, signal-loss is minimized on SE images when motion compensation techniques are used.

The location of signal-loss within the subarachnoid space is determined by the position of the spinal cord, nerve roots, and arachnoid septations.[45] For this reason, signal-loss has characteristic patterns within the cervical, thoracic, and lumbar spinal segments. Signal-loss is commonly observed on both axial and sagittal spine images. During axial imaging, it is increased in prominence when a thin slice thickness is used[45,46] (Figure 1-3). The prominence of signal-loss is also determined in part by how much the CSF moves at any location.[46] From myelographic studies, it is well known that CSF motion is greatest in the cervical spine and least in the lumbar spine.[14,33] For this reason, signal-loss is usually most prominent in the cervical spine, intermediate in the thoracic spine, and least prominent in the lumbar spine.[45]

*References 18, 26, 27, 47, 48, 41.

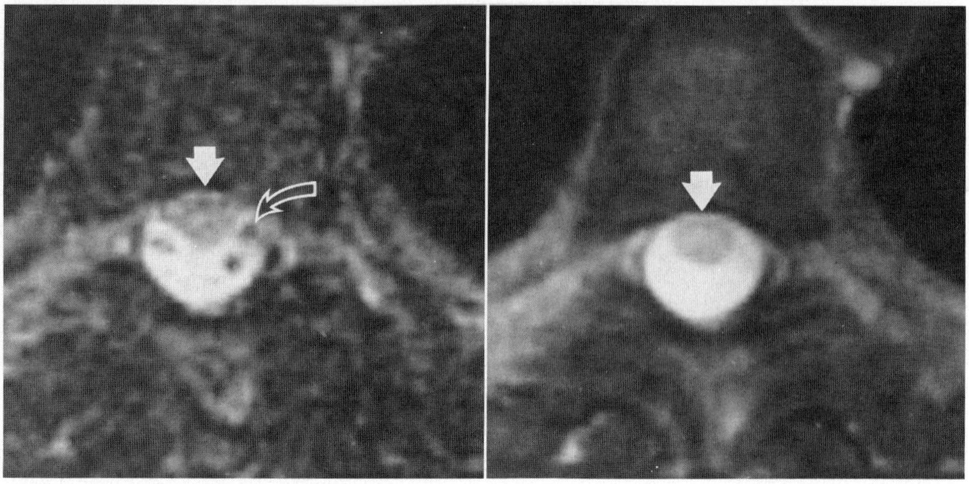

FIGURE 1-3. Effect of slice thickness on prominence of signal-loss. T2W SE 2000/80. **A,** 3 mm slice thickness. **B,** 20 mm slice thickness. Regions of signal-loss occurring secondary to CSF motion *(open arrow)* are very prominent when a thin slice thickness is used but disappear when a thicker slice thickness is used. The CSF-spinal cord interface *(solid arrow)* is also better delineated when a thick slice is used. Note improved image SNR when slice thickness is increased. (From Rubin JB, Enzmann DR. AJNR 1987; 8:297. With permission.)

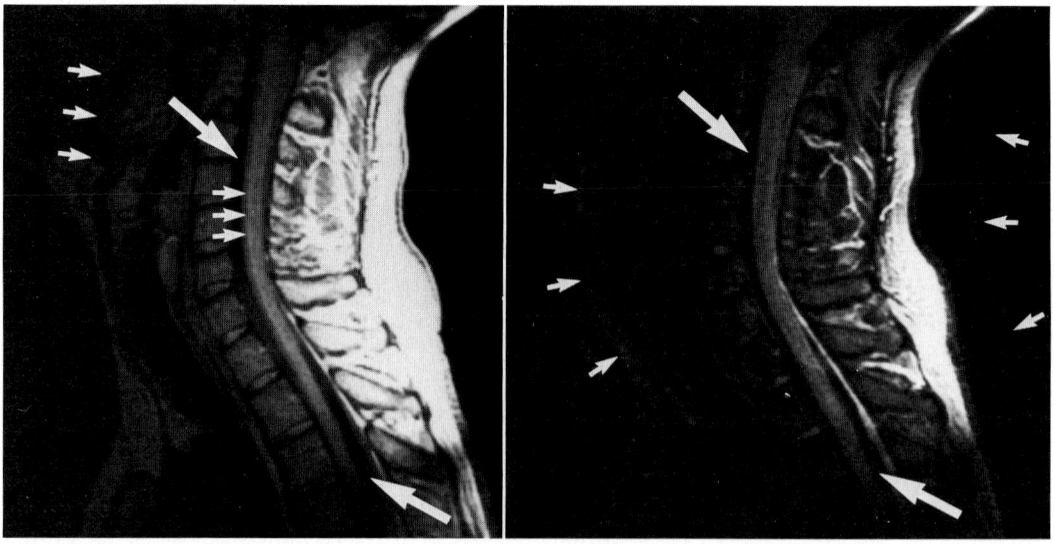

FIGURE 1-4. Sagittal cervical spine signal-loss. **A,** PDW SE 2500/25. **B,** T2W SE 2500/80. Although CSF should be uniformly hyperintense to spinal cord, there are regions of hypointensity anterior to upper cervical spine and posterior to lower cervical spine *(large arrows)*. Signal-loss is more prominent on T2W image than on PDW image. Associated ghosts *(small arrows)* are projected on spinal cord and outside spinal canal. (From Rubin JB, Enzmann DR. AJNR 1987; 8:297. With permission.)

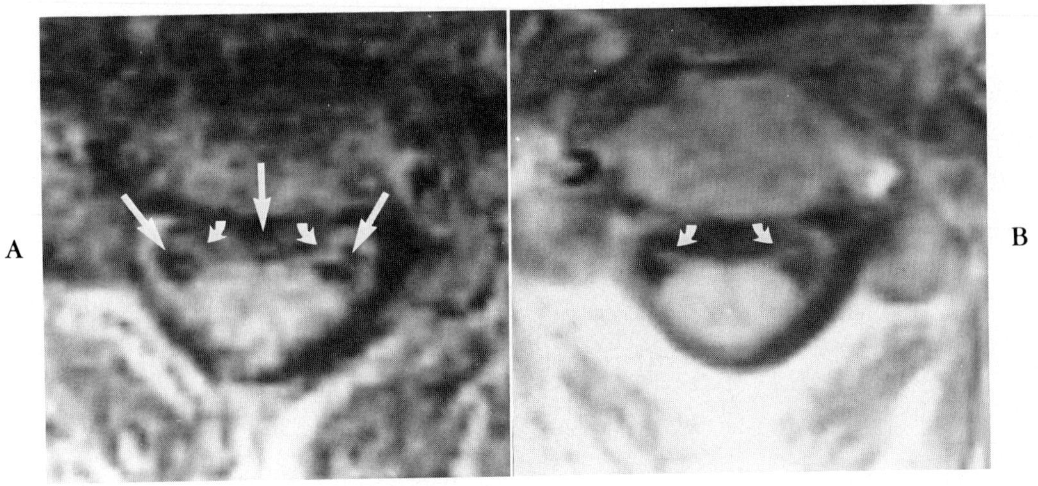

FIGURE 1-5. Axial cervical spine signal-loss. **A**, PDW SE 2000/40. **B**, T1W SE 600/25. Regions of prominent signal-loss are present on PDW image within ventral subarachnoid space and within ventrolateral recesses *(large arrows)*. Note presence of signal-loss between ventral and dorsal nerve roots. Comparison T1W image clearly shows location of nerve roots *(small arrows)*. (From Rubin JB, Enzmann DR. AJNR 1987; 8:297. With permission.)

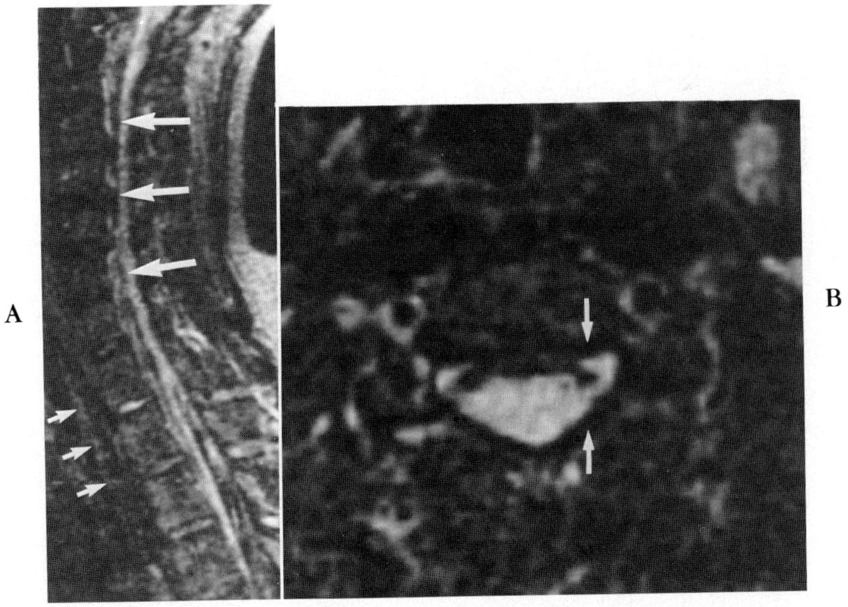

FIGURE 1-6. Signal-loss of CSF simulating abnormal blood vessels in cervical spine subarachnoid space. **A**, Sagittal T2W SE 2000/80. **B**, Axial T2W SE 2500/80. Sagittal imaging plane is through left ventrolateral recess, *(arrows* on B). Signal-loss appears tubular, simulating abnormal blood vessels *(large arrows)*. Associated ghosts are also present *(small arrows)*. (From Rubin JB, Enzmann DR. AJNR 1987; 8:297. With permission.)

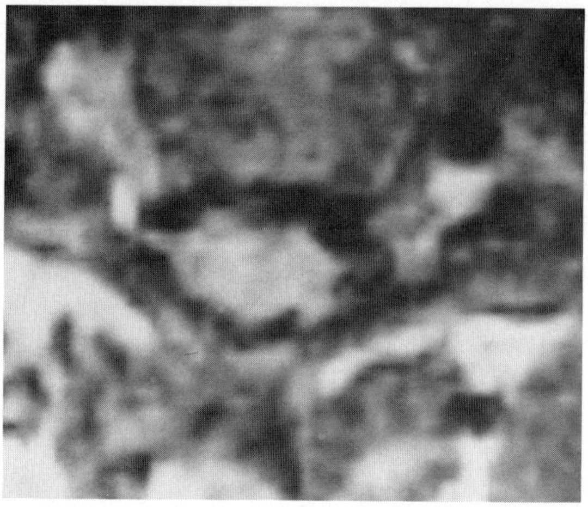

FIGURE 1-7. Reduced conspicuity of cervical spinal cord by nonuniformity of CSF motion. PDW SE 2500/40. Spinal cord margins appear shaggy because of adjacent isointense slow moving CSF. More rapidly moving CSF within remainder of subarachnoid space exhibits signal-loss. (From Rubin JB, Enzmann DR. AJNR 1987; 8:297. With permission.)

In the cervical spine, signal-loss is commonly observed as reduced CSF signal intensity in the ventral and ventrolateral subarachnoid space[45] (Figure 1-4). This occurs because the cervical spinal cord is posterior in the spinal canal secondary to the normal cervical lordosis. Signal-loss may be particularly prominent in the ventrolateral recesses and between the ventral and dorsal nerve roots (Figure 1-5). When sagittal images are obtained through the lateral recesses of the subarachnoid space, the pattern of signal-loss appears linear and often simulates the signal void seen in blood vessels[45] (Figure 1-6). It is therefore important not to mistake cervical CSF signal-loss for pathology, such as the abnormal blood vessels associated with spinal arteriovenous malformation (AVM). At times, slowly moving CSF adjacent to the spinal cord may appear isointense with the spinal cord, giving the cord an abnormal appearance (Figure 1-7).

In the thoracic spine, signal-loss is more prominent in the dorsal subarachnoid space be-

A

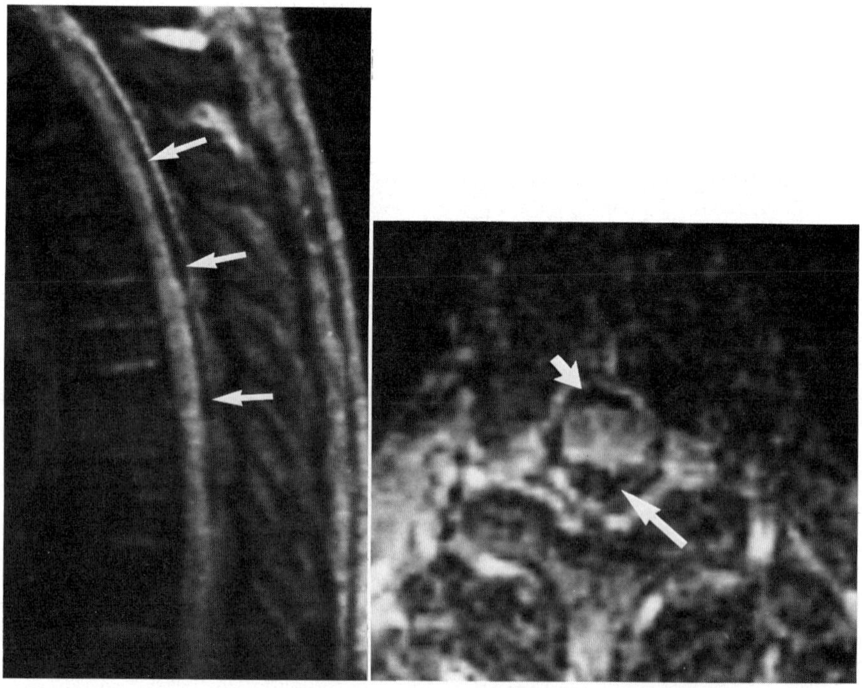

B

FIGURE 1-8. Signal-loss in normal thoracic spine. T2W SE 2000/80. **A,** Sagittal. **B,** Axial. Signal-loss is prominent posterior to spinal cord *(large arrows)* and has tubular appearance on sagittal image. On axial image, signal-loss is also observed ventral to the spinal cord *(small arrow)*. (From Rubin JB, Enzmann DR. AJNR 1987; 8:297. With permission.)

cause the normal thoracic kyphosis causes the spinal cord to assume a relatively anterior position within the spinal canal[45] (Figure 1-8). The pattern of signal-loss posterior to the cord may mimic the abnormal blood vessels feeding or draining a spinal AVM similar to the pattern described in the cervical spine. CSF motion is often highly variable in the dorsal thoracic subarachnoid space because the arachnoid septations in this region may trap CSF and keep it from moving.[31,45] As a result, signal-loss in the thoracic spine is often focal, sometimes simulating the appearance of an intradural-extramedullary mass (Figure 1-9). Prominent arachnoid septations in the thoracic spine are common in children and young adults.[31] Arachnoid septations involute with increasing age; thus thoracic CSF signal-loss is often more uniform in adults.[31,45]

In the lumbar spine, the amount of signal-loss is variable because CSF in this spinal segment may range from stationary to pulsatile.[49] In many adults, relatively little motion is present in the lumbar spine and CSF is observed as high signal intensity on T2W images even without motion compensation techniques (Figure 1-10). When

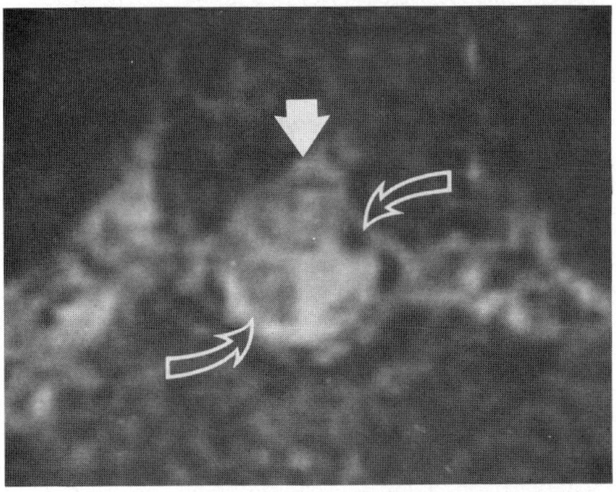

FIGURE 1-9. Signal-loss in normal thoracic spine simulating pathologic lesion. T2W SE 2000/80. Regions of CSF signal-loss appear well-circumscribed and simulate intradural-extramedullary mass *(open arrows)*. Larger region of signal-loss has appearance similar to spinal cord *(solid arrow)*. Corresponding axial and sagittal T1W images demonstrated no abnormalities. (From Rubin JB, Enzmann DR. AJNR 1987; 8:297. With permission.)

A

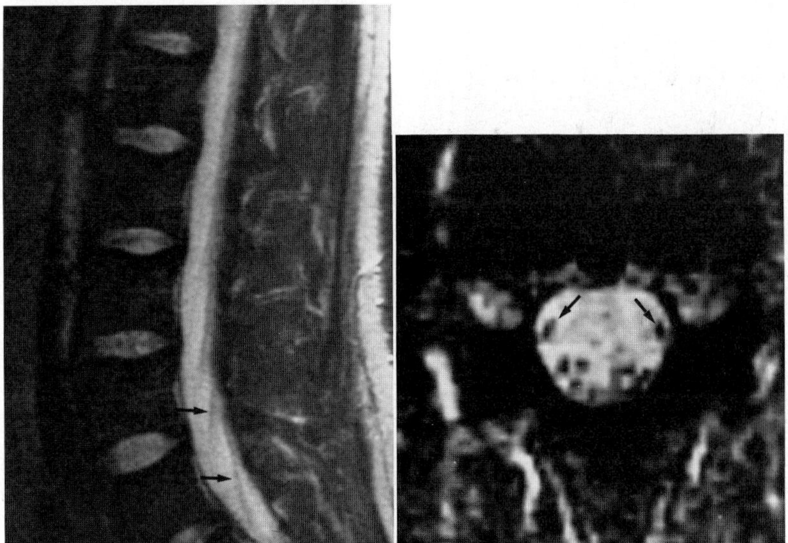

B

FIGURE 1-10. Absence of signal-loss in normal lumbar spine. T2W SE 2000/80. **A,** Sagittal. **B,** Axial. Uniformly high CSF signal intensity permits identification of individual nerve roots *(arrows)*. CSF-thecal sac interface is clearly delineated.

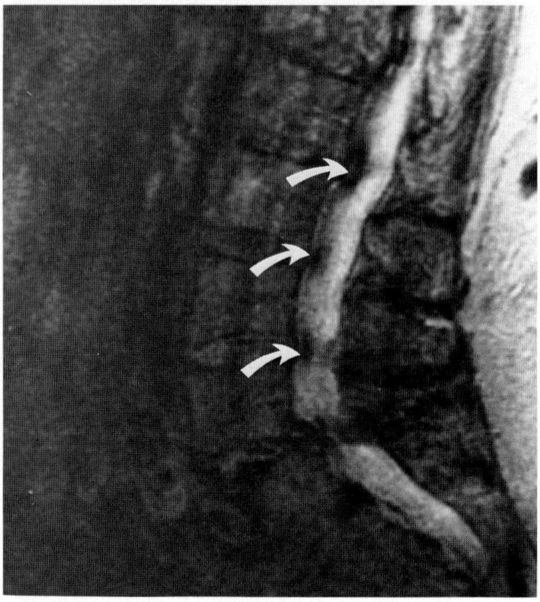

FIGURE 1-11. Focal signal-loss in lumbar spine. T2W SE 2000/80. CSF signal intensity within thecal sac is lower than expected for degree of T2W. In addition, note focal signal-loss adjacent to several bulging lumbar discs *(arrows)*.

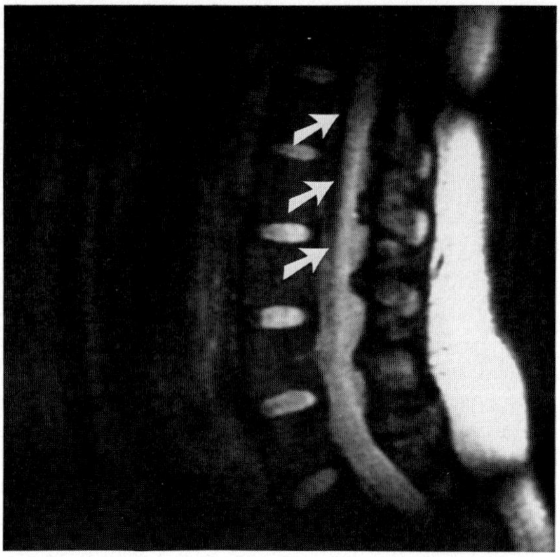

FIGURE 1-12. Signal-loss at level of conus. T2W SE 2500/80. Although CSF in caudal thecal sac is relatively high signal intensity, CSF ventral to conus exhibits prominent signal-loss *(arrows)*, which reduces conspicuity of CSF-thecal sac interface in this region. (From Rubin JB, Wright A, Enzmann DR. Radiology, 1988; 167:225. With permission.)

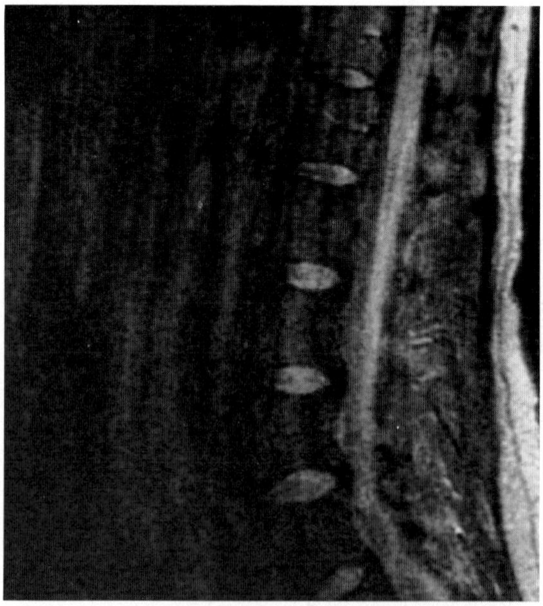

FIGURE 1-13. Prominent lumbar spine signal loss. T2W SE 2000/80. Extensive lumbar signal-loss degrades image quality and reduces conspicuity of CSF-thecal sac interface. Associated CSF ghosts are also present.

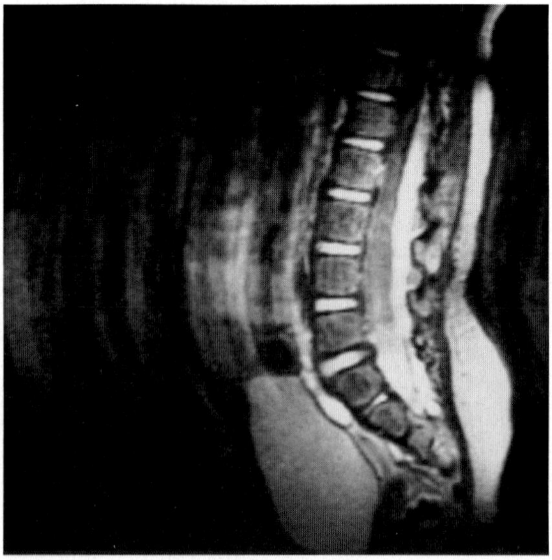

FIGURE 1-14. Prominent lumbar spine signal-loss in child. T2W SE 2500/80. Patient has a tethered cord. CSF signal-loss within thecal sac is more prominent than usually encountered in adults. Ghosts arise from both lumbar CSF and anterior abdominal wall.

CSF is relatively high signal intensity in the lumbar spine, focal regions of signal-loss may be observed adjacent to bulging or herniated discs[49] (Figure 1-11). In adult lumbar spines, CSF signal-loss may be prominent near the level of the conus (Figure 1-12) or extend to the caudal thecal sac[49] (Figure 1-13). In child lumbar spines, signal-loss is usually relatively prominent (Figure 1-14).

Signal-gain

Signal-gain on SE images is recognized as increased signal intensity of moving CSF relative to stationary CSF. Signal-gain may be observed on T1W, PDW, and T2W spine images[48] (Figure 1-15), but is more commonly observed on short-TR pulse sequences (T1W) where it is easily recognized because stationary or slowly moving CSF is low signal intensity. Signal-gain occurs primarily in the cervical and thoracic spinal segments similar to the distribution of signal-loss previously described. It is observed on axial or oblique-axial spine images but not on sagittal spine images, most prominent on single-slice acquisitions or at end slices of multislice acquisitions, and increased in prominence when thin slices are used. The clinical significance of signal-gain is that it alters image contrast and could be mistaken for a pathologic lesion. On T1W images, signal-gain reduces the contrast between CSF and the spinal cord or discs. It could be mistaken for an intradural-extramedullary mass when it is confined to the central part of the subarachnoid space or a herniated disc or epidural tumor when it is peripherally located in the subarachnoid space (see Figure 1-15).

A B

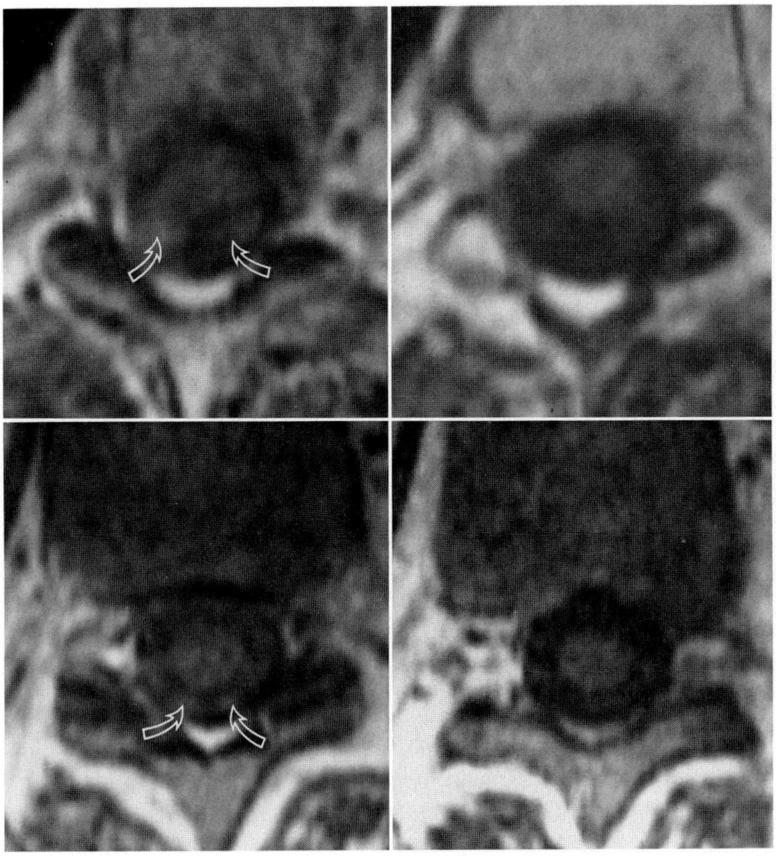

C D

FIGURE 1-15. Thoracic spine signal-gain simulating pathology. T1W SE 800/20. **A,** End-slice. **B,** Adjacent slice to **A. C,** different acquisition, end-slice. **D,** Adjacent slice to **C.** CSF increase in signal intensity on end-slices simulates intradural-extramedullary masses in **A** and epidural disease in **C.** In each case, adjacent slice does not exhibit artifact.

A 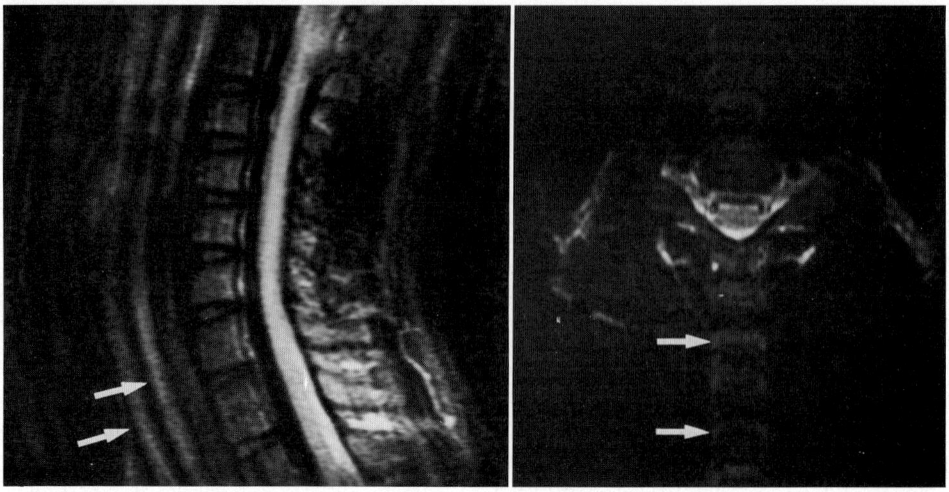 B

FIGURE 1-16. Cervical spine ghost artifacts. **A,** Sagittal SE 800/75. **B,** Axial SE 800/80. Prominent ghost artifacts scattered along phase-encoding axis in both imaging planes *(arrows)* are relatively discrete because patient had a regular heart rate. Shape of ghosts corresponds to pattern of signal-loss within CSF. (From Edelman RR, Rubin JB. MRI flow effects. In: Edelmann RR, ed. Clinical magnetic resonance imaging: a practical text. Philadelphia: W.B. Saunders Co., 1989. In press.)

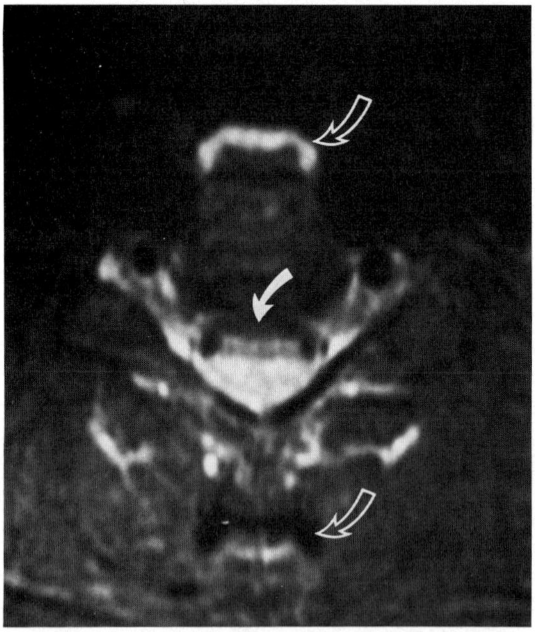

FIGURE 1-17. Cervical spine ghost artifacts. SE 1200/40. Ghost artifacts symmetrically displaced from subarachnoid space along phase-encoding axis *(open arrows)* are either high or low signal intensity depending on whether they add to or subtract from stationary signal intensity. Shape is identical to pattern of signal-loss within subarachnoid space *(solid arrow)*. (From Rubin JB, Enzmann DR. AJNR 1987; 8:297. With permission.)

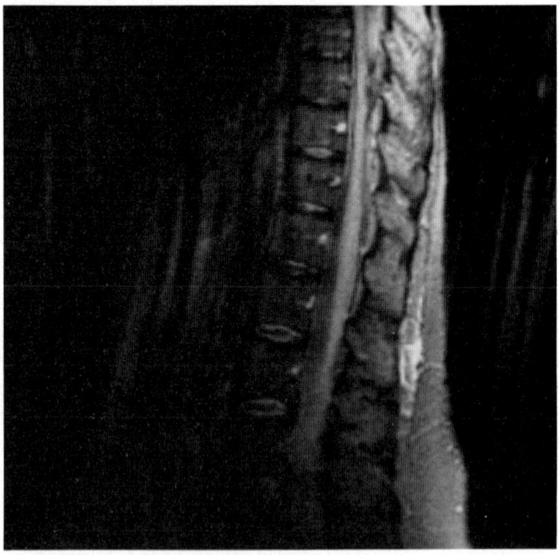

FIGURE 1-18. Thoracolumbar spine ghost artifacts. PDW SE 2000/25. Ghosts in thoracic spine appear similar to those in cervical spine. Thoracic spine ghosts often arise from the heart in addition to thoracic CSF.

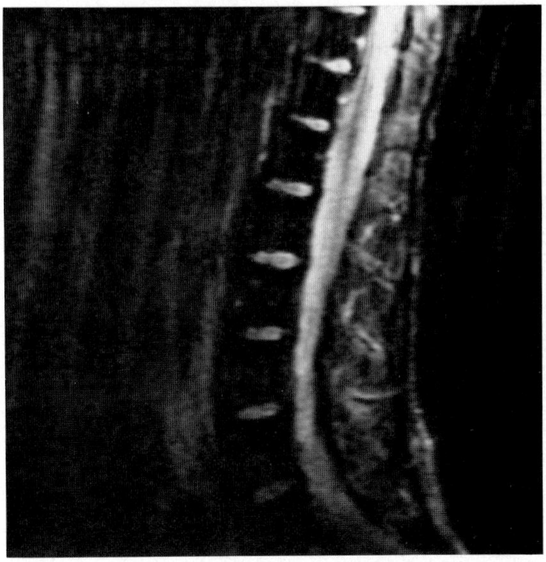

FIGURE 1-19. Lumbar spine ghost artifacts. SE 2500/80. Ghosts in the lumbar spine are most prominent at level of conus and become less intense towards caudal thecal sac.

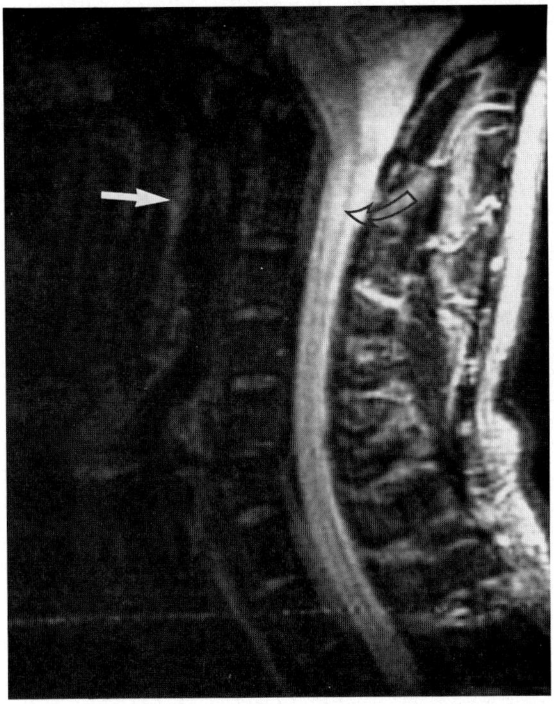

FIGURE 1-20. Ghost artifact simulating spinal cord lesion. SE 2000/80. Ghost superimposed on cervical spinal cord *(open arrow)* simulating an intrinsic cord lesion is recognized as artifact because ghost anterior to spine is identical in shape *(solid arrow)*.

Ghosts

Ghosts on SE spine images resemble the pattern of signal-loss within the subarachnoid space from which they originated[45] and are recognized as CSF signal intensity that is spatially mismapped along the phase-encoding axis[45,46] (Figure 1-16). They may appear as either high or low signal intensity when superimposed onto stationary structures[45,46] (Figure 1-17), are commonly observed on long-TR pulse sequences (balanced or T2W) in which stationary CSF is relatively high signal intensity,[45] and are also prominent when moving CSF signal intensity is elevated by signal-gain on single-slice acquisitions or on end slices of multislice acquisitions. They occur on both axial and sagittal spine images, are relatively discrete when the heart rate is regular[45,46] (see Figures 1-16 and 1-17), and become less discrete when the heart rate is irregular, especially with cardiac arrythmias.[45,46]

Similar to signal-loss and signal-gain, ghosts tend to be prominent in the cervical and thoracic spinal segments (see Figures 1-16 and 1-17) but at times may be quite prominent in the lumbar spine as well[45,49] (Figures 1-18 and 1-19). Ghosts are clinically significant because they degrade image quality and may be mistaken for pathologic conditions.[45] They may be scattered along the phase-encoding axis or clustered in close proximity to the pulsatile CSF from which they arose. Image quality is usually degraded to the greatest extent when they aggregate near the subarachnoid space because the CSF-thecal sac interface and spinal cord are obscured[45,47] (Figure 1-20). Low signal intensity ghosts usually can be recognized as artifacts but could be confused with low signal intensity caused by blood flow, calcium, or hemosiderin. The high signal intensity ghosts may obscure real cord lesions or even simulate pathologic lesions when superimposed on a normal spinal cord (see Figure 1-20). As shown later in this chapter, ghosts are minimized on SE images when flow compensation techniques are used.

Absence of motion artifacts below spinal block

The presence or absence of motion artifacts on SE images may provide useful physiologic information about the CSF motion in the spinal subarachnoid space in cases of suspected spinal

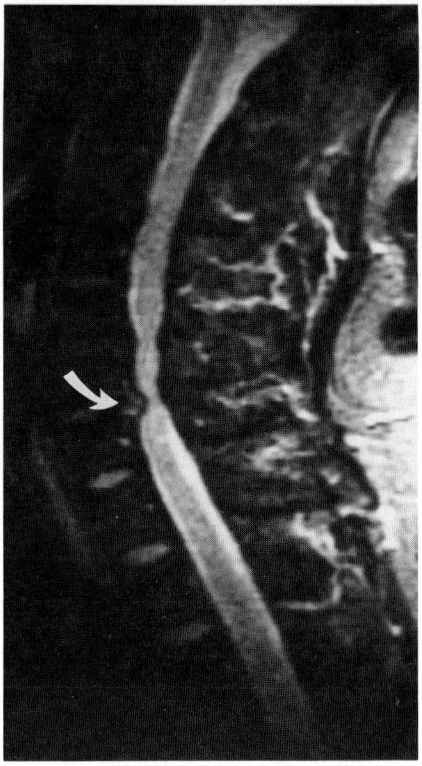

FIGURE 1-21. Reduced CSF motion artifacts caudal to spinal block. SE 2500/80. Large herniated disc *(arrow)* and spinal stenosis cause high-grade spinal block. CSF motion artifacts are absent because CSF motion is prevented from being transmitted beyond block. (From Rubin JB, Enzmann DR. AJNR 1987; 8:297. With permission.)

block. When the subarachnoid space is obliterated by a mass or herniated disc, the absence of signal-loss and ghosts may indicate that the spinal block is high grade[45] (Figure 1-21). Thus MR can provide physiologic information about the degree of spinal block, as well as anatomic information regarding its location and etiology. However, the absence of these motion artifacts does not necessarily mean that a high-grade block is present.[45] Motion artifacts may be absent if the image was inadvertently acquired using a TR that is a multiple of the patient's heart rate, or if multiple, closely spaced echoes were used. The use of a TR that is a multiple of the patient's heart rate causes *inadvertent pseudogating*, whereas the use of multiple closely spaced echoes causes *even echo rephasing*, both of which reduce CSF motion artifacts.[45] When CSF motion is present, these may simulate the appearance of relatively stationary CSF and could lead to a false positive diagnosis of spinal block. As shown later, gating and even echo rephasing are often specifically used to reduce CSF motion artifacts when artifact-free images are desired.

Short-TR Variable Flip Angle/Gradient Echo Imaging

Short-TR variable flip angle/gradient echo pulse sequences are increasingly used clinically in the evaluation of spinal disease.* This increased use is the result of the pulse sequences' ability to generate high signal intensity CSF in a relatively short acquisition time compared with SE imaging.[19,29] High signal intensity CSF is useful clinically in visualizing the CSF-thecal sac interface, which may be impinged on by low signal intensity osteophytes or discs. However, as in SE imaging, the signal intensity of CSF on short-TR variable flip angle/gradient echo images is greatly influenced by motion.[50,51] The term ***variable flip angle*** refers to this category of pulse sequences, which is now available on most commercial imagers.

Although a number of variable flip angle pulse sequences are available,† important differences among them determine what type of image contrast they exhibit and how they are influenced by CSF motion.[42,50,51] The most important distinction is that some sequences are steady-state free precession (SSFP) pulse sequences and some are repeated gradient echo pulse sequences.[42,50] SSFP pulse sequences establish both a longitudinal and transverse steady state magnetization, whereas repeated gradient echo pulse sequences establish only a longitudinal steady-state magnetization.[28,42] To prevent residual coherent transverse magnetization from carrying over from one excitation to the next, the repeated gradient echo pulse sequences employ spoiling pulses that disrupt the transverse steady-state magnetization. The illustrations

*References 11, 19, 20, 29, 50, 51.
†References 10, 22, 28, 30, 50, 51, 55.

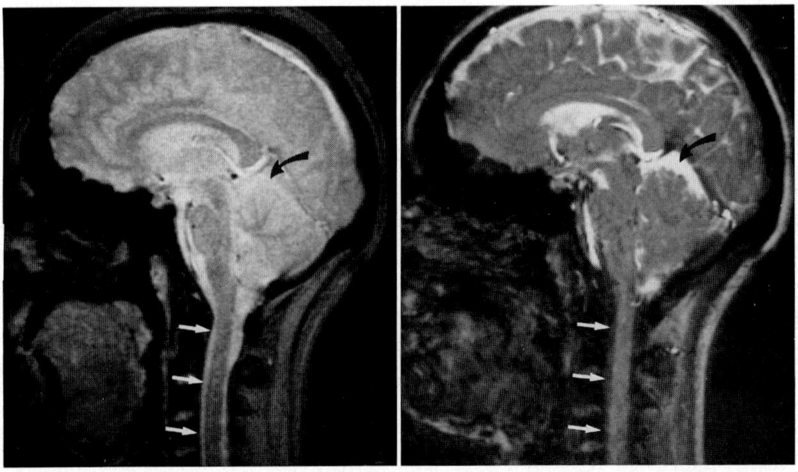

FIGURE 1-22. Signal-loss on variable flip angle images. GRASS 40/15. **A,** 5°. **B,** 75°. Stationary CSF within superior cerebellar cistern is hyperintense compared with white matter on both low and high flip angle images *(curved arrow)*. Moving CSF within fourth ventricle and spinal subarachnoid space is hypointense compared with white matter on high, but not low, flip angle image *(straight arrows)*. (From Rubin JB. Submitted for publication to Radiology.)

used in this text were acquired using the Gradient Recalled Acquisition in the Steady-State (GRASS) pulse sequence, which is a variable flip angle SSFP pulse sequence. The motion artifacts apply equally well to other variable flip angle SSFP pulse sequences but do not necessarily apply to repeated gradient echo pulse sequences.

Variable flip angle images exhibit signal-loss, signal-gain, and ghosts similar to those described for SE images.[50] Most commercially available variable flip angle pulse sequences have a flow compensation option that reduces some of these CSF motion artifacts. All variable flip angle spine images in this text used this flow compensation option, which has the effect of reducing the prominence of ghost artifacts. The following sections focus on signal-loss and signal-gain that persist on flow-compensated, variable flip angle spine images. A later section of this chapter discusses how motion artifacts may be manipulated using imaging parameters to optimize variable flip angle image quality.

Signal-loss

Signal-loss on variable flip angle images is observed as decreased signal intensity of moving CSF compared to stationary CSF[50] (Figure 1-22). It occurs on both sagittal and axial images primarily when intermediate and large flip angles are used. It may be more difficult to recognize signal-loss on variable flip angle images than on SE images because signal-loss is much more uniform on the former. On SE images, low signal intensity, moving CSF within the center of the subarachnoid space, often contrasts with high signal intensity, slow moving CSF at the periphery of the subarachnoid space. During variable flip angle imaging, most of the CSF within the spinal subarachnoid space is uniformly low signal intensity regardless of how much it is moving.[50] Minimally moving CSF (pulsation amplitude 0.5 mm) appears similar in signal intensity to rapidly moving CSF (pulsation amplitude 30 mm). Therefore, signal-loss on variable flip angle cervical spine images is not confined to the ventral and ventrolateral subarachnoid spaces. Even lumbar CSF is low signal intensity when imaged using large flip angles, unless it is completely stationary (Figure 1-23).

The clinical significance of signal-loss during variable flip angle imaging is that it influences the contrast between CSF and adjacent thecal sac, spinal cord, and nerve roots.[51] Signal-loss is

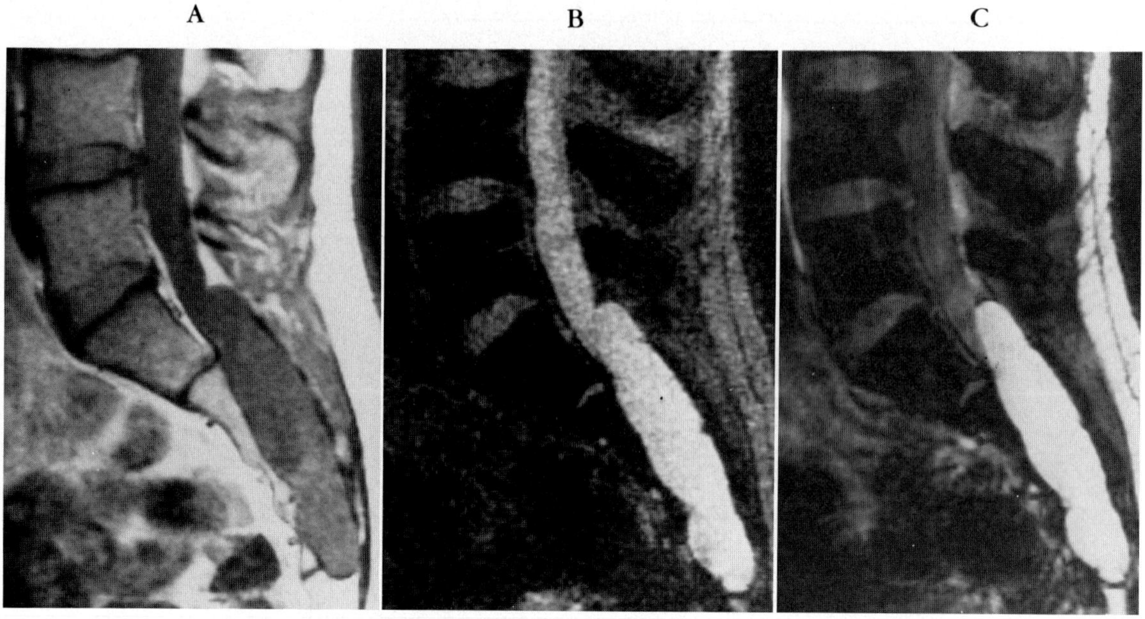

FIGURE 1-23. Signal-loss on sagittal lumbar spine variable flip angle images. **A,** T1W SE 800/20. **B,** GRASS 40/15, 6°. **C,** GRASS 40/15, 90°. Uniform signal-loss is observed within lumbar thecal sac despite minimal CSF motion usually present in this spinal segment. For comparison, stationary CSF within sacral cyst is high signal intensity. (From Rubin JB, Enzmann DR. Submitted for publication to Radiology.)

minimized when small flip angles are used.[50] Signal-loss on variable flip angle images is less likely to be focal, so that this artifact is not usually confused with pathologic lesions. Signal-loss may appear more prominent during sagittal imaging than during axial imaging when identical imaging parameters are used. This is because signal-loss is opposed by signal-gain during axial imaging.[50] However, during axial imaging with large flip angles, signal-loss usually predominates over signal-gain, resulting in low signal intensity CSF similar to the pattern on sagittal images[50] (Figure 1-24). As shown later in this chapter, it is necessary to anticipate the effects of signal-loss on image contrast when selecting imaging parameters for the spine.

Signal-gain

Signal-gain on variable flip angle images is observed as increased signal intensity of faster moving CSF compared to slower moving CSF[50] (Figure 1-25). Unlike signal-loss, it occurs at all but very low flip angles and only on axial or axial-oblique images.[50] Signal-gain is increased in prominence with larger CSF pulsation amplitudes.[50] Therefore, as in SE imaging, it tends to be most prominent in the cervical spine and least prominent in the lumbar spine. It is considerably less prominent at low flip angles, with thick slices, or when interleaved multislice acquisitions are used.[50]

Signal-gain on variable flip angle images occurs simultaneously with and is opposed by signal-loss.[50] As shown later in this chapter, the mechanism for signal-gain on variable flip angle images is similar to the mechanism for signal-gain on SE images. The major clinical significance of signal-gain on variable flip angle images is that it alters image contrast and therefore may be used to advantage in order to achieve a myelographic-type of image contrast.

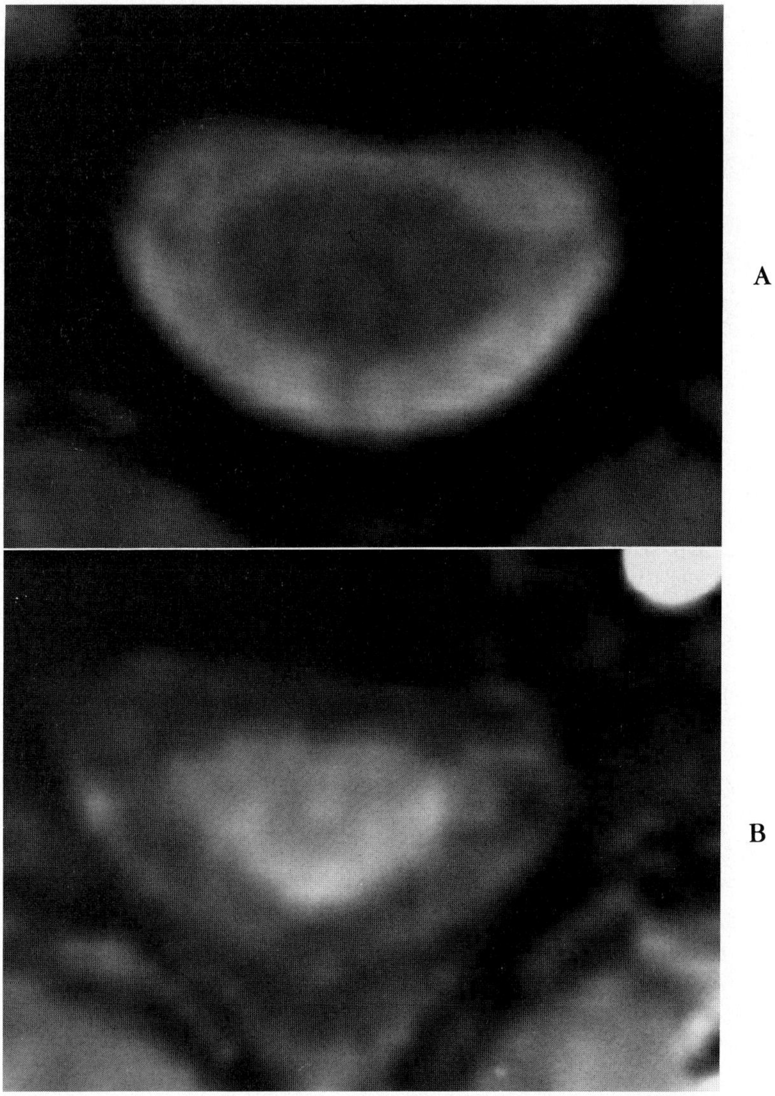

FIGURE 1-24. Signal-loss on axial cervical spine variable flip angle images. GRASS 40/15. **A,** 6°. **B,** 70°. On high flip angle image, oscillatory CSF exhibits signal-loss. Stationary CSF would be hyperintense compared to spinal cord under these conditions. (From Rubin JB. Submitted for publication to Radiology.)

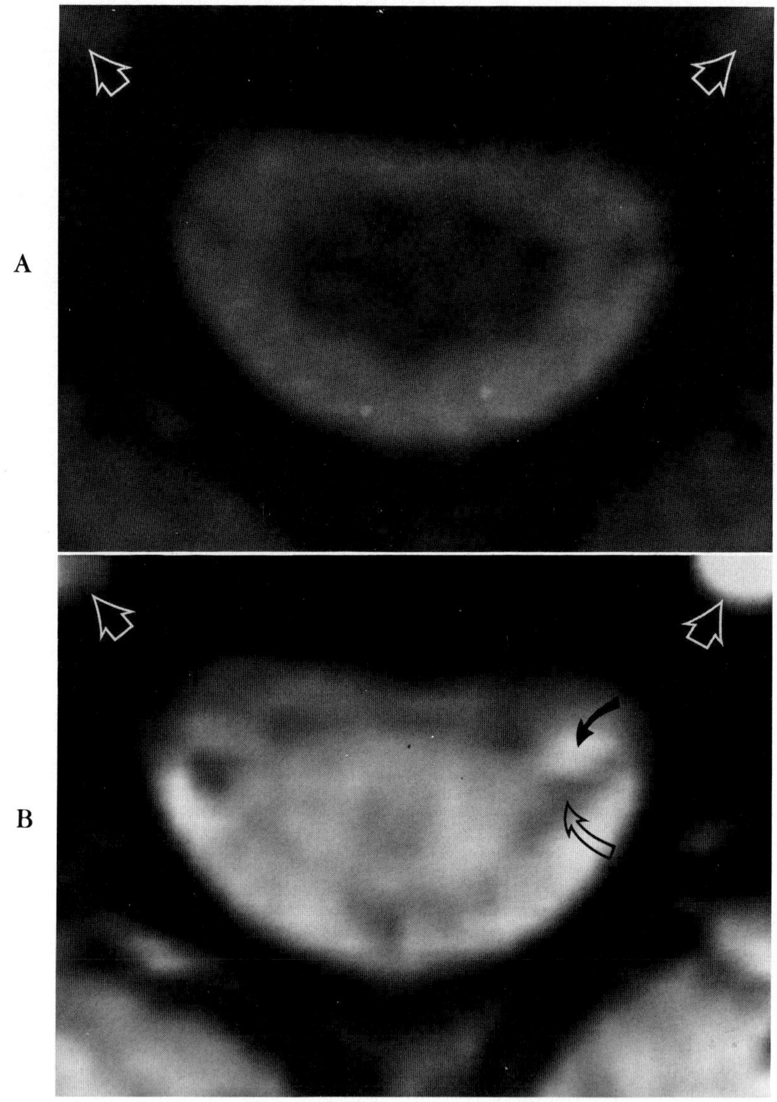

FIGURE 1-25. Signal-gain in axial cervical spine variable flip angle images. GRASS 40/15. **A,** 3°. **B,** 30°. On low flip angle image, CSF within subarachnoid space is uniform in signal intensity and vertebral arteries exhibit almost no entry phenomenon *(straight open arrows).* On higher flip angle image, CSF within subarachnoid space is heterogeneous in signal intensity. Slower moving CSF adjacent to spinal cord exhibits signal-loss *(curved open arrow).* CSF with larger pulsation amplitude exhibits signal-gain *(curved solid arrow).* Under these conditions, entry phenomenon within vertebral arteries is prominent *(straight open arrows).* (From Rubin JB. Submitted for publication to Radiology.)

PHYSICAL BASIS FOR CSF MOTION ARTIFACTS

The physical basis and mechanisms for CSF signal-loss, signal-gain, and ghosts on SE and variable flip angle images are of general interest because similar artifacts arise from moving blood, the heart, the oropharynx, the chest or abdominal wall, and the bowel.[16] This occurs because each of these structures undergoes a cyclic motion similar to spinal CSF.

There are important similarities and differences between CSF motion artifacts (signal-loss, signal-gain, and ghosts) that occur on SE and variable flip angle images. Some motion artifacts arise from the use of imaging gradient pulses and two dimensional fourier transformation (2DFT) reconstruction for spatial localization of signal and occur during both SE and variable flip angle imaging because both pulse sequences use these techniques. Other motion artifacts occur only during variable flip angle imaging because they are dependent on the presence or absence of SSFP, which does not occur during SE imaging.

The physical basis for signal-loss, signal-gain, and ghosts on SE and variable flip angle images is complex because several different flow mechanisms usually operate simultaneously, and each flow mechanism may have the same or opposing effects on CSF signal intensity.[45,50] Furthermore, the manifestations of each flow mechanism are influenced by the characteristics of the flow being imaged, by the pulse sequence used, and by numerous imaging system parameters.[45,50] During imaging of CSF motion, some motion artifacts dominate others in a hierarchical relationship that varies depending on how imaging is performed.[45,50] To clarify these complex

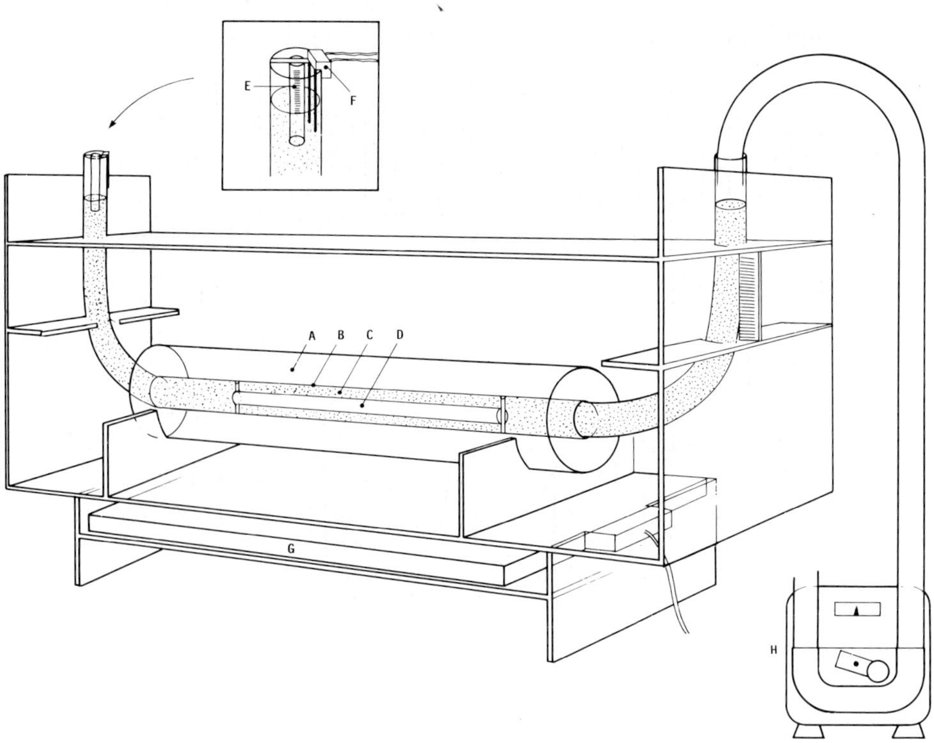

FIGURE 1-26. CSF pulsation spine phantom. Water within phantom subarachnoid space *(C)* is bounded by acrylic walls of phantom thecal sac *(B)* and phantom spinal cord *(D)* and is oscillated by a modified blood pump *(H)* to simulate CSF pulsatile motion. Pulsation amplitude is measured directly on mm scale *(E)*, which displaces volume of water equal to phantom spinal cord *(D)*. Water within phantom spinal cord and phantom perivertebral soft tissues *(A)* is stationary to provide reference signal intensity. Infrared detector *(F)* at water level provides trigger for gating and accurate measurement of pulsation period. Surface coil is positioned below phantom spine *(G)*. (From Rubin JB, Enzmann DR. AJNR 1987; 8:307. With permission.)

relationships, MR images from a phantom spine in which physiologic CSF motion is simulated will be used (Figure 1-26).[46,49,50]

Spin Echo Imaging

In the absence of proton motion, CSF on T2W SE images is hyperintense compared with spinal cord and extradural structures. The relative signal intensity (SI) of different structures on SE images can be calculated in the absence of motion using the following well-known equation[37]:

$$(1) \qquad SI = N_H \cdot (1\text{-}e^{-TR/T1}) \cdot e^{-TE/T2}$$

where N_H is the proton density and TR, TE, T1, and T2 have their usual meaning. The relative contrast between CSF and spinal cord on T2W SE images may be calculated assuming TR/TE = 2000/80 msec, $T1_{CSF} = 3000$ msec, $T2_{CSF} = 2000$ msec, $N_H(CSF) = 1$, $T1_{SC} = 515$ msec, $T2_{SC} = 75$ msec, and $N_H(SC) = 0.77$.[12,61] Under these conditions, SI_{CSF} is 46.7 and SI_{SC} is 26. Therefore, in the absence of CSF motion on T2W spine images, CSF is expected to be approximately 1.8 times higher in signal intensity than spinal cord. This occurs primarily because of the long T2 of CSF compared to spinal cord. However, as shown in the previous section, oscillatory CSF on T2W SE images is not hyperintense compared with spinal cord under these imaging conditions.

Motion influences SE images by two fundamental mechanisms: phase shift effects and time of flight effects.[2,6,7,57,58] Within each category, there are several different flow mechanisms, which will be described in detail in the following sections. These flow mechanisms are related because they arise from the same basic principles governing the interaction of moving protons with the imaging process. They are all distinctly different in the way they are influenced by physiologic or imaging system parameters.

Phase shift effects

Phase shift effects are caused by velocity dependent alterations in the proton precessional phase of moving compared to stationary protons within a nonuniform magnetic field[2,58] (Figure 1-27). The imaging gradients used for spatial localization of signal (G_x, G_y, or G_z depending upon the orientation of flow in relation to the imaging plane) are usually the greatest source of magnetic field nonuniformity that causes

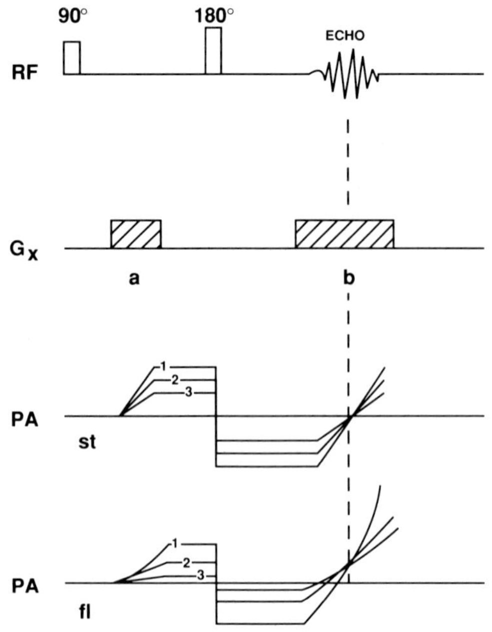

FIGURE 1-27. Phase shift effects. On RF channel, 90° pulse excites protons and 180° pulse refocuses them, leading to generation of a SE. Several imaging gradients spatially localize signal; one is the frequency encoding gradient (G_x), which is turned on at time of expected SE *(b)* so that frequency encoding will occur. A rephasing gradient pulse *(a)* is necessary to permit refocusing of stationary spins when readout gradient pulse *(b)* is applied. Spin-phase graphs are plotted as phase angle (PA), as a function of time *(t)* for stationary *(st)* and constant velocity flowing *(fl)* protons. Whereas phase shift experienced by stationary protons is linear during application of gradient pulses, phase shift of flowing protons is quadratic. As a result, stationary protons are completely refocused at time of SE regardless of position within magnetic field (*1*, stronger region of magnetic field, *3*, weaker region of magnetic field), whereas flowing protons are not. Phase shift experienced by flowing protons is dependent on their velocity (*1*, fastest flow, *3*, slowest flow). (Modified from Rubin JB, Enzmann DR. CSF flow effects during MRI of the central nervous system. In: Magnetic resonance annual 1988. New York: Raven Press, 1988. With permission.)

these effects. The magnitude of phase shift effects depends on proton velocity, gradient pulse amplitude, and gradient pulse duration described by the following equation[58]:

$$(3) \qquad d\Phi_n(t) = \gamma \cdot G_n(t) \cdot n(t) \cdot dt$$

where $d\Phi_n(t)$ is the differential precessional phase of moving protons at position n(t) with respect to stationary protons at position $n = 0$ after a 90° RF pulse, γ is the magnetogyric ratio, G_n is the component of the gradient field along axis n, and n is one of the imaging gradient axes (x, y, or z).

Motion artifacts occurring secondary to phase shift effects are reduced on axial spine images when slice thickness is increased[45] (see Figure 1-3). This occurs because during axial imaging the slice selection gradient amplitude decreases when thicker slices are used.[46]

The manifestations of phase shift effects on MR images depends on how flow varies with respect to time and space.[44,46,48,58] Variations of flow over time occur when proton direction and velocity vary from one moment to the next. Variations of flow over space occur when proton velocity is not equal at each position within a lumen. Phase shift effects, which arise secondary to variations in proton velocity with respect to time, are referred to as temporal phase shift effects.[46] Phase shift effects, which arise secondary to variations in proton velocity with respect to space, are referred to as spatial phase shift ef-

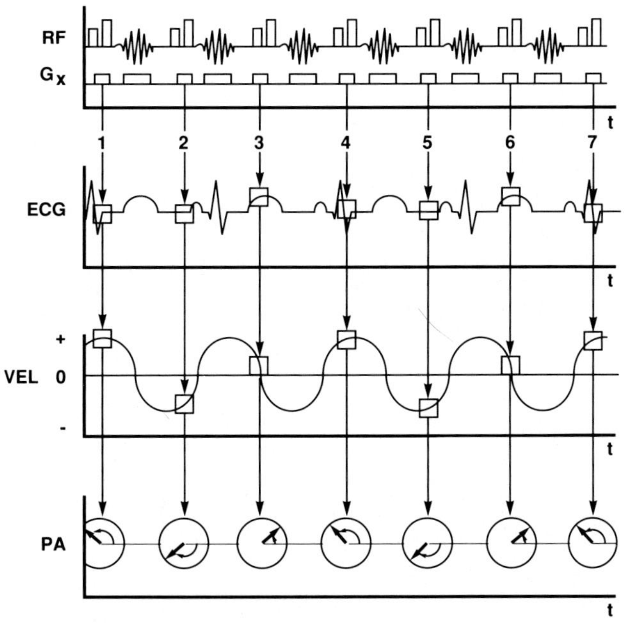

FIGURE 1-28. Temporal phase shift effects. Temporal variations in proton precessional phase occur when proton motion varies as function of time and is not synchronized with MR acquisition. Successive MR excitations *(1-7)* occur at regular time intervals. Timing of excitation and refocusing RF pulses and SE signal are shown on RF channel, although in practice separate channels are used to transmit and receive RF. Readout gradient (G_x) consists of rephasing pulse followed by actual readout gradient pulse. Only phase shift effects of rephasing gradient are illustrated, although both gradient pulses contribute to phase shift effects, which vary as function of time. On successive excitations *(1-7)*, gradients are activated at different phases of cardiac cycle (on Q-wave on first excitation, after T-wave on second excitation, etc.). Different phases of cardiac cycle are associated with different positive *(+)* and negative *(−)* velocities *(VEL)* of CSF within subarachnoid space. Variations in proton velocity lead to variations in proton phase angle *(PA)* on successive excitations. (Modified from Rubin JB, Enzmann DR. CSF flow effects during MRI of the central nervous system. In: Magnetic resonance annual 1988. New York: Raven Press, 1988. With permission.)

fects.[46] In the case of CSF, flow varies over both time and space so that both phase shift effects occur simultaneously.

Temporal phase shift effects. Temporal phase shift effects occur during the imaging of oscillatory CSF because CSF direction, velocity, and acceleration vary as a function of time[46] (Figure 1-28). This leads to variations in proton precessional phase on successive excitations, depending on the proton motion at the time the imaging gradient pulses are applied. The temporal variation in proton phase by itself does not alter signal intensity arising from any given voxel. Rather, the temporal (view to view) variations in phase influence 2DFT image reconstruction according to the Fourier transform frequency shift theorem[8,46] (Figure 1-29). This causes the characteristic artifacts of signal-loss and ghost artifacts[45] (Figures 1-30 and 1-31). The variable relationship between TR and the pulsation period explains why a variable pattern of CSF ghosts may be observed in relation to the spinal canal[46] (Figure 1-32).

Spatial phase shift effects. Spatial phase shift effects occur when proton direction, velocity, and acceleration are the same on successive excitations and there is a distribution of proton velocities within individual imaging voxels.[46,58] These motion artifacts are usually masked by temporal phase shift effects but become visible when temporal phase shift effects are eliminated using gating (described later in this chapter).

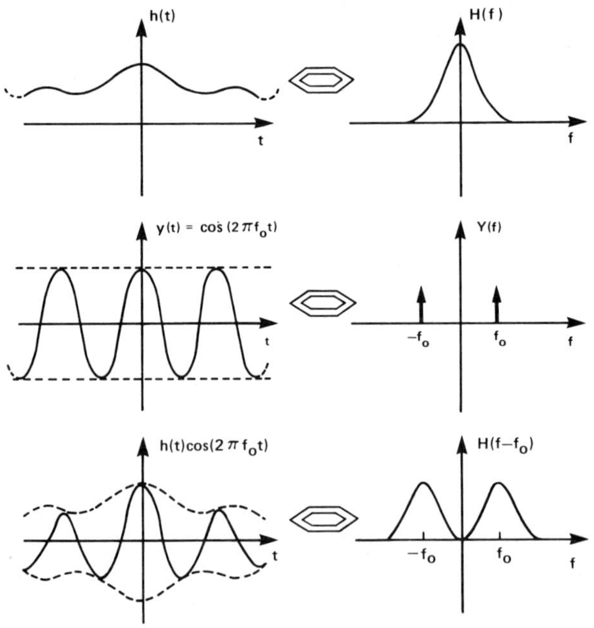

FIGURE 1-29. Fourier transform frequency shift theorem. During 2DFT image reconstruction, fourier transform is applied to first dimension (time axis) and then to second dimension (pseudo-time axis) of spatial fourier plane to localize signal. Fourier transform pairs are shown with pseudo-time domain (left) and frequency domain (right). Phase is pseudo-time function (second spatial fourier variable) during 2DFT imaging. **A,** Fourier transform *H(f)* of pseudo-time function *h(t)* is a frequency distribution. Central peak of frequency distribution is known as *baseband frequency*, which permits spatial localization of signal along the phase-encoding axis. When CSF is stationary, baseband frequency locates CSF along phase-encoding axis of the spatial Fourier plane. **B,** Effect of oscillatory motion on CSF phase may be represented by a cosine function with frequency equal to heart rate. Fourier transform of cosine function is frequency pair $(f_0, -f_0)$. **C,** CSF oscillatory motion causes modulation of proton phase. Effect of this on fourier transform is a frequency shift from baseband frequency, causing appearance of sidebands. Frequency shift from baseband causes signal-loss within pulsatile CSF, and appearance of sidebands causes ghosts, which are symmetrically displaced along phase-encoding axis. (From Rubin JB, Enzmann DR. AJNR 1987; 8:307. With permission.)

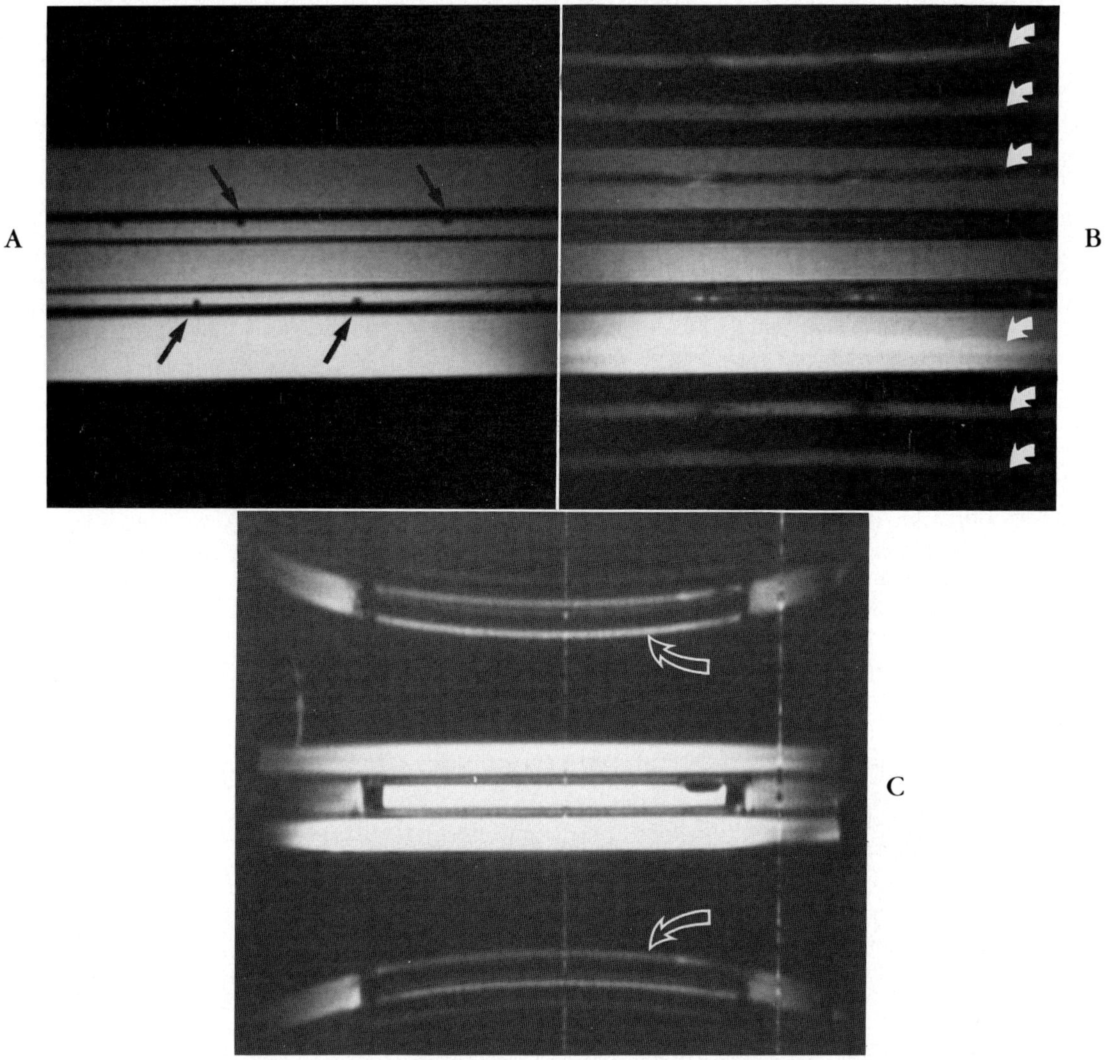

FIGURE 1-30. CSF flow effects in sagittal phantom spine. **A,** Stationary CSF is same signal intensity as water within phantom spinal cord. In absence of CSF motion, multiple phantom extradural defects impinging on thecal sac are well delineated *(arrows)*. Oscillatory CSF: **B,** small field of view; **C,** large field of view. Oscillatory CSF exhibits prominent signal-loss and ghost artifacts *(arrows)*. Ghosts are identical in shape to pattern of signal-loss within subarachnoid space. Signal-loss reduces contrast between oscillatory CSF and phantom extradural defects. (From Rubin JB, Enzmann DR. AJNR 1987; 8:307. With permission.)

A 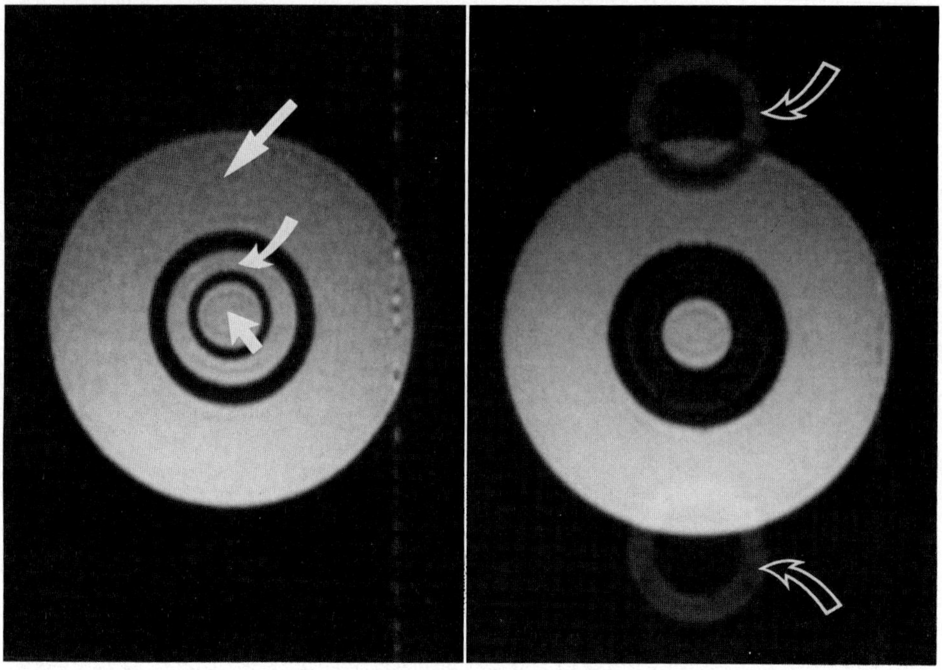 B

FIGURE 1-31. CSF flow effects in axial phantom spine. **A,** Stationary CSF. **B,** Oscillatory CSF. Stationary CSF *(curved arrow)* is same signal intensity as water within phantom spinal cord *(small straight arrow)* and water surrounding phantom spinal canal *(large straight arrow)*. Oscillatory CSF exhibits prominent signal-loss and ghost artifacts *(curved arrows)*. Ghosts either add to or subtract from stationary signal intensity. They are identical in shape to pattern of signal-loss within subarachnoid space. (From Rubin JB, Enzmann DR. AJNR 1987; 8:307. With permission.)

A 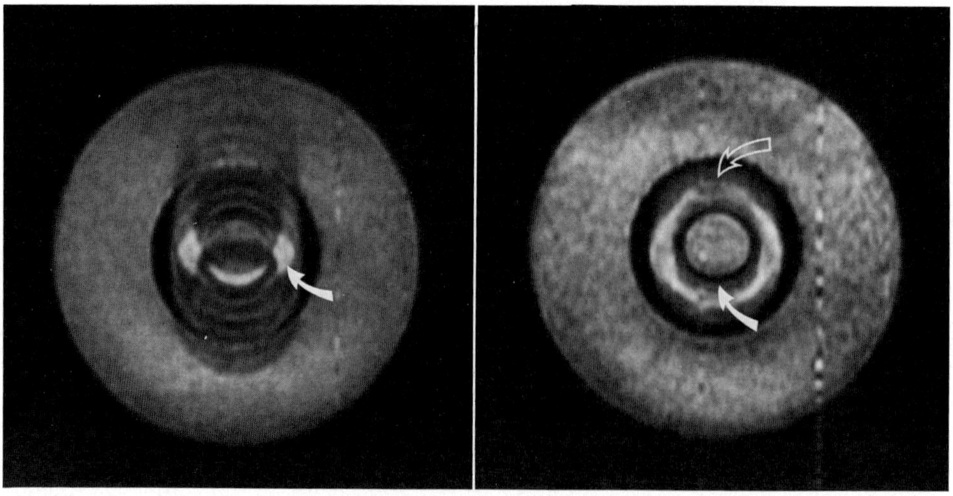 B

FIGURE 1-32. Effect of TR and heart rate on position of ghosts. Axial spine phantom, pulsation period 1060 msec. **A,** TR 1050 msec. When TR is a near integral multiple of the pulsation period, ghosts converge on spinal canal, which obscures margins of phantom spinal cord *(arrow)* and thecal sac. **B,** TR 1060 msec. When TR is set approximately equal to pulsation period, ghosts nearly completely superimpose each other. However, CSF-thecal sac interface *(open arrow)* and CSF-spinal cord interface *(solid arrow)* remain indistinct because of minor variations in the pulsation period. (From Rubin JB, Enzmann DR, Wright A. Radiology 1987; **163:**784. With permission.)

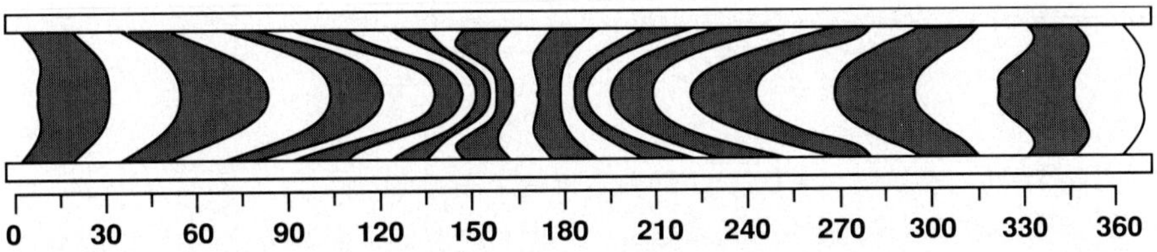

FIGURE 1-33. Schematic representation of CSF flow profile within subarachnoid space at each phase of CSF oscillatory cycle (15° intervals). Shape of flow profile changes markedly at different phases of oscillation. Notice reversal in direction between systole (0°-180°) and diastole (180°-360°). Greatest spatial distribution of velocity occurs at periphery of lumen in most phases of oscillation. (Modified from Rubin JB and Enzmann DR. CSF flow effects during MRI of the central nervous system. In: Magnetic resonance annual 1988, New York: Raven Press, 1988. With permission.)

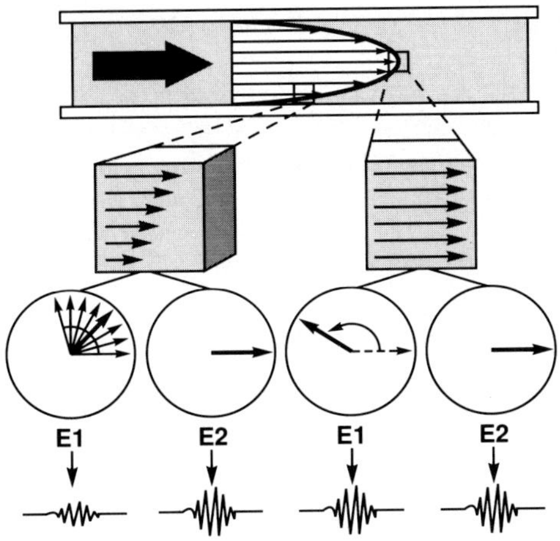

FIGURE 1-34. Spatial phase shift effects during imaging of laminar flow: boundary layer phase dispersion. At any phase of oscillation, spatial distribution of proton velocities may be represented by a specific flow profile. Voxels at periphery of subarachnoid space near boundary layer contain protons with great distribution of velocities that cause phase dispersion and signal-loss on first echo *(E1)* images (boundary layer phase dispersion). Partial even echo rephasing occurs on second echo *(E2)* images, resulting in increased signal. Voxels within center of subarachnoid space contain protons whose velocities are all similar, so that a coherent phase shift occurs without concomitant signal-loss. Even though rephasing occurs on subsequent even echo images similar to periphery of lumen, no change in signal intensity is observed in voxels. (Modified from Rubin JB, Enzmann DR. CSF flow effects during MRI of the central nervous system. In: Magnetic resonance annual 1988. New York: Raven Press, 1988. With permission.)

Spatial phase shift effects cause regions of signal-loss because the differing proton velocities cause an incoherent phase shift (phase dispersion), which is responsible for destructive interference of the signal arising from a voxel.[58] The prominence of spatial phase shift effects depends on the shape of the flow profile because this describes the spatial distribution of proton velocities.[38,40] During constant velocity laminar flow, the flow profile is parabolic. During oscillatory flow, the shape of the flow profile is complex because it continuously changes with the phase of oscillation (Figure 1-33). In both types of flow, the greatest spatial distribution of proton velocity occurs secondary to shear forces acting on flowing protons adjacent to the boundary layer, which consists of slowly moving and stationary protons at fluid interfaces.[38,40]

Signal intensity within the center of a lumen during imaging of laminar flow is not reduced by spatial phase shift effects because in this region the flow profile is relatively flat, so that all protons move at a similar high velocity[58] (Figure 1-34). However, signal intensity is reduced at the periphery of the lumen and in regions of turbulent flow secondary to phase dispersion caused by the varying proton velocities in these regions.[58] Boundary layer phase dispersion occurs near fluid interfaces during imaging of laminar flow[48] (Figure 1-34), resulting in bands of low signal intensity, which silhouette CSF interfaces when temporal phase shift effects are eliminated (Figure 1-35). Turbulent phase dispersion occurs during imaging of turbulent flow[48] (Figure 1-36), resulting in focal regions of signal-loss adjacent to lesions responsible for the

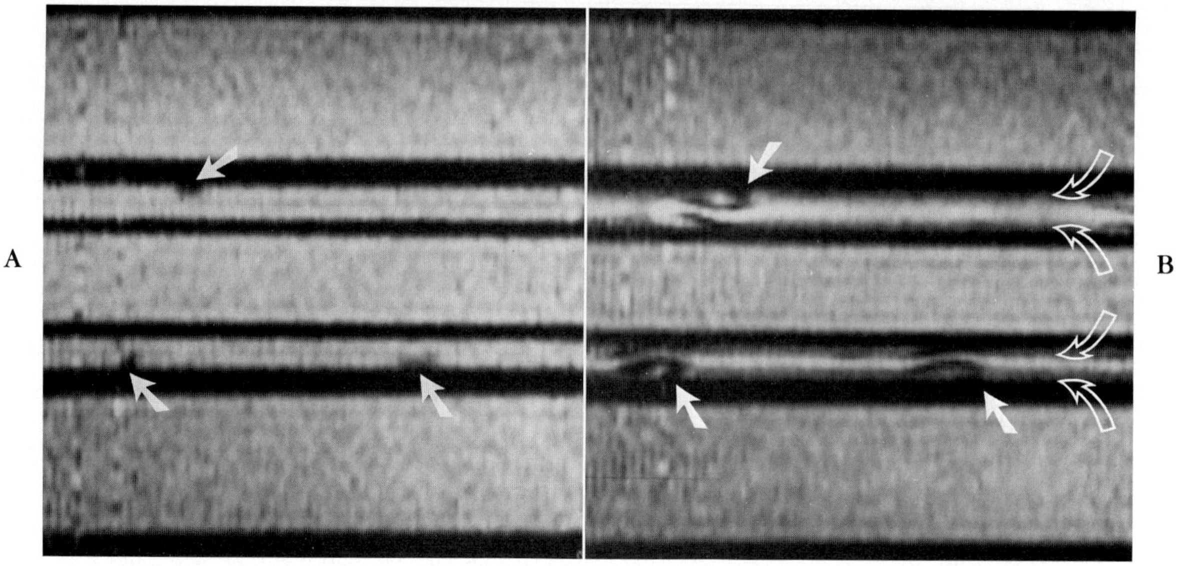

FIGURE 1-35. Boundary layer phase dispersion in sagittal spine phantom. Gated SE 2000/40. **A,** Stationary CSF signal intensity is uniform. Low intensity phantom extradural defects contrast well with stationary CSF *(arrows)*. **B,** Gated oscillatory CSF exhibits bands of low signal intensity at CSF interfaces (boundary layer phase dispersion) *(curved open arrows)* and crescentic bands of low signal intensity adjacent to phantom extradural defects (turbulent phase dispersion) *(solid arrows)*. These were eliminated using flow-compensated imaging gradient pulses.

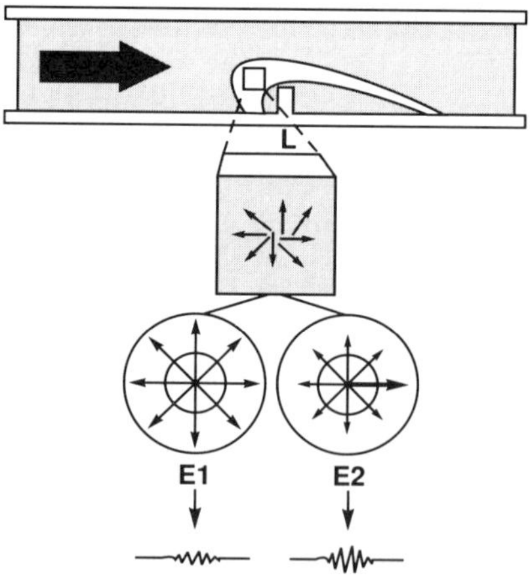

FIGURE 1-36. Spatial phase shift effects during imaging of turbulent flow: turbulent phase dispersion. If extradural lesion *(L)* exists, this creates turbulence that disorganizes orderly pattern of laminar flow. Voxels within regions of turbulence contain large distribution of proton direction and velocity, which causes phase dispersion and prominent signal-loss on first echo *(E1)* images. Less complete even echo rephasing occurs on second echo *(E2)* images in turbulent flow compared to laminar flow because turbulent proton direction and velocity vary greatly between successive echoes. (Modified from Rubin JB and Enzmann DR. CSF flow effects during MRI of the central nervous system. In: Magnetic resonance annual 1988, New York: Raven Press, 1988. With permission.)

turbulence (Figure 1-35). During spine imaging, turbulence is caused by extradural defects which impinge on the thecal sac.

Time of flight effects

Time of flight effects are caused by the movement of protons into or out of an imaging volume while imaging is in progress.[2,6,7,57,60] They alter the signal intensity of moving CSF but do not cause spatial mismapping of the signal. Time of flight effects may be classified into three categories: (1) effective TR prolongation, (2) fast transition phenomenon, and (3) saturation effects.

Effective TR prolongation. Effective TR prolongation occurs when relatively unsaturated protons enter an imaging volume between successive excitations (wash-in), but do not leave that volume before refocusing (wash-out)[7,48,50] (Figure 1-37). This tends to occur at relatively low velocities, which are common in oscillatory CSF. Effective TR prolongation is observed as an increased signal intensity of flowing protons compared to stationary protons when flow travels through the imaging plane (Figure 1-38). It is usually masked by temporal and spatial phase shift effects but becomes visible when flow mechanisms are eliminated, by methods described later in this chapter.[48]

To understand effective TR prolongation, it is helpful to compare it with entry phenomenon, commonly observed as increased signal intensity during the imaging of flowing blood.[2,7] Similar to effective TR prolongation, this flow mechanism results in an increased signal intensity arising from flowing protons secondary to a wash-in of relatively unsaturated protons. However, in the case of flowing blood, the inflowing protons are completely unsaturated because blood continually moves in one direction, so that an endless supply of protons is continually available.

The signal enhancement during the imaging of flowing blood is dependent on the rate of replacement of saturated by unsaturated protons.[2,7] This is influenced by flow velocity, slice

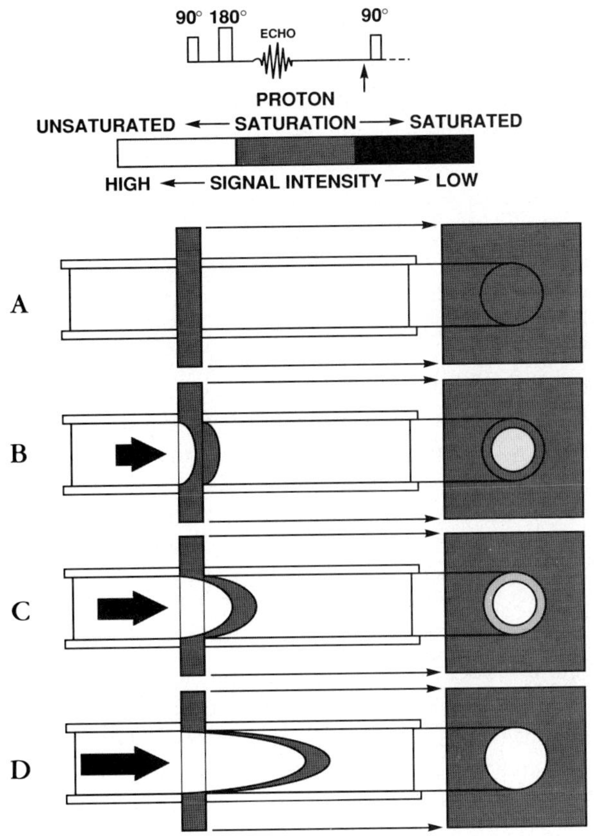

FIGURE 1-37. Effective TR prolongation. Timing of SE pulse sequence is shown at top of figure assuming single echo and single-slice acquisition. Sagittal images *(left)* represent maps of proton saturation just before the next excitation (arrow before to next 90° pulse). Saturation maps show different CSF pulsation amplitudes (stationary and three increasing pulsation amplitudes). Axial images *(right)* represent signal intensity observed on magnitude images for each pulsation amplitude. Protons within imaging plane are relatively saturated compared to protons outside imaging plane because of repetitive excitations. **A,** In absence of CSF motion, protons within lumen are saturated to same extent as protons outside lumen, so no difference between intraluminal and extraluminal signal intensity is observed. **B and C,** When pulsation amplitude is low, central relatively saturated protons within plane exchange with relatively less saturated protons from outside plane before next excitation occurs, effectively prolonging TR of protons, which causes signal enhancement at center of subarachnoid space where oscillation amplitude is greater than at its periphery. **D,** In presence of larger pulsation amplitude, signal enhancement is observed throughout lumen on axial magnitude image. (Modified from Rubin JB and Enzmann DR. CSF flow effects during MRI of the central nervous system. In: Magnetic resonance annual 1988, New York: Raven Press, 1988. With permission.)

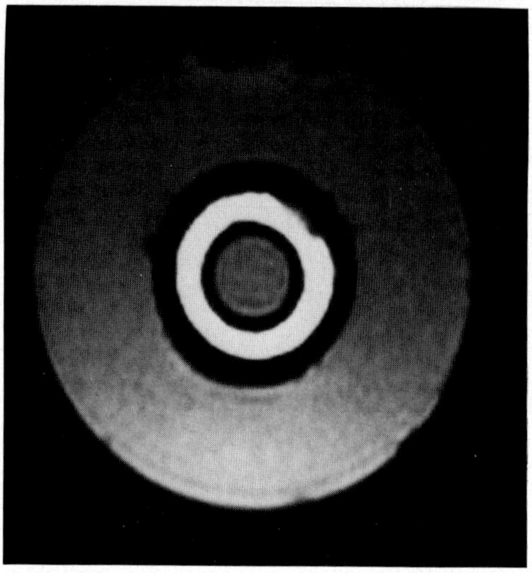

FIGURE 1-38. Effective TR prolongation in axial spine phantom. Gated SE 2000/80. Increased signal intensity of CSF within subarachnoid space is observed relative to stationary water within spinal cord (signal-gain).

thickness, and TR. Entry phenomenon progressively increases in prominence with increasing flow velocity because this leads to more wash-in of unsaturated protons.[2,7] At very low blood flow velocities, only the central protons wash in so that central signal enhancement is observed. At greater velocities, both central and peripheral flowing protons wash in and cause signal enhancement throughout the blood vessel lumen. At even higher velocities, the flow is fast enough to cause wash-out of some or all of these protons before being refocused (fast transition phenomenon, discussed later). Entry phenomena are more pronounced when thinner slice thicknesses are used because more wash-in occurs at any given flow velocity.[2,7] The effect of TR on entry phenomena is slightly more complex. A short TR limits the amount of wash-in of unsaturated protons and reduces entry phenomena, whereas longer TR permits more wash-in to occur and increases entry phenomena. A very long TR permits more wash-in to occur but also permits greater relaxation of stationary protons within the slice, so that the relative difference between them and moving protons is diminished, leading to less prominent signal enhancement of flowing protons.

Effective TR prolongation is related to entry phenomenon but is fundamentally different from it in some important respects.[48,50] During imaging of oscillatory CSF flow, the inflowing protons are in limited supply and partially saturated. This is because the same protons continually leave and re-enter the imaging volume on different excitations. An equilibrium saturation is established so that the effective TR of the protons within the imaging volume is increased and the effective TR of protons outside the imaging volume is reduced from what they would have been if no motion had occurred. This explains a fundamental difference between effective TR prolongation and entry phenomenon: entry phenomenon is proportional to flow velocity, whereas effective TR prolongation is not. The reasons for this difference are discussed later in the chapter.

Fast transition phenomenon. Fast transition phenomenon occurs when flowing protons, excited within an imaging volume, wash out of the imaging volume before the application of the refocusing 180° RF pulse[6] (Figure 1-39). These flowing protons are less saturated at the time of their excitation in comparison with stationary protons in the imaging plane because they washed in since the previous excitation. However, signal-loss is observed instead of signal-gain because their signal is not detected unless refocusing occurs within the imaging volume. During multislice SE imaging, selective refocusing 180° RF pulses are used so that protons, which leave an imaging plane before the application of this pulse, are not refocused. Fast transition phenomenon occurs at higher flow velocities than is encountered in CSF within the normal spinal subarachnoid space.[45,46] CSF velocity is increased in pathologic conditions that narrow the subarachnoid space. Under these circumstances, fast transition phenomenon may be observed in proximity to lesions on axial images as focally reduced CSF signal intensity.

Whereas effective TR prolongation of oscillatory CSF is not dependent on average CSF flow velocity, this is not true of fast transition phenomenon. Fast transition phenomena progressively increase with increasing flow velocity because a larger proportion of protons leave the imaging volume without being refocused as velocity increases.[6] Initially, only the central protons wash out showing signal-loss, whereas the

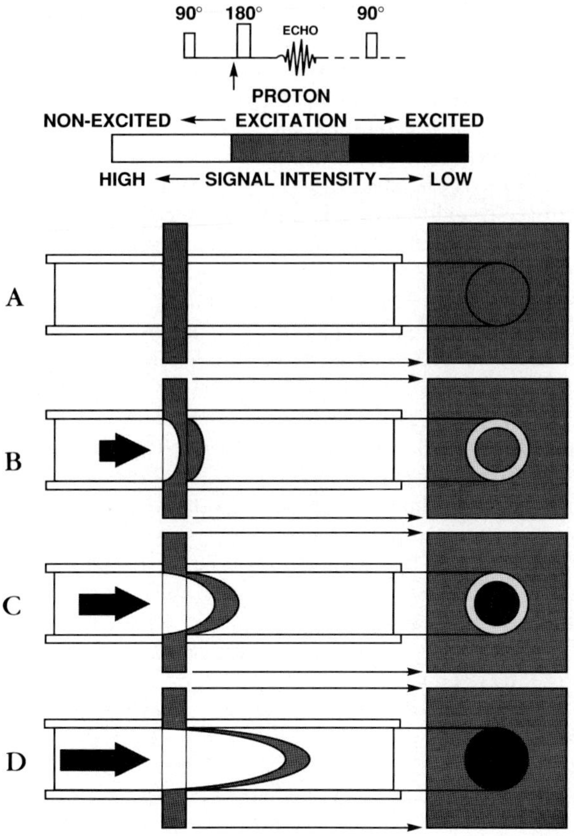

FIGURE 1-39. Fast transition phenomenon. Timing of SE pulse sequence is shown at top of figure assuming single echo and single-slice acquisition. Sagittal images *(left)* represent maps of proton saturation just before refocusing (arrow before 180° refocusing pulse). Saturation maps show different CSF velocities (stationary and three instantaneous velocities). To exhibit fast transition phenomenon, CSF velocities must be large enough to cause excited protons to leave the imaging plane between time they are excited and time refocusing occurs. Axial images *(right)* represent signal intensity observed on magnitude images for each CSF velocity. Protons within imaging plane are relatively saturated compared to protons outside imaging plane because of repetitive excitations. **A,** In absence of flow, excited protons within imaging plane are all present at time of refocusing. **B,** In presence of relatively rapid flow, only some excited protons wash out of imaging plane before they can be refocused. Remainder contribute to overall signal intensity. The two populations of protons average a signal intensity that is not much different than signal intensity of stationary protons. **C and D,** In presence of faster flow, excited protons wash out of imaging plane before they can be refocused, causing protons to appear as low signal intensity on axial magnitude images. (Modified from Rubin JB, Enzmann DR. CSF flow effects during MRI of the central nervous system. In: Magnetic resonance annual 1988, New York: Raven Press, 1988. With permission.)

peripheral protons exhibit signal enhancement because they do not wash out. At greater velocities, all the flowing protons wash out and global signal-loss is observed. Fast transition phenomena are more pronounced when longer TEs and thinner slices are used because they permit a larger proportion of flowing protons to wash out from an imaging volume at any given flow velocity.

Saturation effects. Saturation effects occur when multislice imaging is used and when flow travels through multiple imaging planes.[48] Under these circumstances, flowing protons, which were previously excited in one plane of the imaging volume, travel to a neighboring plane in time for its excitation (Figure 1-40). This shortens the effective TR of some of the flowing protons because they may be excited several times in different slices during a single TR interval.[48] Saturation effects are observed as variable degrees of signal-loss of flowing protons compared to stationary protons[48] (Figure 1-41). They are easily recognized during spine imaging when temporal phase shift effects and spatial phase shift effects have been eliminated using the methods described later in this chapter. The pattern of signal intensity caused by saturation effects is often complex.

Short-TR Variable Flip Angle/Gradient Echo Imaging

In the absence of proton motion, CSF on T2W variable flip angle images is hyperintense compared with spinal cord and extradural structures. The relative signal intensity (SI) of different structures on variable flip angle images can be calculated in the absence of motion using the following equation[37]:

(3)

$$SI = \frac{k \cdot [1 - e^{-TR/T1}] \cdot \sin\beta \cdot N_H \cdot e^{-TE/T2^*}}{1 - e^{-TR/T1} \cdot e^{-TR/T2^*} - \cos\beta \cdot [e^{-TR/T1} - e^{-TR/T2^*}]}$$

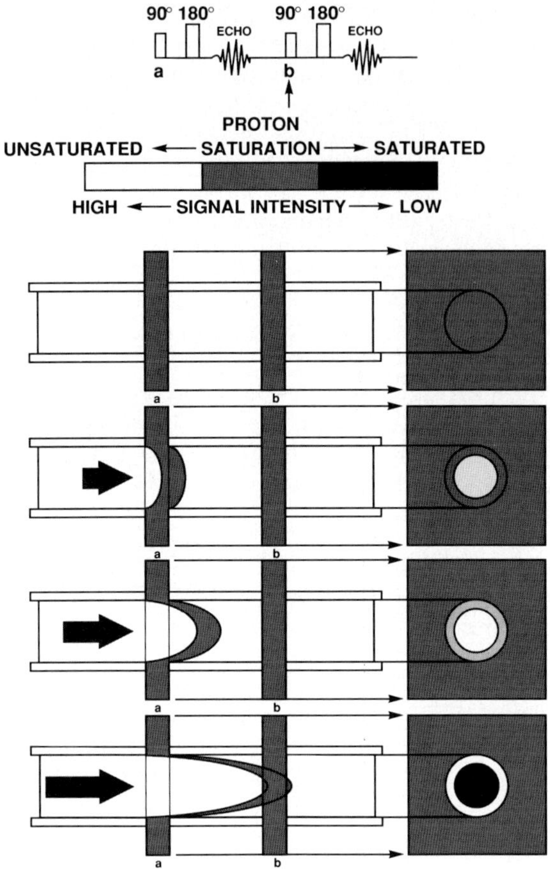

FIGURE 1-40. Saturation effects. Timing of SE pulse sequence is shown at top of figure assuming single echo and two-slice acquisition, *(a, b)*. Sagittal images *(left)* represent maps of proton saturation just before excitation of second slice (arrow before second 90° excitation pulse, *b*). Saturation maps show different pulsation amplitudes (stationary and three increasing pulsation amplitudes). To exhibit saturation effects, CSF velocities must be large enough to allow excited protons to move between adjacent imaging slices before second slice is excited. Axial images *(right)* represent signal intensity observed on magnitude images of slice *b* for each pulsation amplitude. In absence of flow, no protons move between the two imaging planes. In presence of CSF motion, signal-gain is observed secondary to effective TR prolongation if velocity is not fast enough to move protons between the two slices in time for excitation of the second slice. In presence of faster flow, protons excited in slice *a* move to slice *b* by the time it is excited, which lowers effective TR of these protons so they appear reduced in signal intensity on axial magnitude image of slice *b*. When gating is used during imaging of oscillatory flow, this sequence is strictly repeated and luminal signal may be high on one slice, *a*, and low on an adjacent slice, *b*, as occurred here. (Modified from Rubin JB, Enzmann DR. CSF flow effects during MRI of the central nervous system. In: Magnetic resonance annual 1988. New York: Raven Press, 1988. With permission.)

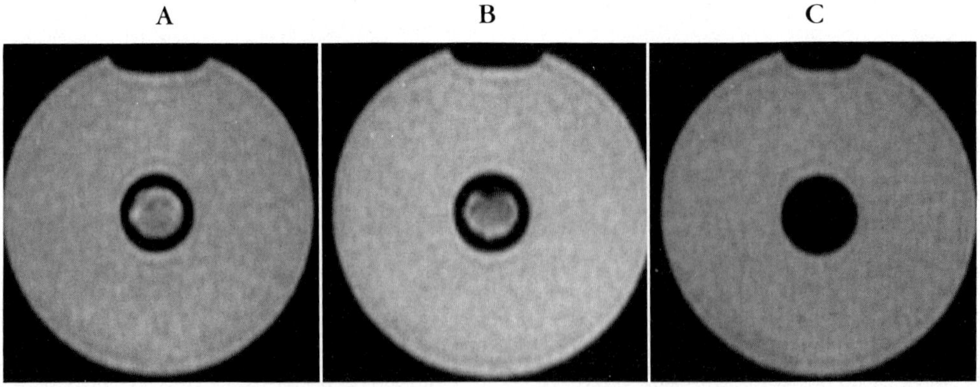

FIGURE 1-41. Saturation effects in axial oscillatory phantom. Gated SE 2000/80. **A,** Middle slice. Signal intensity of oscillatory water on middle slice is isointense with stationary water because velocity at this phase of oscillation is too low to cause saturation effects. **B,** Adjacent slice to **A. C,** Adjacent slice to **B.** Signal intensity of oscillatory water on adjacent slices is hypointense compared with stationary water because greater flow velocity at these phases of oscillation permits saturation effects to occur.

where β is the flip angle used, k is a constant of proportionality, T2* is the transverse magnetization decay time (described in detail later), and TR, TE, N_H, and T1 have their usual meaning. For example, the relative contrast between CSF and spinal cord on T2W variable flip angle images may be calculated assuming TR/TE = 200/80 msec, flip angle = 90°, $T1_{CSF}$ = 3000 msec, $T2^*_{CSF}$ = 800 msec, N_H(CSF) = 1, $T1_{SC}$ = 515 msec, $T2^*_{WM}$ = 57 msec, and N_H(spinal cord) = 0.77. Under these conditions, SI_{CSF} is 21 and SI_{WM} is 6. Therefore, in the absence of CSF motion, CSF is expected to be approximately 3.5 times higher in signal intensity than spinal cord. However, as discussed previously, oscillatory CSF is lower in signal intensity than spinal cord under these imaging conditions.

Motion influences variable flip angle images by the same fundamental mechanisms previously described for SE imaging: phase shift effects and time of flight effects.[50] In the absence of flow compensation, phase shift effects (temporal and spatial) are prominent on variable flip angle images just as they are on SE images. These motion artifacts are reduced or eliminated on variable flip angle images by flow compensation similar to SE images. Although phase shift effects appear similar on both SE and variable flip angle images, some of the time of flight effects do not occur on variable flip angle images. Fast transition phenomena do not occur because a gradient echo is used instead of a 180° RF refocusing pulse. This means that excited protons are refocused regardless of how rapidly they leave the imaging volume. Saturation effects do not occur because gating cannot be used on variable flip angle acquisitions when the TR is shorter than the heart period.

In the following sections, flow compensation is assumed to be used during routine variable flip angle imaging in the spine. Under these conditions, temporal and spatial phase shift effects (boundary layer phase dispersion, turbulent phase dispersion, and ghosts) are not prominent. The two flow mechanisms that remain—disruption of the steady state and effective TR prolongation[50]—will be described in detail. Disruption of the steady state is an important flow mechanism on variable flip angle images that does not occur on SE images because of fundamental differences between the two pulse sequences. Effective TR prolongation is similar to that observed on SE images but is usually more prominent on variable flip angle images for the reasons described in the following section.

Disruption of the steady state

Signal-loss during variable flip angle imaging occurs because as protons move along the imaging gradients they are driven towards a different steady state at each position.[42] Under these circumstances, protons cannot establish a steady state and instead become saturated.[42] Therefore, flow-induced disruption of the steady state causes a reduction of the signal intensity on magnitude images (Figures 1-42 and 1-43). In contrast, stationary protons have a very high signal intensity because their steady state is maintained. Motion along the frequency encoding or slice selection gradient is more likely to cause disruption of the steady state than motion along the phase-encoding gradient because of the lower amplitude and duration of the phase-encoding gradient. Flow-induced disruption of the steady state occurs with even small amounts of motion.[42] During imaging of constant velocity flow, signal-loss occurs with velocities as small as 1 mm/sec.[42] This explains why signal-loss is usually observed throughout the subarachnoid space rather than occurring only in the regions of greatest CSF motion. As discussed later in this chapter, adjustment of the various imaging parameters alters the prominence of this motion artifact and allows the desired image contrast to be achieved.

Effective TR prolongation

Signal-gain during variable flip angle imaging of oscillatory CSF occurs secondary to effective TR prolongation, which is similar to that which occurs during SE imaging.[50] It may be prominent on variable flip angle images, particularly when single-slice acquisition is used (see Figure 1-43), and it results from the establishment of an equilibrium saturation of protons within and adjacent to the imaging volume, already described. During imaging, protons within the imaging volume continually exchange with protons adjacent to the imaging volume. After a number of excitations, the in-flowing protons are partially saturated and the out-flowing protons return before they have regained full magneti-

A B C D

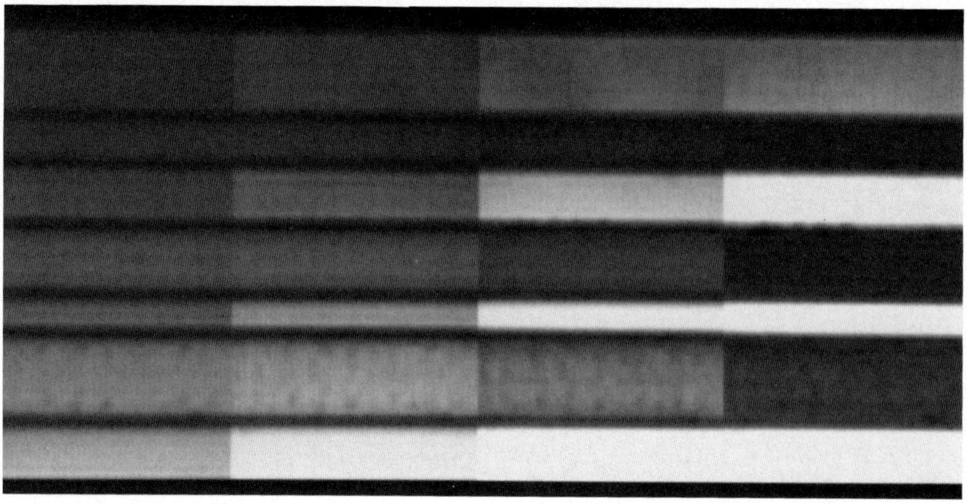

FIGURE 1-42. Flow-induced disruption of steady state during variable flip angle imaging in sagittal oscillatory flow phantom. GRASS 22/12. **A,** Flip angle 3°. **B,** Flip angle 8°. **C,** Flip angle 45°. **D,** Flip angle 90°. In three tube phantom, pulsation amplitude is 10 mm in large tube, 18 mm in intermediate tube, and 40 mm in small tube. Stationary water surrounds tubes for reference signal intensity. At low flip angles, no signal-loss of oscillatory compared with stationary water is observed. However, at larger flip angles, signal-loss becomes pronounced secondary to disruption of the steady state. Note that amount of signal-loss is independent of pulsation amplitude. (From Rubin JB. Submitted for publication to Radiology.)

A B C D

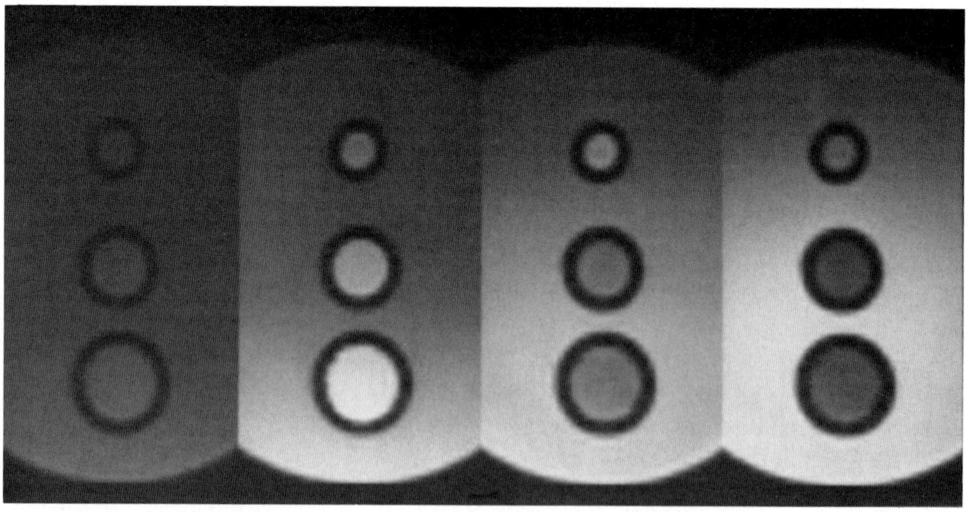

FIGURE 1-43. Effective TR prolongation during variable flip angle imaging in axial oscillatory flow phantom. GRASS 22/12. **A,** Flip angle 3°. **B,** Flip angle 8°. **C,** Flip angle 45°. **D,** Flip angle 90°. (Note same phantom and pulsation amplitudes as in Figure 1-42.) At low flip angles, oscillatory water is isointense with stationary water regardless of pulsation amplitude. At larger flip angles, signal-gain is observed secondary to effective TR prolongation at all pulsation amplitudes but it is greatest at highest pulsation amplitude. At still larger flip angles, opposing signal-loss secondary to disruption of the steady state predominates in tubes with low pulsation amplitude. (From Rubin JB. Submitted for publication to Radiology.)

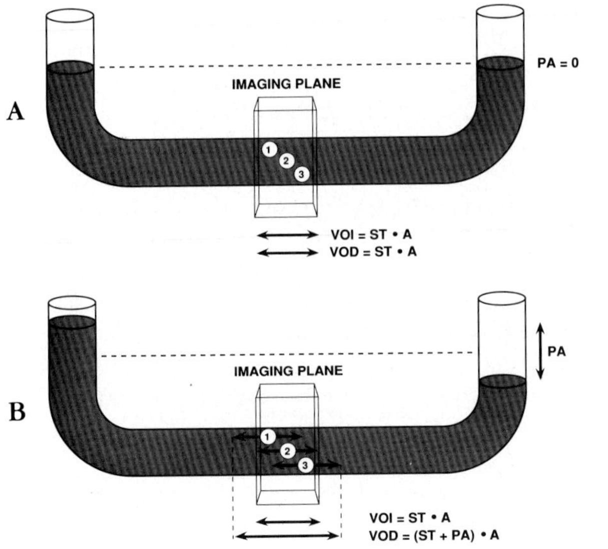

FIGURE 1-44. Schematic diagram of flow-dependent effective TR prolongation during single-slice imaging of oscillatory water. **A,** Stationary water. **B,** Oscillatory water. Protons *(1)* at left edge of slice, *(2)* within center of slice, and *(3)* at right edge of slice. When water is stationary, protons remain in slice and are excited on every excitation. Effective TR is equal to actual TR used during imaging. When water is oscillatory, protons within slice exchange with protons outside slice so that not every proton is excited on every excitation. Effective TR of protons within slice is prolonged compared to actual TR used for imaging. Amount of flow-dependent effective TR prolongation is related to likelihood that any proton will be in slice on any excitation. It is dependent on relationship between volume of RF irradiation *(VOI)* and volume of proton distribution *(VOD)*, which is determined by slice thickness *(ST)*, pulsation amplitude *(PA)*, and cross-sectional area of the lumen **(A).** (From Rubin JB. Submitted for publication to Radiology.)

zation. The resultant equilibrium saturation is determined by the relative number of exchanging protons outside the imaging volume compared to the relative number inside the imaging volume (Figure 1-44).[50]

Effective TR prolongation is not proportional to velocity, but rather is proportional to the relative volume of protons outside the imaging slice that exchange with protons within the imaging slice.[50] The volume of protons within the imaging slice is referred to as the volume of RF irradiation (VOI), and the total volume of exchanging protons is referred to as the volume of proton distribution (VOD). The VOD is proportional to pulsation amplitude but is independent of average CSF velocity. Therefore increasing the pulsation amplitude increases signal-gain because of its effect on the VOD and not because of its effect on average flow velocity.[50] In contrast, reducing the pulsation period (which increases average flow velocity) has no effect on signal-gain because it does not alter the VOD.[50] Therefore effective TR prolongation is proportional to the VOD and not dependent on average CSF velocity.[50] Signal-gain is reduced when thicker slices are used because the VOI is proportional to the slice thickness.[50] The use of effective TR prolongation to improve image contrast on axial variable flip-angle images will be discussed later in the chapter.

ALTERATION OF IMAGE CONTRAST BY CSF MOTION ARTIFACTS

This section summarizes the determinants of image contrast on SE and variable flip angle images, reviews the clinical utility of the different types of image contrasts, and closely examines how each kind of image contrast is altered by CSF motion. The next section discusses how high quality SE and variable flip angle images may be obtained by eliminating CSF motion artifacts.

In the absence of motion, the contrast of SE and variable flip angle images is determined by the relative weighting (T1, T2, or PD) of the pulse sequence used and on the T1, T2, and PD of each tissue.[61] During SE imaging, TR and TE are the most important determinants of image contrast. During variable flip angle imaging, flip angle is the most important determinant of image contrast, followed by TR and TE.[30,65] On relatively T1W images, stationary CSF is hypointense relative to spinal cord because CSF has a longer T1 relaxation time than white matter. On relatively T2W images, stationary CSF is hyperintense relative to spinal cord because CSF has a longer T2 relaxation time than white matter. On relatively PDW images, stationary CSF is hyperintense relative to spinal cord because CSF has a higher proton density than white matter.

T1W images are excellent for the anatomic delineation of normal CSF interfaces because low signal intensity CSF contrasts well with medium signal intensity discs, epidural lesions, and spinal cord. Therefore, T1W images are useful in the evaluation of disc disease (herniated discs), epidural disease (tumor, blood, or infection), and spinal cord morphology (cord widening secondary to inflammatory lesions or neoplasm vs. atrophy secondary to previous trauma or demyelination). Spinal cord cavities (caused by syrinx or tumor cysts) are also well demonstrated on T1W images because these contain either CSF or fluid, which has a longer T1 than adjacent normal spinal cord. T1W images are of limited utility in the delineation of low signal intensity structures that interface with CSF. For example, osteophytes are usually relatively inapparent on T1W images because there is little contrast between them and the low signal intensity CSF.[17,45]

T2W and PDW images provide an alternative CSF contrast in which CSF is hyperintense relative to extradural structures and spinal cord (myelographic effect) (Figure 1-45). This facilitates the identification of low signal intensity osteophytes impinging on the subarachnoid space.[45] T2W images are also used for the detection of solid intrinsic spinal cord lesions, usually detected on T1W images only when they are bulky enough to deform the normal spinal cord contour. Solid spinal cord lesions are not usually detected on T1W images by virtue of their signal intensity because the T1 of these lesions is not sufficiently different from the T1 of normal white matter. On T2W images, lesions are readily visualized as regions of high signal intensity relative to spinal cord because they usually have a long T2 relative to normal white matter. Of the various types of image contrast, T2W and PDW contrasts are degraded to the greatest extent by CSF motion artifacts.[45,46] Therefore, when T2W or PDW imaging is needed for the evaluation of intrinsic cord disease and extradural disease, CSF motion compensation techniques become essential.

Spin Echo Imaging

During SE imaging, TR and TE are major imaging system determinants of image contrast.[61] T1W images are obtained using a short TR and short TE (i.e., TR/TE 800/20 msec) and T2W images are obtained using a long TR and

A

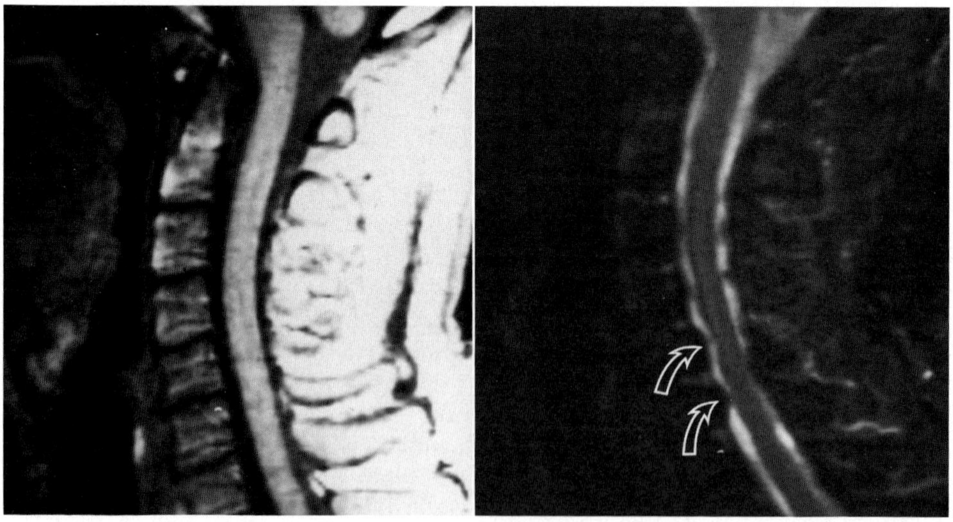

B

FIGURE 1-45. Utility of myelographic contrast in spine imaging. **A**, T1W SE 800/20. **B**, T2W SE 2200/80 (gated). Poor contrast between CSF and extradural structures on T1W image makes evaluation of extradural disease difficult. On T2W image, high signal intensity CSF contrasts well with low signal intensity cortical bone and disc so that osteophytes *(arrows)* are easier to detect. To obtain image of this quality, it is necessary to use methods to eliminate CSF motion artifacts.

long TE (i.e., TR/TE 2000/80 msec). To obtain true PDW images, TR should be at least three times the expected longest T1. For SE imaging where CSF has a long T1 (≥3000 msec), this is not practical because excessive imaging times would be required. Instead, balanced images are usually obtained using the same TR used for T2W images and a short TE (i.e., TR/TE 2000/20 msec). To save time, balanced and T2W images are customarily obtained as different echoes of the same long TR acquisition (i.e., TR/TE 2000/20, 80 msec).

Signal-loss on SE images alters image contrast by reducing CSF signal intensity from what it would have been if CSF was stationary.[45,47,48] On T2W SE spine images, stationary CSF has the highest signal intensity on the image. The spinal cord, the anulus, and other extradural structures are all of lower signal intensity on these images and are visualized only in relief because of the high signal intensity CSF. Therefore a reduction in CSF signal intensity by motion leads to a loss of contrast on T2W SE images (Figure 1-46), thus reducing their diagnostic value, particularly in the evaluation of extradural disease. In contrast, on T1W SE images, signal-loss does not usually influence image contrast because CSF is already one of the lowest signal intensity substances on the image. At times, signal-loss may actually increase contrast between CSF and spinal cord on T1W SE images (Figure 1-47). It is recognized as a motion artifact under these conditions only when the CSF motion within the subarachnoid space is nonuniform (see Figure 1-47).

Signal-gain alters image contrast on T1W, PDW, and T2W SE images by increasing CSF signal intensity. When temporal phase shift effects are not prominent, signal-gain increases CSF signal intensity above what it would have been if CSF was stationary. When temporal phase shifts are prominent, signal-gain increases CSF signal intensity above what it would have been if signal-loss alone had occurred.[46,48] Signal-gain increases the contrast between CSF and spinal cord on end slices of axial T2W or PDW acquisitions by making the otherwise low signal intensity CSF hyperintense to spinal cord. In

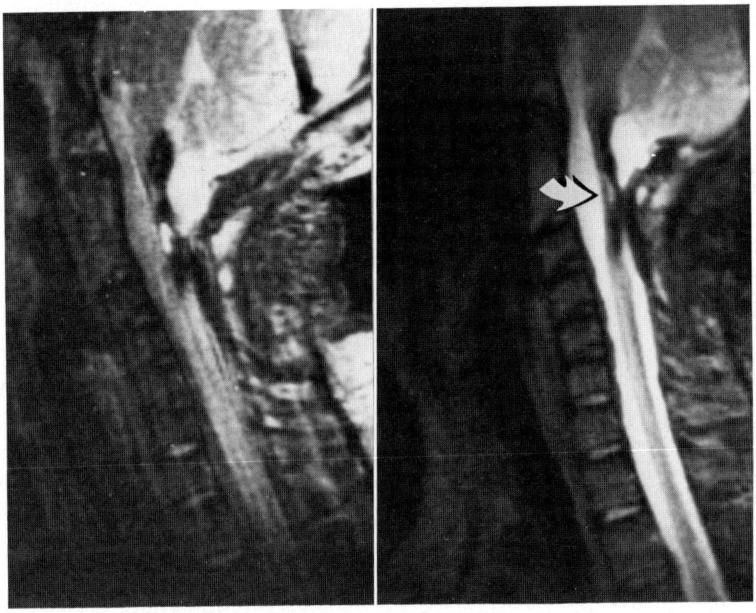

FIGURE 1-46. Loss of T2W image contrast secondary to CSF motion artifacts. **A,** T2W SE 2000/80. **B,** Gated T2W SE 2200/80. Spinal cord glioma, postoperative. Signal-loss and ghosts markedly degrade conventional T2W image quality, making evaluation of spinal cord abnormalities difficult. When CSF motion artifacts are eliminated, postoperative changes such as hemosiderin deposition *(arrow)* are more easily visualized. (From Young S. Nuclear magnetic resonance imaging. New York: Raven Press, 1988. With permission.)

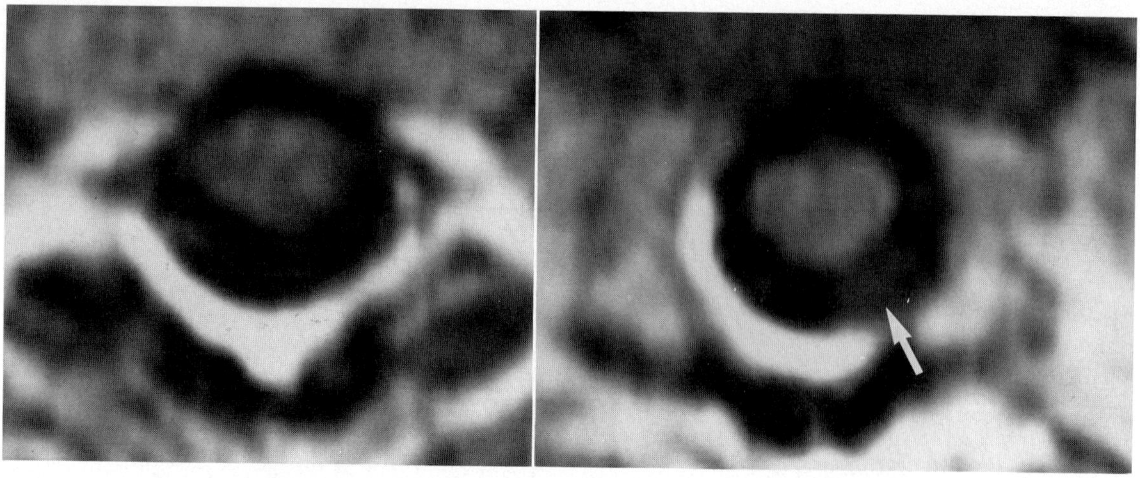

FIGURE 1-47. Improvement of T1W image contrast secondary to CSF motion artifacts. T1W SE 800/20. **A,** Uniform CSF motion. **B,** Nonuniform CSF motion. When CSF motion is uniform within subarachnoid space, CSF signal intensity is reduced, which improves contrast between CSF and spinal cord. When some regions of CSF are more stationary than others *(arrow)*, contribution of signal-loss to image contrast on T1W images is evident.

comparison, signal-gain reduces the contrast between CSF and spinal cord on end slices of axial T1W acquisitions by making the otherwise low signal intensity CSF isointense with spinal cord (see Figure 1-15). This is observed only when temporal phase shift effects on T1W images are not prominent. The presence of signal-gain makes more signal available for spatial mismapping by temporal phase shift effects so that ghost artifacts are often increased in prominence when signal-gain occurs.[46,48] Signal-gain is rarely observed on interior slices of multislice acquisitions because it is reduced by saturation effects.[46,48]

Ghosts alter the image contrast of SE images by superimposing spatially mismapped CSF signal intensity onto other structures in the image.[45] This spatially mismapped CSF signal intensity may either add to or subtract from the signal of structures on which it is superimposed[46] (see Figure 1-17). T2W image contrast is affected to a much greater degree than T1W image contrast. Ghosts markedly reduce T2W SE image quality because stationary CSF is very high signal intensity and all of this signal is available for spatial mismapping. When CSF signal is superimposed onto other structures on T2W images, it obscures the relatively small amount of signal intensity already there.[45,46] Image noise is increased and image contrast is reduced when ghosts are scattered randomly along the phase-encoding axis of T2W spine images. Ghosts have much less effect on T1W SE images because stationary CSF is relatively low signal intensity and there is relatively little signal available for spatial mismapping. When small amounts of CSF signal are superimposed onto other structures on T1W images, they contribute little to the overall signal intensity so that no significant alteration of image contrast is observed.

Short-TR Variable Flip Angle/Gradient Echo Imaging

Important differences between variable flip angle and SE imaging relate to how the SE is formed in each pulse sequence. During SE imaging, both a gradient echo and a 180° RF refocusing pulse are used to form the SE. In contrast, during variable flip angle imaging, only a gradient echo is used to form the SE. The 180° refocusing pulse used during SE imaging markedly reduces inhomogeneities in the magnetic field caused by nonuniformity of the magnet or induced by adjacent tissues of different tissue magnetic susceptibility. Absence of this 180° RF pulse during variable flip angle imaging causes prominent magnetic susceptibility artifacts to occur because the gradient echo alone cannot correct for these inhomogeneities in the magnetic field.[64]

Magnetic susceptibility artifacts commonly

A 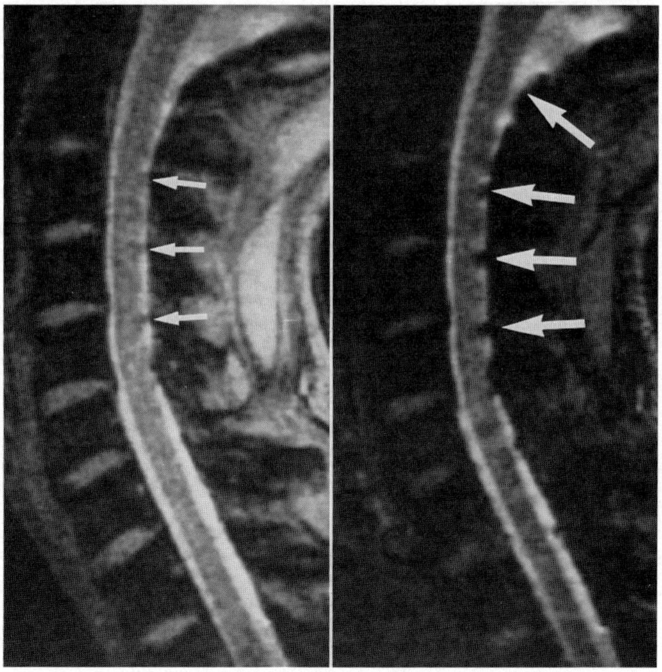 B

FIGURE 1-48. Magnetic susceptibility artifacts in sagittal cervical spine variable flip angle images. **A,** GRASS 80/15. **B,** GRASS 80/40. There is increased CSF-spinal cord contrast on more heavily T2*W image, although degraded by artifacts of low signal intensity in posterior subarachnoid space adjacent to base of spinous processes *(large arrows)*. Magnetic susceptibility artifacts are less prominent on shorter TE image *(small arrows)*. (From Rubin JB. Submitted for publication to Radiology.)

occur at air-water and bone-water interfaces and cause focal regions of low signal intensity. During imaging of the spine, these artifacts interfere with the visualization of the spinal canal and its contents. Magnetic susceptibility artifacts interfere with the production of high quality T2W variable flip angle images. The term T2*W is applied to variable flip angle images that appear similar to T2W images but differ from them because a gradient echo was used, which does not compensate for nonuniformities of the magnetic field. When very uniform magnetic fields are used, T2*W images are similar to T2W images except in regions where differences in tissue magnetic susceptibility are prominent.

During variable flip angle imaging, flip angle is the major determinant of image contrast followed by TR and TE.[30,65] T1W images are obtained using a long TR, short TE, and large flip angle (i.e., TR/TE 400/20 msec, FA 45 to 90°), whereas T2*W images are obtained using a short TR, long TE, and small flip angle (i.e., TR/TE 80/40 to 60 msec, FA 5 to 25°). Unfortunately, magnetic susceptibility artifacts become unacceptably prominent during spine imaging with long TEs because of dense bone in the posterior elements[19,20,51] (Figure 1-48). These tend to be less prominent on axial spine images (Figure 1-49). PDW imaging can provide myelographic contrast without prominent magnetic susceptibility artifacts. PDW images are obtained using a short TR, short TE, and low flip angle (i.e., TR/TE 25/15 msec, FA 5 to 25°) and do not exhibit prominent magnetic susceptibility effects because of the short TE used. Fortunately, variable flip angle PDW images may be obtained rapidly compared to the acquisition times necessary for PDW SE images. In addition to their use in the evaluation of extradural disease, intrinsic cord lesions may sometimes be visualized using PDW images when the lesion contains more water than adjacent normal spinal cord.

Signal-loss on variable flip angle images alters spine image contrast by reducing CSF signal intensity from what it would have been if CSF was stationary.[50,51] Myelographic contrast is achieved during variable flip angle imaging of stationary CSF using both small and large flip

A 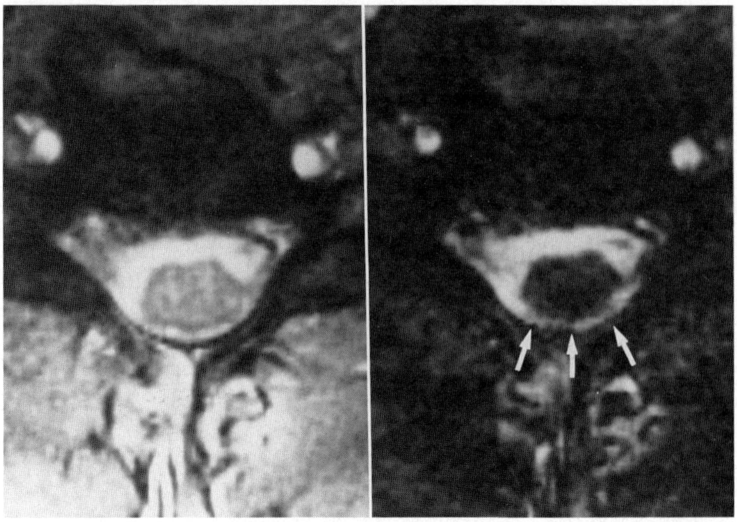 B

FIGURE 1-49. Magnetic susceptibility artifacts in axial cervical spine on variable flip angle images. **A,** GRASS 80/15. **B,** GRASS 80/30. Increased CSF-spinal cord contrast on more heavily T2*W image. Magnetic susceptibility artifacts are slightly less prominent *(arrows)* on these axial images than on sagittal images in Figure 1-48. (From Rubin JB. Submitted for publication to Radiology.)

angles[43] (Figure 1-22 and 1-23). However, CSF motion causes signal-loss on variable flip angle images when intermediate or large flip angles are used, leading to a loss of the expected myelographic contrast[50] (Figure 1-24). CSF motion has no significant effect on CSF signal intensity when small flip angles are used.[50] Therefore, during variable flip angle imaging, *low flip angle* images are relatively *motion insensitive*, whereas *high flip angle* images are *motion sensitive*.[50] CSF signal-loss during variable flip angle imaging reduces the diagnostic efficacy of high flip angle imaging in the assessment of extradural disease. The signal-loss of moving CSF on variable flip angle images is much more uniform than the signal-loss of CSF on SE images because variable flip angle imaging is more sensitive to motion than SE imaging.

As described previously, signal-loss on variable flip angle images is caused by flow-induced disruption of the steady state. Although there is no way to prevent the steady state from being disrupted by CSF motion, it is possible to minimize the effects of CSF motion on image contrast by manipulating imaging parameters, of which the most important is the flip angle.[50,51] Use of low flip angles reduces the prominence of signal-loss of moving CSF relative to stationary CSF. Low flip angle images are relatively insensitive to most kinds of motion.[50] The only disadvantage of this approach is an associated reduction in image signal to noise (SNR).

Low flip angle imaging used clinically as a method to reduce motion-induced signal-loss requires knowing the optimum flip angle to use for any particular set of imaging conditions[50,51] (Figures 1-50 and 1-51). Determination of the optimum flip angle is complex because it is influenced by a number of factors that vary depending on the imaging conditions[50,51] (Figures 1-52 and 1-53). The flip angle needed to achieve the best possible myelographic contrast between CSF and spinal cord or extradural structures depends on imaging plane, TR, slice thickness, number of slices, the amplitude of CSF motion, T1, T2*, and proton density.[50,51] By optimizing these imaging parameters, it is possible to achieve acceptable image contrast and SNR in reasonable imaging times. Techniques to minimize signal-loss on variable flip angle images by manipulating imaging parameters are described in the next section of this chapter and in Chapter 2.

Signal-gain on variable flip angle images alters

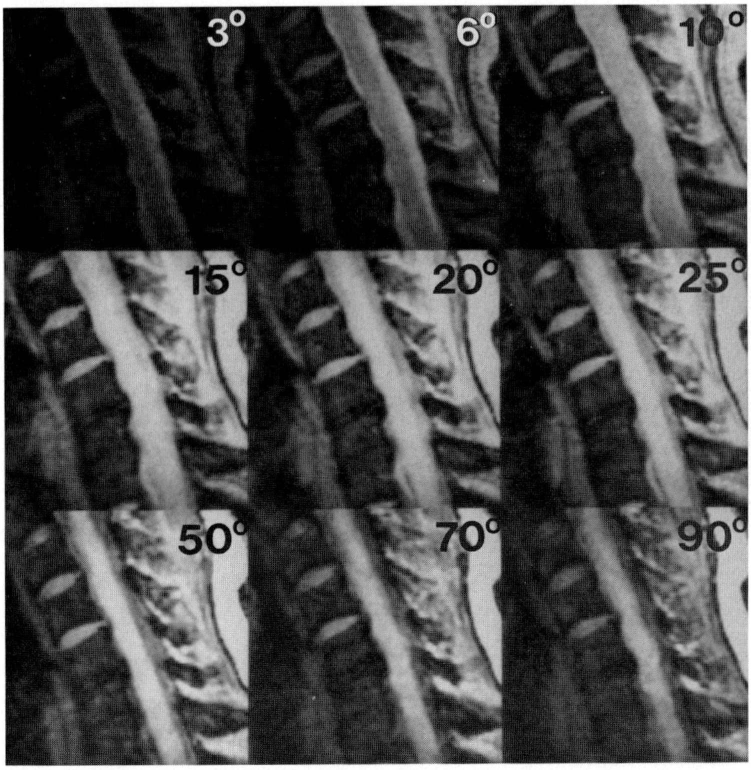

FIGURE 1-50. Effect of flip angle on CSF signal-loss in sagittal cervical spine on variable flip angle images. GRASS 40/15. Flip angles are indicated on individual images. CSF is hyperintense compared with spinal cord when low flip angles are used. As flip angle is increased, CSF signal intensity becomes heterogeneous and then hypointense compared to spinal cord. This empirical approach determines flip angle at which peak myelographic contrast occurs. (From Rubin JB. Submitted for publication to Radiology.)

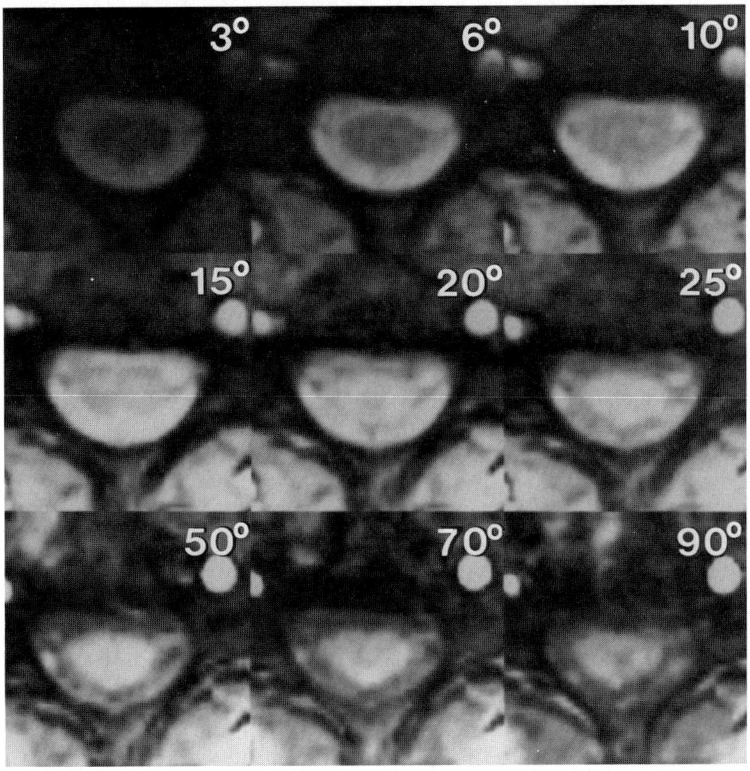

FIGURE 1-51. Effect of flip angle on CSF signal-loss in axial cervical spine on variable flip angle images. GRASS 40/15. Flip angles are indicated on individual images. CSF is hyperintense compared with spinal cord when low flip angles are used. As flip angle is increased, CSF signal intensity becomes heterogeneous and then hypointense compared to spinal cord. Flip angle at which peak myelographic contrast occurs is slightly higher for axial imaging than for sagittal imaging (compare with Figure 1-50). (From Rubin JB. Submitted for publication to Radiology.)

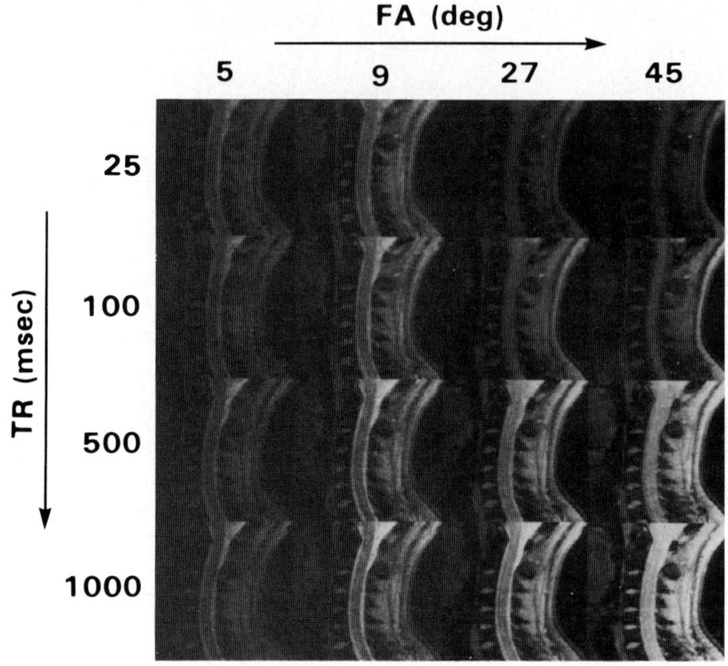

FIGURE 1-52. Effect of flip angle, TR, and number of slices on sagittal cervical spine variable flip angle images. GRASS, TR (25, 100, 500, and 1000 msec) and flip angle (5°, 9°, 27°, and 45°) are indicated on individual images. All images TE 15 msec. Images obtained with TR of 25 msec are single-slice acquisitions, whereas images obtained with TRs of 100-1000 are interleaved multislice acquisitions. CSF signal intensity and CSF-cord contrast peak depend on both TR and flip angle. On short-TR images (25 msec), maximum CSF signal intensity occurs at relatively low flip angle (9°), whereas maximum CSF-cord contrast occurs at lower flip angle (5°). As TR is prolonged, flip angle at which CSF signal intensity and CSF-cord contrast peak and flip angle range over which acceptable image contrast is obtained increases. Maximum CSF signal intensity and CSF-cord contrast are observed with TR of 1000 msec and flip angle of 27°, although acceptable SNR and contrast also occur at shorter TRs and lower flip angles. Increasing TR at very low flip angle (5°) does not increase either CSF signal intensity or CSF-cord contrast. (From Rubin JB. Submitted for publication to Radiology.)

image contrast by increasing CSF signal intensity above what it would have been if CSF was stationary similar to the signal-gain on SE images.[50,51] During axial T2*W or PDW variable flip angle imaging, signal-gain increases the myelographic effect, which accentuates delineation between CSF and spinal cord, nerve roots, and extradural structures.[50,51] Therefore on PDW and T2*W variable flip angle axial spine images, it is desirable to minimize flow-induced signal-loss and maximize flow-induced signal-gain.

Signal-gain on variable flip angle images is caused by effective TR prolongation of moving protons within the imaging volume. It is possible to maximize the prominence of signal-gain on variable flip angle imaging by manipulating imaging parameters.[50,51] Signal-gain is influenced by numerous imaging parameters including imaging plane, TR, slice thickness, and number of slices.[50,51] As with signal-loss, to exploit this motion artifact clinically, it is necessary to optimize the flip angle for any combination of these imaging parameters[50,51] (see Figures 1-52 and 1-53). For example, signal-gain permits use of a larger flip angle, and this improves the contrast between CSF and extradural structures and has the added benefit of increasing the overall image SNR. How to maximize signal-gain on variable flip angle images by manipulating imaging parameters is discussed in the next section of this chapter and in Chapter 2.

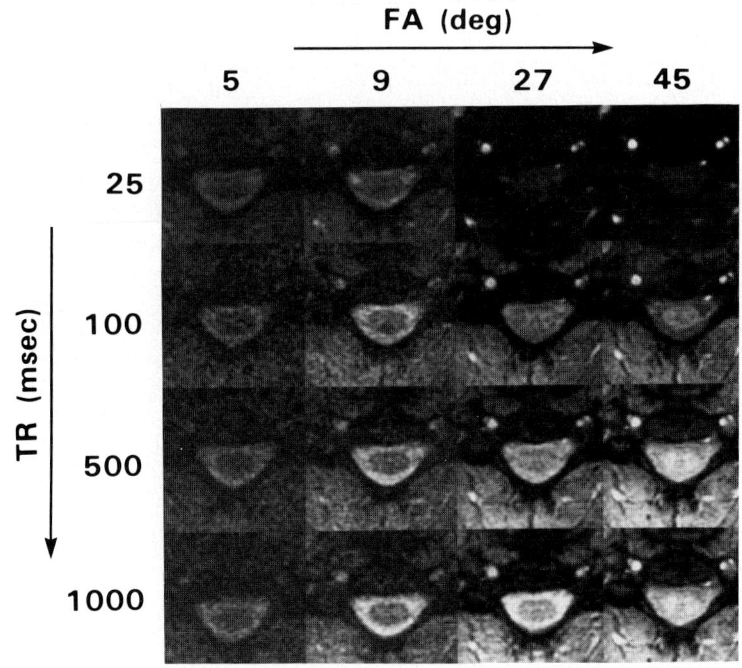

FIGURE 1-53. Effect of flip angle, TR, and number of slices on axial cervical spine variable flip angle images with same acquisition parameters used in Figure 1-52. CSF signal intensity and CSF-cord contrast peak depend on both TR and flip angle. On short-TR (25 msec) images, both maximum CSF signal intensity and CSF-cord contrast occur at low flip angle (9°). TR influences axial CSF signal intensity and CSF-cord contrast similar to the way it affects sagittal images. Maximum CSF signal intensity and CSF-cord contrast are observed with TR of 1000 msec and flip angle of 27°. Increasing TR at very low flip angle (5°) does not increase either CSF signal intensity or CSF-cord contrast. (From Rubin JB. Submitted for publication to Radiology.)

REDUCING CSF MOTION ARTIFACTS ON CLINICAL IMAGES

Some motion artifacts observed on SE and variable flip angle images arise from the same mechanism and are amenable to the same kind of flow compensation techniques. Other motion artifacts occur only on variable flip angle images for reasons previously described. Therefore, different approaches are necessary to optimize image quality on variable flip angle images compared with SE images. These techniques are discussed in the following sections.

Spin Echo Imaging

This section describes how motion compensation techniques may be applied to SE imaging to reduce signal-loss and ghost artifacts. Available techniques include CSF gated acquisition, flow compensation gradients, a combination of these two techniques, and reversal of the imaging gradient orientation.

CSF gated acquisition

Temporal phase shift effects (signal-loss and ghost artifacts) on SE images may be reduced by using CSF gating, which synchronizes MR acquisition with the oscillatory motion of CSF so that temporal variations in CSF direction, velocity, and acceleration on successive excitations do not occur[48] (Figure 1-54). When temporal phase shift effects are eliminated by this method, spatial phase shift effects become unmasked[48] (Figures 1-55 and 1-56). Only the cardiac-dependent temporal phase shift effects are eliminated by CSF gating.[48] Fortunately, respiratory-dependent temporal phase shift effects are not usually prominent. Respiratory-dependent phase shift effects may be reduced

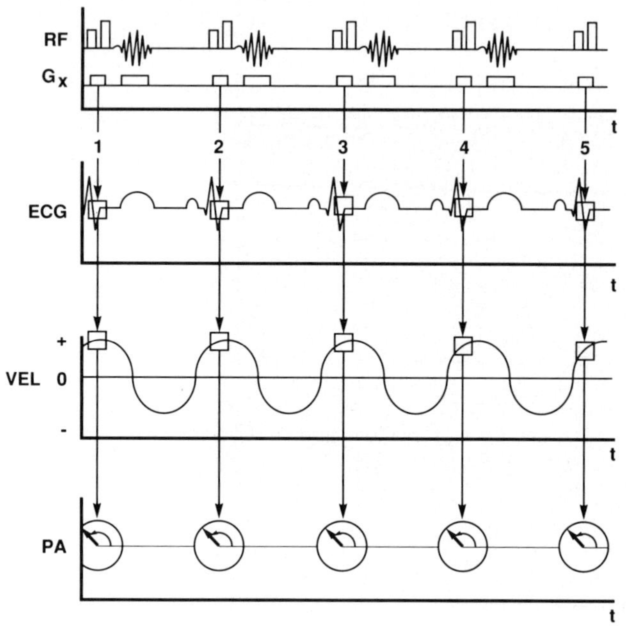

FIGURE 1-54. CSF grated acquisition. The same schematic diagram conventions are used as in Figure 1-28. Successive MR excitations *(1-5)* gradients are activated at same phase of cardiac cycle (Q-wave of *ECG*). Therefore gated imaging of oscillatory flow proton effectively simulates constant velocity flow because velocity *(VEL)* is constant on successive excitations, causing phase shift *(PA)* of flowing protons on successive excitations to be constant. Temporal phase shift effects are eliminated because modulation of proton precessional phase is effectively prevented by this method. (Modified from Rubin JB, Enzmann DR. CSF flow effects during MRI of the central nervous system. In: Magnetic resonance annual 1988. New York: Raven Press, 1988. With permission.)

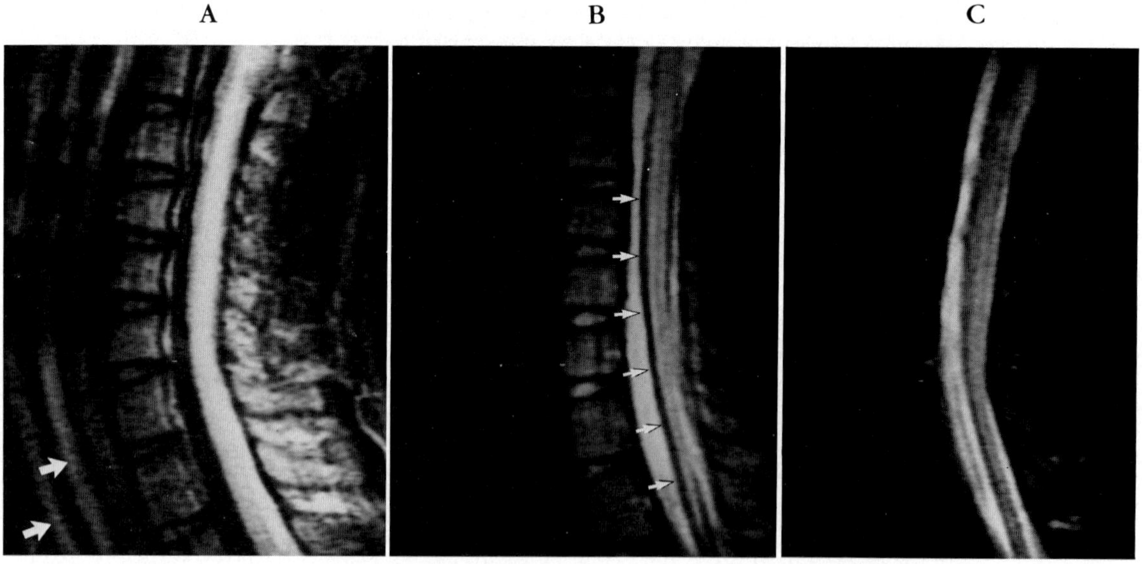

FIGURE 1-55. CSF gated acquisition in sagittal cervical spine. **A,** Non-gated SE 800/75. **B,** Gated SE 2100/80, trigger delay 0 (systolic gated). **C,** Gated SE 2100/80, trigger delay 400 msec (diastolic gated). Prominent CSF motion artifacts (signal-loss and ghost artifacts) *(arrows)* are present on non-gated image. Most CSF motion artifacts are eliminated by gating, although a prominent band of low signal intensity (boundary layer phase dispersion) *(arrows)* silhouettes the CSF-spinal cord and CSF-thecal sac interface on systolic (**B**) but not diastolic (**C**) images. This occurs secondary to higher systolic CSF velocities, which increase spatial distribution of proton velocities at CSF interfaces (spatial phase shift effects). At times, boundary layer phase dispersion may be prominent on diastolic gated images.

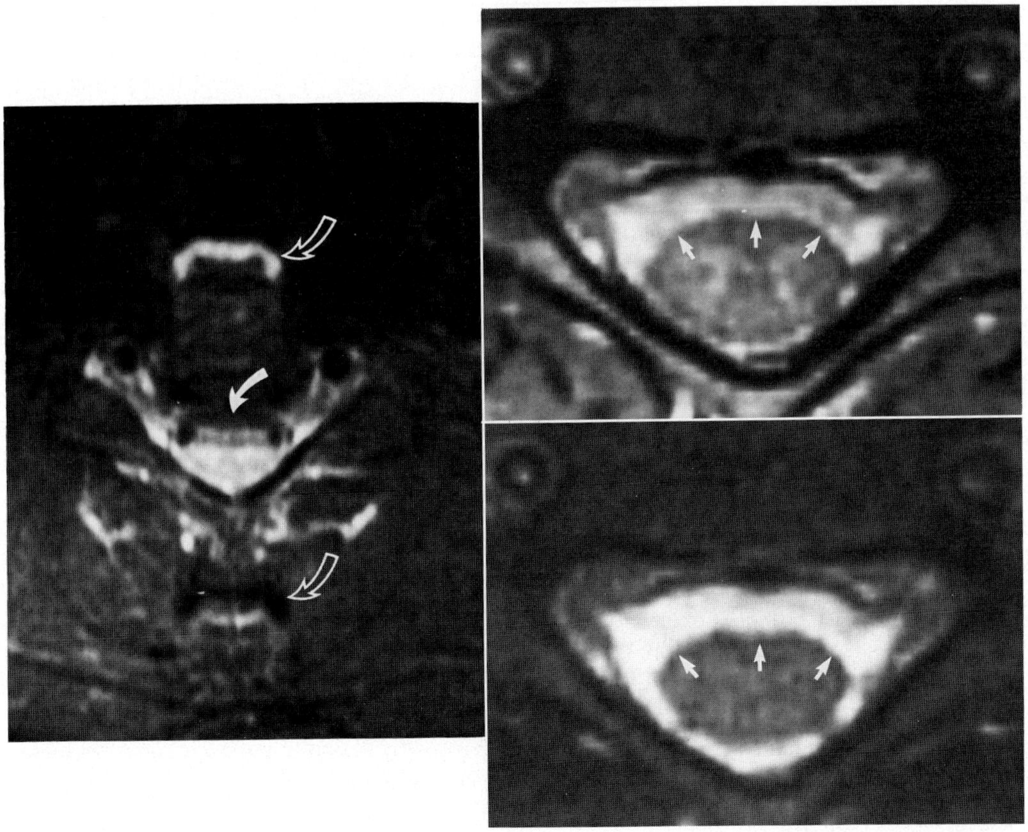

FIGURE 1-56. CSF gated acquisition in axial cervical spine. **A,** Non-gated SE 1200/25. **B,** Gated SE 1200/25 (first of four echoes). **C,** Gated, SE 1200/100 (fourth of four echoes). Gated acquisition trigger delay 400 msec. Prominent CSF motion artifacts consisting of signal-loss *(open arrows)* and ghost artifacts *(solid arrows)* are present on non-gated image. Most CSF motion artifacts are eliminated using gating except for boundary layer phase dispersion, which persists as thin rim of low signal intensity silhouetting CSF interfaces on gated images *(arrows)*. (From Rubin JB, Enzmann DR, Wright A. Radiology 1987; **163**:784. With permission.)

by respiratory-ordered phase encoding, although this prolongs acquisition time.[3] Techniques to eliminate spatial phase shift effects are discussed in the next section of this chapter.

Unfortunately, direct MR gating to CSF motion in humans is difficult and invasive.[48] However, indirect gating may be performed using a variety of triggering signals.[48] The electrocardiogram (ECG) may at first seem to be optimal for this purpose because CSF motion is synchronized with the cardiac cycle. However, cardiac electrical activity is not always followed by an effective cardiac output in certain arrythmias, such as premature ventricular contractions (PVCs), so that gating with an ECG may inappropriately trigger the MR system in the wrong phase of CSF motion. In addition, when gating is used on a large number of patients, the time required to attach multiple electrodes and ensure a satisfactory gating signal reduces clinical throughput.

Peripheral gating overcomes difficulties associated with using the ECG as a trigger by utilizing a signal that measures peripheral blood flow or capillary perfusion.[48] An infrared detector may be used to measure capillary perfusion in a fingertip or toe, or a peripheral doppler may be used to measure radial arterial blood flow. These signals are synchronized with cerebral perfusion, which is responsible for CSF motion, and therefore they function as a "hardware arrythmia filter" because MR acquisition is triggered only after an effective cardiac output.[48] In addition, they overcome the problem of reduced throughput because only a single lead that can be placed quickly is used.

To implement CSF gating clinically, it is helpful to understand the timing relationships between CSF motion and each triggering signal.[48] The ECG *R* wave and cardiac contraction precede caudal CSF motion (CSF systole). Peripheral gating signals are detected an average of 250 msec after the ECG *R* wave in most individuals. The delay from the ECG *R* wave to peak CSF systole is approximately 200 msec. Therefore, peripheral gating triggers MR acquisition shortly after peak CSF systole, whereas ECG gating triggers MR acquisition before CSF systole. In spine imaging, there is no particular advantage to triggering data acquisition before the CSF systole.

Effective TR and TE used during CSF gating determines the T2W of gated images.[48] Long effective TRs of 1800 to 2500 msec are achieved by gating on every other or every third heartbeat. New gating algorithms are becoming available that make optimized multislice gated imaging efficient and practical by reducing the errors associated with gating multiple slices across several heart periods. When used with late echo times (TE 80 msec), gating to every other or every third heartbeat provides heavily T2W images free of spatially mismapped CSF signal intensity that arise from cardiac-dependent temporal phase shift effects[18,48] (see Figures 1-55 and 1-56). Gated images with shorter effective TRs of 600 to 1000 msec may be obtained by gating to consecutive heartbeats. Gating with short effective TRs may be used with short echo times (TE 20 msec) to improve T1W image quality in cervical spine images when these are degraded by transmitted aortic pulsations that slightly move the neck with each heartbeat. Using CSF gating, single excitation imaging may be possible because image SNR is improved when spatially mismapped CSF signal is eliminated. This is particularly true if optimized slice profiles are available on an imager.

A single-slice diastolic gated image may be obtained using peripheral gating by setting the trigger delay to approximately one half the heart period.[48] Spatial phase shift effects are minimized on diastolic gated images because lower CSF velocities occur during CSF diastole com-

A

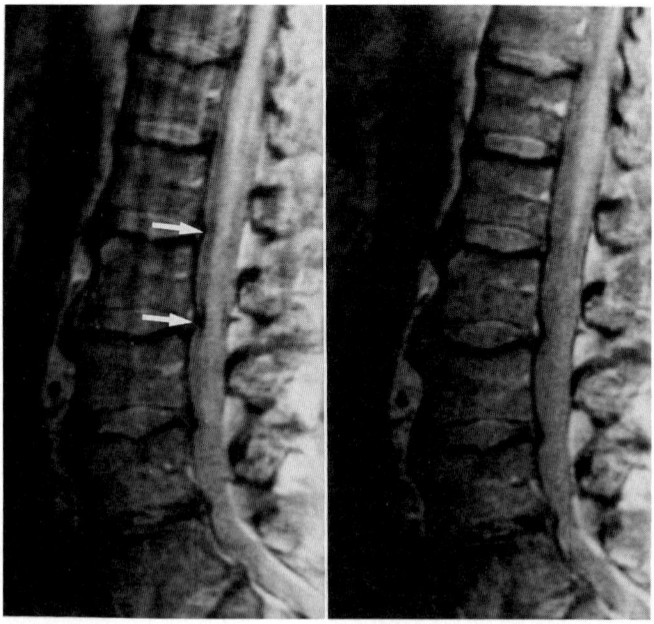

B

FIGURE 1-57. CSF gated acquisition in sagittal lumbar spine. **A**, Non-gated SE 2500/25. **B**, Gated SE 2100/25, trigger delay 400 msec. Crescentic bands of low signal intensity adjacent to bulging discs *(arrows)* occur on conventional SE image secondary to locally increased CSF velocity. CSF ghosts are superimposed on spinal canal and on vertebral bodies. CSF motion artifacts are eliminated by gating. (From Rubin JB, Wright A, Enzmann DR. Radiology 1988; **167**:225. With permission.)

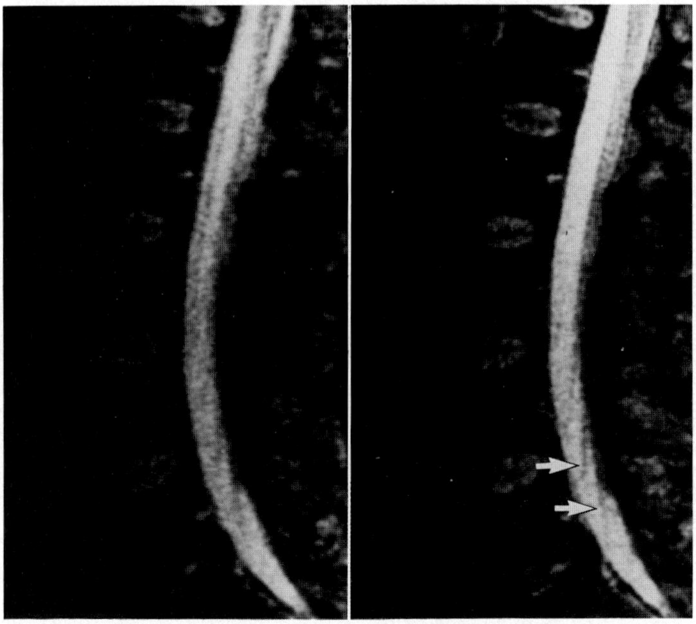

FIGURE 1-58. CSF gated acquisition in sagittal lumbar spine. **A,** Conventional SE 2500/100. **B,** Gated SE 2200/100, trigger delay 400 msec. CSF-thecal sac interface is somewhat indistinct on conventional acquisition compared to gated acquisition. CSF signal intensity is increased by gating despite shorter TR on gated acquisition. Individual nerve roots are better delineated on gated acquisition *(arrows)*. (From Rubin JB, Wright A, Enzmann DR. Radiology 1988; **167**:225. With permission.)

pared to CSF systole (see Figure 1-55). When multislice gated imaging is desired, a trigger delay of 0 msec is used. Some slices will be collected during CSF systole and other slices will be collected during CSF diastole. Slices acquired during CSF systole usually exhibit prominent spatial phase shift effects, which must be compensated for by using techniques described in the next section of this chapter. The only exception to this is in the lumbar spine where CSF velocities are generally so low that gating alone usually eliminates most CSF motion artifacts (Figures 1-57 and 1-58).

Rephasing gradients

CSF gating does not compensate for spatial phase shift effects visible on gated images unless flow compensation gradients are also used.[48] Spatial phase shift effects occur because the routine imaging gradients function as dephasing gradients when there is a large distribution of proton velocities within any voxel[46] (see Figure 1-27). These appear as linear bands of decreased signal intensity in regions of laminar CSF flow, which silhouette CSF interfaces (boundary layer phase dispersion) (see Figure 1-55), or as focal regions of decreased CSF signal intensity involving regions of CSF turbulence (turbulent phase dispersion)[46,48] (Figure 1-59).

For the same reason that a gradient pulse can cause dephasing of these protons, it is possible for other gradient pulses to rephase them. Gradient rephasing may be accomplished by two methods: adding new gradient pulses to a pulse sequence (flow-compensated pulse sequence) or exploiting existing imaging gradient pulses that are used repeatedly in a conventional pulse sequence (even echo rephasing using a short TE echo train). Flow-compensated pulse sequences use added gradient pulses to correct for phase shifts arising from constant velocity, acceleration, or even pulsatility on each echo in any imaging plane[26,27,41] (Figure 1-60). Even echo rephasing relies on repeated use of the imaging gradients to correct for phase shifts arising from constant velocity flow during sagittal spine imaging[47,59] (Figure 1-61). This approach is use-

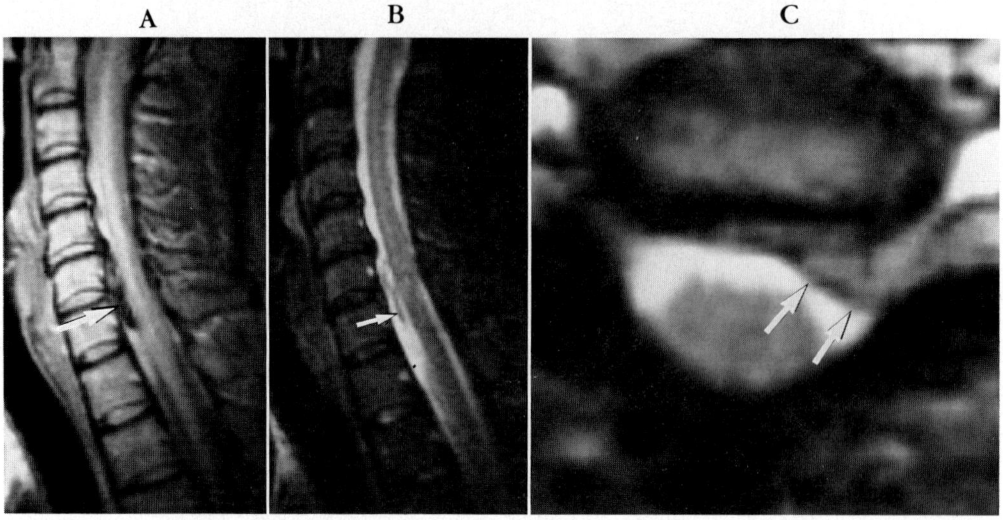

FIGURE 1-59. Reduction of turbulent phase dispersion by even echo rephasing. **A,** Gated SE TR 2300/25. **B,** Gated SE TR 2300/100. Gated trigger delay 400 msec. **C,** GRASS 40/15, flip angle 5°. Gated first echo image exhibits prominent region of low signal intensity in anterior subarachnoid space secondary to turbulent phase dispersion *(arrow)*. This is reduced but not eliminated on fourth echo image *(arrow)*. Left-sided herniated disc responsible for CSF turbulence is demonstrated on GRASS image. This case illustrates how turbulence of CSF may highlight extradural disease. Turbulent phase dispersion is difficult to completely eliminate even when using combined gating and flow compensation gradients.

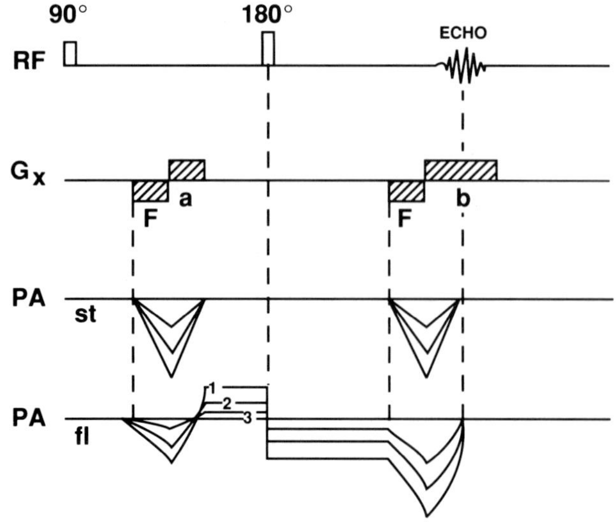

FIGURE 1-60. Flow-compensated imaging using added gradient pulses. Same schematic diagram conventions are used in Figure 1-27, which illustrates phase shift effects. Flow compensating gradient pulses are *(F)* added before rephasing *(a)* and readout *(b)* gradient pulses, which permit rephasing of both stationary *(st)* protons (zero order flow) and constant velocity flowing *(fl)* protons (first order flow) at time of first echo, irrespective of position within the magnetic field (1, stronger magnetic field; 3, weaker magnetic field) or velocity (1, faster flow; 3, slower flow). Additional gradient pulses may be used to compensate for higher order flow terms (acceleration, etc). (Modified from Rubin JB, Enzmann DR. CSF flow effects during MRI of the central nervous system. In: Magnetic resonance annual 1988. New York: Raven Press, 1988. With permission.)

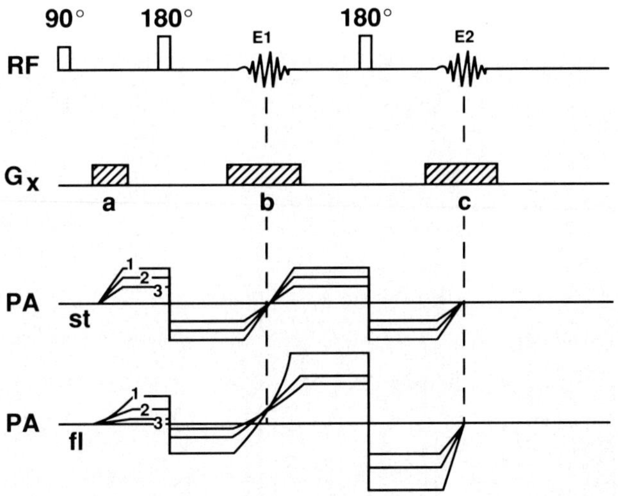

FIGURE 1-61. Flow-compensated SE imaging using even echo rephasing. During conventional SE imaging, stationary *(st)* protons are rephased on both odd and even echoes irrespective of their position with the magnetic field (1, stronger magnetic field; 3, weaker magnetic field). In contrast, flowing *(fl)* protons accrue net phase shifts that persist at time of first echo. Flow-induced phase shifts are eliminated at time of second echo (even echo rephasing) irrespective of flow velocity (1, faster flow; 3, slower flow). Therefore even echo rephasing permits velocity compensation on even echo images of conventional SE pulse sequences. Although CSF motion is not a form of constant velocity flow, shortening the time interval between successive echoes of an echo train and adding enough echoes to achieve latest desired echo permits an approximation of constant velocity flow, which exhibits even echo rephasing during imaging of oscillatory CSF. (Modified from Rubin JB, Enzmann DR. CSF flow effects during MRI of the central nervous system. In: Magnetic resonance annual 1988. New York: Raven Press, 1988. With permission.)

ful if a particular imager does not provide the option to image with flow-compensated gradient pulses. However, both approaches effectively compensate for spatial phase shift effects that are observed on gated spine images (Figures 1-62 and 1-63).

Conventional pulse sequences without flow compensation become velocity compensated on even echoes during imaging of oscillatory flow by using a short TE echo train consisting of four closely spaced echoes (i.e., TE 20, 40, 60, 80 msec), which maximizes even echo rephasing during sagittal imaging[47] (see Figure 1-63). Whereas stationary protons change phase linearly with time, permitting refocusing at odd and even echoes, the phase shift occurring in flowing protons is nonlinear and dependent on flow characteristics.[59] Under the special case of constant velocity flow within an imaging plane the phase shift is quadratic with time, and this permits refocusing of protons at even echoes despite incomplete refocusing at odd echoes (even echo rephasing)[59] (see Figure 1-61). Gating CSF oscillatory flow simulates constant velocity flow because CSF moves in the same direction and at the same velocity on each excitation[48] (see Figure 1-54). Non-gated oscillatory CSF motion approximates constant velocity flow when the time interval between successive echoes is shortened, which permits more complete even echo rephasing.[48] When echoes are widely separated, such as in an asymmetric echo train (TE 25, 80 msec), CSF motion artifacts are prominent because even echo rephasing of CSF does not occur.[47,48]

In general, flow compensation gradient pulses are preferable to the use of even echo rephasing for the following reasons:

1. Odd echo images are not flow compensated
2. Acceleration compensation on even echo images is incomplete
3. Flow compensation is effective only with in-plane flow, such as occurs during spinal sagittal but not axial imaging
4. A slight reduction in image SNR occurs with each refocusing in the echo train from

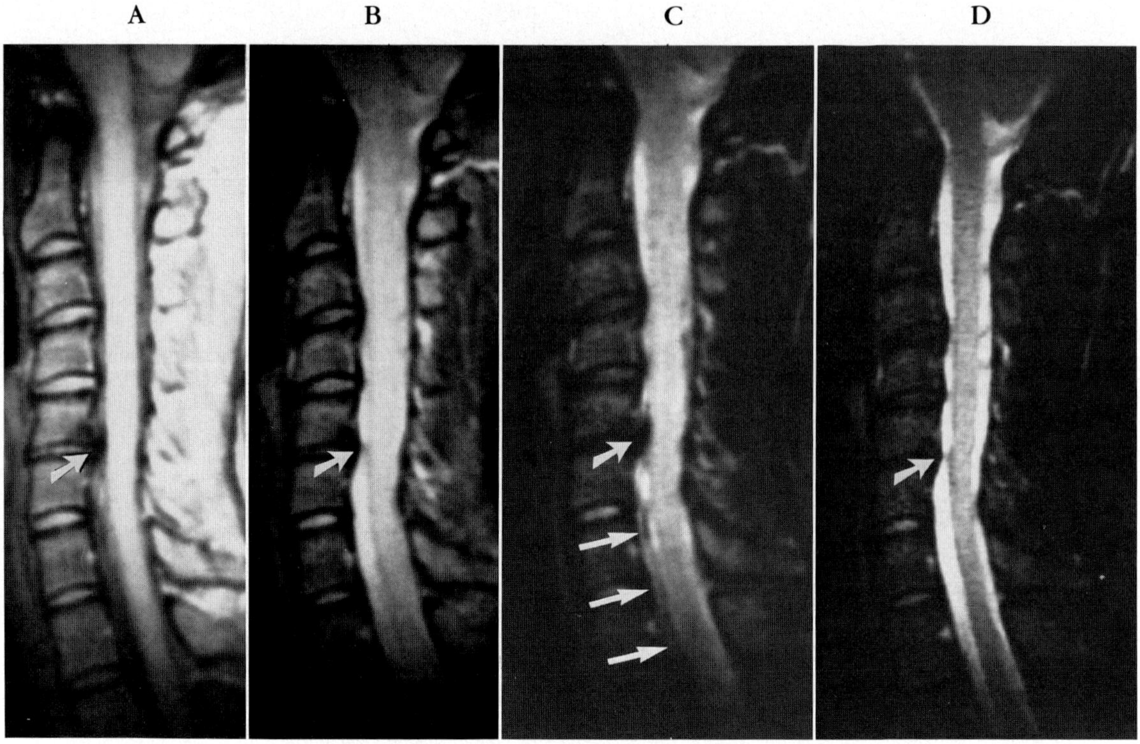

FIGURE 1-62. Even echo rephasing of spatial phase shift effects, SE 2100/25, 50, 75, 100. **A,** TE 25. **B,** TE 50. **C,** TE 75. **D,** TE 100. Spatial phase shift effects are observed as CSF signal-loss on odd echo images *(straight arrows)*. Focal regions of CSF signal-loss occur adjacent to bulging intervertebral discs *(slanted arrows)* on odd echo images because discs narrow anterior subarachnoid space and increase CSF velocity. Spatial phase shift effects are reduced or eliminated on even echo images by even echo rephasing. (From Enzmann DR, Rubin JB, Wright A. Radiology 1987; **163**:233. With permission.)

a propagating error in refocusing arising from imperfect estimation of the magnitude of the 180° RF refocusing pulse.

In contrast, flow-compensated pulse sequences may have constraints arising from the necessity to incorporate additional gradient pulses into a limited amount of imaging time. There may be restrictions on the timing and the number of echoes allowed, the maximum number of slices is reduced, and there may be some reduction in image SNR if the readout gradient is shortened to accommodate the additional gradient pulses.

Combined CSF gating and rephasing gradients

Combining CSF gating with flow compensation gradients during proton density or T2W spinal imaging makes sense because each flow compensation technique reduces or eliminates a motion artifact that arises from a different flow mechanism.[48] A combination of these techniques effectively compensates for both temporal and spatial phase shift effects, whereas either method alone is not as effective[48] (see Figure 1-63). The combination of flow compensation techniques and SE imaging permits generation of artifact-free true T2W sagittal spine images[18,48] (Figures 1-63 to 1-66). Occasionally, a band of high signal intensity within the central region of the spinal cord is observed on sagittal and axial T2W images obtained using combined gating and flow compensation[35] (Figure 1-67). This is not a motion artifact and it should not be confused with pathology. It occurs secondary to truncation errors that arise during 2DFT imaging (Gibb's effect), particularly when a low resolution acquisition matrix (i.e., 128 × 256) is used.[35,36,63]

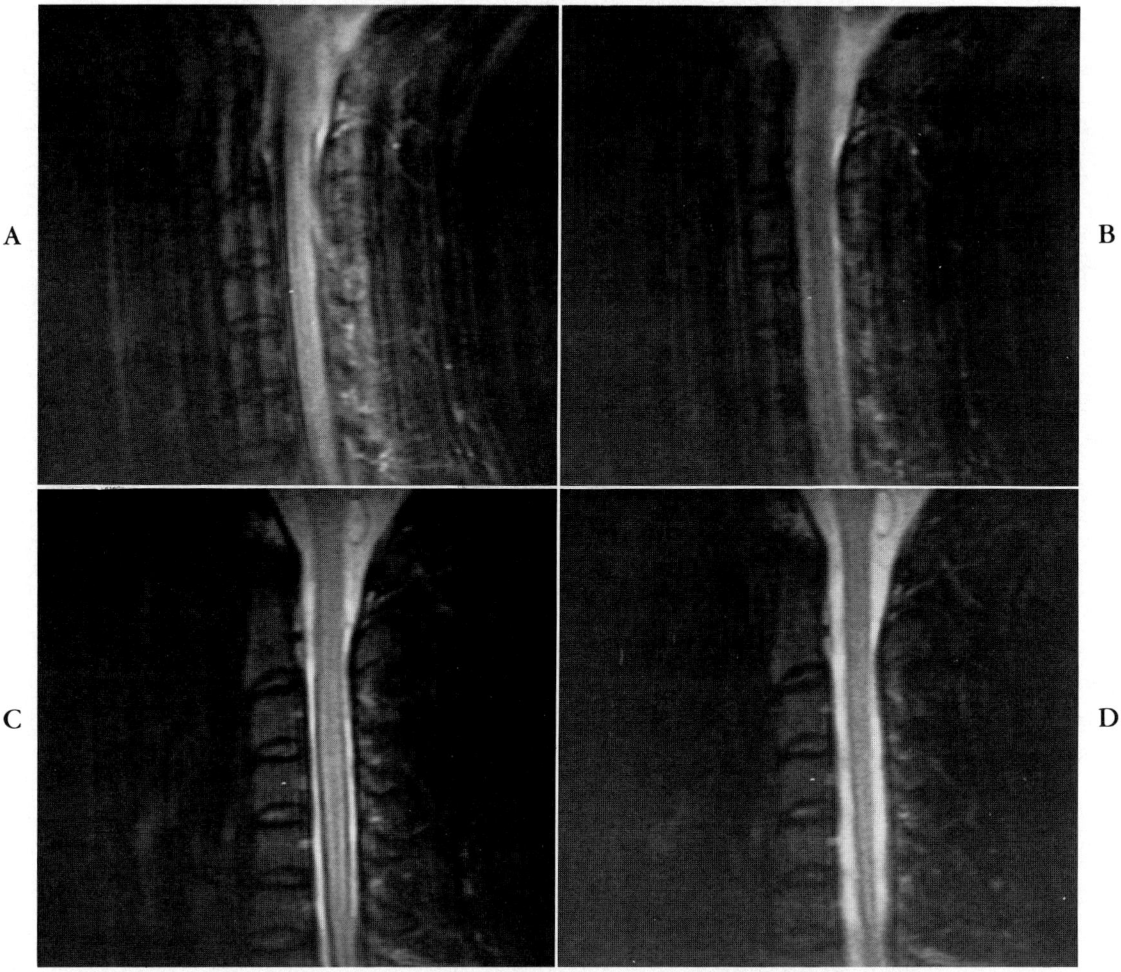

FIGURE 1-63. Comparison of different approaches to CSF motion compensation during sagittal cervical spine imaging. **A,** Conventional SE 1200/40. **B,** Flow-compensated SE 1200/80. **C,** Gated SE 1200/80, trigger delay 200 msec (systole). **D,** Gated and flow-compensated SE 1200/80. Without use of any CSF motion compensation techniques, CSF motion artifacts (signal-loss and ghosts) markedly degrade image quality. Using flow compensation alone, signal-loss and ghosts are reduced but image quality is not optimal because ghosts are not eliminated. Using gating alone, ghosts and signal-loss within center of subarachnoid space is eliminated, but image quality is still not optimal because bands of low CSF signal intensity silhouetting CSF interfaces persist (boundary layer phase dispersion). Using combined gating and flow compensation, all CSF motion artifacts are eliminated, providing a high quality image.

A 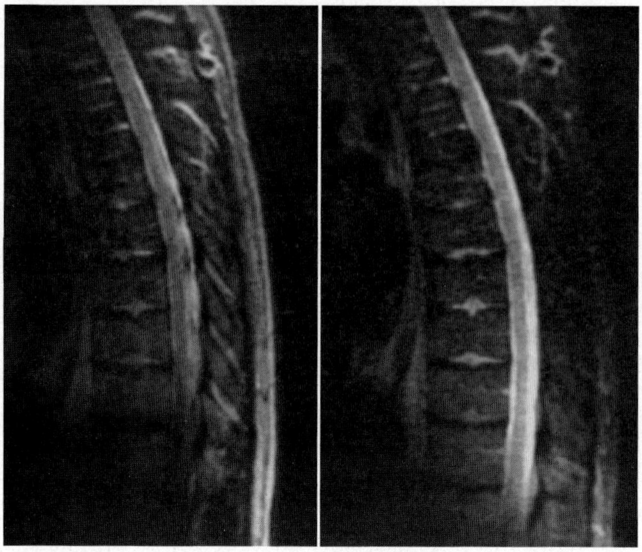 B

FIGURE 1-64. Combined CSF motion compensation in thoracic spine. **A,** Conventional SE 2000/80. **B,** Gated and flow-compensated SE 2200/80. Nonmotion-compensated image is difficult to evaluate because of very heterogeneous CSF signal intensity. Combining gating and flow-compensated SE imaging markedly improves image quality, making image interpretation much simpler.

A 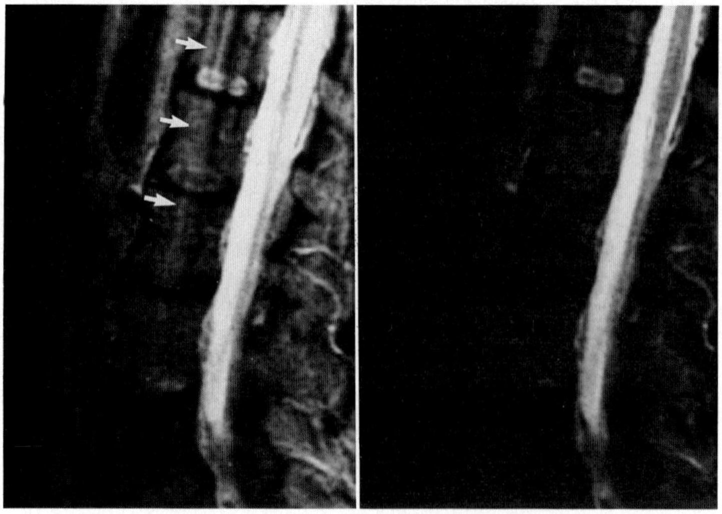 B

FIGURE 1-65. Combined CSF motion compensation in the lumbar spine. **A,** Conventional SE 2500/80. **B,** Gated and flow-compensated SE 2400/80. Ghosts prominent on nonmotion-compensated image *(arrows)* are eliminated using combined gating and flow compensation.

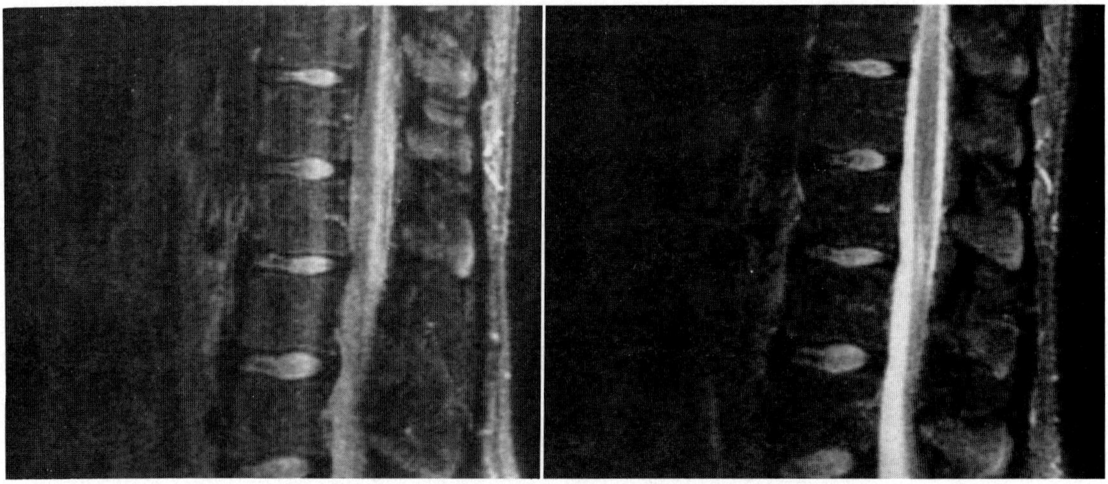

FIGURE 1-66. T2W imaging of conus using motion compensation techniques. **A,** Conventional SE 2500/80. **B,** Gated and flow-compensated SE 2300/80. Small circular surface coil and small field of view were used to improve spatial resolution and SNR. Conus is difficult to evaluate on conventional SE image. Using motion compensation techniques, it is well visualized. Small amount of CSF within cauda equina should not be mistaken for a lesion.

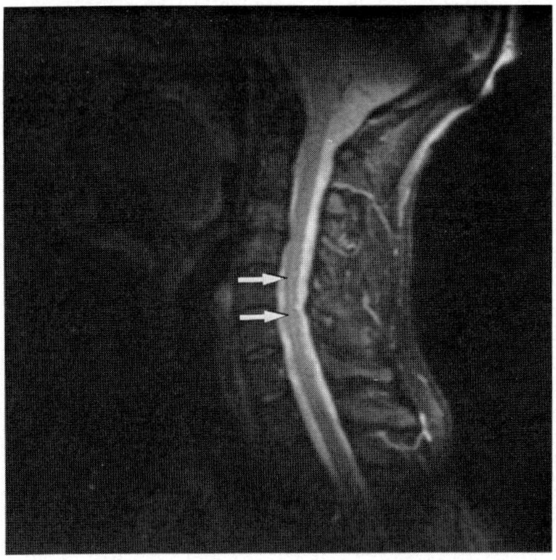

FIGURE 1-67. Truncation (Gibb's) artifact during T2W cervical spine imaging. Gated and flow-compensated SE 2100/80. CSF signal-loss and ghost artifacts are absent. There is a curvilinear band of high signal intensity superimposed on the spinal cord. This is not a ghost artifact, should not be mistaken for pathologic condition, occurs secondary to truncation errors during 2DFT imaging, and is most prominent when low resolution acquisition matrices are used.

Although it is possible to generate high quality sagittal T2W spine images using these techniques, these methods do not eliminate the *saturation effects* that occur during axial T2W spine imaging.[48] Saturation effects are observed as decreased CSF signal intensity on all slices of a non-gated acquisition, or on some slices of a gated acquisition.[48] Saturation effects are troublesome because they impair visualization of low intensity extradural structures by reducing contrast at the CSF thecal sac interface. Entry phenomena and saturation effects may be simultaneously observed in different regions of the subarachnoid space as a result of nonuniformity of CSF flow.[48] Complex patterns of subarachnoid signal intensity may therefore be observed on gated multislice axial spine images that may be misinterpreted as having an anatomic rather than a physiologic basis. For this reason, variable flip angle images are preferable to the gated flow-compensated SE spine images for the evaluation of extradural disease during axial imaging. However, gated axial T2W SE spine images remain useful to confirm the intrinsic cord lesions suspected on the sagittal images.

Reversal of imaging gradient orientation

The greatest source of spatially mismapped signal intensity that creates clinical difficulty is pulsatile CSF. Other sources include the heart, oropharynx, bowel, and anterior chest or abdominal walls because each of these structures undergoes an oscillatory motion.[16,48] Oropharyngeal signal may project over the cervical spine when the patient swallows repeatedly during imaging. Cardiac and chest wall signal may project over the thoracic spine. Bowel and abdominal wall signal may project over the lumbar spine. Surface-coil imaging reduces chest and abdominal wall breathing artifacts during spine imaging because the anterior chest and abdominal walls are positioned further from the sensitive volume of the surface coil and are lower in signal intensity. The difficulty caused by these sources of spatially mismapped signal may be further reduced by switching the orientation of the phase and frequency axes,[48] which causes the spatially mismapped signal to be projected anterior to the spine instead of superimposed on top of it. This also reduces CSF ghost artifacts because of the lower average gradient amplitude and duration of the phase-encoding gradient compared to the readout gradient.

Short-TR Variable Flip Angle/Gradient Echo Imaging

Although it is not possible to gate variable flip angle images when the TR is shorter than the heart period, spatial and temporal phase shift effects may be reduced on variable flip angle images by using flow compensation gradients similar to those previously described for SE imaging. If flow compensation gradients were not used, then variable flip angle images with this flow compensation technique would exhibit more prominent signal-loss and ghosts than they do.[50] In this section the presence of flow compensation gradients is assumed and the technique of optimizing image quality by adjusting the routine imaging system parameters, such as flip angle, TR, TE, slice thickness, and number of slices, is discussed.

Mathematic model

The interaction of motion artifacts with each other and with the various imaging systems and physiologic parameters is complex.[50] One approach to this problem is the use of a mathematic model of variable flip angle imaging that takes all of these factors into account. The model is a useful clinical tool because it combines important relationships into a single set of equations that permits comparison of different imaging strategies.[50,51] In this way, various trade-offs between image quality and acquisition time may be easily evaluated on a computer, rather than in volunteers or patients. The theoretic basis for the model and its validation in patients and phantoms of the spine is fully described elsewhere.[50,51] For the purposes of this chapter, it is not necessary to understand the mathematic basis of this approach. Rather, the model may simply be considered a "black box" into which various questions are posed and from which rational answers are returned. Curves derived from this mathematic model can be used as nomograms to help optimize imaging parameters for individual imaging requirements.

As discussed earlier in this chapter, signal intensity of stationary structures such as spinal cord or stationary CSF on variable flip angle images may be described as[37]

$$(3)\quad SI = \frac{k \cdot [1-e^{-TR/T1}] \cdot \sin\beta \cdot N_H \cdot e^{-TE/T2*}}{1-e^{-TR/T1} \cdot e^{-TR/T2*} - \cos\beta \cdot [e^{-TR/T1} - e^{-TR/T2*}]}$$

where SI is the signal intensity at flip angle β, k is a constant of proportionality, N_H is the proton density, T2* is the transverse magnetization decay time, and TR, TE, and T1 have their usual meaning. This equation assumes ideal rectangular slice-selective pulse profiles, phase inversion on alternate RF pulses, uniform excitation and equal flip angle of all protons, and fully compensated gradient-induced phase shifts of the transverse magnetization.

Signal intensity of oscillatory CSF on variable flip angle images may be described as[50]

$$(4)\quad SI = \frac{k \cdot [1-e^{-TRe/T1}] \cdot \sin\beta \cdot N_H \cdot e^{-TE/T2*}}{1-\cos\beta \cdot e^{-TRe/T1}}$$

where TR_e is the effective TR of the moving CSF described as[50]

$$(5)\quad TR_e = TR_i \cdot \left[1 + \frac{PA \cdot \sin\alpha}{ST \cdot NS}\right]$$

where TR_i is the actual TR used for imaging, PA is the pulsation amplitude of oscillatory CSF, α

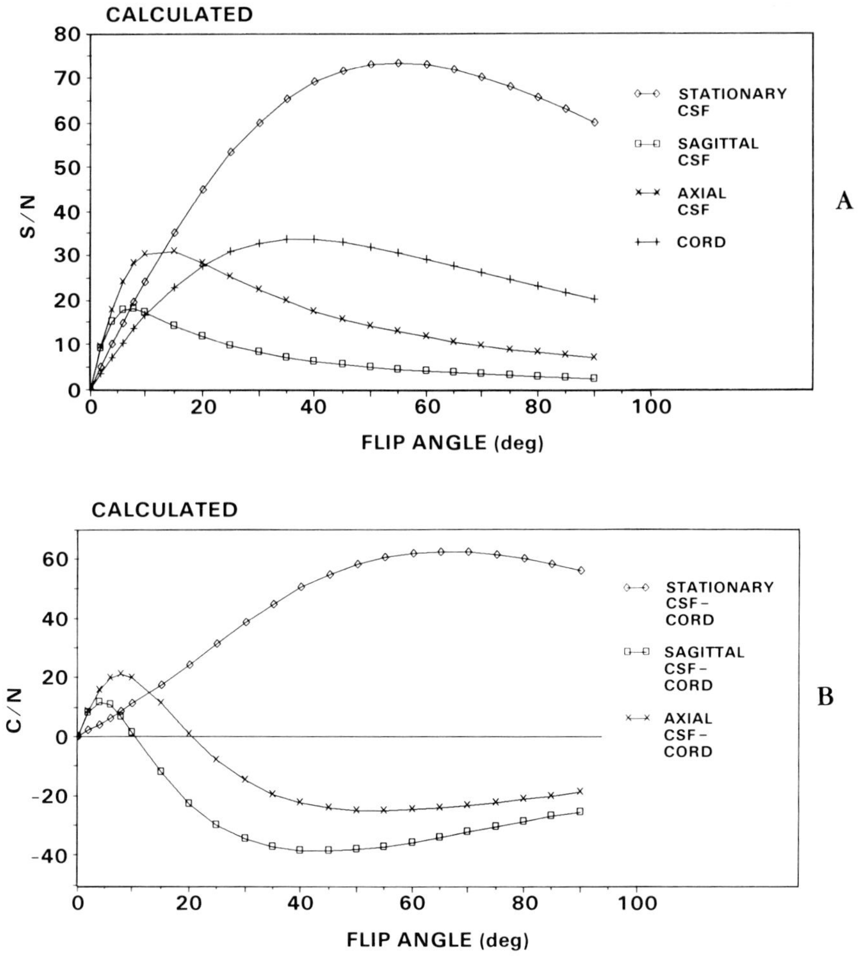

FIGURE 1-68. Calculated cervical spine SNR (**A**) and CNR (**B**) for stationary CSF, sagittal oscillatory CSF, axial oscillatory CSF, and spinal cord during variable flip angle imaging. CNR values are for CSF relative to spinal cord. Flip angle at which peak CSF SNR and CNR occur is dependent on presence or absence of CSF motion and on imaging plane. Stationary CSF peaks at much larger flip angle than oscillatory CSF. Axial oscillatory CSF peaks at slightly larger flip angle than sagittal oscillatory CSF. Stationary CSF is hyperintense to spinal cord at all flip angles. Axial and sagittal oscillatory CSF are hyperintense to spinal cord only at relatively low flip angles. Axial oscillatory CSF CNR peaks at a larger flip angle and is positive over a larger range of flip angles than sagittal oscillatory CSF. (From Rubin JB. Submitted for publication to Radiology.)

is the angle of CSF motion relative to the imaging plane (0°, in-plane, 90°, through-plane), ST is the slice thickness, and NS is the number of slices.

Using the mathematic model to generate curves of stationary CSF, oscillatory CSF, and spinal cord is a useful way to understand the effects of the various imaging and physiologic parameters[50,51] (Figures 1-68 and 1-69). These curves show excellent agreement with actual curves obtained from flow phantoms and volunteers and patients.

Optimizing imaging parameters using the mathematic model

The influence of individual tissue, physiologic, and imaging parameters on the outcome of variable flip angle imaging was previously discussed. Intrinsic tissue parameters include pro-

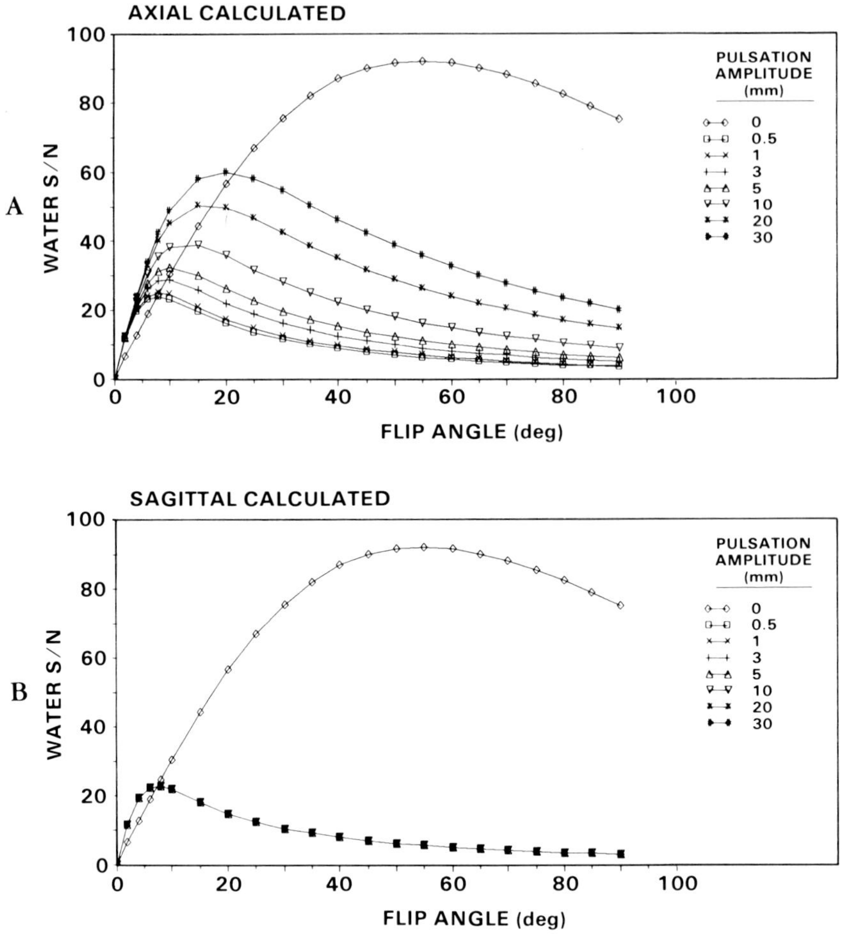

FIGURE 1-69. Calculated oscillatory CSF (water) SNR vs. flip angle for different pulsation amplitudes during variable flip angle imaging. **A,** Axial imaging. **B,** Sagittal imaging. During sagittal imaging, prominent signal-loss occurs at intermediate and large flip angles regardless of pulsation amplitude secondary to flow-induced disruption of the steady state. In contrast, during axial imaging, peak SNR and flip angle at which SNR peaks is proportional to pulsation amplitude. This occurs because signal-gain caused by effective TR prolongation opposes signal-loss during axial imaging. (From Rubin JB. Submitted for publication to Radiology.)

ton density, T1, and T2*. Physiologic parameters include the characteristics and the direction of flow relative to the imaging plane. Imaging parameters include TR, TE, flip angle, single-slice vs. multislice acquisition, slice thickness, and number of slices. Understanding the effects of individual parameters on variable flip angle images is not sufficient to predict the outcome of imaging because interactions between the numerous parameters occur.[50,51] The mathematic model is a useful clinical tool because it simultaneously accounts for each of the opposing factors (motion effects and intrinsic tissue, physiologic, and imaging system parameters[50,51]) that determine the outcome of variable flip angle imaging.

To evaluate different imaging strategies using the mathematic model, a figure of merit must be selected.[51] A figure of merit is a quantitative measure of the desired characteristic of an image that permits images obtained under different imaging conditions to be directly compared. For example, to optimize myelographic contrast on variable flip angle images, CSF-cord CNR is a useful figure of merit because it describes the success of different imaging strategies in achieving myelographic contrast.[51] Figures of merit may also be used to optimize imaging efficiency. For example, CSF-cord CNR per imaging time permits a comparison of the imaging efficiencies of different imaging strategies in achieving a myelographic contrast.[51]

Calculation of figures of merit for each imaging condition using the mathematic model is straightforward.[51] To calculate the signal intensity of any tissue, the intrinsic relaxation parameters for that tissue and the desired imaging parameters are used in conjunction with equation 3. For example, equation 3 may be used to calculate the signal intensity of stationary CSF or spinal cord for any combination of TR, TE, and flip angle. To calculate the signal intensity of moving CSF, equations 4 and 5 are used in conjunction with the intrinsic relaxation parameters of CSF, an assumption about how much CSF is likely to move, and the desired imaging parameters. Contrast is calculated simply as the difference in signal intensity between two regions of interest. Imaging time is calculated as the product of TR, the number of excitations (NEX), and the number of phase-encoding steps (resolution along the phase axis). Image noise is calculated as $1/\sqrt{NEX}$. Using this approach, figures of merit may be calculated for CSF SNR, CSF-cord CNR, and imaging efficiency.

Once the figures of merit for variable flip angle imaging have been chosen, they may be used to evaluate trade-offs between different imaging strategies.[51] In this section, assume that it is desired to optimize myelographic contrast on variable flip angle images. The important trade-off in this case is between imaging efficiency and absolute *image quality*.[51] Imaging efficiency is a measure of how effective a particular imaging strategy is in achieving the desired contrast-per-unit imaging time. Image quality is a measure of how well the imaging strategy achieved the desired image contrast regardless of how efficient it was. In clinical imaging, it is desirable to simultaneously optimize image quality and imaging efficiency. A trade-off occurs because maximum image quality does not usually occur under conditions that have been optimized for maximum imaging efficiency.

Two fundamentally different acquisition protocols may be used for imaging with variable flip angle pulse sequences: sequential *single slice* using a *short TR*, and interleaved *multislice* using a *long TR*. When both single-slice and multislice acquisition protocols are available, the mathematic model and experimental data indicate that the most efficient way to image depends on the number of slices needed[51] (Figure 1-70). The number of slices needed for any acquisition is dictated by slice thickness, the interslice gap, and the anatomic region of interest. For spine imaging, thin sections (3 to 5 mm) and narrow gaps (0.5 to 1 mm) are customarily used to minimize partial volume effects. The number of slices necessary to image the anatomic region of interest varies with the orientation of the imaging plane. Fewer slices are usually needed to image the spine in the sagittal than in the axial plane. When only one or a few slices are needed, the mathematic model indicates that sequential single-slice acquisition is most efficient.[51] When several or many slices are needed, the mathematic model indicates that interleaved multislice acquisition provides better imaging efficiency.[51] Without performing the calculations, it would not be intuitively clear which acquisition protocol was the most efficient.

The mathematic model indicates that the most efficient TR to use with single-slice acquisitions is the shortest possible TR. In contrast, the most efficient TR to use with multislice acquisitions is the longest practical TR.[51] For single-slice acquisitions, the shortest possible TR is typically 20 to 30 msec. Increasing TR to a value greater than the shortest possible TR during single-slice acquisitions improves image SNR and CNR but requires correspondingly longer acquisition times and is less efficient.[51] For multislice acquisitions, the longest practical TR is limited by total imaging time. It is usually desirable to limit each acquisition to 5 to 10 minutes. The minimum TR for multislice imaging is proportional to the number of slices imaged. Assuming that the pulse sequences require 30 msec per slice and 5 slices are needed, the shortest possible TR would be approximately 150 msec.

One way to make the trade-off between imaging efficiency and image quality is to arbitrarily choose a maximum imaging time and calculate the TR from this figure.[51] Using the previous example and assuming an acquisition matrix of 256×256 and NEX of 4, a TR of 300 msec would permit imaging in a period of approximately 5 minutes. Although imaging is less efficient at TR 300 msec compared to TR 150

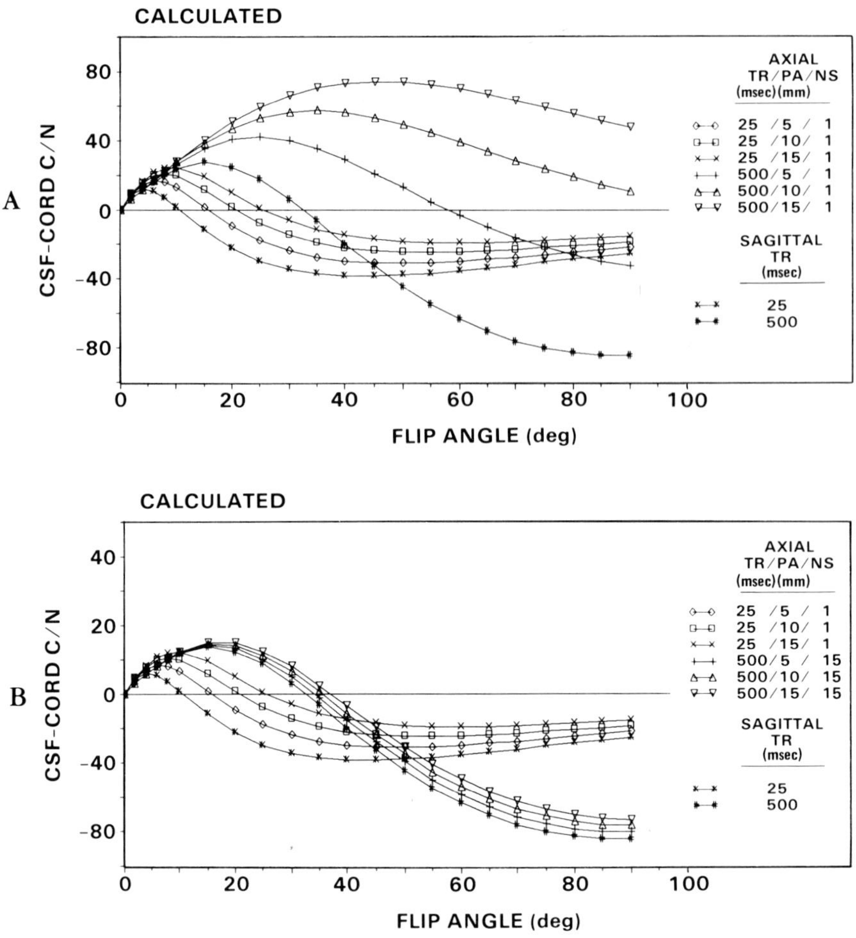

FIGURE 1-70. Calculated oscillatory CSF-cord CNR vs. flip angle for different imaging strategies during variable flip angle imaging. **A,** Single-slice 500/15 vs. single-slice 25/15. **B,** Multislice 500/15 vs. single-slice 25/15. Imaging plane, TR, pulsation amplitude *(PA)*, and number of slices *(NS)* are shown in graph legends. For sagittal imaging, results are independent of pulsation amplitude. Effect of CSF motion on CNR is more pronounced on single-slice long-TR acquisitions than on single-slice short-TR acquisitions because effective TR prolongation is proportional to TR. Effect of CSF motion on CNR is markedly reduced when multiple slices are imaged during long-TR acquisition because effective TR prolongation is inversely proportional to the number of slices. Note CNR is improved on multislice long-TR acquisition compared to single-slice short-TR acquisitions despite reduction in prominence of signal-gain by multislice imaging, because prolonging actual TR overcomes lack of effective TR prolongation by motion. (From Rubin JB. Submitted for publication to Radiology.)

msec, the longer TR image would be higher quality than the shorter TR image. The only disadvantage to longer TR images is that ghost artifacts arising from oropharynx and bowel increase in prominence[51] (Figure 1-71). This occurs because longer TRs increase image SNR and inadvertent patient motion is more likely on longer acquisitions. However, prominent ghosting is usually not a problem at the flip angles used to achieve myelographic contrast.

Once the acquisition protocol and TR have been determined it is necessary to optimize the flip angle for these imaging conditions.[51] Determination of the optimum flip angle to use at first appears very difficult. Without the mathematic model this would be particularly true. However, the model helps calculate curves that simplify the process of determining the optimum flip an-

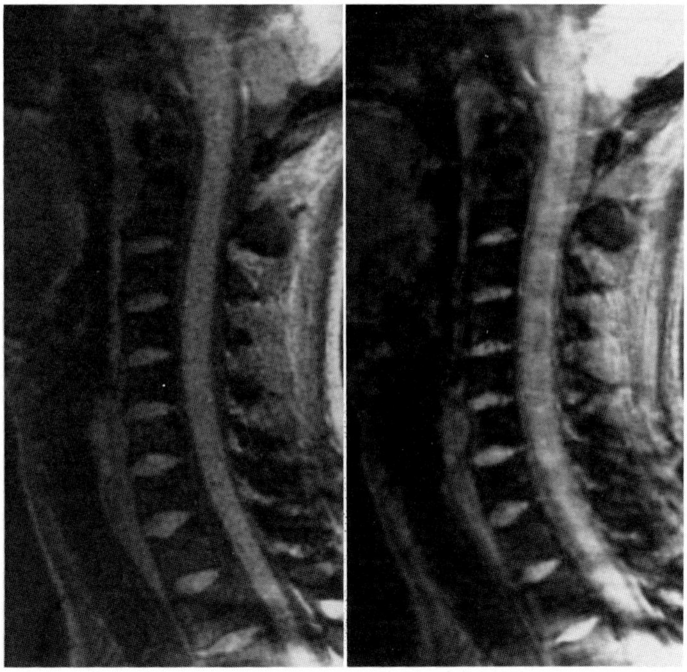

FIGURE 1-71. Ghost artifacts associated with long-TR variable flip angle imaging. **A,** GRASS 25/12, flip angle 90°. **B,** GRASS 1000/12, flip angle 90°. Using these parameters, both images appear relatively T1W. SNR and ghost artifacts are increased on long TR image compared to short TR image. Ghosts originate from the oropharynx rather than from CSF. This occurs because more signal intensity is available for spatial mismapping when overall image SNR is increased by prolonging TR. In addition, oropharyngeal motion is more likely to occur on longer acquisitions. Ghosts on long TR acquisitions are not usually this prominent when PD or T2*W images are obtained using lower flip angles because image SNR is not this great when lower flip angle is used.

gle to use under different circumstances. The optimum flip angle to use for the selected TR and number of slices depends on the imaging plane.[51] Curves are provided for single-slice axial imaging, multislice axial imaging, and sagittal imaging (Figure 1-72). Note that the same curves are used for both single-slice and multislice sagittal imaging. The multislice axial curve is calculated assuming that the maximum number of slices possible is acquired for any given TR. To use these curves as nomograms to find the optimal flip angle for any TR, simply find TR on the x axis and follow this up to the uppermost curve on the y axis. Different curves correspond to different flip angles, as indicated in the curve legend. The uppermost flip angle curve at any given TR is the optimum flip angle to use for that TR and number of slices.

The mathematic model provides some insight into trade-offs among different imaging strategies.[51] Note that as TR is prolonged the maximum possible contrast-to-noise ratio (CNR) increases (Figure 1-72 and 1-73). The flip angle at which optimum CNR is achieved also increases with increasing TR. CNR increases with TR faster for single-slice axial than multislice axial imaging because effective TR prolongation is more prominent when the volume of RF irradiation is reduced. Long TR multislice axial imaging provides better CNR than short TR single-slice axial imaging, because the longer TR more than compensates for the decrease in effective TR prolongation. Single-slice and multislice sagittal curves are identical because all of the flow is within the imaging plane and additional slices do not alter flow effects unless some of the flow passes through those planes. Multislice axial imaging is similar to sagittal imaging because effective TR prolongation is minimized when the volume of RF irradiation is large compared to

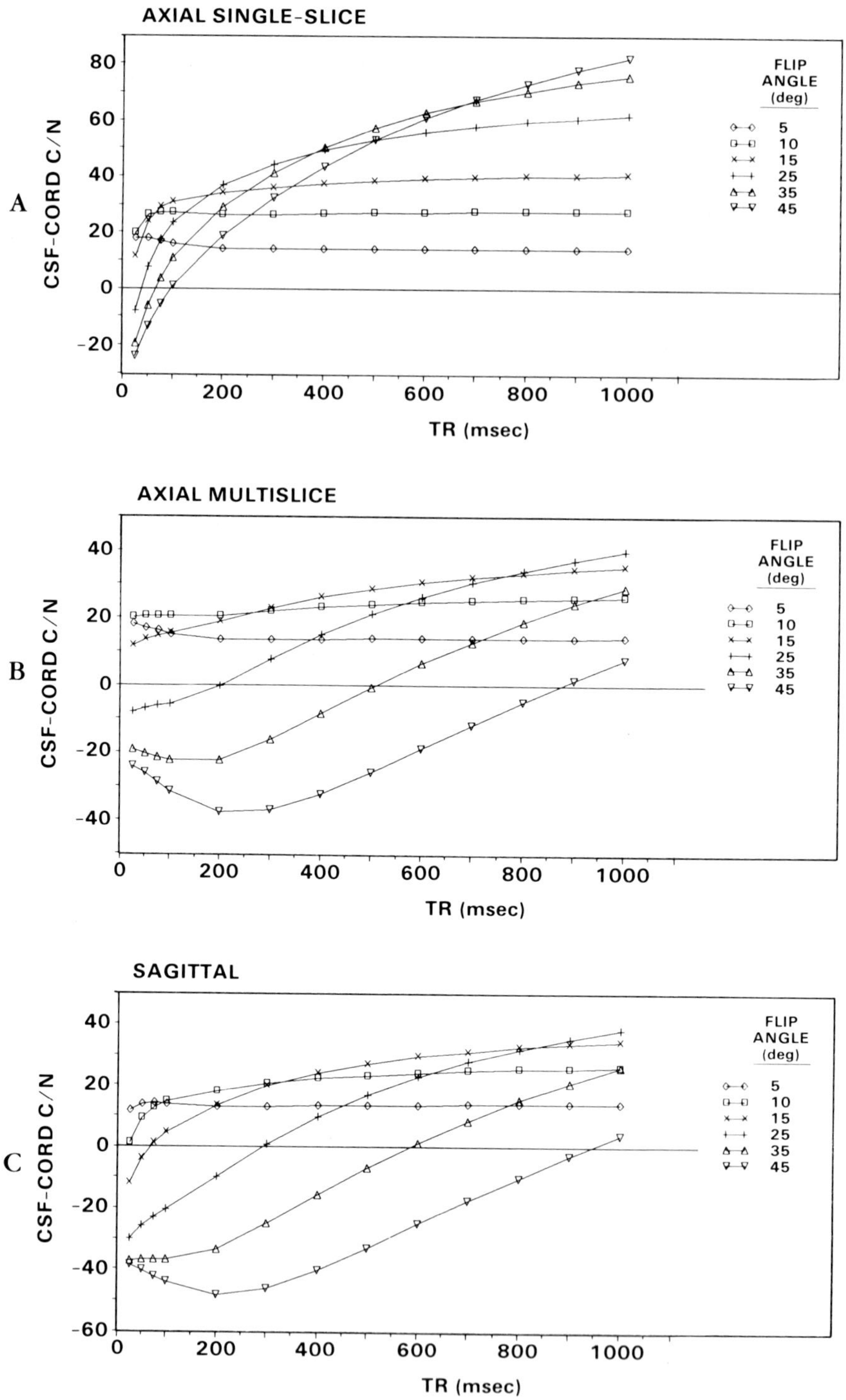

FIGURE 1-72. Calculated oscillatory CSF-cord CNR vs. TR for different flip angles during variable flip angle imaging. **A,** Single-slice axial acquisition. **B,** Multislice axial acquisition. **C,** Sagittal acquisition. Same curves apply to single-slice and multislice. In all three imaging strategies, CSF-cord CNR increases with increasing TR and increasing flip angle. Axial single-slice CSF-cord CNR increases more rapidly than sagittal CSF-cord CNR because of flow-induced effective TR prolongation and occurs only during axial imaging in which CSF flow is perpendicular to the imaging plane. Axial CSF-cord CNR is similar to sagittal CSF-cord CNR when multislice acquisition is used because flow-induced effective TR prolongation is inversely proportional to the number of slices. When short TRs are used, axial multislice CSF-cord CNR is greater than sagittal CSF-cord CNR because only a limited number of slices can be acquired in an interleaved format. On each graph the optimal flip angle for any TR is the uppermost flip angle curve at that TR. (From Rubin JB. Submitted for publication to Radiology.)

A B
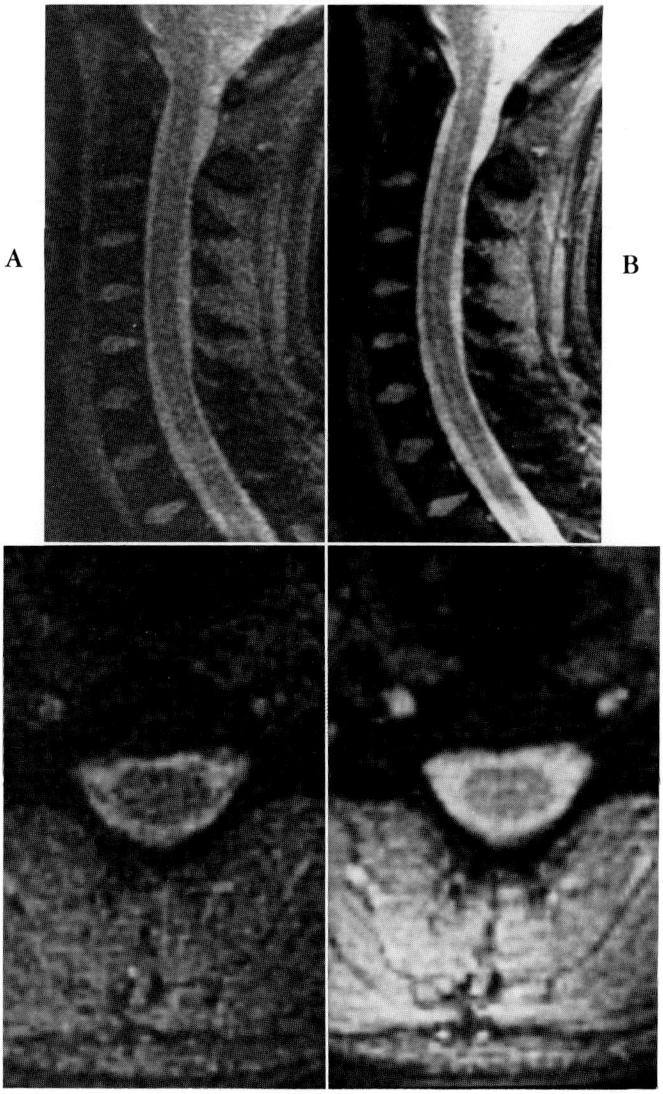
C D

FIGURE 1-73. Comparison of different imaging strategies for sagittal cervical spine variable flip angle imaging. **A,** Sagittal single-slice GRASS 100/15, flip angle 9°. **B,** Sagittal multislice GRASS 100/15, flip angle 27°. **C,** Axial single-slice GRASS 100/15, flip angle 9°. **D,** Axial multislice GRASS 1000/15, flip angle 27°. Optimal flip angles were determined using mathematic model. Although similar myelographic effect is observed on all images, longer TR acquisitions were more efficient and yielded greater CSF SNR and CSF-cord CNR. (From Rubin JB. Submitted for publication to Radiology.)

the volume of proton distribution. Note that there are still differences between curves when short TRs are used because the number of possible slices in this range is limited.

Increasing TE increases the T2*W of variable flip angle images similar to its effect on SE images. CSF cord contrast increases as images become more T2*W. Unfortunately, as described earlier in this chapter, variable flip angle images are degraded by magnetic susceptibility artifacts when TE is prolonged. Therefore, T2*W images are of limited use in the spine. Under most circumstances, particularly in the evaluation of extradural disease, PDW images are a suitable replacement for the reasons previously described. Therefore to minimize magnetic susceptibility artifacts, the optimum TE is the shortest TE possible.[51]

MEASURING CSF MOTION ON CLINICAL IMAGES

Sometimes it is useful to exploit the flow sensitivity of MR to actually measure the amount of CSF motion in a patient's spine. Potential clinical applications include assessment of the degree of a spinal block and estimation of the amount of CSF motion within spinal cord cavities. An estimate of the amount of motion within spinal cord cavities may be helpful in distinguishing syrinx from tumor cysts of the spinal cord. An estimate of CSF motion may also be useful in the preoperative assessment of syrinx cavities before shunting. These clinical applications are described in greater detail in later chapters of this book.

Approaches to CSF Flow Imaging

There are many methods currently available for quantitating flow using MR.* These flow effects fall into two major categories: phase sensitive methods and time of flight methods. Phase sensitive methods rely on the accumulation of different phase shifts between moving and stationary protons but are difficult to apply clinically because of eddy currents. Time of flight methods rely on the physical movement of protons into or out of an imaging plane. These methods do not have problems with eddy currents; however, they are prone to other kinds of errors because their quantitation of flow is based on measurements of signal intensity. Flow is only one of many factors that influences signal intensity; other factors include the distance of a region of interest from a surface coil and the setting of the receiver gain.

Some flow techniques are particularly suited to measuring the velocity of rapidly flowing blood, whereas other methods function best at the lower velocity range found in CSF. Flow techniques are useful clinically only if they can be performed in relatively short acquisition times. Flow imaging methods that require many separate acquisitions to time-resolve flow at different phases of the cardiac cycle are not efficient and are generally reserved for research purposes. In the next section, a simple and rapid method proven useful in imaging CSF motion in the spine is described.

*References 5, 9, 15, 21, 32, 34, 39, 42, 60, 62.

Differential Flip Angle CSF Flow Imaging

Differential flip angle (DFA) CSF flow imaging consists of two different methods for imaging CSF motion. The technique is fully described and validated elsewhere.[52,53] Sagittal DFA provides qualitative flow images of CSF in the sagittal plane (Figures 1-74 and 1-75) and axial DFA provides quantitative flow images in the axial plane (Figures 1-76 and 1-77). These techniques are useful because:

1. They overcome many of the limitations of other flow techniques for the evaluation of CSF
2. They are clinically efficient because they require only several minutes of acquisition time
3. They are well-suited to the velocity range of CSF.

The sagittal DFA technique is sensitive to CSF with a pulsation amplitude (peak-to-trough oscillatory excursion) as small as 0.5 mm.[52] The axial DFA technique is quantitative over the full physiologic range of CSF pulsation amplitudes, from less than 1 mm to over 40 mm.[52] Furthermore, the axial DFA technique does not rely on absolute signal intensity measurements, so it is not affected by differences in surface coil distance or alterations in the receiver gain.

DFA CSF flow imaging is performed by collecting two or three variable flip angle images at different flip angles.[52,53] Sagittal and axial DFA acquisitions differ in imaging plane, TR, flip angles, slice thickness, and method of processing. Sagittal DFA images are collected using a short TR (25 to 100 msec) at a low flip angle (6°) and an intermedite (30°) or high flip angle (80°) using a 5 mm slice thickness (see Figures 1-74 and 1-75). Axial DFA images are collected using a longer TR (200 to 250 msec) at either two (10° and 30°) or three (10°, 20°, and 30°) different flip angles using a slice thickness of 10 mm (see Figures 1-76 and 1-77). Sagittal DFA images are processed using a normalized subtraction of the larger flip angle image from the smaller flip angle image. Axial DFA images are processed by performing a linear regression on the signal intensity data plotted as $SI/\sin\beta$ vs. $SI/\tan\beta$, where SI is the signal intensity and β is the flip angle. This may be performed on individual regions of interest taken from the operator's console or may be performed on whole images on a pixel by pixel basis. The pulsation amplitude is calculated from the linear regression by first calcu-

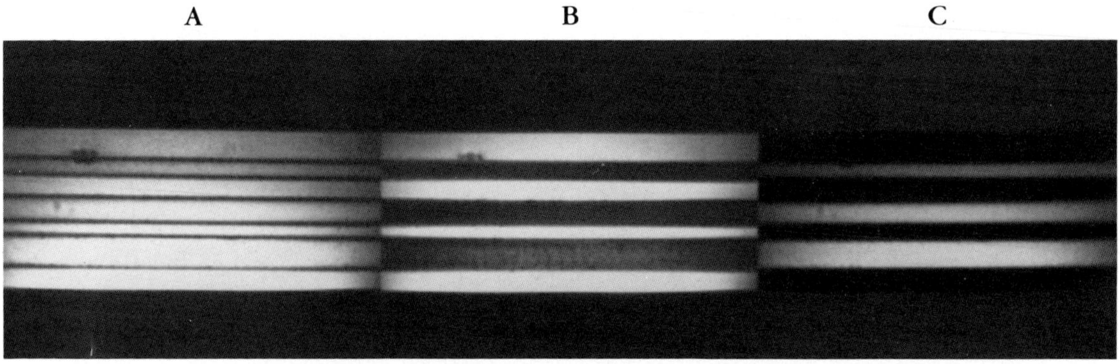

FIGURE 1-74. Sagittal-DFA flow imaging in oscillatory CSF phantom. **A**, GRASS 22/12, flip angle 5°. **B**, GRASS 22/12, flip angle 90°. **C**, Sagittal-DFA image (normalized subtraction of **B** from **A**). Pulsation amplitude is 10 mm in the large tube, 18 mm in the intermediate tube, and 40 mm in the small tube. Sagittal-DFA image combines information from flow-insensitive low flip angle image with flow-sensitive high flip angle image to generate flow map of in-plane pulsatile CSF motion. Moving water within three tubes is high signal intensity, whereas stationary water surrounding tubes is low signal intensity. Signal intensity of stationary water is lower than that of air, providing wide dynamic range and excellent separation between moving and stationary water. This technique is sensitive to pulsatile motion as small as fraction of millimeter. Allowing for surface coil signal gradient, signal intensity is identical within all three tubes (even though they contain CSF moving at different pulsation amplitudes) because this method is not quantitative. (From Rubin JB. Submitted for publication to Radiology.)

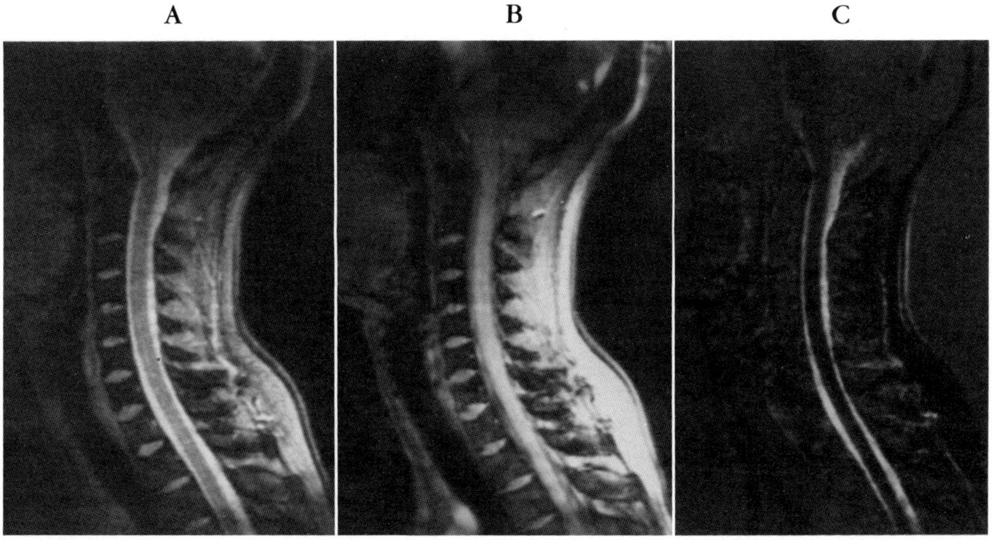

FIGURE 1-75. Sagittal-DFA CSF flow imaging in normal cervical spine. **A**, GRASS 40/15, flip angle 6°. **B**, GRASS 40/15, flip angle 80°. **C**, Sagittal-DFA image (normalized subtraction of **B** from **A**) demonstrates in-plane CSF motion within anterior and posterior subarachnoid spaces. Sagittal-DFA technique permits rapid screening for presence or absence of motion, functioning as a flow map "scout view." Technique does not quantitate in-plane motion. If documented in any region of sagittal-DFA image, motion at that location can be quantitated by using axial-DFA technique. (From Rubin JB. Submitted for publication to Radiology.)

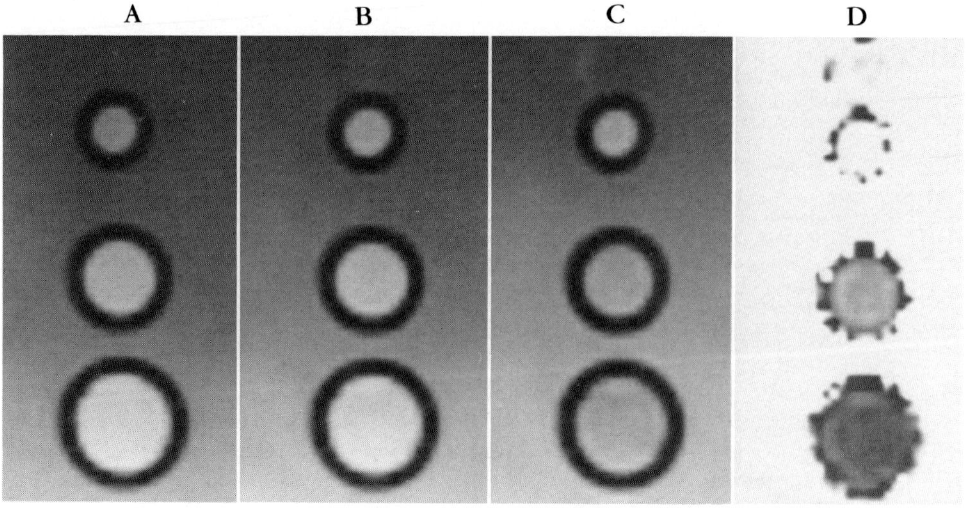

FIGURE 1-76. Axial-DFA flow imaging in oscillatory CSF phantom. **A,** GRASS 250/15, flip angle 10°. **B,** GRASS 250/15, flip angle 20°. **C,** GRASS 250/15, flip angle 30°. **D,** Axial-DFA image calculated from images (**A-C**) using equations described in the text. Pulsation amplitude is 4 mm in the large tube, 7 mm in the intermediate tube, and 16 mm in the small tube. On GRASS images, signal intensity of pulsatile water increases with increasing flip angle when pulsation amplitude is large but decreases with increasing flip angle when pulsation amplitude is small because effective TR prolongation is proportional to pulsation amplitude. Axial-DFA image represents a quantitative pulsation amplitude flow map in which signal intensity in any voxel is equal to the pulsation amplitude (in millimeters) perpendicular to imaging plane. Signal intensities measured within tubes using this method are 4.3, 7.7, and 16.5 for large, intermediate, and small tubes, which agree with actual pulsation amplitudes. Stationary water is high signal intensity because axial-DFA calculation does not apply to completely stationary water that exhibits steady state behavior. (From Rubin JB. Submitted for publication to Radiology.)

lating the effective TR prolongation caused by CSF motion as[52]

(6) $$TR_e = -\ln(S) \cdot T1_c$$

where TR_e is the effective TR prolongation, S is the slope of the signal intensity curve plotted as SI/sinβ vs. SI/tanβ obtained by linear regression, and $T1_c$ is the T1 of CSF (3000 msec). From this, the pulsation amplitude of CSF is calculated as[52]

(7) $$PA = \left[\frac{TR_e}{TR_i} - 1\right] \cdot \left[\frac{ST \cdot NS}{\sin\alpha}\right]$$

where PA is the pulsation amplitude of CSF motion in mm, TR_i is the actual TR used for imaging (recommended value, 250 msec), ST is the slice thickness used (recommended value, 10 mm), NS is the number of slices used (recommended value, 1), and α is the flow angle relative to the imaging plane (recommended value, 90°, flow perpendicular to the imaging plane). Note that the calculation is valid only for CSF and not for other tissues, which means that if the technique is applied to whole images, only the signal intensity of the CSF provides meaningful information.

In clinical application, the sagittal DFA technique is used first as a localizer of CSF motion or "scout view" (see Figure 1-75). On sagittal DFA images, moving CSF is high signal intensity and stationary CSF is very low signal intensity. The method shows moving CSF as high signal regardless of how much it moves, as long as it has a pulsation amplitude (peak-to-trough oscillation) of at least 1 mm (see Figure 1-74). Once regions of moving CSF are identified, the axial DFA technique may be used to quantitate

A B C D

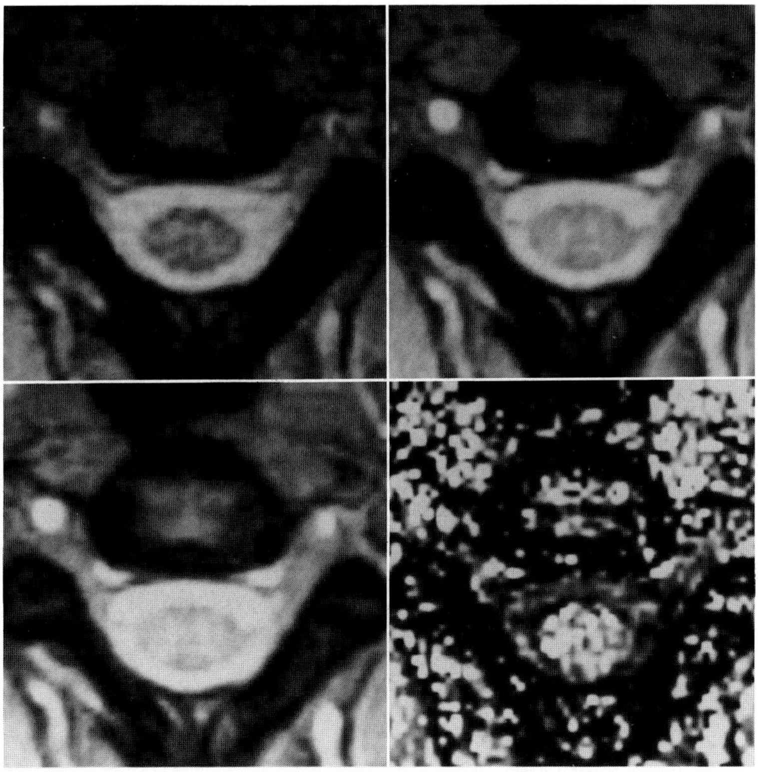

FIGURE 1-77. Axial-DFA CSF flow imaging in normal cervical spine of patient in Figure 1-75. **A,** GRASS 250/15, flip angle 10°. **B,** GRASS 250/15, flip angle 20°. **C,** GRASS 250/15, flip angle 30°. **D,** Axial-DFA image calculated from **A-C.** CSF pulsation amplitude measured 13 mm in the anterior subarachnoid space. Thin band of low signal intensity silhouetting spinal cord and nerve roots occurs secondary to low pulsation amplitude CSF. Pattern of CSF motion within subarachnoid space is complex because of nonuniformity of CSF motion. Pulsation amplitude of CSF measured 18 mm between left ventral and dorsal nerve roots. Only voxels containing CSF can be meaningfully interpreted on axial-DFA images. Signal intensity of the spinal cord is much higher than CSF because its short T1 is interpreted as long, effective TR by calculations. (From Rubin JB. Submitted for publication to Radiology.)

the amount of CSF motion at this level (see Figure 1-77). On axial DFA images, signal intensity of CSF is a quantitative measure of its motion. For example, if a cursor is placed on the image and reads "15", it means that the CSF pulsation amplitude is 15 mm at this location. When significant amounts of CSF motion are present, CSF appears intermedite signal intensity on axial DFA images (see Figure 1-77). When less than 1 mm of motion is present, CSF appears low signal intensity on axial DFA images (Figure 1-78). These techniques will be used in later chapters to illustrate various kinds of normal and abnormal CSF motion.

REFERENCES

1. Adolph RS, Fukusumi H, Fowler NO. Origin of cerebrospinal fluid pulsations. Am J Physiol 1967; 212:840.
2. Axel L. Blood flow effects in magnetic resonance imaging. AJR 1984; 143:1157.
3. Bailes DR, Gilderdale DJ, Bydder GM, et al. Respiratory ordered phase encoding (ROPE): a method for reducing respiratory motion artifacts in MR imaging. J Comput Assist Tomogr 1985; 9:835.
4. Bergstrand G, Gergstrom M, Nordell B, et al. Cardiac gated MR imaging of cerebrospinal fluid flow. J Comput Assist Tomogr 1985; 9:1003.
5. Bradley WG, Kortman KE, Burgoyne B, et al. Flowing cerebrospinal fluid in normal and hydrocephalic states: appearance on MR images. Radiology 1986; 159:611.
6. Bradley WG, Waluch V, Ka-Siu L, et al. The appearance of rapidly flowing blood on magnetic resonance images. AJR 1984; 143:1167.

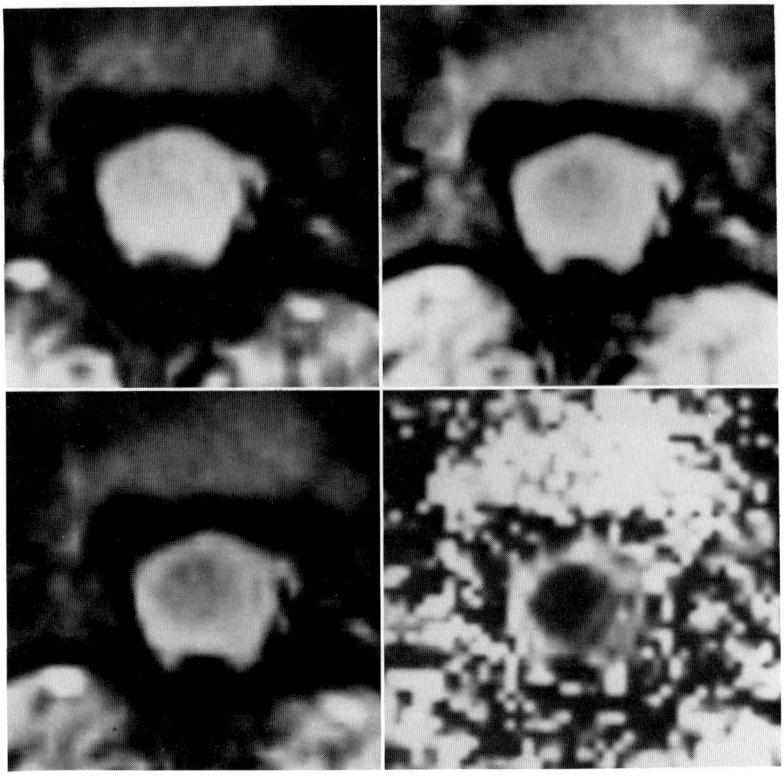

FIGURE 1-78. Axial-DFA flow imaging in cervical spinal cord glioma. **A,** GRASS 250/15, flip angle 10°. **B,** GRASS 250/15, flip angle 20°. **C,** GRASS 250/15, flip angle 30°. **D,** Axial-DFA image calculated from **A-C.** On GRASS images, signal intensity within cystic glioma decreases with increasing flip angle because signal-loss is unopposed by signal-gain. On axial-DFA image, fluid within tumor cyst is very low signal intensity (measured value approximately equal to zero) indicating no significant motion. In comparison, CSF is often pulsatile within syrinx cavities.

7. Bradley WG, Waluch V. Blood flow: magnetic resonance imaging. Radiology 1985; 154:443.
8. Brigham EO. The fast fourier transform. Englewood Cliffs, N.J.: Prentice Hall, Inc., 1974.
9. Bryant DJ, Payne JA, Firmin DN, et al. Measurement of flow with NMR imaging using a gradient pulse and phase difference technique. J Comput Assist Tomogr 1984; 8:588.
10. Buxton RB, Edelman RR, Rosen BR, et al. Contrast in rapid MR imaging: T1- and T2-weighted imaging. J Comput Assist Tomogr 1987; 11(1):7.
11. Bydder GM, Payne JA, Collins AG, et al. Clinical use of rapid T2-weighted partial saturation sequences in MR imaging. J Comput Assist Tomogr 1987; 11(1):17.
12. Condon B, Patterson J, Jenkins A, et al. MR relaxation times of cerebrospinal fluid. J Comput Assist Tomogr 1987; 11(2):203.
13. Cutler RWP, Page L, Galicich J, et al. Formation and absorbtion of cerebrospinal fluid in man. Brain 1968; 91:707.
14. DuBoulay GH. Pulsatile movements in the CSF pathways. Br J Radiol 1966; 39:255.
15. Edelman RR, Wedeen VJ, Davis KR, et al. Multiphasic MR imaging: a new method for direct imaging of pulsatile CSF flow. Radiology 1986; 161:779.
16. Ehman RL, McNamera MT, Brasch RC, et al. Influence of physiologic motion on the appearance of tissue in MR images. Radiology 1986; 159:777.
17. Enzmann DR, Rubin JB, Wright A. Cervical spine MR imaging: generating high-signal CSF in sagittal and axial images. Radiology 1987; 163:233.
18. Enzmann DR, Rubin JB, Wright A. Use of cerebrospinal fluid gating to improve T2-weighted images, I. The spinal cord. Radiology 1987; 162:763.
19. Enzmann DR, Rubin JB. Cervical spine: MR imaging with a partial flip angle, gradient-refocused pulse sequence. I. General considerations and disk disease. Radiology 1988; 166:467.
20. Enzmann DR, Rubin JB. Cervical spine: MR imaging with a partial flip angle, gradient-refocused pulse sequence, II. Spinal cord disease. Radiology 1988; 166:473.
21. Feinberg DA, Crooks LE, Hoenninger J, et al. Pulsatile blood velocity in human arteries displayed by magnetic resonance imaging. Radiology 1984; 153:177.

22. Frahm J, Haase A, Matthaei D. Rapid NMR imaging of dynamic processes using the FLASH technique. Magn Reson Med 1986; 3:321.
23. George CR, Jacobs G, MacIntyre WJ, et al. Magnetic resonance signal intensity patterns obtained from continuous and pulsatile flow models. Radiology 1984; 151:421.
24. Gilland O, Chin F, Anderson WB, et al. A cinemyelographic study of cerebrospinal fluid dynamics. AJR 1969; 106:369.
25. Grover T, Singer JR: NMR spin-echo flow measurements. J Appl Physiol 1971; 42:938.
26. Haacke EM, Lenz GW. Improving MR image quality in the presence of motion by using rephasing gradients. AJR 1987; 148:1251.
27. Haacke EM, Patrick JL. Reducing motion artifacts in two-dimensional fourier transform imaging. Magn Reson Imaging 1096; 4:359.
28. Hawkes RC, Patz S. Rapid fourier imaging using steady-state free precession. Magn Reson Med 1987; 4:9.
29. Hedberg MC, Drayer BP, Flom RA, et al. Gradient echo (GRASS) MR imaging in cervical radiculopathy. AJNR 1988; 9:145.
30. Hendrick RE, Kneeland JB, Stark DD. Maximizing signal-to-noise and contrast-to-noise ratios in FLASH imaging. Magn Reson Imaging 1987; 5:117.
31. Jirout VJ, Fisher J, Nadvornik F. Anatomic and pneumographic studies of the posterior arachnoid space of the normal thoracic spine. ROFO 1964; 101:395.
32. Jolesz FA, Patz S, Hawkes RC, et al. Fast imaging of CSF flow/motion patterns using steady-state free precession (SSFP). Invest Radiol 1987; 22:761.
33. Lanc B, Kricheff II. Cerebrospinal fluid pulsations at myelography: a videodensitometric study. Radiology 1974; 110:579.
34. Le Bihan D, Breton E, Lallemand D, et al. MR imaging of intravoxel incoherent motions: application to diffusion and perfusion in neurologic disorders. Radiology 1986; 161:401.
35. Levy LM, Di Chiro G, Brooks R, et al. Spinal cord artifacts from truncation errors during MR imaging. Radiology 1988; 166:479.
36. Lufkin RB, Pusey E, Stark DD, et al. Boundary artifact due to truncation errors in magnetic resonance imaging. AJR 1986; 147:1283.
37. Mansfield P, Morris PG. NMR imaging in biomedicine. In: Waugh JS, ed. Advances in magnetic resonance, (suppl 2). New York; Academic Press, 1982.
38. McDonald DA. Blood flow in arteries, ed 2. Baltimore: Williams and Wilkins, 1974.
39. Moran PR, Moran RA, Karstaedt N. Verification and evaluation of internal flow and motion: true magnetic resonance imaging by the phase gradient modulation method. Radiology 1985; 154:433.
40. Patel JP, Ramesh NV. Basic hemodynamics and its role in disease processes. Baltimore: University Park, 1980.
41. Pattany PM, Phillips JJ, Chiu LC, et al. Motion artifact suppression technique (MAST) for MR imaging. J Comput Assist Tomogr 1987; 11:369.
42. Patz S, Hawkes RC. The application of steady-state free precession to the study of very slow flow. Magn Reson Med 1986; 3:140.
43. Perkins TG, Wehrli FW. CSF signal enhancement in short TR gradient echo images. Magn Reson Imaging 1986; 4:465.
44. Perman WH, Moran PR, Moran RA, et al. Artifacts from pulsatile flow in MR imaging. J Comput Assist Tomogr 1986; 10(3):473.
45. Rubin JB, Enzmann DR. Imaging of spinal CSF pulsation by 2DFT MR: significance during clinical imaging. AJNR 1987; 8:297-306.
46. Rubin JB, Enzmann DR. Harmonic modulation of proton MR precessional phase by pulsatile motion: origin of spinal CSF flow phenomenon. AJNR 1987; 8:307.
47. Rubin JB, Enzmann DR. Optimizing conventional MR imaging of the spine. Radiology 1987; 163:777.
48. Rubin JB, Enzmann DR, Wright A. CSF gated MR imaging of the spine: theory and clinical implementation. Radiology 1987; 163:784.
49. Rubin JB, Wright A, Enzmann DR. Lumbar Spine: motion compensation for cerebrospinal fluid on MR imaging. Radiology 1988; 166:225.
50. Rubin JB. Cerebrospinal fluid flow effects on GRASS MR. I. Significance and theoretical basis. (Submitted for publication.)
51. Rubin JB. Cerebrospinal fluid flow effects on GRASS MR. II. Optimizing spine image contrast. (Submitted for publication.)
52. Rubin JB. Differential flip angle CSF flow imaging. I. Theoretical basis and clinical implementation. (Submitted for publication.)
53. Rubin JB, Enzmann DR: Differential flip angle CSF flow imaging. II. Clinical application. (Submitted for publication.)
54. Schultz CL, Alfidi RJ, Nelson AD, et al. The effect of motion on two-dimensional fourier transformation magnetic resonance images. Radiology 1984; 152:117.
55. van der Meulen P, Groen JP, Cuppen JJM. Very fast MR imaging by field echoes and small angle excitation. Magn Reson Imaging 1985; 3:297.
56. Valk PE, Hale JD, Crooks LE, et al. MRI of blood flow: correlation of image appearance with spin-echo phase shift and signal intensity. AJR 1986; 146:931.
57. von Schulthess GK, Fisher M, Crooks LE, et al. Gated MR imaging of the heart: intracardiac signals in patients and healthy subjects. Radiology 1985; 156:125.
58. von Schultness GK, Higgins CB. Blood flow imaging with MR: spin phase phenomena. Radiology 1985; 157:687.
59. Waluch V, Bradley WG. NMR even echo rephasing in slow laminar flow. J Comput Assist Tomogr 1984; 8:594.
60. Wehrli FW, MacFall JR, Axel L, et al. Approaches to in-plane and out-of-plane flow imaging. Noninv Med Imaging 1984; 1:127.
61. Wehrli FW, MacFall JR, Shutts D, et al. Mechanisms of contrast in NMR imaging. J Comput Assist Tomogr 1984; 8(3):369.
62. Wehrli FW, Shimakawa A, McFall JR, et al. MR imaging of venous and arterial flow by a selective saturation recovery spin-echo method. J Comput Assist Tomogr 1985; 9:537.
63. Wood ML, Henkelman RM. Truncation artifacts in magnetic resonance imaging. Magn Reson Med 1985; 2:517.
64. Young IR, Khenia S, Thomas GT, et al. Clinical magnetic susceptibility mapping of the brain. J Comput Assist Tomogr 1987; 11(1):2.
65. Young IR, Payne JA, Collins AG, et al. MRI: The development of T2 contrast with rapid field echo sequences. Magn Reson Med 1987; 4:333.

2
Spine Imaging Techniques

Dieter R. Enzmann
Jeremy B. Rubin

Spine MR scanning requires balancing several parameters to obtain the appropriate contrast, signal-to-noise ratio (SNR), and spatial resolution. In addition, because of the prominence of cerebral spinal fluid (CSF) pulsation, motion compensation techniques become important in certain diagnostic situations and the specific MR scanning technique will be a function of suspected pathologic condition and site. To ensure an optimal MR study, an accurate, detailed clinical history is essential, especially in nonroutine diagnostic problems. The history will determine MR pulse sequence selection for the suspected pathologic condition and the site of spine involvement. Monitoring the study is encouraged so that the scanning technique can be modified as findings unfold. An iterative and flexible spine scanning approach requires significant physician input, which greatly improves the accuracy and quality of the MR study. Optimal spine MR examinations require attention to details regarding hardware and software.

SURFACE COILS

MR machines have a variety of coils that detect the NMR signal from the body. The coil acts as an antenna, has the primary purpose of transferring the NMR signal arising in body tissue to the receiver preamplifier, and efficiently detects the NMR signal when tuned to the correct proton resonance frequency. Transmission of the signal to the preamplifier is most efficient when the impedance of the coil and the preamplifier are matched. The largest coil, the "body" coil, is designed to make maximum use of the available imaging volume and to be uniformly sensitive to NMR signals arising from the body. It is used to both transmit and receive RF signal. The body coil is limited in spine imaging because

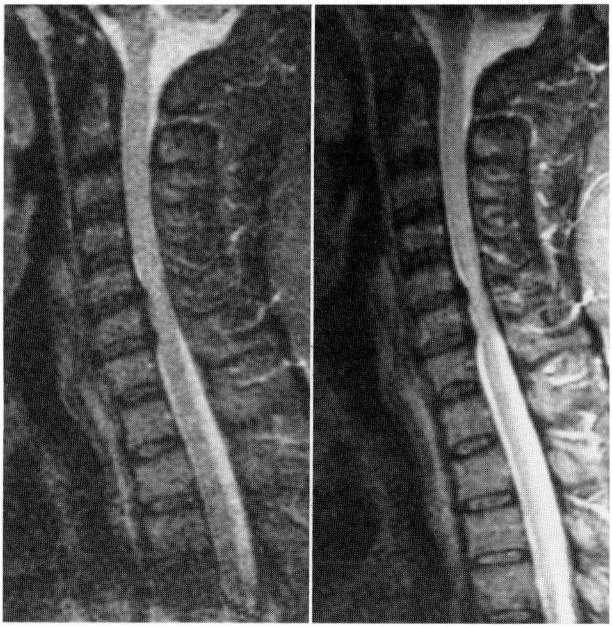

FIGURE 2-1. **A,** Sagittal view of cervical spine using gated acquisition (SE 2000/80) comparing body coil and **B,** surface coil placed posteriorly to the neck. All parameters—256 x 256; NEX 2; FOV 24 cm—were held constant for both images. Higher SNR in image **B** is major attribute of a surface coil.

of its low SNR and consequent loss of detail (Figure 2-1).

It may be difficult to localize a specific vertebral body level in the spine when a small field of view (FOV) is used with a surface coil. A low resolution image using the body coil can be helpful in identifying C_2 or L_5 to permit precise localization of a specific vertebral level (Figure 2-2). A somewhat distorted and expanded view of the spine can be obtained with large FOVs and larger surface coils. The poor quality of such images is of little concern because they are used simply for localization, not diagnosis.

The most useful type of coil for spine imaging is the local coil, a general term for the more common term *surface coil*. Its physical configuration can range from a flat plate to a complex shape conforming to a body part such as the neck. The most common local coil "receives" only, which means that the large body coil is used to transmit RF signals because of its uniformity and the local coil is used to receive the NMR signal from its sensitive volume in the body. All local coils detect NMR signals from only a limited portion of the body, the "sensitive volume."[8] The size of the sensitive volume is important because it determines many characteristics of the coil that are relevant to clinical imaging. The sensitive volume determines the region of the body that can be imaged and what the SNR will be in the image. It is roughly hemispheric from the coil with the width equal to the diameter of the coil and the depth equal to one half the diameter (Figure 2-3). A smaller sensitive volume yields a more limited view of the anatomy but a higher SNR (Figure 2-4). With higher SNR, a smaller pixel size can be used to improve spatial resolution. The increased SNR results from (1) an increase in signal because of the close proximity of the coil to the area of interest and (2) a reduction in patient-generated thermal noise.[16] Noise reduction is achieved because noise is proportional to the volume of tissue generating signal; this is reduced with smaller coils.[16] In the spine, the implication is clear: the better localization of the area of interest, the smaller the surface coil that can be used. This allows higher image quality because of increased SNR. A higher SNR allows use of a smaller pixel size, thus better resolution (see Figure 2-2).

As a result of the usual state of clinical histories or prescan clinical localization, the initial pixel size-FOV-SNR trade-off is usually in favor of a larger FOV. Nevertheless, the basic concept is that once a lesion is localized, higher SNR images can be obtained by switching to a smaller surface coil, which means that holding all other parameters constant, simply switching to a surface coil with a smaller sensitive volume will

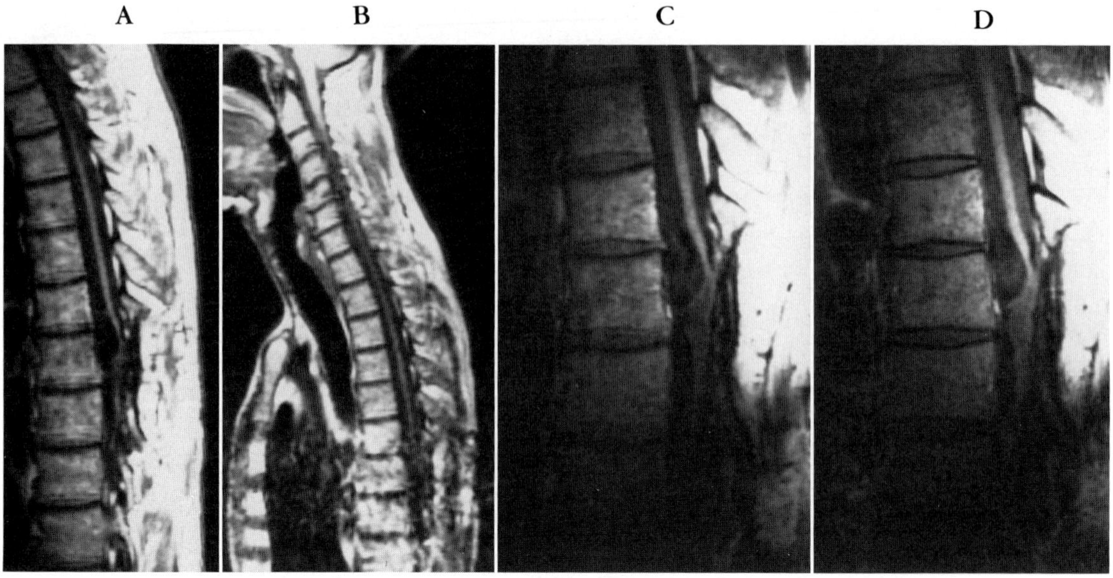

FIGURE 2-2. Series of three sagittal T1W scans of patient with postoperative arachnoiditis illustrates use of various coil techniques to help localize and characterize cord lesion. **A,** T1W scan (SE 800/20, FOV 32 cm) identifies lesion in midthoracic cord, but exact location cannot be determined because there are no specific landmarks to help count vertebral bodies accurately. **B,** Problem is solved by use of low resolution scan using body coil. T1W image (SE 400/20, FOV 48) includes C_2 and allows correct count of vertebral bodies. Poor image quality does not detract from limited purpose of localization. **C** and **D,** Once area of pathology is identified, small surface coil can be placed directly over lesion and high resolution image (SE 800/20, FOV 20 cm) obtained depicting pathology in greater detail. Cord atrophy and dorsal and ventral adhesions in canal are well seen at T_7. Note higher SNR and thus higher spatial resolution by small surface coil image in **C** and **D** compared to larger surface coil image in **A.**

improve image quality (see Figure 2-4). The rationale for choosing local coils therefore is to select one with a sensitive volume just large enough to cover the area of interest but no larger.

Another factor in choosing a surface coil is how it interacts with the body. "Coupling" refers to how the coil and body interact to induce a current in the coil's circuit.[2] The purpose of a coil is to transfer energy from the body to the MR instrument. The interaction of the coil and body and its electronic characteristics determine the efficiency with which this is accomplished. One such electronic characteristic is coupling with the body, i.e., how the coil is loaded by tissue. Loose coupling describes a situation in which significant amounts of air can be present between the coil and body (i.e., cervical spine), resulting in coupling that is position-sensitive because of air gaps and therefore relatively inefficient. This sets certain impedance match requirements. This type of coil is preferable for cervical spine imaging, whereas a "tightly coupled" coil would be the choice in the lumbar region. In the lumber area, coupling is less position-sensitive because there are no significant air gaps. The coil would be fully loaded with tissue in the lumbar spine and have different impedance match requirements.

Differing impedance matches are handled in two ways: either the local coil is adjustable or it is preset. Choice of the preset coil is important because it is not optimized to the patient, whereas the adjustable coil may be used in many situations because it is tuned and matched for each site in each patient. Set-up time is somewhat longer with these coils, but energy transfer may be improved. Proper choice of surface coils is basic to all spine scanning. Surface coil technology and development will continually undergo improvement and require reassessment because of their importance in spine imaging.

A B

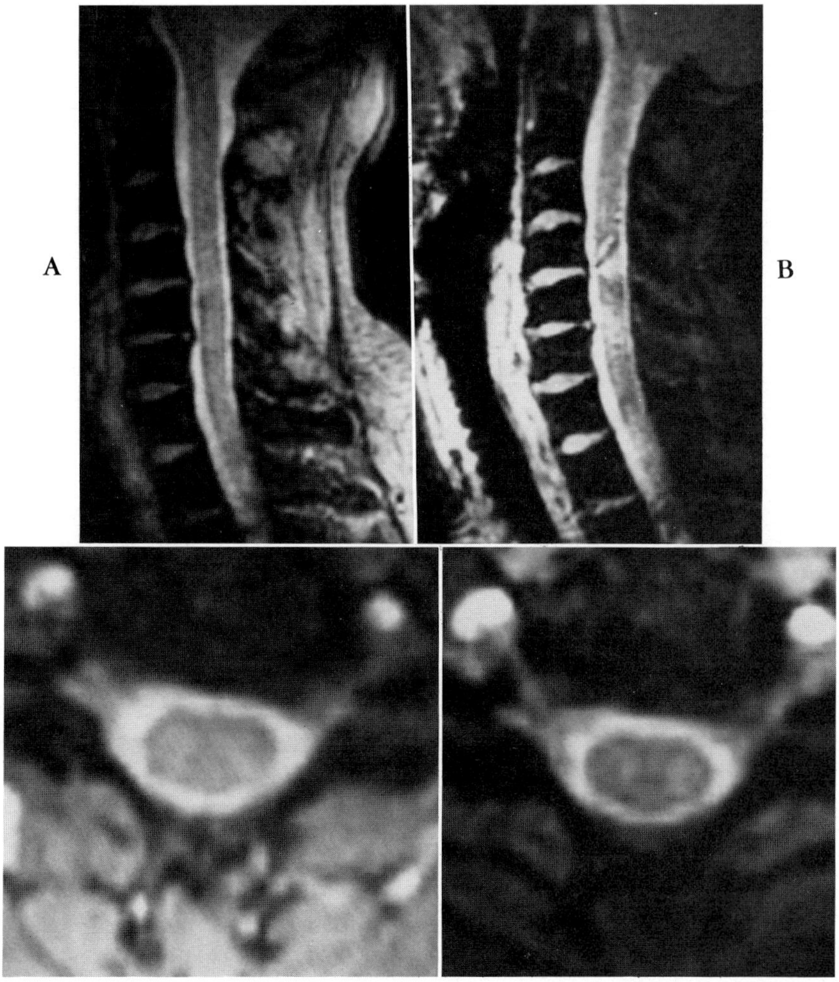

C D

FIGURE 2-3. Choice of surface coil determines sensitive volume and orientation for imaging—in cervical spine, choice between posteriorly located surface coil vs. one placed anteriorly. Depending on individual anatomy and area of interest, one choice may prove superior to another in specific patients; for many patients results are nearly equivalent for cervical disc disease. **A** and **C**, Posteriorly placed coil in this patient resulted in lower SNR of cord and CSF compared to **B** and **D** anteriorly placed coil in set of variable flip angle/gradient echo scans. **A**, Brightness distribution more even with posterior coil. Difference in SNR is simply function of how close anatomic area of interest is to the specific coil. **B**, Anterior coil yields high SNR from disc, cord, and CSF but also results in more artifact overlying the cord. **D**, Use of anterior coil is appropriate for anatomy around vertebral body or larynx. One major drawback of anterior coil in cervical spine is that high signal is generated from larynx and oropharynx and, if patient swallows a great deal of this high signal will then be mismapped across image, obscuring areas of interest at level of discs and spinal canal (see Figure 2-25). Posterior coil will suffer less from this problem because less signal emanates from region of larynx or oropharynx and thus less signal is available to be mismapped.

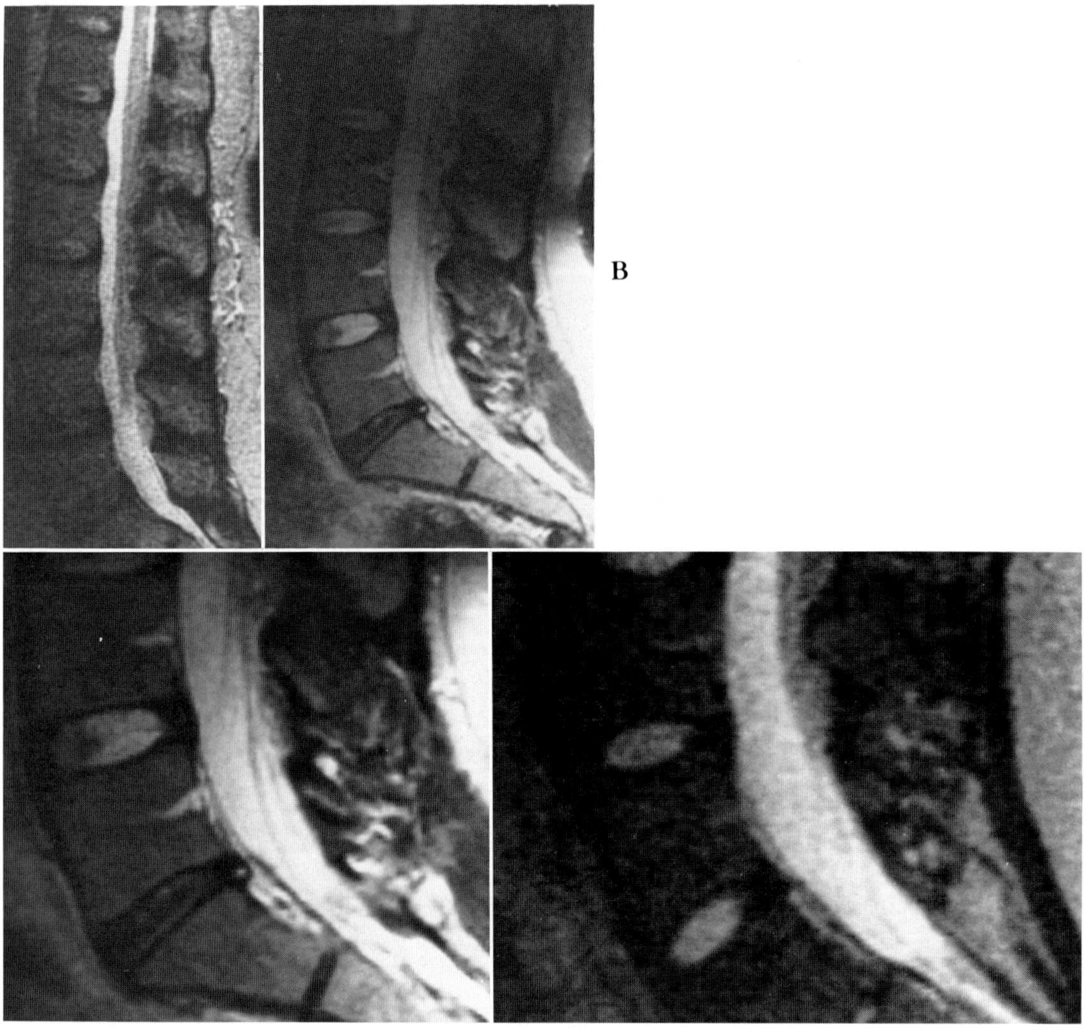

A B C D

FIGURE 2-4. Surface coil chosen initially depends on extent of anatomy that needs to be investigated. **A,** With larger surface coil, entire lumbar spine and conus region seen on one image (SE 2000/80, FOV 24 cm). Good contrast allows adequate depiction of conus and cauda equina. **B,** Use of smaller surface coil with same FOV (24 cm) yields higher SNR and results in significant improvement in anatomic detail without changing spatial resolution (pixel size .94 mm). Note that large part of the FOV has little signal. **C,** Greater detail appreciated in visualization of L_5, S_1, and S_2 nerve roots when image (**B**) is optically magnified (x 2). **D,** Compare with similarly magnified (x 2) image (**A**) of L_4 to S_1 obtained with larger surface coil. SNR and root depiction greatly improved with smaller coil (**C**). Proper choice of surface coil is important technique for increasing SNR without attendant time penalty associated with other methods. Particularly relevant for pediatric congenital spine abnormalities where very small surface coils can be used.

SIGNAL-TO-NOISE RATIO

Signal-to-Noise Ratio vs. Resolution

A fundamental trade-off between spatial resolution and SNR impinges on most MR imaging parameter decisions. For any particular diagnostic purpose, a balance between spatial resolution and SNR is needed. These two critical factors are balanced at the expense of one another; i.e., an increase in spatial resolution decreases the SNR and vice versa. However, a desired spatial resolution cannot be achieved without sufficient SNR to maintain diagnostic image quality. The trade-off pushes spatial resolution to a point where SNR remains acceptable; beyond that point, SNR becomes insufficient and image quality deteriorates.[4] In clinical imaging, awareness of strategies capable of boosting SNR is needed. One major limitation is scanning time. Many methods for increasing SNR increase scanning time so this has to be balanced with clinical reality and the patient's ability to remain immobile.

Tissue Volume and Resolution

The NMR signal emanating from tissue is directly proportional to the tissue volume; i.e., the number of protons in a voxel emitting the signal:

$$S \alpha\ V \alpha\ Dx \cdot Dy \cdot Dz$$

where S is signal intensity, V is volume, Dx is dimension in X axis, Dy is dimension in Y axis, and Dz is dimension in Z axis. The signal is proportional to slice thickness and the in-plane dimensions of the pixel; i.e., voxel volume. This means that a thicker slice has a higher SNR. The major counterbalancing factor is partial volume artifact, which must be at an acceptable level and limits the use of thick slices. SNR drops 70% from a 10 mm slice to a 3 mm slice. Spine imaging can stress an MR system because the most common and useful slice thicknesses are in a 2 to 5 mm range (see Figure 2-7). The thickest slice should be compatible with the suspected disease process and the anatomy being investigated should be used.

The in-plane spatial resolution (i.e., pixel size) is governed by the matrix size, which is measured along the frequency encoding and the phase-encoding axes. Pixel dimensions can be calculated by dividing the FOV (in centimeters) by the matrix size for the appropriate axis. On current machines, the frequency encoding axis is usually set at 256 points (although 512 points may be an option), whereas the phase-encoding axis usually allows a choice between 128, 192, and 256 phase-encoding steps. Use of the 256 × 128 matrix doubles the SNR compared to a 256 × 256 matrix; i.e., the voxel volume is doubled, one side being twice as long as the other. While the scanning time is halved, the spatial resolution is also reduced. These effects result simply from changes in voxel volume. In a 256 × 128 matrix the pixel is asymmetric, whereas in a 256 × 256 matrix the in-plane pixel dimension is symmetric. The latter is preferred because the asymmetric pixel size causes images to appear somewhat blurred. In addition the use of a 128 matrix size makes the spine image susceptible to the Gibbs phenomenon[10,16] (see Chapter 1), which refers to image brightness oscillations at the site of sharp steps in image contrast (Figure 2-5) inherent in the two-dimensional fourier transformation (2DFT) method of image reconstruction. Pixel size and slice thickness interact in a predictable way; significant SNR loss can occur whenever voxel volume is reduced by either decreasing slice thickness or decreasing pixel size. This is the essence of the fundamental trade-off between SNR and resolution. As spatial resolution increases, the voxel volume decreases and so does SNR, with the effect being nearly linear in most of the clinically relevant ranges. Image quality can be improved by maximizing SNR for a desired resolution. Two common methods are available for increasing SNR without decreasing resolution: increasing the number of excitations (NEX) and increasing repetition time (TR).

Number of Excitations

$$S \alpha \sqrt{NEX}$$

where S is signal intensity and NEX, the number of excitations.

Increasing the NEXs in MR imaging has the effect of signal averaging. SNR is increased by the square root of the number of excitations. For most standard scans NEX is 2. For higher resolution applications, NEX may be increased to 4 or 6. In going from 2 to 4 NEX, one can achieve

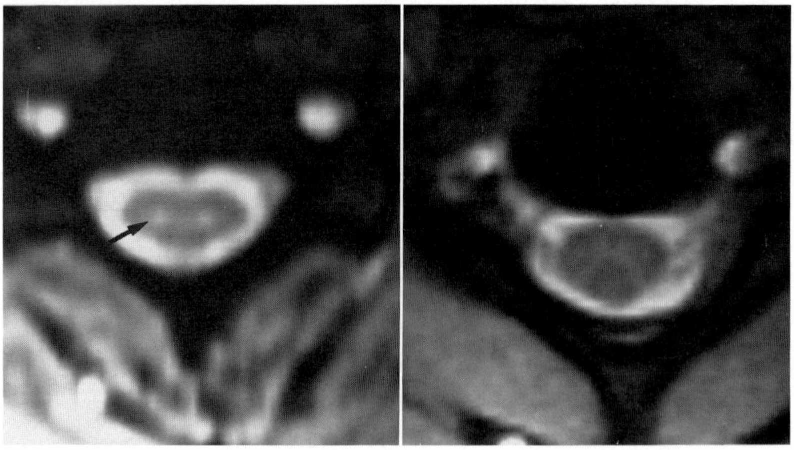

FIGURE 2-5. **A,** Axial, variable flip angle/gradient echo scan using 256 x 128 matrix (GRASS 22/12, 7°) shows Gibbs artifact characterized by horizontal area of increased signal in middle of spinal cord *(arrow)*. Central signal is artifactual and does not represent any structure within spinal cord. **B,** Area of high signal disappears when 256 x 256 matrix is used.

a 41% increase in SNR; from 2 to 6 NEX, it is a 73% increase; and from 4 to 6, a 22% increase is achieved. The penalty is longer scanning time, which is directly proportional to NEX. This method of increasing SNR is practical with shorter TR scans, usually ≤1000 msec. With longer TRs, higher SNR may reduce the need for signal averaging, thus allowing a reduction in scanning time. Long TR scans could trade-off some SNR to use a NEX of 1, cutting imaging time by 50% from the more usual NEX 2 scan (see Figure 2-8).

Repetition Time (TR)

The SNR of an image is proportional to TR. Although SNR increases with increasing TR, the effect is one of diminishing returns; i.e., as a TR increases, the increment in SNR decreases. The exact increment depends on the T1 of the tissue of interest. There are two penalties with this approach to increasing SNR: (1) reduced contrast on T1W images as TR is increased and (2) longer imaging time, which is directly proportional to TR. There are limits to increasing TR because image contrast will change in character starting with T1W images, going to "balanced images" (approximation of proton density), and ultimately to T2W images. So there are practical limits to increasing TR for T1W images. TRs above 1000 msec are less useful for spine imaging because of decreasing cord-CSF contrast.

Understanding trade-offs between increasing TR and increasing NEX to achieve a higher SNR helps in clinical imaging. At 1.5 T for neural tissue (assuming T1 800, T2 70 msec), it is often efficacious to increase TR when TR is in the low range rather than increase NEX since the gains in SNR are greater per unit of imaging time. For example, going from a TR of 400 to a TR of 800, the improvement is 66% in SNR compared to increasing NEX from 2 to 4 for a TR of 400 where improvement in SNR is only 41% for equal scanning time. Another example is to compare going from 2 to 6 NEX for a TR of 400, yielding a 73% increase in SNR. This can be compared to going from a TR of 400 to a TR of 1000, yielding an 88% increase in SNR but using a shorter scanning time. The cost, of course, is contrast. This trade-off is workable for T1W images where grey-white differentiation in the cord is not particularly useful for diagnosis and where cord-CSF contrast is still acceptable at higher TRs.

Variable Bandwidth (BW)

The SNR of an image is inversely proportional to the square root of the bandwidth:

$$\text{SNR} \; \alpha \; \frac{1}{\sqrt{\text{BW}}}$$

A method for increasing SNR in a heavily T2W

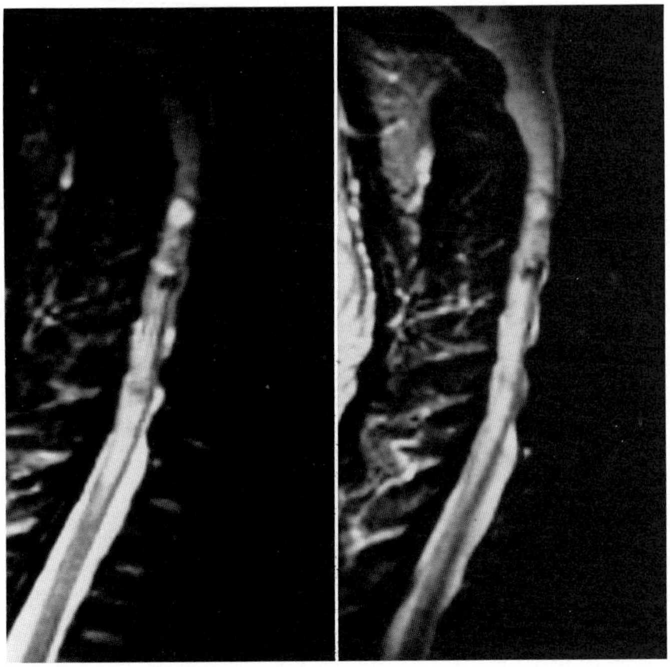

FIGURE 2-6. Sagittal T2W scans (SE 2300/80) obtained using both gating and first order motion compensation (gradient moment nulling technique). Images compare incremental improvement in SNR of second echo image when reduced bandwidth sequence is used. **A,** Normal bandwidth and **B,** reduced bandwidth resulting in higher SNR in second echo. Note better definition of tumor and its internal pattern on higher SNR variable bandwidth image **B.**

image is a variable bandwidth pulse sequence, which uses a normal bandwidth for the first echo and a reduced bandwidth (30% to 50% range) for the second echo, resulting in decreased noise and therefore an increased SNR (Figure 2-6). The advantage of a variable bandwidth pulse sequence is that it increases SNR without increasing scanning time. The disadvantage is a more prominent chemical shift artifact. Variable bandwidth pulse sequences are useful in the spine in the sagittal view where chemical shift artifact on the second echo is not significant and is unlikely to cause diagnostic difficulty. They are less useful on axial T2W images, especially in the lumbar spine, where chemical shift artifact may be bothersome because of epidural fat.

Scan Time

Scanning time is equal to the number of phase-encoding steps × NEX × TR. It is desirable to minimize scan time for a given application. Spatial resolution (phase-encoding axis), NEX, and TR are all determinants of scanning time, which puts practical limits on scanning time parameters. For T1W images of the spine, increasing TR is often the best first step for increasing SNR. Higher NEXs are used after TR has been exploited. Decreasing the number of phase-encoding steps can compensate for other factors that increase scan time, but it also reduces spatial resolution. A 256 × 256 matrix is recommended, although a 256 × 192 matrix may be an acceptable alternative. A 128 matrix size is not recommended, in part because it is susceptible to the Gibbs phenomenon, which can result in artifacts within the spinal cord (see Chapter 1). On T1W images, low signal can be seen within the cord, whereas on T2W or T2*W images high signal can be seen in the cord on sagittal and axial images (see Figure 2-5). The artifactual signal in the cord reflects the signal intensity of CSF in the image. Variable flip angle/ gradient refocused scans will show high signal artifact because of high signal CSF (see Figure 2-5). A high resolution technique is normally recommended for spine imaging. Nevertheless, decreasing spatial resolution is a useful option to reduce scanning time when patient motion is a problem. It is also a method of increasing patient throughput.

Slice Effect, Slice Gap

Slice selection techniques in MR imagers have been imperfect with significant "cross talk" occurring between adjacent slices; therefore a small gap between slices is often used to minimize this effect. To counteract the problem, many pulse sequences use interleaved slice data acquisition. This means in the first pass, for example, slice 1, 3, 5, 7, 9, etc. data are acquired, and on a second pass, slice 2, 4, 6, 8, 10, etc. data are acquired. This reduces but does not eliminate the effect of "cross-talk," which will manifest as alternating bright and somewhat darker images in a series of T1W images. Slices obtained during the second pass will show a lower SNR because of partial saturation of the protons from the first pass of data acquisition. This is one reason for choosing gaps between slices. The decrease in SNR in the adjacent slice is more severe when the interslice gap is small and is more noticeable with shorter TRs. For example, an adjacent slice can have a 43% reduction in SNR with a TR of 400, but only 14% SNR reduction with a TR of 800. A longer TR allows a longer interval between data acquisition for adjacent slices and thus more time for longitudinal relaxation to recover. With very long TR images, such as those normally used for T2W images (TR ≤ 2000 msec), the slice effect is minimal because of the longer time allowed for longitudinal magnetization to recover before adjacent slices are sampled.

The slice gap must also be considered when determining the anatomic volume to be scanned, especially axial spine views. Even when improvements are made in slice selection techniques so that this problem is minimized, slice gaps will still be used to survey or cover an anatomic region because the number of slices available will still be limited by TR. TR and TE are major determinants of the number of slices available for a pulse sequence, and this will vary between machines and type of pulse sequence. A reference table giving distances covered by various combinations of slice thicknesses and interslice gaps is often helpful (Table 2-1). The total distance to be scanned can be determined

TABLE 2-1
Distances for Slice/Gap Combinations (mm/mm)

Slices (no.)	3/0	3/.5	3/1	3/1.5	3/3	5/0	5/1	5/2.5	5/5	10/0	10/1	10/.5
2	3	4	4	5	6	5	6	8	10	10	11	15
3	6	7	8	9	12	10	12	15	20	20	22	30
4	9	11	12	14	18	15	18	23	30	30	33	45
5	12	14	16	18	24	20	24	30	40	40	44	60
6	15	18	20	23	30	25	30	38	50	50	55	75
7	18	22	24	27	36	30	36	45	60	60	66	90
8	21	25	28	32	42	35	42	53	70	70	77	105
9	24	29	32	36	48	40	48	60	80	80	88	120
10	27	32	36	41	54	45	54	68	90	90	99	135
11	30	36	40	45	60	50	60	75	100	100	110	150
12	33	40	44	50	66	55	66	83	110	110	121	165
13	36	43	48	54	72	60	72	90	120	120	132	180
14	39	47	52	59	78	65	78	98	130	130	143	195
15	42	50	56	63	84	70	84	105	140	140	154	210
16	45	54	60	68	90	75	90	113	150	150	165	225
17	48	58	64	72	96	80	96	120	160	160	176	240
18	51	61	68	77	102	85	102	128	170	170	187	225
19	54	65	72	81	108	90	108	135	180	180	198	270
20	57	68	76	86	114	95	114	143	190	190	209	285

from an initial sagittal image and then an appropriate slice thickness and gap combination can be chosen to cover the desired anatomy. For example, if a total distance of 85 mm needs to be investigated then a decision must be made whether image contrast or partial volume artifact is of primary concern. If contrast is more important, a TR is chosen first, which determines the maximum number of slices. If the maximum number of available slices is 14, a 5 mm slice with a 2.5 mm gap would cover the distance (see Table 2-1). Alternatively, if partial volume artifact is the limiting factor because of the small size of the lesion, a thin slice/small gap technique should be chosen that will require more slices and thus a longer TR. For a 3 mm/1.5 mm gap combination, 20 slices are necessary and this will determine the TR (see Table 2-1).

T1W IMAGES

T1W images are heavily influenced by differences in the longitudinal relaxation time (T1) of different tissues. Generally obtained with a TR range of 400 to 1000 msec and a TE range of 15 to 25 msec, these images are used primarily for morphologic delineation of anatomy rather than the detection of abnormal signal from pathologic tissue (Figure 2-7). In the spine they are used for a wide variety of disease processes, but most often they are used as the initial sagittal scan in a spine imaging protocol (see Table 2-2). T1W images provide good contrast for cord, CSF, vertebral body, and the nucleus pulposus. They provide poor contrast between CSF, anulus, ligaments, and osteophytes (Figure 2-8) (see Chapter 10). In the axial view, they can provide internal differentiation of gray and white matter

A B

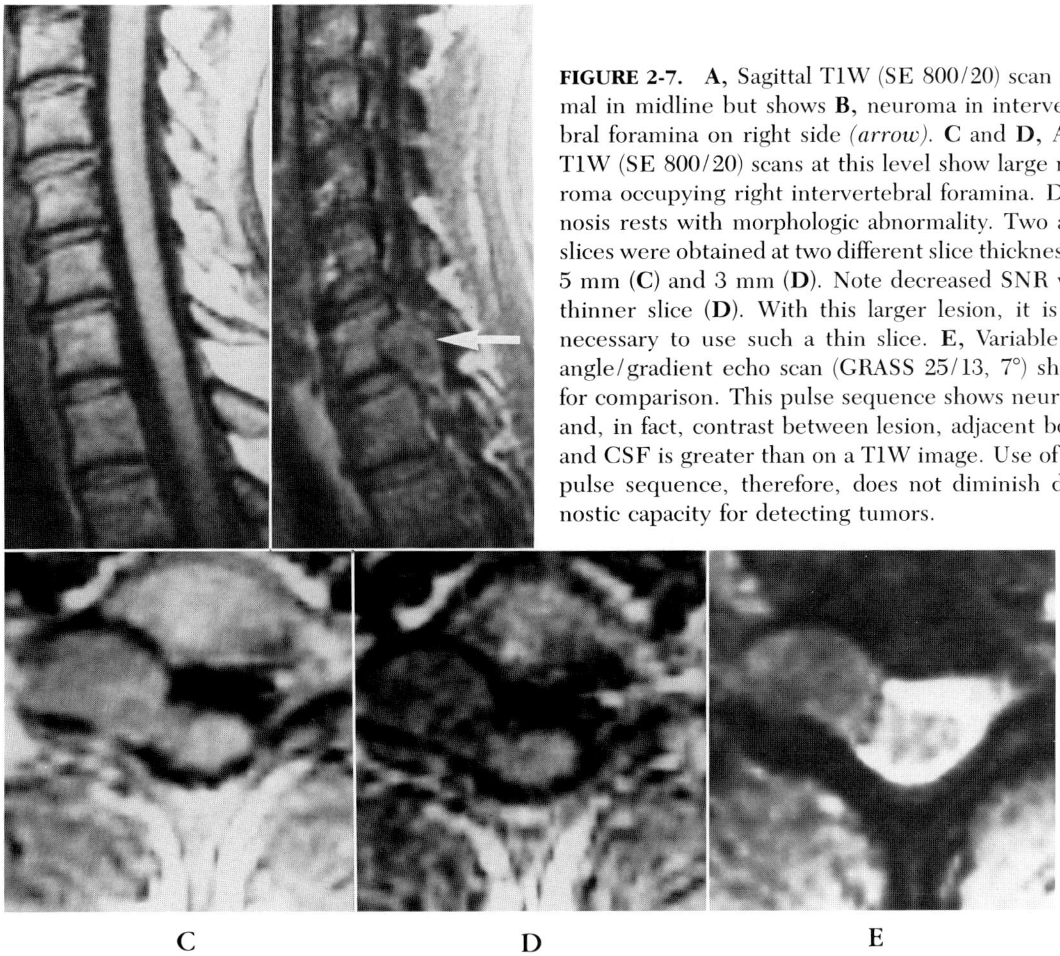

C D E

FIGURE 2-7. **A,** Sagittal T1W (SE 800/20) scan normal in midline but shows **B,** neuroma in intervertebral foramina on right side *(arrow).* **C** and **D,** Axial T1W (SE 800/20) scans at this level show large neuroma occupying right intervertebral foramina. Diagnosis rests with morphologic abnormality. Two axial slices were obtained at two different slice thicknesses, 5 mm (**C**) and 3 mm (**D**). Note decreased SNR with thinner slice (**D**). With this larger lesion, it is not necessary to use such a thin slice. **E,** Variable flip angle/gradient echo scan (GRASS 25/13, 7°) shown for comparison. This pulse sequence shows neuroma and, in fact, contrast between lesion, adjacent bone, and CSF is greater than on a T1W image. Use of this pulse sequence, therefore, does not diminish diagnostic capacity for detecting tumors.

TABLE 2-2
Spine Protocols

	Footnote	Seq number	Plane	Slice	Gap	FA	TR	TE	NEX	Matrix	FOV	Gating	FC	Phase	NPW	PreSat
Generic Initial			S	3	1	–	800	20	2	256	24	–	–	A/P	–	–
Localizer	1	If motion artifact											–	S/I	on	–
Disc																
Cervical		1	S	3	1		800	20	2	256	24	–	–	A/P	–	–
	2	2	S	5 single		5°	40	16	8	256	24	–	on	A/P	–	–
		3	A	5	0	7°	25	16	8	256	24	–	on	R/L	–	–
	3	4 Same as no. 3 but offset by 2 mm from C_4-C_7														
		5	A	5	1	15°	600	16	2	256	24	–	on	R/L	–	–
		6 Same as no. 5 but offset by 2 mm from C_4-C_7														
Thoracic		1	S	3	1		800	20	2	256	24-32	–		A/P	–	–
	4	2	S	5 single		5°	25	16	8	256	24-32	–	on	A/P	–	–
		3	A	3	1		800	20	2	256	24	–	–	R/L	on	on
	5	4 opt	A	5	0	7°	25	16	8	256	24	–	on	R/L	–	–
Lumbar		1	S	3	1		800	20	2	256	24-30	–		A/P	–	–
	6	2	Ax-oblq	3	1		>2000	20,80	2	256	24	on	–	R/L	–	–
		3	Ax-oblq	3	1		1000	20	2	256	24	–	–	R/L	on	on
				Prescribe each disc from sagittal view												
	7 For severe stenosis as determined by seq #1															
		2a	A	3	1		>2000	30,80	1	256	24	on	on	R/L	on	–
	8 For suspected lateral discs or postoperative changes															
		2b	S-oblq	3	1		800	20	2	256	24	–	–	S/I	on	–
Lumbar postoperative disc		1	S	3	1		800	20	2	256	24-30	–		A/P	–	–
		2	Ax-oblq	3	1		1000	20	2	256	24	–	–	R/L	on	on
						Infuse GdDTPA										
		3	S	3	1		800	20	2	256	24-30	–		A/P	–	–
		4	Ax-oblq	3	1		1000	20	2	256	24	–	–	R/L	–	–
Extraaxial Tumor		1	S	3	1		800	20	2	256	24-32	–	–	A/P	–	–
		2	A	5	1		1000	20	2	256	24	–	–	R/L	–	on
						Infuse GdDTPA										
	9	3	S	3	1		800	20	2	256	24-32	–	–	A/P	–	–
		4	A	5	1		1000	20	2	256	24	–	–	R/L	–	on
Spine Metastases		1	S	3	1		800	20	2	256	24-32	–	–	A/P	–	–
		2	A	5	1		1000	20	2	256	24	–	–	R/L	–	on
	10	3	S	3	1		1400(TI 150)	40	2	256	24-32	–	–	A/P	–	–
Cord Tumor		1	S	3	1		800	20	2	256	24-32	–	–	A/P	–	–
	11	2	S	5 single			>2000	30,80	1	256	24	on	on	A/P	–	–

	12	If motion artifact							2	256	24	on		R/L	on	–
	13	3	S	5		5°	25	13	8	256	24	–	on	A/P	–	–
		4	A	5	1		800	20	2	256	24	–	–	R/L	–	on
					Infuse GdDTPA											
	14	5	S	3	1		800	20	2	256	24-32	–	–	A/P	–	–
		6	A	5	1		800	20	2	256	24	–	–	R/L	–	on
Cord-MS		1	S	3	1		800	20	2	256	24	–	–	A/P	–	–
	15	2	S	5	1		>2000	30,80	1	256	24	on	on	A/P	–	–
	16	If motion artifact							2	256	24	on	on	S/I	on	–
	17	3 opt	S	5	1	10°	400	13	2	256	24	–	on	A/P	–	–
	18	4	A	5	0	7°	25	13	8	256	24	–	on	R/L	–	–
Pediatric Dysraphism		1	S	3	1		800	20	2	256	20-24	–	–	A/P	–	–
		2	A	5	1-5		800	20	2	256	16	–	–	R/L	–	on
Syrinx		1	S	3	1		800	20	2	256	24-32	–	–	A/P	–	–
		2	A	3	1		1000	20	2	256	24	–	–	R/L	–	on
	19	3	A	3	1		2000	20,80	2	256	24	–	–	R/L	–	–

*1. If motion artifact (swallowing, cardiac, abdominal wall) obscures area of interest, switch phase and frequency axes and utilize a phase wrap correction option (NPW); this usually requires NEX 2.
2. Usually only a midline slice is necessary for the lateral myelographic view. At most 3 slices are needed.
3. Sequences #3 and #4 are for the sequential, single-slice mode. Sequences #5 and #6 are for the multislice. See the variable flip angle section for optimizing these parameters using the nomograms. These can be obliqued but this is usually not necessary. 5 mm slices are used because this is often a limitation of these pulse sequences.
4. See 2.
5. Optional: This sequence provides further information with regard to dural and cord impingement by a herniated disc. The single-slice mode is sufficient for the limited anatomy to be covered. See 3.
6. The axial slices are obliqued so that they are parallel to the individual disc spaces (see Figure 8). This can be done for T1W or T2W axial images. May use presaturation if allowed, but limits the number of slices, (i.e. disc spaces that can be studied). Perform either sequence #2 or #3.
7. For severe lumbar stenosis, stacked slices rather than obliqued slices are more informative.
8. Sagittal oblique views through the foramen are recommended for the assessment of lateral discs and recurrent disc with postoperative changes.
9. Post contrast scans 5-10 min after infusion. Mandatory for leptomeningeal mets.
10. A STIR sequence can be used to increase sensitivity to vertebral body mets. Can also consider using "fat" and "water" images to increase sensitivity.
11. Gate to as many heart beats as necessary to yield TR >2000 msec. Asymmetrical echoes can be used with flow compensation enabled. If flow compensation not available use even echo train: 20, 40, 60, 80 msec. NEX 1 may be sufficient.
12. If motion artifact is a problem, switch phase and frequency axes, increase NEX to 2, and use phase wrap correction option (NPW).
13. Single or multislice mode of variable flip angle scan depending upon the anatomic area to be covered. Can be useful for further characterizing tumor and possible hemorrhagic components (i.e., slow flow AVMs [see Chapter 11]). Useful to confirm findings on sagittal T2W scan. If the sagittal gated study is suboptimal, try partial flip angle scan with TR 300-500 and flip angle of 10° to 15°, NEX 2-4.
14. Postcontrast scans at same locations as precontrast scans. For tumor follow-up only precontrast and postcontrast T1W images may be needed. GdDTPA necessary for suspected hemangioblastoma and noncryptic AVMs.
15. See 11.
16. See 12.
17. Sagittal variable flip angle scan used to confirm the presence of plaques seen on T2W scan—sequence #2.
18. Single-slice mode just through plaques for confirmation.
19. Ungated T2W to sensitize images to fluid motion. Slices to be in same positions as in sequence #2. This allows accurate correlation with the T1W images for morphology.

Abbreviations: *A*, Axial; *AP*, Anteroposterior; *FA*, Flip angle; *FC*, Flow compensation; *FOV*, Field of view; *NEX*, No. of excitations; *NPW*, No. phase wrap; *oblq*, Oblique slice; *opt*, Optional; *PreSat*, Spatial saturation; *R/L*, Right/left; *S*, Sagittal; *S/I*, Superior/inferior; *TE*, Echo time; *TR*, Repetition.

A 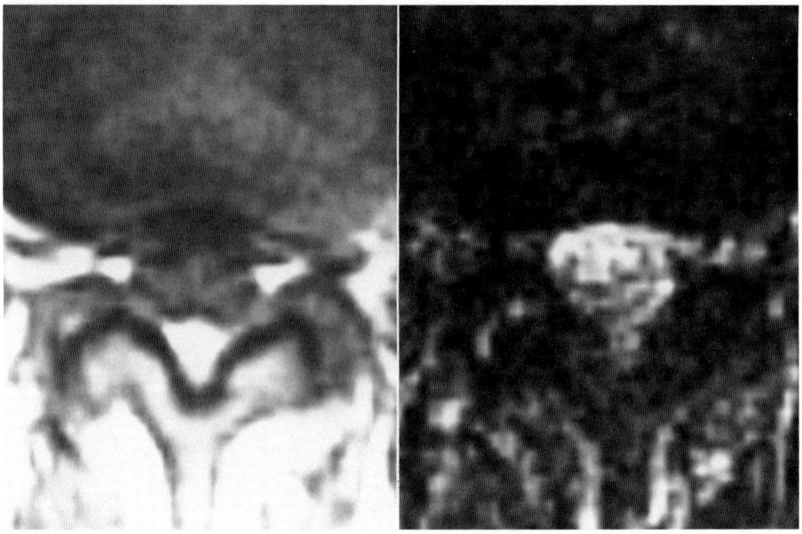 B

FIGURE 2-8. Comparison of axial T1W and T2W images of lumbar spine: **A,** Axial T1W image (SE 800/20) shows area of low signal in anterior half of spinal canal and area of higher signal in posterior half of spinal cord. Contrast between anulus, ligament, potential osteophyte, and CSF is poor. CSF is darker than normal because of prominent pulsation. **B,** Gated axial T2W image (SE 2200/80, NEX 1) clearly delineates dural sac and individual lumbar nerve roots at this lumbar level. Axial T2W lumbar spine scan is useful in delineating outline of dural sac or impingement thereon; this may not always be clear on T1W axial image.

within the normal cord, but this has not been of great diagnostic value. In spinal cord assessment, T1W images are sensitive to deviations from normal cord size and can provide important signal intensity information in detecting fat tissue or hemorrhage of varying ages. They can therefore play a diagnostic role in detecting abnormal signal indicative of tumors (teratoma, spinal lipomatosis), infection (epidural abscess), and hemorrhage (epidural hemorrhage).

An axiom that holds true for any MR scan is that an abnormality must be visualized in two planes or on two different pulse sequences to verify the finding as real and not artifactual. A host of physiologic and machine specific factors can cause artifacts. Confirmation of an abnormality, especially if it has unusual characteristics, is essential (Figure 2-9).

Oblique Planes

The two most useful oblique views are (1) the off-axial view, in which the slice is oriented parallel to the disc space and (2) the sagittal oblique, in which the slice is oriented perpendicular to the intervertebral foramina (Figures 2-10 and 2-11). Oblique T1W images are used primarily for the evaluation of disc disease. The off-axial views provide a more accurate assessment of the disc and its relationship to the dural sac and nerve roots, especially in the lumbar spine. Axial oblique views are useful with T2W images as well (see Figure 2-10). Sagittal oblique views of the foramina rely on fat tissue to provide contrast for disc and nerve roots (see Figure 2-11). For this reason T1W images are preferred for this scanning orientation. In selected patients, especially those with suspected lateral disc herniations, sagittal oblique views of the disc and foramina may help clarify the diagnosis. Many MR machines allow multiple different oblique angles to be obtained within a single pulse sequence. The off-axial oblique will likely become the standard for lumbar disc diagnosis (as it has with computed tomography [CT]), whereas the sagittal oblique will be used selectively in both the cervical and lumbar spine.

At present, only the variable flip angle/gra-

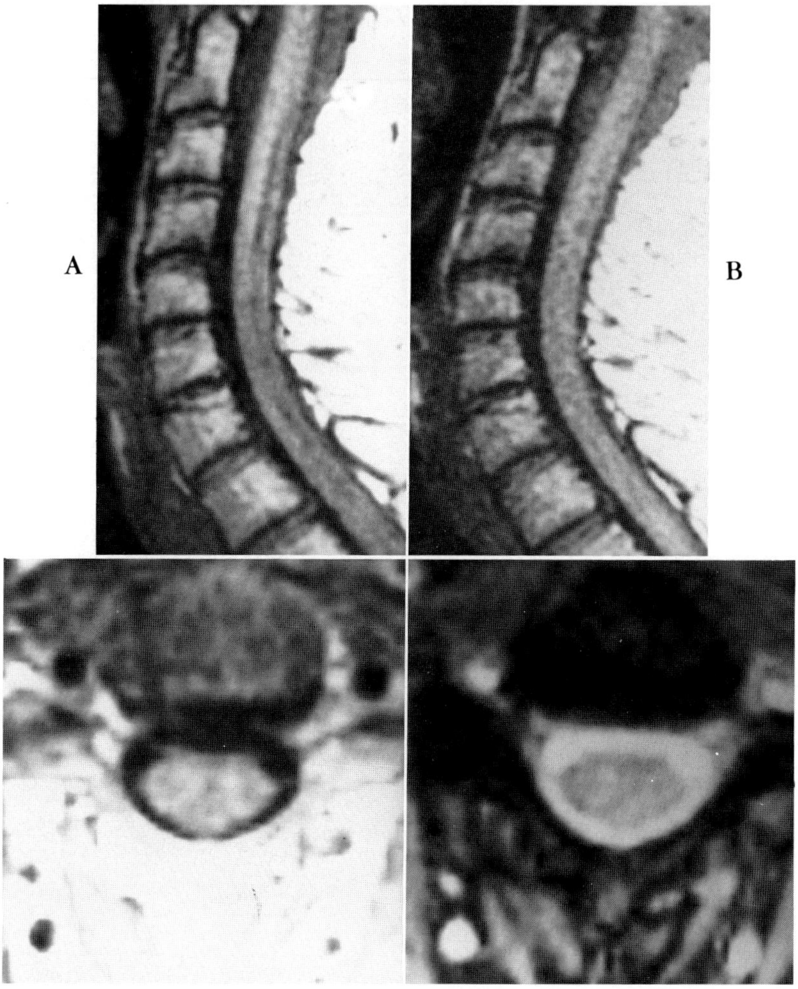

FIGURE 2-9. T1W artifact. Sagittal T1W scan of 58-year-old male presenting with myelopathy shows finding suggestive of lesion but confirmed as artifact by other views. **A,** Sagittal T1W scan (SE 800/20) shows long, linear, low signal intensity abnormality through midcervical cord that is not enlarged. Finding was not obvious artifact caused by either flow effect or Gibbs phenomenon. **B,** Repeat sagittal T1W scan (SE 800/20) performed after axial scans (**C** and **D**) shows finding on initial sagittal scan is artifact. Etiology of artifact not clear. **C,** Axial T1W scan performed immediately after initial sagittal scan (**A**) shows no low signal abnormality within cervical cord. **D,** Axial T2*W scan (GRASS 25/16, 7°) performed after axial T1W scan (**C**) also shows no abnormality within cord. A sagittal T1W scan was repeated (**B**) after these axial scans.

A

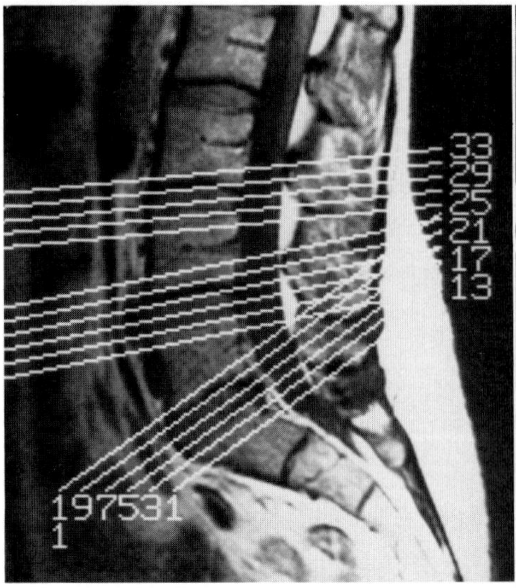

B

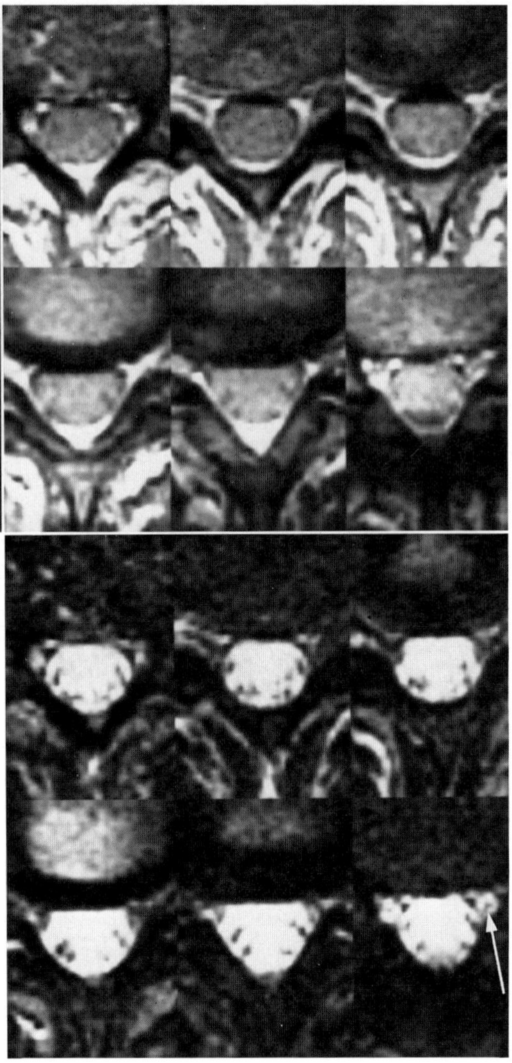

C

FIGURE 2-10. Oblique views obtained by orienting imaging plane parallel through disc space; a technique adopted with CT. **A,** Angle of plane can be varied individually for each disc space, and planes can be prescribed directly from sagittal image. **B** and **C,** Axial T2W (SE 2100/20, 80; NEX 1) were obtained at L_4-L_5 level with 3 mm sections starting at L_4 pedicle and ending at L_5 pedicle. **B,** Set of six first-echo images (TE 20) yields sufficient T1 information to delineate bone, fat, and dural sac. **C,** Set of second echo images (TE 80) provides T2W information showing nerve roots within dural sac and even within individual root sleeves *(arrow).*

dient echo pulse sequences allow practical isotropic three-dimensional imaging from which oblique planes can be generated.[11] Their contrast characteristics do not recommend them above T1W or T2W images in the lumbar spine. Three-dimensional imaging in the cervical spine has not matched two-dimensional single-slice or multislice results with variable flip angle scans, although this could be a future development.

Chemical Shift

Chemical shift occurs in images because fat and water protons precess at slightly different rates.[1,15] This is expressed as 3.5 parts per million because this varies with field strength. With the 2DFT method of image reconstruction, one axis defines a proton's position by its precessional frequency. Fat and water, despite being in the same voxel, have different frequencies and thus will be mapped differently. Fat signal is mismapped into adjacent pixels, resulting in dark lines where fat signal has shifted out of a voxel and bright lines where it has shifted into a voxel and added to water signal already present in it. This artifact appears whenever fat generates sufficient signal, which can occur even with T2W pulse sequences (Figure 2-12). The chemical shift artifact is more severe when stronger gradients are used, such as with thin slices; is easy to recognize because dark and bright lines are found in tandem and are perpendicular to

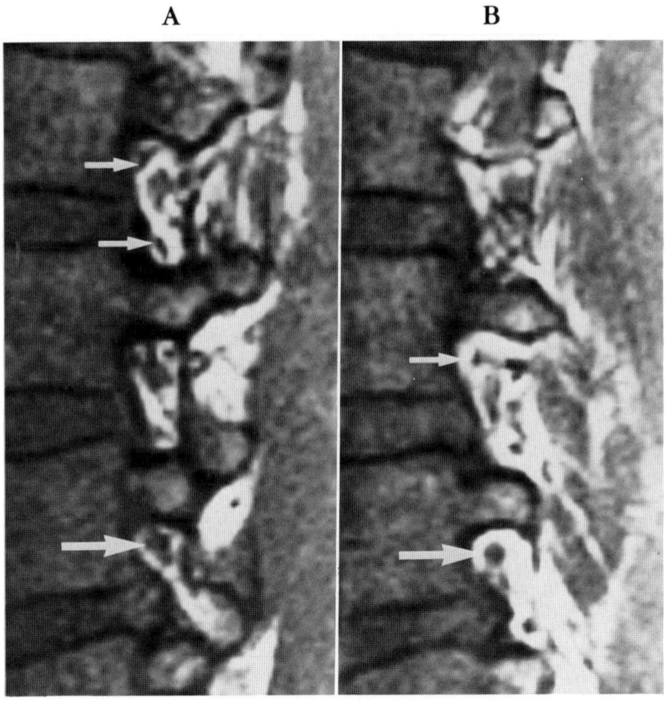

FIGURE 2-11. Sagittal oblique T1W sequence (SE 800/20) of lumbar spine. Images were obtained perpendicular to long axis of the foramen with **A** more medial than **B.** Note excellent delineation of nerve root *(large arrows)* afforded by perineural fat. Other multiple small round areas of intermediate signal within fat represent vessels, primarily veins (*small arrows*). Lowest disc (L_4-L_5) shows mild bulging into foramen without compression of L_4 nerve root.

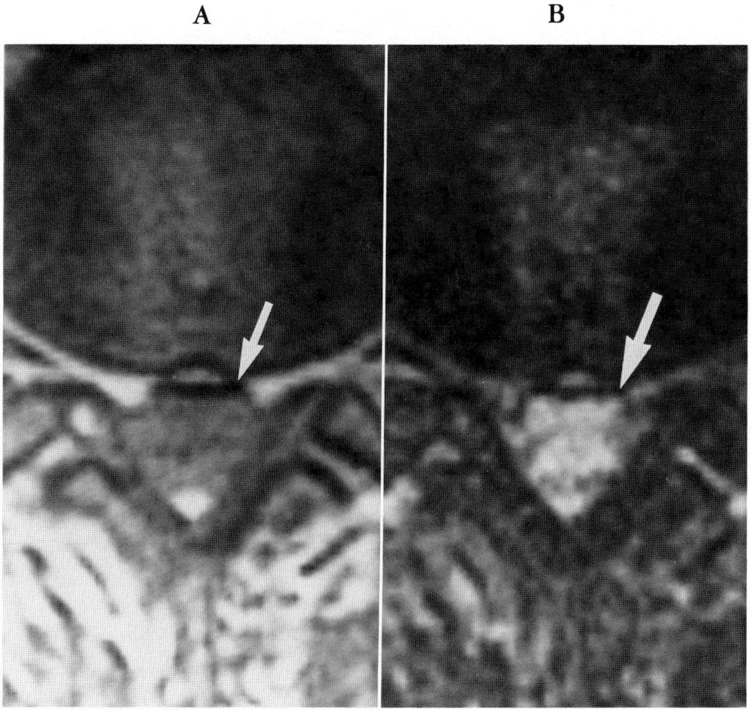

FIGURE 2-12. Axial view of lumbar spine shows chemical shift effect even on long TR, long TE scans (gated, TR 2300, TE 20 [A] and 80 [B]). Note thin black line on first (**A,** *arrow*) and second (**B,** *arrow*) echo images between canal and black line representing posterior vertebral cortical margin. Black line is a chemical shift artifact because fat signal in this area is mismapped anteriorly. Black line is not dura. Signal between the two black lines could be mistaken for small disc bulge.

the frequency axis; and may cause some diagnostic difficulty. One problem area can be thoracic disc disease (see Chapter 10); in the lumbar area on the axial view this phenomenon may simulate a small central disc bulge or herniation (see Figure 2-12).

Fat and Water Suppression

Numerous techniques to generate images that represent only water protons or only fat protons[2,15] vary from image subtraction to selective excitation techniques. The end-point desired is an image composed of only water or only fat protons (Figure 2-13). This may be useful in special circumstances, such as when differentiation of the amount of water and fat signal in marrow has diagnostic utility. On water-only images, the bone detail of the vertebrae is better visualized than with conventional T1W images because the chemical shift artifact is eliminated.

MR Contrast Medium

T1W images are the key in the use of MR contrast agents that shorten the T1 relaxation time of tissue. The contrast medium that is currently available and most likely will have the greatest initial impact in the spine is Gadopentate Dimeglumine (GdDTPA),[17,18] a gadolinium ion chelate that is strongly paramagnetic and has the ability to shorten the T1 relaxation time of the hydrogen proton, even in low concentrations. Its effects are best visualized on T1W images where contrast enhancement is visualized as marked increases in signal intensity of tissue. The contrast agent is injected intravenously at a dose of 0.1 millimole/kg (.2 ml/kg) up to a maximum dose of 20 ml. The injection rate should not exceed 10 ml/minute. Scanning can begin approximately five minutes after injection to allow time for equilibration. Although there are sequential changes in signal intensity of the contrast enhancement over time, a relatively long interval of time (1 hour) is available for

A, B

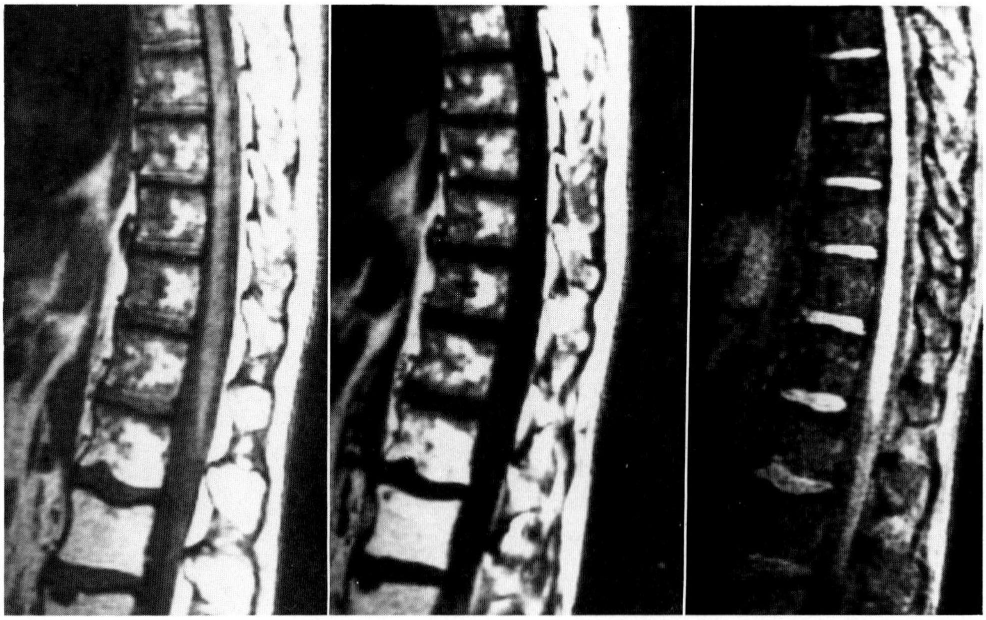

C

FIGURE 2-13. **A,** T1W sagittal image (800/20) of thoracolumbar region compared with **B,** fat-only image (SE 800/20) and **C,** water-only image (SE 800/20). Note that on fat-only image, cord composed of water protons is not visualized. Sphingolipids are not detectable. Fat signal from marrow is pjrominent because of previous radiotherapy, which increases marrow fat content. Vertebral body heterogeneity results from previous metastatic disease. Water-only image highlights cord, cauda equina, and disc spaces. Significant signal is seen in marrow on water images.

scanning while the enhancement effect is still present.

The use of GdDTPA clinically parallels the use of intravenous iodinated contrast medium with CT. GdDTPA does not normally cross the blood-brain barrier but does so when the barrier has abnormal permeability. It is a marker in the CNS for an abnormal blood-brain barrier and therefore has major application in the detection and follow-up of intramedullary spinal cord tumors. Other indications are hemangioblastomas and leptomeningeal carcinomatosis (see Chapter 8). Contrast enhancement effect is prominent enough that venous structures show enhancement. This enhancement can represent a blood pool effect, which is applicable for use in the detection of spinal cord arteriovenous malformations (AVMs) (noncryptic) (see Chapter 11). Arterial structures do not normally exhibit enhancement because of the rapidity of blood flow and its attendant flow effects causing signal loss. Tissues that do not have a blood-brain barrier will show enhancement compared to neural tissue; this is the basis for use in diagnosing extramedullary tumors such as meningiomas and neurinomas (see Chapter 8). Avascular tissue will not show enhancement compared to vascularized tissue without a blood-brain barrier. GdDTPA can be used to differentiate avascular disc material from postoperative fibrosis (see Chapter 10). Although no doubt there will be ultimately a wide variety of MR contrast agents available, those that cross the blood-brain and blood-meningeal barriers will have major application in spine imaging.

CSF Flow on T1W Images

CSF flow effects are prominent on T2W images but can also be seen on T1W images. A common CSF flow effect is the in-flow phenomenon where unsaturated protons flow into an imaging slice, resulting in higher signal; the effect is seen on end-slices and is usually easily recognized (Figure 2-14). The area of interest, therefore, should not be in an end-slice position. CSF pulsation decreases CSF signal intensity on T1W images even though it is already normally low (see Figure 2-33). The explanation is the same as for T2W images (see Chapter 1). The lower signal can make distinction between CSF, ligament, osteophyte, and anulus difficult (see Figure 2-8). A T2W image may be necessary to clarify T1W image findings.

A

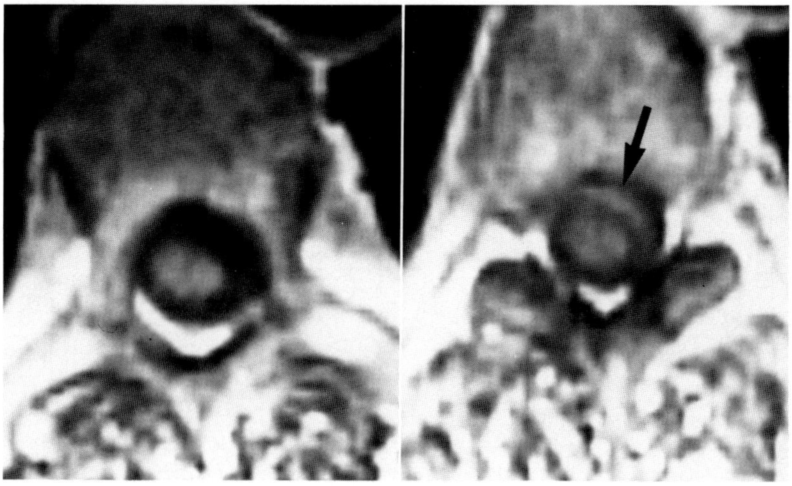

B

FIGURE 2-14. Important phenomenon caused by CSF pulsation is that of in-flow of unsaturated protons into the end-slice of an imaging volume. In-flow is seen as area of increased signal intensity. In the spine, this may be seen as area of increased signal where low signal would be expected, as in subarachnoid space *(arrow)*. On these two T1W images (SE 1000/20), **B,** end slice and **A,** 2 cm from end slice, the semicircular area of increased signal *(arrow)* represents in-flow of unsaturated protons and should not be mistaken for pathologic lesion such as an epidural mass. *Continued.*

C 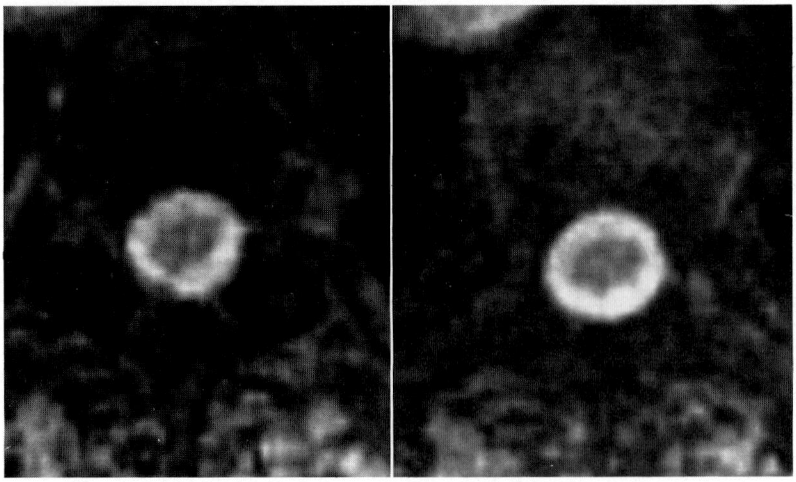 D

FIGURE 2-14, cont'd. **C** and **D**, Companion set of partial flip angle, gradient refocused images at same levels illustrate normal cord and normal subarachnoid space in high thoracic region.

INVERSION-RECOVERY PULSE SEQUENCES

Inversion-recovery pulse sequences have application in the spine primarily as techniques for lipid suppression to detect bone lesions. For spine imaging these sequences usually have short inversion times, thus the acronym, *STIR* (short inversion time, inversion recovery).[9] The inversion time (TI) is specifically selected to nullify fat signal using the following relationship[9]:

$$TI_{(null)}\ T1 * 1n2$$

In addition, the polarity in STIR images is usually reversed so that lipid is displayed as black. STIR images may be helpful in investigating vertebral body disease, such as metastases (Figure 2-15), and the results are similar to T2W images where fat is low signal and lesions are of high signal but higher sensitivity may be possible. STIR images may have some scanning time advantage and better fat suppression compared to routine spin-echo (SE). Specific water and fat suppression techniques using selective saturation of each signal can yield similar results with similar scanning times (see metastatic section of Chapter 8). The extent to which these techniques are duplicative or complementary still has to be determined by clinical experience.

T2W IMAGES

T2W images reflect differences between tissue transverse relaxation times, T2, and are used primarily because of their sensitivity to pathologic tissue within the cord and spine. T2W images provide superior sensitivity to pathologic tissue at the expense of a lower SNR. In the brain, conventional T2W images fall in the category of long TR, long TE (TR 2000 to 2500 msec, TE 70 to 80 msec), but in the spine a conventional SE technique is plagued by motion artifacts, limiting its effectiveness (Figure 2-16). The reason for the motion artifacts is the presence of pulsatile CSF, which causes two artifacts with the 2DFT method of image reconstruction: CSF signal loss and phase shift images dispersed in the phase-encoding direction. Motion artifacts degrade image quality sufficiently so that motion compensating techniques need to be employed to obtain artifact-free T2W images of the spine. See Chapter 1 for a detailed discussion of motion artifacts.

Some type of motion compensation method is necessary to obtain an artifact-free T2W image of the spine,[12,13] particularly where CSF pulsation has the greatest amplitude; i.e., the cervical and thoracic spine. It may even be useful in the lumbar spine because CSF pulsation in some

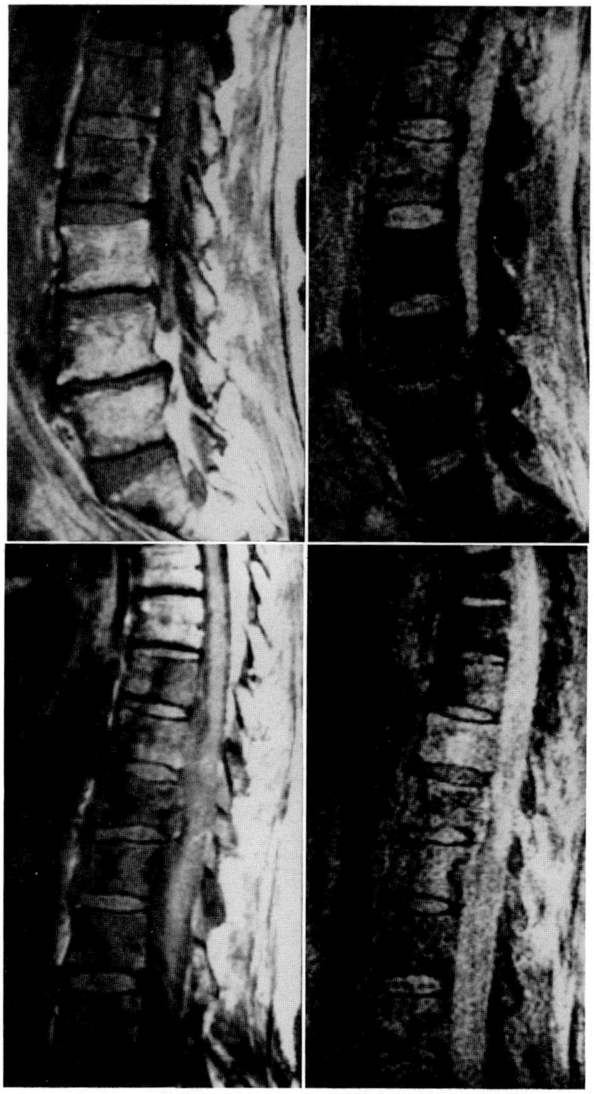

FIGURE 2-15. **A** and **C**, Comparison of T1W scans (SE 800/20) with **B** and **D**, STIR scans (IR 1400/40, TI 100) in patient with metastatic breast carcinoma. **A**, Lumbar spine sagittal T1W scan shows abnormal low signal intensity of L_1 and L_2 indicative of metastatic disease. **B**, On STIR image these two vertebrae show increased signal in L_1 and L_2 compared to more normal marrow signal seen in L_3-L_5. **C**, In thoracic spine, vertebral body signal intensity is quite inhomogenous on T1W scan. Many vertebrae show abnormal low signal intensity. Upper vertebrae show increased signal intensity because of marrow replacement by fat due to radiation therapy. **D**, STIR image shows abnormal high signal in areas corresponding to low signal on T1W image (**C**). Abnormal soft tissue within spinal canal is better appreciated on T1W scan, **C**, compared to STIR image, **D**. STIR images show increased contrast between neoplastic tissue and normal marrow in vertebrae but are of lower SNR. Contents of spinal canal are better appreciated on T1W scan in part because STIR sequence is susceptible to flow effects that are more prominent when CSF is of high signal.

patients can be quite prominent in this region.[14] When seeking subtle lesions within the cord, artifact-free T2W images are necessary to visualize areas of abnormal increased signal intensity within the cord, particularly in disease processes such as multiple sclerosis, transverse myelitis, small AVMs, subtle tumors, and infections (Figure 2-17). Whenever a disease process does not cause a detectable increase in cord diameter, an artifact-free T2W image will be crucial for its detection. Both sagittal and axial views will be needed to confirm such a lesion. Motion compensation techniques allow CSF to be displayed as uniform high signal, producing high contrast that increases the conspicuity of the cord and lesions within it (see Figure 2-17). Motion compensation techniques are a prerequisite for accurate diagnosis of a wide variety of diseases.

In addition to detecting cord lesions, motion-compensated T2W images provide high cord-CSF contrast to highlight extradural lesions such as disc disease. Because contrast between anulus, ligament, and CSF may be poor on T1W images, images with high signal CSF are desirable to provide better contrast. This type of image can be obtained with different techniques and does not require true T2 weighting. Gated or flow-compensated SE sequences in the lum-

A, B

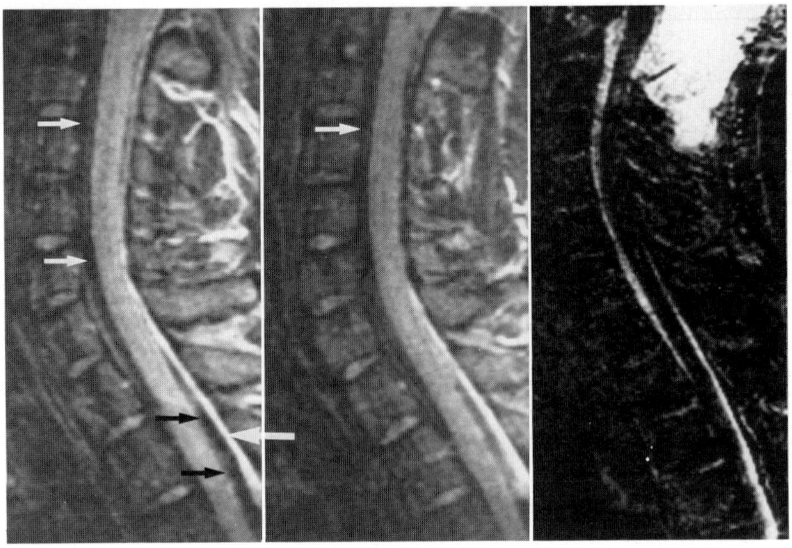

C

FIGURE 2-16. Ungated T2W images (SE 2000/80) of adjacent midline slices **A** and **B** show two major artifacts caused by CSF pulsation: signal-loss at sites of CSF motion and phase-shift images (ghosts) projected in phase-encoding axis—anterior to posterior. Areas of signal-loss result in signal "voids" seen anterior to cervical cord extending from C_2 to C_7 *(small white arrows)* and posterior to cord extending from T_1 to T_3 *(black arrows)*. Note area of increased signal dorsal to cord starting at C_6 and extending to T_3 in posterior spinal canal. High signal emanates from relatively static CSF in this location *(large white arrow)*. Unless some type of motion compensation technique is employed, these areas of normal CSF pulsation will result in artifacts. Using DFA technique (see Chapter 1), sites of pulsatile CSF can be mapped and displayed as high signal. **C,** In normal patient, DFA technique delineates moving CSF in same areas where signal voids are visualized on non-gated study (**A** and **B**).

A, B

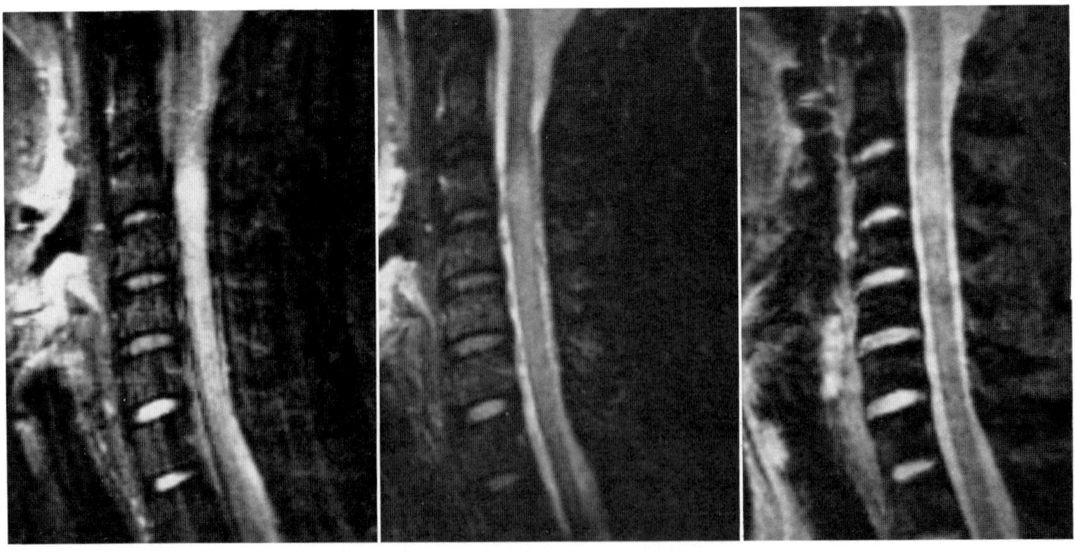

C

FIGURE 2-17. Comparison of sagittal scans. **A,** Non-gated (SE 2000/80), **B,** CSF gated (SE 1900/80), and **C,** variable flip angle/gradient echo scans (GRASS 400/15, 15°) in multiple sclerosis patient who has plaque at C_3 level in cervical cord. Plaque can be visualized on all scans, but gated scan, **B,** has less signal inhomogeneity in the cord and thus better lesion delineation. (From Enzmann DR, Rubin JB. Radiology 1988: 166:467. With permission.)

A, B

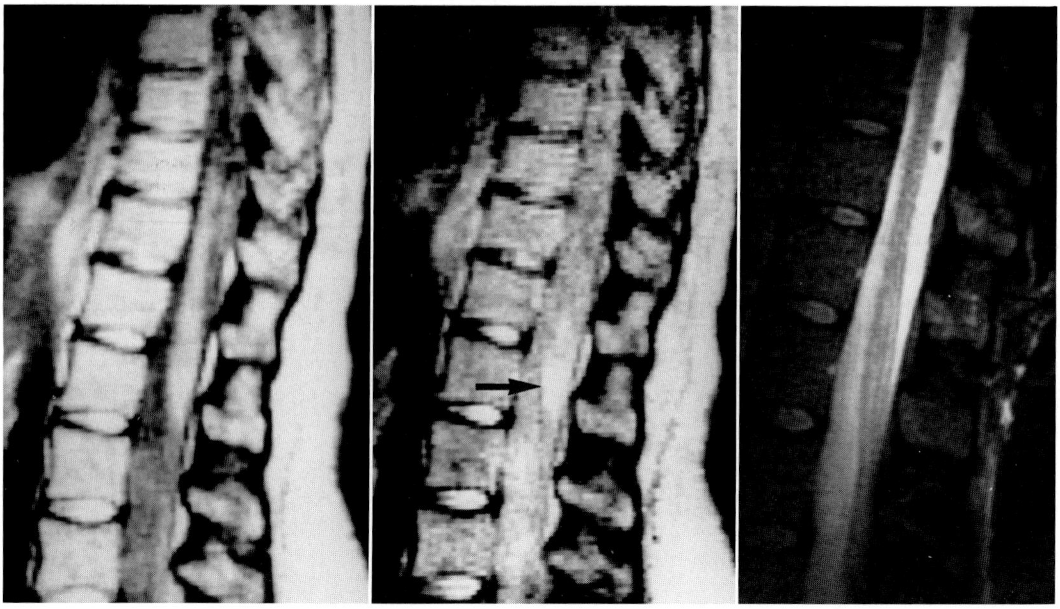

C

FIGURE 2-18. Area where high signal from CSF can be expected because of differential motion is below conus and within cauda equina. This is normal finding and should not be mistaken for a pathologic condition. Sagittal T2W (SE 1500/40, 80) obtained on a midfield machine (.5T) shows high signal near conus on second echo (TE 80) image (*arrow*, B). **A,** First echo image (TE 40) shows conus of normal size. **B,** High signal on T2W second echo *(arrow)* was secondary to relative lack of motion of CSF within cauda vs. CSF around it—moving CSF around it was of lower signal intensity. **C,** Gated T2W scan (SE 2100/100) eliminated differential motion and difference in signal intensity. (From Enzmann DR, Rubin JB, DeLaPaz R, et al. Radiology 1986; 161:773. With permission.)

bar region provide high CSF signal and excellent definition of individual lumbar and sacral nerves in sagittal and axial views. These same sequences are effective in sagittal cervical and thoracic imaging areas in which high signal CSF can be achieved with variable flip angle/gradient echo scans.[5] In cervical and thoracic axial imaging, variable flip angle scans are more successful in generating high signal CSF[5,6] than is gating and flow compensation (see Figures 2-19 and 2-20).

CSF Motion

Signal-loss and phase shift artifacts caused by CSF pulsation can result in false positive and false negative imaging studies.[7] Once understood, however, the effect of CSF motion can be used to diagnostic advantage. Although signal-loss and phase shift images are usually seen in combination, there are times when signal-loss is more noticeable and phase shift images can be difficult to detect. This occurs especially when fluid motion is complex and not primarily of a cranio-caudal pulsatile nature. Moving CSF in conventional SE imaging causes a signal-loss. Thus CSF that is identical in every way except for the degree of motion will have different signal intensities on SE imaging if no motion compensation techniques are employed (Figure 2-18). Stationary CSF will have a higher signal intensity compared to moving CSF even if that motion is minimal[7] (see Figure 2-18). Remembering this will prevent false positive interpretations. The lack of normal areas of signal loss in the spinal canal can also be important because it may signify some type of block that dampens CSF pulsations.

As new pulse sequences are introduced, many will have motion compensation schemes integral to them, and it is important for the operator to know exactly what motion is being compensated. There are times when it is useful to disable the motion compensating techniques to uncover motion effects for their diagnostic value (see Chapter 12, Syrinx).

A 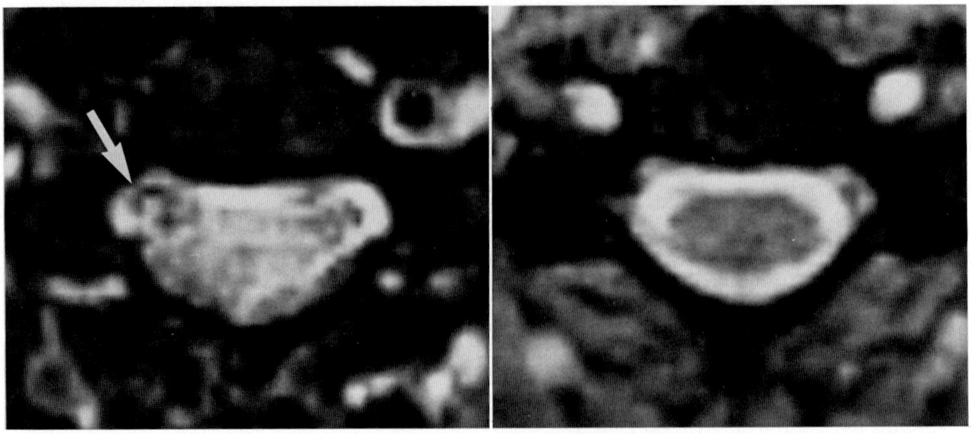 B

FIGURE 2-19. Comparison of axial gated T2W (SE 2100/80) image with axial variable flip angle/gradient echo scan (GRASS 25/12) using low flip angle of 7°. **A,** Gated image exhibits inhomogeneous high signal intensity in CSF surrounding cord. Several areas of signal loss are still present, especially in anterolateral recesses where turbulent flow is present around nerve roots *(arrow)*. Delineation of cord and other structures is suboptimal. **B,** Variable flip angle scan using very low flip angle makes it very insensitive to CSF motion. Short TR allows a steady state to occur resulting in higher and uniform high signal CSF within entire subarachnoid space, even though pulsation amplitude differs markedly between anterior and posterior locations. Partial flip angle scan provides fast and easy way to duplicate findings seen with positive contrast CT spine scans.

CSF MOTION COMPENSATION

CSF Gating (Peripheral Trigger)

One method to compensate for CSF pulsation is that of cardiac gating, or more accurately, peripheral gating, because data acquisition is synchronized to the peripheral pulse[13] (see Chapter 1). This method is simple to employ and effective in minimizing or eliminating ghost artifacts and areas of signal loss in sagittal images of the cervical and thoracic spine (see Figure 2-17). The technique can be employed as either a single-slice or a multislice sequence. Although the gating technique is effective in the sagittal view it is more limited in its application to axial imaging (Figure 2-19). In the axial view, CSF gating eliminates ghost artifacts but does not consistently eliminate areas of signal loss caused by turbulence-induced intravoxel dephasing (see Figure 2-19). Therefore homogeneous high signal CSF can be achieved consistently in the sagittal view but only inconsistently in the axial view. In a multislice mode in the axial view, only a few slices timed in diastole achieve homogeneous high signal CSF. Technical details of this difference between sagittal and axial imaging are discussed in Chapter 1.

Although CSF gating yields similar results as flow compensating gradients, gating has an advantage of correcting for motion unsharpness, which can be a problem with transmitted aortic pulsations in the neck. When multislice gating is performed and synchronization is not achieved for all slices (as may happen with gating to every other or every third beat to gain T2 weighting), it can be inferior to flow compensating gradients when the heart rate fluctuates during this period. A newer method of gating that provides for synchronization of each slice to every beat avoids this problem.

In the cervical region the combination of gating, flow compensation (at least first order), and variable bandwidth option yields excellent results for sagittal T2W images. In the thoracic spine, because of mismapped cardiac signal, gating in combination with phase/frequency axis switching and a no phase wrap option yields good results for sagittal T2W images. Many of the motion compensation, SNR enhancement, and aliasing correction techniques cannot be used simultaneously. Trade-offs need to be made and these may be machine specific. One should be familiar with the trade-offs to optimize a T2W pulse sequence for SNR and minimal artifact.

Echo Train

The choice of echoes with or without CSF gating is an important variable. Asymmetric echoes with a relatively long interval between echoes is inferior to a symmetric echo train (such as 20, 40, 60, and 80 msec vs. a 20, 80 msec asymmetric pair).[13] Again, details are described in the CSF flow section of Chapter 1. In short, CSF gating technique converts CSF pulsatile flow to constant velocity flow, which in turn exhibits the phenomenon of even echo rephasing.[13] Even echo rephasing is a characteristic of constant velocity flow and can be well visualized in spine images (see Figure 1-62). The practical aspect is that the most homogeneous depiction of high signal CSF and the most accurate measurement for cord size or extradural defect size is seen on even echoes. Odd echoes may show loss of signal at CSF boundaries that can accentuate extradural deformities. The addition of flow compensating gradients eliminates the need to favor even echo trains.

Motion Compensating Gradients (Gradient moment nulling)

Newer pulse sequences have specific motion compensating gradients in various axes to correct for motion in those axes. In general, the slice-select gradient and the read-out gradient are stronger than the phase-encoding gradient; the former two usually require specific compensating gradients, whereas the latter does not. Motion compensation can be for first order (constant velocity), second order (acceleration), and third order (jerk or pulsatility) motion characteristics. The desired effect of compensating gradient wave forms is such that any moving proton experiencing these gradients will result in a net phase shift of zero compared to stationary protons.

Pulse sequences can incorporate compensating gradients for all three orders of motion effects but because these complex gradient wave forms take time to generate, compensating for the higher orders of motion prolongs TE and limits the number of interleavable slices. From a practical point of view, first order motion compensation appears sufficient for spine imaging, which can be achieved by a relatively simple gradient wave form in the ratio of 1:-2:1 that balances the phase of both stationary protons and those moving at constant velocity (see diagram in Chapter 1). Although CSF clearly does not move at a constant velocity, first order motion compensation is valid enough when one considers only the very short time interval between the slice-select gradient and the read-out gradient. To the extent that this may not be true in some situations, the less successful this simple motion compensation technique will be.

Motion-compensated pulse sequences achieve good results in both sagittal and axial views. Nevertheless, the results in the axial projection, although better than gating alone, are still inconsistent and not always optimal (Figure 2-20). They do not solve the problem of uniform high signal CSF in axial cervical and thoracic images. This solution seems to lie with variable flip angle scans.

In the sagittal view, motion compensating gradients appear capable of approaching the image quality produced by CSF gating with even echo rephasing. An advantage of gradient motion compensation is that it does not require an external device, as does gating. In some patients, the addition of gating to gradient flow compensation adds little to image quality (Figure 2-21). In other patients the combination of flow compensation and gating improves the SNR (Figure 2-22). In a few patients, neither flow compensation nor gating alone are as effective as their combination (Figure 2-23). The combination of CSF gating and gradient compensation appears to yield more consistent and better results, which is not surprising because first order motion compensation assumes constant velocity flow and CSF gating essentially converts pulsatile flow into constant velocity flow. The addition of gating places no further restrictions on TE and slice number. Gating also reduces motion unsharpness; something not achieved by gradient flow compensation alone.

Phase-Encoding Axis

As previously mentioned, one of the most disturbing effects of motion is the ghost artifacts generated by the 2DFT method of image reconstruction. Ghosts are projected in the phase-encoding direction, may arise from pulsating CSF on T2W images, or may arise from the oropharynx, larynx, heart, or anterior abdominal wall on either T1W or T2W images. When ghost artifacts overlie an area of interest, one simple method for dealing with them is to change the

A 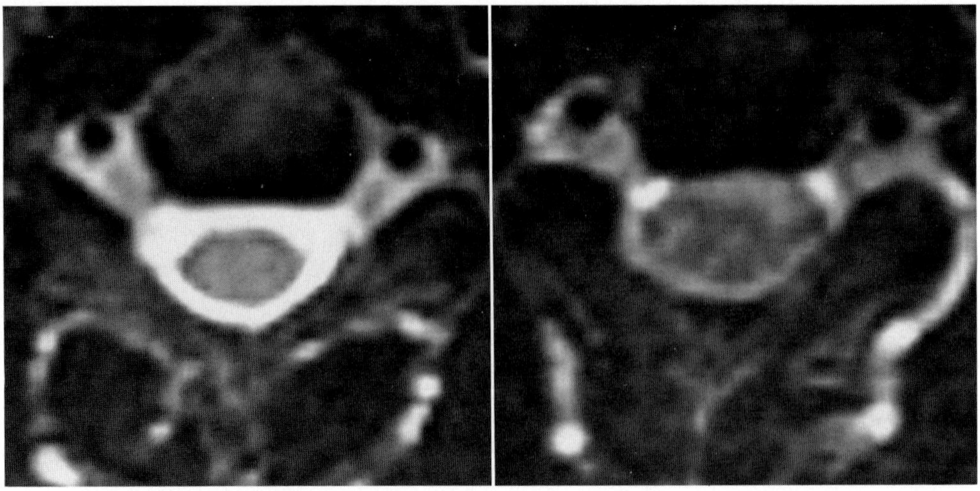 B

FIGURE 2-20. Axial T2W images using combination of CSF gating and flow compensation by gradient moment nulling method (SE 2100/80). **A,** Some levels achieve very high quality, high contrast images of cervical cord and subarachnoid space. **B,** Other levels in this multislice technique, lose signal in subarachnoid space, resulting in poor cord delineation and inaccurate assessment of subarachnoid space. Combination of gating and flow compensation in axial view, therefore, is inferior to variable flip angle/gradient echo scans for consistently achieving high signal CSF and high CSF-cord contrast.

A 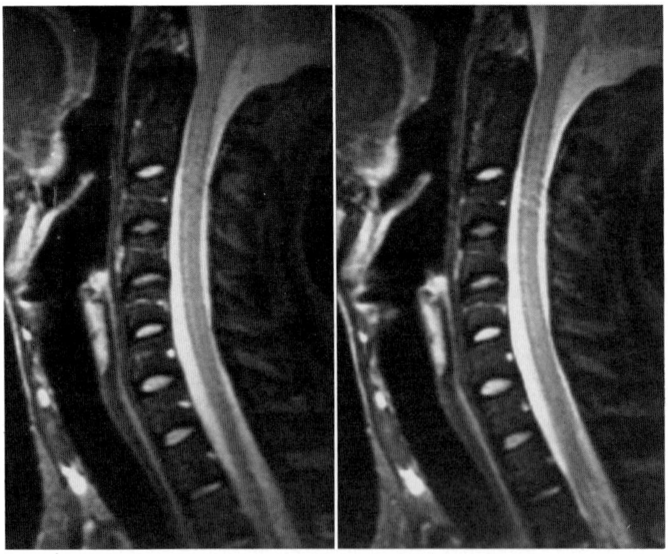 B

FIGURE 2-21. Using anterior surface coil, T2W sagittal (SE 2100/80) scans were generated using **A,** gradient moment nulling technique and **B,** combination of gradient moment nulling plus peripheral gating. Both techniques produced "lateral myelographic" image consisting of high signal CSF and a lower signal cord. Results are comparable.

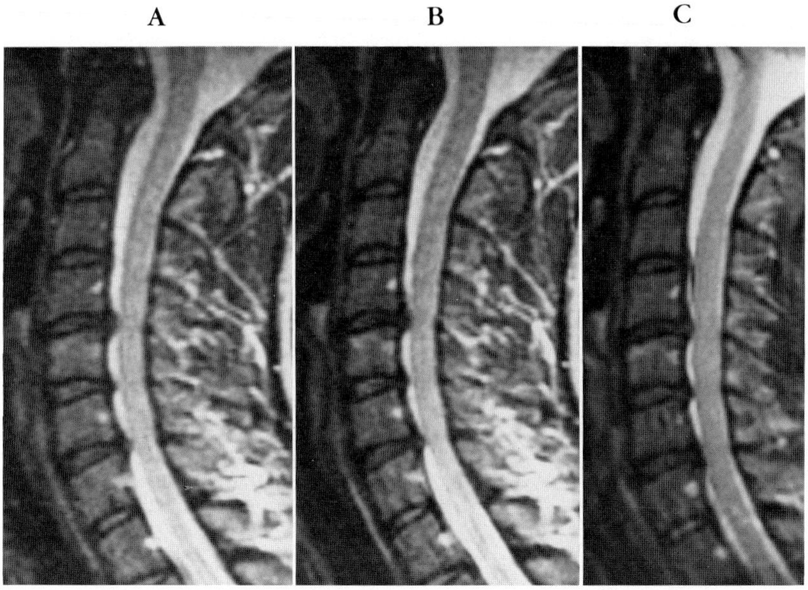

FIGURE 2-22. Series of T2W scans obtained with **A**, gating alone (SE 1900/80), **B**, first order gradient flow compensation alone (SE 2000/80), and **C**, combination of gating and flow compensation (SE 1900/80). All methods were effective in generating artifact-free T2W sagittal images but combination image had higher SNR.

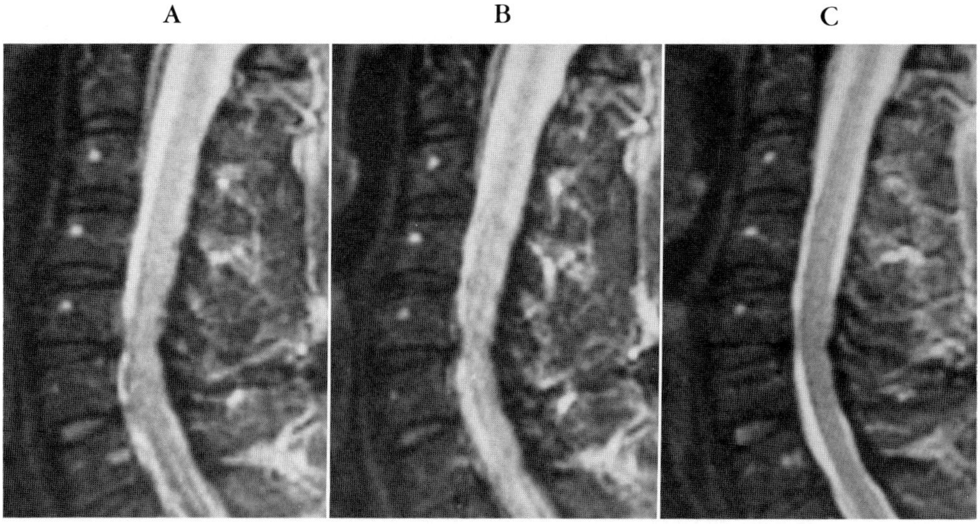

FIGURE 2-23. Series of sagittal T2W images of cervical spine obtained using **A**, gating alone (SE 2300/80), **B**, first order gradient moment nulling alone (SE 2400/80), and **C**, combination of gating and gradient flow compensation (SE 2300/80). CSF gating alone in some patients and flow compensation alone in other patients may be sufficient to provide diagnostic images but both methods may fail individually. Highest success rate is obtained with combination of peripheral gating and flow compensation.

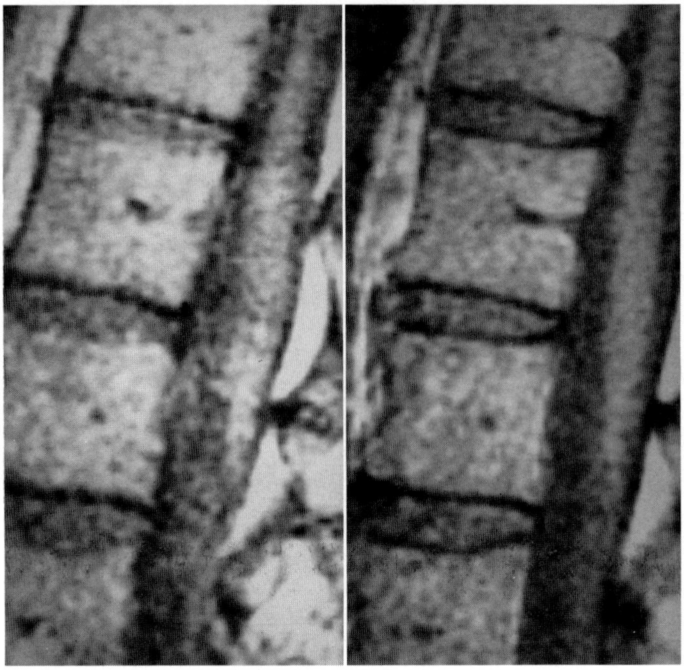

FIGURE 2-24. Sagittal T1W images (SE 800/20) show potential value of switching phase-encoding axis from **A,** perpendicular to spinal cord, to **B,** parallel to spinal cord. **A,** "Ghost" artifact from abdominal motion obscures conus medullaris. When phase axis is switched "ghost" shift artifacts are projected in a superior-inferior direction, **B** and the conus is better visualized. Note relative increase in signal intensity of CSF in **B** compared to **A,** which is another manifestation of this same phenomenon.

phase-encoding direction so to redirect the "ghosts" into the other axis, thus clearing up the area of interest.

Although other areas may be obscured, selected areas of interest can be cleaned up with this method (Figure 2-24). This is a useful technique to remember, but it is not without diagnostic side effects. In swapping the phase-encoding axis and the frequency encoding axis, one also changes the direction of the chemical shift artifact caused by fat in bone marrow (Figures 2-25 and 2-26). This can be a problem in the thoracic spine, because the shift in bone marrow fat signal can obscure subtle disc herniations[3] (see Chapter 10). Although the problem is less critical in the cervical region, the posterior bony margin of these vertebrae can be obscured, making disc herniations more difficult to delineate on the sagittal view. The shift of the bone marrow fat signal has the additional effect of falsely narrowing the size of the anterior subarachnoid space.

Moving CSF signal is mismapped in the phase-encoding direction and this is evident even on T1W images (see Figure 2-26). When the phase-encoding direction is perpendicular to the cervical or thoracic spinal canal it has the effect of decreasing CSF signal, thus increasing CSF-cord contrast. With this orientation, CSF moves parallel to the frequency encoding axis resulting in greater phase shifts. When the frequency encoding direction is switched perpendicular to the cervical or thoracic cord, the quantity of mismapped CSF signal is less because there is little motion along its axis. The signal that is mismapped is superimposed back on the spinal canal (the phase direction) in another location, resulting in lower cord-CSF contrast (see Figure 2-26). With variable flip angle scans, switching the phase and frequency axes may minimize the need for flow compensation (Figure 2-27).

If the area of interest is the status of the vertebral body end-plates, the desired effects would

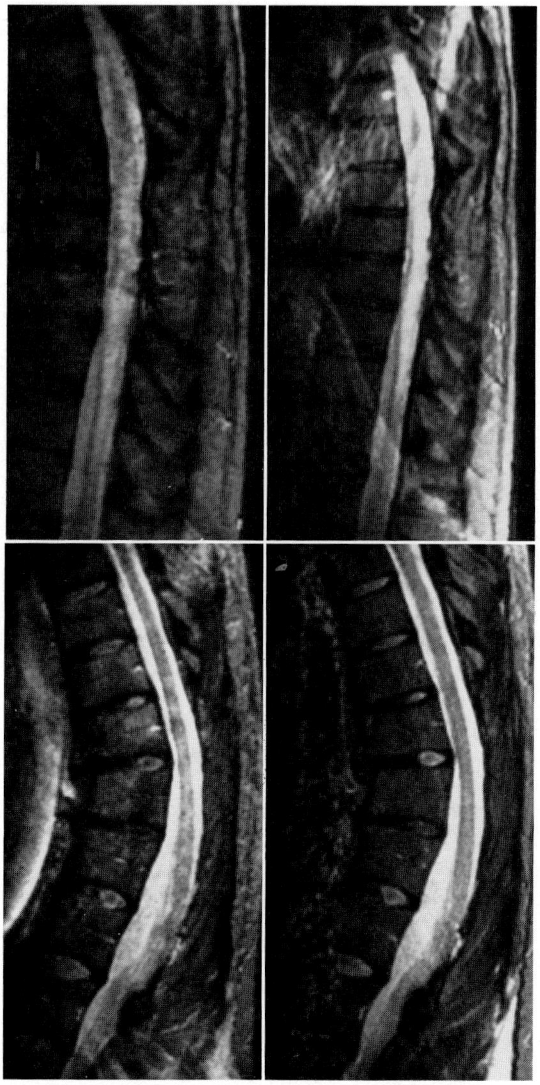

FIGURE 2-25. Comparison of effects of switching phase and frequency encoding axes on a T2W sequence (gated SE 2200/80) in the thorax. **A,** When the phase-encoding axis is oriented anteroposteriorly, it causes mismapped signal from cardiac motion to be superimposed on midthoracic spinal cord, obscuring anatomic detail. **B,** Midthoracic cord region is better visualized when phase-encoding axis is switched to superior-inferior orientation, leaving midthoracic cord region free of artifact. Penalty, however, is "phase wrap" from adjacent tissue above and below area of interest that obscures superior and inferior portion of image. There are techniques available for reducing phase wrap artifact but they may not be implementable when both gating and gradient flow compensation techniques are used simultaneously to reduce CSF flow artifact. On T1W sequences this is usually not a problem because flow compensation and cardiac gating are not used. In another patient an alternative approach was used. **C,** T2W image using CSF gating plus gradient flow compensation (SE 2100/80; NEX 1) and phase-encoding axis perpendicular to the spine. Image is average quality but cord signal is inhomogeneous because of mismapped signal from the heart. **D,** Artifact reduced by using only CSF gating (SE 2100/80), but switching phase direction parallel to spine and using no phase wrap option that necessitated use of NEX 2. Technique allowed accurate assessment of cord signal intensity that was being investigated for subtle abnormalities.

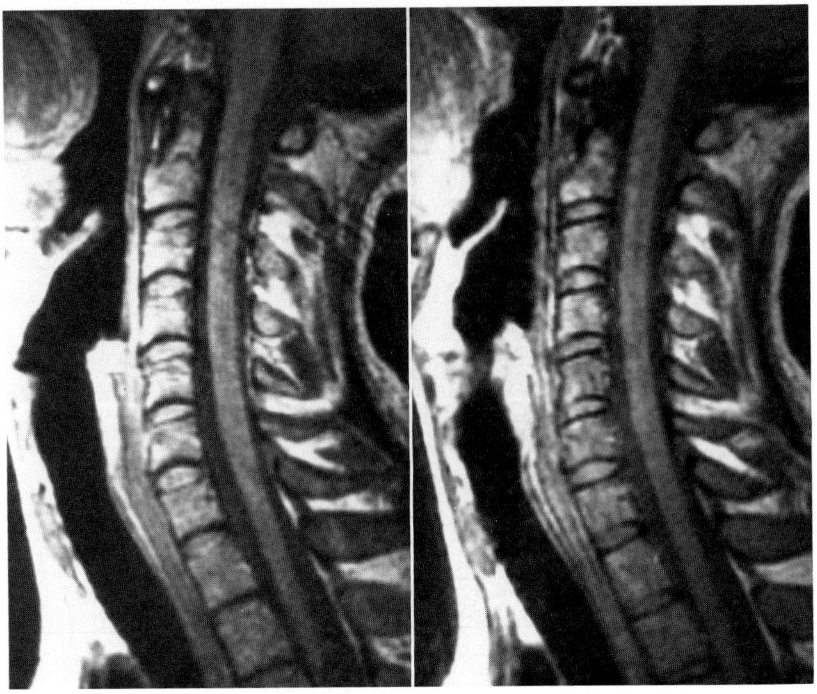

FIGURE 2-26. Lateral T1W images (SE 800/20) of cervical spine using anterior neck coil. Subtle but definite differences between images obtained with phase-encoding axis **A,** in anteroposterior compared to **B,** superior-inferior direction. **A,** Chemical shift artifact, i.e., mismapping of marrow fat signal results in obscuration of the superior end-plate of each vertebral body. There is good contrast between cord and CSF in anterior subarachnoid space because mismapped signal from CSF is spread out in an AP direction. Note also well-delineated posterior margin of the vertebral body. **B,** When phase-encoding axis is switched to superior-inferior, chemical shift artifact is directed anteroposteriorly, resulting in obscuration of posterior cortical margin of the vertebral body. Superior and inferior bony end-plates are well seen. With this axis orientation, contrast between cord and CSF decreases in anterior subarachnoid space. CSF motion, therefore, causes reduced signal from CSF even on T1W images. Because CSF signal intensity is low it is not readily seen as ghost artifact, as it is on T2W images where signal is high. Amount of CSF moving in relationship to perpendicular frequency encoding axis is small and therefore less signal is mismapped, resulting in higher signal from CSF space, which reduces cord-CSF contrast. In addition, CSF signal that is mismapped will be superimposed back on the spinal canal and cord because of superior-inferior orientation of the phase-encoding axis. Because it is often useful to switch phase and frequency encoding axes it is important to recognize the effects of this technique.

be just the opposite. Bony end-plates are seen best with the phase-encoding direction parallel to the cord because fat signal is displaced posteriorly (the frequency axis), allowing good depiction of the end-plates. With the phase-encoding direction perpendicular to the spinal canal, the frequency encoding direction causes the chemical shift to appear in a cranio-caudad direction that results in obscuration of one of the end-plates because of superimposed fat signal. Depending on the purpose of imaging and the structures that need to be accurately delineated, this fundamental relationship of the phase- and frequency encoding axes and the effect on bone marrow and CSF signal need to be kept in mind. If a water-only image is generated, this chemical shift effect of axes swapping is not necessary, because no fat signal is available to be mismapped. This sequence, therefore, provides good bone detail.

Another effect of changing phase direction is phase wrap if tissue is present outside the FOV.

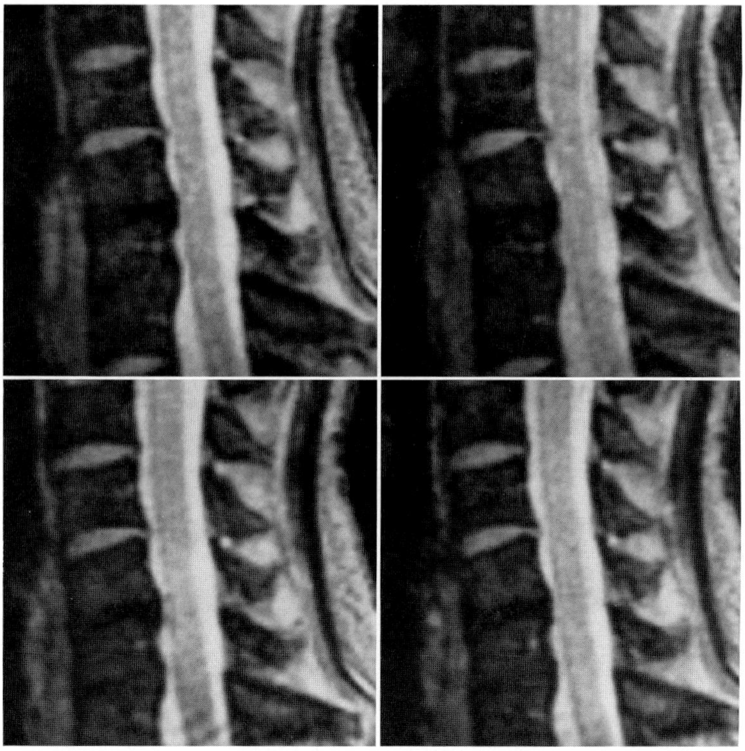

A B C D

FIGURE 2-27. Effect of first order gradient nulling flow compensation and phase axis switching with variable flip angle/gradient echo scan (GRASS 40/20, 5°). **A,** Enabled flow compensation (first order) achieves high CSF-cord contrast. **B,** Disabled CSF-cord contrast decreases. Note lower CSF signal intensity anterior and posterior to cord and reduced cord-CSF contrast. **C,** With flow compensation disabled and frequency cord phase axes switched, high signal CSF is obtained. High signal CSF can be achieved even with flow compensation disabled when frequency encoding axis is switched perpendicular to spinal canal. In this situation, moving CSF does not accumulate large phase differences because CSF motion is perpendicular to the frequency axis, i.e., a strong gradient. Phase-encoding gradient is relatively weak causing less phase shift. **D,** Enabling flow compensation in addition to axes switching does not greatly improve contrast. Axes switching causes some linear artifacts with this particular pulse sequence (**C** and **D**). In general, best results with variable flip angle scans are obtained with flow compensation enabled and phase-encoding axis perpendicular to spine.

This tissue gets mapped into the image as a result of the aliasing problem (see Figure 2-25), and becomes a truncation artifact caused by undersampling. There are methods to eliminate phase wrap, such as sampling with a larger FOV and displaying only a portion of it. The penalty for using it is usually small, although imaging time may increase if larger NEXs are required. The technique of reducing phase wrap works well for T1W images. There may be limitations on its use with T2W images when gradient nulling flow compensation is employed (see Figure 2-25). If CSF gating is the only flow compensation method used, it can be combined with phase wrap correction techniques and with phase and frequency axes switching (see Figure 2-25). It may be necessary to consult the instruction manuals for different machines to determine which of the many artifact compensation techniques operate simultaneously and which are mutually exclusive.

Spatial Saturation Techniques

Spatial saturation techniques are used in spine imaging for removing ghost artifacts when they arise from a moving structure (i.e., larynx or heart) or moving blood, venous or arterial, and may obviate the need for switching phase and frequency axes. The basis for this technique is that saturated, dephased protons give off virtually no signal and thus cannot cause "ghost" artifacts. Therefore in the regions showing motion (hence the term *spatial saturation*) the protons are exposed to 90° pulses and dephasing gradients to eliminate their signal. Such "saturation slabs" (thick slices) are placed anatomically to cancel signal from moving structures. For example, in thoracic spine imaging they could be placed anteriorly to negate signal arising from the heart. In the neck, anterior placement over the larynx and oropharynx would eliminate ghosts arising from swallowing motion. In axial imaging, they would be placed cranially and caudally to the imaging volume to eliminate ghost signal from blood in arteries and veins entering the imaging volume; i.e., the entry phenomenon. Spatial saturation techniques are applicable for both T1W and T2W images. Eliminating ghosts arising from blood vessels can be of value in axial thoracic and lumbar spine imaging. The price paid for this benefit is fewer available slices because saturation slabs require time that could otherwise be used to obtain more slice data.

Variable Flip Angle Scans

The variable flip angle pulse sequence has a complex interaction with pulsatile CSF flow, explained in detail in Chapter 1. This type of sequence can circumvent the problems of CSF motion because at very low flip angles, CSF signal intensity is independent of motion. The problem of motion therefore is circumvented entirely when very low flip angles are used (see Figure 2-18). This then is another method of CSF motion compensation.

VARIABLE FLIP ANGLE/GRADIENT ECHO PULSE SEQUENCES

Variable flip angle/gradient echo pulse sequences are characterized by a variable flip angle (less than a 90° RF pulse) and a gradient refocused echo. These sequences, of which there are several versions, have already proven to be of significant value in spine imaging. There are several important technical features that distinguish the many variations of this type of sequence. The type most useful for spine imaging takes advantage of a steady state in the transverse plane of magnetization.

Variable flip angle/gradient echo pulse sequences have several important characteristics. Contrast is controlled primarily by choice of flip angle rather than by TR and TE as in conventional SE imaging (see Figures 1-50, 1-51, 2-28, and 2-31). They can be fast because gradient refocused echos allow the use of very short TRs; as a result, motion artifacts related to long scanning times may be reduced (Figure 2-29). Images are of lower SNR than conventional SE images. The substitution of the gradient refocused echo for the 180° refocusing pulse in SE makes these pulse sequences more sensitive to magnetic field inhomogeneities and magnetic susceptibility effects, which can degrade image quality by causing inhomogeneous brightness in the image. Occasionally this feature can be used to diagnostic advantage in identifying parenchymal hemorrhage (see Chapter 11). For pulse sequences to be useful in generating myelographic images of the spine in both sagittal and axial views, at least first order motion compensation is necessary in the slice-select and frequency encoding axes. Without first order motion compensation, CSF signal is mismapped, just as in a SE sequence, and signal intensity in the subarachnoid space is reduced (see Figure 2-27).

As a general rule, SNR and contrast is primarily controlled by choice of flip angle, especially with shorter TRs (see Figure 2-28), whereas in conventional SE imaging, TR and TE have the greatest effect. Although these sequences can be used to generate T1W images, their greatest utility in the spine lies in producing images with high CSF signal. The flip angle range useful for spinal imaging depends on TR. The choice of TR depends on whether one desires to use the pulse sequence in a single-slice or multislice mode. For the multislice mode, a longer TR is necessary to permit the interleaving of slices. The optimal flip angle increases as TR increases (Figure 2-30). One disadvantage of the multislice mode is that motion will degrade all of the images. In rapid sequential single-slice scanning, motion may degrade only one slice.

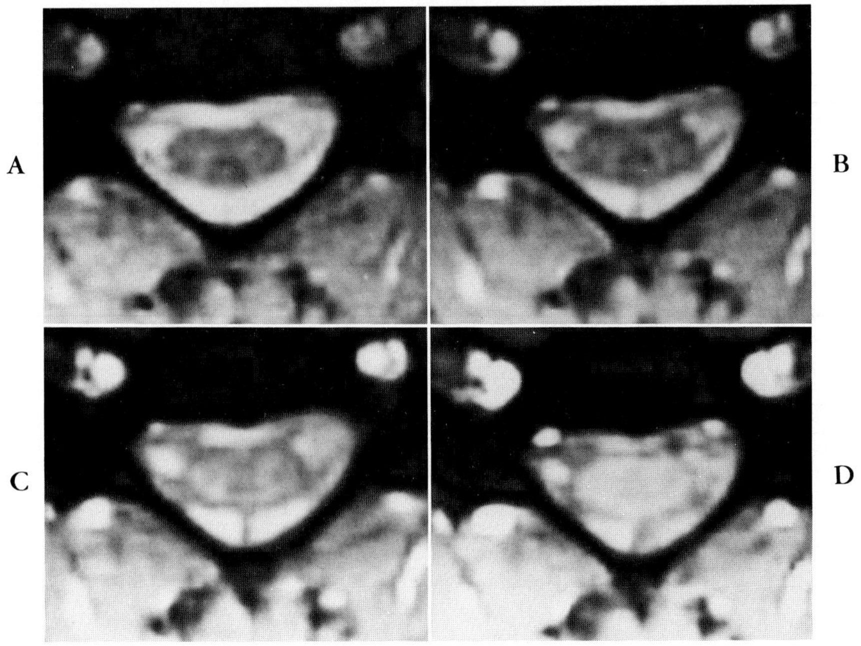

FIGURE 2-28. Axial, variable flip angle/gradient echo scans (GRASS 22/12) show flip angle dependence of CSF signal intensity and CSF-cord contrast. Flip angles: **A,** 3°; **B,** 6°; **C,** 10°; and **D,** 18°. As flip angle is increased, signal intensity within subarachnoid space becomes more inhomogeneous with irregular areas of low signal intensity appearing around cord and around both ventral and dorsal roots, **D.** Best results are achieved with lower flip angles, which are less sensitive to CSF motion. As flip angle is increased, sensitivity to CSF motion increases and signal intensity of CSF decreases. (From Enzmann DR, Rubin JB. Radiology 1988; 166:467. With permission.)

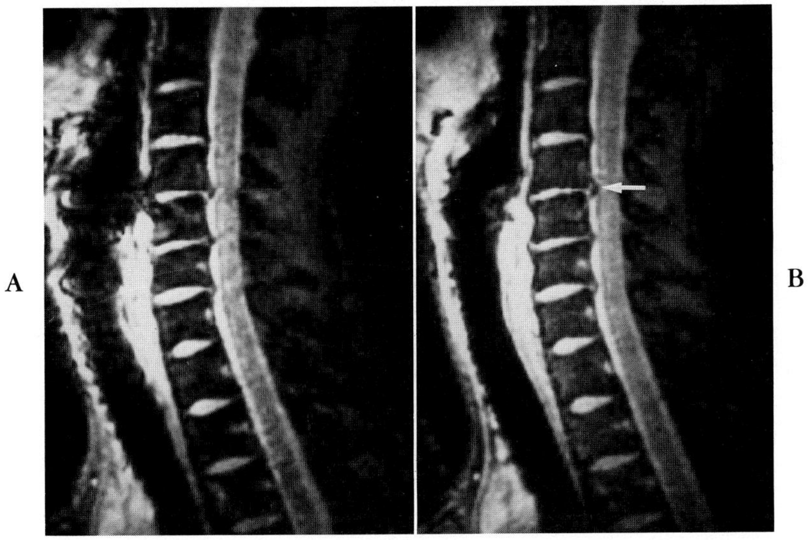

FIGURE 2-29. Comparison of long and short TR techniques when using variable flip angle/ gradient refocused scan in patient with repetitive swallowing. **A,** Despite higher SNR of longer TR technique (GRASS 300/15, 10°), **B,** short TR scan (GRASS 40/13, 5°) provides superior assessment of cord because of fewer motion artifacts. Longer scanning time resulted in greater motion artifact in oropharynx and larynx, causing obscuration of cord because of mismapped signal in phase-encoding direction (anterior to posterior). Although shorter TR scan has lower SNR it also has less motion artifact, and herniated disc at 4-5 is better visualized *(arrow)*. Motion artifacts are accentuated because anterior neck surface coil results in large amount of signal being generated by larynx. Use of posteriorly situated surface coil would lessen effect of swallowing.

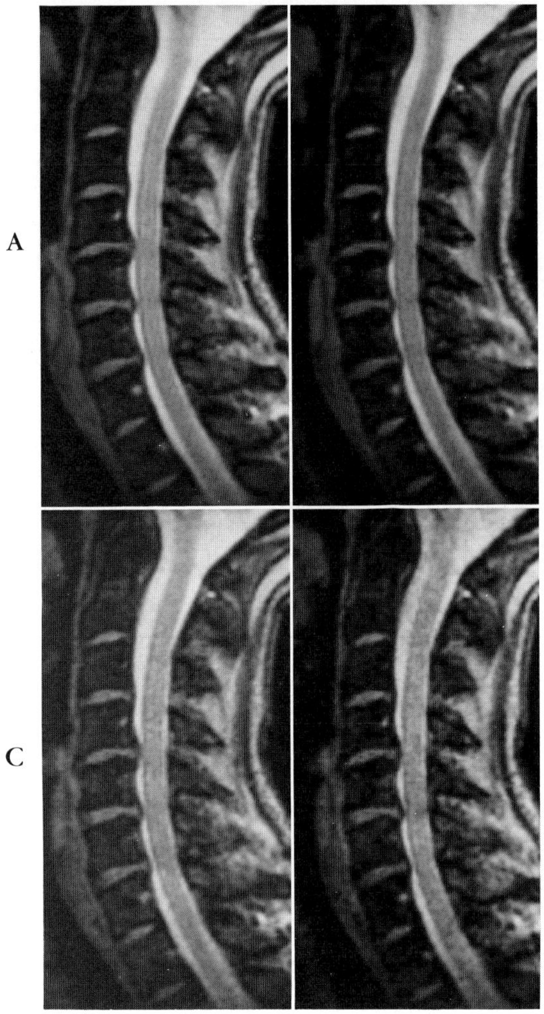

FIGURE 2-30. Series of sagittal variable flip angle/gradient echo scans of cervical spine:
A, TR 1000; TE 15; flip angle, 25°; NEX 2
B, TR 600; TE 15; flip angle, 20°; NEX 2
C, TR 300; TE 15; flip angle, 10°; NEX 2
D, TR 30; TE 15; flip angle, 5°; NEX 8
SNR of entire image increases with increasing TR and flip angle. CSF-cord contrast is maintained at longer TR's with larger flip angles. All scans provide adequate information for diagnosing disc disease.

Single-Slice vs. Multislice Mode (Nomograms)

Physiologic CSF motion alters the contrast of variable flip angle spine images for the reasons described in Chapter 1. Flow effects make myelographic contrast, which is useful in the evaluation of extradural disease, difficult to achieve. To obtain myelographic contrast, it is necessary to adjust imaging parameters so that detrimental flow effects are minimized. This is not straightforward because the effects of flow are dependent on interactions between several imaging parameters. Fortunately, the mathematic model described in Chapter 1 provides a rational means to optimize imaging parameters on variable flip angle images for nearly any imaging condition (Figure 2-31). Curves generated from this model may be used as nomograms to select the best combination of imaging parameters for any imaging condition, but they apply only to variable flip angle SSFP pulse sequences, described in Chapter 1.

Some variable flip angle pulse sequences acquire single slices sequentially, whereas others acquire multiple slices in an interleaved format (Figure 2-32). When both acquisition formats are available, the best method depends on the number of slices needed. During sagittal spine imaging, there are times when a single slice will be sufficient. During axial imaging, numerous slices are usually desired. The single-slice sequential acquisition format is more efficient when only one or a few slices are needed, whereas the multislice interleaved acquisition

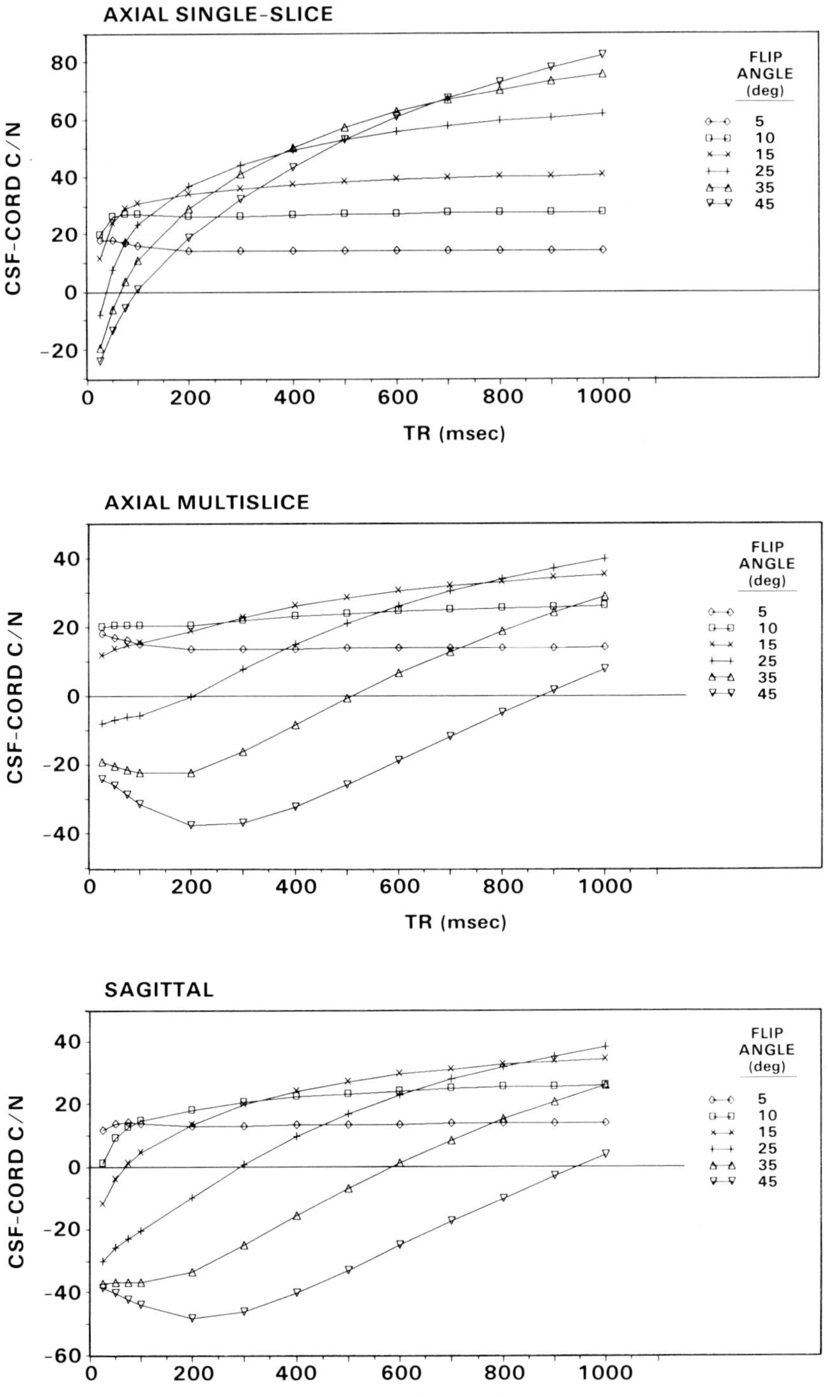

A

B

C

FIGURE 2-31. Nomograms permitting selection of optimal flip angle for each imaging plane (axial and sagittal) and acquisition protocol (single-slice, multislice). **A,** Axial single-slice. **B,** Axial multislice. **C,** Sagittal single-slice or multislice. Find desired TR on X axis. Trace upwards to find uppermost curve on Y axis. Each curve corresponds to different flip angle as shown in graph legend. Uppermost graph at each TR is optimal flip angle to use for this TR and acquisition protocol.

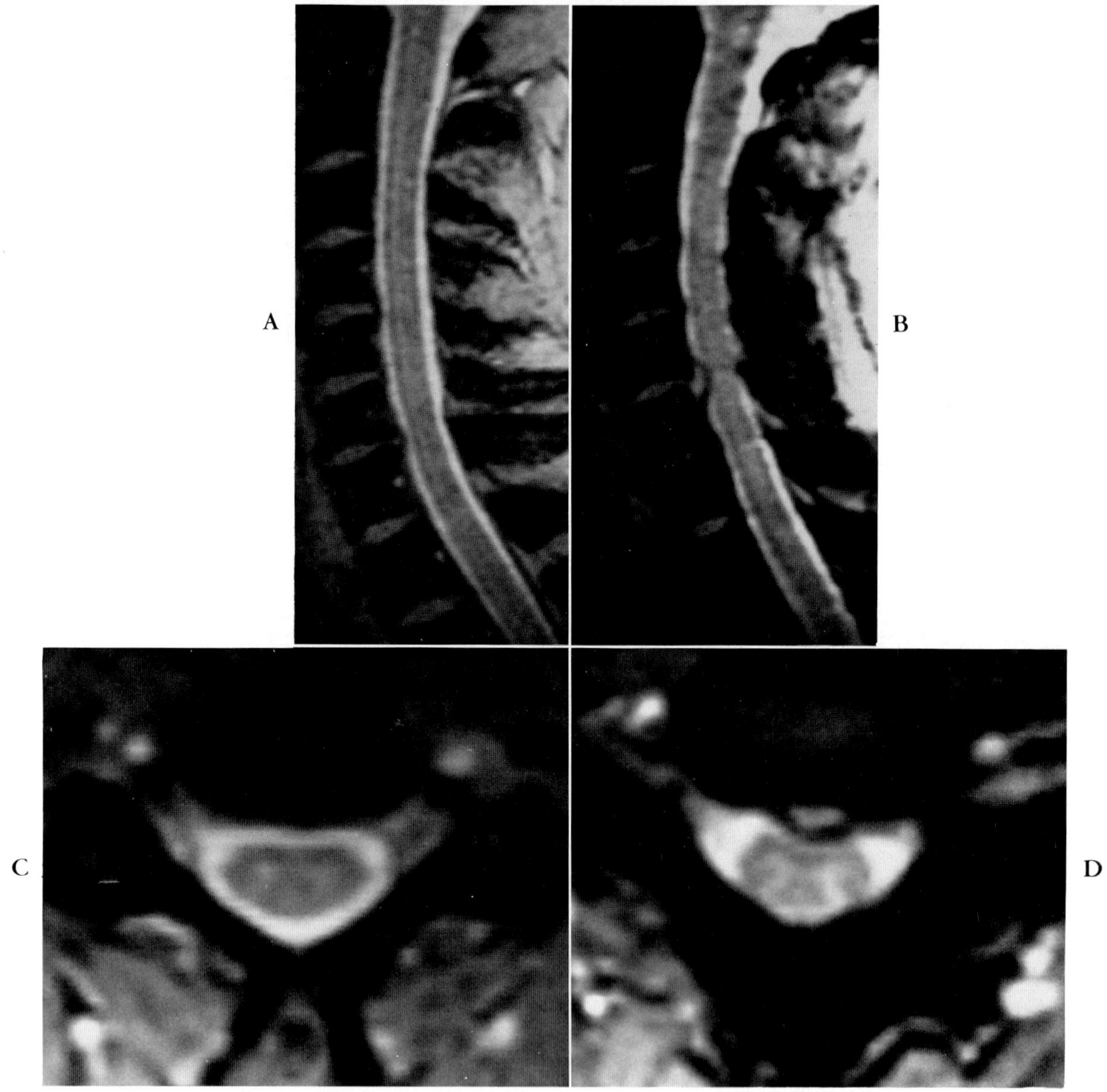

FIGURE 2-32. **A** and **B**, Sagittal and **C** and **D**, axial of multislice version of variable flip angle/gradient echo pulse sequence. Sagittal scans demonstrate **A**, normal and **B**, C_5-C_6 disc using following parameters: 500/15; NEX 2; matrix 256 x 192, and flip angle, 20°. Corresponding axial scans in **C**, normal and **D**, herniated disc used 600/20; NEX 4; matrix 256 x 192; and flip angle 15°. Multislice version of partial flip angle sequence demonstrated high CSF cord contrast and good SNR. (Courtesy of Dr. Burton Drayer.)

format is more efficient when many slices are needed, for reasons described in Chapter 1.

The most efficient TR for imaging depends on whether single-slice or multislice imaging will be used. The shortest TR allowed by the pulse sequence is generally the most efficient when single-slice sequential imaging is used.[5,6] Clearly, a longer TR will be necessary to image several slices in an interleaved format, in which case the most efficient TR is the shortest TR that will yield the desired number of slices. For example, if the variable flip angle pulse sequences require 30 msec per slice and 15 slices are desired, then a TR of 450 msec would be necessary. Increasing TR above these minimum values for both single-slice and multislice imaging increases the overall image SNR and CNR at the expense of prolonged imaging time (see Figure 2-31). Therefore longer TRs provide improved image quality even though their imaging efficiency is not as great as short TR acquisitions. Image SNR is also improved by increasing the NEX.

Once acquisition format and TR have been chosen, it is necessary to select the optimum flip angle for these parameters. This is greatly simplified using curves from the mathematic model described in Chapter 1 that can be used as a nomogram to find the optimal flip angle (see Figure 2-31). Locate the graph corresponding to the imaging plane and acquisition protocol (single-slice vs. multislice) desired. Different graphs are used for each imaging plane and are provided also for axial single-slice and multislice acquisitions. The same graph is used for both acquisition protocols during sagittal imaging. Each graph consists of a series of curves that correspond to a different flip angle. To find the optimal flip angle for any given TR, simply find the TR on the X axis and trace upwards on the Y axis to the uppermost flip angle curve at that TR. The flip angle of each curve is given in the graph legends. For example, the optimal flip angle for sagittal imaging with a TR of 600 msec is 15°.

Once the acquisition protocol, number of slices, TR, and flip angle have been selected, it is necessary to select the best TE. Longer TEs permit more heavily T2*W images to be obtained, but long TE images are usually associated with prominent magnetic susceptibility artifacts for the reasons described in Chapter 1. Because it is possible to achieve myelographic contrast without using long TEs, the shortest TE is usually the best choice to minimize susceptibility artifacts.[6]

Cord Pathology

Variable flip angle pulse sequences have many counteracting factors and thus need to be tailored not only for axial and sagittal imaging but also for disc vs. cord pathology. For the diagnosis of intrinsic cord disease it is not recommended that a variable flip angle scan be the primary pulse sequence. Its role is probably best as a confirmatory scan. For the sagittal view, a motion-compensated, conventional T2W SE scan is usually superior (see Figures 2-17 and 2-33) because it reflects true tissue T2 relaxation time changes. Variable flip angle scans at best are dependent on T2*, not true tissue T2, and usually exhibit mainly features of a proton density image.

T2* is the time decay constant for the FID, is machine specific, and differs from T2, which is tissue specific and relatively independent of machine or field strength. T2* is always shorter than T2, since it is greatly influenced by inhomogeneities in the magnetic field and by magnetic susceptibility effects. With the appropriate imaging parameters, variable flip angle scans can reflect proton density and show some T2* weighting with long TEs. The assumption is that for many disease processes involving the spine and cord, T2* and T2 are positively and closely correlated. Because T2* is correlated with the true tissue T2 relaxation time, such pulse sequences can be used to detect lesions in a way similar to conventional SE T2W sequences. To the extent lesions such as multiple sclerosis plaques are visible on proton density images, they can be visualized by high SNR variable flip angle scans (see Figure 2-33). A high SNR scan is necessary to detect cord lesions. A useful TR range is 400 to 800 msec; usually at least a NEX of 2 is necessary. A range of optimal flip angles can be derived from the nomograms provided for optimizing cord-CSF CNR (see Figure 2-31); having good cord-CSF contrast improves the conspicuity of cord lesions. In general, however, variable flip angle scans are inferior to SE images for subtle lesion detection in the cord. Both types of images are susceptible to various arti-

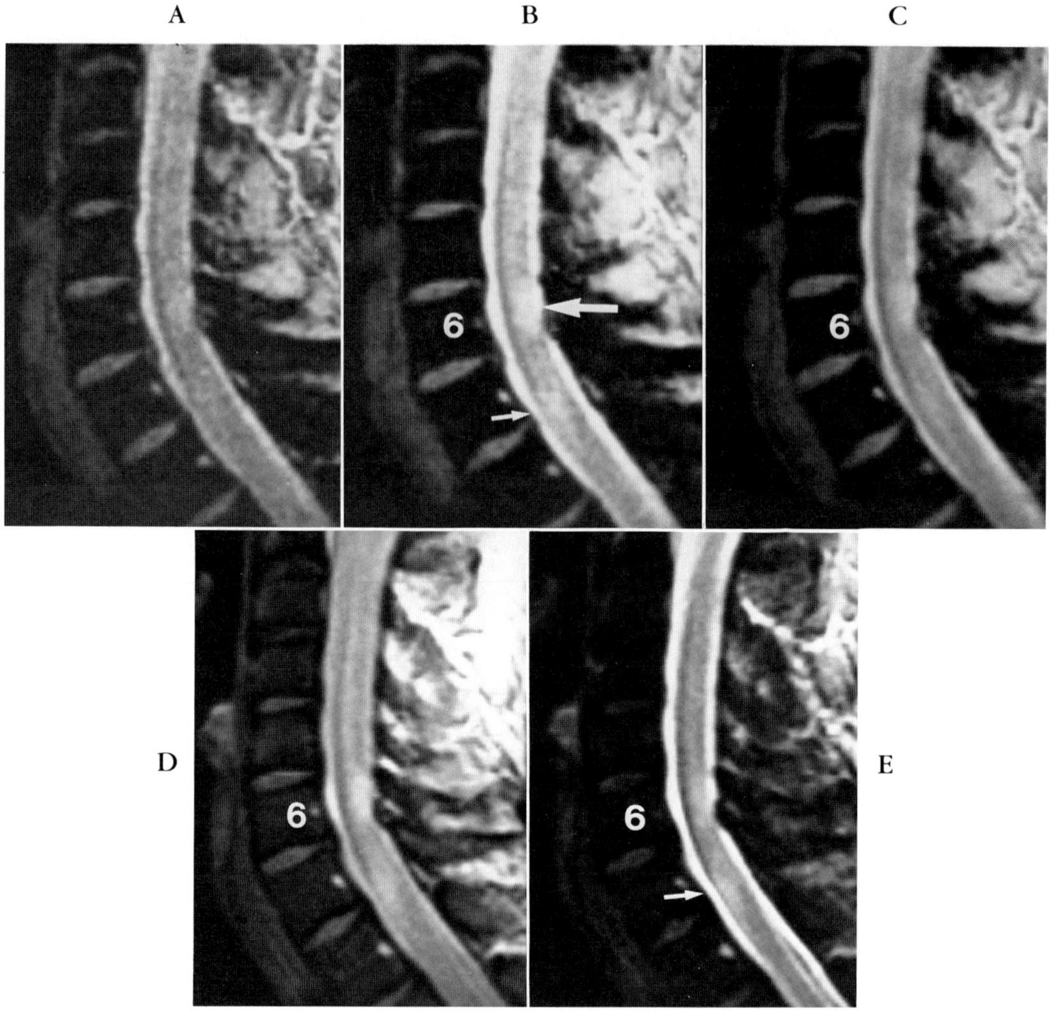

FIGURE 2-33. Comparison of **A, B,** and **C,** variable partial flip angle scans and **D** and **E,** CSF gated/flow-compensated scan in detection of multiple sclerosis plaques in cervical cord. All pulse sequences utilized first order flow compensation by gradient moment nulling technique. **A,** Plaque in posterior cord at level of C_6 barely detectable on partial flip angle scan using short TR (GRASS 40/13, 5°; NEX 8). **B,** When SNR was significantly improved with a longer TR (GRASS 300/15, 10°; NEX 4), posterior MS plaque at C_6 was better visualized *(large arrow)* and second plaque was suggested more anteriorly in cord at C_7-T_1 *(small arrow)*. **C,** Although SNR is higher in third variable flip angle scan with still longer TR (GRASS 600/15, 15°; NEX 2), lesion contrast was reduced. **D,** Flow-compensated plus gated study (gated SE 2400/30, 80) showed both plaques clearly on first echo (TE 30) and **E,** second echo scans (TE 80). In fact, balanced image (approximate proton density [PD] image) (**D**) shows plaque at C_6 level to better advantage than more heavily T2W; TE 80 image (**E**). The second plaque at C_7-T_1 level is better seen on more heavily T2W image (**E**), *(arrow)*. Variable flip angle scans with short TE reflect primarily PD. It is, therefore, not surprising that cord lesions are seen as well as they are, since PD image with conventional SE method (**D**) also showed lesion to good advantage. Despite detectibility of lesions on variable flip angle scans, visualization of lesion on first and second echo of T2W scan provides higher level of diagnostic confidence.

facts, and detecting a lesion on both sequences can increase diagnostic confidence.

Signal inhomogeneity on variable flip angle images caused by magnetic susceptibility artifacts is usually related to bony structures in the spine. This is accentuated when trying to increase T2*W by lengthening TE. Therefore increasing sensitivity by increasing TE has definite limits. Increasing TE causes variability in the signal intensity of the cord, potentially obscuring subtle areas of increased signal intensity (long T2*) representing lesions or causing false areas of relatively high signal. This disturbing magnetic susceptibility artifact is somewhat less evident on axial views because of fewer bone-soft tissue interfaces.[6] The axial view can be useful in detecting abnormal signal within the cord. One workable solution for the diagnosis of spinal cord lesions that do not alter cord morphology is a motion-compensated T2W SE scan in the sagittal view and axial variable flip angle scans through the suspected lesion(s) to confirm their presence and to further characterize them.[6]

Pitfalls

Using pulse sequences to generate myelographic images in the cervical and thoracic spine is generally quite successful. It is important, however, to remember that CSF contrast can change with CSF motion and that signal intensity differences could represent CSF motion differences rather than anatomic abnormalities. On images where contrast is related to CSF motion, the hazards of the conceptual leap of extrapolating true anatomy from such an image must be remembered. Apparent lesions may be nothing more than altered CSF motion (see Figures 2-18, 2-36, and 2-37).

Slice Thickness

Variable flip angle/gradient echo scans in both single-slice or multislice modes put significant stresses on the machine, particularly the gradients. They therefore have some limitations that require trade-offs between TR, TE, slice thickness, field of view, and number of slices. To examine the entire cervical spine in a reasonable scanning time currently requires the use of 5 mm slices. Fortunately axial images have such high contrast between CSF, cord, and disc that the risk of partial volume artifact is reduced (see Chapter 10, Disc). To minimize pitfalls from partial thickness artifact and still cover the entire cervical spine one solution is to do two sets of stacked 5 mm slices through the cervical spine with the second set of slices offset from the first by 2 mm. In this way, a routine cervical spine study includes all of the relevant axial views. In the diagnosis of thoracic disc disease usually only selected levels are studied, as determined from the sagittal T1W scan. In the investigation of cord disease, axial levels are chosen from sagittal T1W or sagittal T2W images. In situations where partial volume artifact is a diagnostic problem, a limited number of 3 mm slices usually can be obtained.

Flip Angles for Vascular Flow

The use and interaction of flip angles with TR for imaging CSF has been discussed (see Chapter 1). Flip angles, however, may also be chosen to highlight vessels, both arterial and venous, to make a diagnosis more complete (Figures 2-34 and 2-35). As a general rule, increasing the flip angle makes the pulse sequence more sensitive to higher velocities of flow, i.e., vasculature rather than CSF. Understanding this relationship can be a diagnostic advantage to identifying vessels (Figure 2-35). Applications include delineation of vessels associated with a spinal cord AVM or arterial feeders to the nidus of a spinal cord hemangioblastoma (see Chapter 8). Variable flip angle/gradient refocused scans have enormous utility in the imaging of the spinal canal and spinal cord, but basic concepts and the interactions between flip angle, flow, SNR, and contrast must be understood.

Chemical Shift Amplitude Modulation

When water and fat protons are present within the same voxel they will cause phase dispersion within that voxel because even at the identical magnetic field they will precess at different frequencies; i.e., they will accumulate phase at different rates. In conventional SE imaging this phase difference is corrected by the 180° refocusing RF pulse. In gradient echo scans this is not the case. Therefore there will be periodic times determined by the TE when water and fat are in phase, yielding a higher signal

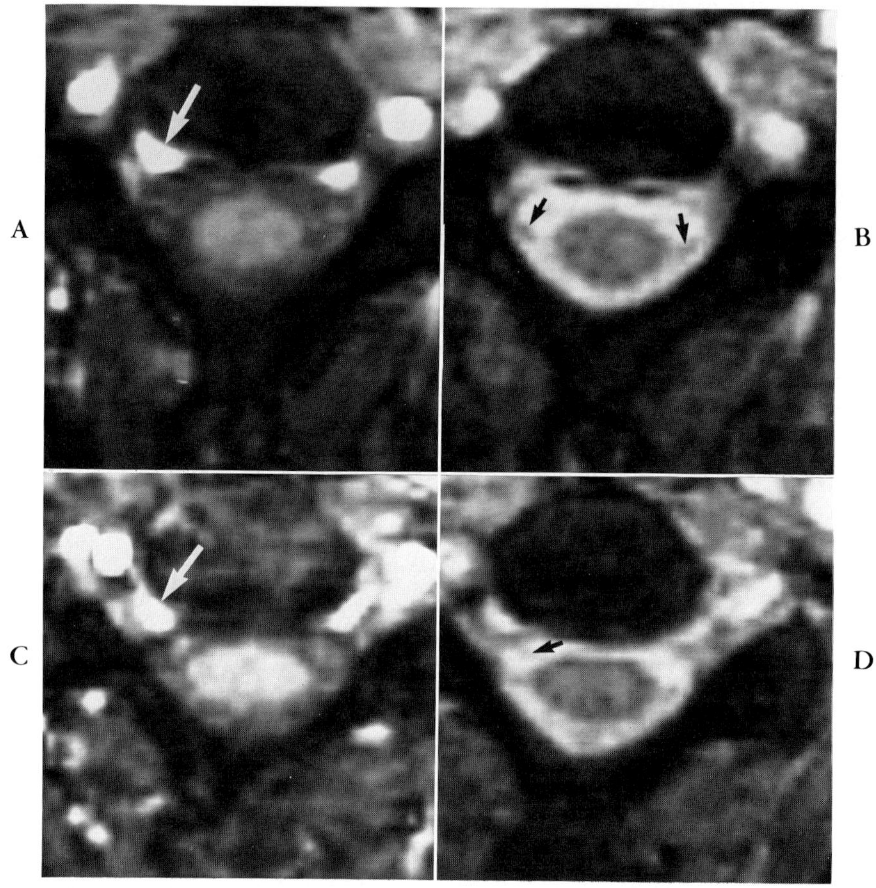

FIGURE 2-34. Comparison of two different flip angles in axial view of cervical spine using variable flip angle/gradient echo scan (Grass 25/13). **A** and **C**, Images obtained with flip angle of 33° whereas images **B** and **D** are at exact same level but obtained with flip angle of 7°. At higher flip angle CSF is lower signal than cord but high signal is seen in both arteries and veins (*arrow* **A** and **C**). Note venous structures in anterolateral recesses of spinal canal (**A**, *arrow*) extending through intervertebral foramina parallel to exiting nerve (**C**, *arrow*). High signal in intervertebral foramina on low flip angle scan (**B** and **D**) can represent either traversing vein or epidural fat. Small linear defects in CSF (*arrows*, **B** and **D**) are dorsal and ventral nerve roots. Cord-CSF contrast clearly depends on flip angle.

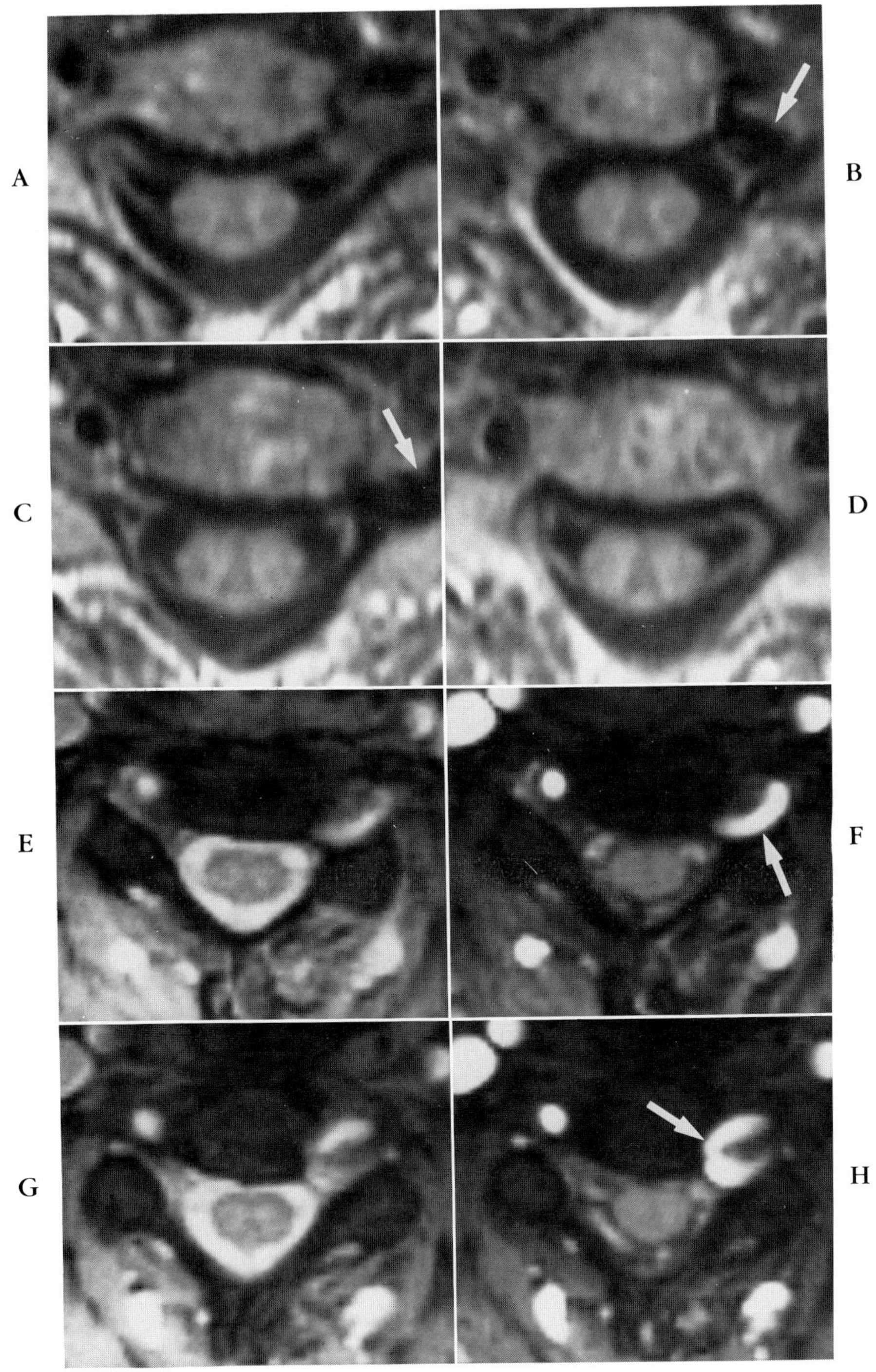

FIGURE 2-35. **A-D,** Axial T1W scan (SE 800/20) shows widened intervertebral foramen on left with unusual configuration of soft tissue and large area of low signal intensity within (*arrows*, **B** and **C**). **E** and **G**, In same region, variable flip angle/gradient echo (GRASS 25/13) images using low flip angle, 7°, show usual high contrast between cord and CSF and widened intervertebral foramen. Increased signal in foramen was nonspecific. **F** and **H**, Nature of structure in foramen clarified by images at same levels but with higher flip angle, 33°, used to highlight vascular structures (*arrows*). Although high CSF-cord contrast was lost, vascular structures are better delineated and nature of lesion in foramen is clear—a tortuous vertebral artery.

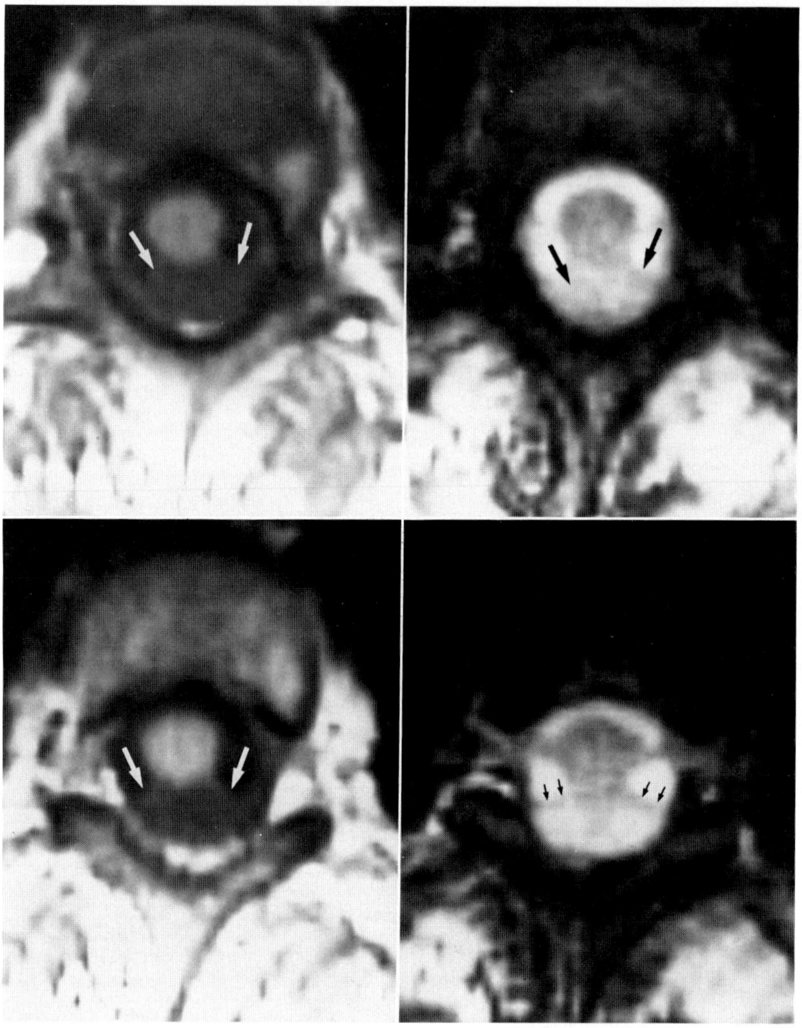

FIGURE 2-36. Differences in CSF signal intensity in cervical and thoracic spine caused by motion. Differences can occur on (**A** and **C**) T1W images (SE 1000/20) and on **B** and **D**, variable flip angle/gradient echo images, GRASS 22/12. In normal cervico-thoracic junction, areas of relatively higher signal intensity dorsal to spinal cord can be expected, even on T1W images because of decreased motion of CSF trapped in dorsal arachnoid septations (*arrows* **A** and **C**). Phenomenon will also be present on variable flip angle/gradient refocused echo scans, because in single-slice mode they are sensitive to in-flow phenomenon (*arrows*, **B**). On these sequences, less pulsatile CSF will show lower signal intensity on axial views because of less in-flow phenomenon. This should not be mistaken for a mass dorsal to the spinal cord (**B**). The location's extent and sometimes spiculated nature (*arrows*, **D**) of this intermediate signal area behind cord should clear up any diagnostic confusion.

A B C D E, F G

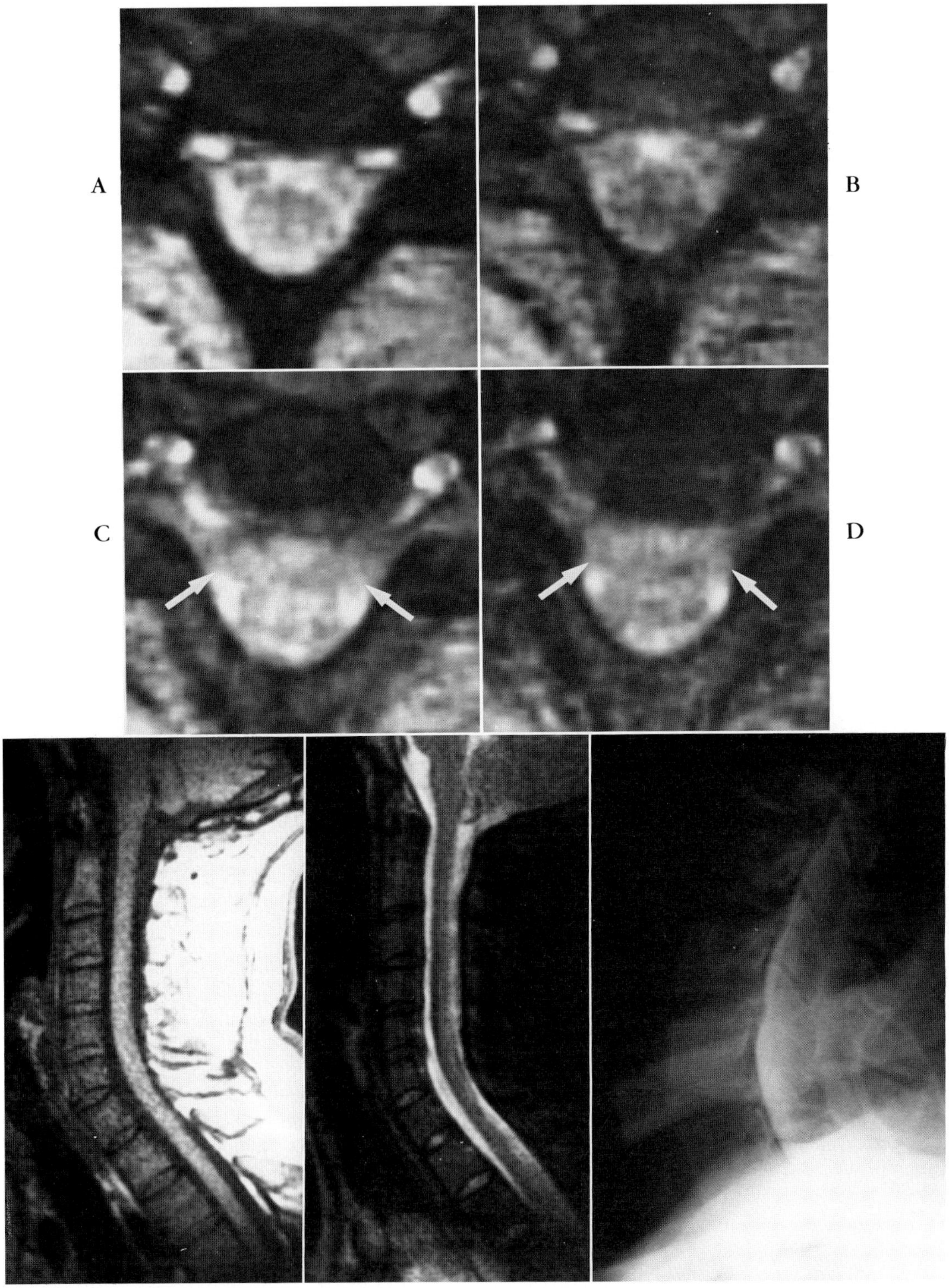

FIGURE 2-37. Sensitivity of variable flip angle/gradient echo scans to motion in axial view when used in single-slice mode can sometimes lead to confusing findings that require sagittal and axial correlation. **A-D,** Series of variable flip angle scans (Grass 25/12, 7°) at C_6-C_7 cervical level suggest possibility of either anterior mass or extradural defect on axial views *(arrows)*. Finding unusual in that it had intermediate signal intensity and was not well circumscribed. Highest CSF signal lateral to cord rather than in anterolateral recesses was unusual (**C** and **D**). Importance is that **E,** sagittal T1W (SE 800/20) and **F,** sagittal gated T1W (SE 2000/80) did not confirm presence of a mass anterior to cord at that level. **G,** Lateral view of water soluble contrast myelogram also confirmed lack of any significant extradural defect or mass in that region. Findings on axial variable flip angle scan represent flow phenomenon rather than true anatomic defect. This type of correlation between views is mandatory whenever pulse sequence is used that has known sensitivity to CSF motion.

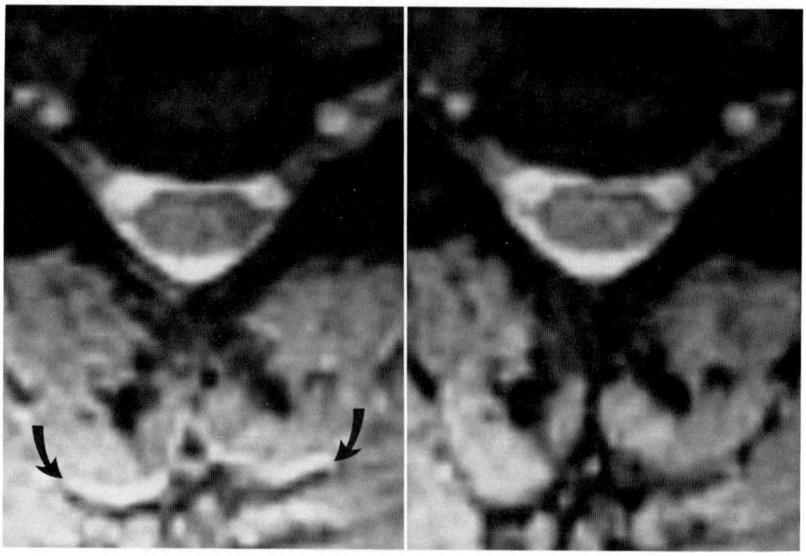

FIGURE 2-38. Axial variable flip angle/gradient echo scans (GRASS 25/14.4, 16.1) demonstrate chemical shift amplitude modulation effect by changing TE from **A**, 14.4 msec to **B**, 16.5 msec. **A**, In water-plus-fat image note chemical shift artifact at boundary of fat and water in fascial planes of posterior neck *(arrows)*. **B**, In water-minus-fat image bright lines caused by chemical shift disappear because of destructive interference within voxel at these fascial planes. There is no significant difference in delineation of nerve in the neural foramen. Although this is potential concern for the neural foramen considering the angle of the foramen compared to frequency encoding axis and amount of fat, this effect is not clinically important in cervical spine imaging.

from a voxel, or when they are out of phase, yielding a lower signal from a voxel.[19] At fat-muscle or fat-nerve interfaces the voxels containing both tissues can change in relative intensities depending on the TE chosen (Figure 2-38). This destructive interference caused by phase dispersion occurs at water-fat boundaries. A TE that accentuates boundary effects may seem preferable in the investigation of disc disease. Although these dark boundary lines are artifactual, they sometimes are helpful in depicting muscle anatomy. In delineating neural structures in the cervical intervertebral foramina, however, this boundary effect of chemical shift amplitude modulation does not appear to be clinically important.

SPINE MR PROTOCOLS

There are numerous combinations of imaging parameters that are available for spine imaging. There is no one correct way to perform an individual study. The protocols listed in Table 2-2 are a good starting point for the various disease types listed and provide an idea of what type of pulse sequences are useful. In applying the protocols, time can be saved by reducing spatial resolution by decreasing the matrix size. For example, the 256 × 192 matrix size may be a good compromise because the 256 × 128 matrix produces blurred images but is certainly an effective means to reduce imaging time and increase patient throughput.

Table 2-2 lists imaging parameters in columns and individual pulse sequences by row under the various clinical categories. The abbreviations are listed in alphabetical order. For many pulse sequences, specific footnotes are included that expand on pertinent points with regard to the pulse sequence.

The protocols reflect the authors' bias toward high resolution spine imaging.

REFERENCES

1. Dixon WT. Simple proton spectroscopic imaging. Radiology 1984; 153:189.
2. Edelman RR, McFarland E, Stark DD, et al. Surface coil MR imaging of abdominal viscera. I. Theory, technique, and initial results. Radiology 1985; 157:425.
3. Enzmann DR, Griffin C, Rubin JB. Potential false-negative MR images of the thoracic spine in disk disease with switching of phase- and frequency-encoding gradients. Radiology 1987; 165:635.
4. Enzmann DR, O'Donohue J. Optimizing MRI for detection of small tumors in the cerebellopontine angle and internal auditory canal. AJNR 1987; 8:99.
5. Enzmann DR, Rubin JB. Cervical spine: MR imaging with partial flip angle, gradient-refocused pulse sequence. I. General considerations and disc disease. Radiology 1988; 166:467.
6. Enzmann DR, Rubin JB. Cervical spine: MR imaging with a partial flip angle, gradient-refocused pulse sequence. II. Spinal cord disease. Radiology 1988; 166:473.
7. Enzmann DR, Rubin JB, DeLaPaz R, et al. Benefits and pitfalls in MRI scanning resulting from CSF pulsation. Radiology 1986; 161:773.
8. Fisher MR, Barker B, Amparo EG, et al. MR imaging using specialized coils. Radiology 1985; 157:443.
9. Johnson G, Miller DH, MacManus D, et al. STIR sequences in NMR imaging of the topic nerve. Neuroradiology 1987; 29:238.
10. Levy LM, Bichiro G, Brooks R, et al. Spinal cord artifacts from truncation nerves during MR imaging. Radiology 1988; 166:479.
11. Matthaei D, Frahm J, Haase A, et al. Three-dimensional flash MR imaging of thorax and abdomen without triggering or gating. MRI 1986; 4:381.
12. Rubin JB, Enzmann DR. Harmonic modulation of proton MR precessional phase by pulsatile motion: origin of spinal CSF flow phenomenon, II, (Dyke Award). AJNR 1987; 8:307.
13. Rubin JB, Enzmann DR, Wright A. CSF-gated MR imaging of the spine: theory and clinical implementation. Radiology 1987; 163:784.
14. Rubin JB, Wright A, Enzmann DRJ. Lumbar spine: motion compensation for cerebrospinal fluid on MR imaging. Radiology 1988; 166:225.
15. Sepponen RE, Sipponen JT, Tanttu JI. A method for chemical shift imaging: demonstration of bone marrow involvement with proton chemical shift imaging. J. Comput Assist Tomogr 1984; 8:585.
16. Schenck JF, Hart HR, Foster TH, et al. High resolution magnetic resonance imaging using surface coils. In: Kressel HY, ed. Magnetic resonance annual 1986. New York: Raven Press, 1986.
17. Sze G, Abramson A, Krol G, et al. Gadolinium-DTPA in the evaluation of intradural extramedullary spinal disease. AJNR 1988; 9:153.
18. Valk J. Gd-DTPA in MR of spinal lesions. AJNR 1988; 9:345.
19. Wehrli FW, Perkins TG, Shimakawa A, et al. Chemical shift-induced amplitude modulations in images obtained with gradient refocusing. Magn Reson Imaging 1987; 5:157.

3

Physical Basis and Anatomic Correlates of MR Signal in the Spine and Cord

Robert L. DeLaPaz

Understanding the physical basis of MR images is essential for intelligent interpretation of clinical studies. This chapter focuses on the physical, biochemical, anatomic, and physiologic properties of the spine and spinal cord relevant to MR imaging. General principles that apply to all MR imaging systems are discussed with specific examples taken from a General Electric Signa 1.5 Tesla imaging unit.

BASIC PRINCIPLES

Magnetic Field Strength

There is a relatively consistent appearance of clinical spine images across the range of magnetic field strengths currently in use (0.15 to 1.5 Tesla), in spite of T1 prolongation and greater signal-to-noise ratio (SNR) at high field and specific technical differences between imaging systems. However, subtle field-dependent effects on relaxation times, inherent magnetic properties of the tissue (magnetic susceptibility) and proton-electron interactions (paramagnetic effects) may be significant on spine MR images in certain circumstances, especially at higher magnetic fields.

T1

The T1 in tissues and biologic solutions is prolonged at higher field strength, approximately two- to three-fold over the range of clinical imaging fields. The typical change in T1 values is from 200 to 300 msec at 0.15 Tesla to approximately 600 to 800 msec at 1.5 Tesla.[2] The increase in T1 is not a simple linear function of field strength and varies from tissue to tissue. This field-dependent variability might be expected to significantly alter MR image contrast through changes in T1 relationships between tissues and because there is little change in T2 over the clinical range of field strengths. However, field-dependent T1 prolongation has little effect on MR image contrast in most clinical applications because field-dependent T1 prolongation in most tissues is roughly parallel. However, the increasing ratio of T1 to T2 also has no practical significance in most clinical MR imaging.

T1 differences between tissues reflect differences in water and fat content. As in MR imaging of other tissues, increases in water content are often subtle on T1W images. For instance, noncystic lesions in the spinal cord with prolonged T1 are often difficult to see on T1W images when no mass effect is present. Conversely, marked dessication occurs with disc degeneration, which appears as low signal in T1W images largely because of low proton density. T1W images are most useful in the spine where water and fat interfaces are present because the short T1 of fat produces high signal and sharp contrast against adjacent water-containing tissue. Neoplastic infiltration of fatty bone marrow and fatty replacement of normal marrow are best seen on T1W images.

T2

T2 relaxation times vary little over the range of clinical MR imaging field strengths. T2 values for most tissues are between 30 and 90 msec.[2] Relevant to spine imaging are the T2 values for neural tissue (70 to 90 msec),[2] vertebral bone marrow (55 to 65 msec),[11] and fatty tissue (50 to 60 msec).[12] Abnormalities of the spine and spinal cord cause T2 variations from normal, which in most cases are parallel to changes in tissue water content. Spinal cord lesions and tumor infiltration of bone marrow result in abnormally prolonged T2, whereas disc degeneration and fatty infiltration of vertebral marrow accelerate T2.

T2*

Differences in tissue magnetic susceptibility and subtle effects of paramagnetic substances become more important as magnetic field strength increases, especially as they affect T2W images. Magnetic susceptibility is simply the inherent ability of a substance to become magnetized. In tissue, magnetic susceptibility varies at the microscopic level, being homogeneous in pure fluids and inhomogeneous in complex tissues. At interfaces between cellular structures or tissues with different magnetic susceptibilities, small magnetic field gradients are produced. These subtle, microscopic gradients cause a loss of phase coherence within image voxels because water protons diffuse across them during image acquisition and because of spatially dependent phase shifts induced in static protons. Protons in different magnetic environments within the voxel precess at different rates, resulting in rapid phase dispersion and loss of signal from the voxel. The longer the interval between signal acquisitions (echoes) in a pulse sequence, the more time is allowed for loss of phase coherence and consequent loss of signal. The time constant for this loss of phase coherence is *T2**, which is a measure of transverse magnetization and a function of T2, machine magnetic field inhomogenieties (B_0), and local tissue magnetic susceptibility inhomogeneities. T2* effects differ from T2 relaxation in that they are strongly dependent on field strength. Phase dispersion increases (T2* is accelerated) as the square of local magnetic susceptibility differences (gradients) and as the square of the applied magnetic field. Spin echo (SE) images are less sensitive to T2* than variable flip angle/gradient echo images because the 180° pulse used to produce the echo corrects for phase incoherence, whereas the gradient echo does not. Thus, magnetic susceptibility effects are generally seen on T2W SE images only at long interecho delays (long TEs) and at high field. With gradient echo imaging, however, T2* effects are prominent and may be seen at lower magnetic fields.[33] Maps of magnetic susceptibility changes (T2′ maps; "T2 prime" maps) isolated from B_0 inhomogenieties may aid tissue characterization by identifying sharp susceptibility gradients such as those adjacent to trabecular bone or ferric iron in hemosiderin[24a]. In spine MR imaging, magnetic susceptibility effects are relevant to tissue contrast in the cord and in vertebral bone marrow.

The direct effect of a paramagnetic substance on proton relaxation is marked acceleration of both T1 and T2 caused by unpaired electrons, which have very large magnetic moments (approximately 650 times larger than protons because of unit charge and very small mass).[17] These large moments accelerate relaxation because their interactions with adjacent protons are much stronger than proton-proton interactions. However, electron-proton dipole-dipole interactions are very localized, falling off as the sixth power of the radius from the electron, and thus occur over very short distances (a few angstroms). When a paramagnetic substance, such as ferric iron (Fe^{3+}) within ferritin, is not homogeneously distributed through tissue and is isolated from direct interaction with water protons, its effect is similar to magnetic susceptibility inhomogeniety and results in T2* acceleration. Paramagnetic T1 acceleration is reduced in this situation. Thus, paramagnetic substances in tissue may have direct effects on proton relaxation and produce high signal on T1W images (short T1 effect) and low signal on T2W images (short T2 effect). They may also be isolated from tissue protons and affect image contrast indirectly to produce little change on T1W images but marked signal loss on T2W images, especially gradient echo images. The latter effect, because of ferric iron (Fe^{3+}) in ferritin, may contribute to the low signal seen in vertebral bone marrow on T2W images.

SPINAL CORD

Water Content

The water content of spinal cord gray matter and white matter is similar to that of cerebral gray matter and white matter. Gray matter has approximately 12% more free water than white matter and therefore has a slightly greater proton density and longer relaxation times (T1 and T2) than white matter. The presence of myelin in the white matter also influences the MR differences between gray and white matter. The protons in the membrane lipids of myelin do not produce signal on MR images but they do cause a shortening of relaxation times in the adjacent water protons, thus enhancing T1 and T2 differences between gray and white matter.[26] This effect is clearly seen on heavily T2W SE images that show high signal in the central gray matter and low signal in surrounding white matter regions of the cord (see Figures 3-3 and 3-4). T1W axial images of the spinal cord do not demonstrate gray-white boundaries as well as T2W images. This is partly due to the typically lower contrast of T1W images but also due to properties of the tissue that are not well understood, especially in the dorsal column white matter. This will be discussed later in detail. As in the brain, most abnormalities of the spinal cord cause increases in free water content resulting in low signal on T1W images and high signal on T2W images accompanied by disruption of normal internal architecture.

White Matter Anatomy

Spinal cord white matter is typical of CNS white matter, which is characterized by the presence of axons and myelin-forming oligodendroglial cells and by the absence of neuronal cell bodies. Most of the axons are myelinated. Fibrous astrocytes are also found.

Spinal cord white matter is organized into bundles, or tracts, of axons each with a major motor or sensory function (Figure 3-1). Most of the tracts are myelinated, some are unmyelinated, and some are mixed. The major types of tracts are propriospinal, which interconnect different levels of the cord, and long ascending and descending tracts, named for the cells of origin and destination. The dorsal funiculi contain many propriospinal fibers traveling just a few segments and longer fibers extending almost the entire length of the cord. A special category of such fibers comprises the fasciculi gracilis and cuneatus in the dorsal funiculus. They are long ascending pathways to the brain carrying sensory information, including discriminative touch, joint position, pressure, and vibration. The fasciculus cuneatus fibers originate from the upper body and extremities and therefore are present only from the midthoracic level cranially. The lateral and ventral funiculi contain several long tracts and large numbers of propriospinal fibers, many of which are myelinated. The major ascending (sensory) tracts are the dorsal and ventral spinocerebellar tracts in the lateral funiculus and the spinothalamic and spinoreticular tracts in the ventrolateral funiculi. The major descending (motor) tracts are the lateral corticospinal, rubrospinal, and medullary reticulospinal tracts in the medial portion of the lateral funiculus and the ventral corticospinal, vestibulospinal, pontine reticulospinal, and tectospinal tracts in the ventral funiculus.[32]

Gray Matter Anatomy

Spinal cord gray matter, like other CNS gray matter, is characterized by the presence of neuronal cell bodies and the bulk of dendrites. The neuronal cell bodies are not uniformly distributed in gray matter. In some areas the cell bodies form layers, especially in the dorsal horns (see

Figure 3-1). In other areas, neuronal cell bodies having similar functions form clusters or columns. Between neuronal cell bodies there is the neuropil, a tangle of neuronal cell processes, mostly dendrites, and associated neuroglial processes. Gray matter contains axons, both myelinated and unmyelinated, but in a smaller proportion than in white matter, and oligodendroglia and protoplasmic astrocytes. Furthermore, gray matter is also more vascular than white matter.[32]

The gray matter of the spinal cord forms an H-shaped structure in cross section that is surrounded by the various white matter tracts (see Figure 3-1). The relative proportion of gray matter to white matter varies with segmental level; it is greatest in the cervical and lumbar enlargements and smallest in the midthoracic cord. This is related to the larger number of neurons needed for control of the upper and lower extremities. The crossbars of the H-shaped gray matter form the gray commissures, which pass anterior and posterior to the central canal. Fibers cross through these commissures between the gray matter on the two sides of the cord. Within each half of the cord the gray matter is divided into the dorsal and ventral horns. The dorsal horn contains sensory synapses and may be subdivided into horizontal layers, known in older terminology as the marginal zone, substantia gelatinosa of Rolando, nucleus proprius, cervix, and base. The intermediate region contains the cell group known as the intermediate nucleus. The ventral horn includes a number of motor neuron nuclei, as well as many interneurons, and a commissural nucleus in its medial portion. An alternative to the traditional terminology has been suggested by Rexed,[32] which gives ten numerical labels to zones of the gray matter.

Vascular Anatomy

Blood is supplied to the spinal cord through radicular arteries, which are branches of the vertebral arteries and aortic intercostal and lumbar arteries (Figure 3-2). These vessels form the single anterior spinal artery and the paired posterior spinal arteries. The anterior spinal artery is formed at the cranial end by paired branches of the distal vertebral arteries. The vascular pattern of radicular branches to the rest of the spinal cord is extremely variable. In general, there are two to three branches to the cervical cord with the most consistent large branch entering the cervical canal at C_6. Vascularity to the midthoracic cord is variable with a watershed region often found at approximately the T_4 cord level. A consistent lower thoracic major artery, the arteria radicularis magna (artery of Adamkiewicz) enters from the left side in 75% of cases, usually between T_9 and L_2 (85%) and less frequently between T_5 and T_8 (15%).[10]

The anterior spinal artery courses along the ventral median sulcus. The caliber of the anterior spinal artery varies with the segmental level of the cord, being largest at the conus and smallest at the midthoracic level. Branches of the anterior spinal artery penetrate the cord from the ventral median sulcus to supply the ventral funiculi, the ventral horns, and the base of the dorsal horns (see Figure 3-2). The anterior spinal artery also contributes to the vascular supply of the lateral columns and, by way of anastomoses with the posterior spinal arteries, the dorsal part of the cord. Important tracts supplied by the anterior spinal artery include the corticospinal and the spinothalamic tracts.[32]

The dorsal radicular arteries form the posterior spinal arteries, located along the dorsolateral surface of each side of the cord. The posterior spinal arteries also derive a part of their vascular supply from branches of either the posterior inferior cerebellar arteries or the vertebral arteries. The posterior spinal arteries supply blood to the dorsal funiculi and dorsal horns, and they provide anastomotic connections with branches from the anterior spinal artery.[32]

Veins of the spinal cord run longitudinally in the pia accompanying the spinal arteries. Radicular veins, which run with the nerve roots, drain the pial veins into the internal vertebral venous plexus, which lies in the epidural space surrounded by fat. Within this dense plexus of veins, the anterior longitudinal vertebral sinuses are two large venous channels that lie in the anterolateral gutters of the spinal canal on the posterior surfaces of the vertebral bodies and discs. This internal vertebral venous plexus drains into the dorsispinal branches of the paired intercostal veins. In addition, there are the basivertebral veins within the central vertebral bodies that communicate between the internal and the external venous plexus. The functional significance of the vertebral venous system is two-fold. Changes in intraabdominal and intra-

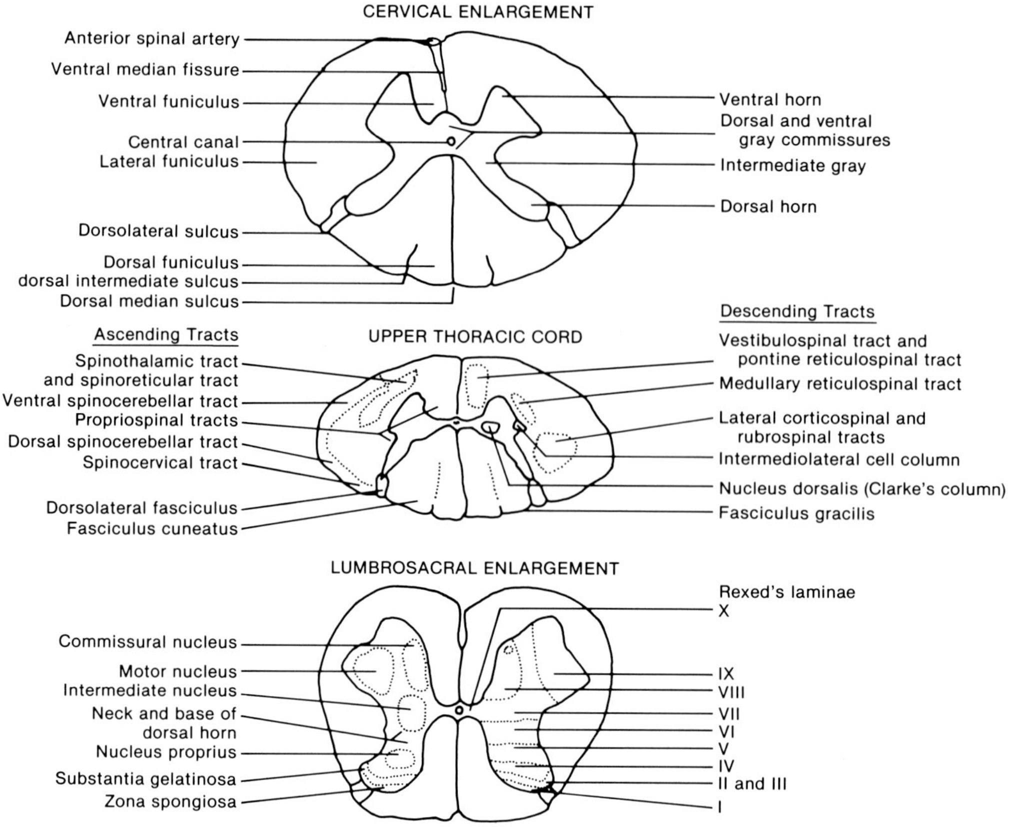

FIGURE 3-1. Cross-sectional anatomy of the spinal cord. **A,** General external and internal landmarks of cervical spinal cord. **B,** Major ascending and descending white matter tracts and special gray matter nuclei of thoracic spinal cord. **C,** Major gray matter nuclei and Rexed's laminae of lumbosacral enlargement. Laminae I to VI occupy the dorsal horn with lamina II equivalent to the substantia gelatinosa. Part of lamina VII corresponds to the intermediate region. Lamina VII also forms part of the ventral horn. Medial part of the ventral horn in enlargements includes lamina VIII. Motor neurons in the ventral horn are classed as lamina IX and zone around the central canal is lamina X.[32] (Modified from Willis WD, and Grossman RG, Medical Neurobiology, ed 3. St Louis: the CV Mosby Co, 1981. With permission.)

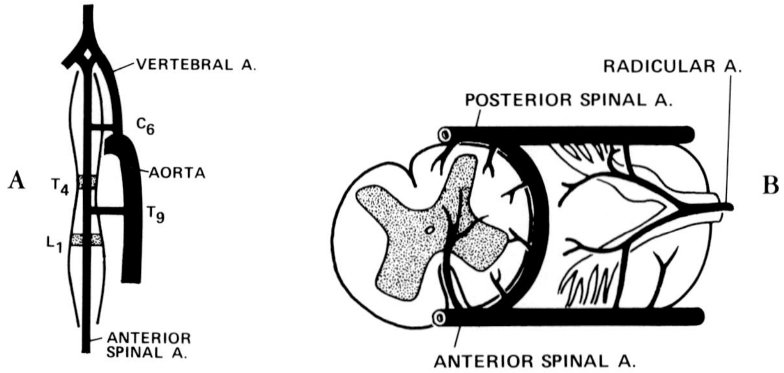

FIGURE 3-2. Vascular supply to the spinal cord. **A,** Schematic representation of systemic blood supply to spinal cord, which arises primarily from branches of vertebral arteries and thoracolumbar aorta. Precise levels of major radicular branches that form anterior spinal artery and paired posterior spinal arteries (not shown) are widely variable. Watershed zones within cord between major radicular arteries lie at approximately T_4 and L_1 cord levels. **B,** Normal local arterial supply to spinal cord includes multiple penetrating arterioles from anterior and posterior spinal arteries and their anastomotic connections with systemic blood supplied via radicular arteries. Accompanying veins are not shown. (Modified from Willis WD, Grossman RG. Medical neurobiology, ed 3. St Louis: the CV Mosby Co, 1981. With permission.)

A

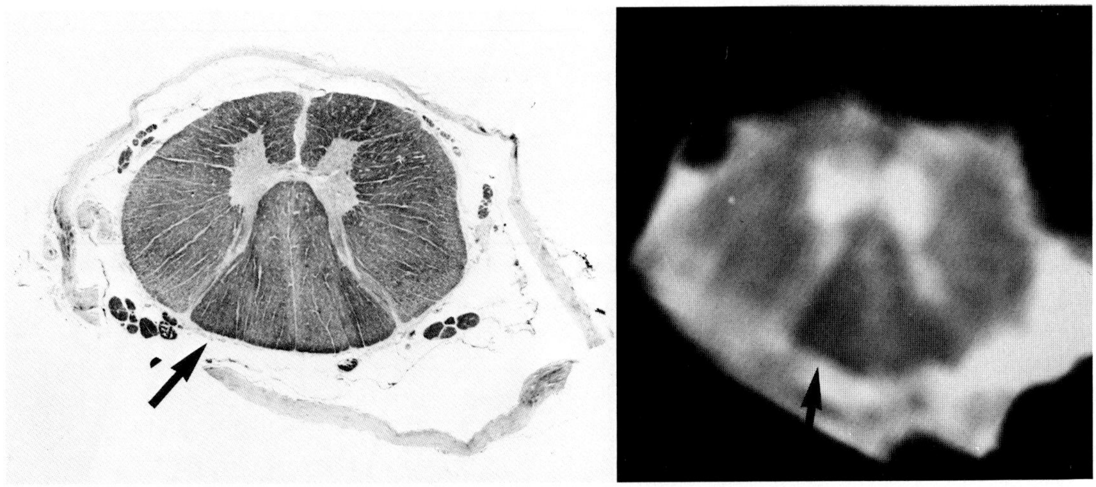

B

FIGURE 3-3. Axial white matter anatomy of the spinal cord. **A,** Luxol Fast Blue stain of white matter in cross section of cervical spinal cord. Note relatively higher density of staining in the fasciculus cuneatus region, medial to dorsal horns of gray matter *(arrow)*. **B,** Axial T2W image of cadaver spinal cord at location of stained section. Note lower signal regions in fasciculus cuneatus, corresponding to denser myelin staining in stained section *(arrow)*.

A

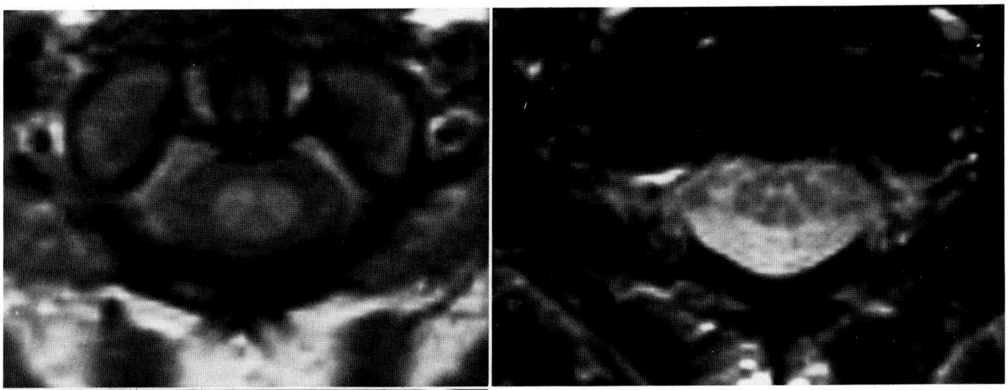

C

B

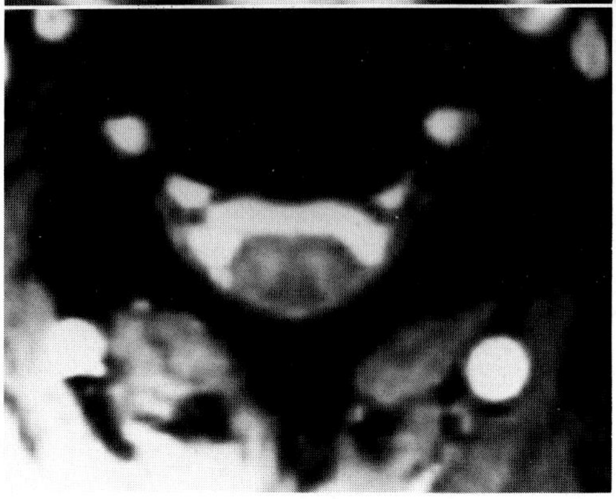

FIGURE 3-4. Axial MR of the spinal cord. **A,** Axial T1W image of cervical spinal cord with characteristic low signal in posterior column white matter. **B,** Axial T2W image of cervical spinal cord with high signal in central gray matter and low signal in surrounding white matter. **C,** Axial variable flip angle/gradient echo (GRASS) image with contrast similar to T2W image but with prominent low signal in posterior column white matter similar to T1W image.

thoracic pressure are communicated to the spinal subarachnoid space by way of these veins and affect CSF pressure. The presence of these veins also acts as a damper to CSF oscillation, which is reduced in the lumbar region compared to the cervical level. The second important aspect of the vertebral veins is the network of interconnections with the azygos system, Bateson's plexus, which provides a parallel drainage channel bypassing superior and inferior vena cava systems. Pelvic carcinomas, particularly of the prostate gland, are believed to spread throughout the vertebral column by entry into this plexus of veins.

Normal Spinal Cord MR

The signal from within the spinal cord directly reflects water content and relaxation times of white matter and gray matter in axial T2W and T2*/proton density-weighted variable flip angle/gradient-echo images. The central gray matter is seen as an H-shaped high signal area surrounded by low signal in the white matter tracts (see Figure 3-4). However, on T1W SE images, low signal in the central gray and high signal in the surrounding white matter are not seen, as might be expected from their relative water content or from brain MR. Instead, intermediate signal is seen in most of the cord cross-section and low signal is seen in the white matter of the posterior (dorsal) and lateral columns. These white matter regions are also seen as low signal on T2W and variable flip angle/gradient-echo images (see Figure 3-4). The physical basis of this signal pattern is not clear. Low proton density in white matter would partially explain low signal on both T1W and T2W images. If we assume that signal from white matter is not from the lipids in myelin but from the water protons adjacent to myelin membranes, as is the case in the brain,[26] signal may be low because water content is relatively low. Experimentally, low signal in the posterior columns is seen on axial MR images (1.5 Tesla) of cadaver cord in regions with slightly denser staining for white matter (especially fasciculus cuneatus of the cervical cord) (Figure 3-3). This is consistent with partial displacement of signal-producing water protons by myelin. Another possible explanation is that the acceleration of water T1 and T2 produced by myelin lipids affects images more through the shortening of T2 than T1. This could result in low signal in areas of very short T2 on the T1W images because of the use of a SE for signal acquisition. The SE produces sensitivity to tissue T2 differences or T2 weighting even on short TR images (e.g., with a T2 of 5 msec, little signal would be produced by a SE at 25 msec, five times the T2). This effect may be more prominent at high magnetic field because of the preferential shortening of T2 (via T2*) through magnetic susceptibility inhomogenieties (microgradients) created by myelin lipids. T2* acceleration best explains the very low signal seen in posterior column white matter on variable flip angle/gradient echo images at high field (Figure 3-4). Thus, low proton density and short T2 may combine to produce low signal in dense myelin, where membrane lipids cause marked shortening of relaxation times in a small population of interstitial water protons. A third possible explanation is that there are paramagnetic substances in these white matter regions such as stored ferric iron (Fe^{3+}) or melanin. A paramagnetic substance isolated from direct water proton interaction (e.g., Fe^{3+} within ferritin) might preferentially accelerate T2* through a magnetic susceptibility effect without significantly shortening T1. However, preliminary studies of cadaver spinal cord show no histologic evidence (Perls' and hematoxylin and eosin [H&E] stains) for iron or melanin in regions corresponding to low signal white matter on MR images at 1.5 Tesla* (see Figure 3-3).

Sagittal T2W and variable flip angle/gradient echo images of the cord generally show homogeneous intermediate to low signal throughout the cord, compared to the high signal of CSF. T2W and variable flip angle/gradient echo sagittal images in the midline may show a thin (approximately 1 mm), longitudinal stripe of high signal along the midpoint of the cord silhouette (Figure 3-5). This represents signal from the central, midline gray matter (intermediate gray commissures, Rexed region X) that surrounds the central canal. Gray matter in ventral horns may be included in this signal by partial volume averaging, depending on slice thickness and position relative to the midline. The central canal is not seen directly (normal diameter, 0.05 mm) except when pathologically enlarged (hydromyelia). Midline sagittal T1W images do not

*Unpublished data courtesy of Robert L. DeLapaz.

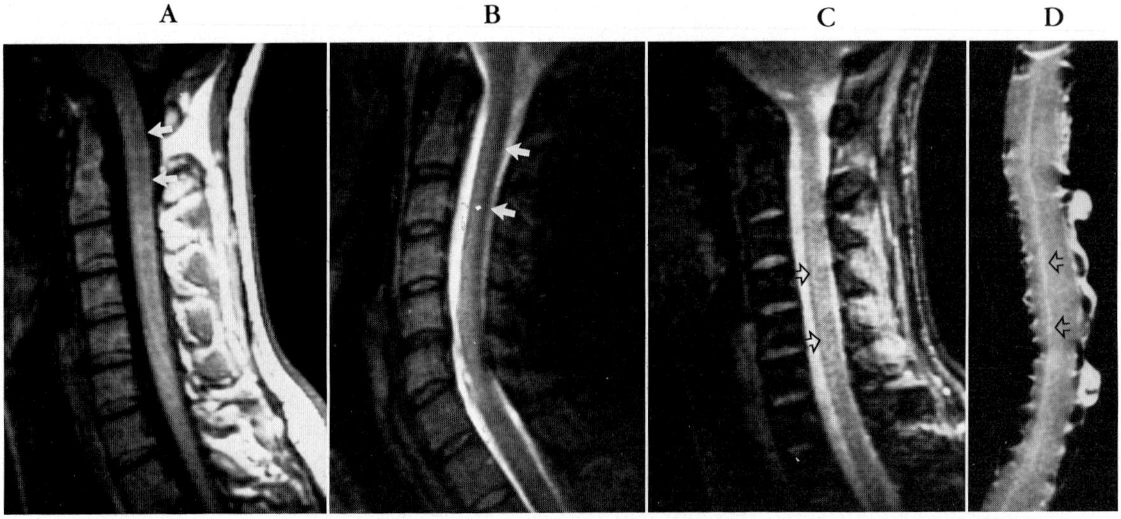

FIGURE 3-5. Sagittal MR of the spinal cord. **A,** Sagittal T1W image of cervical spinal cord with low signal in posterior columns *(arrows)*. **B,** Sagittal T2W image of cervical spinal cord. Low signal is also seen in posterior columns *(arrows)*. CSF motion artifact is present anterior to cord at C_6-C_7. **C,** Sagittal variable flip angle/gradient echo (GRASS) image of cervical spinal cord. Thin longitudinal high signal line corresponds to gray commissures of central cord *(arrows)*. Signal from gray matter in ventral horns may be included in this high signal by partial volume averaging, depending on slice thickness and position. **D,** Sagittal T2W image of cadaver cord specimen. Prominent longitudinal high signal line corresponds to gray commissures of central cord *(arrows)* and, possibly, partial volume averaging of ventral horns.

show a corresponding thin strip of low signal in the center of the cord. Instead, a wide low signal band is seen in the posterior half of the cord (see Figure 3-5). Suggested explanations for this low signal band have included two unlikely causes: central gray matter (inconsistent with axial T1W images) and CSF in the central canal (unlikely, considering the small diameter of the normal central canal and the posterior position of the band). Two forms of artifact may produce longitudinal low or high signal stripes in the central cord under special circumstances: Gibbs artifact (with a coarse image matrix and large pixel size) and phase shift artifact (a mismapped "phase-ghost" image of oscillatory CSF superimposed on the cord in images without flow compensation) (see Chapter 1). The most likely explanation for the longitudinal band on high resolution, flowcompensated T1W images is low signal in the posterior column white matter, corresponding to low signal seen on T1W axial images. Subtle changes in the normal internal architecture of the cord may be seen in ischemic, inflammatory, demyelinating, and early neoplastic disease of the cord.

The outer dimensions of the spinal cord are accurately demonstrated on high resolution, flow-compensated sagittal and axial MR images. T1W images often show the cord margins best because of high contrast against CSF and minimal CSF motion artifacts. In images with improper or no flow compensation, the cord margins may be obscured by CSF motion artifacts. Cord margins may also be obscured by isointense signal in static boundary-layer CSF on T2W or variable flip angle/gradient echo images (see Chapters 1 and 2).

INTERVERTEBRAL DISC

Anatomy

The intervertebral disc is made up of two major components, the central, gelatinous nucleus pulposus and the peripheral fibrous anulus fibrosus (see Figure 3-6). The nucleus is composed of a soft, pulpy, highly elastic material that is an embryologic remnant of the primitive notochord. Histologically, this material is made up of a fine loosely organized mesh of fibrous ele-

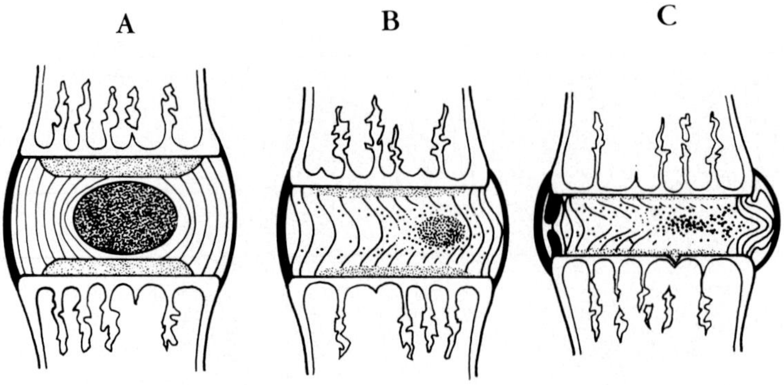

FIGURE 3-6. Intervertebral disc changes with aging and degeneration. **A,** Normal young adult intervertebral disc with well-defined nucleus pulposus, intact anular fibers, and generous cartilaginous end-plates. **B,** Aging disc shows progressive disorganization of nucleus pulposus, splitting of inner anulus fibers, and narrowing of disc space. **C,** Degenerated disc shows severe disorganization of nucleus pulposus and splitting of anulus fibers with bulging of disc margins and osteophyte formation. (Modified from Pritzker KPH. Aging and degeneration in the lumbar intervertebral disc. Orthop Clin North Am 1977; 8(1): 65.)

ments embedded in a gelatinous matrix.[24] A denser fibrous collection, oriented horizontally, is found in the central disc, which becomes more prominent with aging and conforms to the position of the embryonic fissure separating sclerotomes in the perichordal disc.[6] At the superior and inferior margins of the disc, on the bony surface of the vertebral end plates, there are thin (1 mm) cribriform layers of hyalin cartilage. The perforations in this cartilage provide a pathway for diffusion of metabolites and water through the vertebral end plates.[14] The fibers of the nucleus pulposus are more organized adjacent to these chondral plates and become embedded in the cartilage to provide attachment for the nucleus.[24] The nucleus is situated eccentrically within the anulus toward the posterior margin of the disc. The histologic difference between the nucleus and anulus is clear in the healthy disc, but no structural interface is present. The concentrically oriented fibrous lamina of the anulus interlace in a vertical X pattern between the vertebral end plates. The anulus is attached to the margins of the vertebrae at slightly raised traction apophyses by short Sharpey's fiber extensions of the outer lamina.[24]

The disc undergoes marked anatomic change with aging. The nucleus pulposus in infancy is a slightly flattened spheroid of clear gel. During the first two decades, a more fibrous collagen matrix develops that merges with the anulus fibrosus peripherally and progressively encroaches on the central gelatinous nucleus. In the young healthy disc there is a sharp transition between nucleus and anulus that becomes less distinct with aging. During the next several decades, nuclear involution occurs, with progressive loss of water content and fragmentation. As the reduction of the nuclear material progresses, the disc becomes a mass of fibrous tissue. With further aging, in the fifties and sixties, multiple radial fissures develop in the thinned-out, bulging disc anulus. This bulging elevates the periosteum from the vertebral bodies at the disc margin, leading to osteophytic spurring. The degenerated disc represents the extreme endpoint of this aging process. In the degenerated disc, the nucleus pulposus is a combination of necrotic debris, fibrocartilage, and gelatinous residue. The cartilaginous end-plate is indistinguishable from the nucleus. The anulus fibrosis is disorganized, especially in the inner layers, with cartilaginous metaplasia, desiccation, and development of marked concentric and radial fissures through which nuclear material may herniate.[5,25]

Anatomic changes in the neural foramina accompany aging and degeneration of the intervertebral disc. These changes are seen most easily in the lumbar spine (Figures 3-7 and 3-8). As disc height is lost, posterior bulging of the disc anulus and associated marginal vertebral body hypertrophy encroach on the inferior neural foramen, impinging primarily on vascular

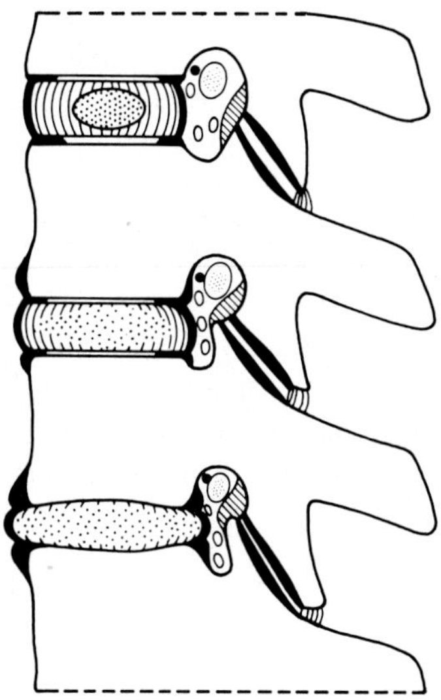

FIGURE 3-7. Neural foramen changes with aging and degeneration. **A,** Normal disc with intact nucleus pulposus, anulus fibrosus, apophyseal rings, and cartilaginous end-plates. Spinal nerve *(speckled)* is positioned in superior part of neural foramen with sinuvertebral nerve (recurrent sensory and autonomic fibers) *(solid)* and radicular artery ventral and radicular veins inferior to it. Ligamentum flavum *(striped)* lies ventral to the facet joint. **B,** With aging, disc height is reduced and nuclear and anular degeneration cause posterior disc margin to impinge on structures in inferior part of the neural foramen. Hypertrophy and superior displacement of superior articular process of facet (projecting from the inferior vertebral body) with ligamentum flavum hypertrophy impinge on contents of superior part of the neural foramen. Osteophytic hypertrophy of vertebral bodies also occurs at anular attachments. **C,** Severe degeneration of disc and facet produce severe crowding of neural foramen contents with direct nerve root compression in extreme cases.

structures. Facet elements, especially the superior articular process (forming the inferior facet surface) hypertrophy and dislocate slightly to encroach on the superior neural foramen. Eventually, these structures may impinge on the exiting spinal nerves in the superior foramen and, combined with disc herniation and lateral recess narrowing, cause radicular symptoms.

Water Content

The fibrocartilage forming the intervertebral disc varies in water content from a high level in the central nucleus pulposus to a low level at the disc margin in the anulus fibrosus. Fibrocartilage is a dense connective tissue with poorly defined margins where typical cartilage cells and pericellular matrix (ground substance) are found among abundant fibrous elements. Collagen fibers and elastic fibers are randomly distributed in the matrix of the higher water content central nucleus and become progressively more organized into a concentric lamellar pattern in the peripheral anulus where fibrous elements predominate. The matrix and chondrocyte intracellular water comprise the major water-containing structures within the intervertebral disc. This matrix is a highly proteinaceous solution of complex carbohydrates; chondromucoprotein, the main constituent, is a copolymer

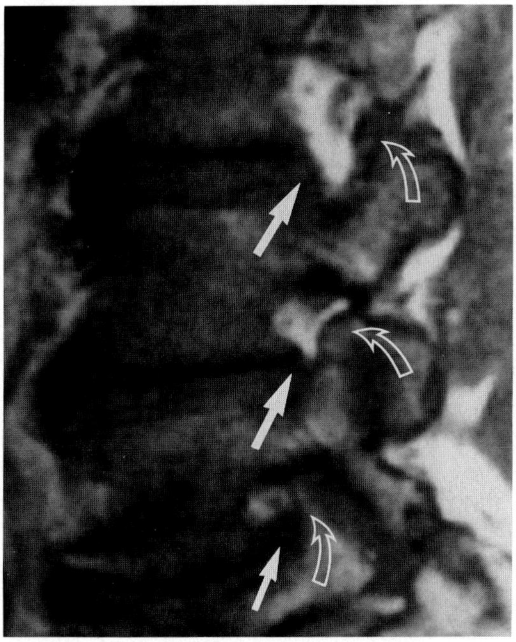

FIGURE 3-8. Disc and foramen changes with aging and degeneration. Sagittal T1W image of lumbar spine shows three stages of disc degeneration. Progressive loss of height is seen from superior disc through inferior disc *(arrows)*. Increasing encroachment on neural foramina by disc and posterior vertebral elements, especially hypertrophic facet structures *(open arrows)*, is also seen.

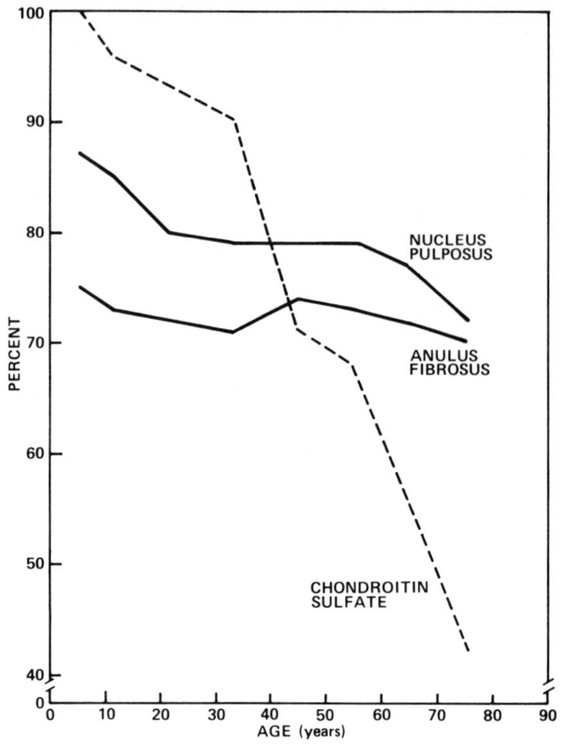

FIGURE 3-9. Disc water content changes with aging. Solid lines represent water content of intervertebral disc components as a percent of fresh weight. Dashed line represents relative chondroitin sulfate content of nucleus pulposus (as indicated by galactosamine content in proteinpolysaccharide light fraction). (Adapted from Gower WE. Age-related variations in protein polysaccharides from human nucleus pulposus, anulus fibrosus, and costal cartilage. J Bone Joint Surg 1969; 51-A(6):1154.)

of a mucoprotein core with 15 to 20 polysaccharide side chains. The side chains are formed by chondroitin sulfate (a galactosamine and glucuronic acid polymer) and keratosulfate (a polymer of alternating units of galactose and glucosamine).[5,22] Relaxation properties of this material are similar to a highly proteinaceous fluid, with a slight additional relaxation enhancement by strongly acidic sulfate groups.[17]

With aging, the water content decreases from a high in the young disc of 90% of fresh weight to approximately 70% in the aged or degenerated disc[15] (Figure 3-9). The anulus has significantly less water than the nucleus but also shows a decrease with aging from approximately 78% in the young to 70% in the aged or degenerated disc.[15] The nucleus changes histologically from a viscous hydrostatic structure in the young to a desiccated fibrous mass, with altered collagen and noncollagenous protein. Combined with this loss of the gelatinous nucleus pulposus, there is a progressive fibrocartilaginous metamorphosis of the anulus fibrosus. The result is a loss of distinction between nucleus and anulus associated with an overall decrease in water content.[25] The inner layers of the anulus blend with the disorganized fibrocartilage of the nucleus and the outer layers are split by deposits of ground substance.[15] The end stage of this process is a degenerated disc that is a mix of necrosis, fibrocartilage, and gelatinous residue.

Biochemistry

The biochemical explanation for age-related changes in the disc is based on the physical properties of the major mucopolysaccharide with its chondroitin sulfate and keratosulfate side chains. The chondroitin sulfate side chains have net negative charges at normal pH, which cause the macromolecule to be spread out by mutual repulsion of these branches. Adjacent mucopolysaccharides become intermeshed and the resultant extracellular fluid space of the nucleus pulposus is dominated by their interlocking domains.[25] Water and small molecules (e.g., glucose and urea) diffuse through this macromolecular milieu allowing avascular maintenance of nutrition and waste disposal. Solvent trapped between these macromolecules is extremely difficult to squeeze out because its removal would force negative charges together. In the healthy disc, this negatively charged gel resists compression (as much as 1600 lbs.) and also shows a tendency to imbibe water against a pressure gradient (as much as 250 mm Hg), to maximize separation of the side chains.[5] With aging, proteoglycan content of the nucleus pulposus decreases and the ratio of keratin sulfate to chondroitin sulfate increases due to a decline in the chondroitin sulfate.[15] There is a one- to two-fold decrease in the length of the negatively charged chondroitin sulfate side chains, resulting in reduced ability to resist compression and imbibe water. The loss of gel properties of the nucleus transfers mechanical stress to the fibrocartilaginous anulus, accelerating its degeneration.[5,22] The direct role of the decline in chondroitin sulfate on MR appearance of the aging disc has not been defined but might be expected to cause

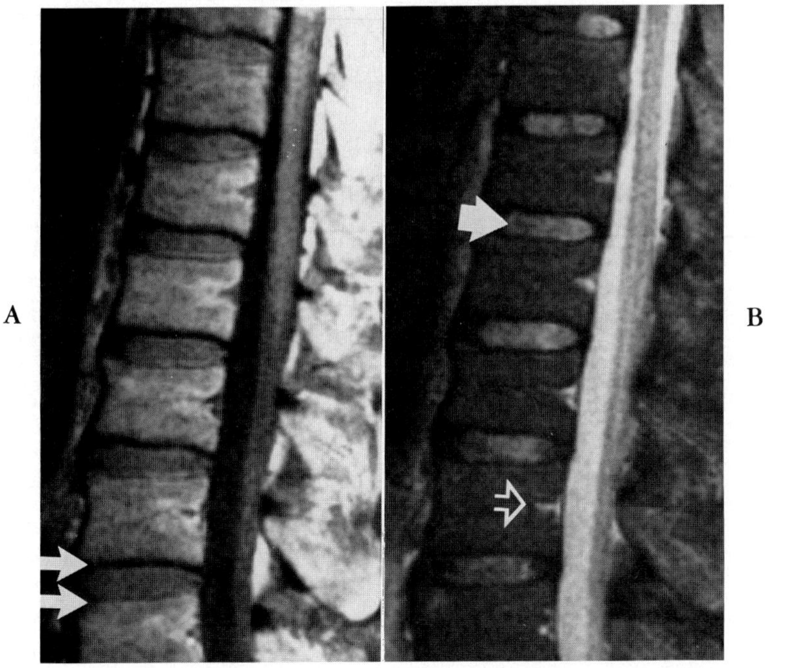

FIGURE 3-10. Sagittal MR of intervertebral disc. **A,** T1W sagittal image of the thoracolumbar spine. Uniform, intermediate intensity signal is seen in all intervertebral discs, which are of normal height. Low signal in posterior, outer anulus blends with low signal in posterior longitudinal ligament, dura, and CSF. Asymmetry of low signal at vertebral end-plates, wide superiorly and narrow inferiorly *(arrows)*, is caused by chemical shift artifact at fat-water interface between marrow and disc. **B,** T2W sagittal image of the thoracolumbar spine. High signal is seen in intervertebral discs with central intranuclear cleft at several levels *(arrow)*. A wider band of low signal is seen in anterior disc anulus than posteriorly, reflecting normal eccentric, posterior position of nucleus pulposus. Triangular high signal in posterior vertebral bodies represents entry point of basivertebral veins *(open arrow)*.

slight prolongation of relaxation times because of the reduction in acidic sulfate groups. The declining water content in the nucleus and anulus is the critical determinant of the MR appearance of aging and degenerated discs.

Intervertebral Disc MR

The typical appearance of the disc on MR is low signal on T1W and high signal on T2W images reflecting the high water content and long relaxation times of the disc compared to the adjacent bone marrow[23] (Figure 3-10). In the normal disc, the decrease in water content radially from the central nucleus to the anulus is seen as a decline in signal on T2W images. The transition is relatively sharp in the young disc and becomes less distinct with aging and degeneration. The indistinct separation of the nucleus and anulus in the older disc reflects a progressively wider zone of fibrosis between the gelatinous nucleus and the fibrous anulus. The thickness of low signal in the normal anulus on sagittal images is often greater anteriorly, reflecting the normal eccentric, posterior position of the nucleus pulposus. A central, horizontal line of low signal is seen on T2W sagittal images (reminiscent of contrast diskograms) in over 90% of patients more than 30 years old.[1] This intranuclear cleft probably represents degenerative fibrosis along the course of the embryonic fissure separating sclerotomes in the primitive notochord.[6] At the outermost margin of the disc, low signal is seen on both T1W and T2W images. This represents the dense fibrous bands of the outer anulus and, along the posterior disc margin, the fibrous posterior longitudinal ligament, which cannot be distinguished from the outer anulus.

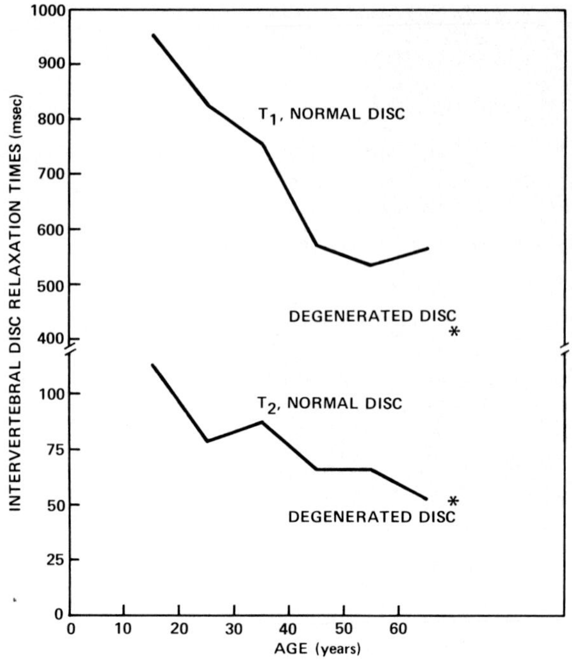

FIGURE 3-11. Disc T_1 and T_2 changes with aging and degeneration. Measurements of T_1 and T_2 in central disc on sagittal images at 0.26 Tesla in 107 normal *(solid lines)* and 18 surgically confirmed degenerated discs *(asterisks)*. Differences between T_1 of normal and degenerated discs were statistically significant at all ages. Differences between T_2 of normal and degenerated discs were significant until seventh decade. (Adapted from Jenkins JPR, et al. MR imaging of the intervertebral disc: a quantitative study. BR J Radiol 1985; 58:705.)

The superior and inferior margins of the disc are also low signal in T1W and T2W images, representing the low proton density of the vertebral end-plates. The hyalin cartilage at the end-plate is not seen as a distinct structure. On images with the frequency encoding gradient oriented parallel to the long axis of the spine, the thickness of the low signal at the two end-plates may appear asymmetrical; wide at one end-plate, narrow at the other. This is caused by the chemical shift artifact at the fat-water interface between vertebral marrow and disc. It is often more prominent on T1W images because of the high signal in marrow fat (see Figure 3-10).

With aging and degeneration, the decrease in water content of the nucleus is paralleled by decrease in both T1 and T2 relaxation times[18] (Figure 3-11). The effect of declining water content and relaxation times is most apparent on T2W images where older and degenerated discs show markedly lower signal than healthy discs.

VERTEBRAL BONE MARROW

Water and Fat Content

Bone marrow may be divided into red (active, hematopoietic) and yellow (inactive, fatty) marrow. Normal active myeloid tissue consists of a spongelike, gelatinous framework or stroma, which is intimately connected with blood vessels and has free cells within it. These cells consist of primitive and phagocytic reticular cells attached to agyrophilic fibers. A distinguishing characteristic of this stroma is the constant presence of fat stores within the reticulocytes. In the normal adult over age 30, 40% to 60% of vertebral red marrow volume is occupied by fat.[13] In yellow marrow, fat occupies most of the tissue. With prolonged starvation or wasting diseases the fat may acquire a peculiar gelatinous appearance known as serous fat atrophy.[4] Between fat cells in yellow marrow there are only blood vessels, reticular fibers, scattered fixed macrophages, and primitive reticular cells. The latter are probably the main local source of new blood cells when the yellow marrow is transformed back into red marrow during periods of increased hematopoietic demand. Small nodules of lymphatic tissue also occur regularly in the bone marrow.[4]

Changes with Aging

In the embryo and newborn, only red marrow is found. With aging the red marrow is progressively converted to yellow marrow, so that in the normal adult approximately equal amounts of red and yellow marrow are found distributed throughout the body. This conversion progresses from the distal to the proximal appendicular skeleton. Vertebrae, ribs, sternum, diploe, and often the proximal epiphyses of the femur and humerus contain red marrow in the adult. In addition to this redistribution of red and yellow marrow there is a slow increase in the fat content of vertebral marrow with aging. In a study of the L_2 vertebral body marrow in 109 cadaver specimens, red marrow, as a percentage of vertebral body volume, declined by nearly half (60% to 30%) betweeen the first de-

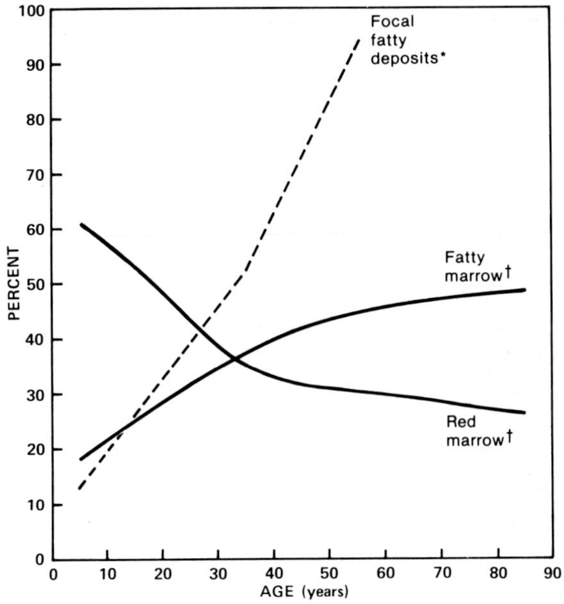

FIGURE 3-12. Vertebral bone marrow changes with aging. Solid lines represent mean values for red (hematopoietic) and fatty (yellow) marrow as a percent of vertebral body volume, measured at L_2 in 109 cadaver specimens. Dashed line represents percent of 72 patients with 0.5 to 1.5 cm diameter focal fatty deposits (high signal on T1W images at 1.5 Tesla) on MRI of cervical, thoracic, and lumbar spine. (*Data from Hajek PC, et al. Focal fat deposition in axial bone marrow: MR characteristics. Radiology 1987; 162:245. †Data from Dunnill MS, et al. Quantitative histologic studies on age changes in bone. J Path Bact 1967; 94:275.)

cade and the eighth decade. Fatty marrow more than doubled during this period from 20% to 50% (Figure 3-12). No differences were seen between males and females.[13] And no difference in rates of conversion in the different levels of the spine were observed.[21]

Normal Bone Marrow MR

MR signal in vertebral bodies is produced by both water and fat protons in marrow. The high fat content of normal adult marrow produces relatively short relaxation times resulting in high signal on T1W images and low signal on T2W images compared to the normal intervertebral disc and CSF (see Figure 3-10). Normal adult marrow at 0.35 Tesla shows T1 relaxation times of approximately 500 msec and T2 relaxation times of approximately 55 msec.[11] T2 relaxation times are close to those of fatty tissue elsewhere in the body, but the T1 is considerably longer than the subcutaneous fat T1 of approximately 250 msec at the same field strength.[12] This difference is probably a result of the contribution of both fat and water protons to MR signal from the marrow (Figure 3-13). The presence of paramagnetic ferric iron (Fe^{3+}) in transferrin, ferritin, and hemosiderin may also contribute to the relatively short relaxation times seen in normal marrow. Ferric iron within ferritin should have an effect that is most prominent on T2W images through acceleration of T2* caused by magnetic susceptibility gradient effects. Experimentally, the ferric iron core of ferritin produces little T1 relaxation enhancement while causing a marked enhancement of T2 relaxation.[20] The separate contributions of water and lipid protons can be identified or enhanced with special pulse sequences that suppress water or fat signal. Examples of signal suppression in Figure 3-13 illustrate water-suppressed images with uniform lack of signal in discs with high signal from fat in the bone marrow. Conversely, the fat-suppressed image shows high signal from water in the discs and reduced but not absent, intermediate signal from marrow, indicating only partial suppression of the net signal from marrow. Normal marrow appears relatively homogeneous, without a trabecular pattern, because the small volume of low proton density trabecular bone is dominated by marrow signal (a partial volume averaging effect). However, the presence of trabecular bone may contribute to reduced signal on T2W images at high field through magnetic susceptibility gradients at the multiple marrow-bone interfaces resulting in T2* acceleration.[11] A more recent study at 0.26T of 66 patients with degenerative disc disease, aged 14 to 77 years, using a different method of relaxation time calculation, showed isolated declines in T1 but an overall less precise correlation between vertebral body relaxation times and age (both T1 and T2).[18a] Dense cortical bone at the vertebral margins is seen as low signal on T1 and T2W images. Chemical shift artifact at the fat-water (marrow-disc) interface of the vertebral end-plate may obscure or widen the low signal cortical margin, as previously noted (Figure 3-10).

As fat content increases in aging vertebral marrow, a parallel decline in relaxation times

A B C D

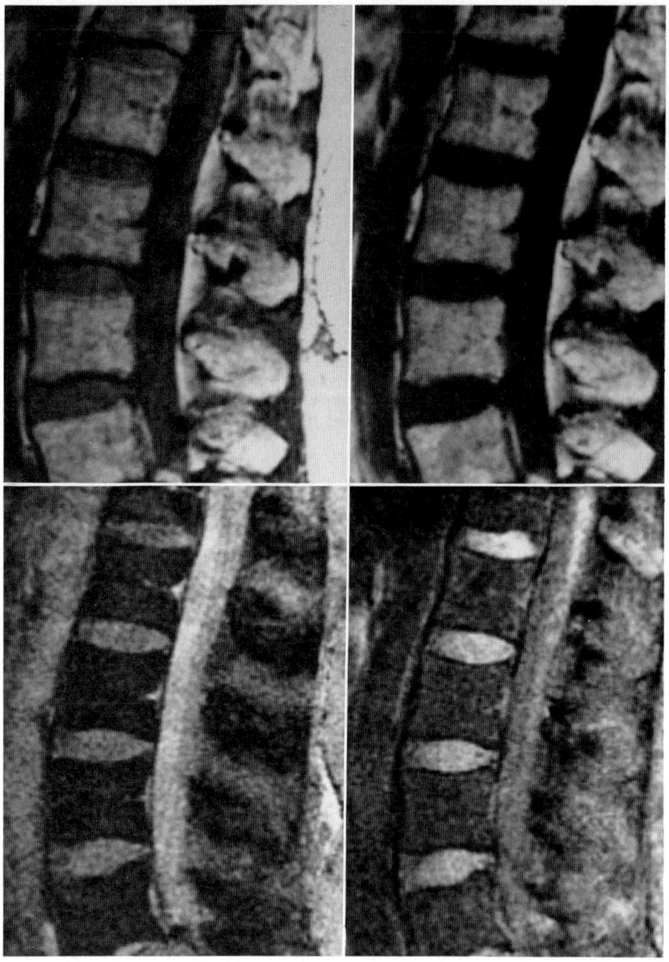

FIGURE 3-13. Fat and water suppression. **A,** Sagittal T1W image of lumbar spine. **B,** Sagittal water-suppressed image shows lack of signal from water in discs and CSF with prominent signal from fat in the vertebral bodies. **C,** Sagittal T2W image of lumbar spine. **D,** Sagittal fat-suppressed image shows prominent signal from water in discs and conus and intermediate signal from vertebral bodies and posterior spinal elements. CSF signal is reduced by motion effects.

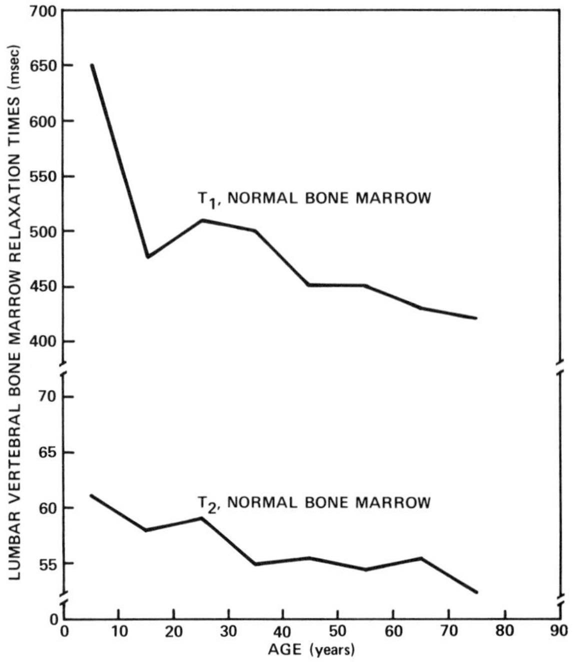

FIGURE 3-14. Vertebral bone marrow T_1 and T_2 changes with aging. T_1 and T_2 relaxation times of lumbar vertebral bone marrow measured on MR images at 0.35 Tesla in 212 patients. (Adapted from data in Dooms GC, et al.: Bone marrow imaging: magnetic resonance studies related to age and sex. Radiology 1985; 155:429.)

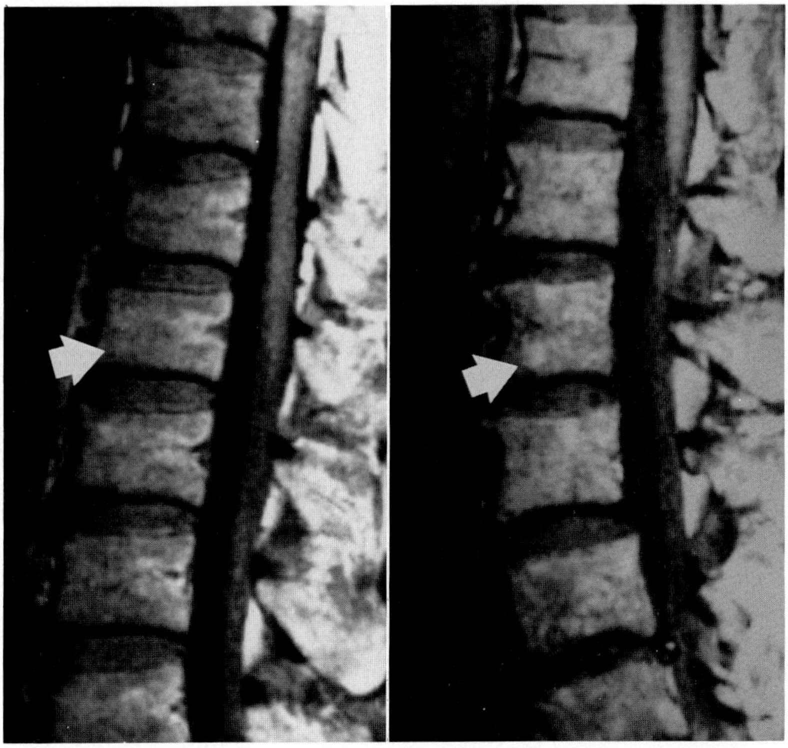

FIGURE 3-15. **A,** Sagittal T1W image of 42-year-old male shows uniform signal in marrow of anterior vertebral bodies *(arrow)*. Higher signal fatty changes are present adjacent to basivertebral veins. **B,** Sagittal T1W image of 63-year-old female shows multiple high signal foci *(arrow)* representing focal fatty deposits in aging vertebral marrow.

occurs. A study of 212 patients in three age groups (1 to 10, 21 to 40, and 51+ years), performed at 0.35 T, showed a decline in T1 from 652 to 427 msec and a decline in T2 from 61 to 54 msec[11] (Figure 3-14). The effect of these changes on MR images is a steady increase in marrow signal on T1W images and a decline in signal on T2W images. No overall difference between males and females is seen although the decline in T2 may be slower in older females because of accelerated loss of trabecular bone.[11]

Focal areas of fatty replacement (0.5 to 1.5 cm diameter) are also seen in normal marrow with increasing age. MR studies of cadaver spines have shown that areas of histologic fatty replacement correspond to high signal on T1W images and intermediate to low signal on T2W images.[16] In one series of 159 MR studies, a clear increase in the frequency of focal fatty marrow with age was seen. These marrow changes were present in only 13% of cases in ages 0 to 10 years, 52% in ages 31 to 40 years, and 93% in ages 51 to 60 years[16] (Figures 3-12 and 3-15). No difference between the sexes or between cervical, thoracic, or lumbar levels was seen. The pathogenesis of these focal changes is probably local ischemia in marrow resulting in degeneration and fatty replacement of functional red marrow.[16] A similar mechanism is probably also responsible for focal fatty changes at vertebral end-plates adjacent to degenerated discs—*discogenic vertebral sclerosis*[29] (Figure 3-16). An MR study of 58 degenerated discs at 1.5 Tesla showed abnormalities of the adjacent end-plates in 50%.[9] In 24 degenerated discs, MR showed high signal on T1W and T2W images, which is consistent with fatty marrow change and possibly hemorrhage and edema in nonhematopoietic marrow. Plain films showed normal vertebral bodies. One case showed low signal on both T1W and T2W images with sclerosis on plain films. Four studies showed low signal on T1W and high signal on T2W images. This finding is nonspecific and may be seen with infection or

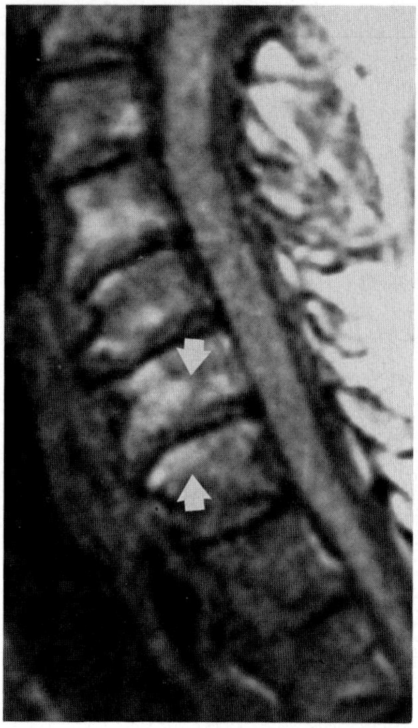

FIGURE 3-16. Vertebral marrow change with degenerative disc disease. Sagittal T1W image of cervical spine shows high signal "discogenic" changes in the marrow adjacent to degenerated discs *(arrows)*.

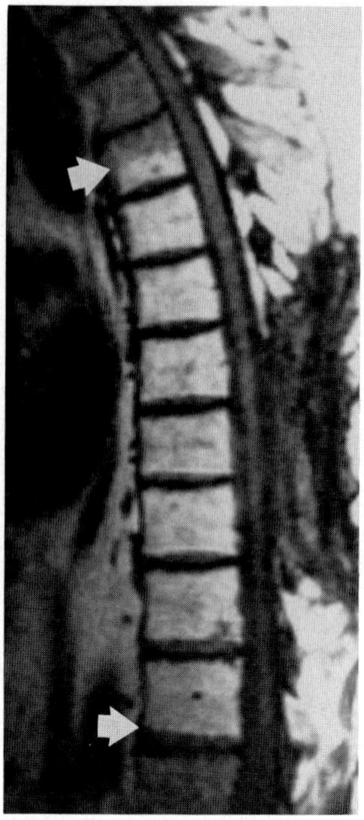

FIGURE 3-17. Bone marrow radiation change. High signal in vertebral marrow on sagittal T1W image represents radiation-induced fatty change, which conforms precisely to margins of the treatment port *(arrows)*.

metastatic tumor. The presence of the adjacent degenerated disc makes infectious discitis unlikely, and metastases restricted to the end-plate are unusual.

Abnormal Bone Marrow MR: Increased Fat

The precursors of blood cells are especially sensitive to ionizing radiation. The decrease in hematopoiesis resulting from irradiation occurs because of an inhibition in mitoses. The net effect on marrow histology is to decrease the proportion of active, red marrow and increase the amount of inactive, yellow marrow in the irradiated regions.[3] High signal on T1W images, consistent with fatty marrow change, has been reported in marrow exposed to 4000 to 5790 rad (40 to 57.9 Gy) at 2 months to 10 years after irradiation[27] (Figure 3-17). This high signal is very homogeneous and appears to be a permanent change in the marrow. Experimental histopathologic studies of irradiated marrow suggest that fatty marrow degeneration may be seen on MR images within weeks after as little as 2000 rad (20 Gy).[27] Other conditions that can result in conversion of normal vertebral hematopoietic marrow to fatty marrow that may appear on T1W images include decreases in intramedullary blood supply (focal fatty change), starvation, aplastic anemia, and chemotherapy.[4,7,16,19]

Focal high signal on T1W images accompanied by high signal on T2W images is characteristic of benign intravertebral hemangiomas. Histologically, these lesions are composed of angiomatous elements mixed with abundant adipose tissue in a region of thickened trabeculation.[28]

Abnormal Bone Marrow MR: Decreased Fat

Replacement of normal marrow by high water-content tissue produces lower signal on T1W images and higher signal on T2W images.

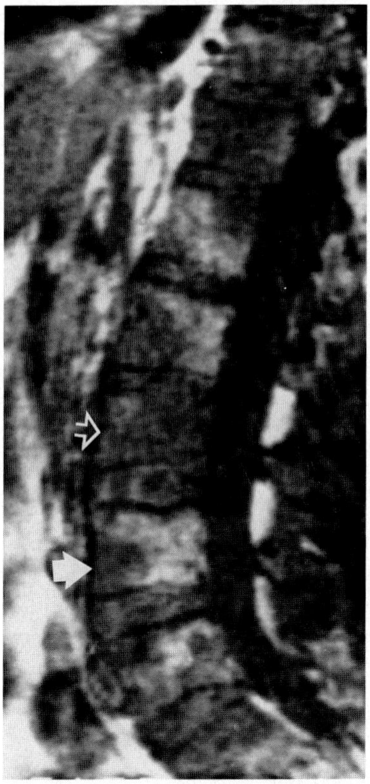

FIGURE 3-18. Extensive metastases. Extensive metastatic replacement of normal marrow by breast carcinoma is seen on this T1W sagittal image as irregular low signal within high signal normal marrow *(arrow)* and as complete replacement of vertebral marrow *(open arrow)*.

This signal pattern is most frequently seen with focal metastatic tumor, but may also be seen diffusely throughout the marrow with myelophthisic disorders such as multiple myeloma, myelofibrosis, and extensive metastatic disease. The most frequent metastatic tumors to the spine (breast, lung, and prostate) all show similar focal low signal on T1W images with isointense to high signal on T2W images[8] (Figure 3-18). The ratio of relaxation times in the lesion to those in normal marrow may be helpful in separating malignent from nonneoplastic lesions.[31] Marrow in the central vertebral body and pedicles is most frequently involved. T1W images generally provide more consistent sensitivity and higher conspicuity against normal marrow than T2W images.[8] Marrow replacement on T1W images shows focal low signal with osteogenic sarcoma metastases, diffuse patchy low signal with leukemia, and uniform low signal with neuroblastoma.[7] In circumstances of accelerated red cell loss, such as with sickle cell anemia, inactive, fatty marrow is converted to active, red marrow and signal is diffusely reduced on T1W images.[19]

Hemochromatosis: Increased Iron

The majority of iron in marrow is within erythrocyte hemoglobin, with smaller smounts of ferric iron associated with plasma transferrin, ferritin, and hemosiderin. The presence of this paramagnetic material may contribute to the relatively short relaxation times seen in normal marrow. The effect of this material is especially pronounced in hemochromatosis when excess iron in ferritin is deposited in the liver and bone marrow. MR images of vertebral marrow show very low signal on T2W images with less effect on T1W images. This suggests that the mechanism of the ferritin effect is via magnetic susceptibility inhomogeneity, preferentially shortening T2 and T2*.[20,26]

REFERENCES

1. Aguila LA, Piraino DW, Modic MT, et al. The intranuclear cleft of the intervertebral disk: magnetic resonance imaging. Radiology 1985; 155:155.
2. Beall PT, Amtey SR, Kasturi SR. NMR data handbook for biomedical applications. New York: Pergamon Press, 1984.
3. Bloom MA. Bone Marrow. In: Bloom W, ed. Histopathology of irradiation from external and internal sources, National nuclear energy series, vol 22-I. New York: McGraw-Hill, 1948.
4. Bloom W, Fawcett DW. A textbook of histology, ed 9. Philadelphia: WB Saunders, 1968.
5. Brown MD. The pathophysiology of disc disease. Orthop Clin North Am 1971; 2(2):359.
6. Clarke LP, Schnitzlein HN, Murtagh FR, et al. MRI: imaging anatomy of the lumboscaral spine. Magn Reson Imaging 1986; 4:515.
7. Cohen MD, Klatte EC, Baehner R, et al. Magnetic resonance imaging of bone marrow disease in children. Radiology 1984; 151:715.
8. Daffner RH, Lupetin AR, Dash N, et al. MRI in the detection of malignant infiltration of bone marrow. AJR 1986; 146:353.
9. De Roos A, Kressel H, Spritzer C, et al. MR imaging of marrow changes adjacent to end plates in degenerative lumbar disk disease. AJR 1987; 149:531.
10. Djinjian R. Vascular malformations. In: Shapiro R, Myelography, ed 4. Chicago: Year Book Medical Publishers, 1984.
11. Dooms GC, Fisher MR, Hricak H, et al. Bone marrow imaging: magnetic resonance studies related to age and sex. Radiology 1985; 155:429.

12. Dooms GC, Hricak H, Margulus AR, et al. MR imaging of fat. Radiology 1986; 158:51.
13. Dunnill MS, Anderson JA, Whitehead R. Quantitative histologic studies on age changes in bone. J Path Bact 1967; 94:275.
14. Eyring EJ. The biochemistry and physiology of the intervertebral disk. Clin Orthop 1969; 67:16.
15. Gower WE. Age-related variations in protein polysaccharides from human nucleus pulposus, anulus fibrosus, and costal cartilage. J Bone Joint Surg 1969; 51A(6):1154.
16. Hajek PC, Baker LL, Goobar JE, et al. Focal fat deposition in axial bone marrow: MR characteristics. Radiology 1987; 162:245.
17. James T. Nuclear Magnetic Resonance in Biochemistry. New York: Academic Press, 1975.
18. Jenkins JPR, Hickey DS, Machin M, et al. MR imaging of the intervertebral disc: a quantitative study. Br J Radiol 1985; 58:705.
18a. Jenkins JPR, Stehling M, Sivewright G, et al. Quantitative magnetic resonance imaging of verebral bodies: a T1 and T2 study, Magn Reson Imaging 7:17, 1989.
19. Kangarloo H, Dietrich RB, Taira RT, et al. MR imaging of bone marrow in children. JCAT 1986; 10(2):205.
20. Koening SH, Brown RD. Relaxometry of ferritin solutions and the influence of the Fe^{3+} core ions. Magn Reson Med 1986; 3:755.
21. Kricun ME. Red-yellow marrow conversion: its effect on the location of some solitary bone lesions. Skeletal Radiol 1985; 14:10.
22. Lipson SJ, Muir H. Proteoglycans in experimental intervertebral disc degeneration. Spine 1981; 6(3):194.
23. Modic MT, Pavlicek W, Weinstein MA, et al. Magnetic resonance imaging of intervertebral disk disease: clinical and pulse sequence considerations. Radiology 1984; 152:103.
24. Parke WW, Schiff DCM. The applied anatomy of the intervertebral disc. Orthop Clin North Am 1971; 2(2):309.
24a. Pelc NJ, Shmikawa A, Boyko OB. A method for mapping of T2' and for improved T2 measurements, Society of Magnetic Resonance in Medicine Abstracts, 7th Annual Meeting, p. 746, 1988.
25. Pritzker KPH. Aging and degeneration in the lumbar intervertebral disc. Orthop Clin North Am 1977; 8(1):65.
26. Pykett IL, Rosen BR. Nuclear magnetic resonance: in vivo proton chemical shift imaging. Radiology 1983; 149:197.
27. Ramsey RG, Zacharias CE. MR imaging of the spine after radiation therapy: easily recognized effects. AJNR 1985; 6:247.
28. Ross JS, Masaryk TJ, Modic MT, et al. Vertebral hemangiomas: MR imaging. Radiology 1987; 165:165.
29. Sobel D, Zyroff J, Thorne RP. Diskogenic vertebral sclerosis: MR imaging. J Comput Assist Tomogr 1987; 11(5):855.
30. Stark DD, Moseley ME, Bacon BR, et al. Magnetic resonance imaging and spectroscopy of hepatic iron overload. Radiology 1985; 154:137.
31. Sugimura K, Yamasaki K, Kitagaki H, et al. Bone marrow disease of the spine: differentiation with T1 and T2 relaxation times in MR imaging. Radiology 1987; 165:541.
32. Willis WD, Grossman RG. Medical neurobiology, ed 3. St Louis: CV Mosby Co, 1981.
33. Young IR, Khenia S, Thomas DGT, et al. Clinical magnetic susceptibility mapping of the brain. J Comput Assist Tomogr 1987; 11(1):2.

4

Atlas of Normal Anatomy

Robert L. DeLaPaz

This chapter is composed of full-page illustrations that serve as an introduction and a quick reference for normal anatomy of the spine. It is organized with the most frequently studied and more complex level of the spine presented first, the cervical, followed by the lumbar and thoracic levels. The section on the cervical spine discusses many structures in general terms that also apply to the lumbar and thoracic levels.

CERVICAL SPINE ANATOMY

The cervical spine is composed of two complex vertebrae, C_1 and C_2, which support the cranium and provide for rotation of the head, and five "conventional" vertebrae, C_3-C_7, which form a column with a moderate lordotic curvature in the typical supine MR imaging position. The lateral masses of the C_1 vertebral body, the *atlas*, support the cranium at the articular condyles of the basiocciput on either side of the foramen magnum. The ring shape of C_1 forms the superior part of the spinal canal and pivots around the *odontoid process*, or *dens*, of C_2 with head rotation. The C_2 vertebral body, the *axis* or *epistropheus*, articulates with the lateral masses of C_1 and projects the odontoid process superiorly in the midline. The anterior arch of C_1 articulates with the odontoid process at a synovial joint and is firmly secured to it by a complex set of ligaments (discussed later). The remaining cervical vertebral bodies are approximately rectangular in coronal and sagittal cross section with a cuplike depression on the superior surface, formed by lateral ridges of bone, the *uncinate processes*. The superior (cephalad) vertebral body sits on the intervertebral disc in this depression. The disc extends laterally and up between the superior vertebral body and the uncinate processes. By early adulthood this portion of the disc degenerates partially to form the *uncovertebral "joints" of Luschka*, which function as articular junctions between vertebrae but do not have the characteristics of true joints.[1,4,8] The disc is seen as moderately low signal on T1W images (lower than vertebral marrow, higher than muscle) and as moderately high signal (greater than marrow, lower than cerebrospinal fluid [CSF]) on T2W and variable flip angle/gradient echo images. The margins of the uncinate processes are compact bone and appear as low signal on all pulse sequences. This low signal allows the uncinate processes to be discriminated from higher signal disc on T2W and variable flip angle/gradient echo images. The base of the uncinate process often contains an extension of vertebral bone marrow (see Figures 4-5 to 4-7) and may appear isointense with disc on T1W images (e.g, SE 600-1000/20). Conversely, very low signal in the severely degenerated disc or in the normal disc on short TR T1W images (e.g., SE 200-400/20) may make the disc indistinguishable from the dense cortical portion of uncinate processes.

The posterior vertebral elements form the *neural arch*, which is composed of the pedicles, *articular pillars*, lamina, and spinous processes. The *pedicles* are relatively short and connect the vertebral body with the articular pillars, which lie between the facet joints. The *facet joints*, or *zygoapophyseal joints*, are arthrodial (gliding, planar) synovial joints with articular cartilage lining the superior and inferior surfaces. The joint is formed by bony processes projecting from the superior and inferior vertebral articular pillars that meet in an oblique coronal plane approximately 45 degrees from the vertical. This is closer to the axial plane than the lumbar and thoracic facets and, with more ligamentous laxity, allows a greater degree of anterior posterior sliding motion along the joint. Some confusion often arises concerning the use of the terms "superior" and "inferior" as they describe parts of the adjacent vertebrae or structures of the joint itself. The articular processes are named for their relationship to the vertebrae of origin so that the articular process projecting from the superior vertebra extends inferiorly and is therefore called the *inferior articular process*. The articular process projecting superiorly from the inferior vertebra is thus called the *superior articular process*. The joint surfaces are named for their relationship to the joint plane. The inferior articular process forms the superior surface of the facet joint, the *superior facet*. The superior articular process forms the inferior surface of the facet joint, the *inferior facet*. In axial images through the facets, because the superior joint surface lies posterior to the inferior surface, the posterior bony elements are part of the more superior neural arch (the inferior articular process) and the anterior elements are part of the inferior neural arch (the superior articular process) (see Figures 4-8 and 4-9). The signal from compact cortical bone immediately under the joint surfaces of the facets is low on T1W SE, T2W SE, and variable flip angle/gradient echo images. Higher signal from bone marrow is often seen on T1W SE images within the central lamina and articular process. The signal from marrow within these elements is lower on T2W SE images and is equal to cortical bone on T2*W variable flip angle/gradient echo images (see Figures 4-8 and 4-9). The signal from articular cartilage is usually low and barely distinguishable from the articular cortical bone on T1W and T2W SE images, whereas on T2*W variable angle/gradient echo images it is seen as high signal, clearly distinct from bone (see Figures 4-17 to 4-19). Fluid may accumulate in degenerated facet joints and can be seen as high signal on T2W SE and variable flip angle/gradient echo images.

The *lamina* of the neural arches project posteriorly and medially from the articular pillars to meet at the base of the spinous process in the midline. They form an ovoid cross section to the posterior cervical spinal canal paired with a more flattened anterior margin against the posterior vertebral body and intervertebral discs. Measurements of the anteroposterior (AP) dimensions of the spinal canal, thecal sac, and spinal cord on MR images agree closely with those from plain film, myelography, and CT scanning. The average AP diameter of the bony *spinal canal* tapers slightly from approximately 18 to 20 mm at C_1 to C_2 to 15 to 17 mm from C_3 through C_7.[4,9] The *thecal sac* AP diameter is 10 to 14 mm and the spinal cord is 6 to 9 mm through the cervical region.[6,10] These dimensions vary in concert so that the normal cervical spinal cord diameter is approximately 40% to 50% of the spinal canal and 60% to 80% of the thecal sac diameter (see Figures 4-8 and 4-9). The internal architecture of the cord can be seen on T1W, T2W, and variable flip angle/gradient echo images and is discussed in more detail in Chapter 3. The spinous processes of the vertebral bodies project posteriorly and inferiorly from the midline junction of the lamina. A spinous process is not present on the neural arch of C_1 and the largest is at C_7.

The major ligamentous structures stabilizing the cervical spine are the atlantoaxial complex, the anterior and posterior longitudinal ligaments, and the ligamentum flavum, interspinous ligament, and the supraspinous ligament.[7] A complex set of ligaments stabilizes the *medial atlantoaxial articulation*, which is composed of the synovial junction between the dens and the anterior arch of C_1 and between the dens and the posterior stabilizing ligaments. The most important of these posterior ligaments is the *cruciform ligament*, which lies in the coronal plane immediately behind to the dens. Its name is derived from vertical and horizontal arms extending from the level of the upper dens in the shape of a cross. The horizontal arms form the *transverse ligament*, which extends between the lateral masses of C_1 behind the dens and holds the dens tightly against the anterior arch of C_1. The vertical arms of the cruciform ligament extend superiorly to the foramen magnum and inferiorly to the body of C_2, running immediately beneath the tectorial membrane (discussed later).[7] The dens is linked directly to the basiocciput by the apical and alar ligaments. The *apical ligament* extends from the tip of the dens to the anterior margin of the foramen magnum, the *basion*. The *alar ligaments* extend laterally from the superior-lateral dens to the medial surfaces of the *occipital condyles*.[7] The vertebral bodies are stabilized by the anterior and posterior longitudinal ligaments. The *anterior longitudinal ligament* (ALL) runs from C_1 to the sacrum along the anterior and anterolateral surface of the vertebral bodies and intervertebral discs. It terminates superiorly in the ligament linking the anterior arch of C_1 with the basiocciput, the *anterior atlanto-occipital membrane*. The *posterior longitudinal ligament* (PLL) runs from C_2 to the sacrum along the posterior surface of the vertebrae and discs. The PLL is tightly adherent to and blends with the posterior anulus of the disc and adjacent edges of the vertebral bodies. It is narrowed and elevated away from the midvertebral body surface allowing a 1 to 2 mm gap that is filled with connective tissue and the anterior internal venous plexus. The cephalad extension of the posterior longitudinal ligament, from C_2 to the foramen magnum, is called the *tectorial membrane* (see Figures 4-1 to 4-3). It inserts, with the superior arm of the cruciform ligament, through the foramen magnum at the level of the hypoglossal canal.[7] The major ligaments stabilizing the posterior vertebral elements are the ligamentum flavum and interspinous and supraspinous ligaments. The *ligamentum flavum* is a discontinuous structure that extends the length of the spine and is formed by segments linking the vertebral lamina. It forms the posterior soft tissue wall of the spinal canal. The *interspinous ligament* links the spinous processes from inferior to superior surfaces along most of their posterior extension.

The *supraspinous ligament* links the spinous processes at their posterior tips. Because most ligaments are dense fibrous (collagen) structures they appear as low signal on T1W, T2W, and variable flip angle/gradient echo images. They are often indistinguishable from cortical bone and other fibrous structures i.e., the anulus fibrosis of the intervertebral disc, the PLL, or the dura. The ligamentum flavum is an exception to this rule, probably because of its high content of elastic fibers,[3] and often appears as intermediate signal on T1W SE and T2W SE images and as high signal on T2*W variable flip angle/gradient echo images (see Figure 4-17).

The *neural foramina* of the cervical spine are formed by the pedicles above and below. Cervical neural foramina may be as long as 1.5 cm (spinal canal to exit), prompting the term, *neural canal*.[8] However, in this discussion the more conventional terms, *neural foramen* and *neural foramina*, will be used to describe the entire structure from medial inlet to lateral exit. The anterior margin of the neural foramen is formed by the vertebral body and uncinate process medially and the transverse process laterally. The posterior margin is formed by the articular pillar and articular processes. With degenerative change, bony hypertrophy of the uncinate process and the superior articular process often encroaches on the contents of the neural foramen. The neural foramen is oriented approximately 30 degrees anterolateral as it exits from the spinal canal, in contrast to the lumbar and thoracic neural foramina that exit almost directly laterally (see Figures 4-8, 4-9, 4-17, 4-18, 4-19, 4-24 and 4-25). The exiting ventral and dorsal spinal nerve roots are within the neural foramen. The *dorsal root ganglion* enlargement lies posterior within the neural foramen, just medial to the junction of the dorsal and ventral roots where they form the spinal nerve.[7] These neural structures lie in the center of the long axis of the foramen in the axial plane and in the mid to superior foramen in the sagittal plane. Connective tissue, fat, and vascular structures surround the exiting nerve roots. There is less fat around the nerve roots in the cervical spine, than in the lumbar and thoracic spine. Most of the space around the nerve roots is occupied by an extensive venous plexus (discussed later). The relationship of the neural foramina to the numbered exiting nerve roots is shown in Figure 4-26 and is best understood by the "over-under rule." The nerve roots exit over the same numbered vertebral bodies (pedicles) in the cervical spine, but because there are eight sets of cervical nerve roots and only seven vertebrae, the eighth nerve root exits under C_7 and from there down in the thoracic and lumbar spine, the nerve roots exit under the same numbered vertebral body (pedicle). In most circumstances variable flip angle/gradient echo axial images are the most useful for visualizing structures of the neural foramina (see Figures 4-8 and 4-9) and T1W SE images, as a supplement, are usually the most useful sagittal images. Oblique images may be required to best visualize the cervical neural foramina in the sagittal plane, although sufficient information is often available from routine orthogonal sagittal images (see Figure 4-4, **B**).

The vascular anatomy of the cervical spine consists of an extensive venous plexus and the bilateral vertebral arteries. The *internal venous plexus* lies in the epidural connective tissue of the spinal canal. It is most prominent along the posterior surface of the midvertebral bodies where the posterior longitudinal ligament is elevated away from the bone and the basivertebral vein enters the vertebral body. Signal in this plexus is variable but is usually seen as low signal in the vascular channels on axial and sagittal images. The internal venous plexus communicates with the *external venous plexus* through the neural foramina laterally, around the lamina posteriorly, and through the basivertebral veins anteriorly. The *basivertebral vein* penetrates the posterior midportion of the vertebral body in the midline and forms a Y-shaped channel within the body. Its branches communicate with the *anterior external venous plexus* along the anterolateral surface of the vertebral body. The entry point of the basivertebral vein is often prominent on midline sagittal MR images. It appears as low signal on T1W SE images and as high signal on T2W SE and variable flip angle/gradient echo images (see Figures 4-1 to 4-3). The Y-shaped channel through the vertebral body is usually seen best on T1W axial images through the midvertebral body. The lateral extension of the venous plexus in the neural foramen is prominent in the cervical spine and fills or empties with changes in spine position.[8] With flexion of the cervical spine, the neural foramen widens and the venous plexus expands as the superior vertebra displaces slightly anteriorly on the inferior one. With extension, the foramen narrows and the venous plexus is compressed around the nerve roots. The importance of this plexus for MR imaging is that blood in the plexus is often high signal on variable flip angle/gradient echo images, similar to the adjacent CSF in the thecal sac (see Figures 4-8 and 4-9). The vertebral arteries ascend anterolateral to the neural foramina (Figures 4-8 and 4-9), and travel, from the C_6 through C_2 levels, through a foramen in the transverse process of the vertebral body, the *foramen trasversarium*. Immediately above C_2 the vertebral artery turns posterior and superior to travel up over the neural arch of C_1, behind the articular pillar, and into the foramen magnum. The artery sometimes passes through a variably present foramen formed on the superior surface of C_1 by a thin bony arch, the *ponticulus*.[7] The arterial supply to the cervical spinal cord from the vertebral arteries is discussed in Chapter 3. The vertebral arteries are seen as low signal vascular structures on T1W SE and T2W SE sagittal, coronal, and axial images because of rapid blood flow. They are usually seen as high signal on variable flip angle/gradient echo axial images because of inflow signal enhancement (Figures 4-1 to 4-9).

Text continued on p. 144.

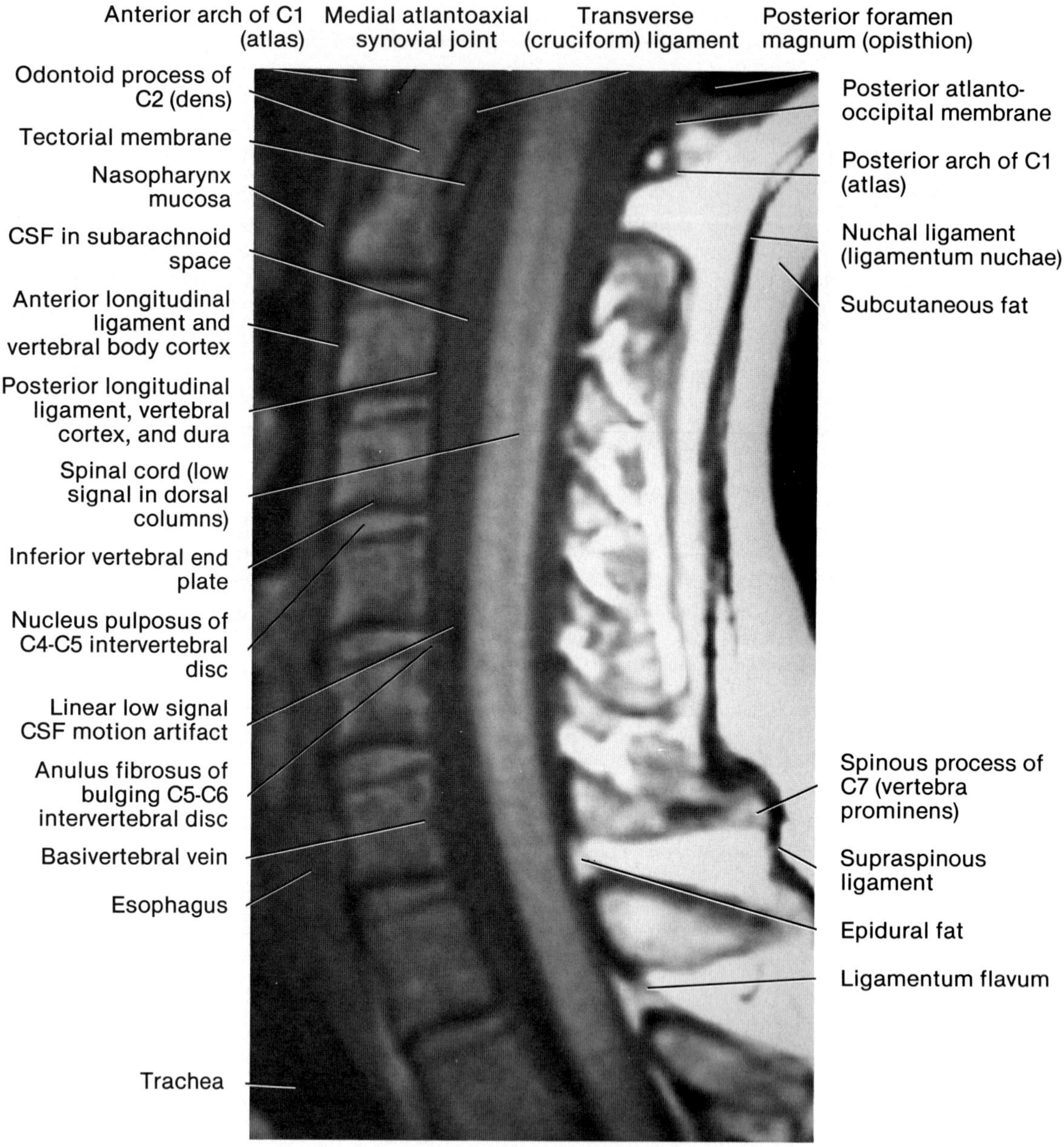

FIGURE 4-1. T1W (SE 800/20) midline sagittal image of the cervical spine.

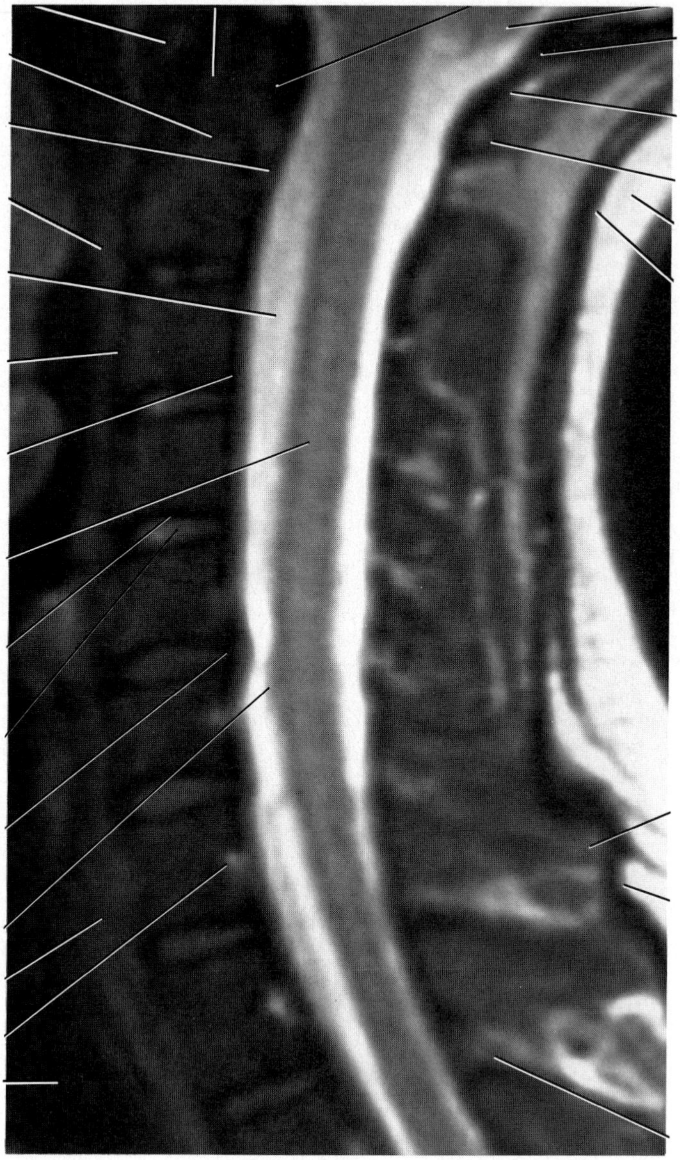

FIGURE 4-2. T2W (SE 2200/80, gated) midline sagittal image of the cervical spine.

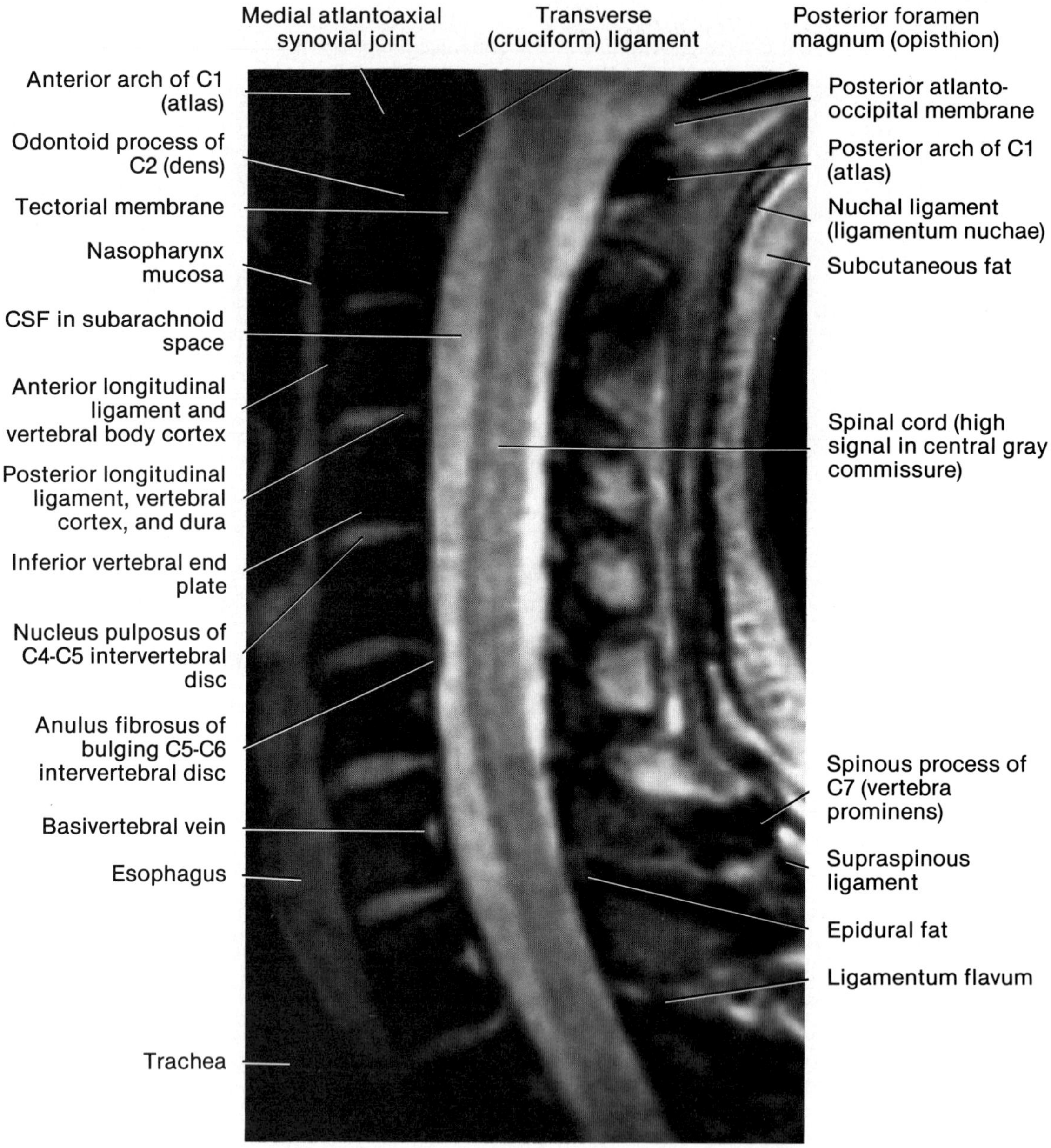

FIGURE 4-3. GRASS (40/20/7) midline sagittal image of the cervical spine.

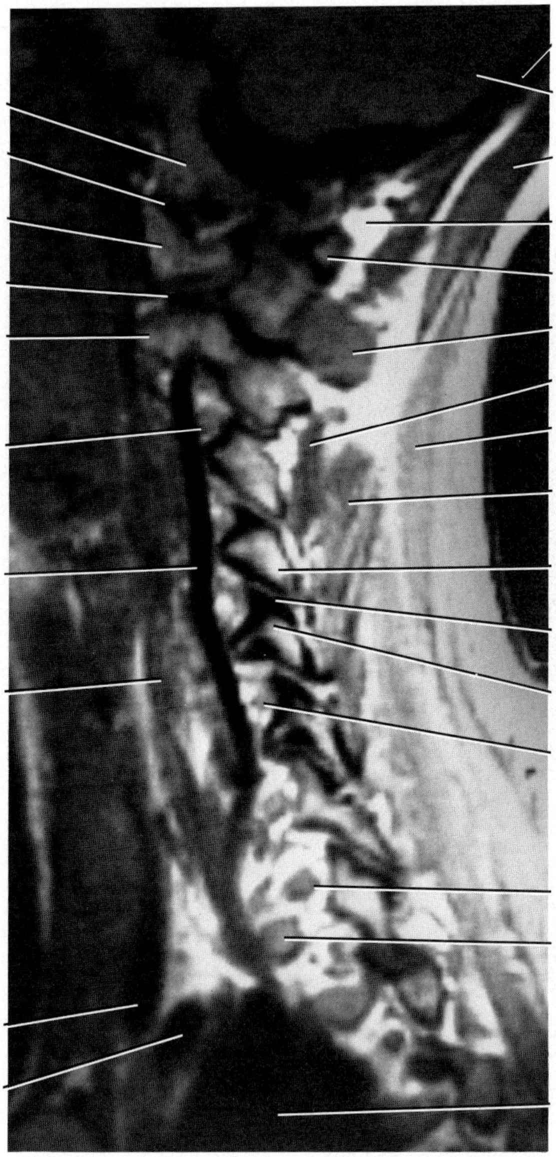

FIGURE 4-4. **A,** T1W (SE 800/20) lateral sagittal image of the cervical spine. *Continued.*

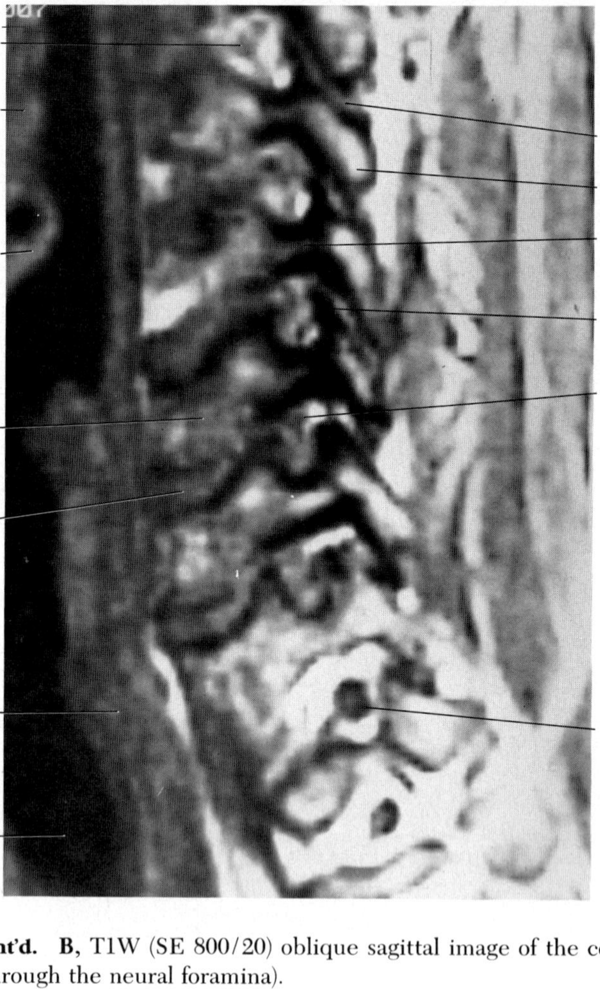

FIGURE 4-4, cont'd. B, T1W (SE 800/20) oblique sagittal image of the cervical spine (along the pedicles, through the neural foramina).

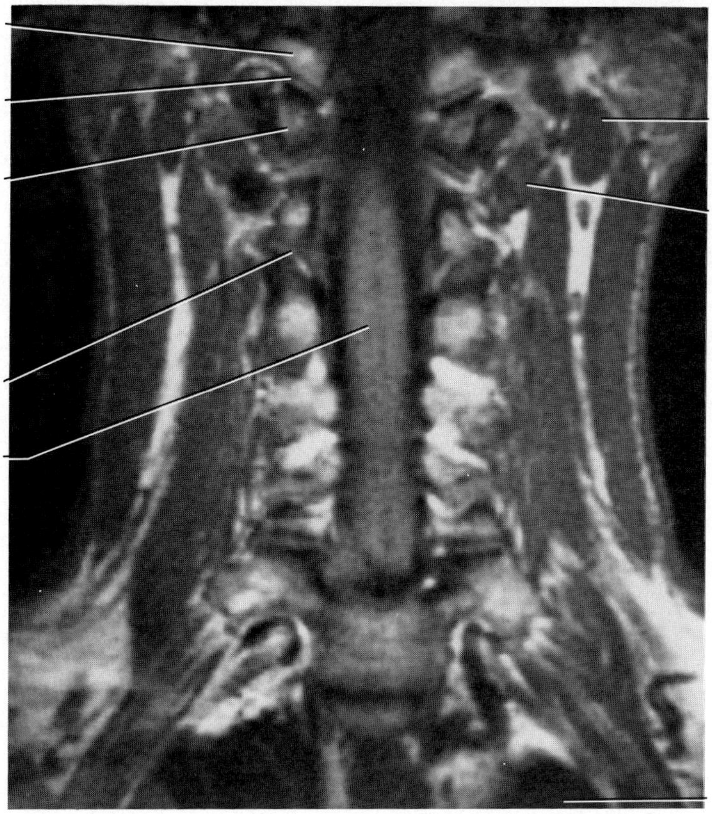

FIGURE 4-5. T1W (SE 800/20) posterior coronal image of the cervical spine.

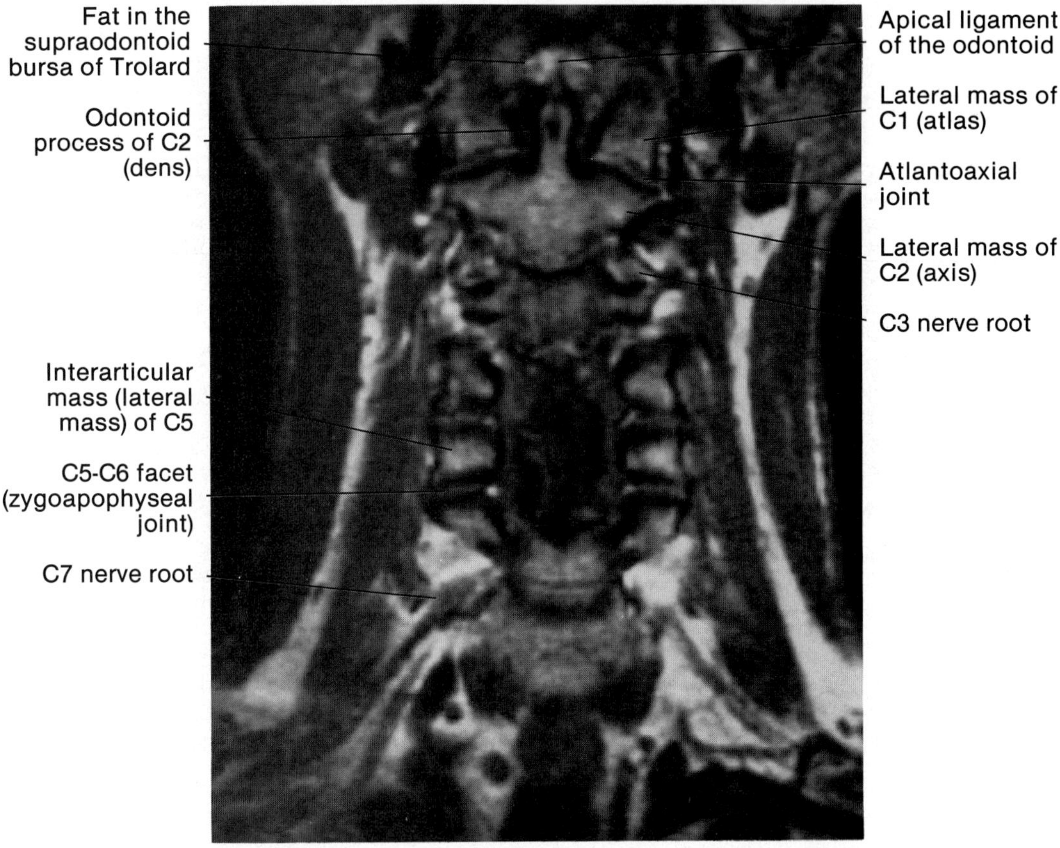

FIGURE 4-6. T1W (SE 800/20) midcanal coronal image of the cervical spine.

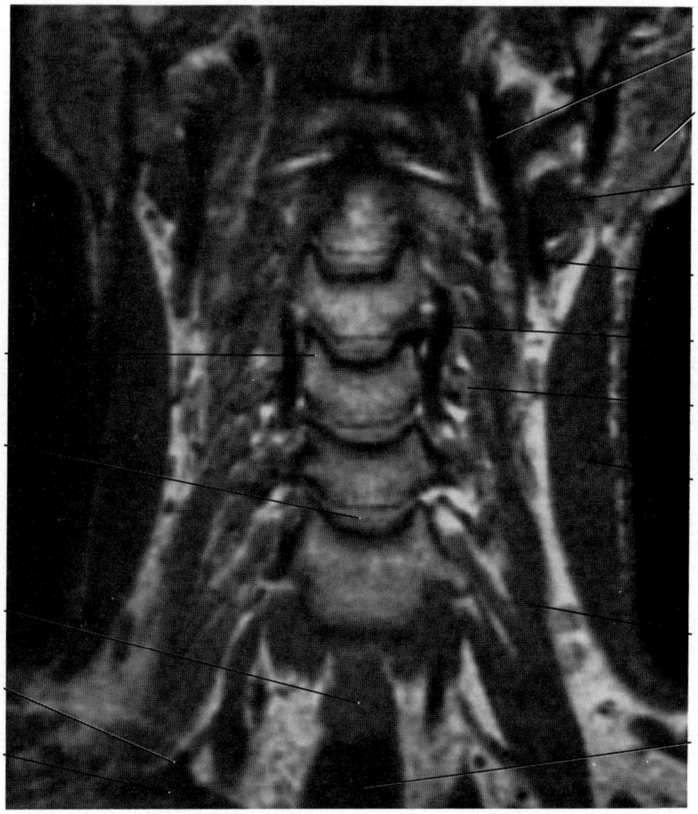

FIGURE 4-7. T1W (SE 800/20) anterior coronal of the cervical spine.

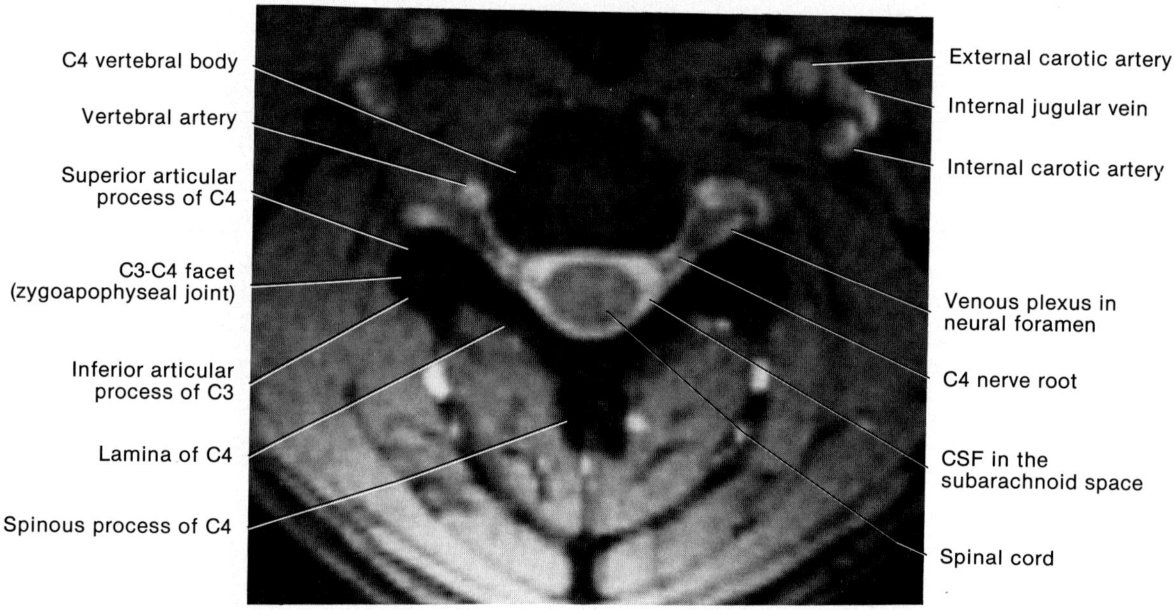

FIGURE 4-8. **A,** GRASS (40/20/7) axial image through the C3-C4 level.

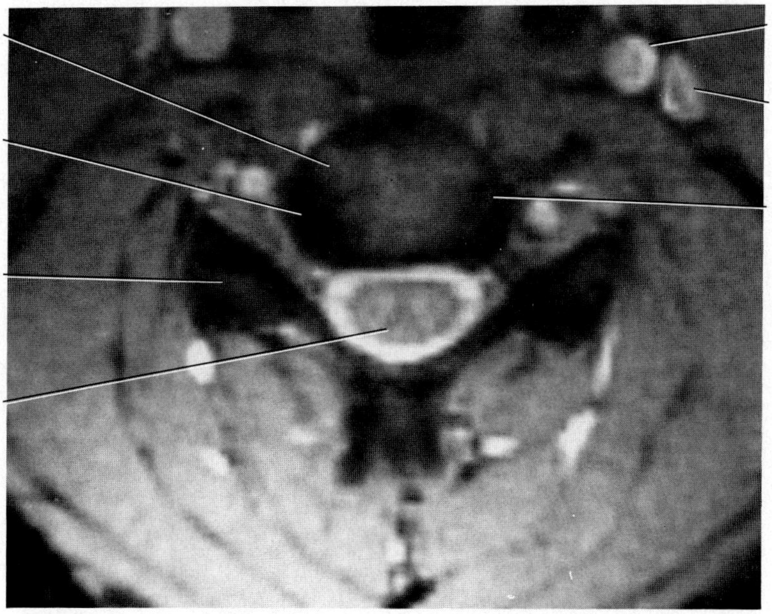

FIGURE 4-8. **B,** GRASS (40/20/7) axial image through the C4-C5 level.

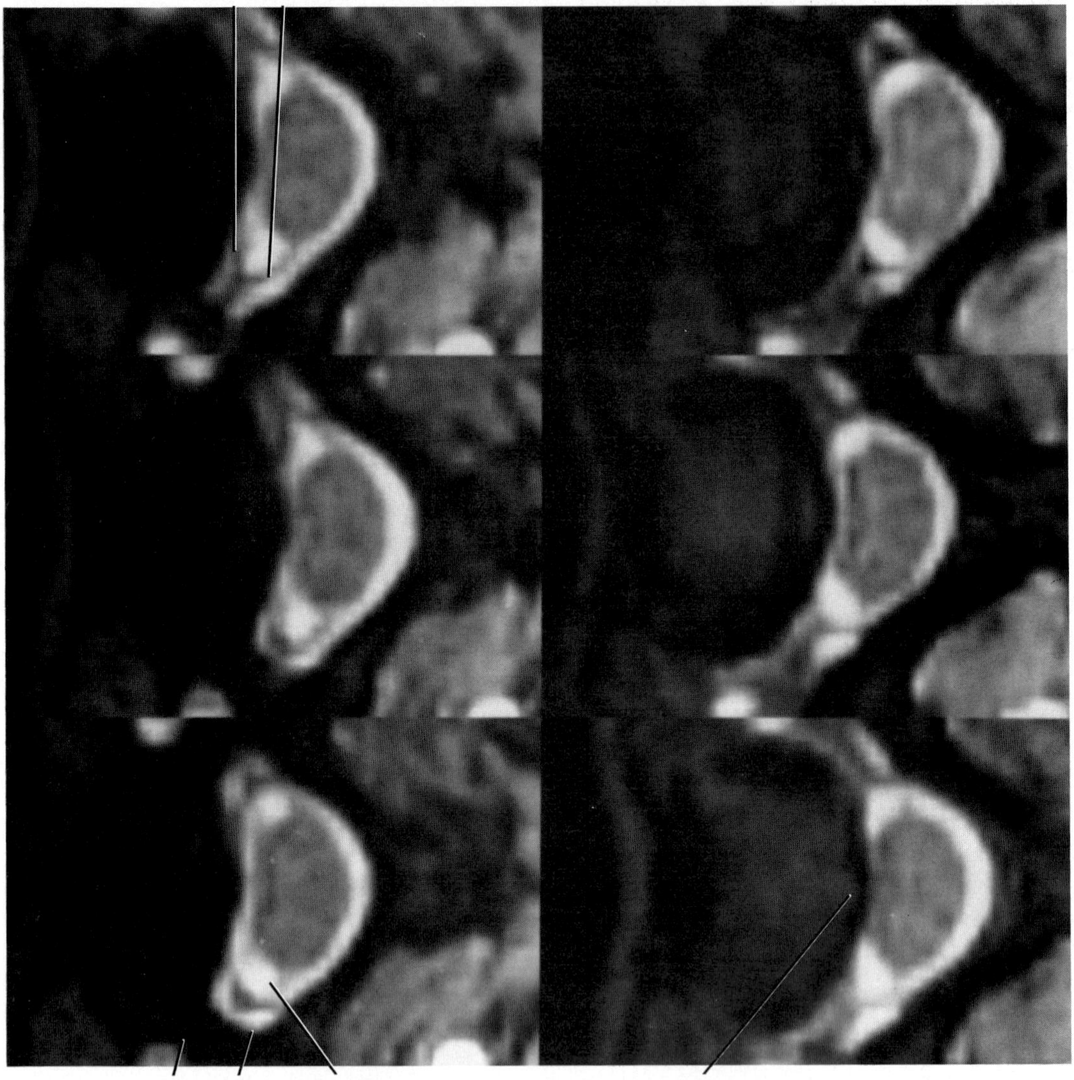

FIGURE 4-9. GRASS (40/20/7) interleaved axial images through the C5-C6 level.

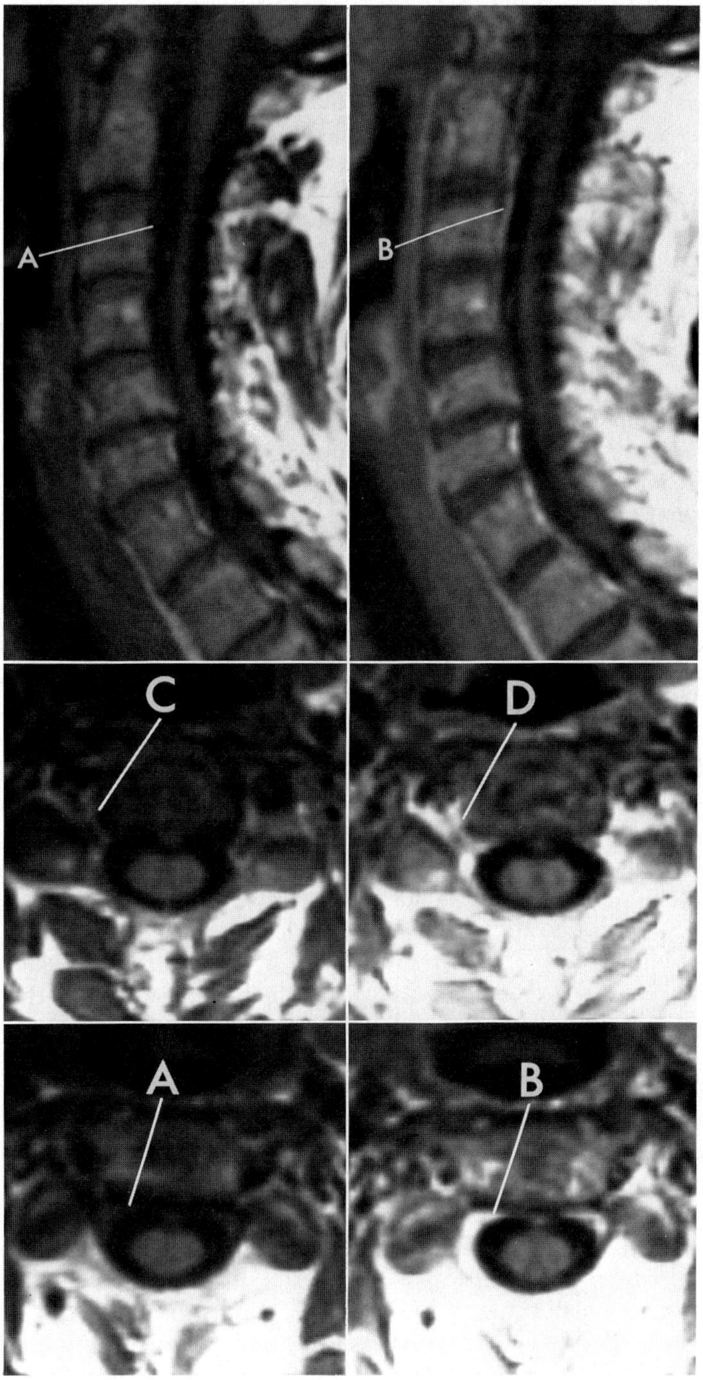

I II III IV V VI

FIGURE 4-9, cont'd. T1W (SE 800/20) images pre-GdDTPA (**I**, **III**, **V**) and post-GddTPA (**II**, **IV**, **VI**) of the cervical spine in sagittal (**I**, **II**) and axial planes (**III-VI**). *A*-Anterior epidural tissues before contrast injection (adjacent to a midline disc herniation). *B*-Enhancement of the anterior internal venous plexus after GdDTPA injection. *C*-Nerve root and adjacent tissues in the neural foramen before contrast injection. *D*-Enhancement of the venous plexus in the neural foramen after GdDTPA injection.

LUMBAR SPINE ANATOMY

The vertebral bodies of the lumbar spine are approximately rectangular in sagittal and coronal cross secion with flat superior and inferior end-plates. The central portion of the vertebral body is formed by trabecular bone supporting a matrix of active bone marrow. Signal from the vertebral body is largely dependent on the fat content of this bone marrow so that it appears as moderately high signal on T1W SE images (higher than cortical bone, but lower than subcutaneous fat), intermediate to low signal on T2W SE images (slightly greater than cortical bone), and low signal on variable flip angle/gradient echo images, especially T2*W images (equal to cortical bone), (see Figures 4-1 through 4-9 and 4-17 to 4-19). A more detailed discussion of the appearance of bone marrow can be found in Chapter 3. The end-plates are covered by a fenestrated cartilage layer to which the intervertebral discs attach. The anatomy of the intervertebral discs is discussed in more detail in Chapter 3. The appearance of the vertebral end-plates is usually low signal on T1W SE, T2W SE, and variable flip angle/gradient echo images but is often obscured by chemical shift artifact on T1W SE images that may artifactually widen the low signal at the end-plate or obscure it with overlapping high signal from bone marrow fat. The mechanism for this artifact is discussed in more detail in Chapter 3.

The pedicles of the lumbar spine project posterolaterally and usually contain a small amount of bone marrow extending from the vertebral body, which is seen best on T1W SE images. The facet joints in the lumbar spine are formed by long articular processes and are oriented approximately in the coronal plane. The portion of the articular process that links the articular pillar with the facet joint is known as the *pars interarticularis*. This structure is most important in the lower lumbar spine where the inferior pars interarticularis is separated, usually at L_5, in patients with spondylolysis. This allows anterior displacement of L_5 on S_1, (spondylolysthesis) with consequent distortions of the disc and thecal sac. Spondylolysthesis can be seen easily on midline sagittal MR images and the defect in the pars interarticularis may be seen in sagittal images through the inferior articular process. On axial images, the pars defect is seen as a facetlike gap with cortical bone margins in an abnormal anterior position with a more precisely coronal orientation than the true facet joint. The lumbar facets are best seen in the axial plane and, as elsewhere, the cortical bone forming the articular process is seen as low signal in all MR pulse sequences. The articular cartilage and fluid in the joint is seen as intermediate to low signal on T1W SE images. The cartilage is seen as intermediate to low signal and fluid is seen as high signal on T2W SE images. Both cartilage and fluid are seen as high signal on variable flip angle/gradient echo images (see Figures 4-17 to 4-19).

The lamina in the lumbar spine form an oval cross section to the spinal canal with a slightly greater lateral than AP diameter. In the lower lumbar spine the canal is more triangular, or *trefoil*, in shape with posterolateral indentations in the cross section produced by the superior articular processes. These form the lateral recesses of the canal anteromedial to the facets. These lateral recesses can become markedly narrowed and produce entrapment of individual nerve roots when significant degenerative hypertrophy of facets occurs (see Figures 4-17 to 4-19). The lateral recesses and the central lumbar canal may be further narrowed by posterior protrusion of the intervertebral disc margin and by hypertrophy and folding of the ligamentum flavum at its medial facet capsule insertion. Circumferential narrowing of the lumbar spinal canal to a severe degree by these structures results in spinal stenosis and produces compression of the thecal sac and the cauda equina. The epidural space of the lumbar spinal canal contains a venous plexus, connective tissue, and a large amount of fat. The epidural fat is high signal on T1W images and sharply outlines the low signal venous plexus, thecal sac, and nerve root sleeves in the spinal canal and the neural foramina. Fat is a less useful marker of the epidural space on T2W SE images where its signal decreases and approaches that of other structures and bone (see Figures 4-17 to 4-19). On T2*W variable flip angle/gradient echo images, signal in the epidural fat may be similar to CSF in the thecal sac and nerve root sleeves (see Figure 4-15).

The major ligaments of concern for MR imaging in the lumbar spine are the anterior and posterior longitudinal ligaments and the ligamentum flavum. The anterior longitudinal ligament is tightly adherent to the anterior vertebral body and disc margins. It is seen as a thin, low signal structure, indistinguishable from cortical bone and disc anulus on all pulse sequences in sagittal and axial images (see Figures 4-10 to 4-19). The posterior longitudinal ligament is tightly adherent to the posterior disc margin where it is low signal and indistinguishable from the anulus and adjacent dura of the thecal sac. At the midvertebral level the posterior longitudinal ligament is narrow, lies in the midline, and is elevated away from the posterior vertebral body. This allows room for fat, connective tissue, and the anterior internal venous plexus in the epidural space (see Figures 4-10 to 4-19). The ligamentum flavum is 3 to 5 mm thick (mean: 4.5 mm ± 0.97 in axial plane)[3] in the lumbar spine and more prominent than in the cervical and thoracic spine. As mentioned previously, it is a segmental ligament that inserts on the anterior-inferior surface of the lamina above and on the posterior-superior surface of the lamina below. It merges with and reinforces the medial joint capsule of the facet at its superior end. Because the ligamentum flavum contains 80% elastin and only 20% type I collagen,[3] it appears different from other ligaments on MR images. It is usually intermediate signal on T1W images (greater than cortical bone but less than fat) and on T2W images (greater than cortical bone but less than CSF) but is high signal on T2*W variable flip angle/gradient echo images (equal to CSF, similar to articular cartilage) (see Figure 4-17).

The neural foramina of the lumbar spine are formed by the pedicles above and below and are oriented almost directly lateral. The anterior neural foramen is bordered by the posterolateral vertebral body (superior foramen) and posterolateral disc margin (inferior foramen). The posterior border of the foramen is formed by the articular processes, most prominently by the superior articular process of the inferior vertebral body. Narrowing of the neural foramen by protrusion and superior articular process hypertrophy are discussed in detail in Chapter 3 and illustrated in Figure 3-7. The exiting nerve roots and dorsal root ganglion consistently lie in the superior portion of the lumbar neural foramen and are seen well on both axial and sagittal images. On T1W images, the nerve root sleeves are low signal round structures outlined by high signal fat. Epidural fat is low signal on T2W images and contrasts with high signal from CSF in the thecal sac and nerve root sleeves (see Figures 4-17 to 4-19). Enhancement of dorsal root ganglia signal on T1W images may be seen normally following intravenous administration (0.1 mM/kg) of gadolinium diethylenetriamine penta-acetic acid (GdDTPA) (see Figure 4-20).

The venous plexus of the lumbar spine, as in the cervical spine, is composed of an internal vertebral plexus in the epidural space of the spinal canal that communicates with an external venous plexus surrounding the vertebral body and posterior elements. The anterior internal venous plexus, lying between the thecal sac and vertebral body, is the most prominent portion on MR images. It is seen as multiple low signal vascular channels on both sagittal and axial images with occasional high signal caused by flow enhancement (see Figures 4-10 to 4-19). Individual veins of the plexus can be quite prominent in the axial plane, and should not be mistaken for nerve root sleeves. At the level of the pedicles, nerve root sleeves lie anterolateral to the thecal sac in the lateral recesses of the spinal canal and, more distally, they lie within the superior neural foramen (see Figures 4-17 to 4-19). The venous plexus lies directly anterior to the thecal sac and exits the canal as smaller branches in the inferior neural foramen. A midline septum extending from the posterior longitudinal ligament to the thecal sac often divides the anterior venous plexus into a pair of structures (see Figures 4-17 to 4-19). When the channels of the plexus are less well-defined, they may be hard to distinguish from the anterior thecal sac and posterior disc margin on axial images. This problem may be further complicated by the presence of low signal chemical-shift artifact at the anterior margin of the thecal sac (see Figure 4-17). The basivertebral vein communicates between the anterior internal venous plexus and the anterior external venous plexus. It is best seen on midline sagittal images and appears on T1W images as a low signal triangular defect in the midportion of the vertebral body and as a high signal defect on T2W SE and variable flip angle/gradient echo images (see Figures 4-10 to 4-16). High signal in the basivertebral vein may be seen on T1W images because of flow effects in the vein, fat accompanying the vein into the vertebral body, chemical-shift artifact (water in venous blood vs. epidural or marrow fat), or enhancement with GdDTPA (see Figure 4-20). The arterial supply to the lumbar spine, cord, and cauda equina is from the radiculo-medullary branches of the lumbar arteries and is discussed in more detail in Chapter 3.

The *dura* of the lumbar thecal sac is a dense fibrous (collagen) tissue that surrounds the tip of the conus medullaris and cauda equina nerve roots. An arachnoid membrane lines the inner dural surface with only a thin or potential subdural space separating them. Virtually all the CSF seen in the thecal sac on MR images lies in the subarachnoid space. Arachnoid and dura are not usually distinguishable on MR images and neither can be discriminated from CSF on T1W images. The thecal sac extends to approximately S_2 in most patients and is seen as a tapering structure within a larger volume of epidural fat in the sacral canal (see Figures 4-10 to 4-19). The tip of the *conus medullaris* lies at L_1 and is surrounded by the dorsal and ventral nerve roots that form the *cauda equina*. The *conus tip* may be seen on sagittal images but is usually obscured by the proximal cauda equina (see Figure 4-21). The most reliable way to identify the conus tip is on axial images where it is positioned in the midline, slightly posterior of the midcanal, and surrounded by the array of ventral and dorsal nerve roots. This array often has the shape of a "VW" sign centered on the conus, with the anterior ventral roots forming the "V" and the posterior dorsal roots forming the "W" (see Figure 4-19). More distally, the roots of the cauda equina are distributed in an arc along the posterior half of the thecal sac. Individual roots are usually distinguishable. Centralized clumping and thickening of the roots or margination along the thecal sac are abnormal distributions and usually indicate arachnoid adhesions (e.g., after hemorrhage or infection) or metastatic tumor (e.g., "drop" metastases from primary central nervous system [CNS] tumor or systemic metastases). The conus tip and cauda equina appear as high signal within low signal CSF on T1W SE images and as low signal within high signal CSF on T2W SE and variable flip angle/gradient echo images (see Figures 4-17 to 4-19). The filum terminale lies in the same position as the conus tip relative to the cauda equina nerve roots on axial images and has signal similar to the nerve roots. The anatomy of the filum terminale is discussed in more detail in Chapter 5.

Text continued on p. 169.

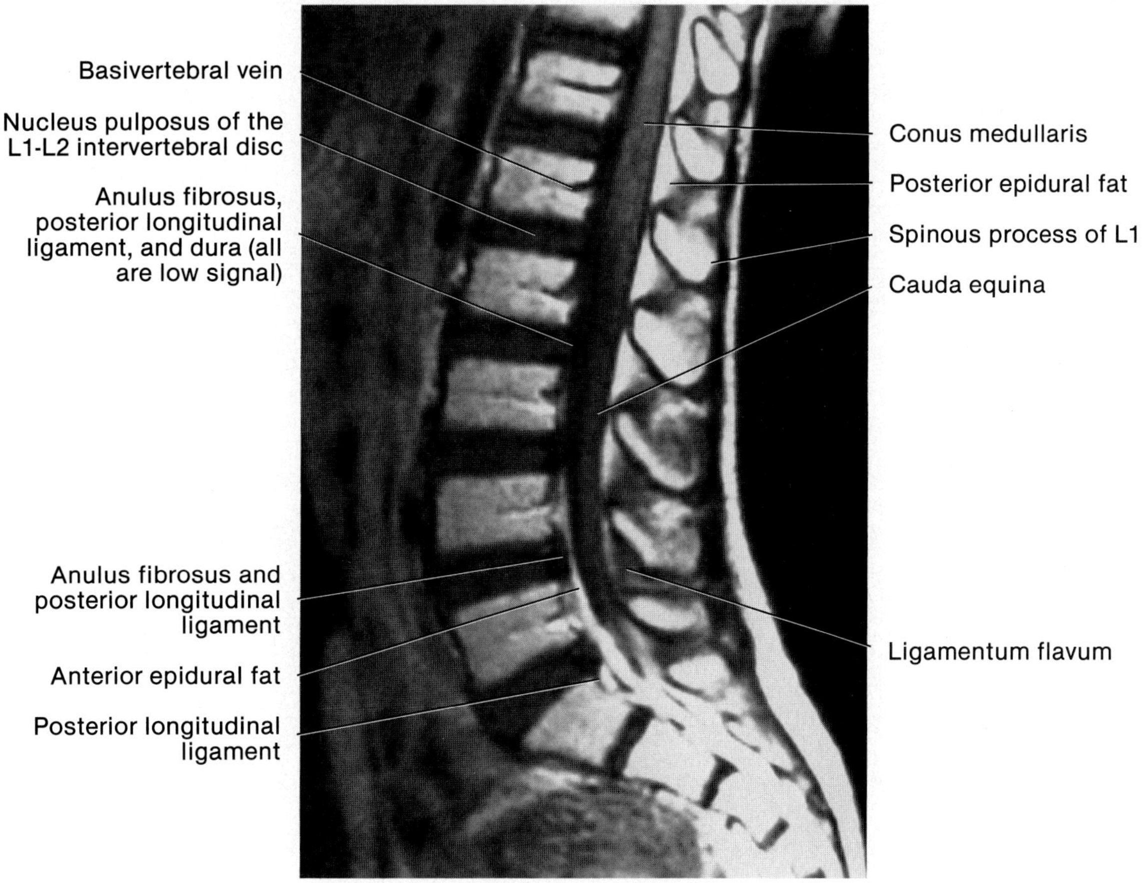

FIGURE 4-10. T1W (SE 800/20) midline sagittal image of the lumbar spine.

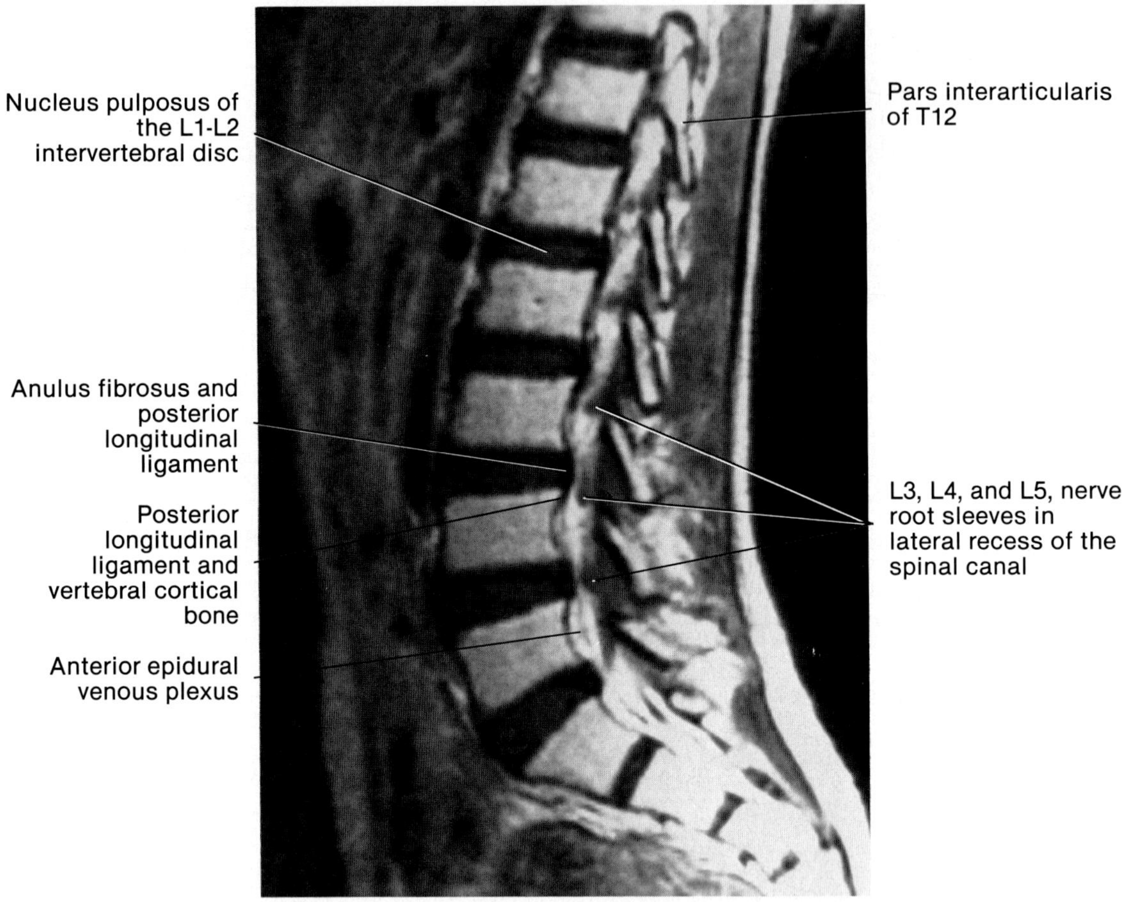

FIGURE 4-11. T1W (SE 800/20) paramedian sagittal image through the lateral recess of the lumbar spinal canal.

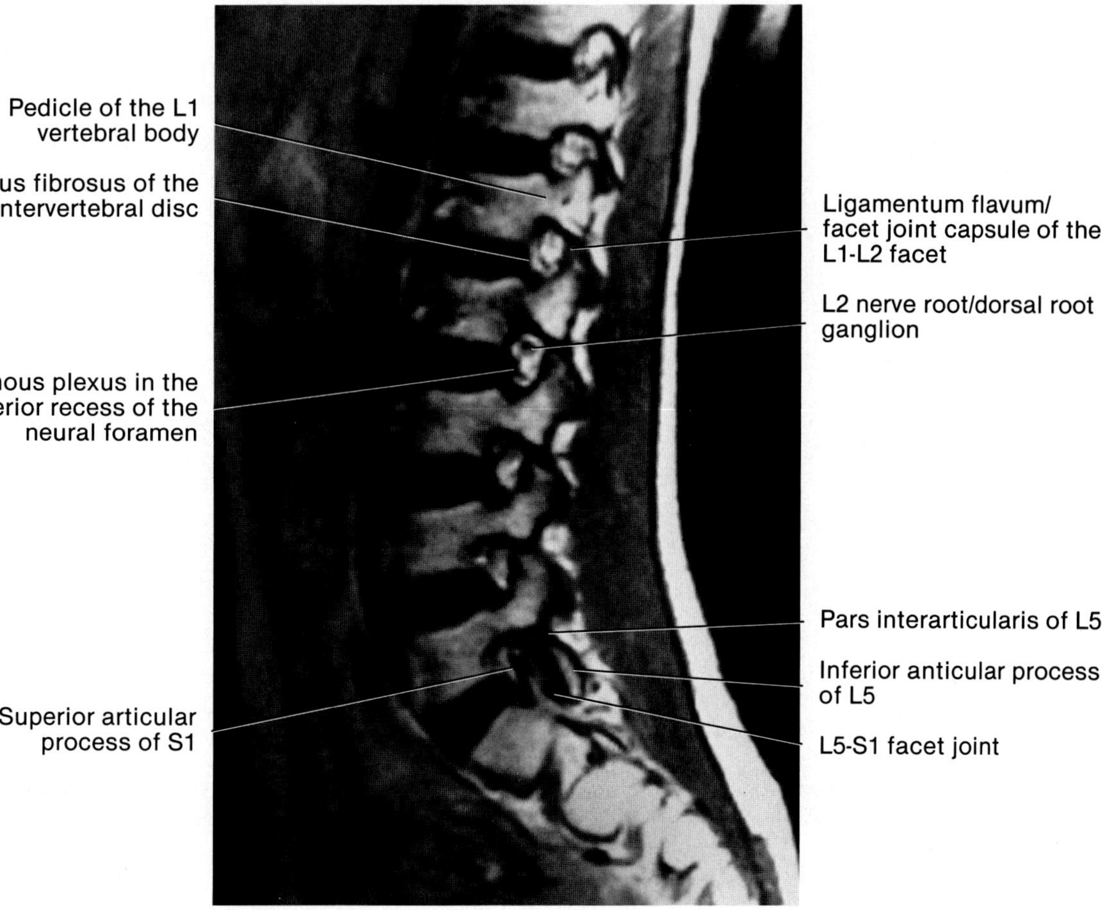

FIGURE 4-12. T1W (SE 800/20) lateral sagittal image through the pedicles and neural foramina of the lumbar spine.

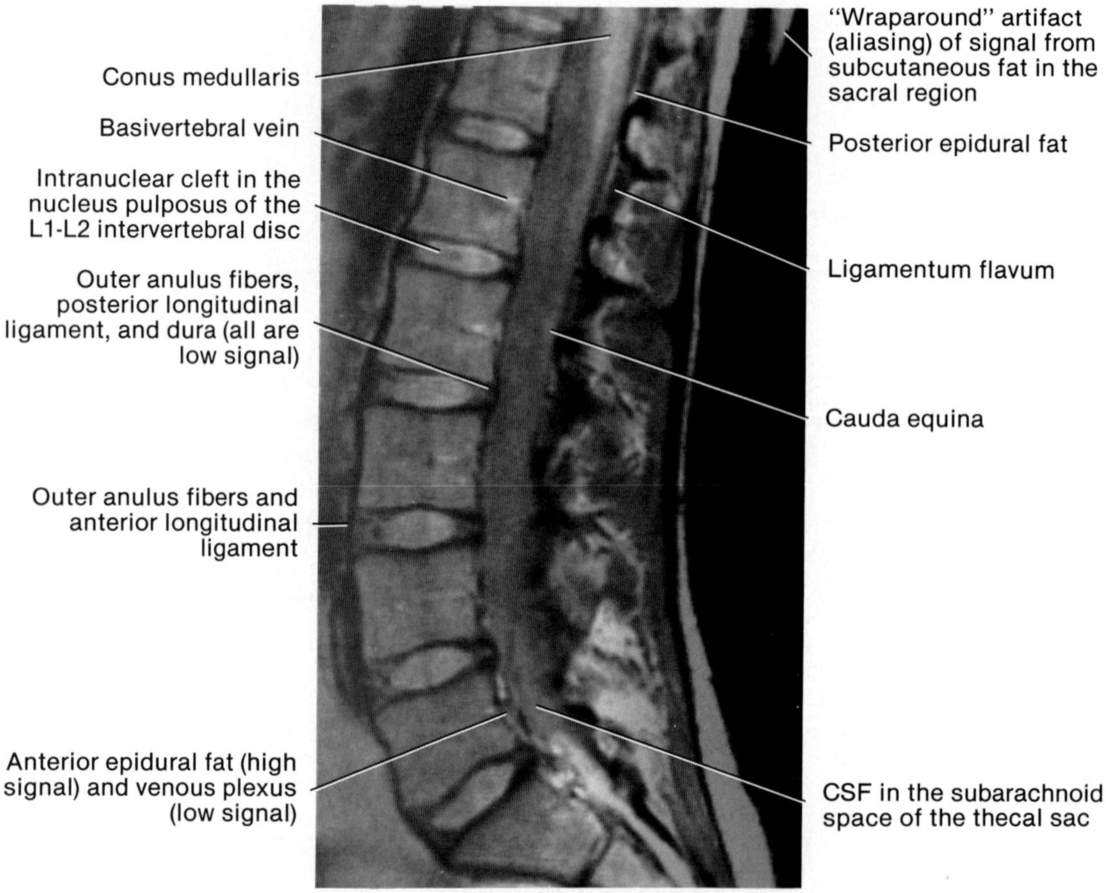

FIGURE 4-13. "T2W" (mixed T1 and T2 contrast, SE 2200/20, gated) sagittal midline image of the lumbar spine.

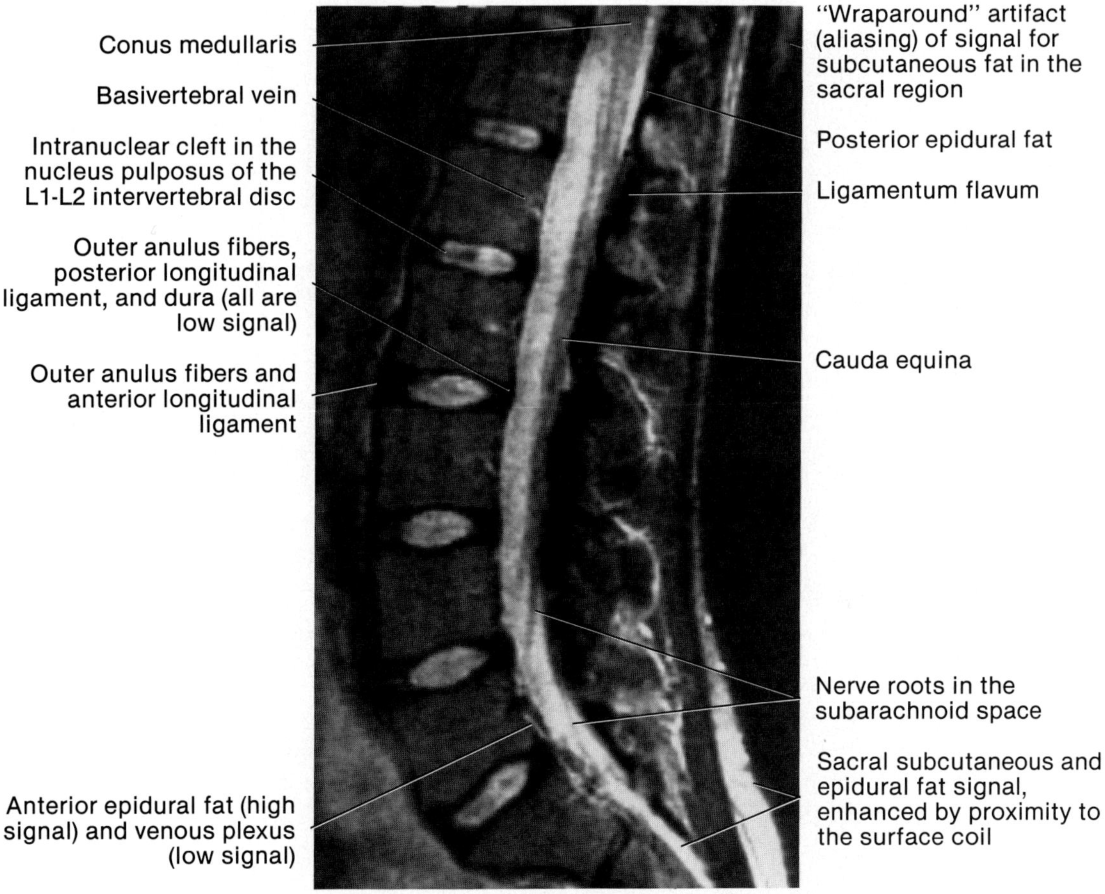

FIGURE 4-14. T2W (SE 2200/80, gated) sagittal midline image of the lumbar spine.

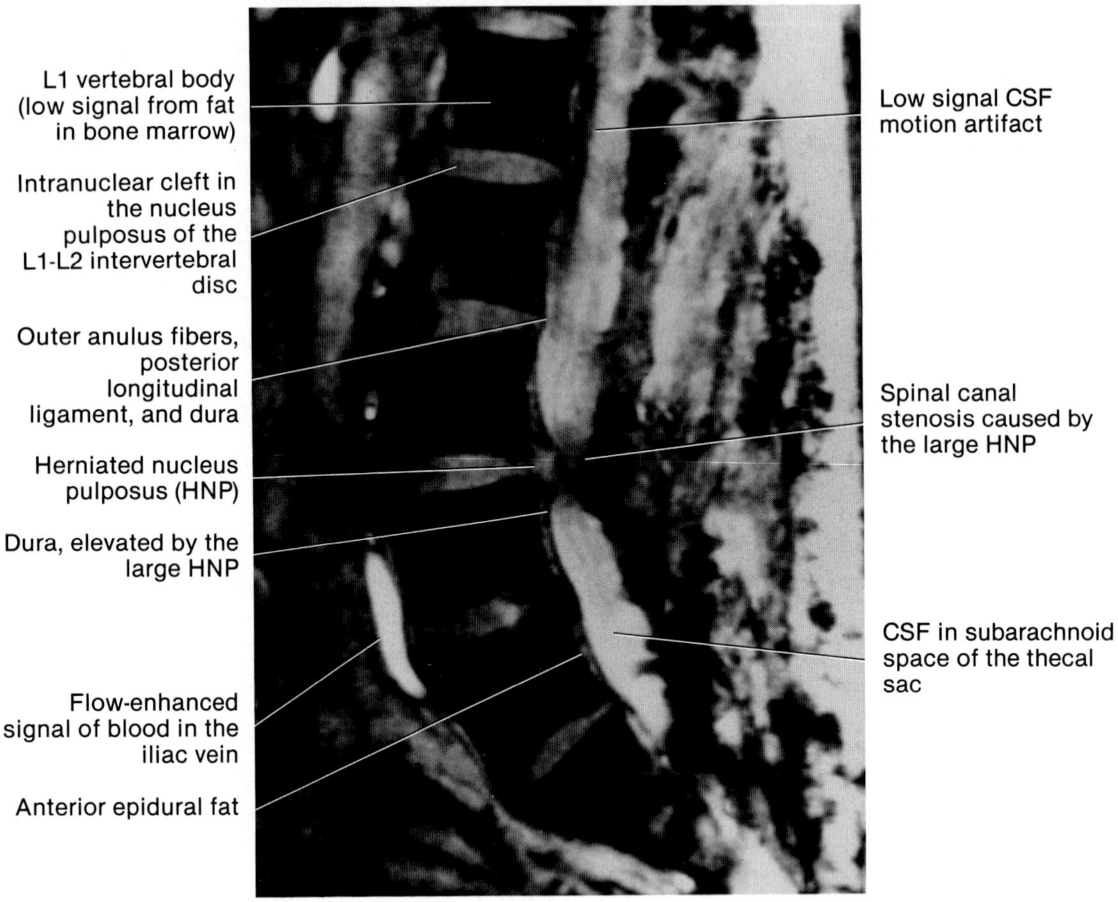
L1 vertebral body (low signal from fat in bone marrow)
Intranuclear cleft in the nucleus pulposus of the L1-L2 intervertebral disc
Outer anulus fibers, posterior longitudinal ligament, and dura
Herniated nucleus pulposus (HNP)
Dura, elevated by the large HNP
Flow-enhanced signal of blood in the iliac vein
Anterior epidural fat
Low signal CSF motion artifact
Spinal canal stenosis caused by the large HNP
CSF in subarachnoid space of the thecal sac

FIGURE 4-15. T2*W GRASS (500/40/30) sagittal midline image of the lumbar spine.

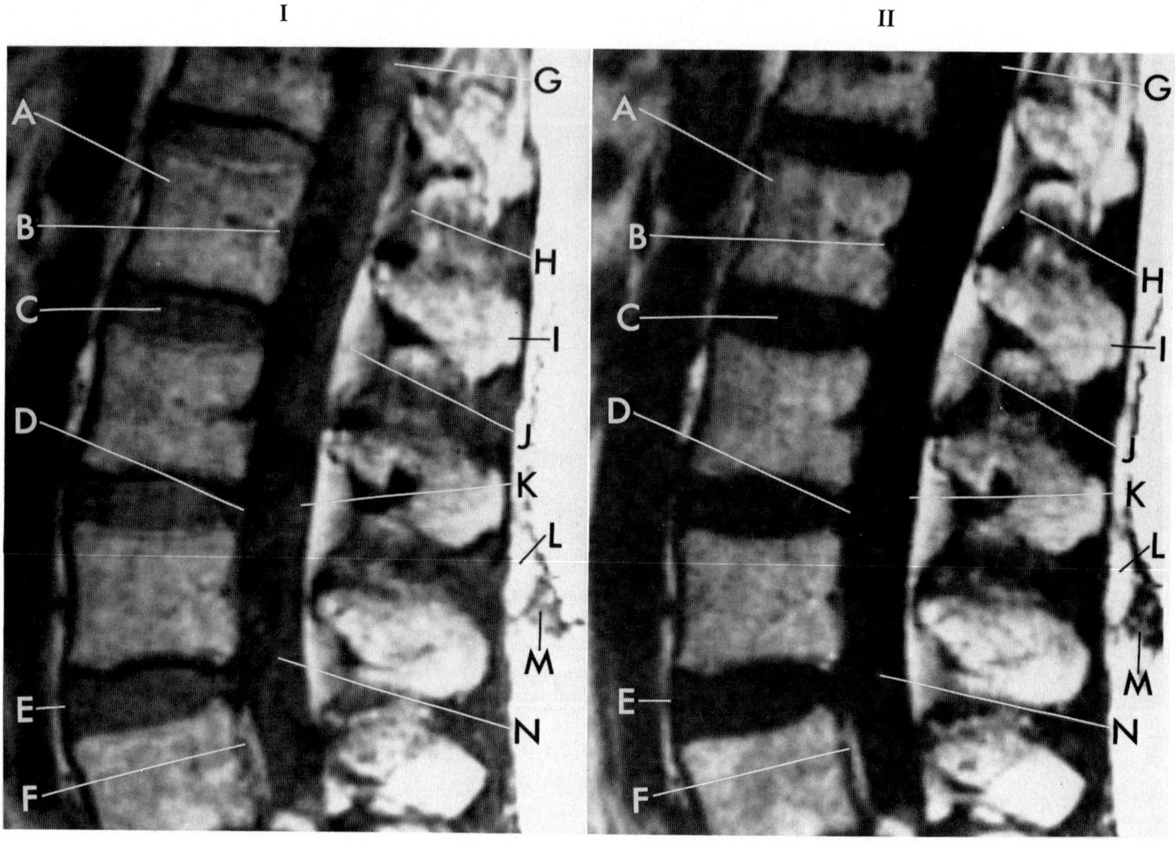

FIGURE 4-16. **I,** T1W (SE 800/20), **II,** water-suppressed (WS), **III,** T2W (SE 2100/80), and **IV,** fat-suppressed (FS) midline sagittal images of the lumbar spine. *A,* L2 vertebral body bone marrow. *B,* Basivertebral vein. *C,* Nucleus pulposus of the L2-L3 intervertebral disc. *D,* Outer anulus fibers, posterior longitudinal ligament and dura (isointense with CSF and nucleus pulposus on the WS image, **II**). *E,* Outer anulus fibers and the anterior longitudinal ligament. *F,* Anterior epidural fat and venous plexus. *G,* Conus medullaris tip/cauda equina (isointense with CSF on the WS image, **II**). *H,* Ligamentum flavum. *I,* Spinous process of L2. *J,* Posterior epidural fat. *K,* Cauda equina (isointense with CSF on the WS image, **II**). *L,* Subcutaneous fat. *M,* Subcutaneous fascia (water signal). *N,* Nerve root in the subarachnoid space (isointense with CSF on the WS image, **II**).

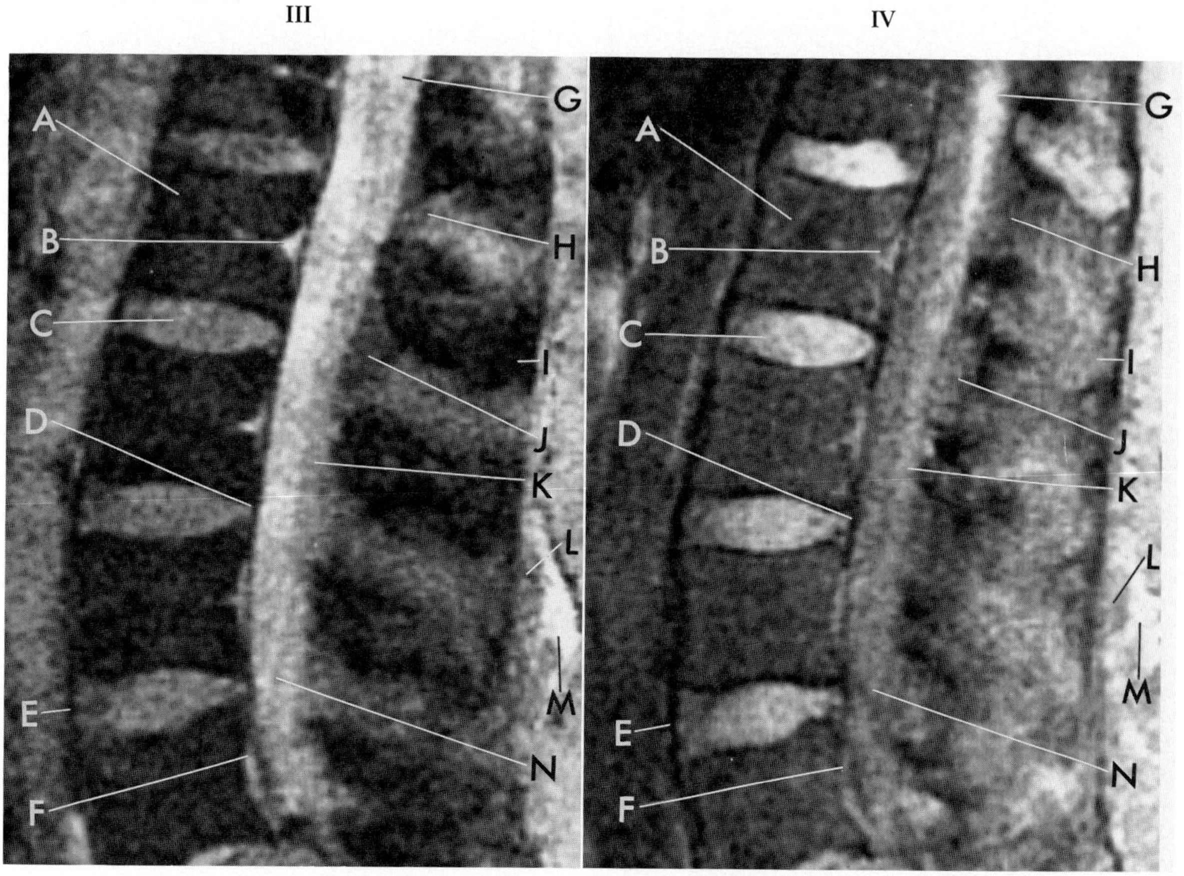

FIGURE 4-16, cont'd. For legend see opposite page.

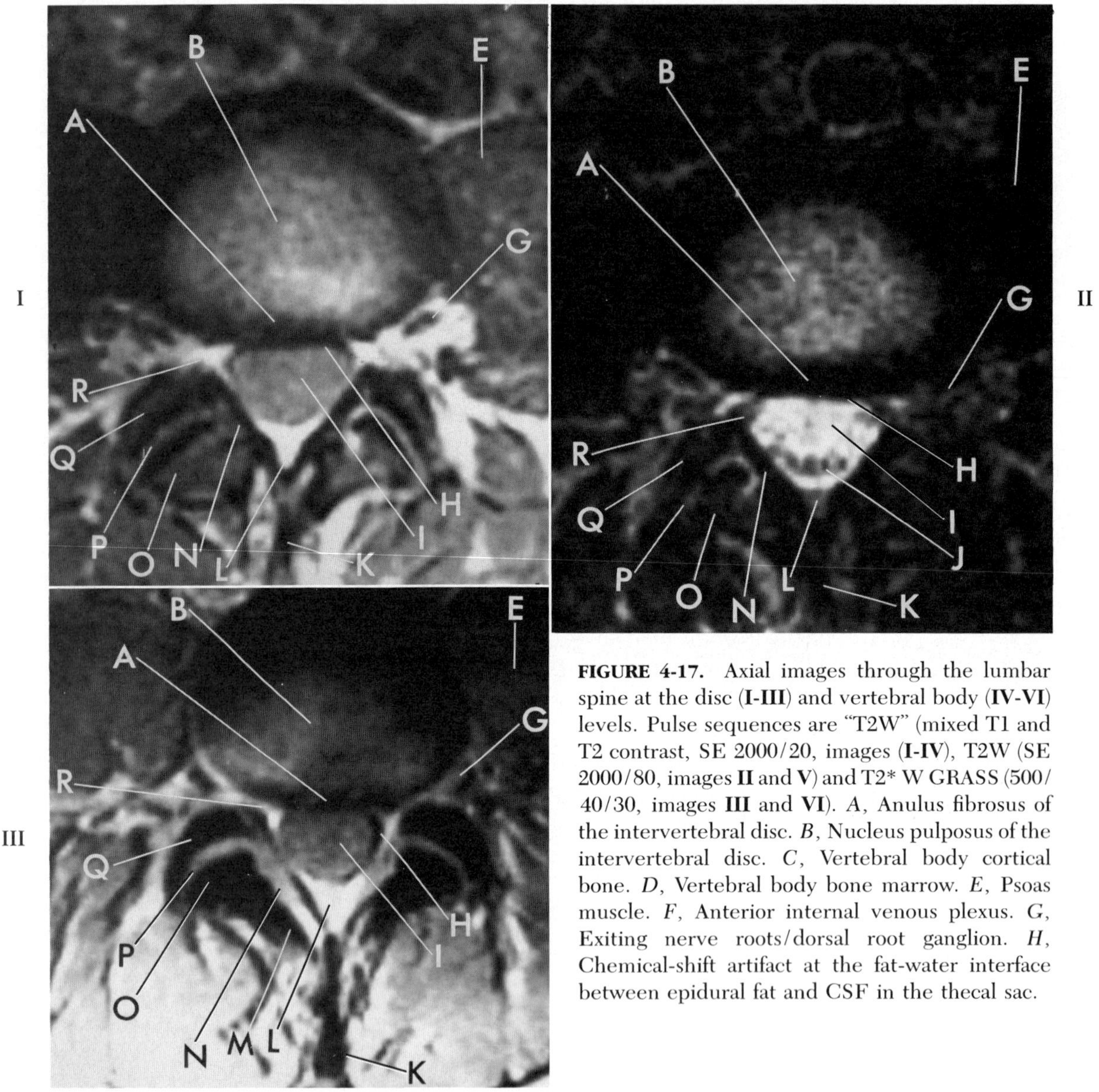

FIGURE 4-17. Axial images through the lumbar spine at the disc (**I-III**) and vertebral body (**IV-VI**) levels. Pulse sequences are "T2W" (mixed T1 and T2 contrast, SE 2000/20, images (**I-IV**), T2W (SE 2000/80, images **II** and **V**) and T2* W GRASS (500/40/30, images **III** and **VI**). *A*, Anulus fibrosus of the intervertebral disc. *B*, Nucleus pulposus of the intervertebral disc. *C*, Vertebral body cortical bone. *D*, Vertebral body bone marrow. *E*, Psoas muscle. *F*, Anterior internal venous plexus. *G*, Exiting nerve roots/dorsal root ganglion. *H*, Chemical-shift artifact at the fat-water interface between epidural fat and CSF in the thecal sac.

IV

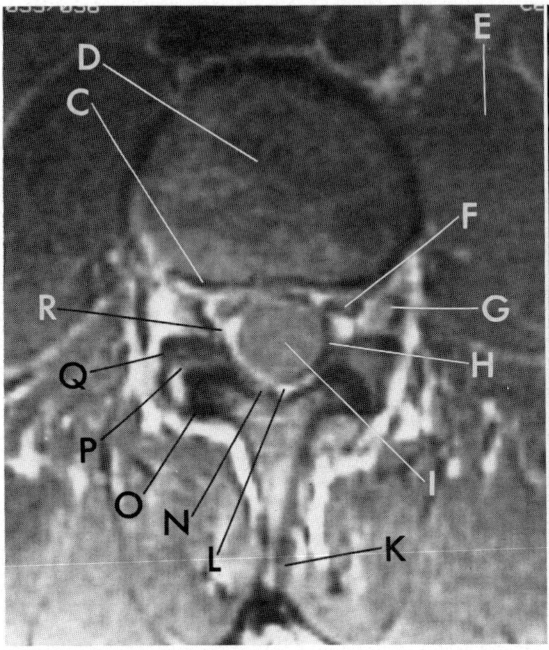

V

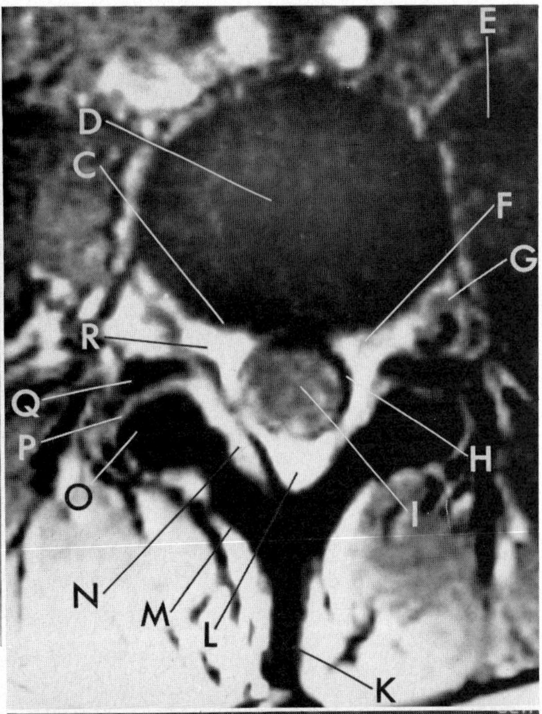

VI

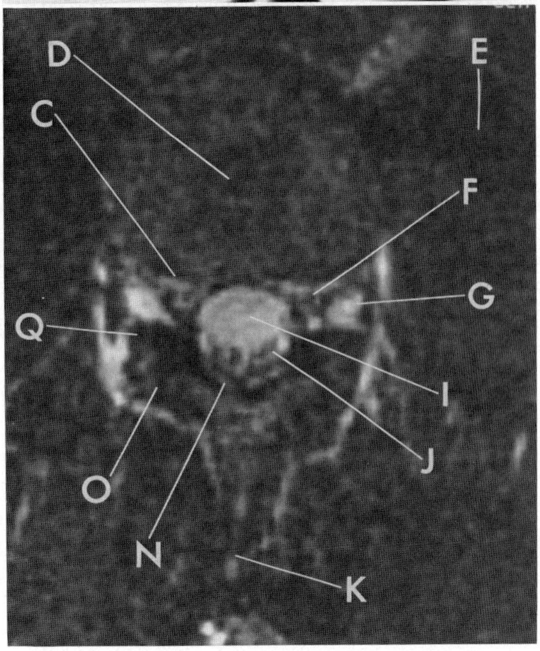

FIGURE 4-17, cont'd. This artifact occurs along the direction of the frequency encoding gradient, which is top-to-bottom in images **I** and **II**, and left-to-right in images **III-VI** (the low signal artifact merges with the low signal of the anulus fibrosus, posterior longitudinal ligament, and dura in images **I** and **II**). High signal chemical-shift artifact is present (see I) at the posterior fat-theca interface, but is obscured by the high signal of the adjacent epidural fat. *I*, CSF in the subarachnoid space of the thecal sac. *J*, Nerve roots of the cauda equina. *K*, Vertebral spinous process. *L*, Posterior epidural fat. *M*, Vertebral lamina. *N*, Ligamentum flavum. *O*, Inferior articular process (from the superior vertebra). *P*, Facet (zygoapophyseal) joint. *Q*, Superior articular process (from the inferior vertebra). *R*, Lateral recess of the spinal canal.

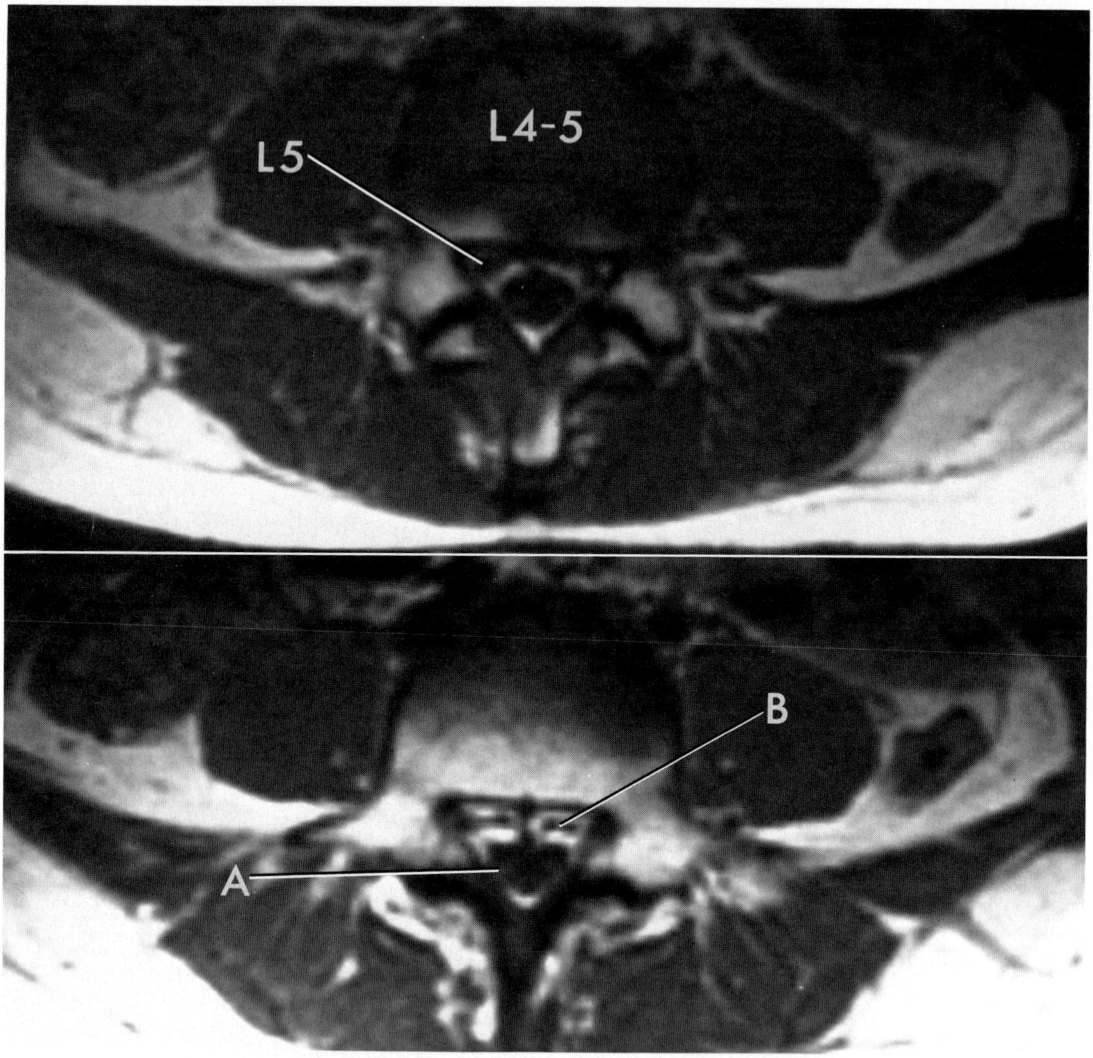

FIGURE 4-18 Serial T1W (SE 800/20) axial 3 mm slices at 4 mm intervals (i.e., 1 mm gap between slices) showing the intraspinal and paraspinous courses of the L5 and S1 nerve roots. *A*, Sacral nerve roots of the cauda equina within the thecal sac. *B*, Anterior internal venous plexus. *C*, Anterior midline fascial septum from the posterior longitudinal ligament to the dura. *D*, Dorsal root ganglion of L5. *E*, L5-S1 facet joint. *F*, Region of upper lumbosacral neural plexus. *G*, Iliac wing. *H*, Sacroiliac joint. *I*, Lower sacral nerve root sleeves within the spinal canal (S2, S3, and S4, lateral to medial, respectively).

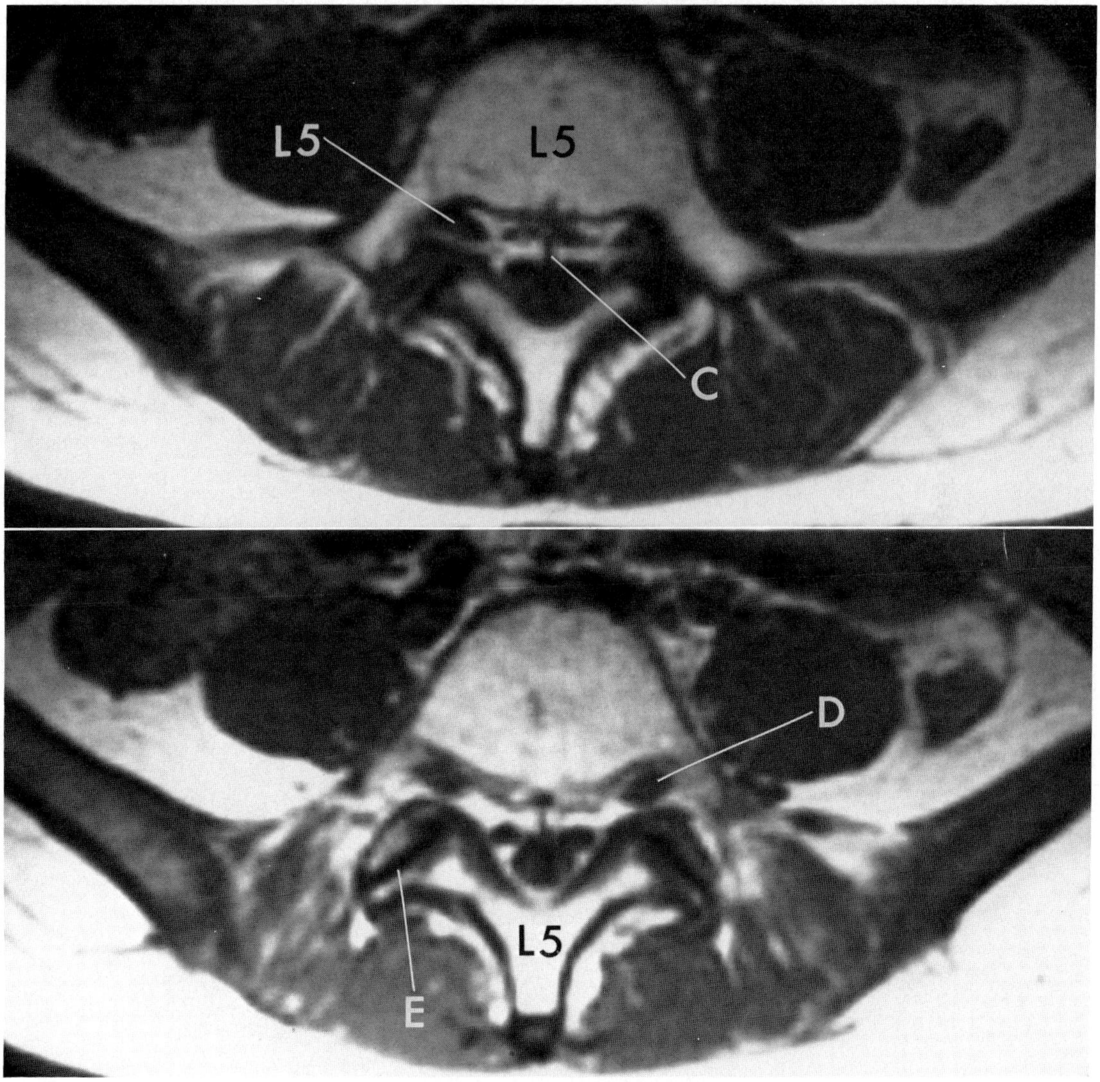

FIGURE 4-18, cont'd. For legend see opposite page. *Continued.*

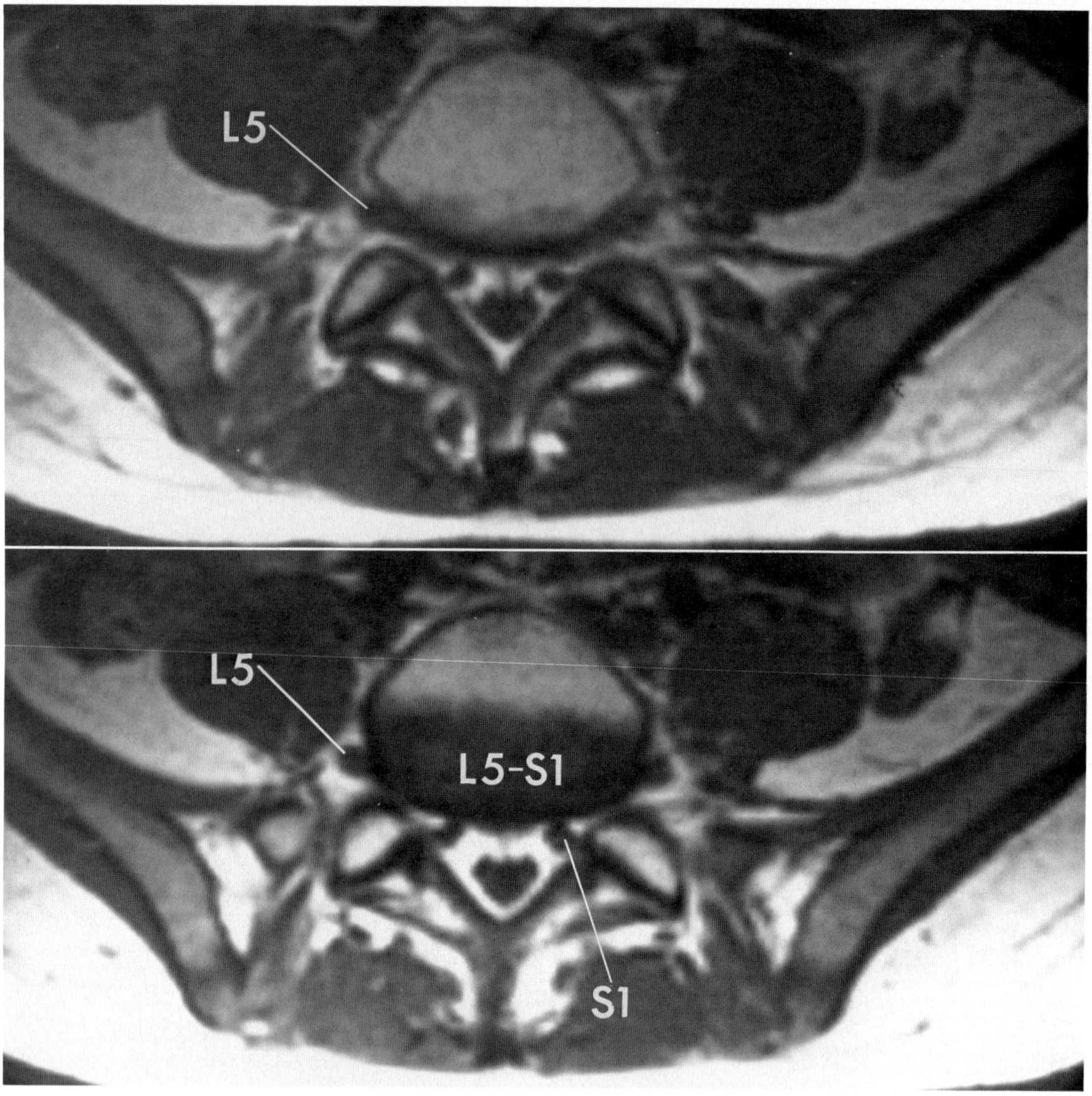

FIGURE 4-18, cont'd. Serial T1W (SE 800/20) axial 3 mm slices at 4 mm intervals (i.e., 1 mm gap between slices) showing the intraspinal and paraspinous courses of the L5 and S1 nerve roots. *A*, Sacral nerve roots of the cauda equina within the thecal sac. *B*, Anterior internal venous plexus. *C*, Anterior midline fascial septum from the posterior longitudinal ligament to the dura. *D*, Dorsal root ganglion of L5. *E*, L5-S1 facet joint. *F*, Region of upper lumbosacral neural plexus. *G*, Iliac wing. *H*, Sacroiliac joint. *I*, Lower sacral nerve root sleeves within the spinal canal (S2, S3, and S4, lateral to medial, respectively).

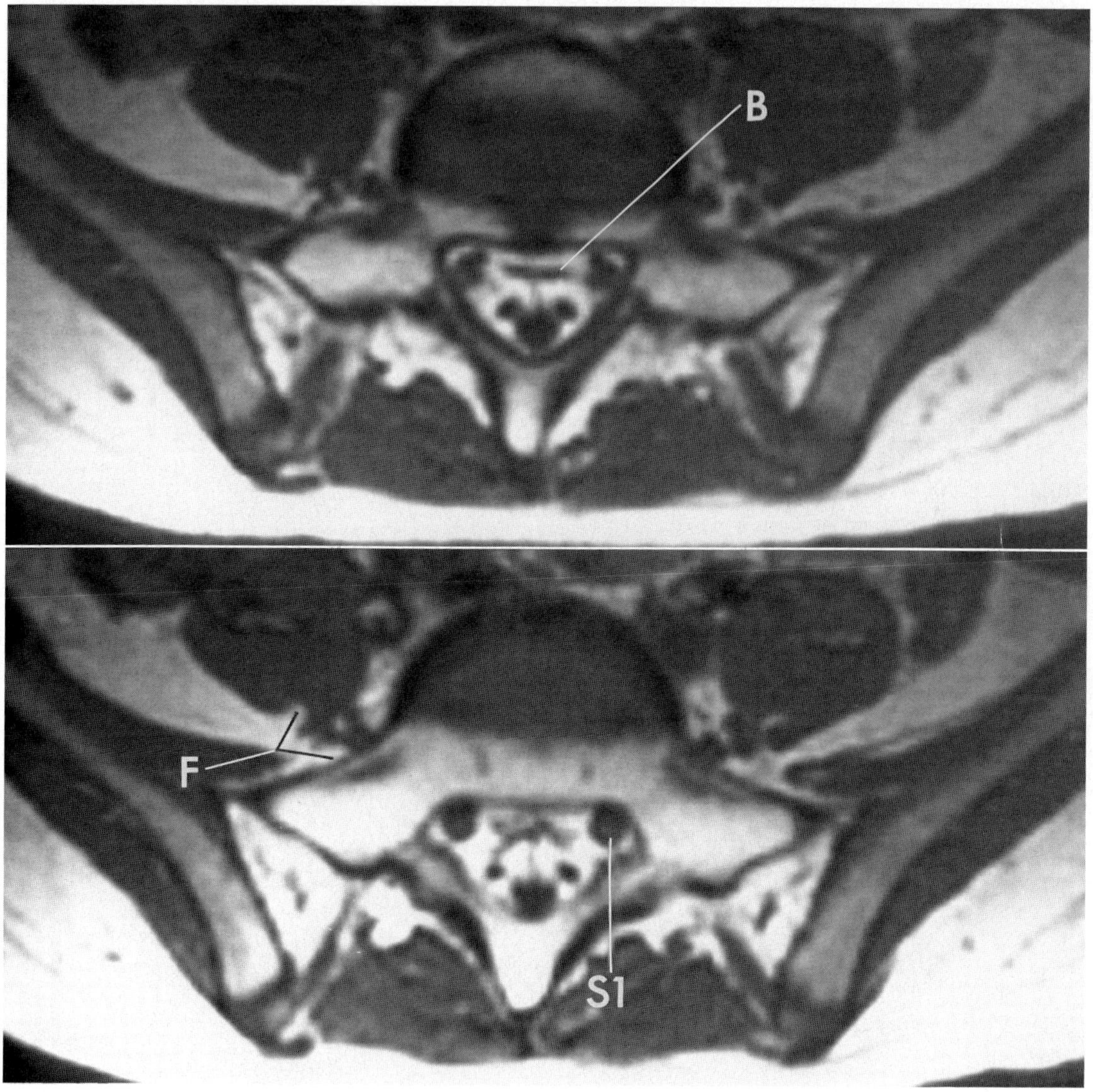

FIGURE 4-18, cont'd. For legend see opposite page. *Continued.*

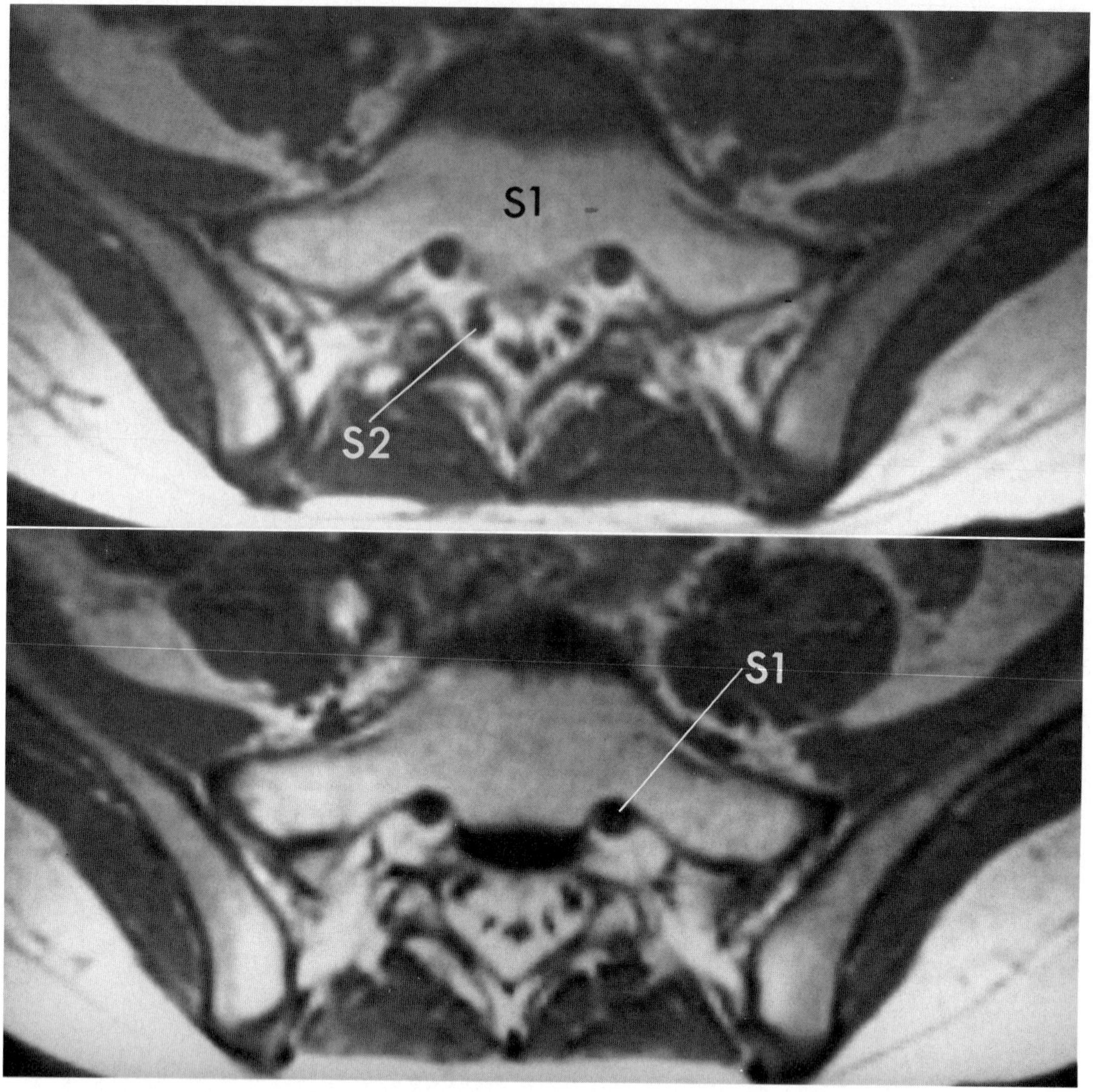

FIGURE 4-18, cont'd. Serial T1W (SE 800/20) axial 3 mm slices at 4 mm intervals (i.e., 1 mm gap between slices) showing the intraspinal and paraspinous courses of the L5 and S1 nerve roots. *A*, Sacral nerve roots of the cauda equina within the thecal sac. *B*, Anterior internal venous plexus. *C*, Anterior midline fascial septum from the posterior longitudinal ligament to the dura. *D*, Dorsal root ganglion of L5. *E*, L5-S1 facet joint. *F*, Region of upper lumbosacral neural plexus. *G*, Iliac wing. *H*, Sacroiliac joint. *I*, Lower sacral nerve root sleeves within the spinal canal (S2, S3, and S4, lateral to medial, respectively).

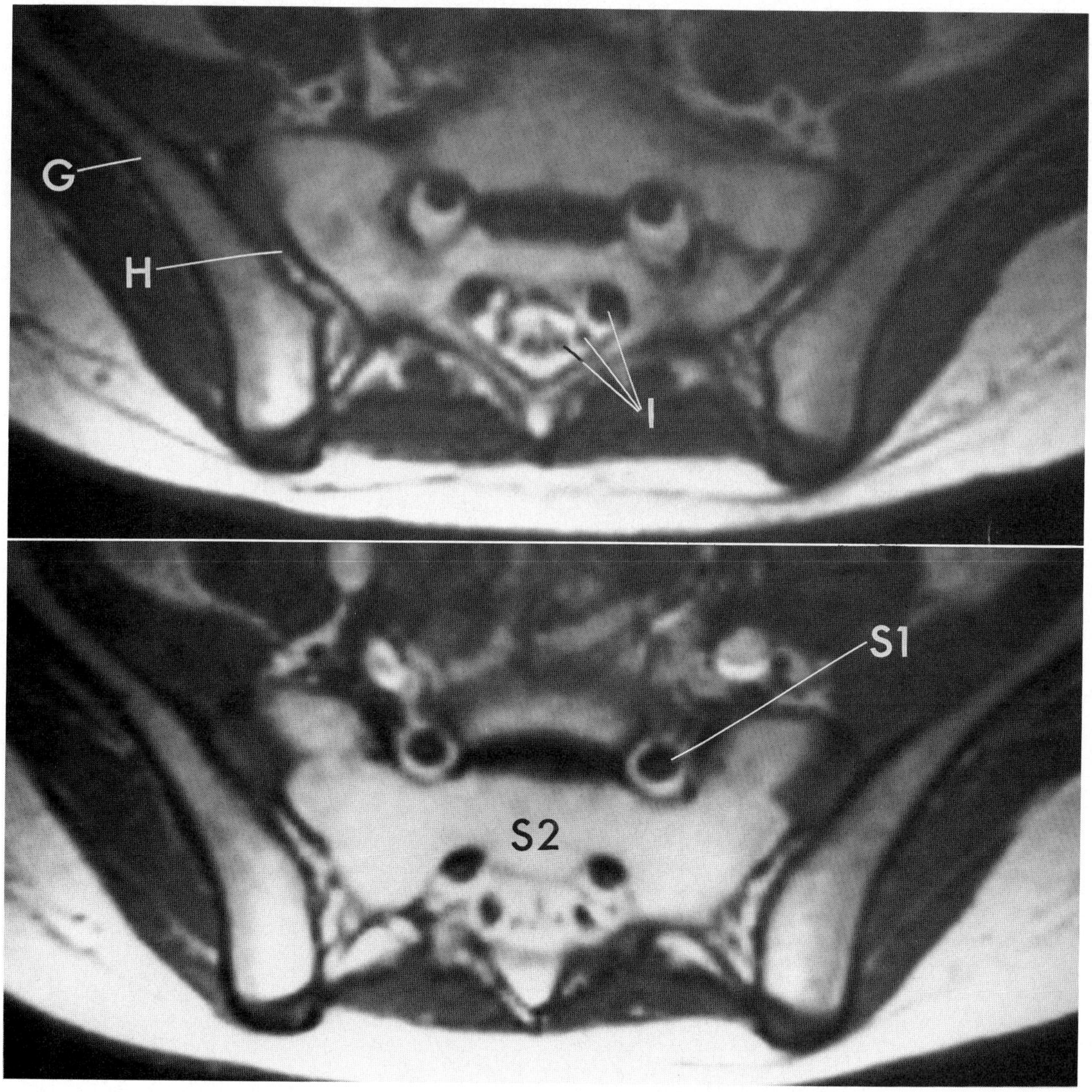

FIGURE 4-18, cont'd. For legend see opposite page.

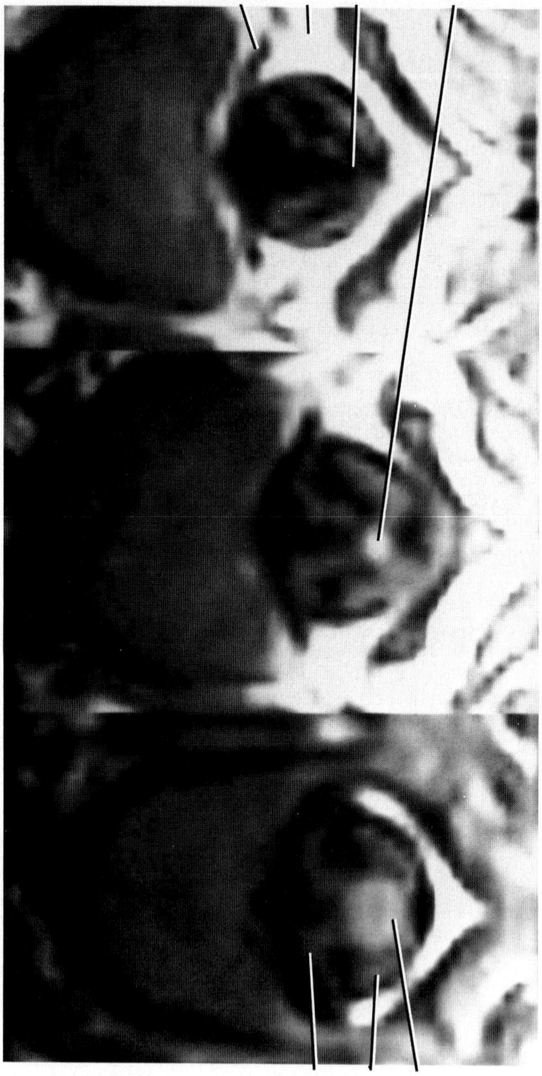

FIGURE 4-19. Serial T1W (SE 800/20) axial 3 mm slices at 4 mm intervals (i.e., 1 mm gap between slices) through the conus medullaris and proximal cauda equina.

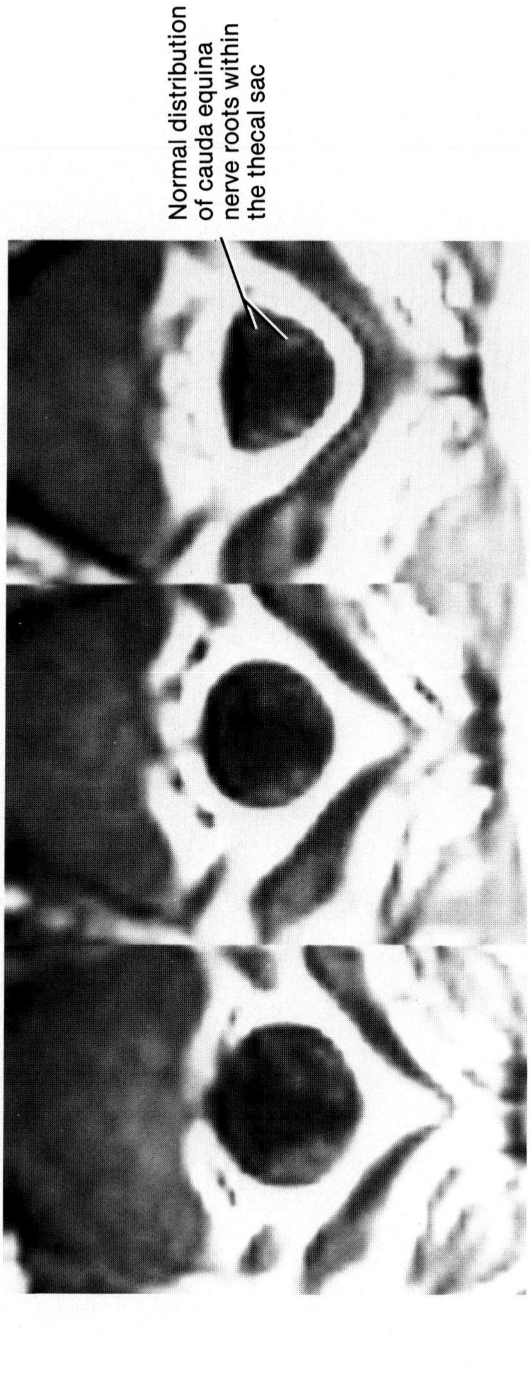

FIGURE 4-19, cont'd.

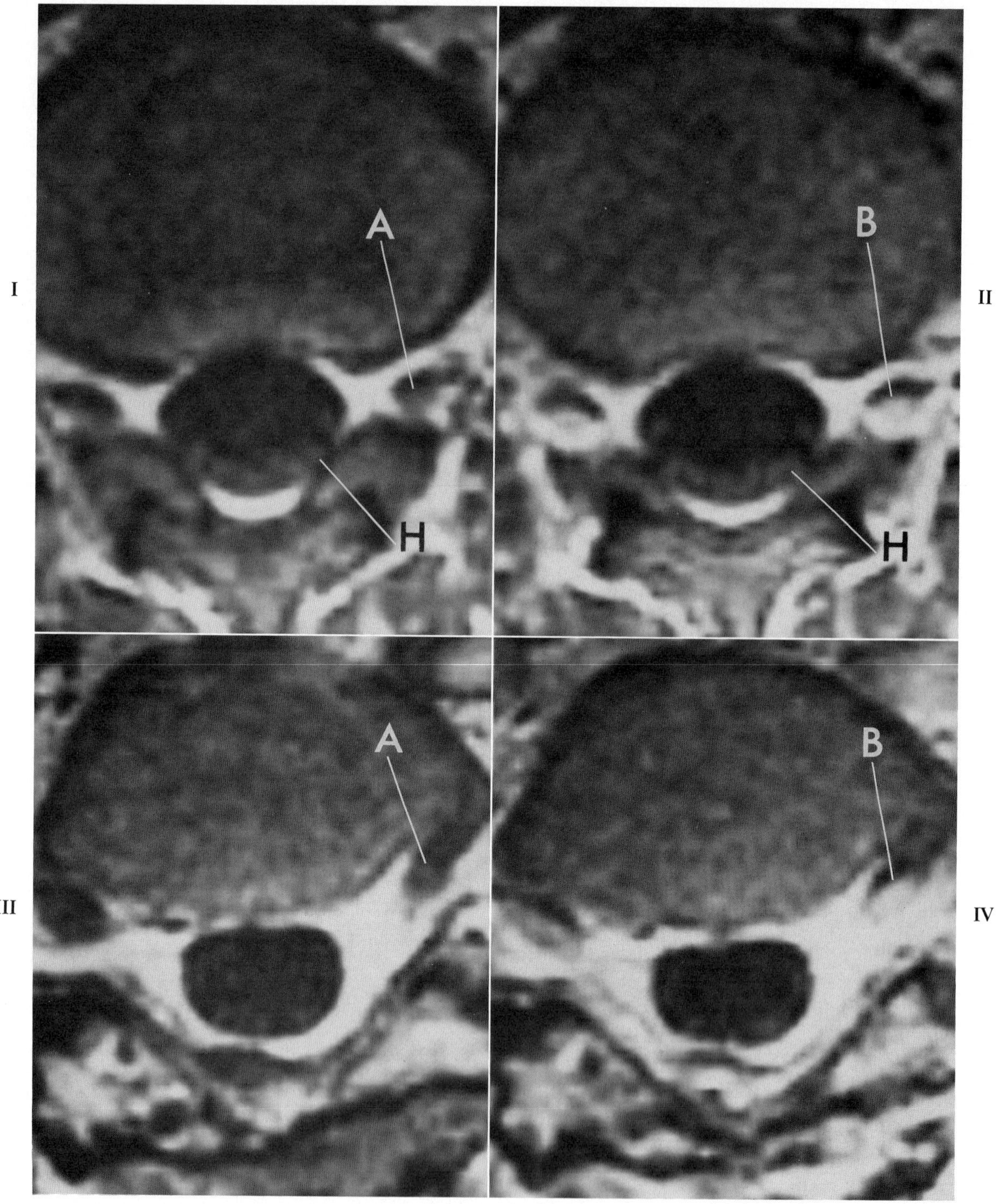

FIGURE 4-20. Axial (**I-IV**) and sagittal (**V-VIII**) T1W (SE 800/20) images pre-GdDTPA (**I, III, V,** and **VII**) and post-GdDTPA (**II, IV, VI,** and **VIII**) contrast enhancement. *A*, Pre-GdDTPA, dorsal root ganglia. *B*, Post-GdDTPA, enhancing dorsal root ganglia. *C*, Pre-GdDTPA, basivertebral vein. *D*, Post-GdDTPA, enhancing basivertebral vein. *E*, Pre-GdDTPA, postoperative fibrosis. *F*, Post-GdDTPA, enhancing postoperative fibrosis. *G*, Conus medullaris. *H*, Normal nerve roots of the cauda equina (no enhancement).

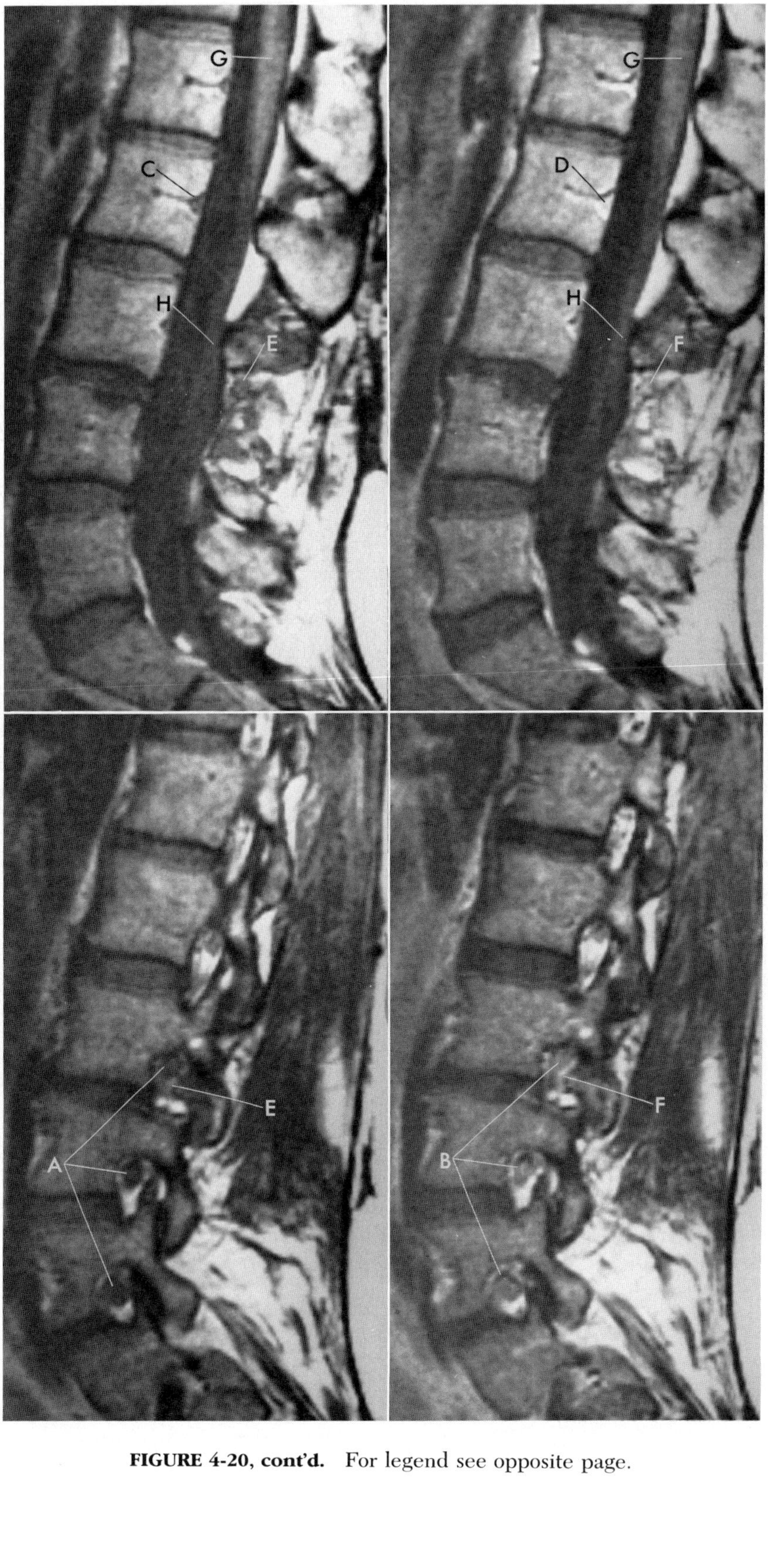

V VI

VII VIII

FIGURE 4-20, cont'd. For legend see opposite page.

I

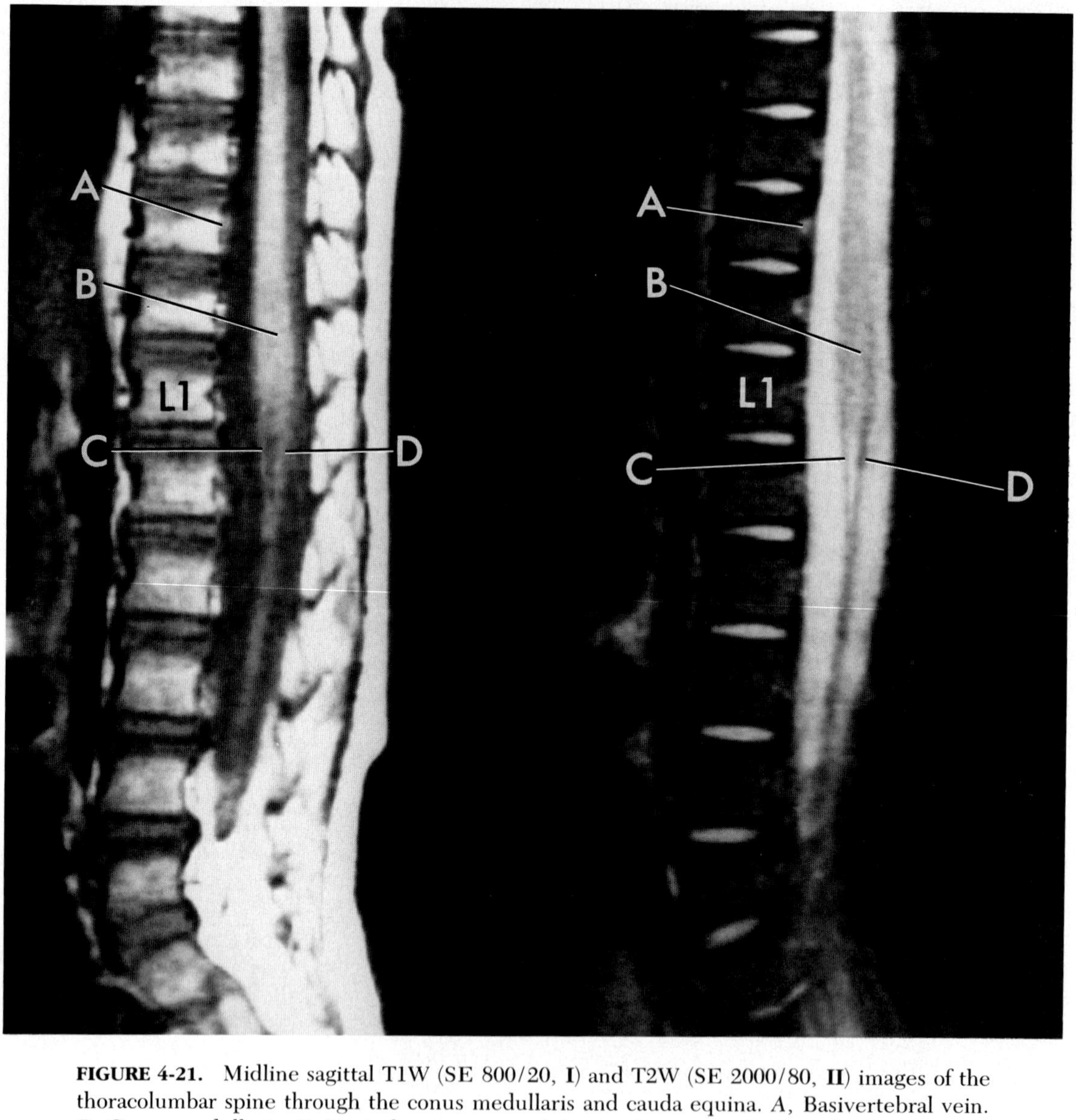

II

FIGURE 4-21. Midline sagittal T1W (SE 800/20, **I**) and T2W (SE 2000/80, **II**) images of the thoracolumbar spine through the conus medullaris and cauda equina. *A*, Basivertebral vein. *B*, Conus medullaris. *C*, Ventral nerve roots of the cauda equina. *D*, Dorsal nerve roots of the cauda equina.

THORACIC SPINE ANATOMY

The thoracic *vertebral bodies*, like the lumbar, are rectangular in sagittal and coronal cross section with flat superior and inferior end-plates that interface with the intervertebral disc via cribriform cartilage layers. The height of each thoracic vertebral body increases progressively in the caudal direction. On sagittal MR images, the *intervertebral discs* in the thoracic spine appear "flatter" than those in the cervical and lumbar spine.

The *pedicles* of the thoracic vertebrae extend from the superior half of the vertebral body and form facets that are directed slightly more posterior and lateral than those in the lumbar spine. The *neural foramina* are directed laterally and the exiting *nerve roots* and *dorsal root ganglia* are approximately centered within them on axial and sagittal images (see Figure 4-23). The lamina are relatively short and form a *spinal canal* that is approximately circular in cross section and of uniform diameter throughout the thoracic spine. The spinal canal is largely filled by the *thecal sac* with a less prominent venous plexus and relatively little epidural fat compared to the lumbar spine (see Figures 4-24 and 4-25). The *spinal cord* is usually positioned centrally within the thecal sac but may be displaced anterior and lateral with curvatures of the vertebral column. The most common displacement is slightly anterior as the cord extends over the normal upper thoracic kyphosis. Scoliosis produces lateral displacement of the cord to the "inside" of the curvature.

The major anatomic difference between thoracic vertebra and those of the cervical and lumbar spine is their articulation with the proximal *ribs*. The upper ten ribs have a head, neck, and tubercle, whereas the eleventh and twelfth ribs lack the neck and tubercle. The second through tenth *rib heads* articulate on their posterior surfaces via arthrodial (gliding) joints at the posterolateral vertebral bodies on demifacets (half of the joint surface on the superior and half on the inferior body). Between the upper and lower joint surfaces of the rib head is the *interarticular crest*, which is joined to the posterior intervertebral disc by an *intra-articular ligament*.[2,5] The first, eleventh, and twelfth rib heads articulate only with the upper part of the same numbered vertebral body, just below the disc level.[1,2] The *tubercles* of ribs one through ten articulate on their posterior surfaces via arthrodial joints with the transverse process of the same numbered vertebrae. On serial axial images, the rib head is seen on the same image as the posterolateral intervertebral disc. The tubercle is usually seen on the same image, depending on slice angulation, as it articulates with the transverse process of the vertebra below the disc level. Because the distal ribs are angled downward, especially in the lower thoracic spine, the more lateral portions of the ribs are seen on successively lower axial images.

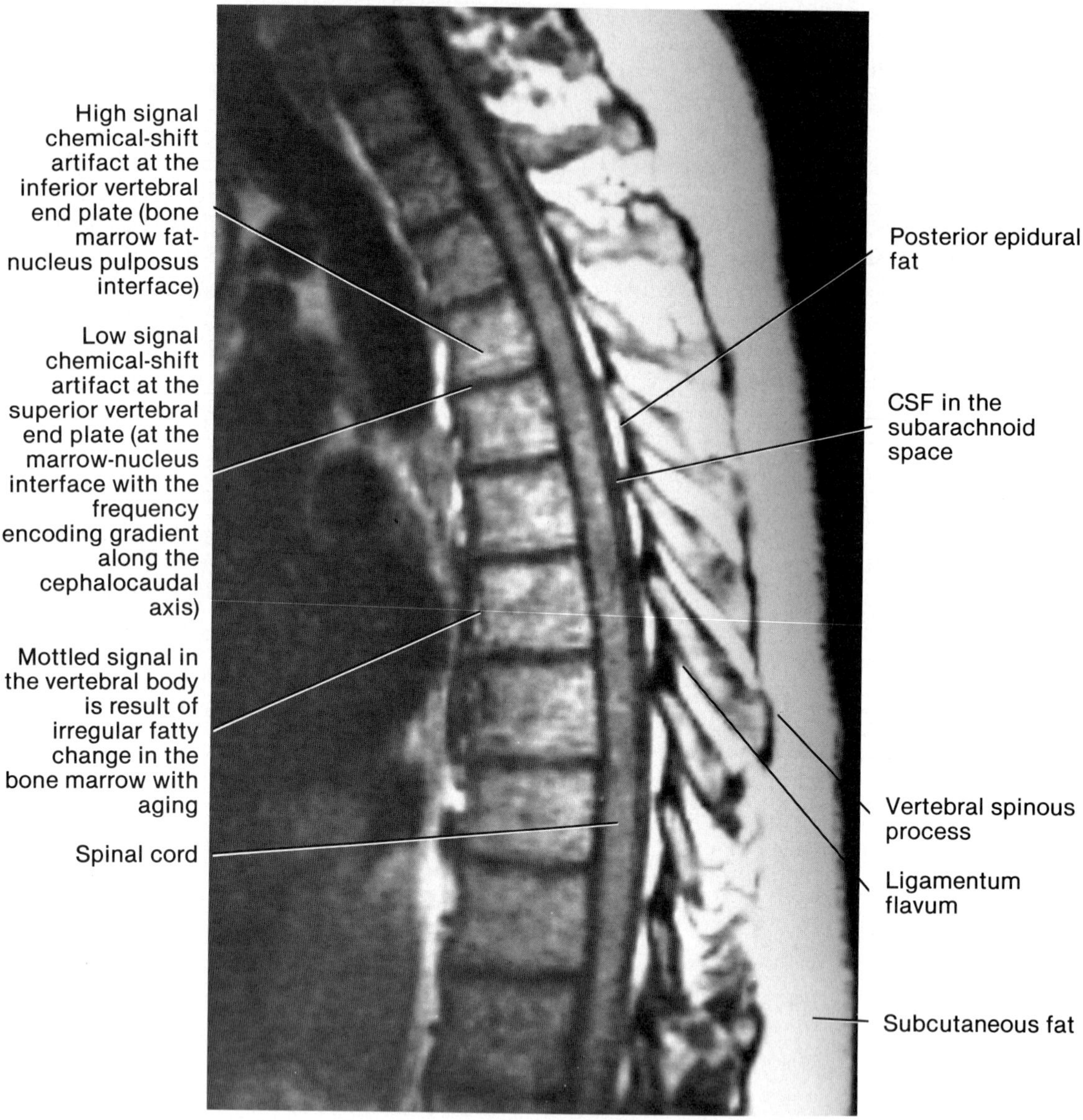

FIGURE 4-22. Sagittal midline T1W (SE 800/20) image of the midthoracic spine.

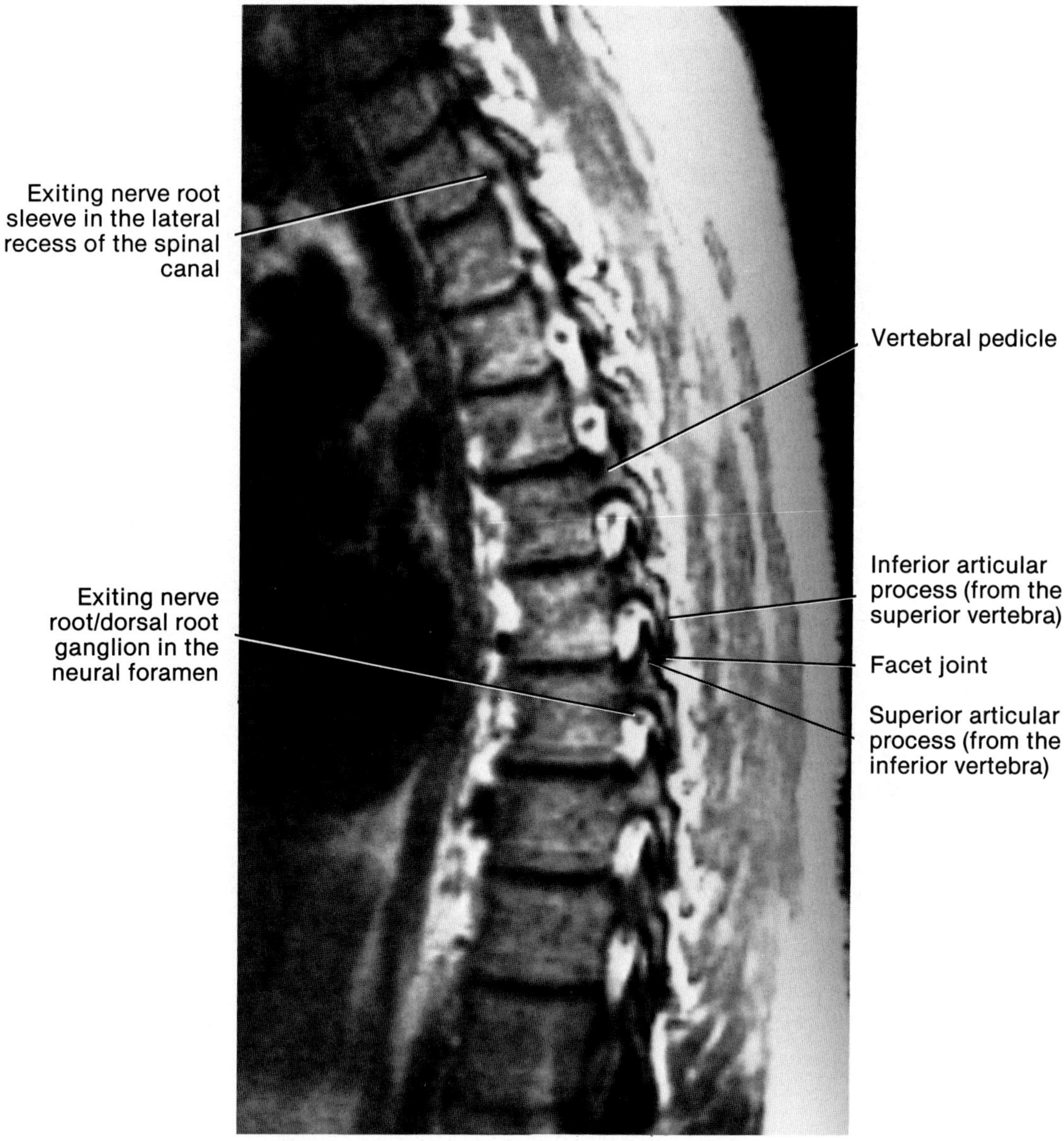

FIGURE 4-23. T1W (SE 800/20) sagittal lateral image through pedicles and neural foramina of the midthoracic spine.

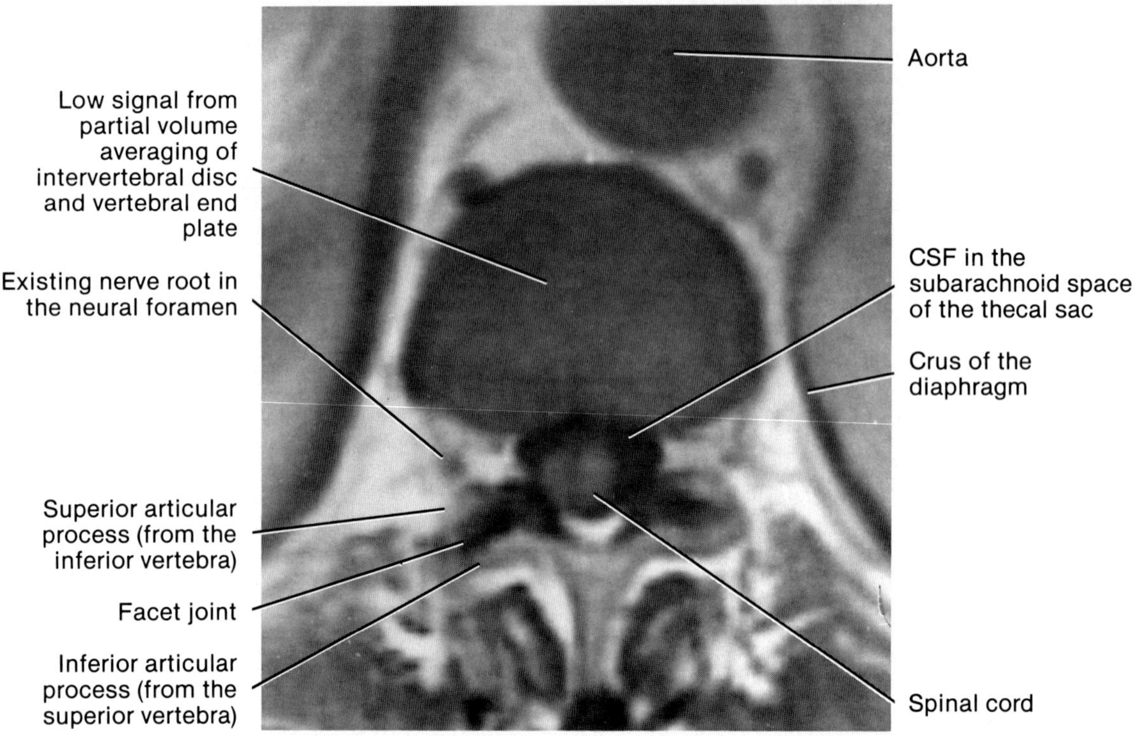

FIGURE 4-24. T1W (SE 800/20) axial image through disc and neural foramina in the lower thoracic spine.

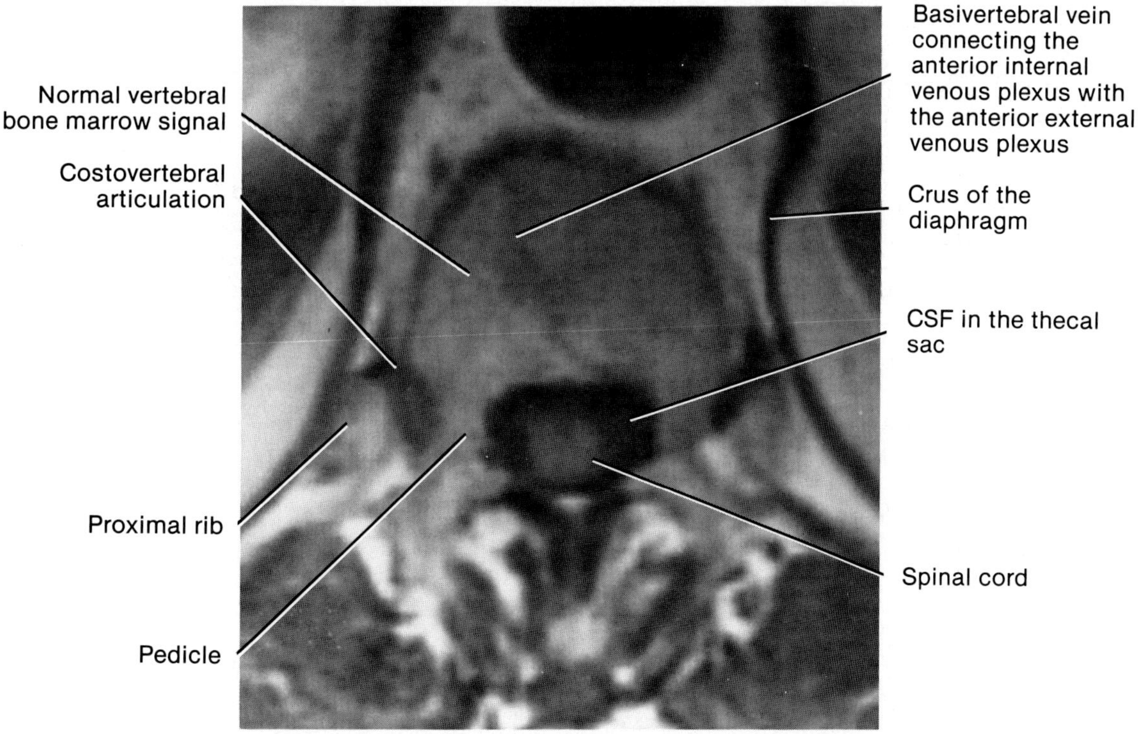

FIGURE 4-25. T1W (SE 800/20) axial image through vertebral body and pedicles in the lower thoracic spine.

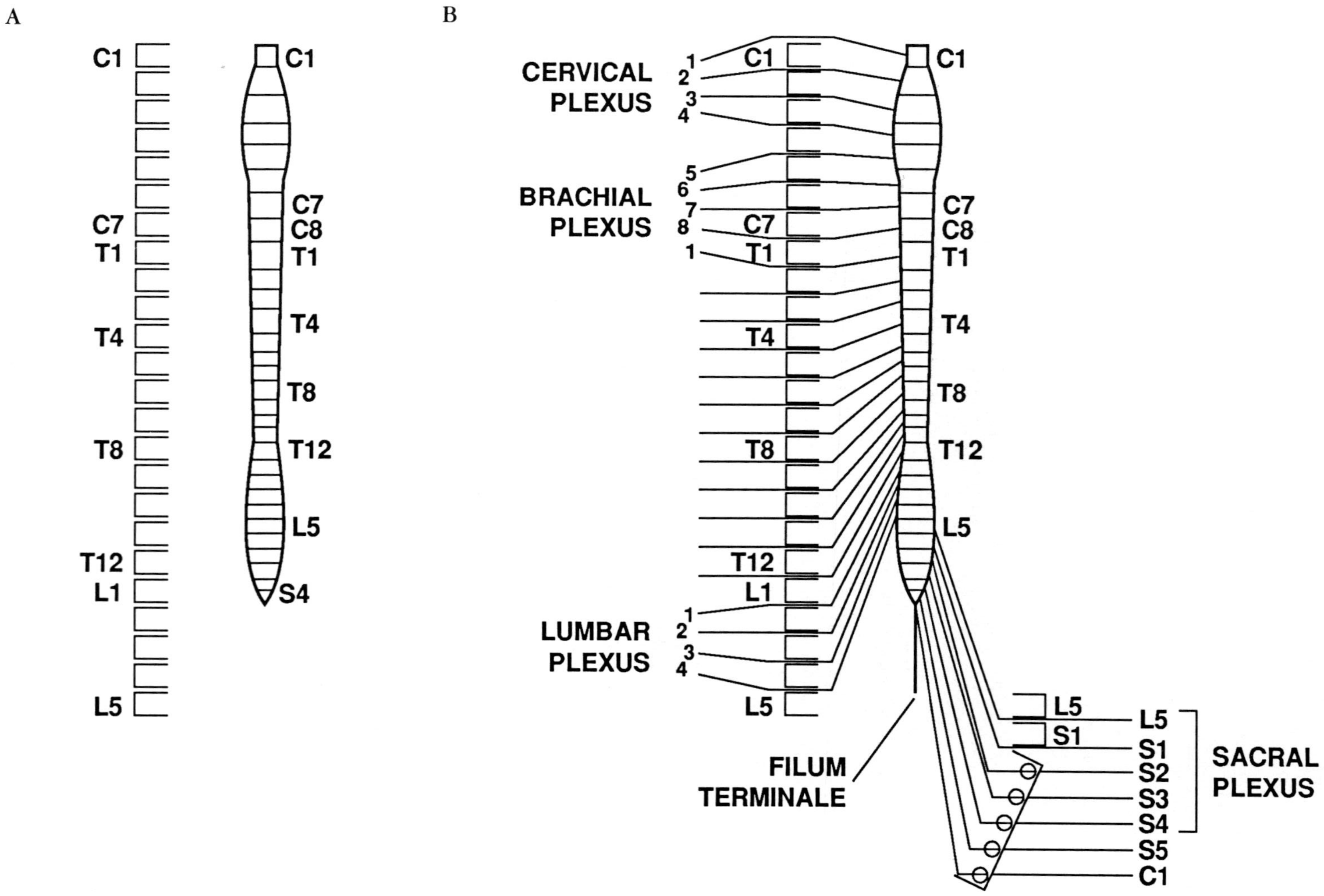

FIGURE 4-26. Diagrammatic representation of the relationship between the vertebral bodies, spinal cord segments, and exiting nerve roots.

REFERENCES

1. Epstein BS. The spine: a radiological text and atlas, ed 4. Philadelphia: Lea & Febiger, 1976.
2. Gray H. Anatomy of the human body, ed 27. Philadelphia: Lea & Febiger, 1959.
3. Greneier N, Kressel HY, Schiebler ML, et al. Normal and degenerative posterior spinal structures: MR imaging. Radiology 1987;165:517.
4. LaMasters DL, deGroot J, Williams AL, et al. Normal cervical spine. In: Newton TH and Potts DG, eds. Computed tomography of the spine and spinal cord. San Anselmo, CA: Clavadel Press, 1983.
5. LaMasters DL, DeGroot J, Williams AL, et al. Normal thoracic spine. In: Newton TH and Potts DG, eds. Computed tomography of the spine and spinal cord. San Anselmo, CA: Clavadel Press, 1983.
6. Nordqvist L. The sagittal diameter of the spinal cord and subarachnoid space in different age groups: a roentgenographic post-mortem study. Acta Radiol [supplement] 1964;227:1.
7. Pernkopf E. Atlas of topographical and applied human anatomy: head and neck, vol. 1. Baltimore-Munich: Urban & Schwarzenberg Inc, 1980.
8. Rauschning W. Correlative multiplanar computed tomographic anatomy of the normal spine. Baltimore: Williams & Wilkins, 1984.
9. Shapiro R. Myelography, ed 4. Chicago: Year Book Medical Publishers Inc, 1984.
10. Thijssen HOM, Keyser A, Horstink MWM, et al. Morphology of the cervical spinal cord on computed myelography. Neuroradiology 1979;18:57.

5

Congenital Anomalies of the Spine and Spinal Cord

Robert L. DeLaPaz

TABLE 5-1
Clinical Signs Suggesting Congenital Spinal Pathologic Conditions

Neurologic Findings

Back pain
Lasègue sign
Gait abnormality
Lower extremity spasticity and hyperreflexia
Lower extremity weakness and hyporeflexia
Lower extremity muscle atrophy
Lower extremity sensory deficits
Bladder (rarely bowel) dysfunction

Dorsal Lumbar Cutaneous Abnormalities

Hypertrichosis
Dimples
Pigmented nevi
Hemangiomas and telangectasias
Dermal sinus
Fluctuant mass (lipomyelomeningocele, myelocystocele)
Soft, compressible mass (lipoma)

Spinal Anomalies

Scoliosis
Sharply angled kyphosis or gibbus deformity
Spina bifida
Widened interpedicular distance
Fused vertebrae and Klippel-Feil deformity

Orthopedic Deformities

Pes cavus, varus and valgus
Sprengel's deformity

Intestinal Anomaly

Neurenteric cyst
Intestinal duplication

MR is ideal for noninvasive evaluation of patients with congenital intraspinal pathologic conditions (Table 5-1). In most cases, MR imaging may be used in place of traditional myelography or cisternography and CT scanning. The essential elements of congential anomalies that must be identified are the internal cord structure, dysraphic bone abnormalities, relationship of the cord to extramedullary lesions such as myelomeningocele or lipoma, the location of nerve roots and filum terminale, and the configuration of the subarachnoid space. MR identifies all of these features without ionizing radiation or without the risks of invasive procedures, contrast reaction, and general anesthesia usually required for evaluation by myelography and CT scanning. MR is the only imaging modality that directly visualizes the internal architecture of the cord for positive identification of syringomyelia, hydromyelia, and intramedullary tumor. MR also delineates the internal architecture of meningoceles and meningeal cysts not opacified by subarachnoid contrast media. Although bony anomalies are still best delineated by plain radiography and CT scanning, high field MR images, especially with variable flip angle/gradient echo techniques, often show bone lesions well by contrast with adjacent soft tissue.

Ultrasound studies of the bifid lumbar spine in infants yield useful information concerning tethering of the cord, lipomyelomeningoceles, and caudal masses.[73,85] However, sonographic studies of structures within the closed osseous spinal canal cannot be performed because of acoustic reflection and shadowing. Although a series of direct comparison has not been done, MR imaging appears to be better than sonography for detailed visualization of congenital spinal lesions and complete evaluation of intraspinal contents.

SPINAL CORD ANOMALIES

Embryology

Spinal dysraphism is a general term for a group of congenital disorders that involve incomplete midline fusion of mesenchymal, bone, and neural elements. The major categories of spinal dysraphic lesions are summarized in Table 5-2 on p. 181.

The spinal cord develops from the embryonic neural tube that is formed by longitudinal folding of the neural plate ectoderm dorsally (Figure 5-1).[20] Between approximately 17 and 21 days of embryonic life (1.5 to 3.0 mm embryo length), this longitudinal "neural groove" deepens. In the next step of development, neurulation, the neural folds converge dorsally and fuse to form the neural tube. Fusion is accomplished by the action of actin myofibrils in microvilli projecting from neuroepithelial cells on either side of the tube.[108] Simultaneously with neurulation, the neural tube separates from the overlying ectoderm, a process called "dysjunction".[61,62] Dorsal cells adjacent to the neural groove separate to

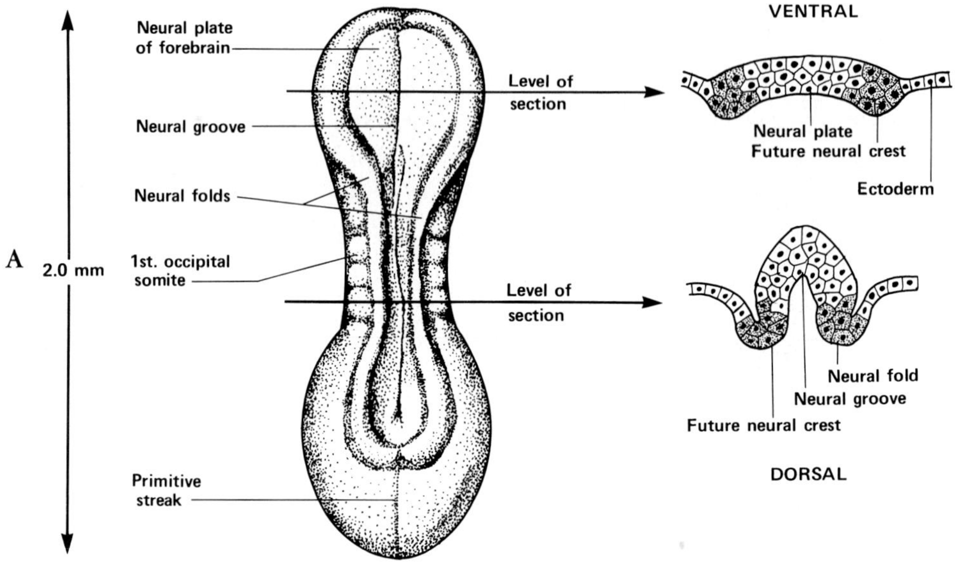

FIGURE 5-1. Closure of neural tube. **A,** Dorsal view of neural plate at 20 days of gestation, just before neurulation. Cross-sections show neural plate at early stage (upper diagram) with shallow neural groove and early differentiation into future dorsal ectoderm, neural tube (future spinal cord), and neural crest (future dorsal root ganglia) cells. At level of cervical somites (lower diagram) cells are further differentiated and neural folds approach midline, deepening neural groove. **B,** Dorsal view of neural tube at 21 days of gestation, early stages of neurulation. Cross-section through level immediately cephalad to fused cervical neural folds and shows nearly closed neural tube and advanced differentiation of neural crest cells into rudimentary dorsal root ganglia. Ectoderm differentiated into distinct cell layer dorsally, just before separation from neural tube and neural crest cells. Anterior and posterior neurospores remain open. **C,** Dorsal view of neural tube at 24 days of gestation, late stages of neurulation. Neural tube almost entirely fused dorsally with only posterior neuropore remaining open. Cross-section through cervical level shows dysjunction with dorsal separation of ectoderm, neural crest, and neural tube cells. Neural crest cells form distinct layer that will become sensory dorsal root ganglia. Neural tube shows early internal differentiation of neuroepithelial cells into future ventral spinal cord (basal plate) and dorsal spinal cord (alar plate). (From Netter FH. In: Crelin ES, Netter FH, Shapter RK. Development of the nervous system: a logical approach to neuroanatomy. CIBA Clinical Symposia 1974; 26[2]:1.)

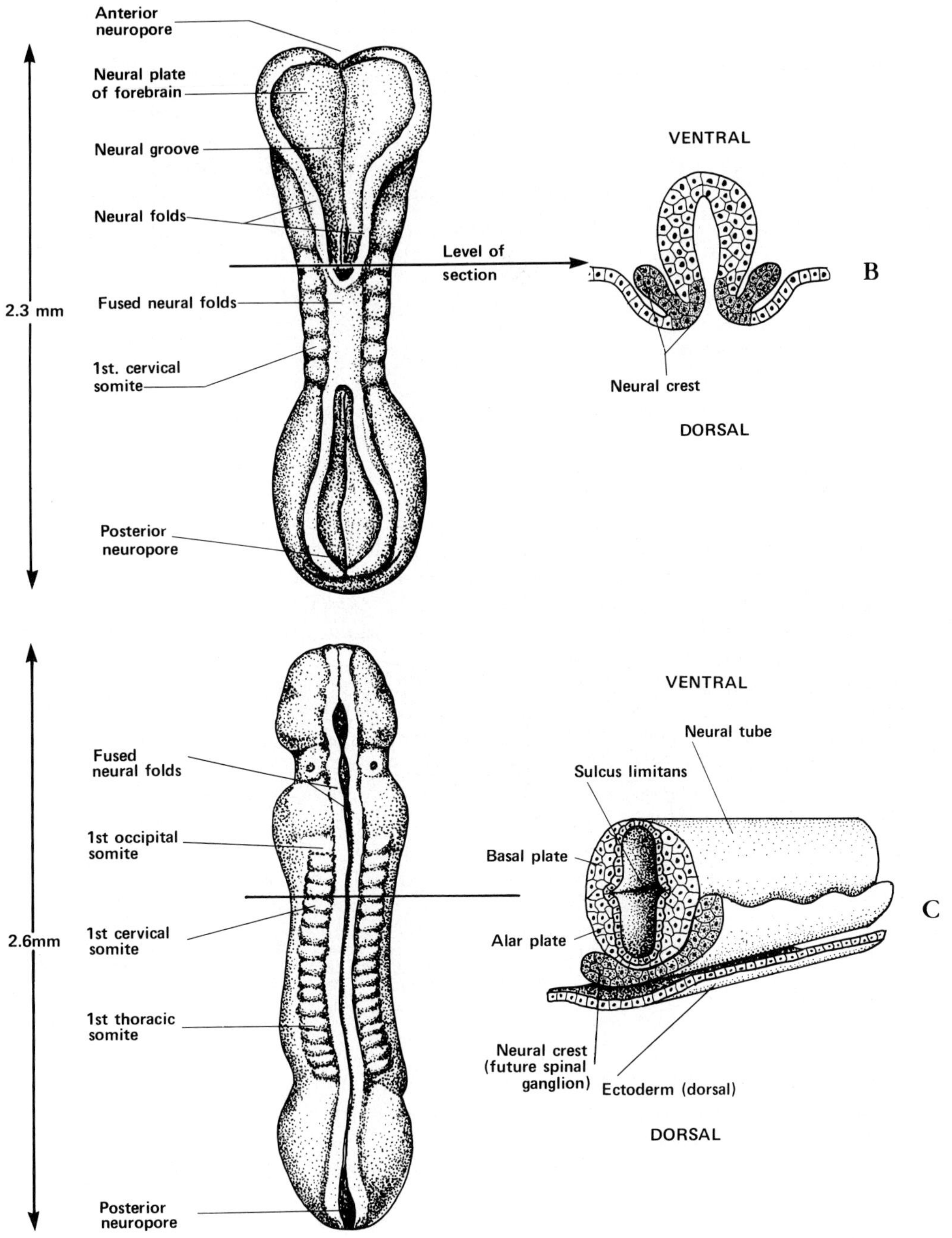
Anterior neuropore
Neural plate of forebrain
Neural groove
Neural folds
Level of section
Fused neural folds
2.3 mm
1st. cervical somite
Posterior neuropore
VENTRAL
Neural crest
DORSAL
B
Fused neural folds
1st occipital somite
1st cervical somite
2.6mm
1st thoracic somite
Posterior neuropore
VENTRAL
Neural tube
Sulcus limitans
Basal plate
Alar plate
Neural crest (future spinal ganglion)
Ectoderm (dorsal)
DORSAL
C

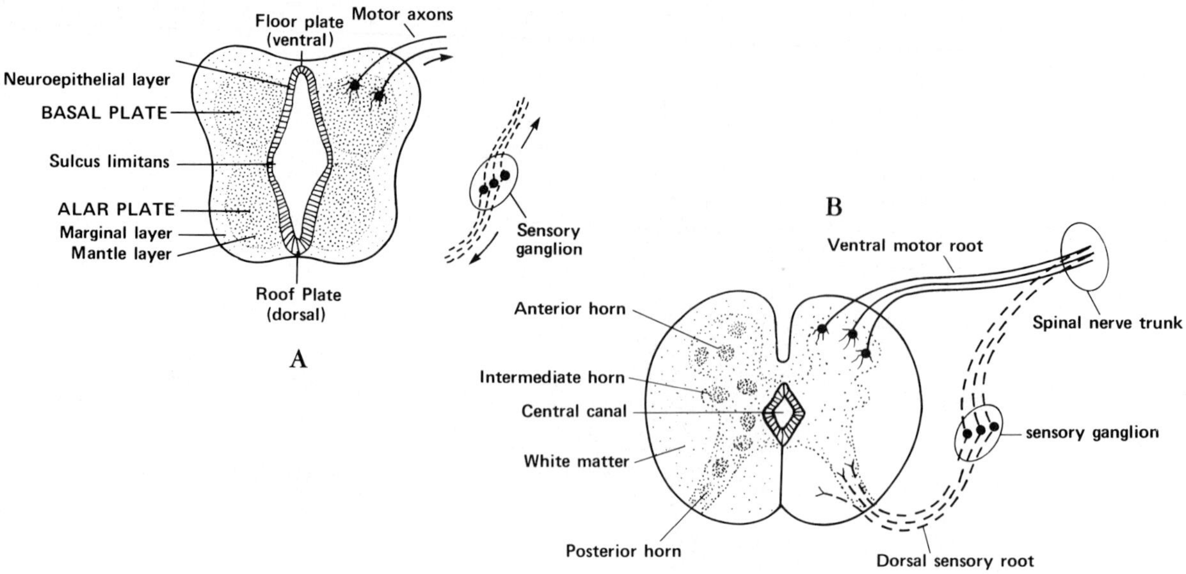

FIGURE 5-2. Spinal cord development. **A,** Early development of internal anatomy of spinal cord. Shortly after neural tube closure, *neuroepithelial layer* gives rise to *neuroblasts* (primitive nerve cells) that migrate laterally to form *mantle layer*, future gray matter of cord. Outer *marginal layer* is future white matter of cord and made up of ascending and descending nerve fibers emerging from primitive neurons of mantle layer. As neuroblasts continue to migrate into mantle layer, ventral and dorsal enlargements occur bilaterally, separated by sulcus limitans, a longitudinal groove on each side of the neural tube. Ventral enlargements form basal plates, which eventually develop into motor areas of cord. Motor neurons in basal plate project axons ventrally to form ventral motor roots. Dorsal enlargements form alar plates, which develop into sensory areas of cord. Sensory neurons in alar plate eventually link with axons from neuroblasts in dorsal sensory ganglia to form dorsal sensory roots. Thin dorsal roof plate and ventral floor plate do not generate neuroblasts but form pathways for nerve fibers crossing between the two halves of cord, eventually forming commissures adjacent to central canal. **B,** Late differentiation of internal spinal cord architecture. Basal plates expand to form anterior motor horns of gray matter, and ventral midline sulcus forms and will later contain anterior spinal artery. Ventral motor roots extend laterally to merge with dorsal roots and form spinal nerve trunk. As alar plates expand to form posterior sensory horns of gray matter, they enlarge medially to compress dorsal portion of neural tube lumen, resulting in small central canal. The two alar plates eventually fuse in midline to form posterior median septum. Axons from neuroblasts in dorsal sensory ganglia enter dorsal cord to end in posterior horns or ascend in marginal layer to sensory centers in the brain. (From Leland J. In: Langman J, ed. Medical embryology, ed 2. Baltimore: Williams & Wilkins Co, 1969.)

become the neural crest, which forms the sensory dorsal root ganglia. The cells of the neural tube form the spinal cord. Closure of the neural tube begins in the upper cervical region and progresses cranially and caudally. The open cranial and caudal ends of the neural tube are called the anterior neuropore and posterior neuropore, respectively. The anterior neuropore closes first, forming the lamina terminalis, at 25 days (4 mm embryo). The posterior neuropore closes at 28 days (6 mm embryo) at approximately the midsacral level.[57]

Development of the cross-sectional anatomy of the spinal cord involves the differentiation of tissue layers within the wall of the neural tube (Figure 5-2). Layering of the neural tube begins with the ependymal layer, the germinal neuroepithelial cells immediately adjacent to the lumen of the neural tube. These cells undergo mitosis and give rise to the precursor cells of neurons and neuroglia, which migrate laterally to form the mantle layer, the future gray matter of the cord. As neurons in the mantle layer differentiate, their projections form the more lat-

TABLE 5-2
Surgical Findings with Spinal Dysraphism

Lesions	Frequency (%)
Traction lesions	65
Lumbosacral lipoma	18
Diastematomyelia associated with bands	18
Meningocele	11
Lumbosacral lipoma with diastoma tomyelia	6
Tight filum terminale	5
Simple traction bands	3
Coccygeal cyst	2
Lipoma in filum terminale	1
Dermal sinus	1
Diastematomyelia without Bands	24
Dermoid cysts	5
Hydromyelia	2
Myelodysplasia	2
	2

(Adapted from James CCM, Lassman LP. Spinal dysraphism: spina bifida occulta. London: Butterworth and Co. 1972. With permission.)

eral marginal layer, the future white matter of the cord. Sensory neurons form propriospinal connections in the marginal layer and ascending tracts that project to the brain. Motor neurons send their axons into the developing ventral roots.[55]

The lumen of the neural tube becomes diamond-shaped as the cord develops. A longitudinal groove on each side of the lumen is called the sulcus limitans. The developing mantle layer dorsal to the sulans limitans is the alar plate, which eventually forms the dorsal horn. Afferent sensory fibers from the neurons of the dorsal root ganglia grow in through the developing dorsal roots to terminate within the alar plate region. The mantle layer ventral to the sulcus limitans is the basal plate, which eventually forms the anterior horn. Axons of the developing motor neurons in the anterior horns form the ventral spinal nerve roots. The midline regions just dorsal and ventral to the central canal are the roof plates and floor plates, respectively, which provide pathways for fibers crossing between the two halves of the cord.

The notochord separates from the primitive gut and neural tube at about 25 days to form the ventral subchordal and dorsal epichordal zones into which the mesenchyme migrates to eventually form the meninges, vertebrae, neural arches, and muscle.

Caudal to the posterior neuropore, the neural tube elongates further by a process called canalization.[57] At this stage the neural epithelium at the caudal end of the embryo fuses with the notochord to form the caudal cell mass in the tail fold (30 days and 7 mm length). Multiple clumps of ependymal cells and multiple microcysts form in this caudal cell mass that coalesce and eventually unite with the neural tube to form the distal conus medullaris and filum terminale. Persistence of ependymal rests and accessory lumina in the conus and filum probably result from this process. In the final phase of caudal spinal cord formation (38 days, 10 mm embryo), retrogressive differentiation produces a decrease in the caudal cell mass.[102] The final result is formation of the conus tip and proximal filum with a focal dilatation of the central canal, the *ventriculus terminalis*.[70] The complexity of these processes of posterior neuropore closure, canalization, and retrogressive differentiation increase the likelihood of an anomalous result and probably account for the greater frequency of congenital abnormalities in the lumbar spine and cord compared to the thoracic and cervical levels.

After the neural tube closes completely, the lengthwise growth of the spinal cord is limited. Elongation of the vertebral canal continues during fetal life and infancy, resulting in termination of the spinal cord at about the L_3 vertebral body in the infant and the L_1 level in the adult.[10] (Figure 5-3).

In general, anomalies of the spine and spinal cord are the result of developmental errors that produce abnormal relationships between mesodermal (vertebral column) and ectodermal (skin and neural elements) tissues.[31] The specific nature of dysraphic anomalies depends on the phase of embryogenesis. Lesions such as lumbar myelomeningoceles, which leave neural tissue exposed to the surface, probably arise from defective neurulation. Lesions such as lumbar lipomeningoceles and caudal diastomatomyelia lying beneath intact skin probably arise after closure of the neural tube during defective canalization and retrogressive differentiation of the caudal cell mass. Sacral teratomas, lipomas wholly within the filum terminale, and tethered spinal cord may also result from abnormal development of the caudal cell mass.[57] Cervical and thoracic lesions probably result from defective dysjunction between the neural tube and overlying ectoderm.[70] Cervical and thoracic dermal sinuses, skin-covered thoracic myelomeningoceles, thoracic lipomeningoceles, and thoracic diastomatomyelia may result from formation of focal neuroectodermal-ectodermal adhesions. Mesenchyme exposed to the interior of the neural tube by a failure of dysjunction appears to form lipomatous tissue, which may explain lipomas and lipomeningoceles at all levels of the spine, as well as the lipoma of the corpus callosum.[70]

TETHERED CORD AND THICKENED FILUM

The tethered cord is defined as an abnormally low position of the conus medullaris tip, below the level of the L_2 vertebral body in adults. Thickened filum terminale is defined as enlargement of the filum to a diameter of 2 mm or greater. These two findings are usually seen in combination but, in some cases, they may occur individually; that is, a tethered cord may occur without a thickened filum and a thickened filum may be present with the conus tip in its normal position.[74]

The conus usually reaches the normal adult level of L_1 to L_2 by approximately 2 months of age. However with individual variation, it may lie as low as L_3 at 2 years or at L_2 to L_3 at 12 years in some normal cases.[10] In general, after 12 years of age, the tip of the conus should not lie below the L_2 level.[30]

The normal adult filum is approximately 20 cm long and less than 2 mm in diameter.[38,93] It is uniform in caliber from the abruptly tapered tip of the conus caudally. The proximal 5 to 6 mm contains the distal central canal, the proximal 5 cm contains neural tissue, and the remainder is made up of fibrous connective tissue. Approximately 15 cm lies within the caudal thecal sac while the distal 5 cm is extradural and inserts on the dorsal surface of the first coccygeal segment.[92] The abnormal filum may be as thick as 5 mm and may show enlargement distally, especially when associated with a lipoma.[38] In the majority of abnormal cases (55%), the filum is thickened by dense fibrosis alone, while in another 23% a thin lipoma is also found and in a small number of cases (3%) a filar cyst (possibly arachnoid in origin) accompanies the thickened filum. In 13% of cases, the pathologic condition overlaps that of the caudal lipoma complex and no true filum is present. Instead, the distal cord is elongated and thinned, ending in a lipoma at the caudal thecal sac.[40]

Embryology

The embryogenesis of the tethered cord is not well understood but is probably the result of failure of involution of the terminal sacral spinal cord during retrogressive differentiation. Normally, caudal to the thirty-second somite, the neural tube becomes atrophic and a ventral remnant forms the filum terminale. With growth of the spinal column, there is lengthening of this structure (Figure 5-3). Failure of either the degeneration of the primitive sacral cord or of the filum and distal nerve fibers to elongate with growth, or both—possibly as a result of insults such as hemorrhage or inflammation—may result in tethering.[70,93]

Vertebral Anomalies

Several vertebral and dural malformations accompany the tethered cord. Spina bifida occulta over one or more segments is present in 33% to 100% of cases.[40,70] Congenital or acquired kyphoscoliosis is present in approximately 25% of cases. Multiple other bony anomalies are also seen, including bifid ribs, additional ribs, spondylolysis and spondylolysthesis, dysplastic vertebral bodies, and widened spinal canal.[70] The dural sac may be widened or constricted by dural and extradural bands. In some cases, the dura is tented posteriorly by the taut filum tethered distally.[70] The filum may be associated with an extradural lipoma, extradural cyst, or meningocele.[78]

Clinical Findings

The tethered cord is usually symptomatic between the ages of 3 and 35. Symptoms usually appear during the adolescent growth spurt.[40,70] The occult tethered cord symptoms may not appear until much later in life, (e.g., eighth decade) and can produce diagnostic confusion if not considered in the differential diagnosis.[50,78]

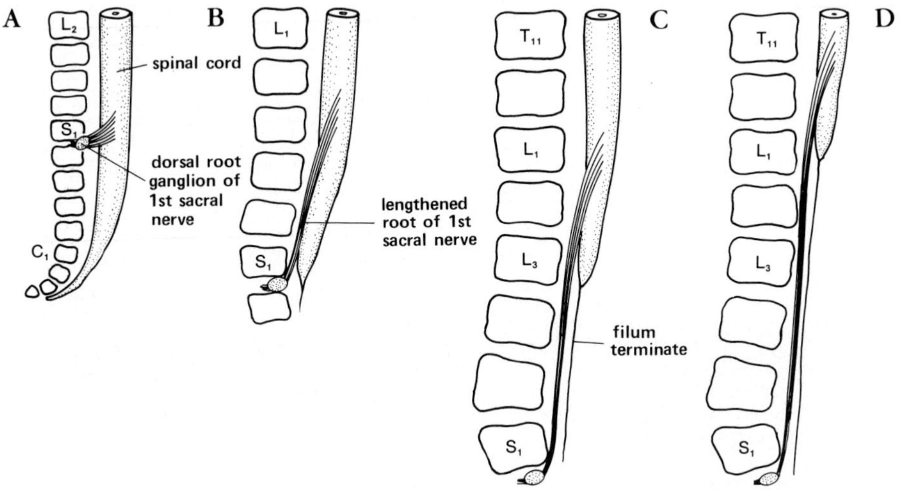

FIGURE 5-3. Differential growth of spine and spinal cord. Schematic sagittal view of caudal spine and cord at different stages of development. **A,** Approximately third month of development. Spine and cord levels correspond directly. **B,** End of fifth month. Growth of spine without lengthening of cord results in elongation of caudal spinal nerve roots and cephalad migration of conus tip. **C,** Term newborn. Conus tip lies at L_3 level and thin filum terminale is present. **D,** Adult. Conus tip lies at L_1 level, with range of normal extending mid-to-inferior L_2 level.

The incidence in males and females is equal and the appearance is sporadic, without a clear familial tendency. Most patients complain of gait difficulty, ranging from a sensation of leg stiffness to true weakness with hyperreflexia, often worse in the morning and after exercise. Approximately 50% also have bladder dysfunction, sensory abnormalities, back pain, hypertrichosis, and associated foot deformities. Bowel dysfunction is uncommon.[70] In cases of thickened filum alone, with the conus tip at L_2 or above, less severe symptoms and signs such as nocturia, pain, and positive Lasègue sign (sciatic pain on hip flexion with knee extension) are more common.[74]

The explanation for clinical symptoms appears to be mechanical, caused by stretching of the distal spinal cord. Evidence for this hypothesis includes the onset of symptoms at the time of development of the lumbar lordosis (which lengthens the spinal canal) and exacerbation with the adolescent growth spurt. Worsening of symptoms typically occurs with movements that produce hip flexion, with prolonged sitting, and with overnight rest that lengthens the spinal column due to normal swelling of the intervertebral discs.[70,78] Additional evidence comes from surgical experience where symptoms are improved or cured with cephalad migration of the cord 0.5 cm to 2.5 cm is seen after sectioning of the filum.[30,50,70,74,78] Experimental, mechanical tethering of the cord in animals demonstrates reduced blood flow and oxidative metabolism in the distal spinal cord.[49,105,113]

MR Imaging

High SNR T1W axial images are the best way to evaluate the filum terminale.[1,23,54,104] This is a fibrous structure but contains sufficient water to produce higher signal than CSF on T1W images, similar to nerve roots. Axial images allow differentiation of the midline filum from the laterally arrayed nerve roots of the cauda equina, especially immediately caudad to the conus tip (Figures 5-4 to 5-6). In most cases, sagittal images do not allow this discrimination because the filum and roots tend to merge into a single longitudinal band of intermediate signal in the posterior thecal sac (see Figure 5-5). Sagittal images also may not show the filum accurately because of partial volume averaging effects with CSF or gaps between slices (see Figure 5-6). Partial volume averaging in axial images is usually not a

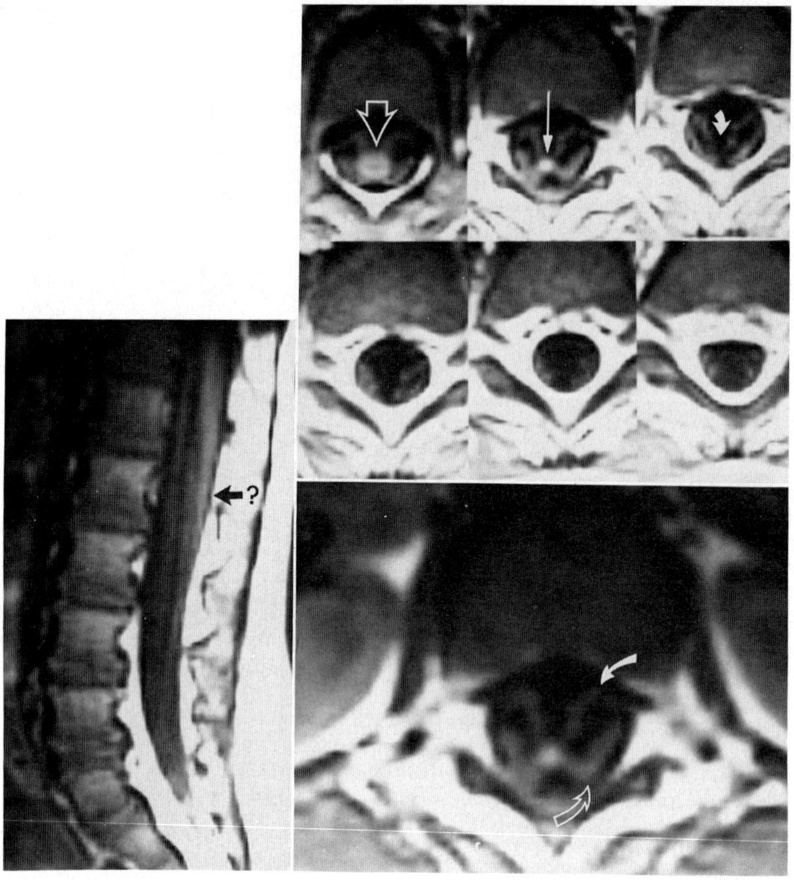

FIGURE 5-4. Normal conus medullaris. **A,** Sagittal T1W image in 19-month-old female suggests tip of conus medullaris is in somewhat low position near L_2-L_3 *(arrow with question mark).* Because conus tip may be obscured by and confused with proximal part of cauda equina, sagittal image alone is not reliable for determining its position. **B,** Multiple T1W axial images through distal cord and proximal cauda equina clearly identify conus medullaris *(open arrow)* and conus tip (straight arrow). Conus tip lies in normal position at L_1-L_2, not in low position suggested by sagittal image. Normal filum terminale lies in center *(curved arrow)* of array of cauda equina nerve roots but is not typically seen as distinct structure unless enlarged (see Figure 5-7). **C,** Magnified T1W axial image through conus tip. Proximal cauda equina nerve roots form typical pattern of "VW" sign with "V" anterior *(solid curved arrow)* and "W" posterior *(open curved arrow).*

significant problem because anatomic change along the filum is of low spatial frequency in the Z axis of the slice. In some cases at surgery, lower sacral roots may be found adherent to the filum.[82] Thus some degree of caution should be exercised in making the diagnosis of a thickened filum if the appropriate clinical picture is not present. Additionally, an ovoid cross section of the enlarged filum may be the result of an adherent root in symptomatic cases, which is helpful information for operative planning. Low SNR images reduce contrast between CSF and the filum making its identification and the diagnosis of the thickened filum problematic.[52,111] With hardware improvements and multiple signal averages, SNR can be improved by simply using thick slices (e.g., 10 mm), which is an expedient solution especially applicable to axial images of the filum.

Axial T1W images are also the best means for localizing the conus medullaris. Serial, contiguous axial images through the distal conus and

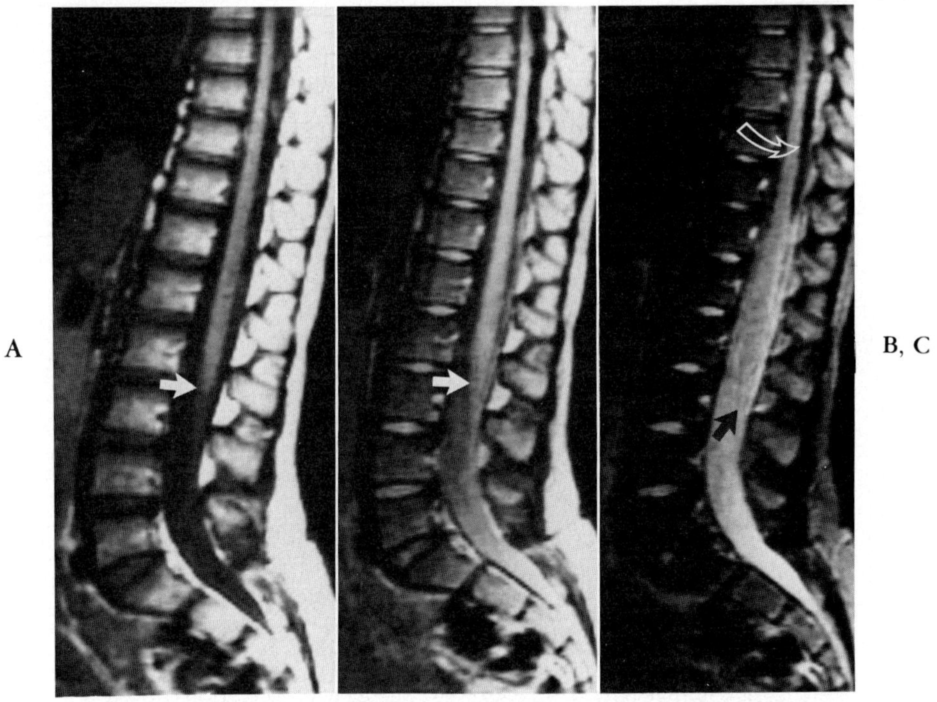

FIGURE 5-5. **A-C,** Sagittal T1W and T2W images (1.5T) of lumbar spinal canal in 6-year-old female with bilateral "shortened heel cords" and lower extremity weakness. T1W image shows tip of conus at L_2-L_3 level *(arrow,* **A**). Short TE (40/2500) T2W image shows conus tip partially obscured by proximal cauda equina *(open arrow).* On long TE (80/2500) image, conus isointense with CSF and not adequately visualized to determine exact position *(arrow,* **B**). CSF motion artifact produces signal void in low thoracic canal posterior to cord *(curved arrow,* **C**).

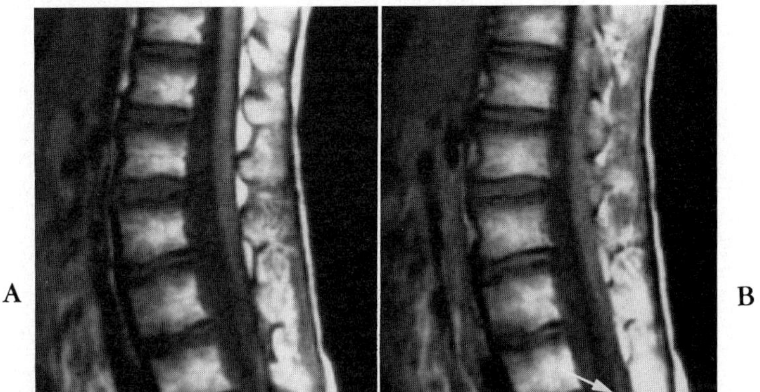

FIGURE 5-6. Tethered cord with filum lipoma. **A** and **B,** Sagittal T1W images in 13-year-old male with neurogenic bladder shows low position of conus with ill-defined tip lying approximately at L_3. **B,** Thickened filum may also be present *(arrows).*

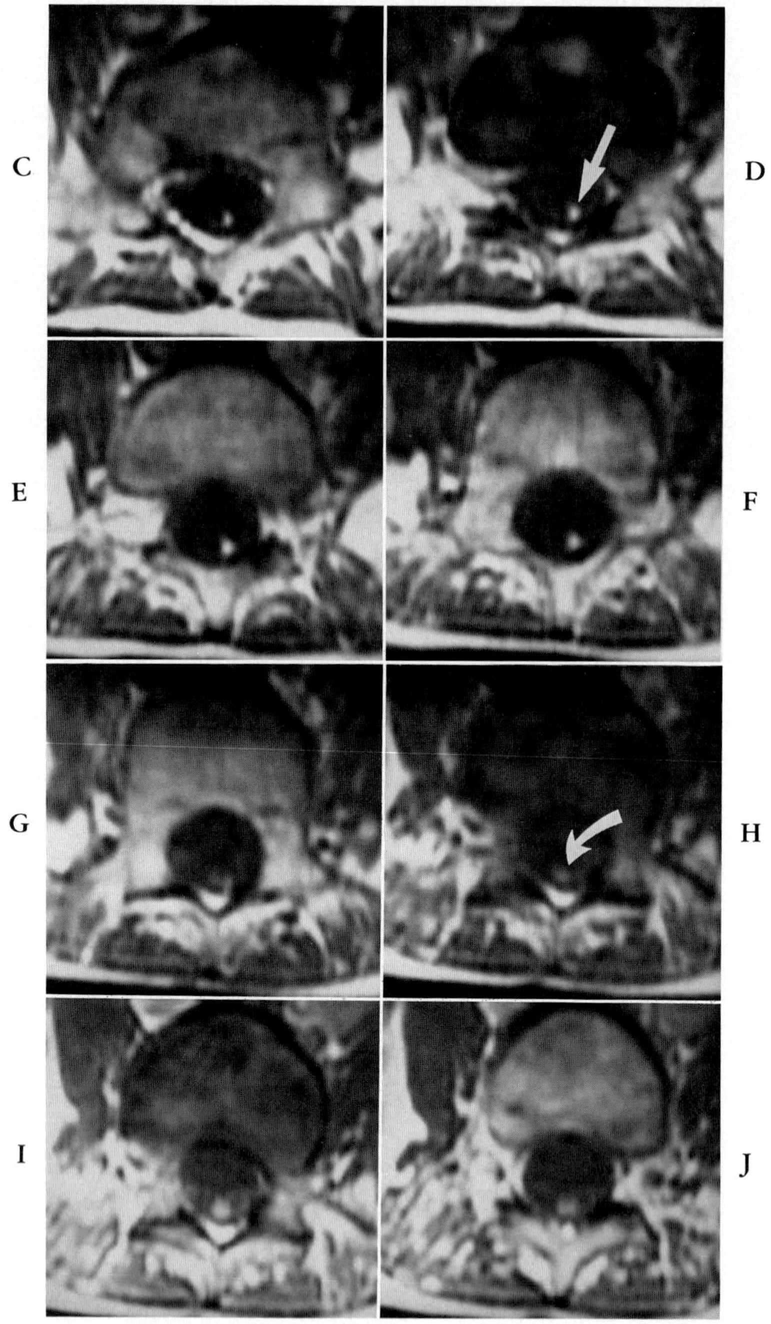

FIGURE 5-6, cont'd. **C-F,** Sequential 5 mm thick axial T1W images, inferior to superior through S_1 and L_5, show thin filum lipoma *(arrows)* not seen on sagittal images (**B,** *between arrows*). **G-J,** Sequential 5 mm thick axial T1W images, inferior to superior through L_5 and L_4 show correct position of conus tip (**H,** *curved arrow*) posterior to L_4 (**A,** *curved arrow*), lower than suggested by sagittal images. This case illustrates importance of obtaining both sagittal and axial images for evaluation of lumbar congenital anomalies.

proximal cauda equina and filum are reliable for precisely localizing the level of the conus tip (see Figures 5-4 to 5-6). On sagittal images the roots of the cauda equina often appear to merge into a single longitudinal structure with the distal cord that obscures the conus tip. For this reason, sagittal images should not be used alone to exclude or confirm tethering of the cord (see Figure 5-5). Axial images also provide positive identification of lipomas of the filum that may be missed on sagittal images (Figures 5-6 and 5-7). The importance of this diagnosis is that a filum lipoma may carry the same clinical significance as a tethered conus or thickened filum terminale. Other lesions may also be missed by sagittal images, such as diastematomyelia (see Figure 5-10).

In good quality flow-compensated T2W images the filum appears as a low signal structure within high signal CSF. T2W images may be used to identify the thickened filum, but on many imaging systems they suffer from low SNR and the imaging time required for high SNR T2W images is usually two to three times longer than high SNR T1W images. CSF motion effects are more prominent on T2W images than on T1W images and may produce artifacts that obscure the filum or decrease signal in CSF reducing contrast with the filum. A major qualitative difference between T2W and T1W images is the relative signal of fat. Because fat is intermediate to low signal on T2W images it can appear similar to filum and nerve roots and may not be easily identified (Figure 5-8). Similar to T1W images, axial T2W images are more useful than sagittal images because the filum has signal similar to the adjacent nerve roots and their differentiation must be based on anatomic position.

A

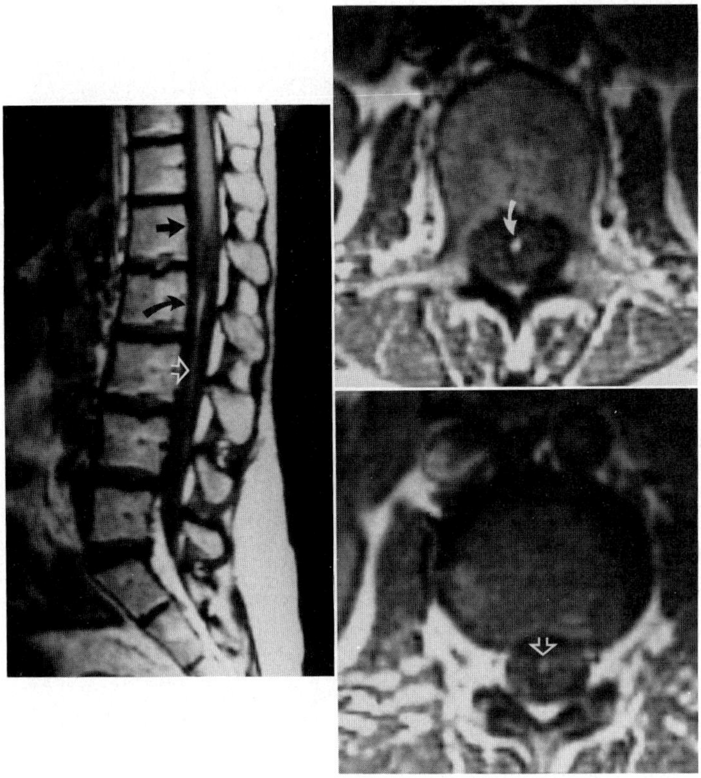

B

C

FIGURE 5-7. Filum terminale lipoma. **A,** Sagittal T1W image in 27-year-old female shows conus tip in normal position at mid-L_1 *(solid straight arrow)*, thin high signal lipoma *(curved arrow)*, and intermediate signal-thickened filum terminale *(open arrow)*. Axial T1W images show the high signal filum lipoma *(arrow,* **B***)* and an intermediate signal-thickened filum terminale *(arrow,* **C***)*. Lipoma and filum both measure approximately 2.5 mm diameter and lipoma appears to replace filum over a short segment.

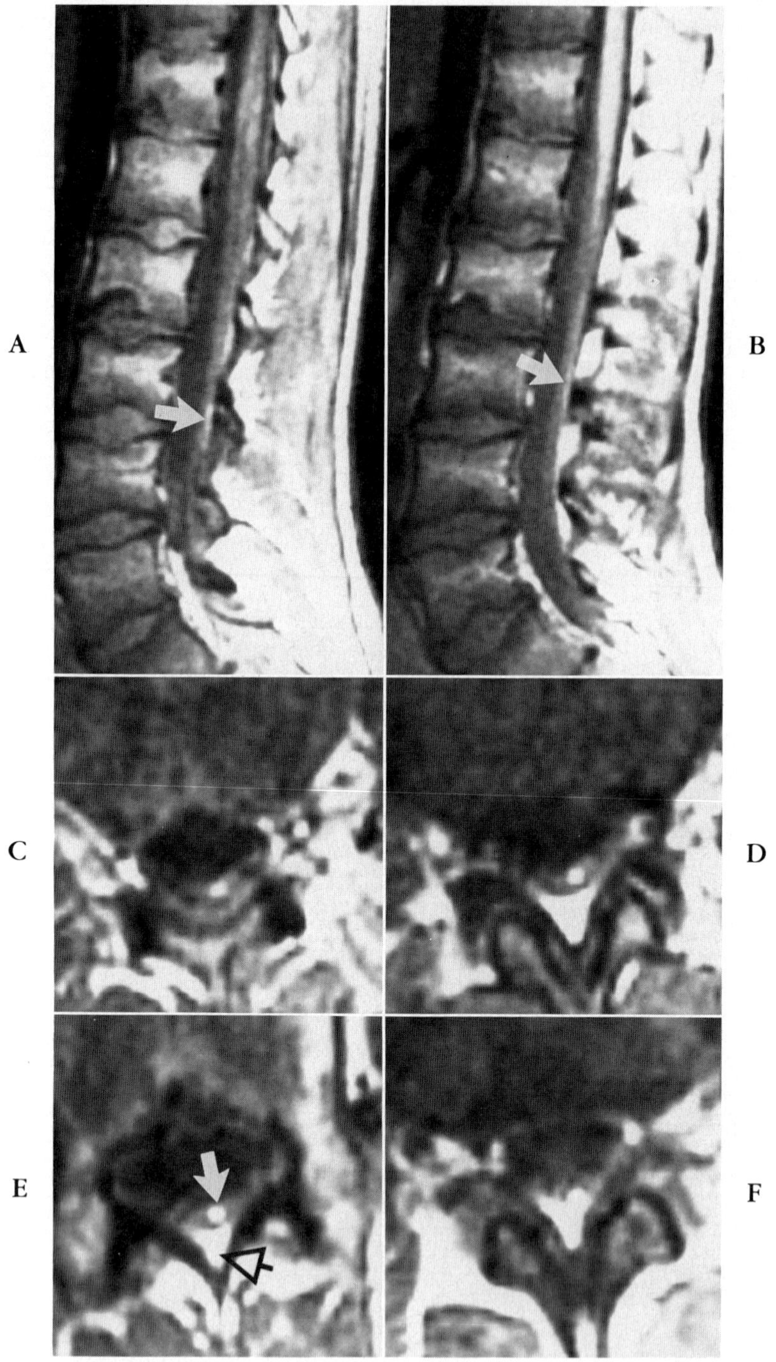

FIGURE 5-8. Filum terminale lipoma in 17-year-old-male. **A** and **B**, Sagittal T1W images of the lumbar spine show linear segments of high signal in the posterior thecal sac in the region of the distal cauda equina (*arrows*), which are difficult to distinguish from epidural fat. **C-F**, Axial T1W images confirm presence of a filum terminale lipoma (**E**, *white arrow*) and clearly distinguish it from the adjacent posterior epidural fat (**E**, *open arrow*1.)

Little experience is available with variable flip angle/gradient echo sequences with T2*-weighting for imaging the filum terminale. The same considerations of low SNR, CSF motion artifacts, and reduced contrast between filum, CSF, and lipoma seen with T2W images are likely to be problems with these images. Thus T1W images, rather than T2W images, should be used to evaluate the filum because they require less imaging time, generally have better SNR and fewer artifact, and produce high contrast between the filum, CSF, and lipomas.

In most cases of tethered cord and thick filum terminale, MR imaging provides sufficient information for diagnosis and surgical planning so that myelography and myelographic CT are not needed. The diagnosis of low position of the conus tip can be made with MR noninvasively in virtually all cases.[1,23,54,104,111] The key advantages of MR over myelography are its noninvasive nature and the positive identification of lipomas. Thin collections of fat in the filum are difficult to diagnose by attenuation values at myelography. The major advantage of MR over CT myelography is its noninvasive character. Nonmyelographic CT scans are not useful for identification of the conus position or thickness of the filum. Sagittal MR images are superior to sagittal reformations of axial CT scans.[75,111] However, CT scans, with or without intrathecal contrast, are very sensitive to low attenuation lipomatous tissue. In a few cases, where the conus is at a normal level and the MR images cannot exclude a thickened filum terminale (e.g., low SNR images), myelography and myelographic CT may be needed to establish the correct diagnosis. Plain radiography and CT may provide more complete characterization of bone anomalies than MR, especially vertebral body malformations, that might be associated with tethered cord or thick filum terminale.[1,52,54]

Sonography is a low-cost technique for diagnosing dysraphic lesions in infants, providing an "acoustic window" exists though a posterior spinal defect.[73] MR has an inherent advantage over sonography by not requiring such a defect for imaging the spinal canal contents. Although MR may also reveal better anatomic detail and tissue characterization, no detailed comparison between MR and sonography for the evaluation of tethered cord and thick filum has been performed.

DIASTEMATOMYELIA

Diastematomyelia is a dysraphic abnormality consisting of a midline, longitudinal cleft through the spinal cord, conus medullaris, or filum terminale. These lesions are rarely present at more than one spinal level. The clefting or myeloschesis of the spinal cord produces two symmetric hemicords, each with a central canal, one dorsal horn and nerve root, and one ventral horn and nerve root. Diastematomyelia is distinguished from diplomyelia, which is a more complete duplication of the cord, with two true hemicords, each containing a central canal, two dorsal and ventral horns, and a complete set of dorsal and ventral roots. Diplomyelia is more a theoretic concept than a description of a pathologic condition because no instance of true, complete diplomyelia has been reported.[12,41,70]

The cleft between the hemicords in diastematomyelia frequently contains a fibrous or osteocartilaginous septum or spur extending anterior to posterior through the spinal canal. This spur or septum is not always present with diastematomyelia and thus is not essential to the pathologic definition.

Embryology

The embryogenesis of diastematomyelia is controversial with the most credible theories focused on whether primary bone and soft tissue abnormalities cause splitting of the cord or whether splitting of the neural tissue induces secondary changes in the surrounding extraneural tissue.[70] Bremer[13] suggests that a persistent accessory neurenteric canal prevents normal midline fusion of prevertebral tissue, vertebrae, cord, and dorsal skin. The normal neurenteric canal extends temporarily from the yolk sac ventrally to the amniotic cavity dorsally before closure of the neural groove. Neural tissue associated with the normal neurenteric canal eventually lies at the tip of the coccyx. The persistence of an accessory neurenteric canal from early embryogenesis may explain the association of multiple segmentation anomalies with diastematomyelia, including hemivertebrae, butterfly vertebrae, spina bifida, skin lesions, dural clefts, and midline cysts and tumors. On the other hand, Herren and Edwards[41] suggest that the primary developmental abnormality with diastematomyelia is caused by the lateral edges of the neural groove turning steeply ventrally as they approach the midline to fuse with the ventral inner surface of the neural plate on either side of the midline rather than with each other, thus forming two separate neural tubes. Depending on the distance separating the two tubes, the mesenchyme may be induced to form only a thin pial layer between the two neural tubes or, with wider separation, arachnoid, dura, and an osteocartilaginous spur or septum.

Morphology

The anatomy of the cord in diastematomyelia spans a range from partial ventral or dorsal clefts to nearly complete duplication of cord structures in each hemicord, short of true diplomyelia.[46,47] The position of the cleft is midthoracic or below (T_9 to S_1) in 85% of cases, exclusively lumbar in 62%, thoracolumbar in 18%, and thoracic in 20%.[42] The cepahlocaudal extent of the cleft is variable, ranging from 1 cm to 9.5 cm or 2 to 15 vertebral segments.[41,46] The two hemicords reunite below the cleft in 91% of cases,[42] but the cleft may extend into the conus, filum terminale, or roots of the cauda equina. Rare cases of isolated bifid filum or cauda equina roots have been reported.[97] The axial diameter of the two hemicords is smaller than the normal cord and they are usually equal in size.[47] In 30% of patients, the hemicords are markedly asymmetric[6] and the smaller one often lies ventral to the larger one.[41] The hemicords are often rotated so that their anatomic ventral surfaces, identified by the split anterior spinal arteries in the prominent ventral sulci, lie along the medial surface and face each other across the cleft. This results in rotation of the nerve roots, orienting the anatomic ventral roots along the medial surfaces and the anatomic dorsal roots along the lateral surfaces. The gray matter of the hemicord usually forms a single dorsal and ventral horn, each giving rise to one set of ipsilateral segmental dorsal and ventral roots.[80,81]

The conus medullaris is usually in a low position with diastematomyelia, lying below L_2 in approximately 75% of cases.[42,97] The filum terminale is also thickened (>2 mm) in 41% of cases and bifid in 9%. Considering the typical clinical presentation, these findings of tethering of the cord may be primarily responsible for the neurologic deficits with diastematomyelia.[70]

The relationship of the meninges to diastematomyelia varies with the degree of separation of the hemicords. In approximately 50% of cases the two hemicords lie within an intact single arachnoid and dural sac and each is surrounded by its own pial membrane.[41,46] There is no fibrous or osteocartilaginous septum extending between the hemicords.[70] In the remaining 50% of cases, the arachnoid and dura form separate sacs around each hemicord that merge into single sacs above and below the level of the cleft in the cord. Most of these cases with duplicated dural sacs also have a fibrous or osteocartilaginous spur or septum extending through the cleft.[70]

Osseous Anatomy

The presence of an osteocartilaginous spur or septum has been reported in 29% to 89% of cases of diastematomyelia.[6,70,97] Spurs attach to the ventral or dorsal walls of the spinal canal and usually lie in the sagittal plane. They may lie off center and divide the spinal canal asymmetrically when it arises from a pedicle or unilateral interlaminar fusion.[70] With partial diastematomyelia and an intact single dural sac, the spur projects only part way into the canal. The spinal level of the spur is L_4 to L_5 in 18% of cases, L_1 to L_3 in 48% of cases, T_7 to T_{12} in 26% of cases, and T_1 to T_6 in 5% of cases.[42] Spurs are double in approximately 5% of cases and usually lie near each other but occasionally may be widely separated, for example, at T_5 and L_4.[43] Cervical lesions[100] and more than two spurs are very rare.[42,47]

Vertebral Anomalies

Segmental anomalies of the vertebral column accompany almost all cases of diastematomyelia.[6,87,112] In 85% of cases, there are anomalies of vertebral bodies, including hemivertebrae (45%), butterfly vertebrae, narrowed disc spaces, and reduced vertebral height.[42,43] Abnormal spinal curvatures, scoliosis or kyphosis, are present in 50% to 60% of patients, usually directly related to segmental anomalies.[42] Scoliosis associated with diastematomyelia accounts for approximately 5% of congenital scoliosis cases,[75,110] and the incidence appears to increase with age.[42] Abnormalities of the lamina are present in 91% of diastematomyelia cases and include thickening, spina bifida, and intersegmental fusions.[70] The combination of spina bifida and intersegmental fusion is present in 59% of cases and usually corresponds to the level of the diastematomyelia.[42] Wide spina bifida and widened interpedicular distance occur in approximately 90% of cases and typically lie near the level of the bony spur.[42,46,51,66,110]

Clinical Findings

Females are predominantly affected, comprising 74%[21,41,66] to 94%[42] of cases. Clinical signs and symptoms of diastematomyelia may occur over a wide range of ages from early childhood to late adulthood, or the lesion may remain silent throughout life. Neurologic symptoms in most patients (88%) are nonspecific and indistinguishable from those caused by tethering of the cord from other causes. In most cases, symptoms cannot be attributed to the smaller of the two hemicords[97] or to the cleft itself,[46] although in some cases the site of the cleft may correlate best with otherwise unexplained symptoms.[70]

Cutaneous, orthopedic, and other findings associated with diastematomyelia are numerous. Cutaneous stigmata occur in 50% to 75% of cases.[43,70,110] The most common associated skin lesion is hypertrichosis, appearing as a patch of long, silky hair, situated close to the level of the diastematomyelia. Nevi and lipomas are associated in 20% to 25%, skin dimples and dermal sinuses in 15%, and hemangiomas and pilonidal cysts in 5% of cases. An orthopedic syndrome of abnormal posture and gait associated with unilateral weakness, deformity, and hypoplasia of the lower leg and foot occurs in 60% of patients.[46] There are significant deformities in the feet, especially clubfoot, in 44% of patients,[110] and Sprengel's deformity is observed in approximately 1% of cases.[70] Midline neurenteric cysts and dermoid tumors may coexist with diastematomyelia and extend into the osteocartilaginous spur.[80] The Chiari II malformation is only rarely associated with diastematomyelia.[42]

MR Imaging

MR images of diastematomyelia can show most of the major pathologic features of a lesion.* The different degrees of duplication of the cord are clearly visualized, especially on axial T1W images[104] (Figures 5-9 and 5-10). Coronal T1W images may also demonstrate the lesion

*References 1, 37, 54, 75, 84, 103, 104.

A, B

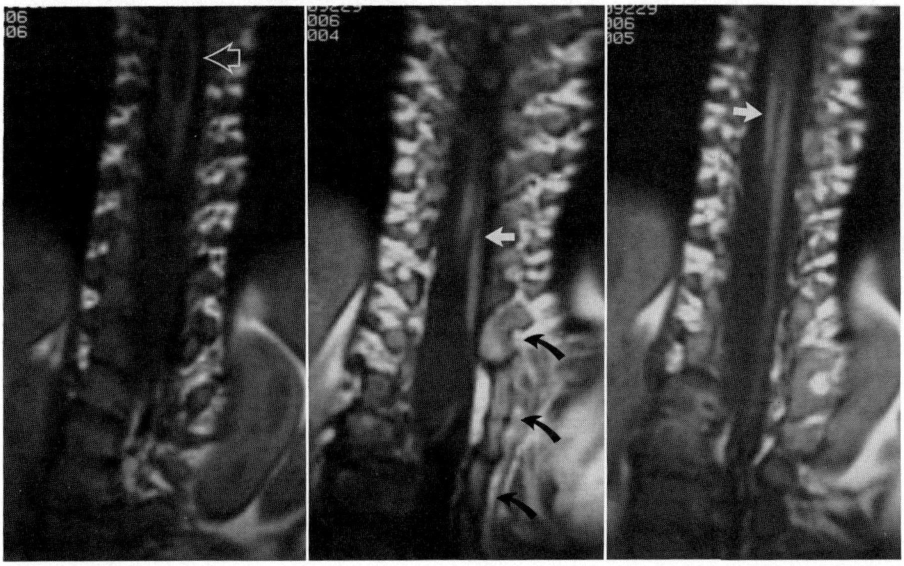

C

FIGURE 5-9. Diastematomyelia with hydromyelia and myelocystocele. Coronal T1W images in 3-year-old female with severe thoracolumbar dysraphism show **A**, cystic fluid collection in midthoracic cord *(arrow)*, probably representing hydromyelia, **B** and **C**, diastematomyelia caudal to cyst extending through most of remainder of cord *(arrows)*, and **C**, vertebral dysraphic anomalies present in lumbar region *(curved arrows)*. *Continued.*

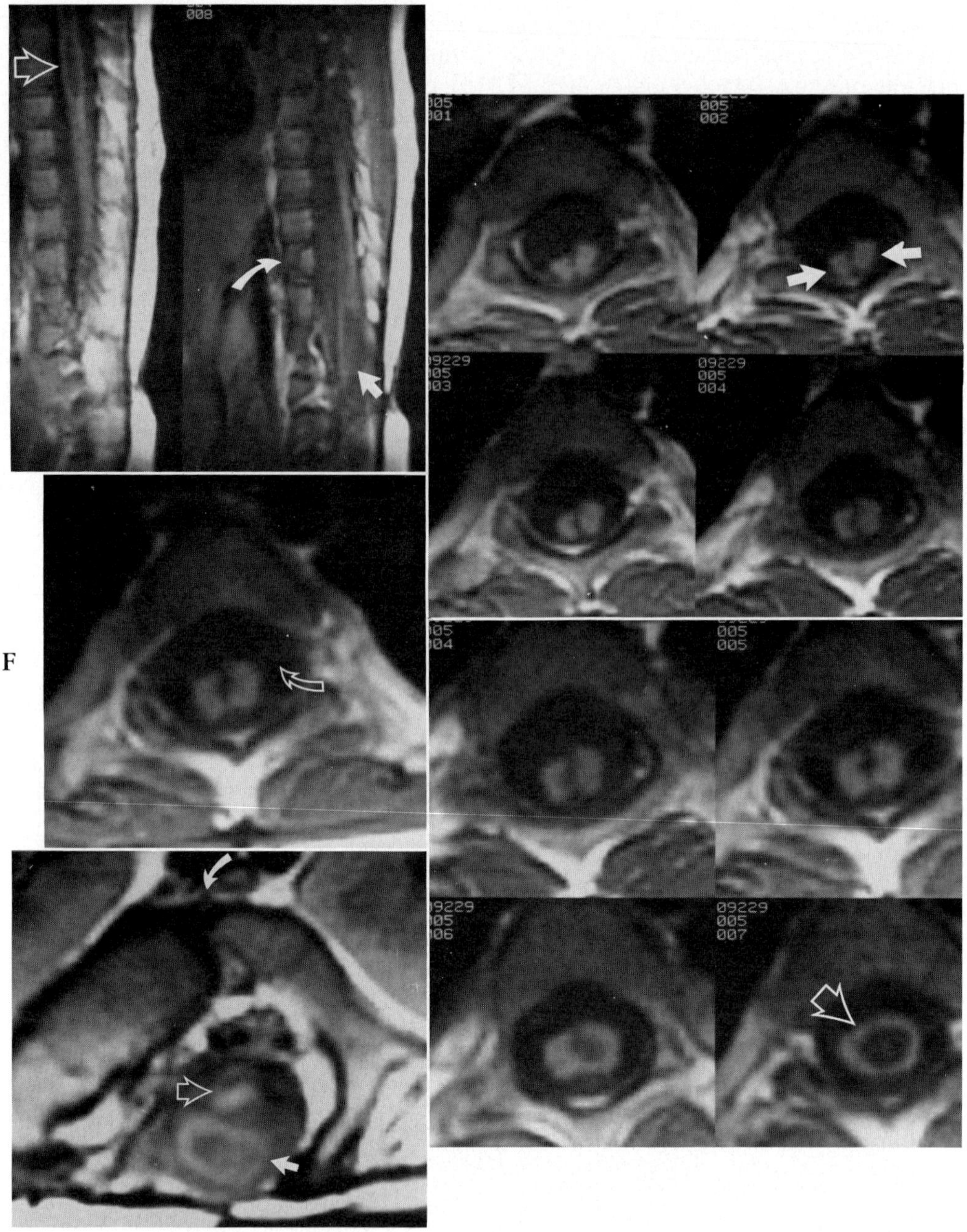

D

E

F

G

H

FIGURE 5-9, cont'd. D, Sagittal T1W images show thoracic hydromyelia *(open arrow)* but not diastematomyelia. Distal cord indistinctly defined and proved to be a myelocystocele on axial images *(closed straight arrow)*. Vertebral dysraphic anomalies are also seen, including a coronal cleft (*curved arrow*). **E**, Sequential axial 5 mm thick T1W images from inferior to superior through midportion of diastematomyelia show the two separate hemicords *(arrows)* without evidence of oseocartilaginous spur or septum. **F**, Magnified T1W axial image shows notched medial surfaces of hemicords representing functional ventral surfaces of each. Thin intermediate signal linear structure traversing CSF space represents nerve roots *(arrow)*. **G**, Sequential axial 5 mm thick T1W images through superior part of diastematomyelia and inferior part of hydromyelia *(arrow)*. **H**, Magnified axial T1W image through distal cord shows large cystic myelocystocele in posterior hemicord *(closed straight arrow)* with second, smaller myelocystocele in anterior hemicord *(open arrow)*. Marked dysraphic changes are also present in vertebral body *(curved arrow)*.

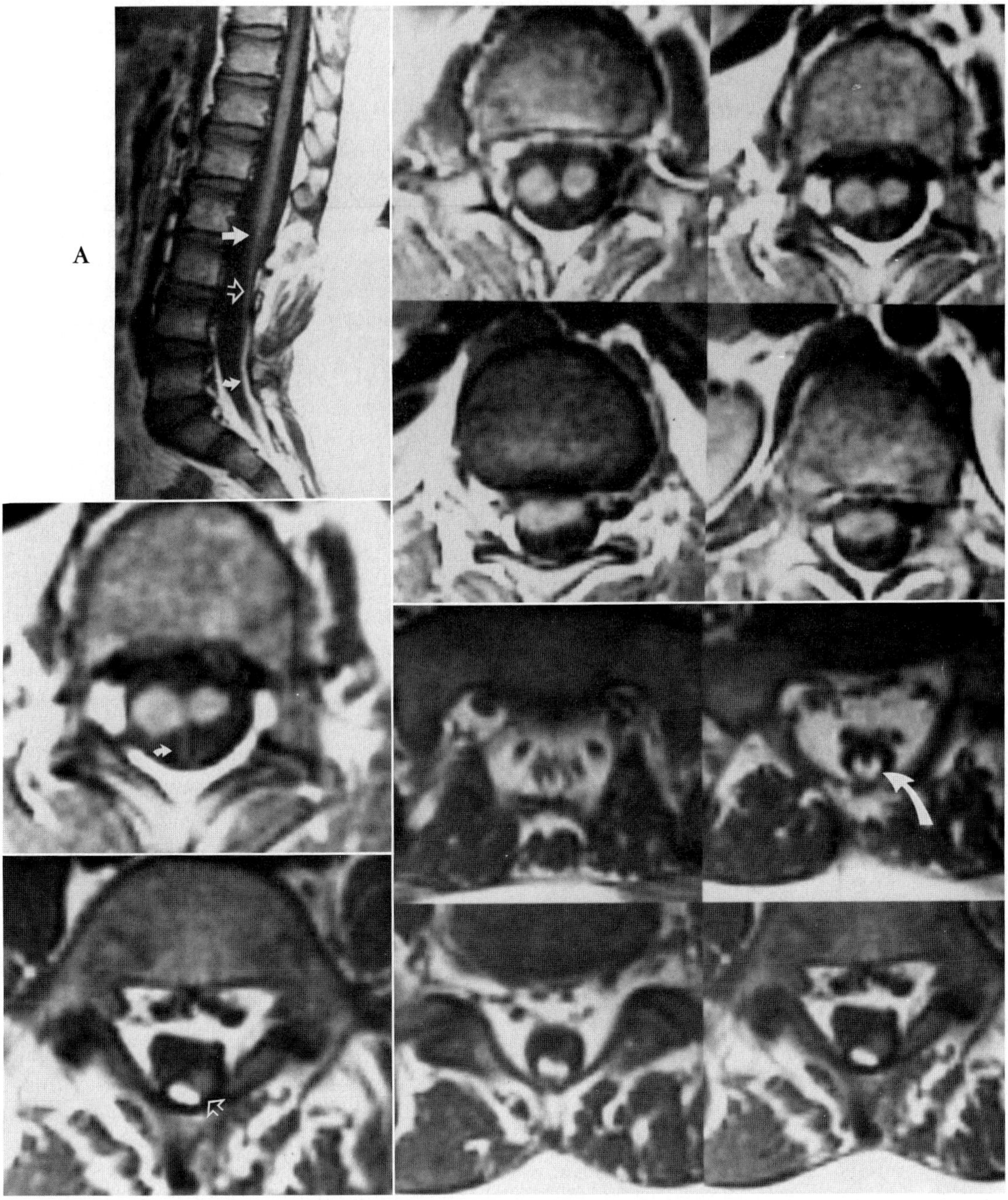

FIGURE 5-10. Tethered cord, diastematomyelia, and lipomeningocele. **A,** Sagittal T1W in 6-year-old male with history of bladder incontinence, normal gait, and no cutaneous lesions. Conus tip appears to lie in relatively low position at L_2-L_3 *(closed straight arrow),* and anterior margin of conus is indistinct. What appears to be thickened filum terminale extends caudally *(open arrow),* and in fact, represents attenuated distal spinal cord. Distal lipoma tethering distal cord is present *(curved arrow).* **B,** Sequential 5 mm thick axial T1W images from inferior to superior at L_1-T_{12}. Diastematomyelia is present in conus at L_1 level—probably accounting for poor definition of anterior conus margin on sagittal image. **C,** Magnified axial T1W image at L_1 shows diastematomyelia with asymmetry of hemicords, right larger than left. Thin, linear low signal structure may represent osteocartilaginous spur extending from lamina *(arrow).* **D,** Sequential 5 mm thick axial T1W images from inferior to superior at S_1-L_5. Caudal lipoma clearly seen as high signal *(arrow)* with notch anterior where it wraps partially around distal cord. Junction of distal cord and lipoma at L_5 level. **E,** Magnified axial T1W image at L_5 shows junction of distal cord and lipoma *(arrow.)*

well, if kyphosis or lordosis is not severe at the level of the lesion (see Figure 5-9). Sagittal T1W images are least useful and may not show the lesion because of their orientation parallel to the cleft between the hemicords (see Figure 5-10).

More subtle features of diastematomyelia can be well demonstrated by MR. The identification of nerve roots exiting the hemicords or thin adhesions may be made on T1W axial images or artifact-free flow-compensated T2W images.[1] With low resolution, low SNR images, supplemental myelography, or CT may be needed to positively identify the nerve roots.[6,52,111] The internal architecture of the cord with dorsal and ventral gray matter in each hemicord may be identified in high quality T2W axial images; but, in general, precise identification of these internal structures is difficult. The precise distinction between diastematomyelia and true diplomyelia may not be critical to surgical planning (e.g., removal of the spur or septum) or symptomatic management of the patient.

The noninvasive identification of tethered cord and thickened filum terminale frequently associated with diastematomyelia[42,97] is an important advantage of MR over myelography and myelographic CT. The major limitation of MR in evaluation of diastematomyelia is difficulty in identifying the composition and extent of spurs and septa separating the hemicords. On T1W images, cortical bone, cartilage, and fibrous elements lying between the hemicords tend to be low signal and isointense with CSF or nonfatty tissues. One exception is high signal on T1W images from marrow in thick bony septa.[54] CSF signal is higher on T2W images and structures in the cleft tend to be low signal. Structures in the cleft may be seen more easily on variable flip angle/gradient echo T2*W images that show dense bone as low signal and cartilage as intermediate signal contrasted against high signal in CSF and fat. Supplementation of MR studies with plain radiographs and CT may be necessary to define extradural tissue separating the hemicords before surgical intervention.[1,54]

VERTEBRAL ANOMALIES

Embryology

The vertebral column and meninges derive from mesenchyme and develop in three stages: membrane formation, chondrification, and ossification.[92,98] At approximately 19 days of gestation, the mesenchyme forms two longitudinal columns lateral to the neural tube called the paraxial mesenchyme. The membranous stage of development begins at about 25 days of gestation when the notochord separates from the primitive gut and neural tube to form the ventral subchondral and dorsal epichondral zones. Mesenchyme then migrates from its lateral position into these zones in a sequence parallel to that of the neural tube, first at the cervical level and then cephalad and caudad from there. The mesenchyme organizes vertically into 42 to 44 pairs of somites that are separated by intersegmental fissures. Medial and lateral sclerotomes form the vertebrae and paraspinous muscles, respectively. After separation of the neural tube from the overlying ectoderm, the mesenchyme migrates dorsal to the neural tube to eventually form the neural arches, ending the membrane development stage at approximately 6 weeks.

During the chondrification stage in the seventh and eighth weeks, the sclerotomes divide in half transversely across the midline sclerotomic fissures and the superior and inferior halves of adjacent sclerotomes fuse along the intersegmental fissure to form the primitive vertebral bodies. This occurs bilaterally and symmetrically with eventual fusion of the two halves across the midline. When this midline fusion occurs, remnants of the notochord persist between the vertebral bodies to eventually form the nucleus pulposus of the intervertebral discs. Ribs are formed in the thoracic region by lateral and ventral migration of portions of each sclerotome. During the ossification stage, from the ninth through twenty fourth week, the chondral vertebral structures ossify and vascularization of the vertebrae occurs.

Formation of the caudal spine proceeds differently from the rest of the spine after normal segmentation and regresses to fusion of most of the sacral and coccygeal segments. The development of this caudal cell mass is more inclined to disorganization than the rest of the spine and is the most frequent site of spinal anomalies.

Vertebral Body Anomalies

Anomalies of the vertebral bodies may result from maldevelopment at any time from the for-

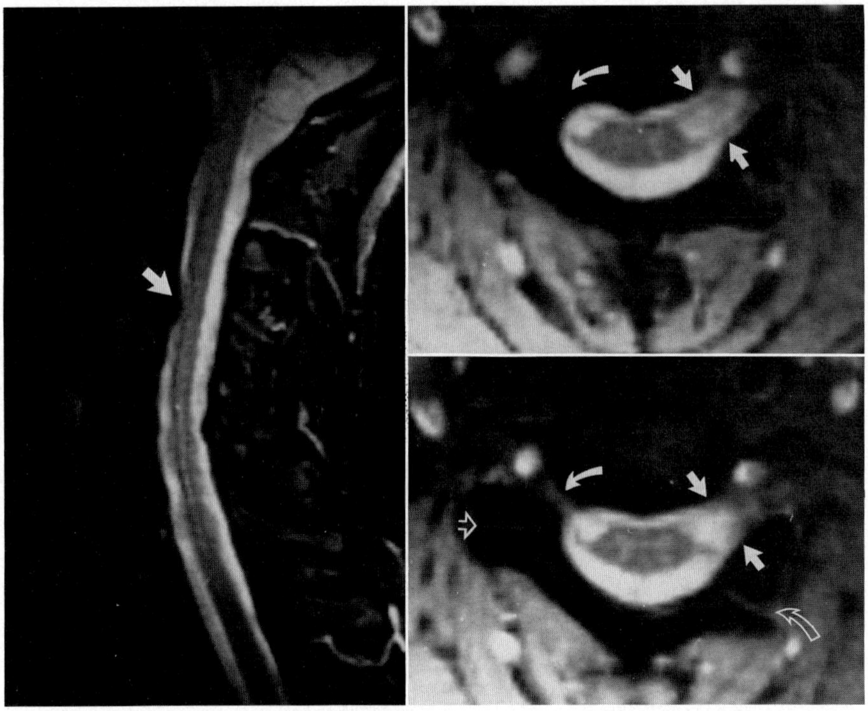

FIGURE 5-11. Congenital absence of pedicle. **A,** Sagittal T2W image in 48-year-old male shows narrowing of C_3-C_4 disc space and prominent posterior protrusion *(arrow),* a nonspecific finding most consistent with disc and/or osteophytic protrusion into spinal canal. Axial GRASS (TE 12 ms, TR 22 ms, flip angle 7°) images at C_3-C_4 show **B,** intact pedicle (*curved arrow*), absence of pedicle *(straight arrows),* **C,** normal neural foramen (right, *curved arrow*), and widening of neural foramen (left, *arrows*). Note wide spacing of low signal nerve roots in left neural foramen. High signal in proximal part of widened left neural foramen represents CSF; but high signal in more lateral portion represents intraspinal venous plexus. Note normal position and orientation of facet joint on right *(open straight arrow).* Left facet joint is posteriorly positioned and abnormally oriented *(open curved arrow).*

mation of the neural tube and notochordal to chondrification or ossification stages. Lesions result from persistence of embryologic clefts, segmental fusions (block vertebrae) (see Figure 5-12), and hypoplasia caused by vascular insufficiency. Persistence of coronal clefts through the vertebral bodies is common in the newborn but usually resolves within 6 months, except when associated with other anomalies such as myelodysplasia and imperforate anus.[19] Less common sagittal clefts are the result of nonfusion of lateral ossification centers and also tend to resolve by 6 months of age (see Figure 5-13). Persistence results in the "butterfly" vertebra malformation.[38,92] Disruption of the normal, symmetric vascular supply to the developing spine in the ossification stage may result in delayed ossification at one level, producing a gibbus deformity, or a hypoplastic hemivertebra. Focal areas of hypoplasia may produce lesions such as absence of a single pedicle (Figure 5-11). Longer segments may also become hypoplastic with compensatory hypertrophy of adjacent segments above and below.[29]

Anomalies of the posterior neural arch are more common than those of the vertebral bodies and are more frequently associated with spinal cord dysraphism.

Klippel-Feil Deformity

Klippel-Feil abnormality of the cervical spine can be clearly demonstrated with MR. The typical appearance is fusion of several cervical vertebrae with partial development of intervertebral disc spaces and narrowed anteroposterior

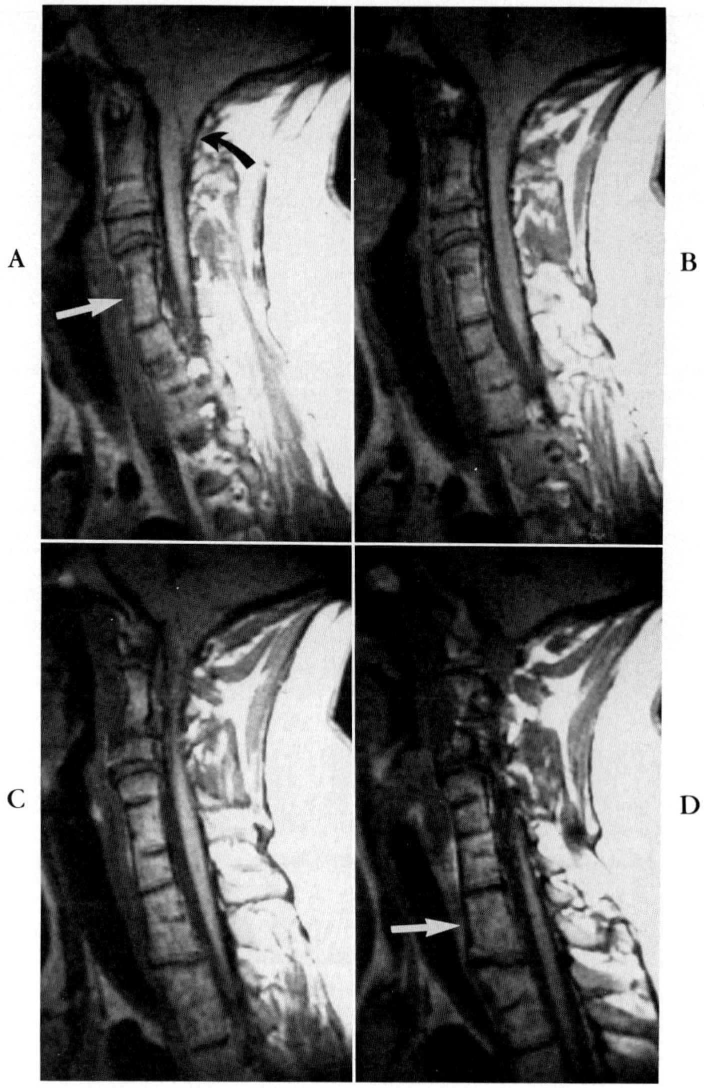

FIGURE 5-12. Chiari I malformation with Klippel-Feil deformity. **A-D,** Sagittal T1W images in 28-year-old female show tonsillar ectopia with distortion of tonsils and cord at cervicomedullary junction indicating Chiari I malformation *(curved arrows)*. Narrowing and fusion of vertebral bodies with partial interspace formation are present at multiple levels from C_4-T_2 (Klippel-Feil deformity, *arrows*). Klippel-Feil deformity occurs in approximately 5% of cases of Chiari I malformation.[70]

diameter of the affected vertebral bodies (Figure 5-12). This appearance, combined with the classic clinical triad (restricted range of cervical motion, short neck, and low hairline and lowset ears) present in 50% of cases, confirms the diagnosis. The cervical abnormality can be visualized with plain films, but the advantage of MR imaging is the noninvasive demonstration of associated anomalies such as Chiari malformation (see Figure 5-12), syringomyelia or hydromyelia, myeloschisis,[69] tethered cord, and agenesis of the corpus callosum.

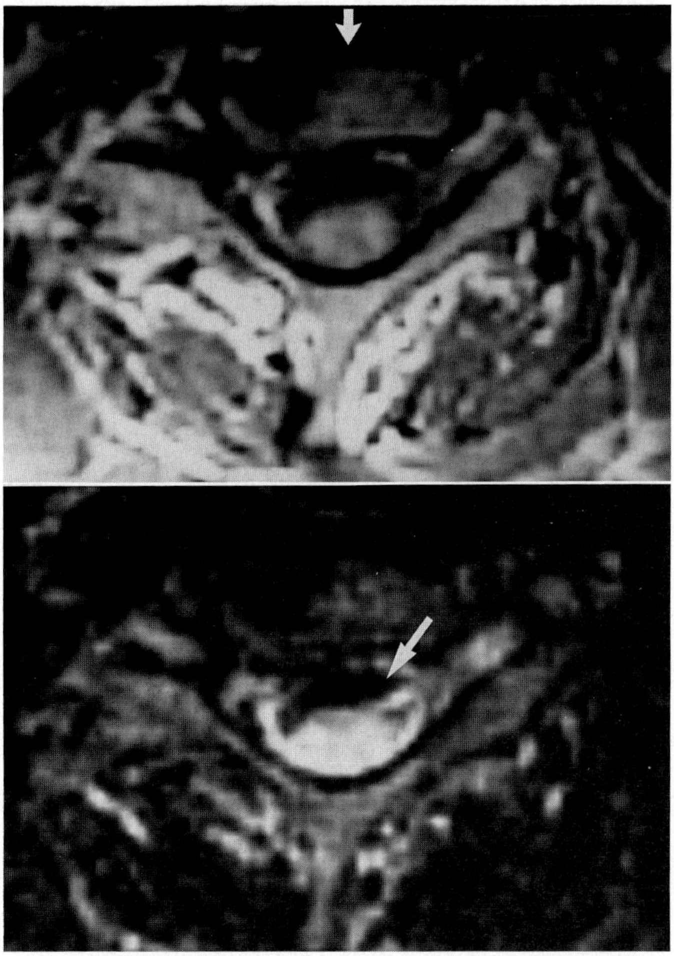

FIGURE 5-12, cont'd. Axial **E,** T1W and **F,** T2W images through C_6 show anteroposterior (AP) narrowing of vertebral body (**E,** *arrow*) with widening of anterior subarachnoid space (**F,** *arrow*). Low signal in subarachnoid space on T2W image (**F,** *arrow*) is caused by oscillatory motion of CSF.

MR Imaging

Plain radiographs and CT remain the best ways to identify anomalous vertebral development. False negative MR studies are frequent with abnormalities of ossification and segmentation.[1,91] Segmentation abnormalities may be seen well with MR if the proper imaging plane is used. Vertebral fusion abnormalities such as "block" vertebrae or multilevel fusion with the Klippel-Feil deformity (see Figure 5-12) are best visualized on sagittal images. Coronal clefts in sagittal and axial planes lie perpendicular to the plane of the abnormality. Individual vertebral body and especially neural arch abnormalities are best imaged in the axial plane (see Figure 5-11). Hemivertebrae and butterfly vertebrae with marked sagittal clefts are easily identified on axial images (Figure 5-13). Subtle degrees of butterfly vertebrae are seen only with coronal images, which show the characteristic butterfly or bow tie configuration seen on plain anteroposterior radiographs (see Figure 5-13).

The role of MR in evaluation of vertebral anomalies is not demonstration of the osseous abnormality, but the noninvasive exclusion or characterization of associated intraspinal lesions such as Chiari I or II malformation, syringohydromyelia, or myelosehis.[91]

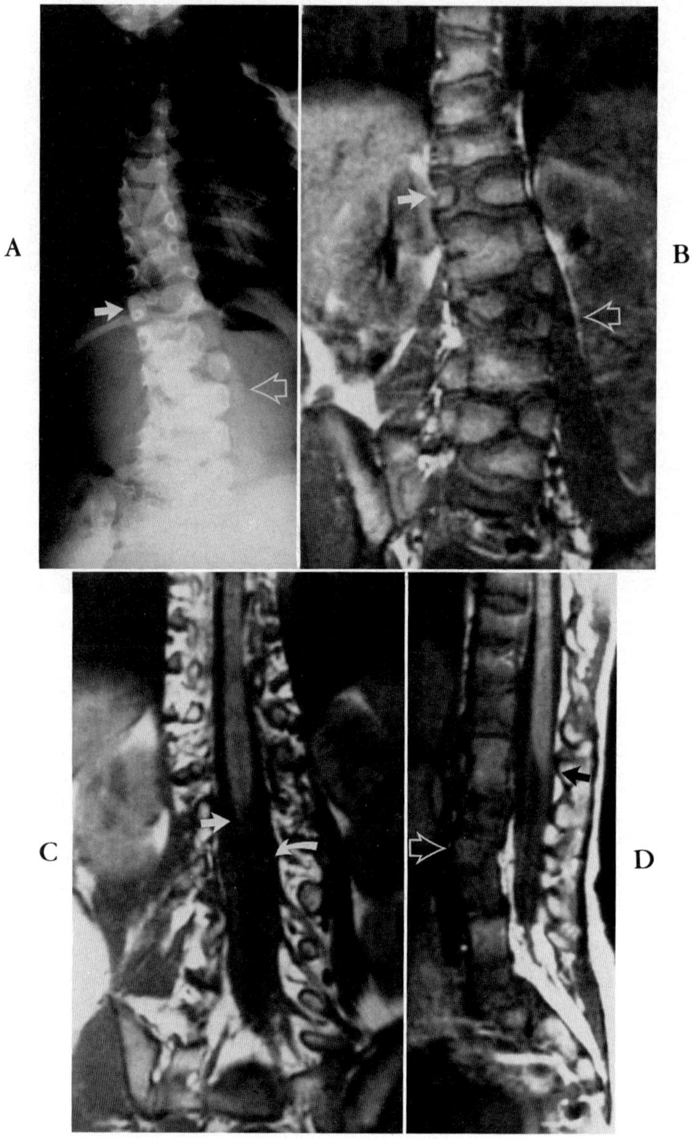

FIGURE 5-13. Congenital scoliosis. **A,** Anteroposterior (AP) radiograph of spine in 4-year-old female with mild bladder dysfunction shows thoracolumbar scoliosis with multiple vertebral anomalies, including bifid vertebra *(arrow)*, and region of markedly disrupted vertebral anatomy in midlumbar spine *(open arrow)*. **B,** Coronal T1W image through thoracolumbar spine shows close correspondence with plain radiograph, specifically bifid vertebra *(arrow)*, and disrupted anatomy in midlumbar region *(open arrow)*. **C,** Coronal T1W image through thoracolumbar spinal canal shows distal cord clearly with conus tip at approximately L_1 level *(arrow)*. Individual nerve roots of cauda equina also seen *(curved arrow)*. No evidence for thickened filum terminale is seen on this image or on axial images (below). **D,** Sagittal T1W image through thoracolumbar spine shows markedly abnormal vertebral anatomy most prominent in midlumbar levels *(open arrow)*. Conus tip at approximately L_1 level *(arrow)* with somewhat abrupt tapering similar to that seen with sacral agenesis. However, bony sacrum appears intact inferiorly and nerve roots of cauda equina can be seen. Filum terminale is not clearly seen and may be partially averaged with posterior group of roots in cauda equina.

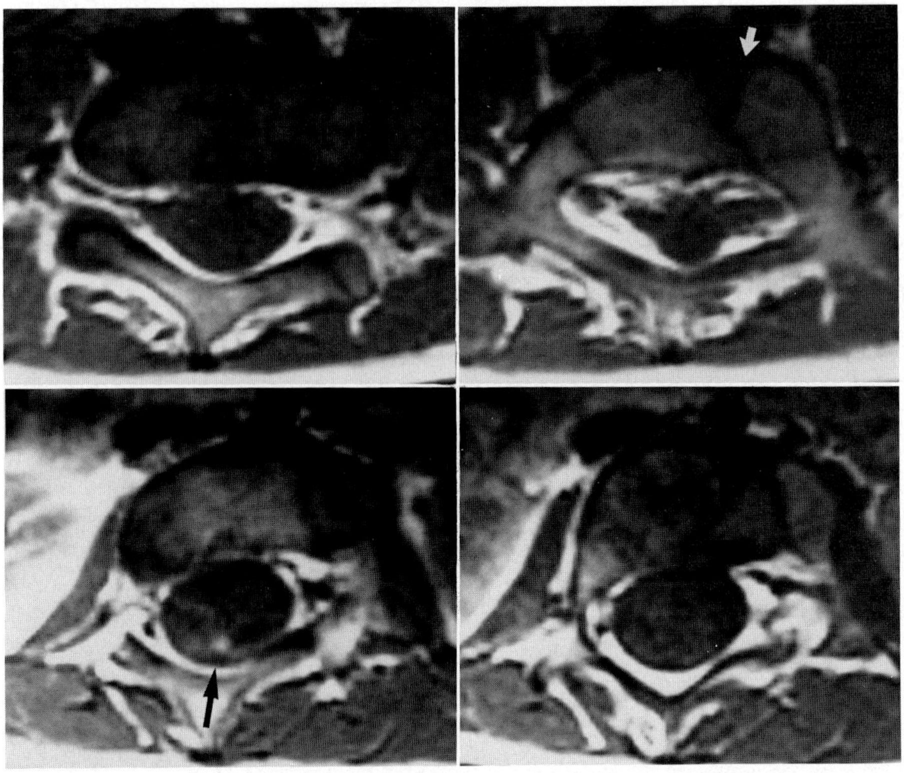

FIGURE 5-13, cont'd. **E** and **F**, Axial T1W images through approximately L_5 level show abnormal ovoid configuration to vertebral bodies and a cleft indicating bifid body *(arrow)*. **G** and **H**, Axial T1W images through the L_1 level show vertebral body disruption similar to L_5 level. Tip of conus *(arrow)* and proximal cauda equina can be seen within thecal sac. No evidence for thickened filum terminale immediately inferior to conus tip (**G**).

SCOLIOSIS

Although 80% to 90% of scoliosis cases are idiopathic and do not require intervention, significant associated abnormalities may be found in the remaining 10% to 20% of cases that require detailed anatomic imaging and surgical correction.[29] Scoliosis is classified as idiopathic, neuromuscular, congenital with vertebral anomalies, congenital with intraspinal pathology, and temporary with traumatic, disc, infectious, or neoplastic (e.g., neuroblastoma) lesions. Imaging of the vertebral column and the intraspinal contents is essential to the proper evaluation of these lesions.

In children with congential scoliosis, intraspinal anomalies occur in approximately 5% to 20% of cases.[32,63] These lesions include Chiari I or II malformation, hydrocephalus, syringomyelia, and hydromyelia, spinal cord tumor, myelomeningocele, lipomyelomeningocele, diastematomyelia, cord atrophy, thickened filum, and tethered cord.[75,104] Diastematomyelia was seen in 16% of cases of scoliosis in one series of 251 cases.[63] Conversely, scoliosis accompanies syringomyelia in 25% to 62% of cases, probably caused by neuromuscular abnormalities produced by syringomyelia.[44,62] Scoliosis was associated with the syringohydromyelia in 40% of myelomeningocele cases studied with MR. These lesions were not correlated with the type of scoliosis, but two cases with the most rapid progression of thoracic scoliosis had the most extensive syrinx and lower lumbar myelomeningoceles.[91] Scoliosis may be present in as many as 25% to 33% of cases of spinal cord tumor.[39] Some authors[103] suggest that left convexity thoracic scoliosis is more likely to be associated with congenital malformations. However, right and left curvatures are found with equal frequency in cases with congenital anomalies. The argument is based on statistics that show right convexity thoracic scoliosis in 73% of idiopathic scoliosis cases not associated with congenital anomalies.[83]

Associated Myelomeningocele

The two basic types of spinal curvature associated with myelomeningocele are congenital and developmental. Congenital scoliosis and kyphosis appear in approximately 30% of patients and arise from associated congenital anomalies such as spina bifida aperta, hemivertebrae, solid bony bars, and unilateral unsegmented bars. In such cases, the arc of curvature is very sharp and the apex of the curve lies at the site of the congenital anomaly.[90] At the level of the myelomeningocele the pedicles rotate outward from the sagittal to the coronal plane as the interpedicular distance widens.[83] As a consequence, (1) transverse processes are directed sagitally and anteriorly, (2) laminae are everted and directed downward and laterally, and (3) facets are rotated into the coronal plane. With these abnormal orientations of the posterior elements, the spine becomes unstable and paraspinous muscle tension causes progressive "jack-knife" kyphosis.[83] Vertebral bodies may be bifid or may appear to be a mass of disorganized ossification centers.[70]

Developmental scoliosis and kyphosis are present in 65% of cases and arise from muscular imbalance and distal pelvic and extremity deformities in the absence of congenital spinal deformities beyond spina bifida.[90] The frequency and degree of developmental scoliosis vary with the level of the primary spinal lesion. Scoliosis with a lateral curvature of 30° or more occurs in 80% of patients with thoracic, 65% with high lumbar (L_1 to L_2), and 25% with low lumbar (L_3 to L_5) spina bifida. Kyphosis with a gibbus of 30° or more or a curvature of 65° or more is seen in 100% of patients with thoracic, 10% with high lumbar, and 18% with low lumbar spina bifida.[99] Patients with uncompensated hydrocephalus and hydromyelia show more rapid progression of developmental scoliosis or kyphosis.[11]

Clinical Findings

Symptoms associated with scoliosis vary widely from none to severe back pain with loss of bladder function and lower extremity sensorimotor deficits. In those cases associated with intraspinal pathologic conditions, symptoms depend primarily on the intraspinal lesion.

MR Imaging

MR images are useful for further characterization of scoliosis after detection of the spinal curvature with plain film radiography (see Figure 5-13). In one series of 28 patients with scoliosis (ages 1 to 17 years) MR showed significant intraspinal abnormalities in 15 (53%) that changed the clinical approach to the patient's condition. The detected abnormalities included tethered cord (7 cases), syringomyelia (5 cases), Chiari I malformation (4 cases), Chiari II malformation (3 cases), spinal cord tumor (2 cases), and diastematomyelia (1 case).[75] MR studies in 30 patients with myelomeningocele revealed thoracolumbar scoliosis in 28 (93%) with severity of curvature ranging from Cobb angles of 7 to 107 degrees. In all of these cases, MR demonstrated a Chiari II malformation.[91]

Detailed imaging of intraspinal lesions with congenital scoliosis is critical to clinical management because many correctable intraspinal lesions must be treated before the scoliosis is treated. In some circumstances, such as intraspinal neurofibroma or syringomyelia, forcible surgical correction of scoliosis may be harmful, producing hematomyelia and paraplegia.[75] MR can characterize the lesion responsible for temporary scoliosis, such as herniated disc, disc infection or osteomyelitis, and trauma, as well as their relationship to the spinal cord.

Depending on the degree of curvature, MR imaging of scoliosis may be accomplished with routine scanning sequences and conventional imaging planes or may require specialized approaches (see Figure 5-13). In many cases, mild degrees of scoliosis (e.g., less than 10 degrees lateral angulation) with curvature in a single plane, usually coronal, can be imaged well with routine sagittal and axial images. The sagittal images may show mild distortion from the oblique orientation of the cord and spine. Routine T1W axial images should be done to compensate for these partial volume averaging artifacts. The entire study of severe scoliosis may be done with axial images alone. Coronal images are occasionally useful but are limited by their tangential orientation to the anterior cordvertebrae-disc interfaces. They are less likely to demonstrate cord impingement by protruding disc and osteophyte or root impingement by facet hypertrophy than axial images. Coronal images also suffer from the same partial volume artifacts as sagittal images when the spinal curvature is oblique to the scan plane or complex and multiplanar. Limited experience is available with the use of longitudinal oblique scans in scoliosis but, ideally, they should be useful with nonorthogonal curvature of the spine; although severe, complex curvatures may not be amenable to scanning in any longitudinal plane. Axial T2W images are useful supplements to T1W images when intramedullary neoplastic or traumatic lesions are suspected. Variable flip angle/fixed gradient echo axial images with short TR, TE, and low flip angle may be useful for evaluating cord position within the spinal canal but should not replace spin-echo (SE) T2W axials for evaluation of the cord itself. T2*W variable flip angle/gradient echo images provide useful images of the bony canal anatomy, but insufficient experience is available to assess their usefulness compared to SE images.

SPINA BIFIDA

The term *spina bifida* describes a dysraphism of the osseous elements forming the spinal canal and usually refers specifically to failure of midline fusion of the dorsal neural arches. *Spina bifida occulta* describes a minimal focal dorsal defect in the lamina, usually a gap of a few millimeters in the midline. Spina bifida occulta occurs in approximately 18% to 34% of the normal population.[4,70,95] The majority are at sites including, in order of frequency, S_1, L_5, C_1, C_7, and T_1.[92] No protrusion of spinal contents occurs through these small defects and the skin is usually intact dorsally. *Spina bifida aperta* (spina bifida cystica) (Table 5-3) refers to a wider defect in the posterior spinal elements with herniation of spinal contents dorsally to form an obvious protrusion. This term encompasses meningocele, myelomeningocele, and rachischisis, which is discussed later.[70,76] Both forms of spina bifida may be accompanied by other forms of dysraphism, including myelodysplasia, syringomyelia, hydromyelia, and diastematomyelia.

TABLE 5-3
Sites of Spina Bifida Aperta

Site	Frequency
Cervical	57 (6%)
Cervicothoracic	4 (0.5%)
Thoracic	68 (7.5%)
Thoracolumbar	57 (6%)
Lumbar	438 (49%)
Lumbosacral	181 (20%)
Sacral	102 (11%)

Modified from Friede, RL: Developmental neuropathology. New York: Springer-Verlag, 1975.

MENINGOCELE

The meningocele is the simplest form of spina bifida aperta with a midline protrusion of dura and arachnoid through a spinal defect into the subcutaneous tissue of the back (Figure 5-14). The incidence of meningoceles is equal in males and females, with a frequency of 1 per 10,000 births or approximately 10% to 33% of spina bifida aperta cases.[57,70,83] The great majority of meningoceles are lumbar and sacral in location but may also be seen in the cervical spine[31] (see Table 5-2 and Figures 5-16 to 5-18). The incidence of Chiari II malformation is high with meningoceles but not present in virtually all cases as it is with myelomeningoceles.[38]

Embryology

The precise mechanism responsible for formation of meningoceles is not known. Lack of coexistence of meningoceles and myelomeningoceles in a study of human embryos suggests that meningoceles are formed earlier in development by a mechanism different from that of myelomeningoceles.[70,77]

Morphology

Basic meningocele may be sessile or pedunculated and varies in size with changes in subarachnoid CSF pressure induced by a change in patient position or the Valsalva maneuver.[70] The meningocele sac is formed by both dura and arachnoid and the contents are subarachnoid fluid. These membranes may fuse posteriorly at the dome of the lesion but are usually separate and distinct at the neck of the sac. The meningocele is always covered by intact skin except where pressure injury causes ulceration and secondary break down. Thin adhesions commonly cross the sac, and dense adhesions obliterate the neck of the sac in some cases.[76]

No neural tissue is contained within a true meningocele. Although normal nerve roots do not traverse the sac, occasional loops of nerve roots may herniate into the sac and become adherent while maintaining a normal origin in the spinal cord and normal exit through the neural foramina.[57,76] The presence of ectopic neural tissue, harmartomatous vessels, smooth muscle, and lipomas takes the lesion out of the category of simple meningocele and places it in that of an epithelized myelomeningocele or lipomyelomeningocele.[70]

Vertebral Anomalies

The degree of spina bifida associated with meningoceles varies from absence of a single spinous process or narrow dehisence of lamina at a single level to absence of multiple neural arches and widening of the adjacent spinal canal. Extensive bony anomalies are rare with meningoceles but common with myelomeningoceles.[76]

MR Imaging

The proper role of MR in mild spina bifida cases, as with vertebral body lesions, is the exclusion or characterization of associated intraspinal abnormalities rather than detailed visualization of the osseous abnormality.[54,103] Plain radiographs are definitive for imaging bone lesion, but many significant features of these lesions can also be shown with MR. Subtle degrees of spina bifida may be indicated by secondary signs on MR images. Absence of the spinous process is easily identified and can be seen on midline sagittal or axial T1W images. Variable flip angle/gradient echo T2*W images may help by showing the cortical bone of the neural arch as low signal in sharp contrast to surrounding soft tissues. A more subtle sign of posterior dysraphism that is seen on midline sagittal T1W images is the loss of normal segmentation of the posterior epidural fat through the levels of the dysraphic anomaly (see Figures 5-7 and 5-8). Continuity of high signal fat over two or more segments on the initial sagittal screening T1W image suggests possible dysraphism and requires acquisition of axial images for confirmation.

MR imaging is the first choice for the initial evaluation and, often, the definitive diagnosis of meningoceles. The critical information is the presence or absence of neural elements within the meningeal pouch, especially if surgical correction is contemplated. High resolution, high SNR T1W MR images often identify loops of cauda equina nerve roots herniating into the meningeal pouch or fibrous adhesions within the pouch, both critical pieces of information for surgical planning.[1,54,104] Identification of the distal cord and abnormalities such as tethered cord or intraspinal mass outside the meningeal pouch are also important for surgical planning. Exclusion or identification of associated abnormalities—Chiari II malformations, hydrocephalus, syringohydromyelia, diastematomyelia, spinal cord tumor—is the other major role for MR in evaluation of meningoceles. Visualization of the overlying cutaneous structures with MR is helpful before surgery, especially for the exclusion of mass lesions or subcutaneous tracts or fistulas.

MYELOCELE AND MYELOMENINGOCELE

The myelocele is a form of spina bifida aperta with a midline, oval plaque of moist, soft, reddish neural tissue that lies exposed at the skin surface and is flush with it (see Figure 5-18). A thick epithelialized fibrous tissue joins the edge of the plaque with the adjacent skin margins.[76] The myelomeningocele (or meningomyelocele) is a myelocele that protrudes beyond the skin surface by expansion of the subarachnoid space ventral to the cord and neural plaque (see Figure 5-18).

Meningoceles and myelomeningoceles with encephalocele, iniencephaly, and anencephaly form a group of disorders known as neural tube defects. The incidence of neural tube defects varies from 1 to 9 per 1000 births.[70] The relative frequencies of each anomaly are 48% spina bifida

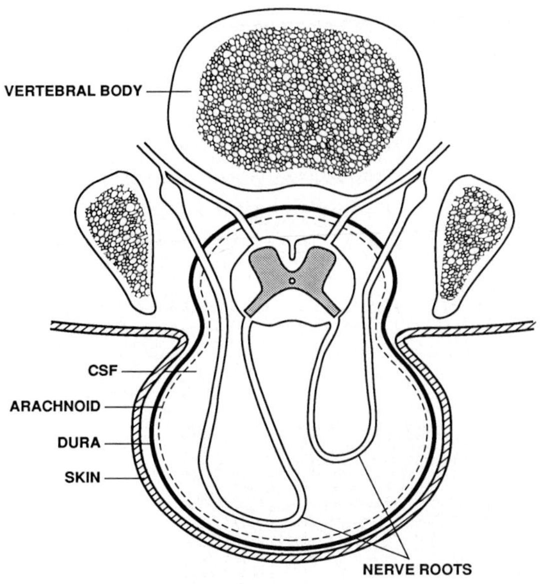

FIGURE 5-14. Meningocele. This diagrammatic representation of a meningocele shows the characteristic herniation of dura and arachnoid through the spina bifida aperta. The skin is intact over the posterior aspect of the dural sac. Loops of nerve roots have herniated into the sac but have normal spinal cord origins and exit normally through neural foramina.

aperta, 48% anencephaly, and 4% encephalocele. The incidence of neural tube defects show familial tendencies, and siblings of patients with myelomeningocele have a frequency of neural tube defects 7 to 15 times greater than the general population (3% to 6% of siblings are effected).[16]

Embryology

The precise embryogenesis of myelomeningoceles is not known. Hypotheses range from failure of the neural tube to close properly to rupture of the already closed neural tube. Data and parsimony suggest that the former hypothesis is most likely. The disturbance probably occurs at or before the 3 mm to 5 mm crown-rump length, producing myeloschisis by leaving the neural plaque in its open, embryonal state. It is not known whether the low position of the spinal cord in myelomeningoceles represents binding of the distal cord to the lesion or a failure of retrogressive differentiation of the lower segments that normally involute.[70] The associated anomalies of hydrocephalus and the Chiari II malformation do not appear at the embryonic period when myelomeningoceles form but develop later in fetal life.[77]

Morphology of Cord and Meninges

The neural placode is a flat remnant of the open embryonic neural plate that usually lies in the midline with its dorsal surface exposed at the skin.[57,76] Because the dorsal surface of the placode is covered with friable vessels, it is also called the "zona medullovasculosa."[70] A midline groove is present on the dorsal surface of the placode in the newborn that probably represents the primitive neural groove. This groove is continuous superiorly and inferiorly with the central canal of the intact spinal cord from which CSF may be discharged.[70] In a few cases, the central canal expands into a small cyst dorsal to the placode called the "terminal myelocele."[28] The membrane at the margins of the placode is referred to as the "zona membranoepitheliosa" and consists of the arachnoid on its ventral surface and partially epithelialized connective tissue on its dorsal surface. The edges of the dura blend with the zona membranoepitheliosa as well.[70] The ventral surface of the placode is lined by pia-arachnoid and faces the subarachnoid space. Nerve roots arise directly from the ventral surface of the placode with the ventral (motor) roots paired medially across the midline and the dorsal (sensory) roots positioned lateral to them. This orientation of the exiting roots can be visualized as if the normal cord were splayed open along the dorsal midline rotating the dorsal and lateral surfaces with their roots ventrally. Strands of dentate ligament may extend from the ventral surface of the placode between the exiting roots.[28]

Paravertebral Myelomeningocele

Lateral lumbar myelomeningoceles appear as skin-covered, asymmetric masses in rare cases, and a lower lumbar vertebra, such as L_5, is a hemivertebra with absence of the pedicle, and arch, which forms a paramedian dorsal defect in the spinal canal. A myelomeningocele herniates through this defect to extend laterally and ventrolaterally around the erector spinae muscle to exit posteriorly in a paramedian location. Contiguous herniation of small bowel and testes through the posterolateral defect may also occur.[70]

Myelocystocele

The myelocystocele is a localized, marked cystic dilatation of the distal cord central canal or, possibly, the ventriculus terminalis[57] (Figure 5-15). Typically, the physical findings are a cystic, skin-covered mass over the lower spine. Vertebral abnormalities such as lordosis, scoliosis, and partial sacral agenesis are common. The myelocystocele can be associated with a ventral or dorsal meningocele to form a myelocystomeningocele. Myelocystoceles are distinguished from myelomeningoceles by ependyma lining the cystic cavity and the absence of a true neural placode dorsally.[57] Myelocystoceles may occur with cloacal extrophy, which is one of the most severe malformations compatible with life.[57,70]

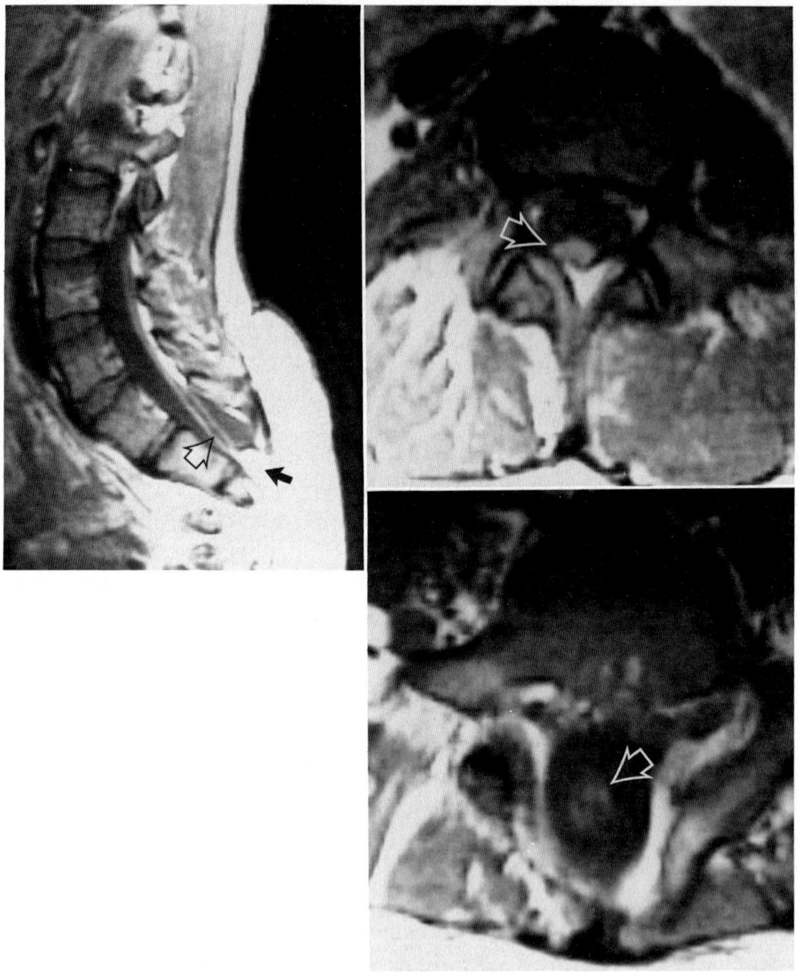

A B C

FIGURE 5-15. Tethered cord with lipoma. Midline sagittal T1W images in 13-year-old female show **A**, tethered cord ending in small sacral lipomyelomeningocele. Distal cord appears to have central cystic cavity *(open arrow)*, probably representing dilatation of central canal or "terminal ventricle." Caudal tip of cord attaches to small lipoma *(closed arrow)*. Scoliosis in midlumbar and upper lumbar canal makes visualization of entire distal cord difficult on a single image. **B**, Axial T1W image at L_4 shows asymmetry of cord with reduced anteroposterior (AP) diameter (arrow). **C**, Axial T1W image through middle of myelomeningocele shows cord as intermediate signal centrally *(arrow)* as it traverses pouch diagonally to insert at posterior-inferior lipoma.

Myelocystoceles are usually not associated with Chiari II malformation.[8] The presence of a large posterior meningeal pouch containing neural elements but without Chiari II malformation should suggest the diagnosis of myelocystocele rather than myelomeningocele.

Vertebral Anomalies

Spinal curvatures associated with myelomeningocele are congenital or developmental. Congenital scoliosis and kyphosis are found in approximately 30% of patients and arise from associated congenital anomalies such as *spina bifida aperta* hemivertebrae, solid bony bars, and unilateral unsegmented bars. Developmental scoliosis and kyphosis are present in 65% of cases and arise from muscular imbalance and distal pelvic and extremity deformities in the absence of congenital spinal deformities beyond spina bifida.

Clinical Findings

Typical symptoms of myelomeningoceles are spastic or flaccid paraparesis, lower-extremity sensory deficits, and neurologically induced orthopedic and urologic disorders. Patients with more cephelad lesions have more severe motor deficits. Gross asymmetry of the neurologic findings raises the question of an associated lesion such as diastematomyelia.[70] Orthopedic abnormalities such as scoliosis, hip dislocation, clubfoot, and pes cavus develop secondary to muscle imbalance in 80% of myelomeningocele patients. Spastic or flaccid neurogenic bladder is found in 90% of cases. The Chiari II malformation is present in 85% to 100% cases of myelomeningocele.[38,59,94] Hydrocephalus associated with aqueductal stenosis or Chiari II malformation and severe enough to require shunting is present in 80% of patients. Hydrocephalus may appear or increase in severity after surgical closure of the dural defect.[38] The incidence of syringomyelia or hydromyelia with myelomeningocele in necropsy studies ranges from 20% to 80% and was 40% in a recent MR series.[70,91]

Surgery

The major reason for imaging myelomeningoceles is surgical planning. The questions to be answered are whether there are spinal cord anomalities or tethering. and what the relationship is between neural tissue (distal cord, placode, and nerve roots) and the dural sac that is to be repaired. Post operative evaluation is important for identification of adhesions, hemorrhage, recurrent tethering of the cord, infarction of the cord and the onset or worsening of hydrocephalus.[70]

MR Imaging

Visualization of the meningeal pouch is noninvasive and direct with MR imaging and the relationship of the distal cord and neural placode to the meningeal pouch can usually be well seen* (Figures 5-16 and 5-21). The transition from intermediate signal cord to the lower signal, fibrous placode can be seen in both sagittal and axial images (see Figure 5-16). Visualization of nerve roots and thin adhesions in the subarachnoid space and, especially, within a myelomeningocele pouch are important for surgical planning. In three series of patients imaged at 0.3T and 0.5T, the major features of myelomeningoceles were well seen but nerve roots were not clearly visualized.[1,52,111] However, high field (1.0 to 1.5T) images with good SNR and high spatial resolution often demonstrate nerve roots and thin adhesions clearly[23,54,104] (sees Figures 5-16, 5-21 and 5-23), providing sufficient information for preoperative evaluation and precluding the need for myelography or CT scanning. If MR images do not adequately characterize the lesion and the fluid surrounding these nerve roots can be filled via an intrathecal contrast injection, myelography or myelographic CT will be needed to complete surgical planning.[1,52,111]

Sagittal and axial T1W images appear to be equally useful for the evaluation of myelomeningoceles. The overall longitudinal anatomy and the relationship of the distal cord to the meningeal pouch are exquisitely demonstrated on sagittal images. Axial images provide supplemental information concerning the lateralization of the meningeal pouch, placement of the distal spinal cord within it, and the location of nerve roots and adhesive bands. Motion-compensated, high SNR T2W images may be helpful by demonstrating the pouch contents, but high quality T1W images generally demonstrate this anat-

*References 1, 9, 23, 52, 54, 75, 91, 104.

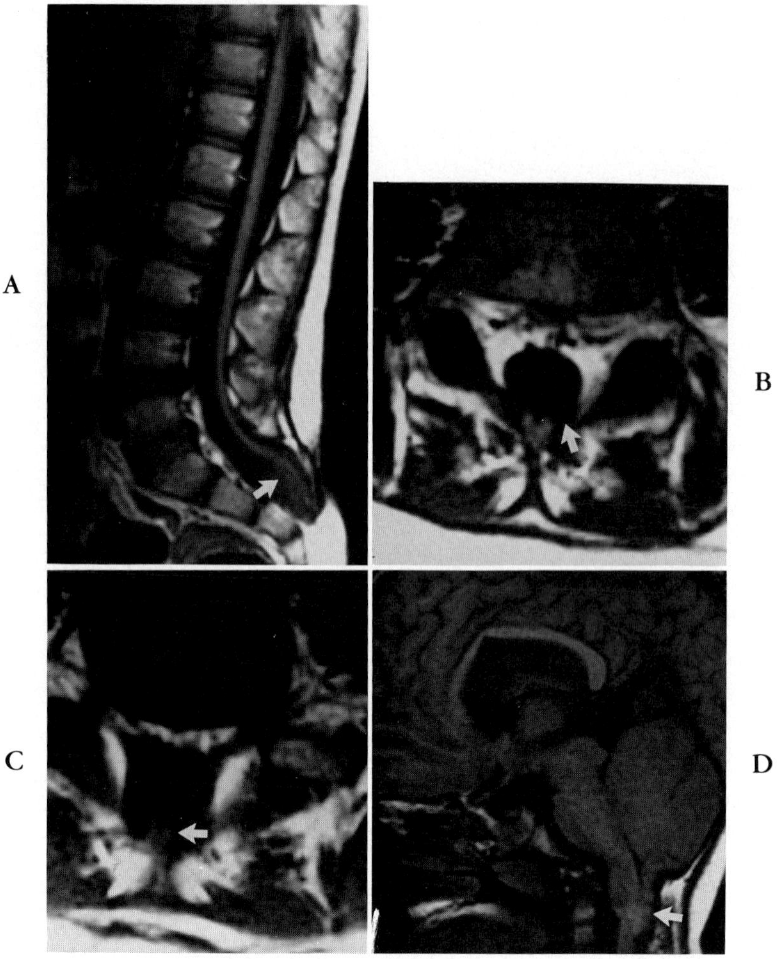

FIGURE 5-16. Sacral myelomeningocele. **A,** Midline sagittal T1W image in 5-year-old male shows tethered cord with thin, elongated caudal portion *(arrow)* entering sacral myelomeningocele. Cord terminates in complex neural placode attached to posterior surface of meningeal pouch. Thin collection of fat interposed between neural placode and cutaneous surface representing small lipomatous inclusion. **B,** Axial T1W image immediately above meningeal pouch. Distal cord tethered posteriorly against superior verge of spina bifida. Cord appears split anteriorly, suggesting partial diastematomyelia. One pair of dorsal spinal nerves extends anteriorly from dorsolateral cord on either side *(arrow)*. Ventral root on left is less distinct. **C,** Axial T1W image through superior part of meningeal pouch shows distal cord *(arrow)* traveling posteriorly in plane of image to neural placode. Low signal line running anterior to posterior through cord suggests diastematomyelia or terminal ventricle. **D,** Sagittal T1W image of cervico-medullary junction shows hydrocephalus and signs of Chiari II malformation, including tonsillar ectopia *(arrow)*, wide foramen magnum, and low position of fourth ventricle. Chiari II malformation appears in virtually all cases of myelomeningocele, and hydrocephalus appears in approximately 80%.

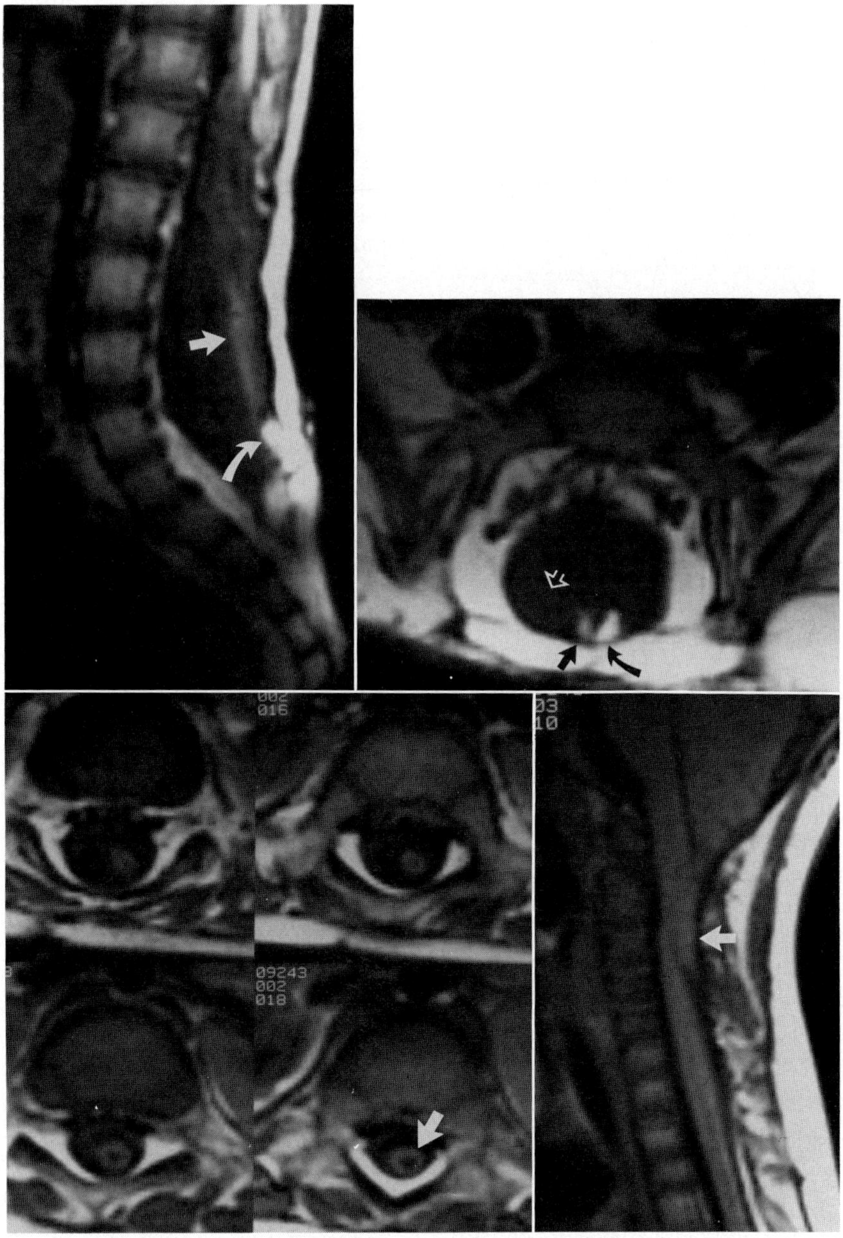

FIGURE 5-17. Lumbar lipomyelomeningomyelocele. **A,** Sagittal T1W images in 5-year-old female show large posterior lumbar dysraphic defect with ill-defined distal spinal cord *(straight arrow)* tethered to caudal lipoma *(curved arrow)*. **B,** Axial T1W image shows distal cord *(closed straight arrow)* adjacent to portion of caudal lipoma *(curved arrow)*. Nerve root extending from ventral surface of attenuated cord anterolaterally through subarachnoid space also seen *(open arrow)*. **C,** Axial T1W images at four levels through distal cord above level of lipoma show low signal in central cord *(arrow)* representing dilatation of distal spinal canal or "terminal ventricle." **D,** Sagittal T1W image at cervico-medullary junction shows typical finding of Chiari II malformation, including tonsilar ectopia *(arrow)*, low position of fourth ventricle, and enlarged foramen magnum.

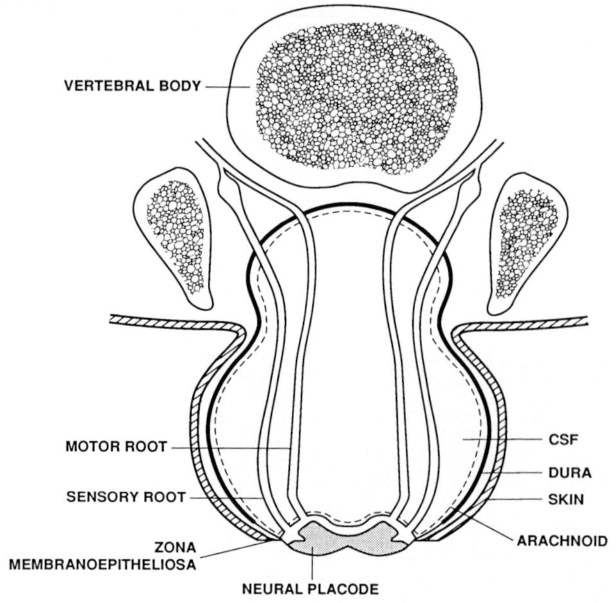

FIGURE 5-18. Myelomeningocele. This diagrammatic representation of a myelomeningocele shows the exposed dorsal surface of the neural placode at the skin surface. This surface is usually covered with friable tissue known as the *zona medullovasculosa*. The midline groove in the placode represents the primitive embryonic neural groove. The arachnoid and dura fuse at the margins of the placode to form the *zona membranoepitheliosa*. The anterior surface of the placode is covered by pia-arachnoid and faces the enlarged subarachnoid space of the meningocele. The nerve roots arising from the ventral surface are grouped into a medial (motor) pair and lateral (sensory) pair. The nerve roots exit normally through neural foramina.

omy more rapidly with fewer artifacts. Minimal experience with variable flip angle/gradient echo images suggest that they are similar to T2W SE images in their utility and susceptibility to motion artifacts. In most cases, good quality T1W sagittal and axial images of myelomeningoceles are adequate for surgical planning.

MR images are especially useful for noninvasive identification of abnormalities associated with myelomeningocele, especially spinal cord lesions that may not be adequately visualized by myelography and CT*. One MR series of 30 patients with myelomeningocele, ages 3 to 32 years, showed the Chiari II malformation in all cases (100%), syringohydromyelia in 12 cases (40%), and hydrocephalus in 10 cases (33%).[91]

Ultrasound has been suggested as a screening technique to evaluate myelomeningoceles in infants with suspected spina bifida.[73,85] However, detailed sonographic studies of structures within the closed osseous spinal canal above the dysraphism are suboptimal because of acoustic reflection and shadowing.[73] Compared with sonography, MR imaging appears to provide more detailed visualization of myelomeningocele contents, as well as complete evaluation of the intraspinal contents above the level of the lesion.

LIPOMYELOMENINGOCELE

Lipomyelomeningoceles consist of lipomas attached to the spinal cord that herniate through a widely bifid dorsal canal to form a subcutaneous fibro-fatty mass associated with meningoceles of various sizes (Figure 5-19).[70] Lipomyelomeningoceles are distinguished from intradural lipomas (discussed later) by the presence of a widely bifid spinal canal and posterior protrusion of the dural sac, lipoma, and tethered cord through the defect.

Embryology

Explanations for the formation of spinal lipomas include suggestions of overgrowth of normally present spinal cord fat cells, perivascular fat cells, and embryonic fatty rests. One hypothesis which best explains the morphology of both intradural lipomas and lipomeningoceles, is that lipomas are formed by premature dysjunction of neuroectoderm from cutaneous ectoderm just before closure of the neural tube,[72] resulting in exposure of the embryologic mesenchyme to the ependymal surface of the neural tube dorsally. Subsequent invagination of mesenchyme prevents final closure of the neural tube and contact with the inner surface of the neural tube induces the mesenchyme to form fat. Conversely, the mesenchyme in contact with the outer surface of the neural tube ventrally is induced to form normal pia, arachnoid, and dura. This hypothesis accounts for the consistent position of lipomas dorsal to the cord or filum, the dorsal myeloschisis (splaying of the dorsal horns) at the cord-lipoma junction (placode), the

*References 1, 23, 52, 54, 75, 104.

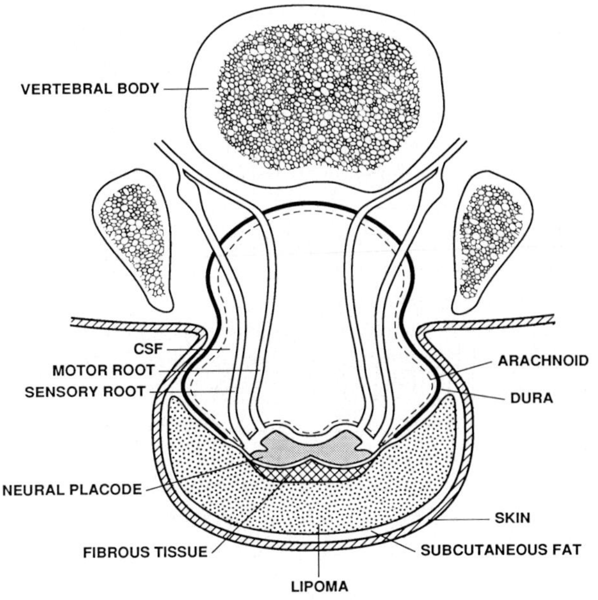

FIGURE 5-19. Lipomyelomeningocele. This diagrammatic representation of a lipomyelomeningocele shows relationships of the lipoma, neural placode, and meningocele. The lipomyelomenigocele differs from the myelomeningocele by the addition of the lipoma posterior to the neural placode and meningocele and the presence of an intact skin covering. The lipoma is similar to but distinct from the subcutaneous fat. There is a variable amount of fibrous tissue at the interface between the lipoma and the neural placode. Nerve roots exit the neural placode as a medical (motor) and lateral (sensory) pair and exit normally through neural foramina as in a myelomeningocele. In the typical lesion, lobulation of the lipoma, rotation of the placode, arachnoid adhesions, and tortuous courses of the nerve roots produce a more complex appearing lesion.

merging of the lipoma with pia, arachnoid, and dura at its lateral margins, and the absence of truly subarachnoid lipomas. Lipomas that appear to lie isolated within the cord, filum, or the central canal of the cord may actually be extensions of the lipomatous tissue from the distal, dorsal meninges invaginating into the pia-arachnoid and so remain extra-arachnoid.[70,72] Meningoceles are also explained as enlargements of the ventral subarachnoid space with the distal cord and lipoma attached to its dorsal aspect with varying degrees of posterior protrusion through dorsal spinal defects. Naidich suggests the unifying term *lipomyeloschisis* for the archetype of these developmental abnormalities.[72]

Morphology

The basic morphology of the spinal lipoma and its junction with the cord placode is similar at all vertebral levels. The bulk of the lipoma, posterior to the placode junction, is composed of uniform adult adipose tissue (yellow fat; rarely, brown fat or mixed yellow and brown fat).[70] Connective tissue strands typically subdivide the lipoma into lobules. Atypical features of lipomas include smooth and striated muscle fibers, angiomatous elements, calcification or ossification,[33,107] ependymal canals (terminale ventricle?), neuroglial islands at the placode junction, and meningeal or enteric cysts with clear or chocolate-colored (hemorrhagic?) fluid contents.[70] Lipomas and lipomeningoceles rarely undergo malignant change.[70]

The lipomeningocele is anatomically analogous to the myelocele or myelomeningocele with the additional components of the lipoma, fibromuscular capsule, and intact skin covering[70] (Figure 5-19). The dorsal lumbosacral subcutaneous mass lies in the midline in 62% of cases, asymmetrically to the left in 33% of cases and asymmetrically to the right in 5% of cases. Asymmetric lipomas are more likely to be associated with large meningoceles.[14,56] The superficial surface of the lipoma is indistinct and merges with the subcutaneous fat; the deep portion extends through the defect in bone and dura (the fibro-osseous fissure or dorsal dural defect) and tightly adheres to the neural placode. The lipoma may extend superiorly along the dorsal myeloschisis, following the open central canal of the cord, to form an intramedullary, intradural extension above the level of the dorsal spinal defect. The spinal cord is almost always in a low position with the conus in the lower lumbar or sacral canal where it terminates in focal dorsal myeloschisis at the neural placode, which is similar to that in simple myeloceles and retains the shape of the embryonal neural placode splayed open dorsally. The ventral face represents the outside of the neural tube, covered by pia mater, that is exposed to CSF in the subarachnoid space. The nerve roots are arrayed with the functional dorsal roots (sensory) situated lateral to the functional ventral roots (motor). The roots exit from the ventral surface, traverse the subarachnoid space to exit through the neural foramina, and do not pass through the lipoma, which is extra-arachnoid and lies dorsal to the placode, although the peripheral portions of the roots may be seen in the epidural and paraspinous fat.[73] With large meningoceles, the lipoma may tether the distal cord to the dorsal surface of the meningocele, resulting in kinking and stretching of the cord over a fibrovascular band at the most cephalad margin of the dorsal spinal defect. This band is usually present at the most cephalad widely bifid dorsal segment.[70] Rotation of the lipoma within the meningocele can produce complicated distortions of cord and nerve root anatomy. Precise delineation of this anatomy in the spinal defect and lipomeningocele is critical to surgical planning, especially when the dorsal roots are rotated into the midline, increasing the risk of surgical trauma.[17] MR imaging shows these complex anatomic distortions and should always be included in surgical planning.

Vertebral anomalies

Lumbosacral lipomyelomeningoceles are almost always associated with focal dorsal defect in the spinal canal.[56,73] At the cephalad margin of the defect, there is usually a progressive transition downward from a shortened spinous process, to a minimal spina bifida, to a widely bifid neural arch, and finally to a widely patent dorsal defect. There is typically a fibrovascular (sometimes cartilaginous) band extending horizontally across the most cephalad widely bifid neural arch that forms the upper margin of the dorsal spinal defect and over which the cord is usually tethered when it herniates into the lipomeningocele.[70] Butterfly vertebrae and segmental anomalies of the vertebral bodies are seen in up to 43% of cases.[70] Sacral asymmetry, confluence of sacral foramina, and partial sacral agenesis are present in approximately 50% of patients.[25,73,89] Unusual bony anomalies include a bony spur at the inferior sacroiliac joint projecting into the sciatic notch, bony "hemispheres" bridging malformed spinous processes that cap the lipoma dorsally, and plaquelike metaplastic bony masses forming part of the lipoma.[70]

Clinical Findings

Symptoms and signs of lipomyeloschisis include weakness and atrophy of the muscles of the lower extremities, disturbances of gait, urinary incontinence, impairment of cutaneous and proprioceptive sensations in the lumbar and sacral segments, and loss of tendon reflexes in the legs. Maldevelopment of the feet with valgus, varus, or cavus deformities, usually unilateral, and scoliosis are the most common associated orthopedic and vertebral column abnormalities.[18]

Symptoms typically appear before the age of 6 months with an obvious, large, fluctuant lumbosacral mass. Neurologic findings are present in only 45% of these large lesions on initial examination because of the early stage of detection but eventually 80% of those not operated on develop progressive deficits.[14] Approximately 50% of children also have cutaneous anomalies, including skin dimples, dermal sinuses, telangectasias, skin tags, patchy hypertrichosis, and skin defects.[14]

Surgery

Lipomyeloschisis may cause neurologic dysfunction in two ways: (1) progressive deposition of fat within a static number of fat cells resulting in increased intracanalicular mass effect and (2) the lipomatous mass tethers the cord, resulting in stretching of the cord, especially during growth spurts.[70]

The goal of surgery therefore is to reduce the bulk of the fatty intracanalicular mass, untether the cord, and reconstruct a closed neural and arachnoid tube to minimize postsurgical scarring and consequent retethering of the cord and placode. Proper preoperative evaluation of lipomyeloschisis is essential for successful surgical correction. The essential surgical anatomy of the lesion can be delineated by MR with supplemental information about the bony anatomy from plain films and CT. The features critical to the surgeon are the following[70]:

1. Presence and site of spina bifida
2. Presence of lipomyeloschisis
3. Side and size of lipoma with its relation to the placode
4. Location of cranial widely bifid laminae where tethering fibrovascular band is located
5. Cranial extent of lipoma and whether extension into central canal is present
6. Side and size of expanded subarachnoid space
7. Relation of placode and dorsal root entry zones to midline

8. Courses and lengths of dorsal and ventral nerve roots

MR Imaging

There are four major advantages of MR over myelography in the evaluation of lipomyelomeningoceles. The two most important advantages are that MR specifically identifies lipomatous collections and noninvasively demonstrates detailed internal anatomy of the lesion,* (Figures 5-17, 5-20, and 5-21). The positive identification of small collections of low density fat may be difficult with myelography.[87,97] Morphology of the distal cord at the neural placode or attachment of the filum to the lipoma is usually well seen with MR. The transition from intermediate signal cord or filum to the lower signal fibrous placode to the high signal lipoma are clearly seen in both sagittal and axial T1W images. These internal morphologic features of the lipoma cannot be seen with myelography. A third advantage of MR derives from the fact that the sacral thecal sac is often truncated by the mass of a large lipoma so that the anatomy around the lipoma cannot be demonstrated by intrathecal contrast material.[87] MR avoids confusion of this compression with a normal high termination of the sacral thecal sac. The fourth advantage is that MR is noninvasive whereas myelography often requires general anesthesia and involves injection of intrathecal contrast material, usually via the lumbar route. Exacerbation of symptoms of lumbar lipoma may follow lumbar puncture.[15] This route may also be precluded in cases of large lipomas, complex lipomeningoceles, low lying conus, dermoid cyst or intraspinal tumor, forcing the use of higher lateral C_1 to C_2 or midline cisternal needle placement for contrast injection. Needle punctures near the cervico medullary junction are relatively high risk procedures requiring specialized training. In addition, cervical or cisternal punctures may be precluded by the presence of tonsilar ectopia with Chiari II malformation. The incidence of Chiari II malformation with tonsilar ectopia is relatively low in cases of simple lipoma alone but is nearly 100% in myelomeningocele with lipomatous inclusions.[14,38,70]

The advantage of MR over nonmyelographic CT in evaluation of lipomeningoceles is not the positive identification of fat, which is done well with CT, but the excellent visualization of intrathecal structures (nerve roots, fibrous bands), which would require intrathecal contrast to be seen with CT. Additionally, fluid collections in cysts and meningeal pouches may not be opacified by intrathecal, subarachnoid contrast material and so would be better visualized by MRI than myelography or myelographic CT.[1] In addition, sagittal MR images are generally superior to sagittal reformations of axial CT scans.[75,111]

*References 1, 9, 23, 52, 54, 75, 91, 104.

DORSAL DERMAL SINUS

The dorsal dermal sinuses are the minimal form of congenital midline defect. These anomalies are epithelium-lined dermal tubes that extend inward from the skin surface for varying depths, frequently deep enough to connect with neural structures or meninges.[67] Dermal sinuses occur with equal frequency in males and females and are usually identified from early childhood to 25 years of age.[58]

Embryology

Dermal sinuses result from incomplete separation (dysjunction) of the cutaneous ectoderm from the neuroectoderm at about the fourth week of fetal development. They are most common in the lumbosacral and occipital regions at the sites of the posterior and anterior neuropores, the last levels of the neural groove to fuse.

Morphology

The stratified squamous epithelium lining the sinus contains hair follicles, sweat glands, and subaceous glands. One half to two thirds of sinuses above the sacrococcygeal region extend intraspinally. Intraspinal extension of sacrococcygeal sinuses is rare.[2,67,70] With intraspinal extension the dermal sinus usually merges with the dura, deeper meningeal layers, or neural structures. Free communication with CSF may be indicated by external leakage of CSF or by meningitis and arachnoiditis.[70] The dermal sinus may also terminate in the cord, conus, filum terminale, or nerve root.[70,96] The inner portion of the sinus enlarges to form dermoid or epidermoid cyst in approximately 50% of cases.[2,67,70] Less frequently, sinus terminates in a teratoma

A 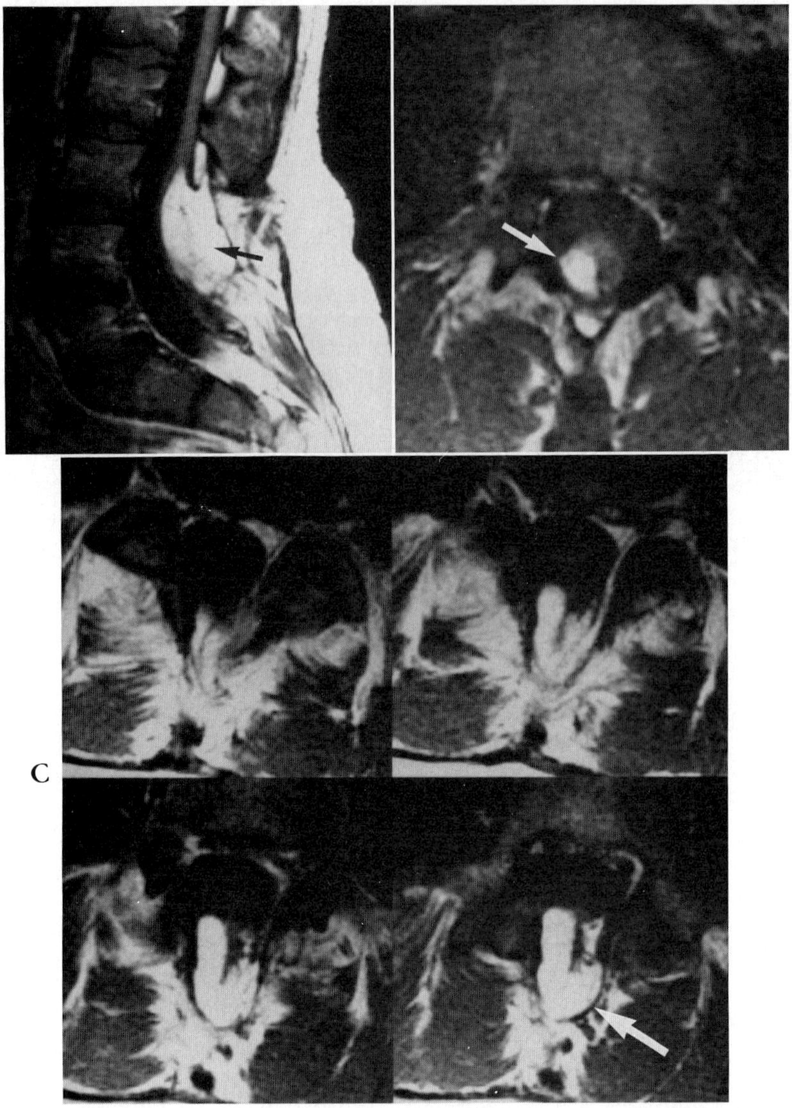 B

C

FIGURE 5-20. Tethered cord and lipomyelomeningocele. **A,** Sagittal T1W image in 15-year-old male shows large, complex lumbar lipoma *(arrow)* with spinal cord tethered to its ventral superior surface at complex placode. **B,** Axial T1W image at cord-lipoma junction shows intermediate signal cord rotated and applied to ventral and left surfaces of high signal lipoma *(arrow)* at midline. **C,** Sequential 5 mm thick axial T1W images, inferior to superior, through central part of lipomyelomeningocele show complex anatomy of lipoma *(arrow)*, which appears to form U-shaped structure within meningocele.

A B C D

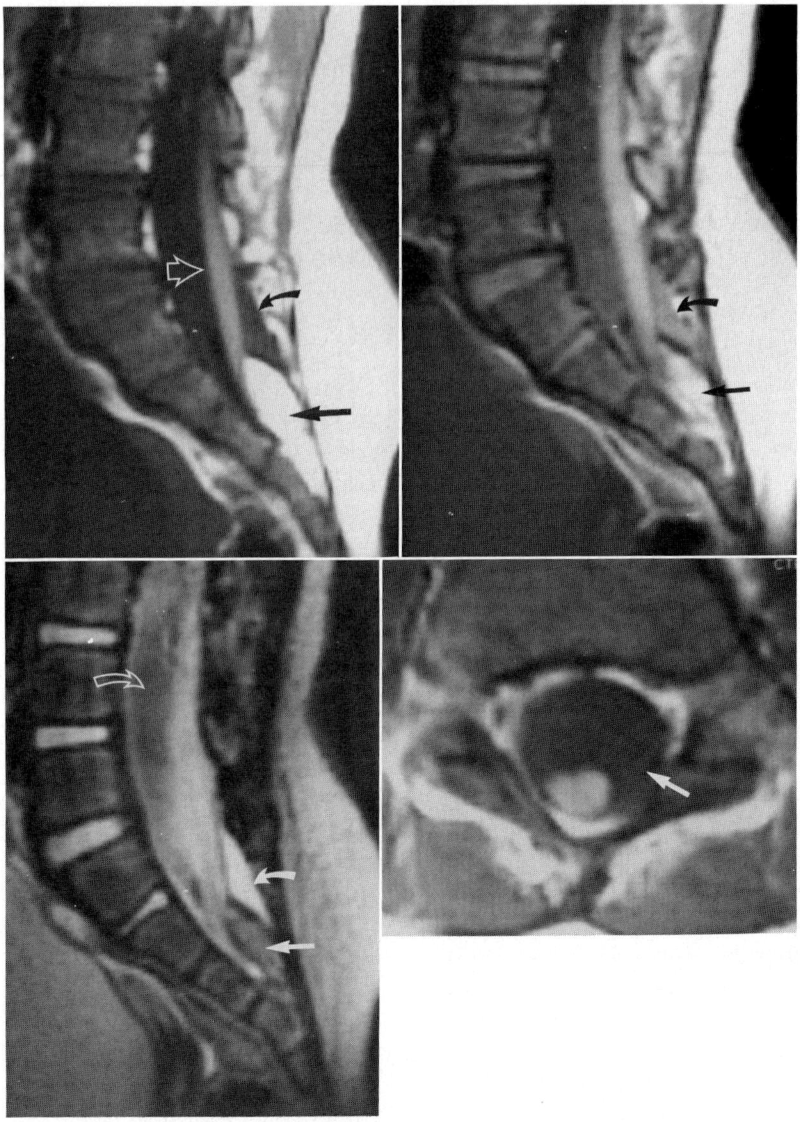

FIGURE 5-21. Tethered cord with lipomyelomeningocele. **A,** Sagittal T1W image (1.5T) in 21-month-old female clearly demonstrates spinal cord *(open arrow)* extending to neural placode *(open arrow)* on ventral surface of large sacral lipoma *(straight arrow)*. Low signal subarachnoid CSF is both anterior and posterior *(curved arrow)* to cord. **B,** Sagittal T2W image (20/2500) shows anatomy well with more complex signal from lipoma *(straight arrow)* and higher signal from CSF *(curved arrow)* than T1W image. **C,** Sagittal T2W image (80/2500) shows anatomy less clearly than T1W images. Fat in lipoma is lower signal *(closed curved arrow)* and CSF higher signal than on T1W images. Cord margin less well defined. CSF is lower signal anterior to cord *(open curved arrow)* because of motion artifacts and higher signal posterior to cord where it is static *(curved arrow)*. **D,** Axial T1W image at L_4-L_5 shows posterior position of tethered cord in spinal canal and elongated dorsal and ventral nerve roots *(arrow)* traversing subarachnoid space anterior to cord.

and occasionally in a fibrous nodule in the dorsal column of the cord.[97] The sinus may continue beyond a dermoid cyst to the conus, or the cord may be adherent to the dura at the site of attachment of the sinus tract.[67,70] Abscesses associated with dermal sinuses usually extend cephalad and caudad to the sinus and may reach considerable distances along the spinal canal. Approximately 3% of spinal abscesses are associated with a dermal sinus.[70]

Vertebral Anomalies

Vertebral anomalies are frequently associated with dermal sinuses, usually minimal midline defects such as a groove in the upper surface of the spinous process or lamina, hypoplastic spinous process, single bifid spinous process, multilevel contiguous spina bifida, or laminar defect along the course of the dermal sinus.[67,70,79]

Clinical Findings

The typical clinical presentation is the result of infection or mass effect. Superficial subcutaneous abscess and meningitis are most common, but deep abscesses in the epidural, subdural, subarachnoid, and subpial spaces also occur.[70] Occasional chemical meningitis occurs as a result of release of cholesterol crystals and other irritating cyst contents into the CSF spaces.[97] The spinal level involved by mass or abscess usually corresponds to the dermatomal level at the ostium of the associated sinus.[70]

Patients with dermal sinuses usually have a midline dimple or ostium that is associated with areas of hyperpigmentation, hairy nevus, or capillary angioma. Hair frequently emerges from the ostium[67] and CSF may drain from the ostium.[97] The cordlike subcutaneous tract can often be palpated.[70] Dermal sinuses may coexist with pilonidal sinuses.[2] The pilonidal sinus is approximately five times more common and is histologically identical but occurs only at the sacrococcygeal level and rarely extends into the spinal canal or causes neurologic symptoms.[79]

MR imaging

The MR appearance of dermal sinuses is that of a thin, low signal midline band of tissue extending through high signal subcutaneous fat.[1,54,75] Associated bony midline defects are best seen on variable flip angle/gradient echo images, which show bone as markedly low signal. The junction of the dermal sinus with the dura is usually indicated by a local outpouching or "beaking" of the thecal sac. Associated dermoid or epidermoid cysts or teratomas are seen as mass lesions with a range of signal characteristics, with the presence of fat identifying teratomas. The high water content of abscesses associated with dermal sinuses will produce low signal on T1W and high signal on T2W images, clearly distinguishable from epidural fat. Because of the high cellular and protein content of these infectious collections, intraspinal lesions will tend to be distinguishable from normal CSF, which will have lower signal on T1W and higher signal on T2W images.

DERMOID AND EPIDERMOID CYSTS

Dermoid cysts are unilocular or multilocular cystic tumors lined by simple or stratified squamous epithelium and skin appendages, such as hair follicles, sweat glands, and subaceous glands.[70] Dermoid and epidermoid tumors compose 1% to 2% of intraspinal tumors in all age groups and 10% of tumors below age 15.[35,36,70]

Embryology

Dermoid cysts usually arise from embryonic cell rests, from focal expansion of a dermal sinus, and, occasionally, from iatrogenically implanted dermal cells (e.g., lumbar puncture in infancy using a hollow needle without a trocar).[70] Single or multiple inclusion dermoid and epidermoid tumors may also arise from tissue inadvertently incorporated into the surgical closure of a myelomeningocele or other dysraphic state. Approximately 80% of lesions are isolated and not associated with a dermal sinus: 41% are single epidermoids, 34% are single dermoids, and 5% are multiple lesions. The remaining 20% of dermoid and epidermoid tumors are associated with dermal sinuses.[35,38,58]

Morphology

Dermoid cysts are filled with cornified, desquamated skin, hair (40%), and secretions of hair follicles and subaceous glands.[7] Epidermoid cysts are lined only by superficial epidermal elements of the skin.[58] Dermoids are extramedullary in 60% of cases and intramedullary in 40%.[35] Intramedullary dermoids predominate in the lumbosacral cord (60%) and are less frequent in cauda equina (20%), lower thoracic (5%), upper thoracic (10%), and cervical (5%) regions.[58] Extramedullary dermoids are usually found in the subdural space (35%) or subarachnoid space (35%) and, less frequently, in the subpial (25%) or extradural (5%) spaces.[70] Epidermoid tumors show a more uniform distribution along the thoracic and lumbar spine: cauda equina (35%), lumbosacral (22%), lower thoracic (26%), and upper thoracic (17%). Epidermoids, especially thoracic lesions, are frequently intramedullary.[58] Teratomas are tumors containing tissue derived from all three germ cell layers and are distinguished from dermoid and epidermoid cysts by the presence of fat within them. Teratomas are discussed in detail in Chapter 8.

Clinical Findings

Dermoids generally appear as symptomatic lesions at a later age than simple dermal sinuses (mean age 28 years)[58] and occur equally in males and females. Epidermoids become symptomatic between 20 and 50 years of age in most cases and are more common in males.[58] The mechanism of presentation for dermoids and epidermoids is spinal block with cord or cauda equina compression in 80% to 90% of cases.[7,35] Large lesions may expand the spinal canal (35%), erode pedicles (20%), and cause scalloping of the vertebral bodies (30%).[70]

MR Imaging

The signal from dermoid and epidermoid cysts is dependent on the water, keratin, collagen, and cholesterol composition of the cyst wall and its contents. Limited experience is available with MR imaging of these lesions in the spine and inconsistent terminology is present in the literature. The term *dermoid tumor* may be used to describe mass lesions containing fat (adult adipose tissue) that produces high signal on T1W images and should not be confused with the true "dermoid cyst," which does not contain fat. Based on the pathology of dermoid cysts, they should be expected to be similar to cysts with high protein content and show signal slightly higher than CSF on T1W images (Figure 5-22) and high signal, similar to CSF on T2W images. Keratin and collagen probably contribute nonspecifically as solutes, causing slight shortening of water proton relaxation times. The role of cholesterol in these cysts is not well understood but may produce high signal on T1W images if the concentration of short T1 lipid protons is sufficiently high. More experience is available with epidermoid tumors, especially intracranial intradural lesions. These cysts tend to have signal similar to CSF on T1W and T2W images with internal architecture not seen in simple cysts. Mass effect from either dermoid or epidermoid cysts compressing or expanding the cord or cauda equina is easily identified on sagittal and axial MR images (see Figure 5-22).

SACRAL ANOMALIES

Sacral anomalies are part of a group of congenital abnormalities referred to as the "caudal regression syndrome," which encompasses different degrees of caudal malformation ranging from complete fusion of the lower extremities (sirenomelia or sympodia), to absence of the distal spine (sacral and lumbar agenesis), and to anal atresia with external genitalia malformation[70] (Table 5-4). The incidence of caudal regression is approximately 1 per 3000 births. Associated nonneurologic abnormalities occur in a minority of cases and include pulmonary hypoplasia and severe renal dysplasia or aplasia (Potter's syndrome).[26,48] A strong association with diabetes mellitus has been observed with 16% of caudal regression patients having diabetic mothers and sacral agenesis occuring in 1% of patients of diabetic mothers.[70] Cardiac malformations occur in up to 22%[48] and mental retardation is present in 30% of patients.[86]

Embryology

Caudal regression occurs because of developmental disturbances before the fourth week of gestation.[48] The embryogenesis of the caudal spine is dependent on normal coordination of development in the notochord and neural tube. Experimental removal of the notochord alone results in abnormal development of vertebral bodies with normal posterior elements and, con-

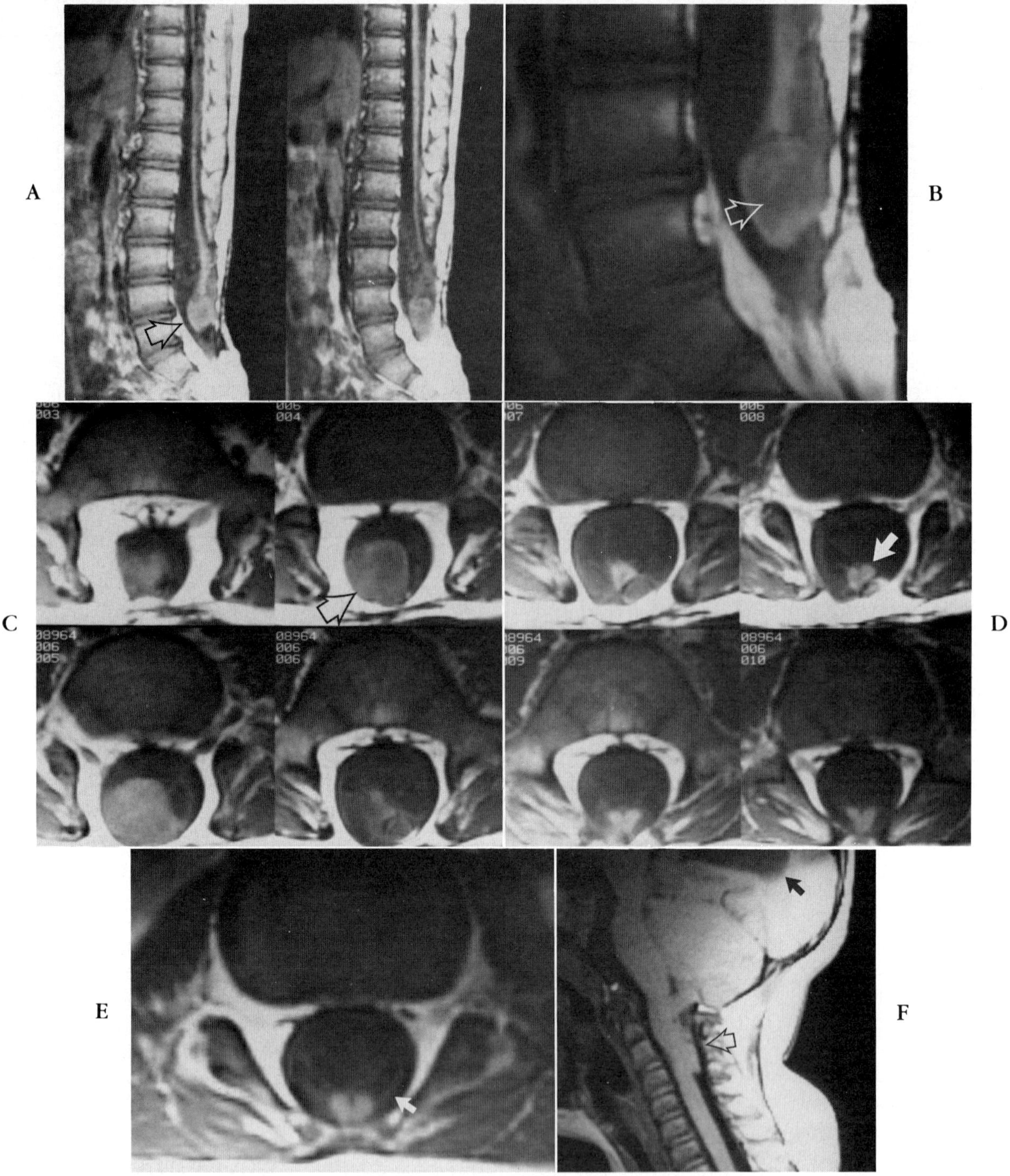

FIGURE 5-22. Tethered cord with lumbar mass. **A,** Sagittal T1W images in 5-year-old male show elongated tethered cord attached to large nonfatty mass *(arrow)*, probably representing dermoid or epidermoid cyst in lumbar spinal canal. Posterior dysraphic defect present from L_2-L_3 level through sacral level. **B,** Magnified sagittal T1W image shows detailed anatomy of mass and its junction with distal cord. Irregular signal within mass indicates complex lesion with low signal suggesting cystic regions *(arrow)*. **C,** Axial T1W images through lumbar mass *(open arrow)* that lies eccentrically in right posterior spinal canal in contact with membranous covering of canal. **D,** Axial images through junction of distal cord and mass show slightly distorted cord *(arrow)* at junction with mass. **E,** Magnified axial view of lumbar cord above mass shows both pairs of ventral and dorsal nerve roots traversing widened subarachnoid space *(arrow)*. **F,** Sagittal T1W image shows hydrocephalus *(closed arrow)* and features of Chiari II malformation, including tonsillar ectopia *(open arrow)*.

TABLE 5-4
Classification of Sacral Agenesis

Type I	Unilateral sacral agenesis (8.7% of cases) Oblique lumbosacral joint, separate ilia, no hip dislocation, and lumbar scoliosis
Type II	Symmetric sacral agenesis (52.2%) Normal or hypoplastic S_1; stable articulations with ilia; 25%, hip dislocation; 50%, scoliosis
Type III	Lumbar agenesis (21.8%) Absent sacrum; ilia articulate with lowest vertebra (stable in 60%); 80%, bilateral hip dislocation; 40%, progressive spinopelvic kyphosis; 4%, scoliosis
Type IV	Lumbar agenesis with fused ilia (17.4%) Absent sacrum; ilia fused or joined at an amphiarthrosis; lowest vertebra is above ilia; 100%, hip flexion contractures but not hip dislocation; 75% to 100%, spinopelvic kyphosis and scoliosis

(From Renshaw, TS. Sacral agenesis: a classification and review of twenty-three cases. J Bone Joint Surg 1978; 60A:373 With permission.)

versely, removal of the distal spinal cord alone produces abnormal posterior elements and intact vertebral bodies.[45]

Vertebral and Iliac Changes

The level of caudal regression is below L_1 in most cases, with the lowest intact vertebra at L_1 to L_5 in 40% of cases and at L_5 or lower in 27%.[70] The lowest intact vertebra may be as high as T_{11} or T_{12} in as many as 33% of cases but is not seen above T_{10}, suggesting that higher levels of agenesis are incompatible with life. Unilateral sacral agenesis may be found in up to one third of patients.[70] Renshaw has classified sacral agenesis into four types, based on the severity of the lumbosacral anomaly and associated abnormalities of the ilia or hips and the presence of kyphosis or scoliosis[86] (Table 5-4).

The thoracolumbar spine above the level of the agenesis is abnormal in 65% of cases. Thoracolumbar vertebral anomalies include hypoplastic vertebrae, hemivertebrae, and unsegmented bars in about equal proportions (22% each).[86] The spinal canal below the lowest intact vertebra may be severely narrowed by bony elements, posterior fibrous bands, or narrowing of the dural sac. Surgical duroplasty may markedly improve neurologic symptoms.[70]

Spinal Cord Anomalies

The caudal spinal cord undergoes anomalous development at and above the segments corresponding to levels of the vertebral agenesis. Distal spinal cord segments are smaller diameter than normal and the gray-white differentiation is abnormal with decreased numbers of anterior horn cells.[70] These dysplastic changes worsen distally and the cord tends to end abruptly at approximately the same segmental level as the spine without gradual tapering to a conus medullaris and filum terminale (Figure 5-23).

Tethered Cord and Myelomeningocele

Tethered cord, thickened filum, lipoma, and diastematomyelia associated with sacral agenesis have been described but are found in only a minority of cases.[70] Myelomeningocele may be associated with sacral agenesis in 35% to 50% of cases,[86,101] although one series demonstrated an incidence less than the random occurrence in the normal population.[48]

Clinical Findings

Patients with lumbar or sacral agenesis have flattening of the buttocks, shortening of the intergluteal cleft, and prominent iliac crests. The gluteal and leg muscles may be severely hypoplastic.[34] Neuromuscular abnormalities associated with sacral agenesis range from minor distal muscle weakness to complete paralysis of the lower extremities. Motor deficits correspond closely to the level of the vertebral termination and usually include the perineum (S_2 through S_5) and leg flexors (L_5 and S_1 myotomes), while sparing the leg extensors and adductors (L_2 through L_4 myotomes).[86] Sensory deficits tend to occur several segments caudal to the motor levels so that perineal sensation may be intact despite complete loss of sphincter control.[86] This persistence of sensation is probably the result of

A, B

C, D

E, F

G, H

I, J

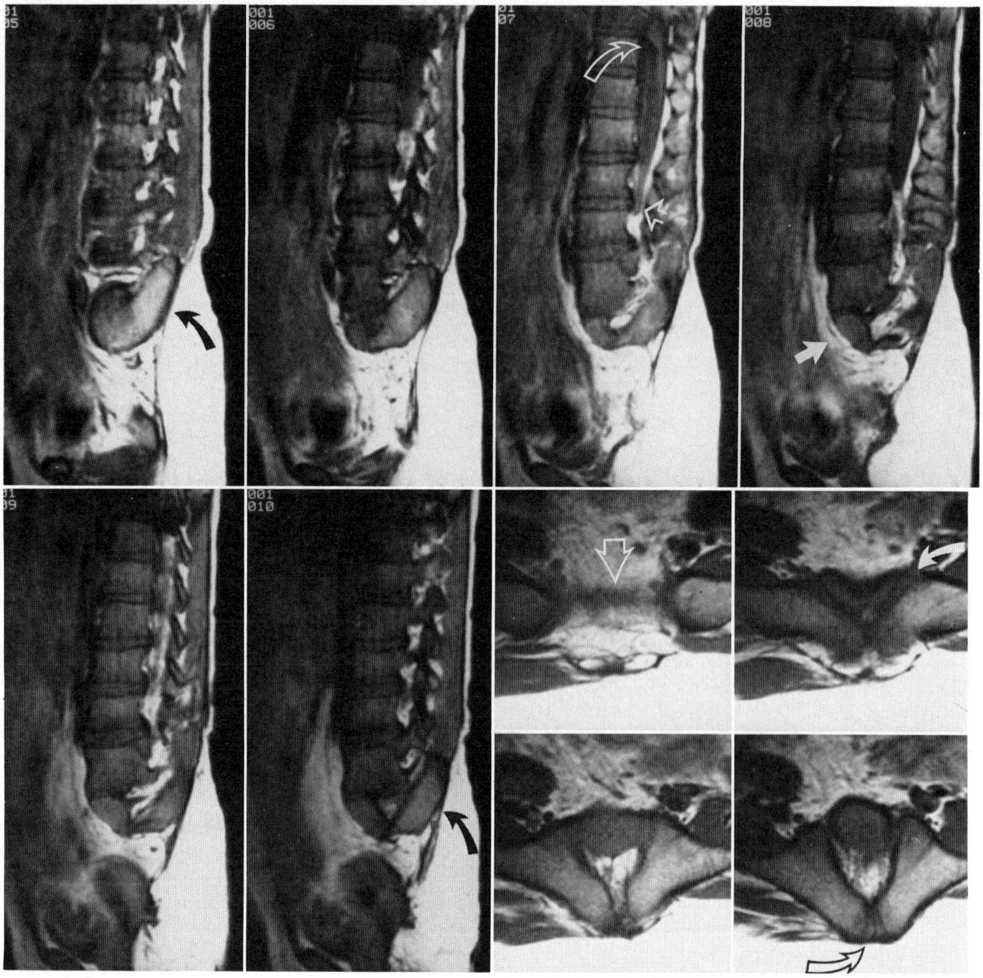

FIGURE 5-23. Sacral agenesis. **A-F**, Sagittal T1W images in 6-year-old male show absence of sacrum below rudimentary S_1 vertebral body (**D**, *arrow*). More lateral sagittal images on either side show bulky masses of medial ilia (**A** and **F**, *curved arrows*). Caudal spinal canal tapers as it approaches S_1 level and narrowing of caudal thecal sac is present (**C**, *open arrow*). **C**, Spinal cord ends abruptly at T_{12} level *(open curved arrow)* without normal tapering to conus tip. Roots of cauda equina appear to extend caudally from ventral and dorsal surfaces of cord termination. Filum terminale lying between ventral and dorsal groups of nerve roots is not seen. **G-J**, Sequential 5 mm thick axial T1W images through caudal spine show **G**, absence of lower sacrum with soft tissue interposed between ilia *(open arrow)*. **H**, Rudimentary S_1 vertebral body *(arrow)* articulates with ilia bilaterally *(curved arrows)*. Articulation of iliac wings posteriorly (**J**, *open curved arrow*) also present, resulting in almost complete obliteration of spinal canal caudally. **K-M**, Axial T1W images through L_5 (**K**), L_4 (**L**), and L_1 (**M**) show narrow caudal spinal canal (**K**, *curved arrow*) and small dural sac (**L**, *open curved arrow*). **K**, Thickened pedicles and articulation of posterior elements with medial iliac wings are also present. Deviation of spinous process to left is caused by fusion to left iliac wing inferior to this image *(small arrow)*. **M**, "W" shape of dorsal cauda equina *(small arrow)*. Filum terminale is not seen as distinct structure. **N** and **O**, Sagittal T1W images in midthoracic spine show widened midthoracic cord with low signal centrally indicating presence of syringomyelia or hydromyelia *(arrows)*. **P**, Note abrupt termination of spinal cord *(open curved arrow)* with exiting nerve roots dorsally and ventrally.

K L M N, O P, Q

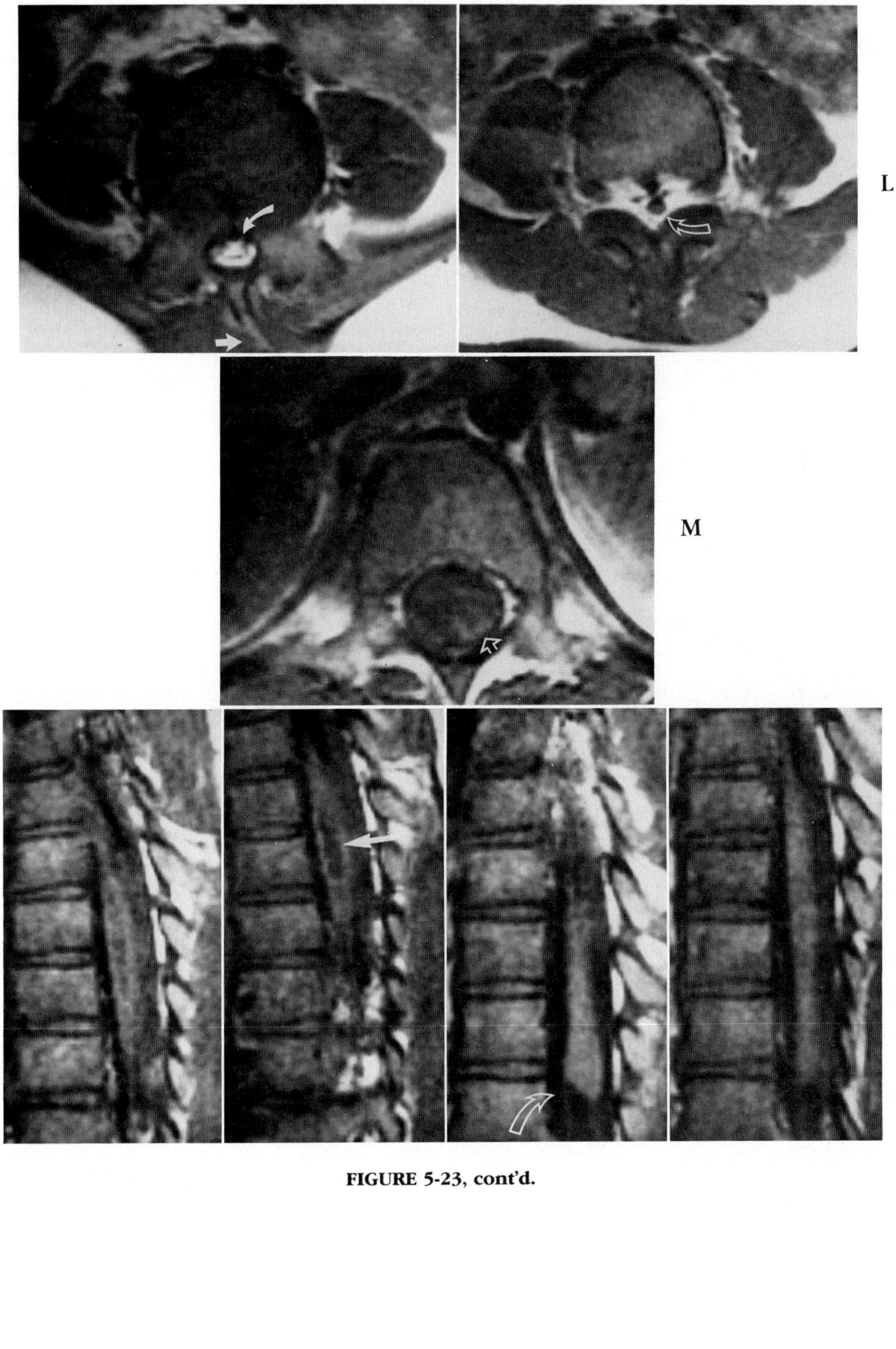

FIGURE 5-23, cont'd.

residual neural crest elements that develop into dorsal root ganglia below the level of vertebral termination and establish connections with the lowest available cord segments.[70] The incidence of neurogenic bladder and lax sphincters is very high when more than one sacral segment is absent.[86] Absence of the coccygeal segments alone is usually asymptomatic. In most cases, the motor and sensory deficits are stable and not responsive to surgical repair, but some progressive deficits may respond well. One series of 106 patients with progressive symptoms and imperforate anus showed sacral anomalies on plain radiographs in 35% with improvement in 53% of those undergoing surgery.[106]

MR Imaging

MR is useful for identification and evaluation of suspected lumbosacral agenesis.[106] Midline, sagittal T1W images provide the most information and clearly demonstrate the absence or truncation of the spine and sacrum. (see Figure 5-23). Subtle bony anomalies such as coccygeal absence or small anomalies of lumbar and sacral vertebra may be missed with MR and better identified by plain radiography, but in most cases these types of anomalies are of little clinical consequence.

MR is the best way to identify spinal cord anomalies associated with sacral agenesis because of the noninvasive, direct visualization of cord tissue. One problem of interpretation may be the determination of the proper level of the cord termination and whether the distal cord is abnormally terminated or tethered. With abrupt, nontapered termination of the cord (see Figure 5-23), projection of the cord to its "true" conus postion is purely speculative and probably not a useful exercise. Identification of the filum terminale may also be difficult when the cauda equina is markedly abnormal with normal and small nerve roots mixed with fibrous bands. It may not be possible to determine the precise nature of the cauda equina elements by their MR appearance or even by gross examination at surgery.

INTRADURAL LIPOMA

Spinal lipomas are collections of fat and connective tissue frequently found at the level of the conus (see Table 5-2) and generally are classified into "intradural lipomas" and "lipomyelomeningoceles." Lipomyelomeningoceles, discussed previously, are always accompanied by spina bifida aperta and meningocele with accompanying tethered spinal cord. Intradural lipomas are probably not truly intradural. Some connection with the dorsal thecal sac usually exists, though they may appear to lie completely within the spinal cord or filum terminale.[27] They usually occur with a normal or minimally bifid vertebral canal.[70]

Embryogenesis

The best explanation for embryogenesis of lipomatous tissue within the spinal canal and cord is that premature dysjunction of neuroectoderm from cutaneous ectoderm exposes embryologic mesenchyme to the ependymal surface of the neural tube dorsally and induces the mesenchyme to form fat. This process was discussed previously under lipomyelomeningocele.

Morphology

Intraspinal lipomas probably form by the same process as lipomyelomeningoceles and should be considered a subset of these lesions in which the dorsal dysraphic defect is minimal.[70,73] The two types of lesions are identical in that the bulk of the lipoma is composed of uniform adult adipose tissue (yellow fat).[70] Connective tissue strands typically subdivide the lipoma into lobules. Intraspinal lipomas tend to involve primarily the cervical and thoracic spinal cord. Typical frequencies are 12% cervical, 24% cervicothoracic, 30% thoracic, 3% thoracolumbar, 2% lumbar, and 4% lumbosacral cord, with 7% of cases involving the entire length of the cord. Other patterns of involvement include 7% conus with cauda equina, 6% cauda only, 1% conus only, and 2% filum only.[33] Almost all intradural lipomas affect the dorsal aspect of the spinal cord. Most lie directly in the midline dorsally (67%) and less frequently posterolateral (23%), lateral (23%), and anterolateral (2%).[33] The lipoma appears to encompass the entire cross section of the cord at some level in 3% of cases, but, in fact, is bordered by an attenuated placode and does not actually replace cord. Intrinsic spinal cord lipomas are not surrounded by the

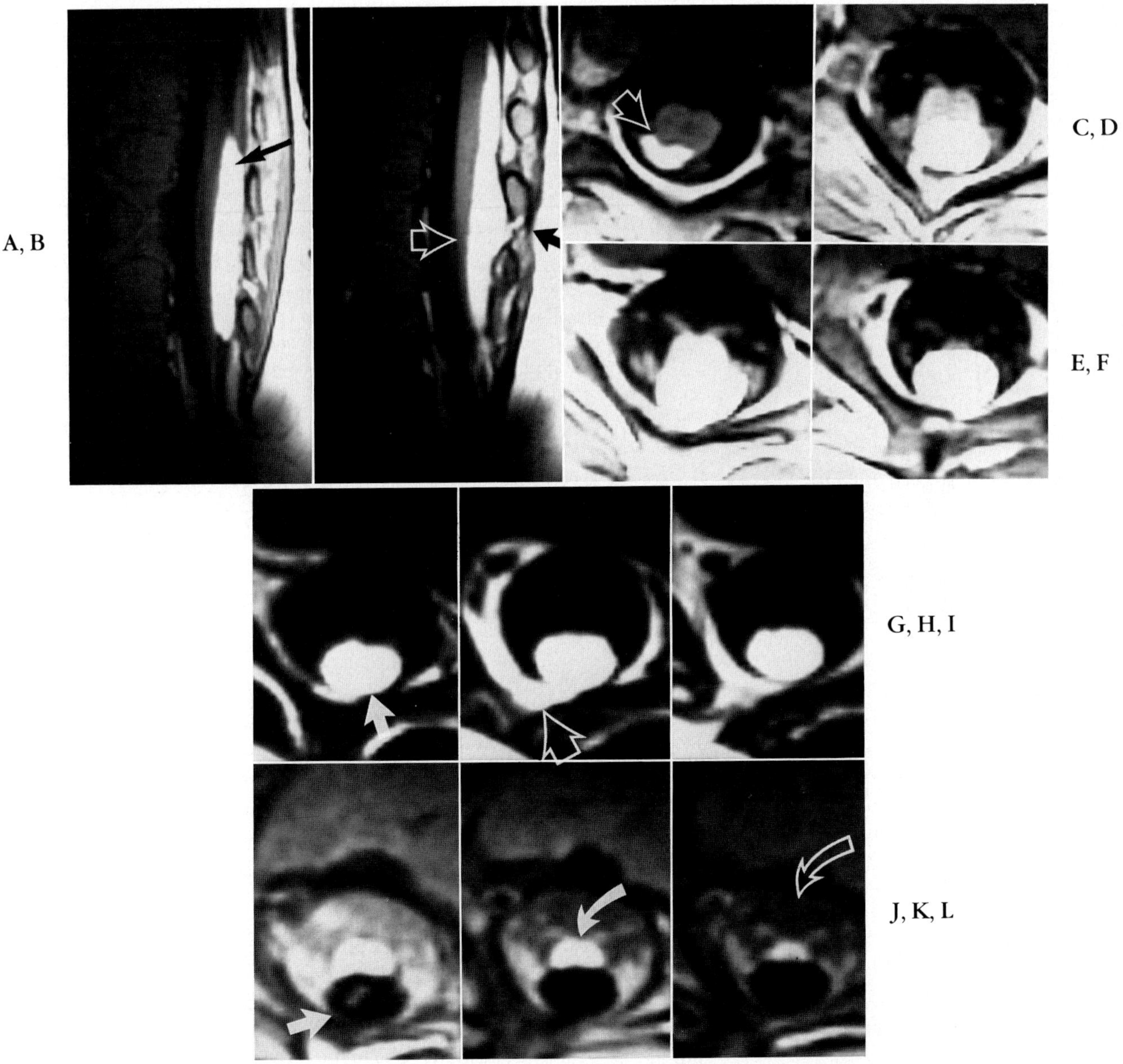

FIGURE 5-24. Intradural lipoma in a 16-month-old female with water-suppressed and fat-suppressed images. **A** and **B**, Saggital T1W images (SE 800/20) of the lumbar spine show a large, high signal intradural mass (**A**, *arrow*) posterior to a low-lying distal spinal cord (the conus tip is at L3-L4; **B**, *open arrow*). A major dysraphic abnormality is not present and minimal posterior, extradural extension of the mass is seen (**B**, *arrow*). These findings are most consistent with an intradual lipoma. **C-F**, Axial T1W images (SE 800/20) through distal cord and lipoma show cord-lipoma interface along the dorsal aspect of the cord at the neural placode (**C**, *arrow*). These images also confirm that the lipoma is largely intradural. Although high signal in the mass is characteristic for lipoma, no chemical-shift artifact is present to positively identify it as fatty tissue. **G-I**, Axial water-suppressed images (image of fat signal only) confirm that the mass is composed of fat. Isolated high signal from intradural lipoma (**G**, *arrow*) and subcutaneous fat (**H**, *arrow*) are contrasted against absence of signal anterior to the lipoma in the spinal cord and CSF. **J-L**, Axial fat-suppressed images (images of water signal only) show absence of signal in the lipoma (**J**, *arrow*) and high signal from water in the spinal cord (**K**, *arrow*) and nerve roots. The intermediate signal anterior to the cord is caused by motion-induced signal loss from the oscillating CSF (**L**, *arrow*).

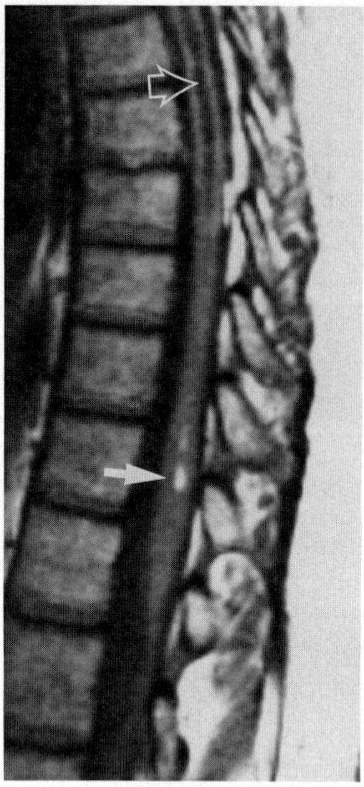

FIGURE 5-25. Conus medullaris lipoma. Sagittal T1W image shows high signal *(closed arrow)* in central conus medullaris indicating presence of intradural, intramedullary lipoma. Conus appears normal otherwise without evidence for myeloschisis. In midthoracic spinal cord, central low signal indicates presence of synrigomyelia or hydromyelia *(open arrow)*.

cord but are actually juxtamedullary in location and 45% have a clear extramedullary component, usually at the upper or lower end of the lipoma.[3,33] The dura is typically displaced posteriorly at the level of the lipoma, may be connected to the lipoma by fibrous strands, and is deficient dorsally when an extradural component of the lipoma is present.[70]

Associated Anomalies

With intradural lipomas, the vertebral column is largely intact but completely normal in only 20% of cases.[33] The most frequent change, seen in 53%, is enlargement of the spinal canal with erosion of pedicles, laminae, and posterior vertebral bodies.[33] Sacral defects, sacral agenesis, Klippel-Feil deformity, and wedged vertebrae are infrequent.[33] Approximately one third of cases are associated with other congenital anomalies, including subcutaneous, extradural, or intracranial lipomas (11%); pilonidal sinuses (3%); cervical ribs (1%); cleft lip (1%); pseudohermaphroditism (1%); absent iris (1%); and cutaneous lesions.[33] Other anomalies, present in about 2% of cases, include patent ductus arteriosis, congenital hydrocephalus, and Chiari I malformation. Only one case of associated Chiari II malformation has been reported.[14,70]

Clinical Findings

Intradural lipomas comprise approximately 1% of primary intraspinal masses. The incidence is slightly greater in males and three age peaks are observed: less than 5 years of age (24%), 10 to 30 years of age (55%), and 40 to 50 years of age (16%).[33] Cervical and thoracic lipomas typically have histories of 3 to 20 years of slowly developing, ascending, spastic monoparesis or paraparesis with cutaneous and deep sensory loss.[33] Radicular pain is uncommon, which helps to differentiate intraspinal lipomas from other intraspinal masses and from intramedullary tumors.[33] Lumbosacral lesions are different, appearing typically with flaccid paraparesis and dysfunction of bowel and bladder sphincters.[33]

MR Imaging

The key advantage of MR over CT and myelography for the characterization of congenital lipomas is the ability to directly visualize the lipoma and its relationship to other soft tissues noninvasively. The fat in congenital lipomas produces signal identical to that of adult subcutaneous fat, and lesions have high signal on T1W images and intermediate to low signal on T2W images.[52,104] In most cases, the intradural lipoma

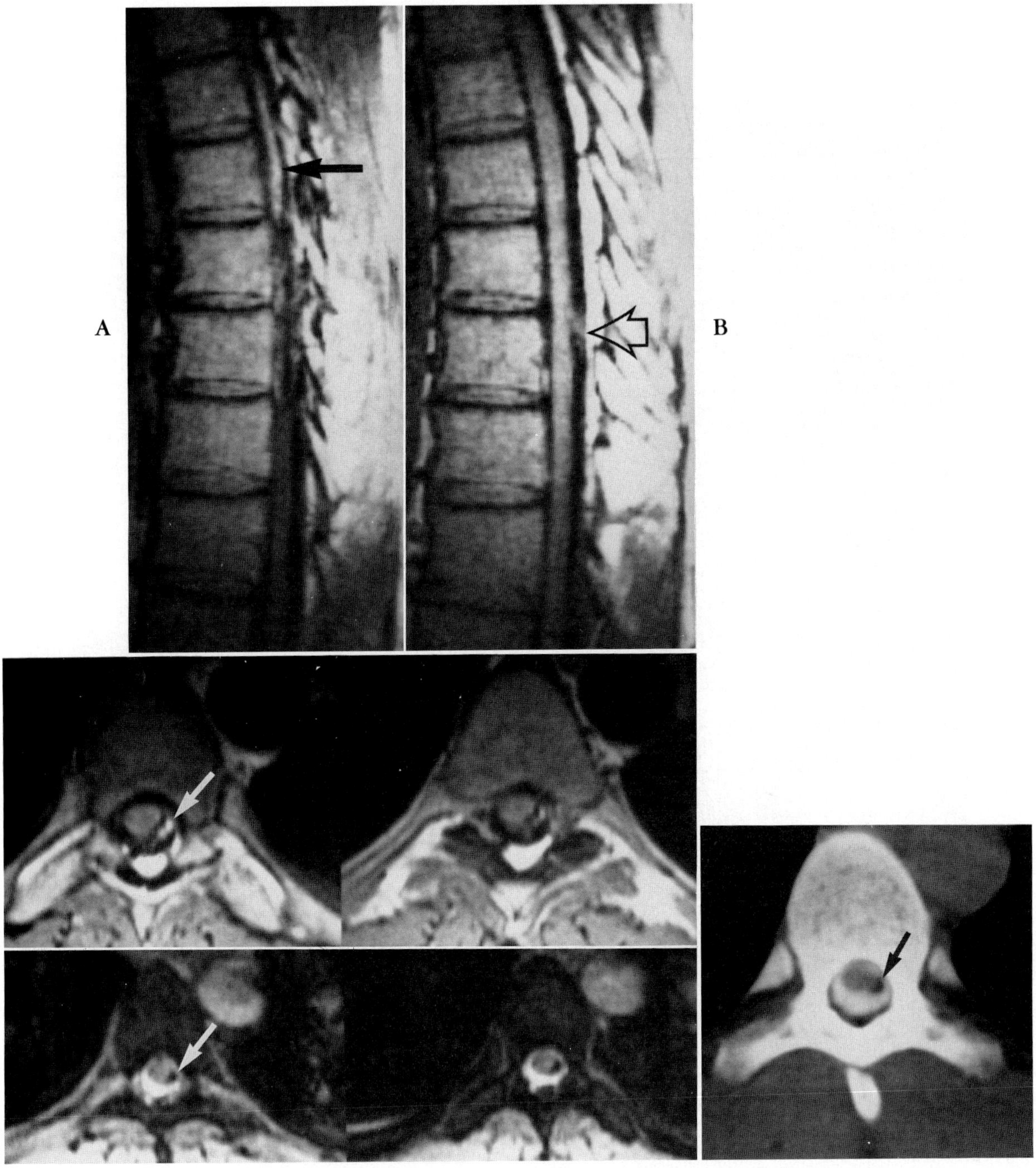

A B C D E

FIGURE 5-26. Thoracic intradural lipoma. Sagittal T1W images in 30-year-old male show **A,** intradural extramedullary lipoma extending over several segments of upper thoracic spine (**A,** *arrow*) and **B,** nonfatty dorsal portion of lesion posterior to cord at lower level *(arrow)*. **C,** Axial T1W images show left-sided intradural lipoma *(arrow)* associated with slight distortion of cord. **D,** Axial GRASS (TE 12 ms, TR 22 ms, flip angle 7°) images show intradural lipoma as low signal *(arrow)*. **E,** Axial metrizamide CT scans show lipoma as low density *(arrow)*.

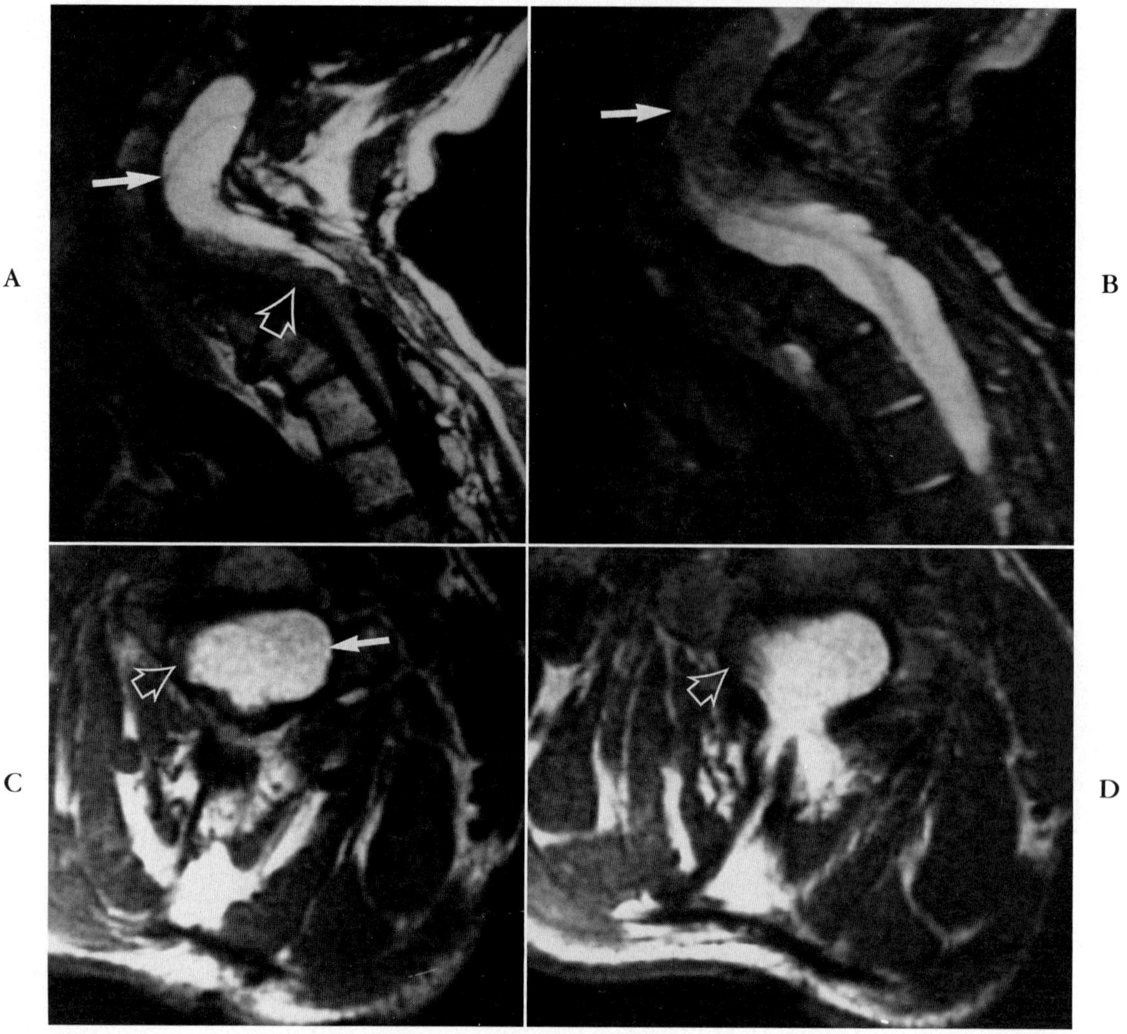

FIGURE 5-27. Cervical intradural lipoma. **A**, Sagittal T1W image in 31-year-old male with progressive quadriparesis shows very large high signal lipoma *(closed arrow)* in cervical spinal canal extending from tip of dens to C_5 level posteriorly. Irregular interface with spinal cord is present inferiorly *(open arrow)*. Disruption of normal anatomy posterior to spinal canal is result of previous laminectomy. Surgery confirmed presence of intradural, extramedullary lipoma with large subdural component. **B**, Sagittal T2W images show lipoma as low signal *(arrow)* contrasting against the high signal CSF and intermediate signal spinal cord. **C** and **D**, Axial T1W images show lipoma *(closed arrow)* occupying most of enlarged spinal canal with dorsal extension. Spinal cord is displaced to right *(open arrows)*.

can be clearly localized within the thecal sac or within the spinal cord (Figures 5-24 to 5-26) on sagittal and axial T1W images. The relationship of the lipoma to the cord or filum is clearly demonstrated by MR but the connection with the overlying meninges is often not seen. Occasionally, the lesion may be so large that the precise relationship to the dura cannot be clearly discerned (Figure 5-27). In these cases, the differential diagnosis must include epidural lipoma, especially in the thoracic spine, when concentric constriction of the thecal sac appears to be present.[109]

In cases where the differential diagnosis of a high signal lesion on T1W images includes hemorrhage, the lipoma can be positively identified by observing the chemical shift artifact, which occurs at fat–water interfaces that are oriented perpendicular to the frequency-encoding gradient and appears as very high signal at one margin and signal void at the opposite margin of the lipoma. It occurs because the difference in resonance frequency between fat and water protons (approximately 200 Hz at 1.5T) results in a small spatial shift or mismapping of the fat signal onto the water signal at one margin (high signal) and separation of signal at the opposite margin (signal void). The width of the artifact is 1 to 2 pixels in most imaging systems, depending mostly on the signal bandwidth used (more prominent with narrow bandwidth). Marked magnetic susceptibility effects from hemorrhage on T2W images may also help to differentiate tissues, especially at high magnetic fields (e.g., 1.5T) using T2*W variable flip angle/gradient echo images. If available, fat-suppressed and water-suppressed images will allow direct identification of signal from water and fat protons, respectively, for a more positive discrimination between hemorrhage and lipoma (see Figure 5-24).

MENINGEAL CYSTS

The classification of spinal cystic lesions is confusing, with a variety of terms used, including cysts, pouches, or diverticula in the thoracolumbar region and Tarlov's perineurial cysts, spinal nerve root perineurial cysts, meningeal diverticula, or occult intrasacral meningocele in the sacral region.[68,71] These lesions are distinct from classic meningocele or myelomeningocele and probably represent various forms of congenital meningeal, nerve root sheath, and arachnoid diverticula. A simplified classification of spinal cysts is presented in Table 5-5.[68] Circumstantial evidence for a congenital origin of all three types of cysts is a familial tendency and a frequent association with other congenital anomalies such as spinal dysraphism. The consistent location of type I cysts at the origin of the dorsal nerve root sheath also suggests a developmental origin.[68]

TABLE 5-5
Classification of Spinal Meningeal Cysts

Type I	Extradural meningeal cyst without spinal nerve root fibers
Type Ia	Extradural meningeal cyst (extradural arachnoid cyst)
Type Ib	Sacral meningocele (occult sacral meningocele)
Type II	Extradural meningeal cyst with spinal nerve root fibers (Tarlov's perineurial cyst, spinal nerve root diverticulum)
Type III	Spinal intradural meningeal cyst (intradural arachnoid cyst)

(From Nabors MW, Pait TG, et al. Updated assessment and current classification of spinal meningeal cysts. J Neurosurg 1988;68:366 With permission).

Clinical Findings

Type I lesions are dural diverticula that occur anywhere along the thecal sac and have a pathologically identifiable pedicle. Those arising above the sacrum (extradural meningeal cysts) contain a pedicle that is usually adjacent to the entrance of the dorsal nerve root. Those in the sacrum (sacral meningoceles) contain a pedicle at the caudal tip of the dural sac, usually adjacent to dorsa sacral or coccygeal nerve roots. Thoracic type I cysts occur more frequently in adolescents whereas sacral lesions are found more often in adults. The duration of symptoms is shorter for thoracic lesions than for sacral lesions, probably because of the greater sensitivity of the cord than nerve roots to extrinsic compression. Types of symptoms are also different with thoracic cysts usually appearing with spasticity and hypesthesia sensory levels caused by cord compression, lumbar lesion with low back pain and radiculopathy, and sacral lesions with radicular symptoms and bowel or bladder dysfunction. Treatment by drainage and occlusion of the ostium is usually sufficient in these cases.[68]

Type II lesions are diverticula of the spinal nerve root sleeves that include Tarlov's perineurial cysts and spinal nerve root diverticula. These cysts are often multiple and may occur at the dorsal nerve roots at any level; they are most prominent and symptomatic in the sacrum. The nerve fibers lie within the cyst wall or freely within the central cyst, surrounded by CSF. The cysts are most frequently symptomatic in adulthood and present with radiculopathy (sciatica) and occasionally bowel and bladder symptoms. Type II cysts do not have a pedicle and must be treated by oversewing or total excision. Simple aspiration is not sufficient.[68]

Type III cysts occur anywhere along the posterior subarachnoid space and are often multiple. Anterior cysts are uncommon. They are often asymptomatic but when symptoms occur they are those of an intradural extramedullary mass lesion. Their origin is probably related to proliferation of arachnoid trabeculae, especially the septum posticum.[68]

MR Imaging

Spinal meningeal cysts appear as masses in the spinal canal or in neural foramina that have low signal on T1W images and high signal on T2W images, similar to CSF. Occasionally, signal may be indicative of chronic hemorrhagic fluid (intermediate to high signal on T1W images and high signal on T2W images), probably caused by trauma. Hemosiderin-laden macrophages have been microscopically identified in the cyst wall in one nontraumatic type III intradural cyst in a patient 3 years old,[68] which might appear as a very low signal margin on T2 or partial flip angle images on high field systems (MRI was not done in this case).

All of the intraspinal cysts probably communicate with the subarachnoid space at some point during their development, and in most, communication can be demonstrated with water-soluble myelographic contrast on CT scans (12 of 14 in one series),[68] (Figures 5-28 and 5-29). This communication is usually through a complex valve mechanism formed by arachnoid remnants that allows predominantly one-way movement of CSF into the cysts, probably accounting for the growth in size and mass effect of these lesions. The result is that CSF is static in these cysts and flow-sensitive MR pulse sequences can be used to differentiate cysts from moving CSF in the subarachnoid space (see Figure 5-31).

Bone erosion occurs with these lesions and is demonstrated as canal widening, pedicle erosion, foraminal enlargement, or scalloping of the posterior-vertebral bodies of the sacrum (Figures 5-30 to 5-31).

The anterior sacral meningocele usually appears as a pelvic mass, which may be confused with other cystic lesions such as ovarian cyst prolapsed into the pouch of Douglas[64] (Figure 5-32). The posterior location of the cyst and the association of an adjacent sacral bony defect specify the cyst as an anterior meningocele. MR imaging is the first choice because of its ability to noninvasively demonstrate the cystic nature of the lesion in multiple planes and define the pedicle with its communication to the thecal sac or root sleeve through the defect in the sacrum. Figure 5-32 illustrates a lesion that appears to be cystic on T1W images with homogeneous low signal similar to lumbar CSF and appears to communicate with the S_2 nerve root sleeve. The T2W images, in this case showed complex high and low signal within the lesion, probably the result of fluid motion effects. Because this patient had neurofibromatosis with multiple intraspinous and paraspinous neurofibromas, the diagnosis of a cystic lesion required confirmation by an ultrasound study. Ultrasound is probably the most reliable and expeditious confirmatory study, although it does not demonstrate the neck of the lesion as clearly as MR, which is an essential feature for surgical planning.[60] Plain film myelography and CT myelography may be useful but are invasive and have a significant false negative rate because the pedicle of the meningocele may be obstructed by adhesions or too narrow to allow entry of intrathecal contrast material. Plain radiographs of the sacrum may be helpful if they show the scimitar sacrum sign, a semicircular erosion of the sacrum highly suggestive of the anterior sacral meningocele.

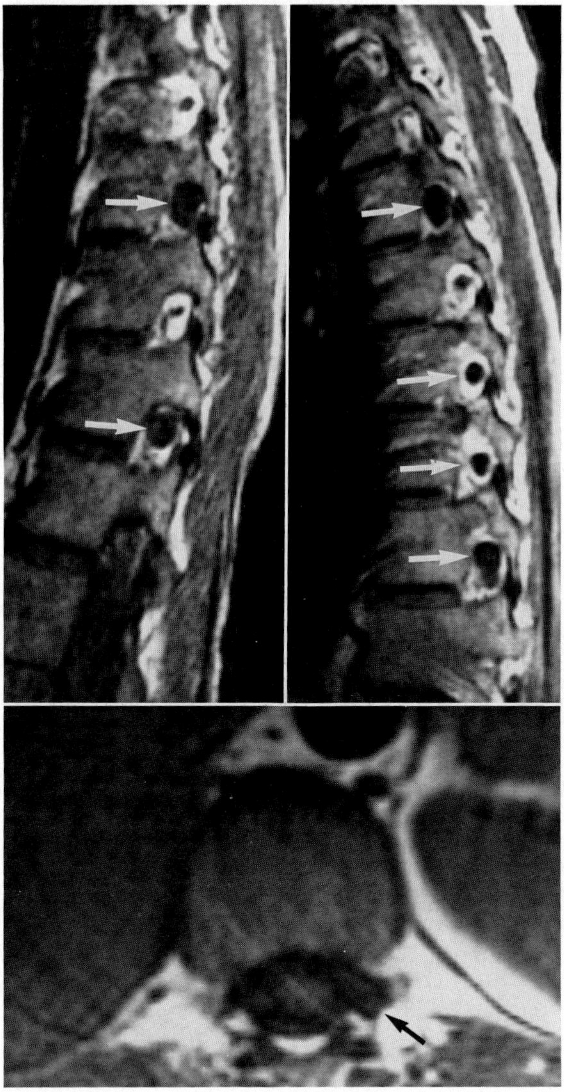

FIGURE 5-28. Thoracic nerve root diverticula. Sagittal T1W images in 43-year-old female show bilateral enlargement of nerve root sleeves (nerve root diverticula) at multiple levels, most prominently **A,** T_9 and T_{11} *(arrows)* and **B,** T_6, T_8, T_9, and T_{10} on right *(arrows)*. Low signal similar to CSF is present. **C,** Axial T1W image at T_{11} shows extension of CSF low signal into enlarged left root sleeve *(arrow)*. Curvilinear high signal artifact superimposed on root sleeve and spinal cord (caused by chest wall motion).

A, B

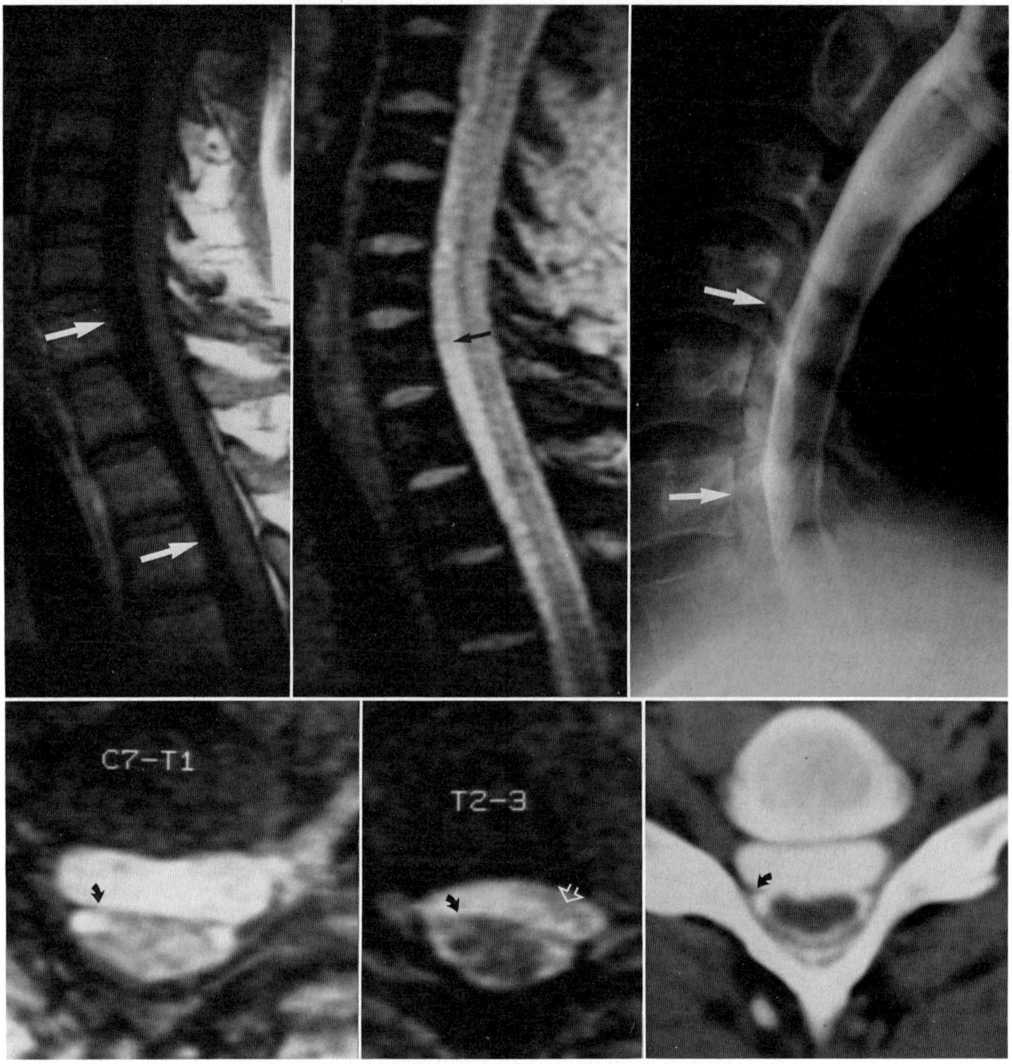

C

D, E

F

FIGURE 5-29. Arachnoid cyst. **A,** Sagittal T1W image in 22-year-old male from C_2-T_4 grossly normal with subtle widening of CSF space anterior to spinal cord, especially in upper thoracic region where it would normally narrow as cord begins to lie in anterior canal *(arrows)*. **B,** Sagittal T2W image from C2-T4 shows slight widening of high signal CSF space anterior to cervicothoracic cord, a more subtle finding than seen on T1W images. Thin, ill-defined line within anterior CSF space may represent anterior margin of thecal sac *(arrow)*, as seen on axial images, **D** and **E. C,** Lateral view from cervical myelogram shows posterior displacement of thecal sac and cord with widening of anterior epidural space *(arrows)*. Slightly increased density in anterior epidural space indicates accumulation of contrast material through a communication with subarachnoid space. Axial T2W images at **D,** C_7-T_1 and **E,** T_2-T_3 show high signal ovoid fluid collection in anterior spinal canal in epidural space; interface between it and thecal sac is clearly seen *(curved arrows)*. Low signal areas *(open arrow)* within fluid collection and thecal sac are result of fluid motion effects. **F,** Axial CT myelogram at C_7-T_1 level shows high density contrast material in anterior epidural fluid collection and thecal sac. Acute angle at lateral junction of epidural cyst and thecal sac *(arrow)* suggests separation of two fluid-filled spaces.

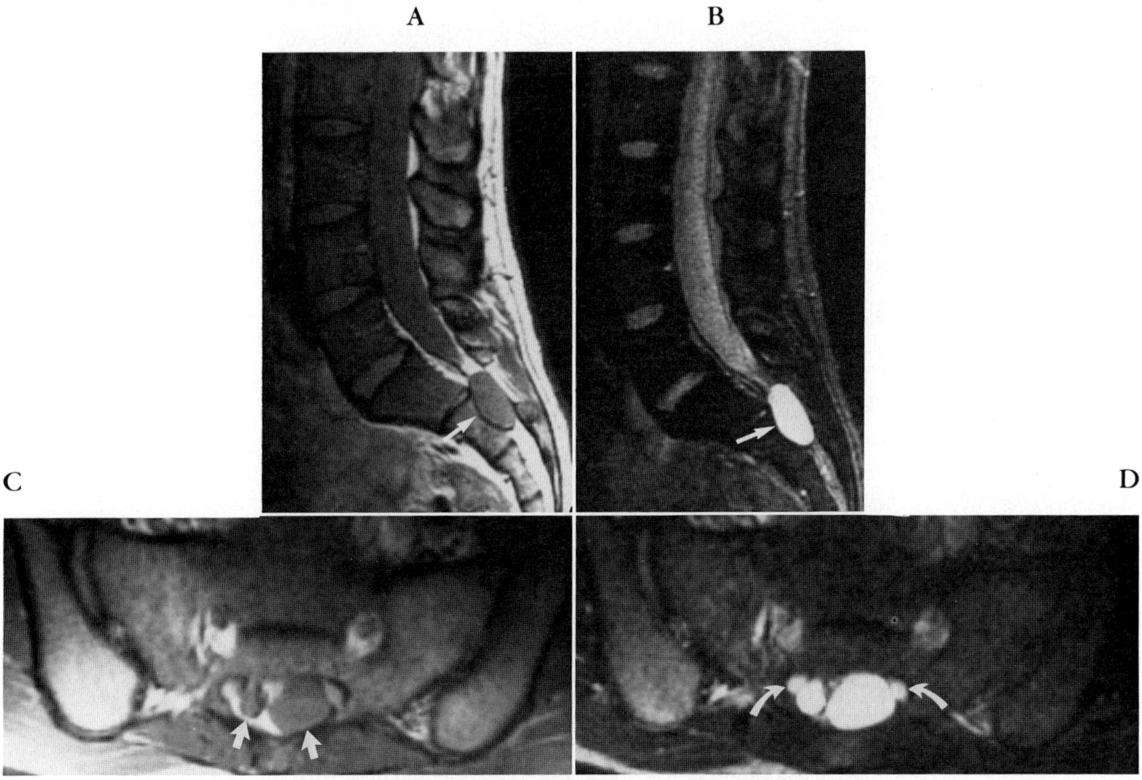

FIGURE 5-30. Sacral Tarlov's perineurial cyst. **A**, Sagittal T1W image in 22-year-old male with symptoms of S_2 root compression. Cystic fluid collection in midsacral canal *(arrow)* with signal similar to CSF. Slight degree of erosion remodeling of sacrum is seen anteriorly *(curved arrow)*. **B**, Sagittal T2W image shows high signal in sacral cyst *(arrow)* compared to CSF, probably because slightly higher protein and solute content and absence of motion effects. **C**, Axial T2W (20/2500) image shows two cysts in sacral canal *(arrows)* with signal intensity similar to nerve root sheaths and bone marrow. **D**, Axial T2W (80/2500) image shows two cysts *(arrows)* seen in **C**, as well as adjacent normal diameter nerve root sleeves *(curved arrows)*.

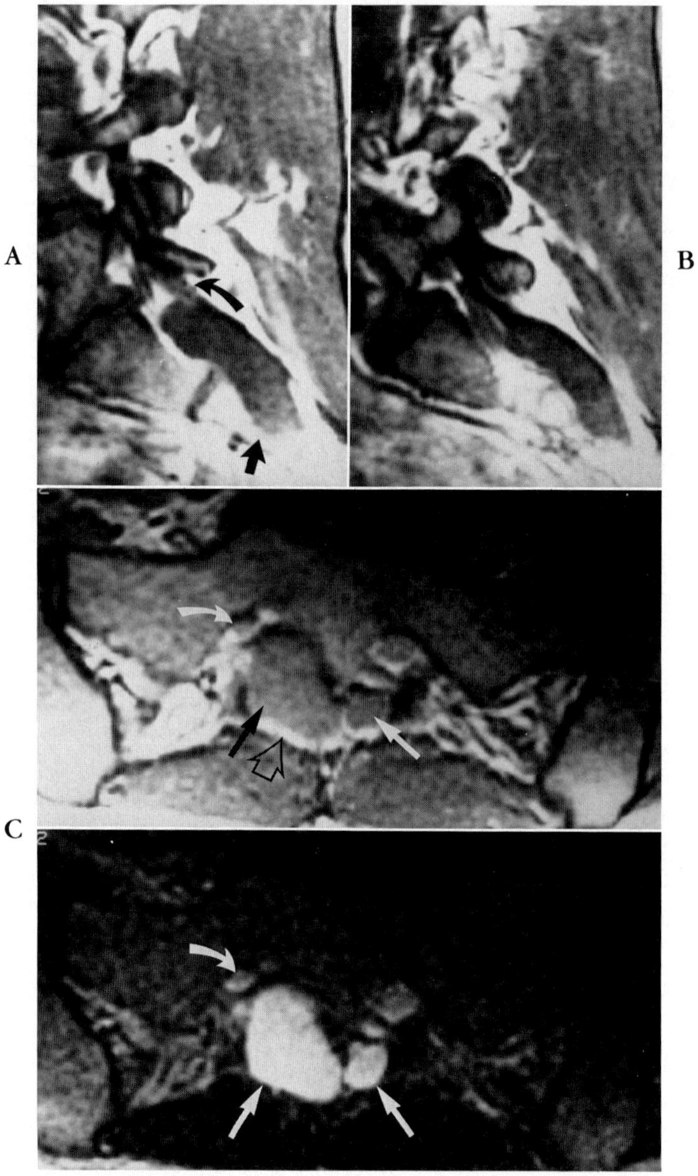

FIGURE 5-31. Sacral Tarlov's perineurial cysts. **A,** Right paramedian sagittal T1W images of lumbosacral spine in 36-year-old female showing low signal (similar to CSF) well-circumscribed Tarlov's cyst in sacral spinal canal. Chronic mass effect from cyst caused enlargement of spinal canal and scalloping of posterior sacral vertebral bodies (*straight arrow*). Superior margin of cyst lies adjacent to right S_1 root sleeve *(curved arrow)* in lateral recess. **B,** Axial T2W 20/2400 image at S_1 shows cystic masses, right larger than left, expanding S_2 neural canals (*straight arrows*). S_1 root sleeve is same intensity as large cyst, adjacent to anterior margin *(curved arrow)*. These Tarlov's cysts are isointense with bone marrow and nerve root sleeves using this pulse sequence. Fat–water interface chemical shift artifact is prominent, producing high signal along posterior cyst margins *(open arrow)* and low signal along anterior cyst margins. **C,** Axial T2W (80/2400) image clearly differentiates Tarlov's cysts with high signal (*straight arrows*) from nerve root sleeves *(curved arrow)* and vertebral marrow. Distortion of neural canals and displacement of nerve root sleeve more prominent on right.

A 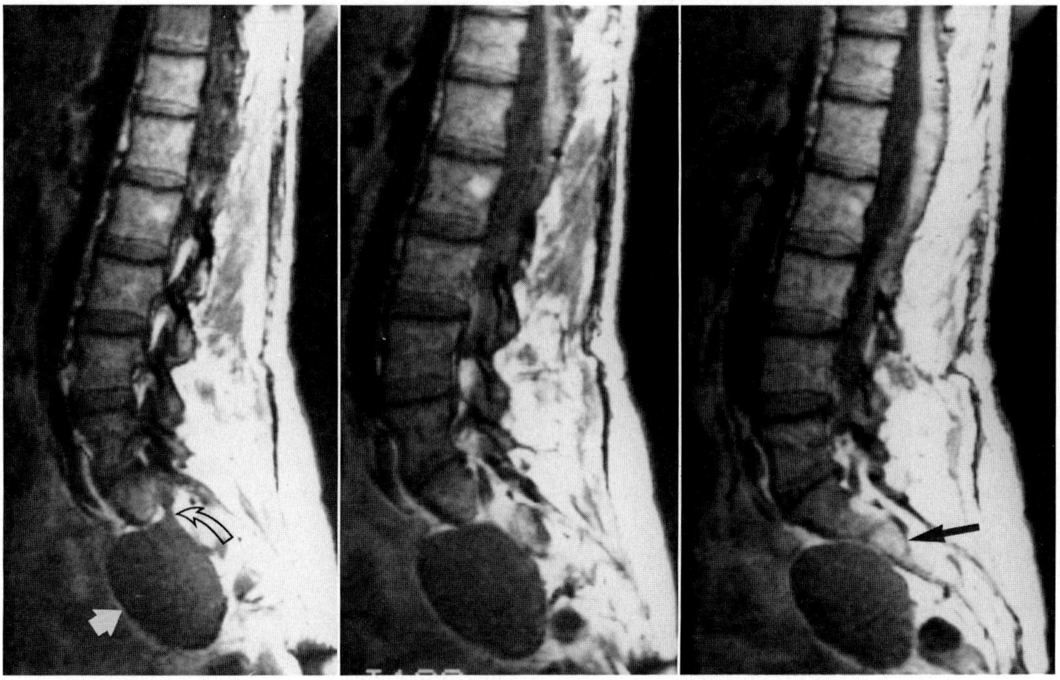 B, C

FIGURE 5-32. Anterior sacral meningocele. **A-C,** Sagittal T1W images in 31-year-old female show left anterior sacral bony defect at S_1-S_2 *(arrows)* through which meningeal pouch extends *(open arrow)*. Meningeal pouch appears extension of left S_1 root sleeve (**A,** *curved arrow*) but not confined to neural foramen or canal as might nerve root diverticulum or Tarlov's perineurial cyst. Pouch extends across midline anterior to intact portion of sacrum *(small arrows)*.

ENTEROGENOUS CYST

Intraspinal enterogenous cyst is a relatively rare finding with only 53 cases reported in the world literature since the cyst was first described in 1934 by Puusepp as an "intenstinoma". Various other names describe the entity, including enteric cyst, neurenteric cyst, gastrocytoma, teratomatous cyst, and archenteric cyst.[5,22,53,65] It has been suggested that teratomatous cysts are distinguished from true enterogenous cysts by the presence of female sex chromatin in the teratomatous cyst.[88] The lesion is defined as a cyst lined by columnar, mucin-secreting epithelium, usually without cilia, similar to that of the gastrointestinal tract. The precise embryogenesis of enterogenous cysts is not known but the end result is interposition of an endodermal rest between the primitive notochord and neuroectoderm that eventually form a cystic mass. Formation may be caused by defect in separation of primitive embryonal layers or by endoderm left behind during caudal migration of Hensen's node with the foregut.[22,65] Enterogenous cysts are usually discovered in patients under 40 years of age, typically in the third decade, and there is a 2 to 1, male to female preference.[22] The most common site of involvement is the cervical spine, usually extending over two to three segments and intradural, extramedullary in location, typically anterior to the spinal cord. Approximately 50% of cases are associated with other congenital abnormalities such as spina bifida, fused vertebrae, hemivertebrae, or anterior spina bifida.[65] A slowly enlarging intraspinal mass with progressive sign of cord compression is typical of enterogenous cysts.[22] In about 50% of cases symptoms are episodic, making it difficult to distinguish this lesion from spinal cord multiple sclerosis on the basis of clinical findings.[65]

MR Imaging

Two recent case reports describe the MR appearance of enterogenous cysts in the cervical spinal canal.[5,65] Lesions in both cases were intradural, extramedullary, and anterior to the spinal cord (Figure 5-33), low signal on T1W images and high signal on T2W images, and consistent with free, nonhemorrhagic fluid contents of the cyst. At 0.35T the T1 relaxation time of the cyst was 2800 ms and the T2 relaxation time was 140 ms, suggesting fluid similar to CSF. Symptomatic cord compression was visualized in one case.[5,65] An enterogenous cyst anterior to the spinal cord with characteristics similar to those in the cases cited is demonstrated in Figure 5-33.

SUMMARY AND RECOMMENDATIONS

MR Advantages

MR is ideal for the noninvasive evaluation of patients with suspected congenital intraspinal pathology and, in most cases, can be used without supplementation by myelography or CT scanning. The noninvasive character of MR is especially important in cases with minimal symptomatology where an invasive evaluation procedure and general anesthesia are difficult to justify. In most cases, a normal high quality MR examination effectively excludes significant pathologic conditions and obviates the use of more invasive procedures for further examination.

MR Disadvantages

MR disadvantages may be largely the result of specific imaging system technical limitations or artifacts. For example, low resolution images (e.g., in-plane resolution greater than 2 mm and slice thickness greater than 5 mm) may not demonstrate small or thin anatomic structures such as syrinx, hydromyelia or thickened filum terminale. Poor choice of pulse sequences may obscure lesions by reducing tissue contrast, such as between the filum terminale and CSF or between neural tissue and CSF in syrinx and hydromyelia. Gross patient motion, phase ghost artifacts from organ motion (e.g., cardiac, abdominal and chest wall, larynx, and tongue) or from

A, B

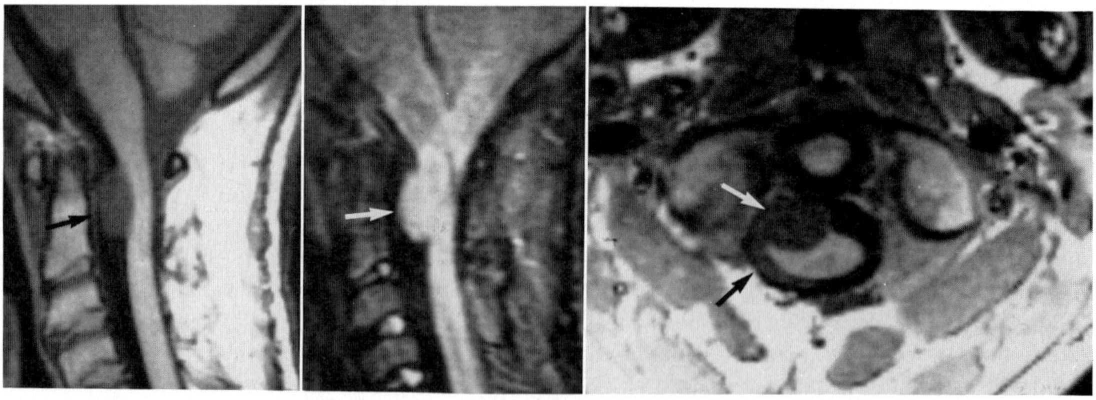

C

FIGURE 5-33. Enterogenous cyst. **A,** Sagittal T1W image of cervical spine shows well-defined, intermediate signal mass *(arrow)* in spinal canal at C_2 level anterior to spinal cord. Cord is deviated posteriorly by mass just below cervico-medullary junction. **B,** Sagittal T2W image shows high signal in mass similar to static CSF, suggesting cyst *(arrow)*. **C,** Axial T1W image shows intermediate signal mass *(arrows)* that indents spinal cord and appears to wrap around cord posterolaterally to right. (Courtesy of Victor Haughton, M.D., Milwaukee, Wis.)

fluid motion (e.g., spinal CSF oscillation or vascular flow, especially aortic on axial images) may obscure anatomy or give false positive signals. If these problems arise, the best solution for poor visualization of syrinx or hydromyelia would be a better quality MR study in both sagittal and axial planes. Poor visualization of the filum terminale, nerve roots, or thin adhesions may be resolved by repeating the MR study but in some cases myelography or myelographic CT may be needed to identify these structures. Another potential disadvantage is poor visualization of fibrous, cartilaginous, or bony spicules and septa associated with diastematomyelia. CT scanning is the best method for imaging these structures.

Ferromagnetic artifacts on MR images may limit their usefulness. Major metallic fixation devices that produce local magnetic artifacts, such as Harrington and Luque rods and Dwyer implants, do not always produce sufficiently large distortions of the image to preclude diagnosis of intraspinal or spinal cord lesions.[103,104]

Practical disadvantages of MR include currently limited availability and cost (rapidly being reduced), length of individual study time (also decreasing), and the need for sedation in very young patients. Sedation and, often, general anesthesia are also needed with myelography and CT. Although the cost of an MR study is greater than the individual costs of myelography and CT the overall cost of the workup of each patient with MR is usually less than the total cost of myelography and CT with sedation, anesthesia and monitoring, as well as overnight hospitalization usually required for multiple studies.

Recommendations for Workup

Considering the wealth and accuracy of information obtainable and the noninvasive nature of MR studies, workup of patients with suspected spinal congenital anomalies should begin with MR imaging. A major advantage of MR over traditional imaging techniques is that, in most cases, a normal study is considered an adequate workup, obviating the need for further, invasive studies. In most pathologic cases, abnormal anatomy is sufficiently well delineated by MR alone for complete preoperative surgical planning.

In general, T1W images (SE sequences with TE 20 to 30 ms and TR 600 to 800 ms) are sufficient for the demonstration of major anatomic features of developmental anomalies. Sagittal images usually provide the most information but should be supplemented with axial images. Coronal plane images are not usually necessary and may be confusing if the lordotic curvature is marked. Coronal images are useful for evaluation of diastematomyelia [Figure 5-9] or tethered cord[9,37] but often do not provide information available on axial images. T2W images, SE sequences with TE 80 to 100 ms and TR 2000 to 3000 ms, should be added when disease within the spinal cord or cystic lesions are suspected. T2W images are more sensitive to subtle degrees of abnormal water content in the cord that might be produced by myelomalacia or neoplasm and are needed for complete evaluation of syringomyelia or hydromyelia (see Chapter 12). Axial gradient echo/variable flip angle images obtained as single slices (TE 15 to 20 ms, TR 30 to 40 ms, flip angle 5° to 10°) may also be helpful in evaluating cord contour, especially in the cervical region, and syringomyelia or hydromyelia because of signal enhancement by CSF oscillatory motion. Gradient echo/variable flip angle images with more sensitivity to T2* (TE 15 to 30 ms, TR 500 to 600, flip angle 10° to 15°) may also be helpful by showing osseous structures as very low signal structure contrasted sharply against adjacent soft tissues.

The utility of intravenous paramagnetic contrast enhancement with MR in evaluation of developmental spinal anomalies has not been demonstrated. It is likely that intravenous gadopentetate (gadolinium diethylenetriamine penta-acetic acid, GdDTPA) will be useful in characterizing nonfatty mass lesions such as hamartoma, neuroma, ependymoma, or astrocytoma, especially in the enlarged cord. The use of gadopentetate as an intrathecal contrast agent has been suggested[24] for differentiating subarachnoid space from cyst or better defining the contents of a myelomeningocele (e.g., nerve roots and adhesions). It is unclear whether this use of intrathecal contrast will have any advantage over myelographic CT, although the ability to directly image in orthogonal and oblique planes with MR may result in better diagnostic utilization of the contrast injection. Gadopentetate is not currently approved for diagnostic use intrathecally.

REFERENCES

1. Altman NR, Altman DH. MR imaging of spinal dysraphism. AJNR 1987;8:533.
2. Amador LH, Hankinson J, Bigler JA. Congenital spinal dermal sinuses. J Pediatr 1955;47:300.
3. Ammerman BJ, Henry JM, De Girolami U, et al. Intradural lipomas of the spinal cord: clinicopathological correlation. J Neurosurg 1976;44:331.
4. Anderson FM. Occult spinal dysraphism: diagnosis and management. J Pediatr 1968;73:163.
5. Aoki S, Machida T, Sasaki Y, et al. Enterogenous cyst of the cervical spine: clinical and radiological aspects (including CT and MRI). Neuroradiology 1987;29:291.
6. Arrendondo F, Haughton VM, Hemmy DC, et al. The computed tomographic appearance of the spinal cord in diastematomyelia. Radiology 1980;136:685.
7. Bailey IC. Dermoid tumors of the spinal cord. J Neurosurg 1970;33:676.
8. Bale PM. Sacrococcygeal developmental abnormalities and tumors in children. Perspect Pediatr Pathol 1984;8:9.
9. Barnes PD, Lester PD, Yamanashi WS, et al. Magnetic resonance in infants and children with spinal dysraphism. AJNR 1986;7:465.
10. Barson AJ. The vertebral level of termination of the spinal cord during normal and abnormal development. J Anat 1970;106:489.
11. Batnitzky S, Hall PV, Lindseth RE, et al. Meningomyelocele and syringohydromyelia: some radiological aspects. Radiology 1976;120:351.
12. Bligh AS. Diastematomyelia. Clin Radiol 1961;12:158.
13. Bremer JL, Dorsal intestinal fistula, accessory neurenteric canal, diastematomyelia. Arch Pathol 1952; 54:132.
14. Bruce DA, Schut L. Spinal lipomas in infancy and childhood. Childs Brain 1979;5:192.
15. Caram PC, Scarcella G, Carton CA. Intradural lipomas of the spinal cord. J Neurosurg 1957;14:28.
16. Carter CO. Clues to the aetiology of neural tube malformations. Dev Med Child Neurol 1974;16(suppl. 32):3.
17. Chapman PH. Congenital intraspinal lipomas: anatomic considerations and surgical treatment. Childs Brain 1982;9:37.
18. Chutorian AM. Spina bifida and cranium bifidum. In: Rowland LP, ed. Merritt's textbook of neurology, ed 7, Philadelphia: Lea & Febiger, 1984.
19. Cohen J, Currarino G, Neuhauser EBD. A significant variation in the ossification centers of the vertebral bodies. AJR 1956;76:469.
20. Crelin ES, Netter FH, Shapter RK. Development of the nervous system: a logical approach to neuroanatomy. CIBA Clinical Symposia 1974;26(2):1.
21. Dale AJD. Diastematomyelia. Arch Neurol 1969; 20:309.
22. D'Almeida AC, Stewart DH, Jr. Neurenteric cyst: case report and literature review. Neurosurgery 1981;8:596.
23. DeLaPaz RL, Floris R, Norman D, et al. MRI of tethered spinal cord and caudal lipoma (abstr). AJNR 1986;7:550.
24. Di Chiro G, Knop RH, Girton ME, et al. MR cisternography and myelography with Gd-DTPA in monkeys. Radiology 1985;157:373.
25. Dubowitz V, Lorber J, Zachary RB. Lipoma of the cauda equina. Arch Dis Child 1965;40:207.
26. Duhamel B. From the mermaid to anal imperforation: the syndrome of caudal regression. Arch Dis Child 1961;36:152.
27. Emery JL, Lendon RG. Lipomas of the cauda equina and other fatty tumors related to neurospinal dysraphism. Dev Med Child Neurol 1969;11(suppl. 20):62.
28. Emery JL, Lendon RG. The local cord lesion in neurospinal dysraphism (meningomyelocele). J Pathol 1973;110:83.
29. Epstein BS. The spine: a radiological text and atlas, ed 4, Philadelphia: Lea & Febiger, 1976.
30. Fitz CR, Harwood-Nash DC. The tethered conus. Am J Roentgenol Radium Ther Nucl Med 1975;125:515.
31. Friede RL. Developmental neuropathology. New York: Springer-Verlag, 1975.
32. Gillespie R, Faithfull DK, Roth A, et al. Intraspinal anomalies in congenital scoliosis. Clin Orthop 1973;93:103.
33. Giuffre R. Intradural spinal lipomas: review of the literature (99 cases) and report of an additional case. Acta Neurochir 1966;14:69.
34. Grand MJH, Eichenfeld S, Jacobson HG. Sacral aplasia (agenesis). Radiology 1960;74:611.
35. Guidetti B, Gagliardi FM. Epidermoid and dermoid cysts: clinical evaluation and late surgical results. J Neurosurg 1977;47:12.
36. Hamby WB. Tumors in the spinal canal in childhood: an analysis of the literature with report of a case. J Nerv Ment Dis 1935;81:24.
37. Han JS, Benson JE, Kaufman B, et al. Demonstrating diastematomyelia and associated abnormalities with MR imaging. AJNR 1985;6:215.
38. Harwood-Nash DC, Fitz CR. Neuroradiology in infants and children, vol. 3. St. Louis: The C.V. Mosby Co., 1976.
39. Hayden JW. Back pain in children. Pediatr Clin North Am 1967;14:611.
40. Hendrick EB, Hoffman HJ, Humphreys RP. Tethered cord syndrome. In: Myelomeningocele, McLaurin RL, ed. New York: Grune and Stratton, 1977.
41. Herren RY, Edwards JE. Diplomyelia (duplication of the spinal cord). Arch Pathol 1940;30:1203.
42. Hilal SK, Marton D, Pollack E. Diastematomyelia in children: radiographic study of 34 cases. Radiology 1974:112:609.
43. Hood RW, Riseborough EJ, Nehme AM, et al. Diastematomyelia and structural spinal deformities. J Bone Joint Surg (AM.) 1980;62A:520.
44. Huebert HT, MacKinnon WB. Syringomyelia and scoliosis. J Bone Joint Surg 1969;51:338.
45. Ignelzi RJ, Lehman RAW. Lumbosacral agenesis: management and embryological implications. J Neurol Neurosurg Psychiatry 1974;37:1273.
46. James CCM, Lassman LP. Diastematomyelia: a critical survey of 24 cases submitted to laminectomy. Arch Dis Child 1964;39:125.
47. James CCM, Lassman LP. Spinal dysraphism; spina bifida occulta. New York: Appleton-Century-Crofts (London: Butterworth & Co.), 1972.
48. Kallen B, Winberg J. Caudal mesoderm pattern of anomalies: from renal agenesis to sirenomelia. Teratology 1974;9:99.
49. Kang JK, Kim MC, Kim DS, et al: Effects of tethering on regional spinal cord blood flow and sensory-evoked potentials in growing cats, Childs Nerv Syst 1987;3:35.
50. Kaplan JO, Quencer RM. The occult tethered conus syndrome in the adult. Radiology 1980;137:387.
51. Kennedy PR. New data on diastematomyelia. J Neurosurg 1979;51:355.
52. Komiyama M, Hakuba A, Inoue Y, et al: Magnetic resonance imaging: lumbosacral lipoma. Surg Neurol 1987;28:259.

53. Kouichi M, Mukawa J, Mekaru S, et al. Enterogenous cyst in the cervical spinal canal. J Neurosurg 1988;68:292.
54. Kuharik MA, Edwards MK, Grossman CB. Magnetic resonance evaluation of pediatric spinal dysraphism. Pediatr Neurosci 1985-86;12:213.
55. Langman J. Medical Embryology, ed 2. Baltimore: Williams & Wilkins, 1969.
56. Lassman LP, James CCM. Lumbosacral lipomas: critical survey of 26 cases submitted to laminectomy. J Neurol Neurosurg Psychiatry 1967;30:174.
57. Lemire RJ, Loeser JD, Leech RW, et al. Normal and abnormal development of the human nervous system. Hagerstown, Md.: Harper & Row Publishers, Inc., 1975.
58. List CF. Intraspinal epidermoids, dermoids, and dermal sinuses. Surg Gynecol Obstet 1941;73:525.
59. McAdams AJ. The Arnold-Chiari malformation: pathology and development considerations. In: McLaurin RL. Myelomeningocele. New York: Grune & Stratton, 1977.
60. McCreath GT, MacPherson P. Sonography in the diagnosis and management of anterior sacral meningocele. J Clin Ultrasound 1980;8:133.
61. McIlroy WJ, Richardson JC. Syringomyelia: a clinical review. Can Med Assoc J 1965;93:731.
62. McLone DG, Mutluer S, Naidich TP. Lipomeningoceles of the conus medullaris. In: Concepts in pediatric neurosurgery, vol. 3. American Society for Pediatric Neurosurgeons. Basel: Karger S, 1982.
63. McMaster ML. Occult intraspinal anomalies and congenital scoliosis. J Bone Joint Surg 1984;66:588.
64. Martin B, de Latour FB. MR imaging of anterior sacral meningocele. J Comput Tomogr 1988;12:166.
65. Miyagi K, Mukawa J, Mekaru S, et al. Enterogenous cyst in the cervical spinal canal. J Neurosurg 1988;68:292.
66. Moes CAF, Hendrick EB. Diastematomyelia. J Pediatr 1963;63:238.
67. Mount LA. Congenital dermal sinuses as a cause of meningitis, intraspinal abscess and intracranial abscess. JAMA 1949;139:1263.
68. Nabors MW, Pait TG, et al. Updated assessment and current classification of spinal meningeal cysts. J Neurosurg 1988;68:366.
69. Nagib MG, Larson DA, Maxwell RE, et al. Neuroschisis of the cervical spinal cord in patient with Klippel-Feil syndrome. Neurosurgery 1987;20:629.
70. Naidich TP, McLone DG, Harwood-Nash DC. Spinal dysraphism. In: Newton TH, Potts DG, eds. Computed tomography of the spine and spinal cord. Clavedel Press, 1983a.
71. Naidich TP, McLone DG, Harwood-Nash DC. Arachnoid cysts, paravertebral meningoceles, and perineurial cysts. In: Newton TH, Potts DG, eds. Computed tomography of the spine and spinal cord. San Anselmo, Calif: Clavedel Press, 1983b.
72. Naidich TP, McLone DG, Mutluer S. A new understanding of dorsal dysraphism with lipoma (lipomyeloschisis): radiologic evaluation and surgical correction. AJNR 1983c;4:103.
73. Naidich TP, Fernbach SK, McLone DG, et al. Sonography of the caudal spine and back: congenital anomalies in children. AJNR 1984;5:221.
74. Nakamura T. Diagnosis and treatment of tethered spinal cord syndrome based on experience of 77 cases. Nippon Seikeigeka Gakkai Zasshi 1984;58:1237.
75. Nokes SR, Murtagh FR, Jones JD, et al. Childhood scoliosis: MR imaging. Radiology 1987;164:791.
76. Northfield DWC. The surgery of the central nervous system. A textbook for postgraduate students. Oxford: Blackwell Scientific Publications, 1973.
77. Osaka K, Tanimura T, Hirayama A, et al. Myelomeningocele before birth. J Neurosurg 1978b;49:711.
78. Pang D, Wilberger JE Jr. Tethered cord syndrome in adults. J Neurosurg 1982;57:32.
79. Perloff MM. Congenital dermal sinus complicated by meningitis: report of a case. J Pediatr 1954;44:73.
80. Perret G. Diagnosis and treatment of diastematomyelia. Surg Gynecol Obstet 1957;105:69.
81. Perret G. Symptoms and diagnosis of diastematomyelia. Neurology 1960;10:51.
82. Piatt JH, Hoffman HJ: The tethered spinal cord with fucus on the tight filum terminale: a review. Neuro-Orthopedics 1987;4:1.
83. Piggott H. The natural history of scoliosis in myelodysplasia. J Bone Joint Surg 1980;62B:54.
84. Powell RG, Marano GD. MRI of congenital spinal lesions. WV Med J 1987;83:375.
85. Raghavendra BN, Epstein FJ. Sonography of the spine and spinal cord. Radiol Clin North Am 1985;23:91.
86. Renshaw TS. Sacral agenesis: a classification and review of twenty-three cases. J Bone Joint Surg 1978;60A:373.
87. Resjo IM, Harwood-Nash DC, Fitz CR, et al. Computed tomographic metrizamide myelography in spinal dysraphism in infants and children. J Comput Tomogr 1978;2:549.
88. Rewcastle NB, Francoeur J. Teratomatous cysts of the spinal canal with "sex chromatin" studies. Arch Neurol 1964;11:91.
89. Roller GJ, Pribram HFW. Lumbosacral intradural lipoma and sacral agenesis. Radiology 1965;84:507.
90. Rozen MJ. Pathophysiology of spinal deformity in myelomeningocele. In: McLaurin RL, ed. Myelomeningocele. New York: Grune & Stratton, 1977.
91. Samuelsson L, Bergstrom K, Thuomas K-A, et al. MR Imaging of syringomyelia and Chiari malformation in myelomeningocele patients with scoliosis. AJNR 1987;8:539.
92. Sarwar M, Kier EL, Virapongse C. Development of the spine and spinal cord. In: Newton TH, Potts DG, eds. Computed tomography of the spine and spinal cord. San Anselmo, Calif: Clavedel Press, 1983.
93. Sarwar M, Virapongse C, Bhimani S. Primary tethered cord syndrome: a new hypothesis of its origin. AJNR 1984;5:235.
94. Sayers MP. The significance of the Arnold-Chiari malformation. In: McLauren RL, ed. Myelomeningocele. New York: Grune & Stratton, 1977.
95. Schut L, Pizzi FJ, Bruce DA. Occult spinal dysraphism. In: Myelomeningocele, McLaurin RL, ed. New York: Grune & Stratton, 1977.
96. Schwartz HG. Congenital tumors of the spinal cord in infants. Ann Surg 1952;136:183.
97. Scotti G, Musgrave MA, Harwood-Nash DC, et al. Diastematomyelia in children: metrizamide and CT metrizamide myelography. AJNR 1980;1:403.
98. Sensenig EC. The early development of the meninges of the spinal cord in human embryos. Contrib Embryol 1951;34:147.
99. Shurtleff DB, Goiney R, Gordon LH, et al. Myelodysplasia. The natural history of kyphosis and scoliosis. A preliminary report. Dev Med Child Neurol 1976;18(suppl. 37):126.

100. Simpson RK, James ER. Cervical diastematomyelia. Arch Neurol 1987;44:331.
101. Smith ED. Congenital sacral defects. In: Congenital malformations of the rectum, anus and genito-urinary tracts, Stephens FP, ed. Edinburgh and London: E & S Livingstone, 1963.
102. Streeter GL. Factors involved in the formation of the filum terminale. Am J Anat 1919;25:1.
103. Sutterlin CE, Grogan DP, Ogden JA. Diagnosis of developmental pathology of the neuraxis by magnetic resonance imaging. J Pediatr Orthop 1987;7:291.
104. Szalay EA, Roach JW, Smith H, et al. Magnetic resonance imaging of the spinal cord in spinal dysraphism. J Pediatr Orthop 1987;7:541.
105. Tani S, Yamada S, Knighton RS. Extensibility of the lumbar and sacral cord. Pathophysiology of the tethered spinal cord in cats, J Neurosurg 1987;66:116.
106. Tunell WP, Austin JC, Barnes PD, et al. Neuroradiologic evaluation of sacral abnormalities in imperforate anus complex. J Pediatr Surg 1987;22:58.
107. Walsh JW, Markesbery WR. Histological features of congenital lipomas of the lower spinal canal. J Neurosurg 1980;52:564.
108. Waterman RE. SEM observation of surface alterations associated with neural tube closure in the mouse and hamster. Anat Rec 1975;183:95.
109. Wiedemayer H, Nau H-E, Reinhardt V, et al. Spinal cord compression by extensive epidural lipoma: a case report. Eur Neurol 1987;27:46.
110. Winter RB, Haven JJ, Moe JH, et al. Diastematomyelia and congenital spine deformities. J Bone Joint Surg (Am.) 1974;56A:27.
111. Wippold FJ, Citrin C, Barkovich AJ, et al. Evaluation of MR in spinal dysraphism with lipoma: comparison with metrizamide computed tomography. Pediatr Radiol 1987;17:184.
112. Wolpert SM, Scott RM, Carter BL. Computed tomography in spinal dysraphism. Surg Neurol 1977; 8:199.
113. Yamada S, Zinke DE, Sanders D. Pathophysiology of "tethered cord syndrome". J Neurosurg 1981;54:494.

6
Trauma

Dieter R. Enzmann
Robert L. DeLaPaz

ACUTE INJURY

MR imaging is important in the evaluation of spine and spinal cord trauma, which involves damage to osseous structures, ligaments, discs, and neural tissue. Fractures of osseous structures are well delineated by plain radiography and x-ray CT. The importance of osseous damage is often not the fractures per se but their relation to spine stability; thus the potential for new or further neural damage. With x-ray studies, ligamentous injury must be inferred from the osseous damage because ligaments are not directly visualized. This is a significant shortcoming because ligaments provide major stability to the spine. MR provides direct visualization of ligaments in spine trauma. Previously, cord and nerve damage was diagnosed primarily by clinical signs and sometimes by CT, thus the direct diagnosis by MR is superior.

An important consideration in the treatment of spine trauma is the determination of the stability of the spine after injury. An unstable spine is one in which a force less than the original traumatic force could cause further neurologic deficit. Although bony structures play a role in stability, the ligamentous structures—anterior and posterior longitudinal ligaments, ligamentum flavum, intraspinous ligaments, and ligaments around the facet joints—are more important. Ligament damage, especially a torn posterior ligament complex, is important to recognize since it does not reconstitute and therefore remains unstable. Treatment is usually some type of fusion procedure. Instability as a result of ligament damage is often assessed indirectly by x-ray criteria, such as a greater than 3.5 mm subluxation of posterior vertebral body margins, or a greater than 11° angulation of adjacent vertebral bodies. Flexion-extension plain films are often used to detect subluxation and ligament injury. MR allows a more direct assessment of ligaments.[9]

Radiologic literature is replete with extensive descriptions of various types of spine fractures that occur in the cervical, thoracic, and lumbar spine as shown by plain film radiography, tomography, and CT. Flexion and extension injuries in the cervical spine, for example, have typical radiographic features that aid in their identification and in assessing their potential stability or instability.[3,16] Flexion injuries can result in subluxed, perched, or locked facets (unilateral or bilateral). Such findings suggest intraspinous ligament disruption. This is especially true for unilateral lesions because they involve a rotatory vector that tears ligaments, resulting in instability. Hyperextension injuries result in retrolisthesis and small anterior avulsion fractures that are associated with disruption of the anterior longitudinal ligament.[20]

Spinal cord damage is related to the type of trauma and is a function of age and preexisting disease. A preexisting narrow spinal canal is associated with a greater degree of cord damage. The canal may be congenitally narrow or narrowed by degenerative changes. Patients with preexisting spondylosis also suffer a greater degree of cord damage after trauma. Patients with ankylosing spondylitis seem to have a propensity for larger epidural hemorrhages. Cord injuries in adults tend to be in the lower cervical spine, whereas children, who have greater laxity in their ligamentous structures, tend to have damage at higher cervical levels. Upper cervical cord damage appears more frequently in children less than 8 years old. Lower cervical cord damage occurs after the age of 8 when the cervical spine assumes adult characteristics.

The incidence of spine injuries in children is less than in adults but up to 20% of pediatric spinal cord trauma shows no x-ray evidence of damage.[7,15,19] Up to 50% of children have a delayed onset of spinal cord symptoms after injury. The delay may be up to 4 days, although at the time of injury there may be transient paresthesia, numbness, or paralysis.[15] This delay in symptoms can have unfortunate consequences because the injury may be compounded by resumption of the physical activity that led to the initial injury. In a study of 42 children with spine trauma but without radiographic signs of instability, eight suffered further injury within a short period of time, 2 to 10 weeks.[18] This reinjury was usually more severe than the original injury and could be related to the same or to a less strenuous activity. The increased elasticity in cervical spines of children shows the limits of conventional imaging techniques and their indirect assessment of the cord.

Spinal cord damage is found in adults even in the absence of x-ray findings.[12] This is most often seen with hyperextension injuries in a patient with preexisting spondylosis. Hyperextension injury results in buckling of the ligamentum flavum impinging upon the cord within the narrowed spinal canal. Cord damage is often manifest as a central cord syndrome and is not visualized directly or indirectly on conventional imaging studies. MR could be useful in the direct assessment of the cord in this group of patients.

CLINICAL PRESENTATIONS

Cord damage assumes four major patterns: anterior cord syndrome, central cord syndrome, Brown-Sequard syndrome, and complete transection. The anterior cord syndrome is characterized by quadriplegia with lower extremities more severely involved than upper extremities. Posterior columns are spared, as indicated by intact proprioception, touch, and deep pressure. The central cord syndrome has quadriparesis with upper extremities involved to a greater degree than lower extremities. Sensory findings are variable but sacral pinprick is usually preserved. This syndrome results from damage to both gray and white matter in the central portion of the cord. Because the descending corticospinal tracts to the arm are more centrally located than in the leg, upper extremities are involved more severely. The Brown-Sequard syndrome is characterized by ipsilateral motor paralysis with contralateral hypesthesia to pain and temperature. The injury is therefore to half of the spinal cord. Complete transection results in total motor and sensory loss below the level of injury.

Any of the spinal cord syndromes that are incomplete have some potential for recovery. Usually assessment after 48 hours provides a good indication of the eventual prognosis for recovery of function. If there is no return of sacral sensation or motor function at 48 hours, permanent paralysis is likely to result. The development of MR criteria for assessing cord damage may modify current methods of prognostication.

PATHOGENESIS AND PATHOLOGY OF CORD INJURY

Injury to the spinal cord may result from direct mechanical forces and compression acting on the cord or from ischemia, a secondary event. Direct mechanical compression may result from bone fragments impinging on the cord as in a compression fracture or odontoid fracture. Cord impingement may be the result of ligament buckling, such as in a hyperextension injury of the cervical spine. Cord damage may also result from secondary vascular changes, especially when these involve the terminal perforating arteries.

Acute gross pathologic changes in the traumatized spinal cord may vary from no gross observable abnormalities to various degrees of swelling, to the most severe form, complete transection. Histologically, even apparently minor degrees of trauma can result in scattered intramedullary hemorrhages and edema in central areas of the cord.[5] Both cytotoxic (intracellular) and vasogenic (interstitial) edema occur in the central cord and spread peripherally and longitudinally with more severe trauma. There is disruption of myelin sheaths and terminal club formation along transected axons.[5] After the acute phase, central zones of mild to moderate injury may progress to local gliosis, which can extend longitudinally.[5]

Experimental animal studies of more severe forms of injury show early central hemorrhage in the cord followed by rapidly progressive central gray matter necrosis.[2,13] This liquefactive necrosis may undergo longitudinal extension several centimeters above and below the site of trauma, and in extreme cases, involve long segments of cord.[5,13] The process is characterized as "pencil shaped" and involves central gray matter and the anterior portion of the dorsal columns.[5] It is postulated that these acute traumatic changes can progress to cavitation of the cord through a progressive self-perpetuating autolytic process. Several mechanisms are proposed for this autolysis, including release of destructive hydrolyzing lysosomal enzymes, enzyme inhibitors, and free radical products, substances that can be toxic to healthy cells at the margin of the injury. When these cells in turn are injured, they release their own lysosomal enzymes and perpetuate the destructive process,[5] which can advance the margin of injury for some distance away from the original site. This necrosis over time can cavitate and form small, glial-lined cavities or cysts. Small cavities can appear as soon as a few weeks after injury. It is postulated that they may coalesce into large cavities forming a posttraumatic syrinx.[5] In some cases, the syrinx cavity may be separated from the site of original trauma by several centimeters of noncystic spinal cord.[5] The incidence of posttraumatic syrinx is 1% to 4% in the pre-MR era; in the post-MR era it is likely to be higher as large series of patients are screened with MR (see Chapter 12).

MR FINDINGS

Acute Injury

Skeletal ligaments

Although cortical bone is seen as an area of low signal, contrast with adjacent soft tissue and marrow allows sufficient depiction of larger fractures[11] (Figure 6-1) that are seen as soft tissue signal insinuating between thin "black" lines of cortical bone, indicating a discontinuity. If insufficient soft tissue intervenes between fracture fragments, the fracture becomes undetectable and is common in small fractures involving the arch and posterior elements of cervical vertebra.[23] Fractures of the odontoid process are detectable primarily by displacement of the dens (Figures 6-2 and 6-3). Undisplaced fractures are difficult to detect directly although soft tissue swelling is present. Fractures can be identified on T1W images but may also be seen on T2W or T2*W images. Fracture fragments, especially retropulsed fragments, in compression fractures are also identifiable (Figure 6-4) and may be determined directly if they have a detectable marrow component within them or indirectly by their mass effect on the dural sac or cord. The marrow component is best seen on T1W images, whereas the latter findings are most evident on T2W or T2*W images (Figure 6-4).

Despite lack of bone detail, vertebral body subluxations are well delineated by MR. The tomographic nature of MR scans show vertebral body offset and facet subluxation, even if unilateral.[11] (See Figure 6-1.) Definition of cortical margins of the cervical vertebrae lateral masses is sufficient to diagnose subluxed, perched, or locked facts. Vertebral body displacement is accurately depicted in Figures 6-1 and 6-5. Ligaments disrupted by such injuries can be directly visualized (see Figure 6-1). "Water" scans, which do not suffer from chemical shift artifact, can delineate ligaments well (Figure 6-5). In one series of patients, ligamentous injury was identified in 78% of patients.[9] Because ligaments normally have low signal intensity, intermediate or high signal intensity on T1W or T2W images within or around ligaments in their normal location is indicative of disruption (see Figure 6-5). Anterior longitudinal ligament disruption may be accompanied by hemorrhage and edema in prevertebral soft tissue[9] that tracks along fascial planes inferiorly and superiorly. Disc herniation can accompany disruption of the posterior or anterior longitudinal ligament. On T1W images, normal intermediate signal intensity of the nucleus pulposus material is identified anterior or posterior to the vertebral body margins (Figures 6-6 and 6-7; see Figure 6-12). Disc herniation may be sufficient to cause a significant extradural defect or cord compression[8] (see Figure 6-6). On T2W images the traumatized disc can show abnormal high signal (Figure 6-8; see Figure 6-11). Prevertebral soft tissue swelling, which is easily detected by T1W and T2W images (see Figure 6-1) often accompanies acute cervical spine fractures. Hemorrhage may be identified in the prevertebral soft tissue as high signal intensity in the cervical spine. Paravertebral soft tissue swelling can be noted in any portion of the spine.

Epidural hematoma can accompany signifi-

A, B

C, D

E, F

G, H

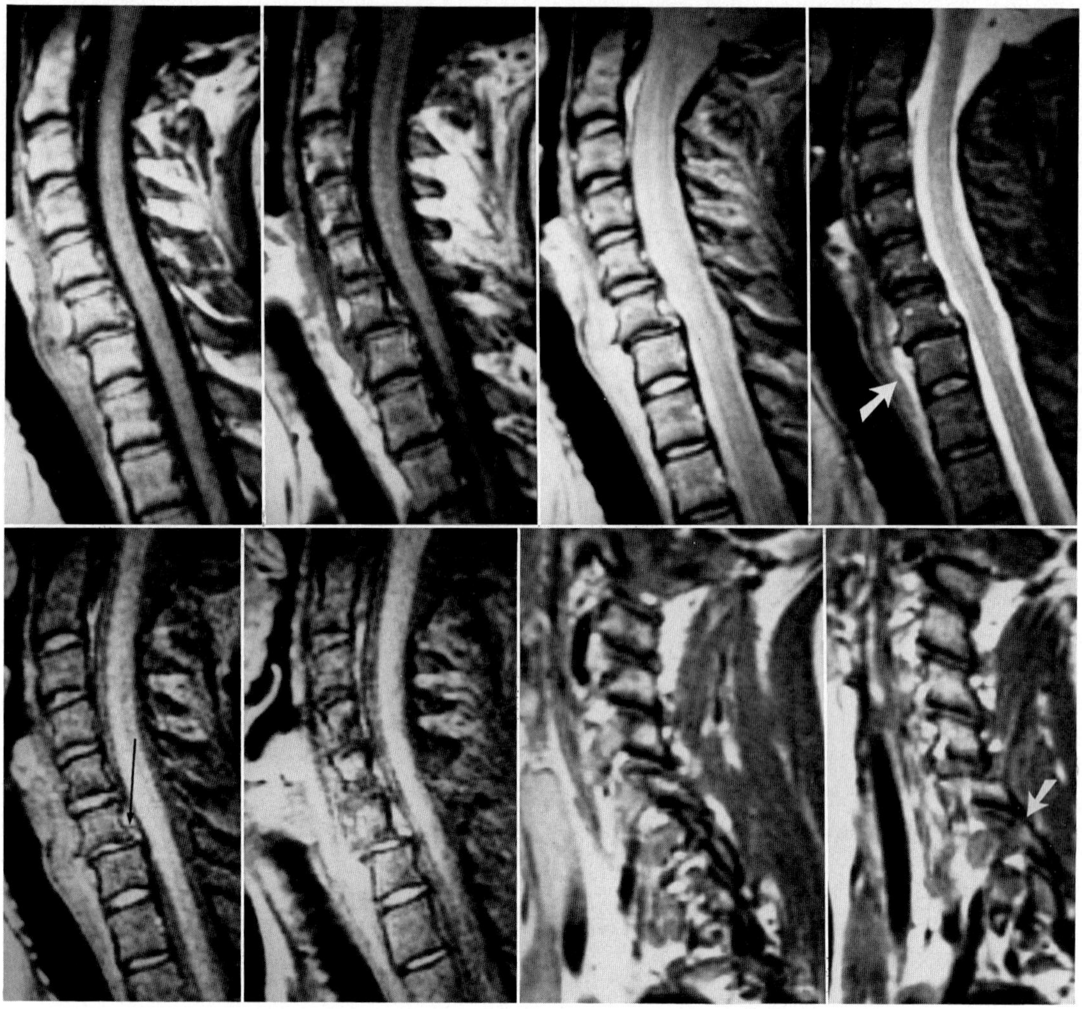

FIGURE 6-1. Unilateral "perched" facet. MR scans of 49-year-old female with rotatory subluxation at C_6-C_7 level, fracture of C_6, and unilateral "perched" facet on right side. **A** and **B,** Sagittal T1W scans (SE 800/20) show mild anterior subluxation of C_6 on C_7. Posterior to C_6 between vertebral body and dural sac is increased soft tissue signal caused by dilatation of epidural venous plexus. Prominence of venous plexus is also noted on T2W scan (**C** and **D**) and "water" scan (**E** and **F**). **C** and **D,** Sagittal T2W scan (SE gated, flow-compensated 2100/30, 80) shows neither abnormal signal in cord nor evidence of cord swelling. Prominence of epidural venous plexus posterior to C_6-C_7 indicates posterior displacement of dura. High signal intensity in prevertebral tissues at C_6-C_7 suggests local edema tracking superiorly and inferiorly *(arrow)*. **E** and **F,** "Water" scans (SE 800/20) confirm that high signal posterior to C_6 represents water, not fat. Linear low signal structure dorsal to C_6 probably represents partial stripping of posterior longitudinal ligament from posterior surface of vertebral body *(arrow)*. Ligament appears intact. Anulus appears disrupted at this narrowed disc space. **G** and **H,** Sagittal T1W scans (SE 800/20) through lateral masses on right show C_6 lateral mass "perched" on C_7 lateral mass *(arrow)*. **I-L,** Axial variable flip angle scans (GRASS 25/16, 7°) through C_6 show rotatory subluxation and high signal in fracture line of right lamina *(arrows)*. **M,** Axial CT scan through C_6 shows rotatory subluxation of vertebral body in relationship to larynx. Fracture through right lamina corresponds to that on MR (**I-L**).

I, J

K, L

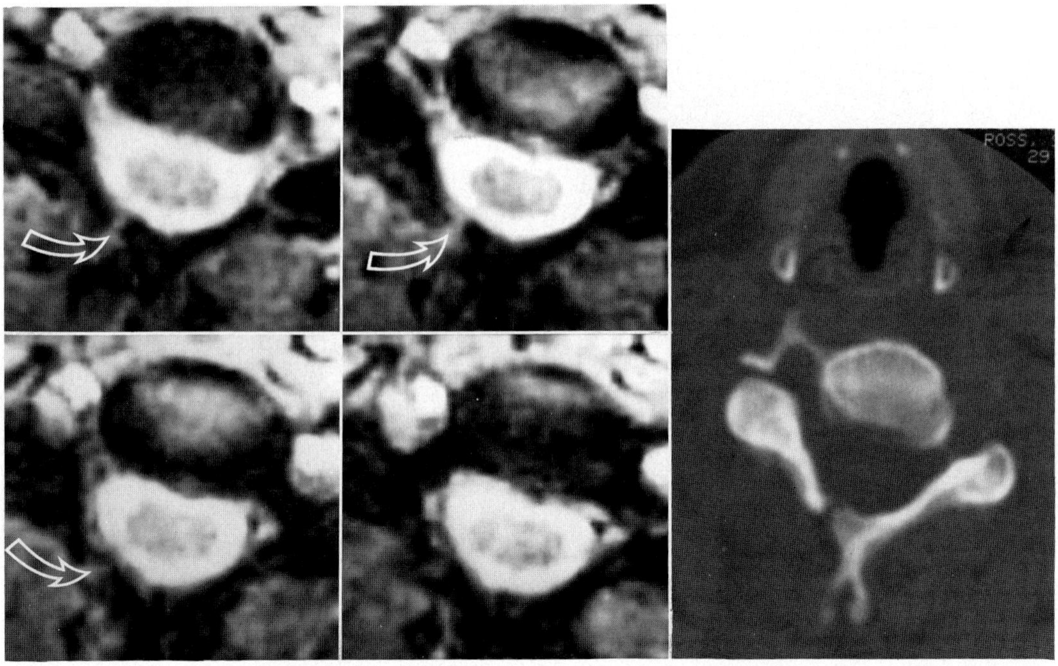

M

FIGURE 6-1. cont'd. For legend see opposite page.

A

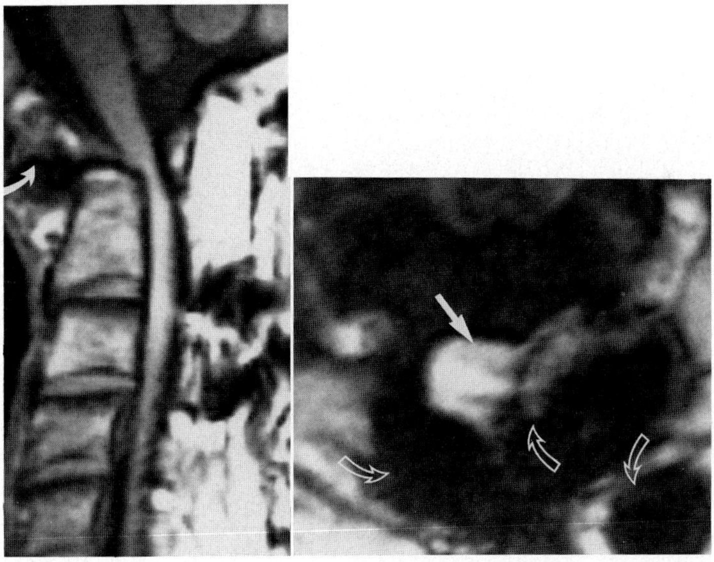

B

FIGURE 6-2. Odontoid fracture and cord compression. **A,** Sagittal T1W scan (SE 800/20) shows displaced, fractured odontoid *(arrow)* with posterior displacement of body of C_2 causing marked cord compression. Prominent irregular areas of low density in posterior cervical spine are metallic artifacts from surgical fusion. **B,** Axial T2*W scan (GRASS 22/12, 7°) did not adequately show severe area of stenosis at C_2 level because of marked susceptibility artifacts *(curved arrows)* caused by posteriorly placed metallic fusion wires. Cord *(straight arrow)* is poorly seen. T1W scan, which has less magnetic susceptibility artifact, better shows degree of cord compression.

A 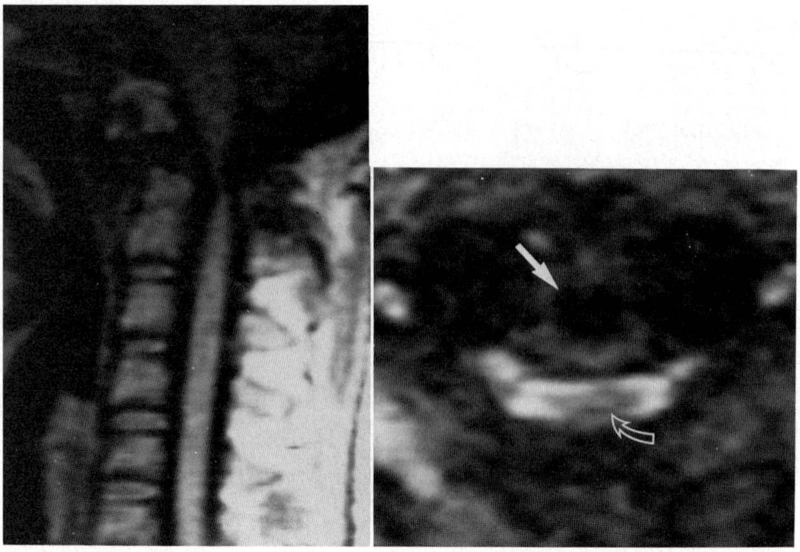 B

FIGURE 6-3. Old dens fracture. MR scan of 23-year-old female, with history of neck injury, right body weakness, muscle wasting, and hyperreflexia. **A,** Sagittal T1W scan shows marked narrowing of spinal canal at C_1 level with severe atrophy of upper cervical cord. Separation between C_1 and dens is difficult to measure. **B,** Axial T2*W scan (GRASS 30/15, 10°) at level of dens *(straight arrow)* shows marked narrowing of spinal canal and flattening of atrophic cervical cord *(curved arrow)*. Note increased soft tissue of intermediate signal intensity around posteriorly displaced dens; it impinges into spinal canal causing cord compression. (Courtesy of Dr. Robert Jahnke.)

A, B 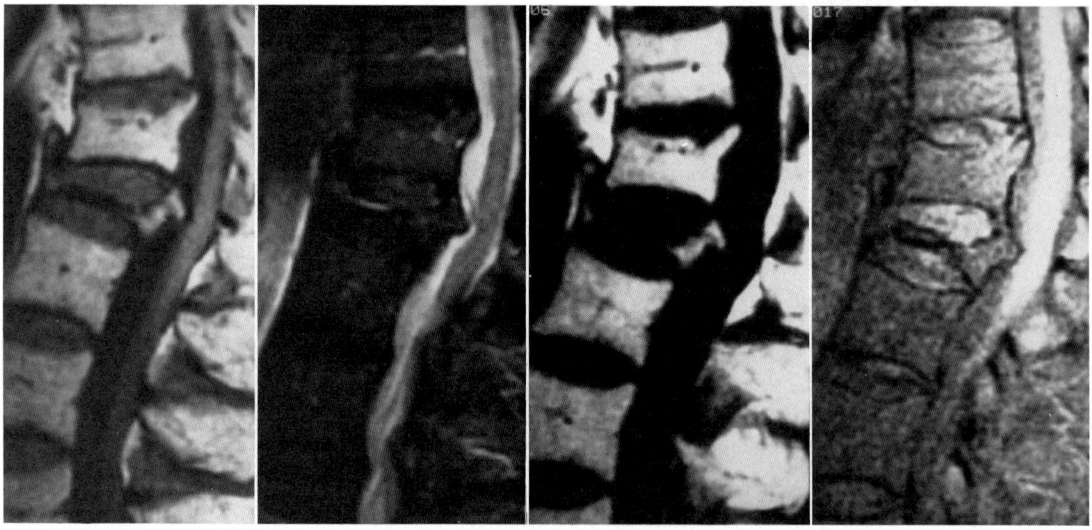 C, D

FIGURE 6-4. Old compression and burst fractures in 76-year-old female. **A,** Sagittal T1W scan (SE 800/20) shows severe compression fracture of L_1 with only thin flat vertebral body remnant and less severe compression fracture at T_{12}. Marrow space remaining in L_1 has normal signal intensity. Retropulsed fragment of L_1 vertebral body impinges on conus. **B,** Sagittal T2W scan (SE, gated 2200/80) confirm impingement of retropulsed fragment on conus. No abnormal, high signal noted within either fractured vertebrae. Marrow signal is within normal limits. **C** and **D,** Sagittal "fat" (SE 800/20) and "water" (SE 800/20) scans confirm normal marrow fat signal (**C**) and lack of abnormal increased water content (**D**). Cortical margins and ligaments are well delineated on "water" scan and appear to be intact at disc spaces.

A, B

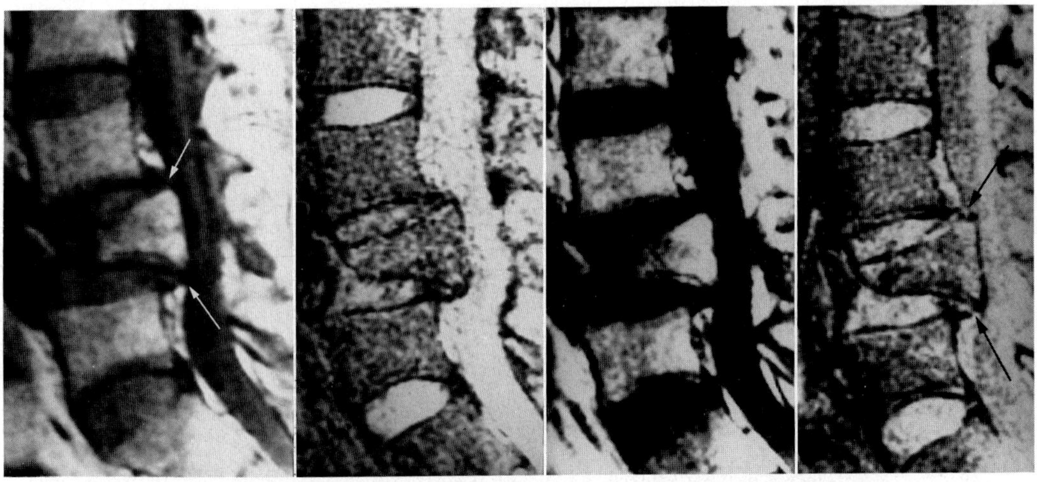

C, D

FIGURE 6-5. Lumbar compression and burst fracture in 23-year-old male three months after injury. **A**, Sagittal T1W scan (SE 800/20) shows compression fracture and anterior wedging and retrolisthesis of L_4. High signal posterior to vertebral bodies of L_3 and L_5. L_4 vertebral body marrow signal is within normal limits. Anulus and posterior longitudinal ligaments appear disrupted *(arrows)*. **B**, Sagittal STIR image (SE 1400/40, TI 100) showed no abnormal high signal in L_4 vertebral body. **C**, Sagittal "fat" (SE 800/20) and **D**, "water" (SE 800/20) scans confirm normal fat content in posterior fractured vertebrae. Part of high signal posterior to L_3 and L_5 vertebral bodies ascribed to presence of fat (**B**). "Water" image shows no abnormal increased signal intensity within fractured vertebrae. Increased signal behind L_3-L_5 vertebral bodies suggests another component of this signal represents dilated epidural venous plexus. Ligaments and anulus are well seen on this water image. Posterior ligament and anulus appear disrupted at L_3-L_4 and L_4-L_5 disc spaces (*arrows*, **D**). This also appreciated on sagittal T1W scan (*arrows*, **A**) but water image, at times, shows ligamentous structures more clearly.

cant subluxation, especially in the cervical region where there is an extensive epidural venous plexus. In the acute stage, hemorrhage may have signal intensity isointense with soft tissue, i.e., cord tissue.[11] Epidural hemorrhage may not have the high signal intensity caused by methemoglobin typically seen in intraparenchymal hemorrhages (Figure 6-9). Epidural hemorrhage is usually not extensive but may impinge on the cord.[11,23]

Compression fractures are more common in thoracic and lumbar vertebrae. The typical deformity of a wedge-shaped vertebral body is well seen on T1W images. In the acute stage marrow signal intensity may be reduced on T1W scans (Figures 6-6 and 6-10). "Fat" images show that the lower signal is a result of decreased marrow fat (see Figure 6-9). "Water" images may show inhomogeneous areas of high signal indicating a higher water content. STIR images, which are very sensitive to abnormal water content, can show heterogeneous high signal (see Figures 6-6 and 6-8). In the acute stage, the abnormal signal intensity on a STIR scan can be homogenous and intense within the vertebral body (see Figure 6-6). After a few months, findings stabilize and compression fractures revert back to a relatively normal marrow signal intensity on T1W, "fat," "water," and STIR images (Figure 6-11; see Figure 6-5). These features allow differentiation of traumatic from pathologic vertebral body compression fractures. Pathologic fractures show low marrow signal on T1W images, absent fat signal on "fat" images, and increased signal on "water" images. These signal abnormalities usually involve the entire vertebra in pathologic fractures, whereas they are more limited in traumatic fractures—except in the very acute stage in severe compression fractures. It apparently requires extensive cancellous bone destruction by neoplasm to result in a compression fracture. This does not present a diagnostic problem because the clinical history is obvious for the severe traumatic compression fracture.

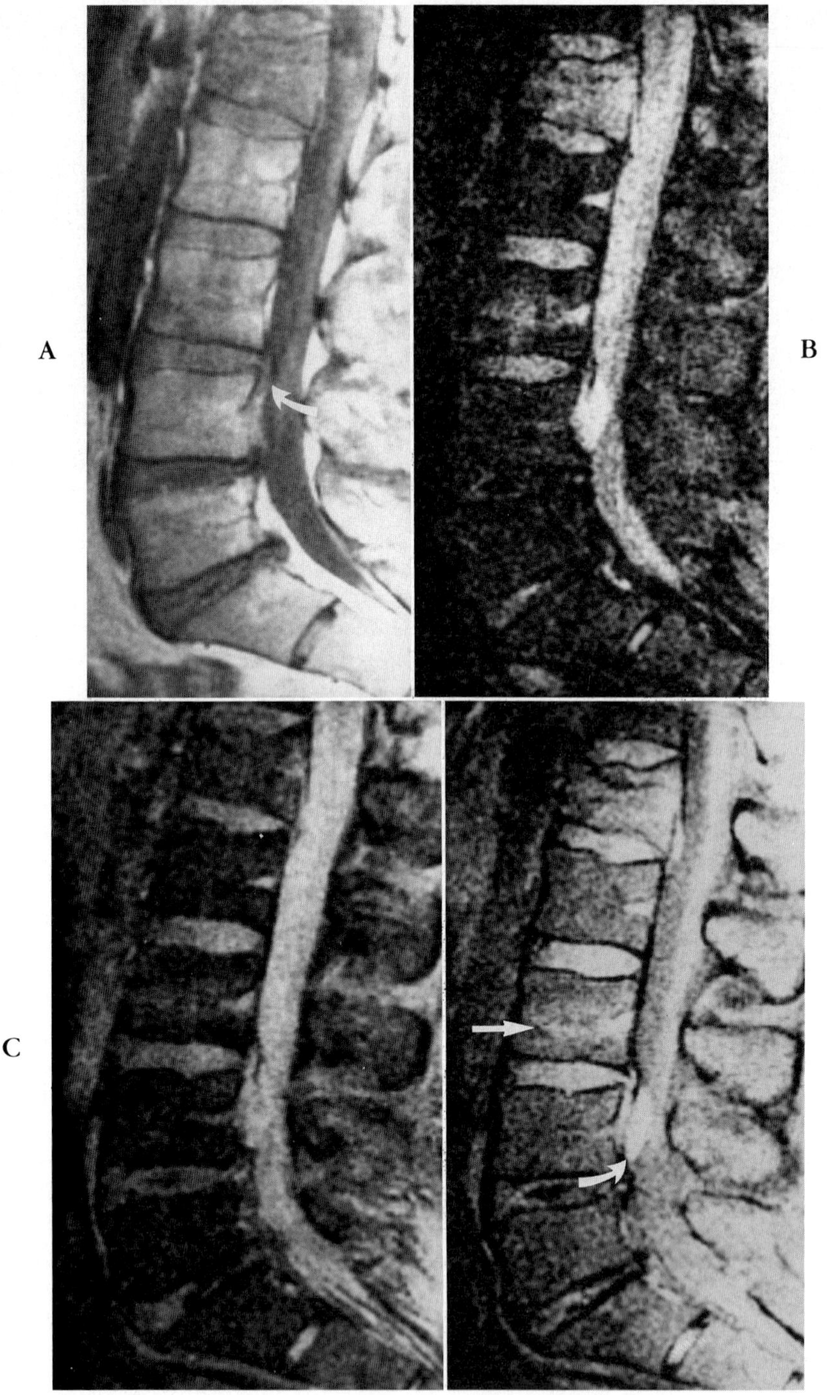

FIGURE 6-6. Traumatic disc herniation and acute compression fracture. Lumbar spine scans of 41-year-old male with acute compression fracture (1 week) of L_1 and traumatic disc herniation with free disc fragment at L_3-L_4. **A,** Sagittal T1W scan (SE 800/20) shows compression fracture of L_1 with some decrease in signal of marrow within this vertebra. Posterior anulus-ligament complex is disrupted at L_3-L_4 *(arrow)*. Significant abnormal tissue is present along the posterior L_4 vertebral body margin. Small midline L_5-S_1 disc herniation is also noted. **B,** Sagittal STIR scan (SE 1400/40, TI 150) shows marked abnormal high signal intensity within L_1 indicative of acute compression fracture. There is also increased signal within midportion of the L_3 vertebral body indicating damage at this level (arrow). Also well seen is marked abnormal

E F G H I J

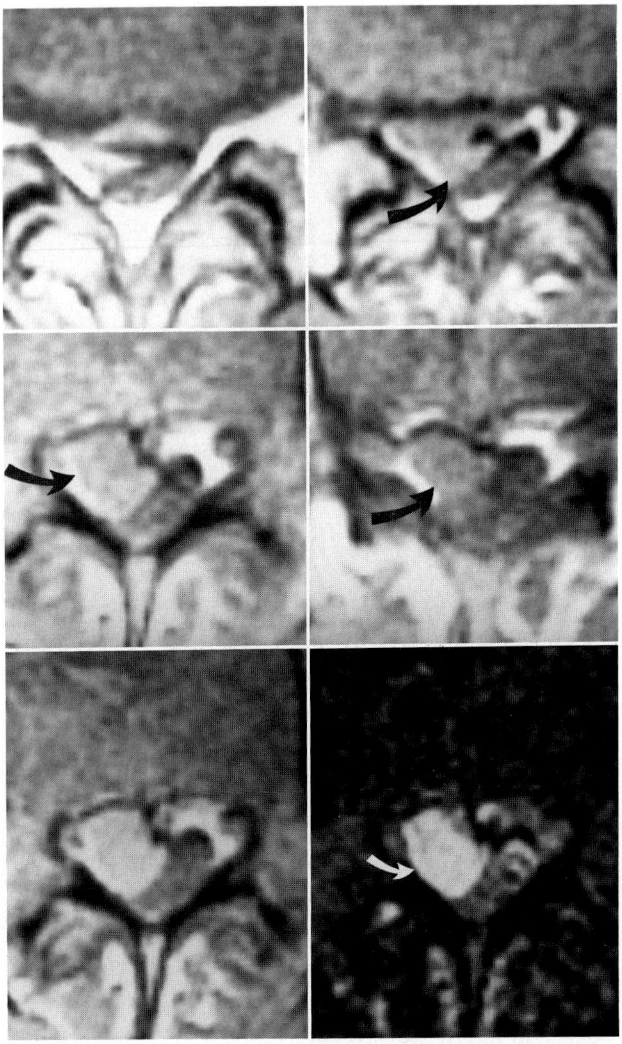

signal intensity of the free disc fragment behind L_4. Disruption of the posterior anulus-ligament complex is also identified by lack of continuity with the posterior superior edge of the L_4 vertebral body. **C**, Variable flip angle/gradient echo scan (GRASS 40/13, FA 5°) shows more subtle increases in signal intensity within L_1 and L_3 vertebral bodies. These changes are not nearly as obvious as on the STIR scan (**B**). Disruption of the anulus-ligament complex and the free fragment are seen, but not as clearly as on the STIR scan (**B**). **D**, Sagittal "water" scan (SE 800/20) shows findings similar to STIR scan (**B**). Abnormal high signal intensity is seen diffusely in the L_1 vertebral body and more focally in the midportion of the L_3 vertebral body. This scan also shows disruption of the anulus-ligament complex at L_3-L_4 and the free disc fragment at L_4. A small soft tissue component is also seen at the L_1-L_2 disc space and this is comparable to the same abnormality seen on (**B**) the STIR sequence. Since the STIR scanning parameters are chosen to suppress fat signal, it is not surprising that the STIR scan should show findings essentially the same as a "water" scan. **E-H**, Axial T1W scans (SE 1000/20) at the L_3-L_4 disc level (cranial to caudal disc) show the large right extradural defect representing the large free disc fragment compressing the dural sac *(arrows)*. On this pulse sequence disc fragment is of higher signal intensity than CSF within the dural sac. **I-J**, An axial T2W scan (SE, gated 2200/20, 80) shows the free fragment to have abnormal high signal intensity on both the first (**I**) and second echo *(arrow*, **J**) images. Marked, abnormal high signal intensity of a herniated disc fragment should suggest a free (sequestered) disc whether traumatic or degenerative in origin. The dural sac shows little high signal because CSF is displaced by the marked compression.

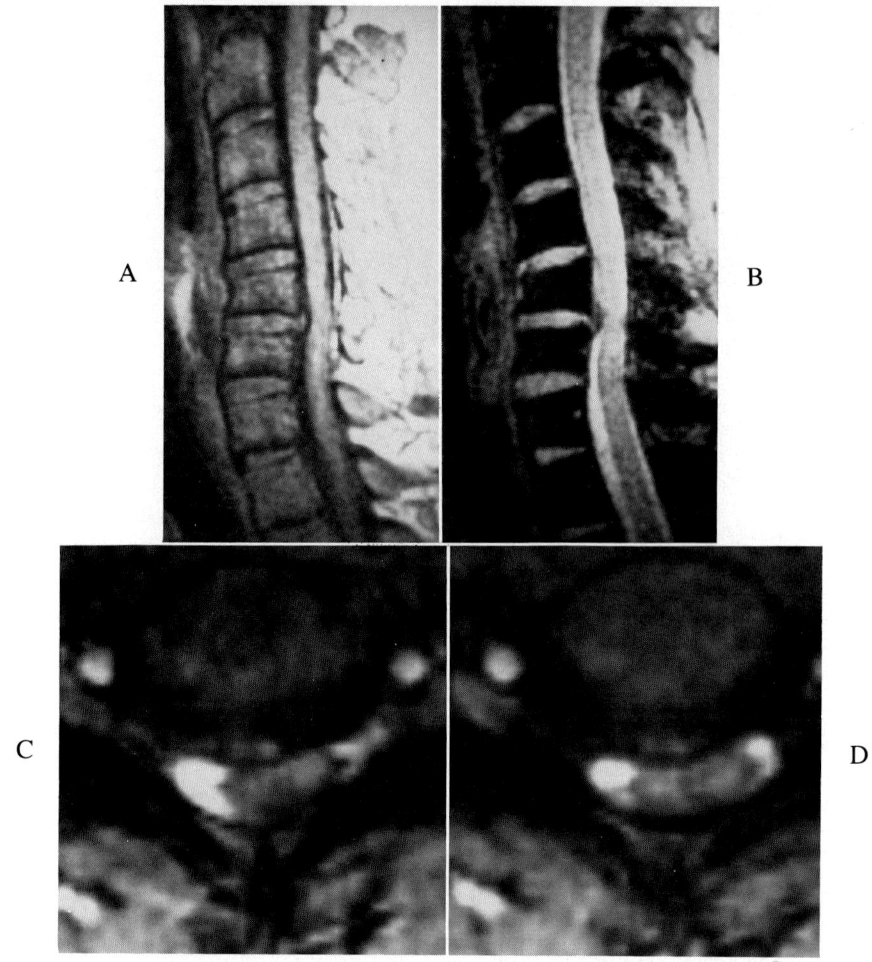

FIGURE 6-7. Traumatic disc herniation. MR scan performed several months after motor vehicle accident. **A,** Sagittal T1W scan (SE 800/20) shows loss of normal cervical lordosis. Disc herniation, evident at C_5-C_6, indents cord and displaces it posteriorly. Remainder of cervical spine shows little degenerative disc disease. **B,** Sagittal T2*W scan (GRASS 40/20, 5°) confirms loss of normal lordosis and displacement of cervical cord at C_5-C_6. Note nucleus pulposus signal intensity is normal on T1W and T2*W pulse sequences. **C** and **D,** Axial T2*W scans (GRASS 25/13, 7°) show typical findings of disc herniation in midline and on right, resulting in moderate cervical spine stenosis with cord deformity. Herniated disc fragment shows intermediate signal intensity similar to that within native disc space.

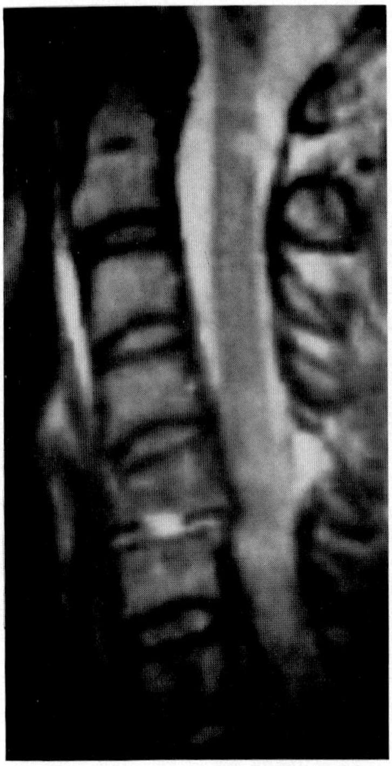

FIGURE 6-8. Acute cervical cord contusion. Acute cord injury in young woman who fell out of a jeep. Sagittal T2W scan (SE 2500/75) shows abnormal high signal intensity within swollen cord at C_5-C_6 level. Disc space is narrowed and has abnormal high signal intensity within it. Abnormal high signal intensity also noted in dorsal spinal canal at same level. Minimal retrolisthesis of C_5 on C_6 but ligaments appear intact. Inferior vertebral end-plate at C_5 is disrupted. (.38T field.) (Courtesy of Dr. Patrick Turski.)

B

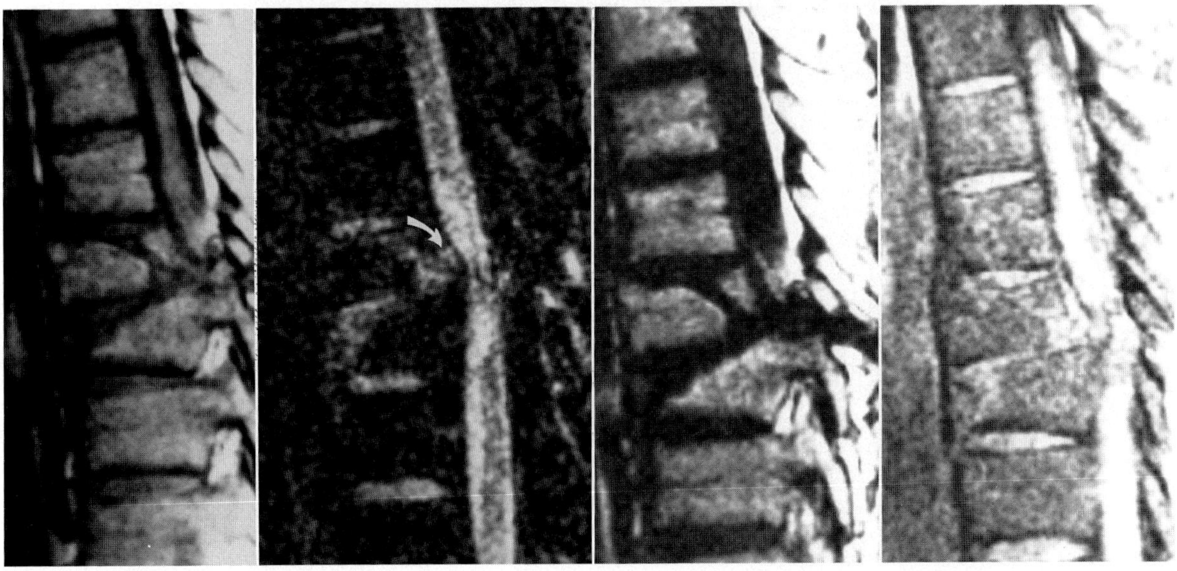

C, D

FIGURE 6-9. Subacute compression fracture. Comminuted compression fracture of T_7 and T_8, 6 weeks after injury in paraplegic patient. **A,** Sagittal T1W scan (SE 800/20) shows multiple compression fracture fragments of T_7 and T_8. Note signal intensity of marrow and disc spaces are within normal limits at this time. **B,** Sagittal STIR scan (1400/40, TI 150) shows minimal abnormal high signal intensity in one small fracture fragment *(arrow)*. Impingement of fracture fragments into spinal canal is evident. **C** and **D,** Sagittal "fat" (SE 800/20, **C**) and "water" (SE 800/20, **D**) scans, show normal marrow and disc space signal intensity. Fat signal in fracture fragments, even small fragments, is normal intensity. *Continued.*

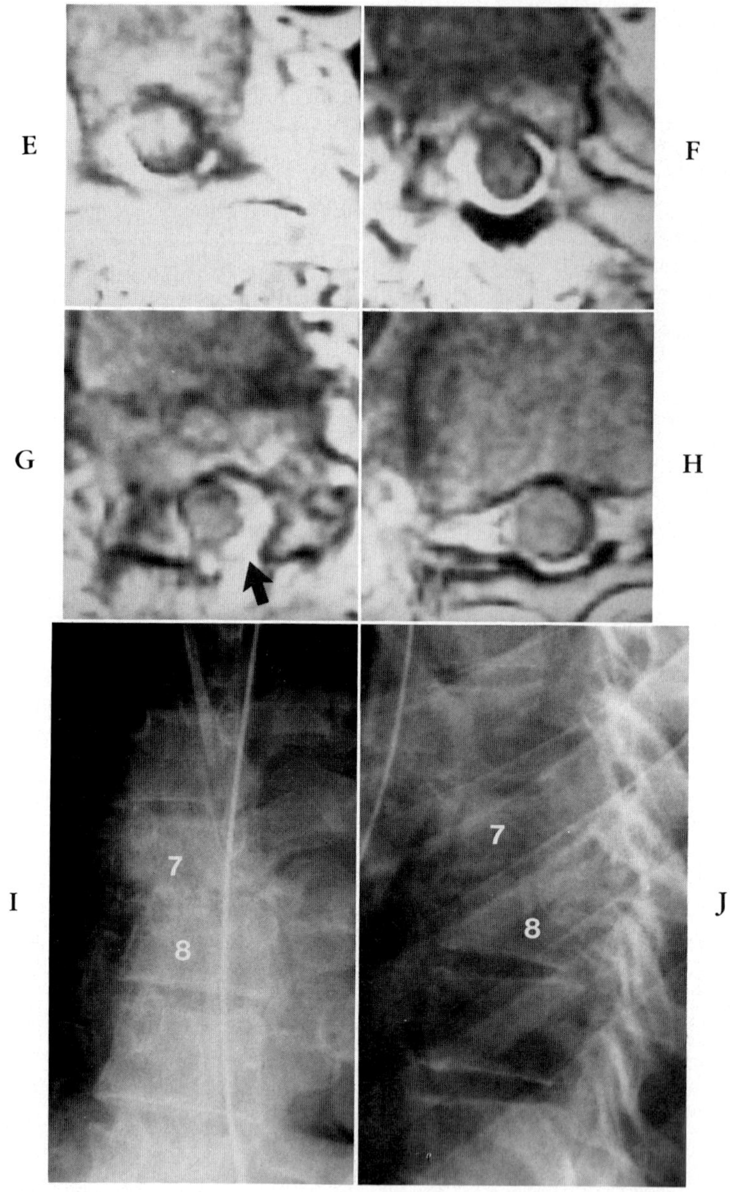

FIGURE 6-9 cont'd. **E-H,** Axial T1W scans (SE 1000/20) show area of high signal in epidural space compressing dural sac and cord toward right, indicative of local hematoma *(arrow)*. Note cord is still enlarged below level of injury (**H**) approximately six weeks after injury. **I,** Anteroposterior (AP) and **J,** lateral plain films show T_7 and T_8 compression fractures and retrolisthesis of T_8 in relation to T_7.

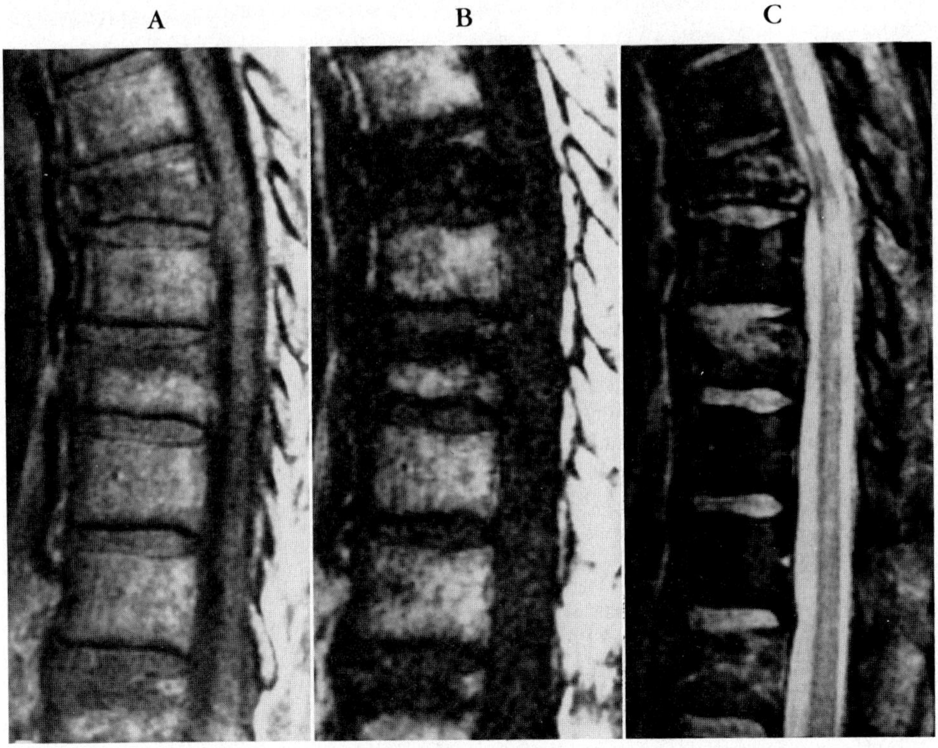

FIGURE 6-10. Acute compression fracture of several vertebrae in 20-year-old male 2 days after a fall. **A,** Sagittal T1W scan (SE 800/20) shows obvious compression fractures of T_7, T_9, and T_{12}. T_7 compression fracture is most severe but all compression fractures show lower than normal signal intensity within marrow of affected vertebral bodies. **B,** Sagittal "fat" image (SE 800/20) shows loss of fat signal in vertebrae with compression fractures. This corresponds to distribution of low signal on T1W image. In acute fracture fat signal may be lost in very early stages. **C,** Sagittal T2W scan (SE gated 2000/80) shows irregular areas of increased signal intensity within fractured vertebrae at T_7, T_9, and T_{12}. Abnormal high signal does not involve vertebrae uniformly nor does it correspond directly to areas of low signal on T1W scan. Although acute compression fractures exhibit abnormal high signal, pattern differs from that in pathologic compression fractures in which abnormality is more uniform throughout vertebrae (see Chapter 10). Compare with Figure 6-6. Note abnormal signal within cord at T_7 lesion.

A, B

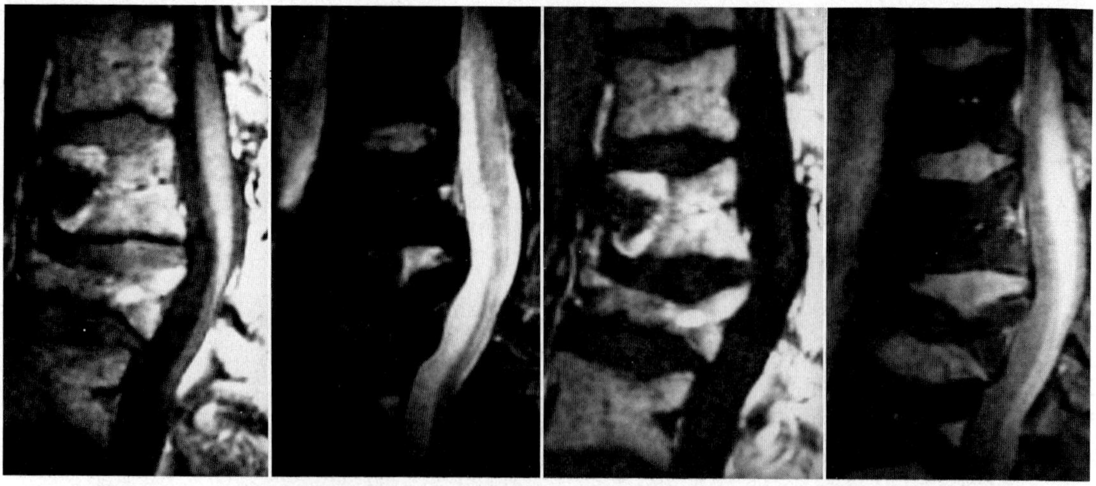

C, D

FIGURE 6-11. Old lumbar compression fractures. **A,** Sagittal T1W scan (SE 800/20) shows compression fractures of L_1 and L_2 with some impingement into spinal canal. Marrow signal remains within normal limits throughout vertebra. **B,** Sagittal T2W scan (SE, gated 2200/80) shows no abnormal high signal within fractured vertebrae and no significant compression of conus or cauda equina. Abnormal high signal is within posterior L_1-L_2 disc space. **C,** "Fat" image shows that significant amount of fat tissue remains in marrow space, even in severely compressed vertebrae, i.e., L_2. **D,** "Water" image shows no abnormal accumulation of water within marrow of either fractured vertebrae. Findings are typical of old, nonpathologic compression fracture.

Spinal cord

MR imaging has a great advantage over other imaging modalities in trauma in that cord damage can be visualized directly. Acute findings on a T1W scan may show focal cord swelling at the site of injury or a normal cord. The cord is usually of normal signal intensity even if it is enlarged (Figure 6-12).[9] On a T2W or T2*W image, the cord can exhibit high or low signal intensity despite a normal T1W scan (Figure 6-13).[2,6,9,23] Cord damage can therefore be subtle, in that the T1W image may be normal but a T2W or T2*W image shows an intramedullary abnormality (see Figures 6-12 and 6-13). In the acute stage (<3 days), the T2W scan is more accurate in detecting cord damage than the T1W scan.[9] In the subacute stage, (>3 days), the T1W image begins to provide more information.[9] This is especially true when there is a hemorrhagic component that appears as high signal as a result of the paramagnetic effect of the methemoglobin.

Acute spinal cord damage assumes two general patterns, hemorrhagic and nonhemorrhagic.[9] The nonhemorrhagic pattern is characterized by normal signal intensity on T1W images in conjunction with abnormal high signal intensity on T2W images. This high signal can be seen extending inferiorly and superiorly from the injury epicenter and usually regresses over a period of seven days to three weeks.[9] This abnormality on the T2W scan can be seen in patients who are neurologically normal. The high signal probably represents edema. This pattern on T2W images indicates a good prognosis in that significant neurologic recovery can occur.[9]

A more serious and ominous finding is that of intramedullary hemorrhage, which represents the second major cord damage pattern.[9] The MR appearance of the intramedullary hemorrhage is similar to that of intracranial hemorrhage and therefore depends upon its age. It may be isointense with the cord in the acute stage and difficult to detect on T1W images; in fact, the T1W image may be normal. There may be no associated skeletal damage.[9] In early stages, hemorrhage may exhibit low signal intensity on a T2W image caused by the deoxyhemoglobin effect,[9] which can be accentuated with a T2*W

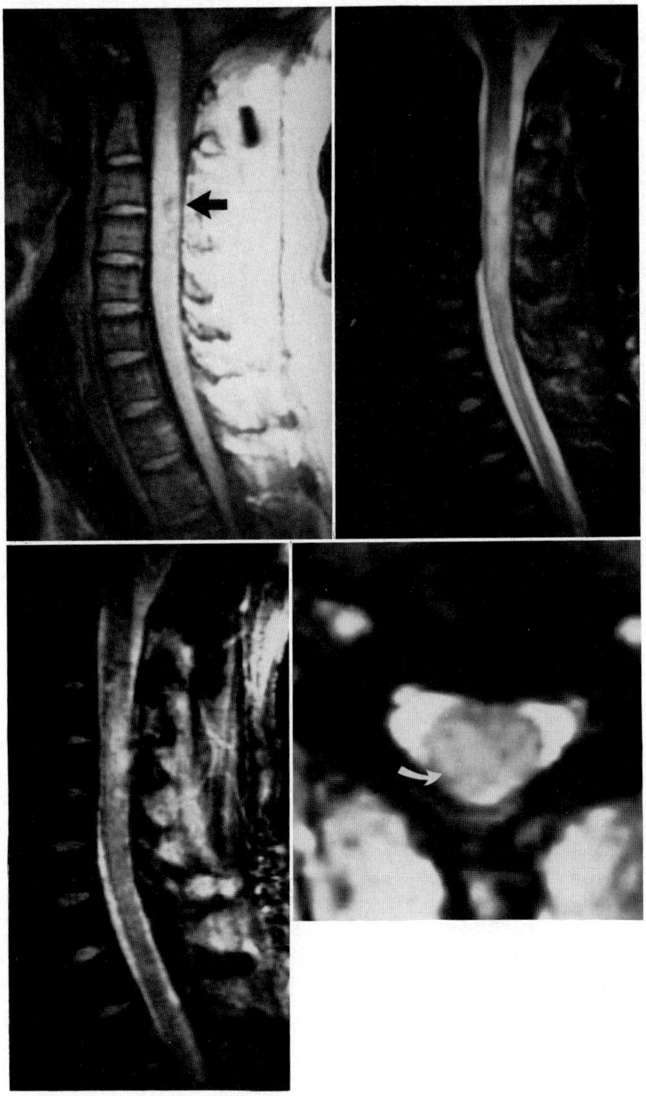

FIGURE 6-12. Cord contusion. MR scans three weeks after gunshot wound to neck. Shrapnel did not enter spinal canal. Patient had quadraparesis and developed central cord syndrome caused by concussive injury. **A,** Sagittal T1W scan (SE 800/20) shows diffuse cord enlargement in upper cervical region with inhomogenous low signal within cord *(arrow)*. No evidence of hematomyelia or epidural hemorrhage. Bullet fragment is seen at C_2 level as rectangular area of signal loss. **B,** Sagittal T2W scan (SE, gated 2600/80) shows extensive area of abnormal high signal within enlarged cord. No evidence of hemorrhage. **C,** Sagittal T2*W scan (GRASS 40/20, 5°) confirms area of abnormal signal intensity within cord, as well as cord swelling. Abnormal high signal intensity in posterior soft tissue of neck is more evident on this scan than on T2W scan (**B**). No magnetic susceptibility effects within cord that would indicate hemorrhage. **D,** Axial T2*W scan (GRASS 40/20, 7°) confirms diffuse cord enlargement and abnormal high signal within cord primarily in central location *(arrow)*. Cord damage resulted from concussion injury without direct contact with bullet. Findings involve central portion of cord and correlate well with developing central cord syndrome.

A, B

C

D

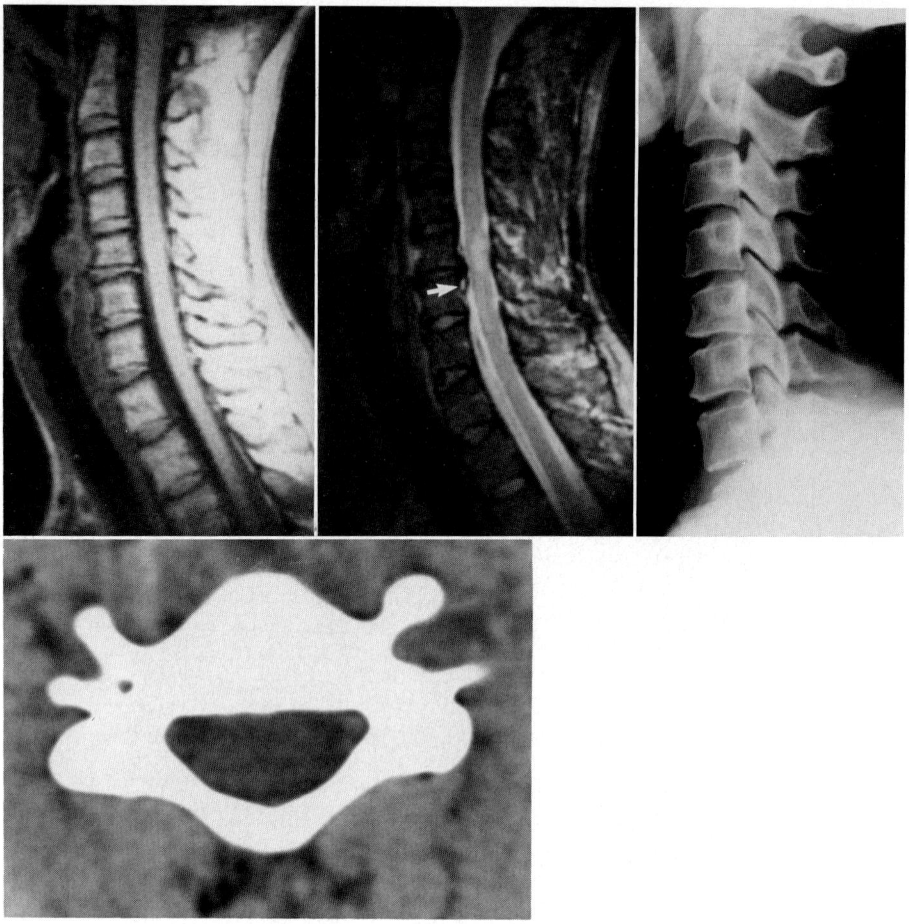

FIGURE 6-13. Cord contusion in 44-year-old female who fell off a horse, causing immediate motor weakness. **A,** Sagittal T1W scan (SE 800/20) shows no significant cord abnormality although traumatic disc herniation is evident at C_5-C_6. No evidence of hemorrhage, and cord signal intensity is within normal limits. **B,** Sagittal T2W scan (SE, gated 1800/80) confirms normal size of cord but shows focal intramedullary area of abnormal high signal intensity at C_5-C_6 level. Abnormal cord signal was evident hours after injury. No evidence of hemorrhage. Dura at C_6 displaced slightly posteriorly with dilated venous plexus *(arrow)* visualized between it and vertebral body. **C,** Lateral cervical spine plain film shows only minimal narrowing of C_5-C_6 disc space. No prevertebral soft tissue swelling and no other evidence of potentially significant cord damage. **D,** Noncontrast CT scan at C_5 shows no fracture and no evidence of cord damage. Significant cord damage can occur even in absence of plain film and CT findings, which would indicate even indirectly an injury to the cord.

image. At a later stage, when sufficient methemoglobin has accumulated, the hemorrhage has high signal intensity on T1W and T2W images. At a late stage only the residual hemosiderin effect remains as evidence of intramedullary hemorrhage (see Figure 6-17). The presence of spinal cord hemorrhage indicates a poor prognosis in that it is associated with a lack of any significant neurologic recovery.[9] The hemorrhagic nature of cord contusion caused by an experimental compression injury was studied with MR and shows similar findings.[2,6] The incidence of intramedullary hemorrhage in trauma has not been determined, but hematomyelia may be more common than previously thought, appearing in 5 of 27 patients in one series.[9] Obviously the most serious injury is complete cord transection, easily diagnosed on T1W scans that show discontinuity of the cord in the acute stage (Figure 6-14).

A 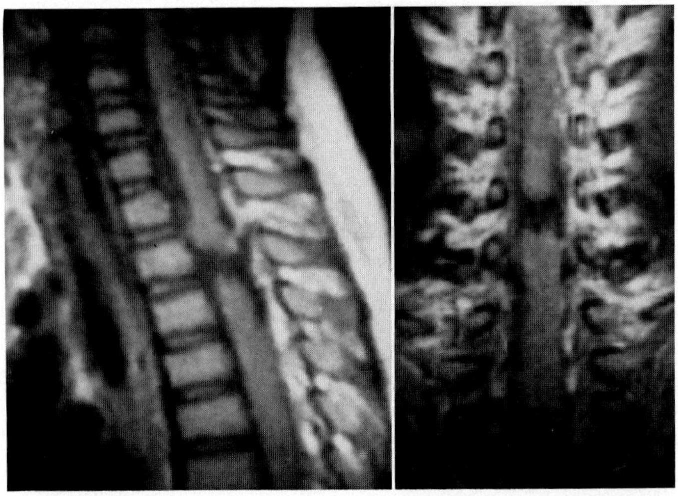 B

FIGURE 6-14. Cord transection. Cervical trauma in 8-year-old female resulting from bicycle/ auto accident. Sagittal T1W scan (SE 500/30) shows complete transection of cord in upper thoracic spine. **A,** Note gap between sheared ends of cord because they have retracted somewhat. Coronal T1W scan (SE 600/30) confirms transection of cord and retraction of cord remnants. **B,** Injury resulted in complete motor and sensory loss below transection. (Courtesy of Dr. Patrick Turski.)

The end stage of cord damage has varied findings. Limited cord damage may leave minimal residua. With central cord damage a thin well-defined area of low signal can be seen on T1W scans (Figure 6-15). Cord damage may cause only focal cord atrophy, which exhibits abnormal signal on T2W scans (Figure 6-16. With more severe damage, long segments of cord are atrophic and abnormal signal intensity on T1W and T2W images. Hematomyelia leaves characteristic hemosiderin residua (Figure 6-17).

MR vs. CT

When MR and CT are compared in acute spinal trauma MR is more useful in assessing spinal cord compression, traumatic disc pathology, and posttraumatic intramedullary abnormalities and soft tissue hemorrhage.[9,23] The most impressive advantage of MR compared with normal x-ray studies is the detection of cord pathology. CT is more accurate in detecting neural arch fractures and assessing the number of displaced fragments.

Life support systems, respirators, and metallic immobilization frames, for example, may cause logistic problems with MR that can be reduced by different magnet designs, i.e., permanent and resistive magnets. MR may also be limited by the ambiguous identification of acute hemorrhage, but this is also difficult with CT in the spinal canal as a result of beam hardening artifact. The importance of this identification is controversial, in that surgical evaluation of acute traumatic hematomas has resulted in variable clinical improvement.[5] The clinical impact of early and correct diagnosis of traumatic intraspinal hemorrhage by MR has not been assessed.

Late Sequelae

MR can show progressive changes in the cord following trauma.[21] Early scans may show small "cystic" areas in the cord. Fluid in these cysts is low signal intensity on T1W scans and high signal intensity on T2W scans. In the early stages these "cysts" may actually represent microcystic change in an area of myelomalacia. Eventually, several of the smaller cystic regions may coalesce to form a larger cyst, which may progress to a more typical syrinx. These changes parallel typical pathologic changes, which show small areas of cavitation that then merge into larger cysts. The MR appearance of such cysts on a T1W scan may be a well-circumscribed low signal area

A 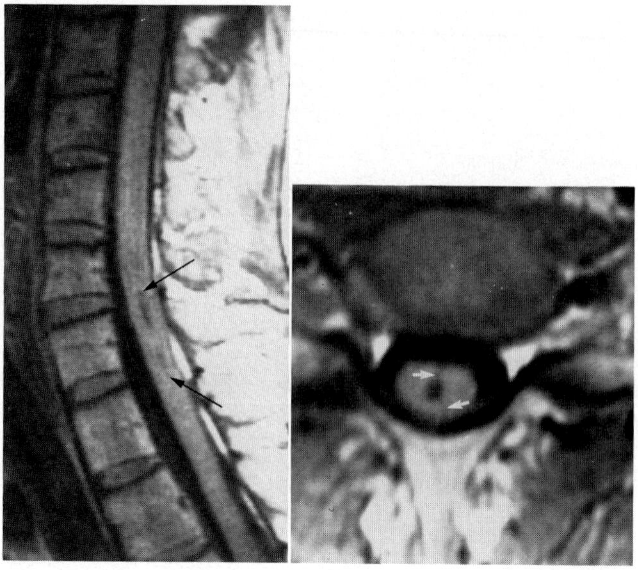 B

FIGURE 6-15. Old cord infarction–contusion. Residua of cervical spine trauma as a result of diving into shallow water 20 years earlier. Patient has decreased motor strength, pain sensation, and position sense in upper extremities with sparing of lower extremities. MR and clinical findings are those of central cord syndrome. **A,** Sagittal T1W scan (SE 800/20) shows thin, central area of low signal intensity at C_7 level. Lesion has linear shape extending for slightly more than length of one vertebral body height *(arrows)*. **B,** Axial T1W scan (SE 1000/20) at C_7 level shows focal well-defined area of low signal intensity in central cord. Two small linear extensions *(arrows)* of low signal intensity extend to anterior median sulcus and region of fasciculus gracilis just left of posterior median sulcus. These MR findings are probably secondary to ischemic change and represent infarction; they are MR correlate of central cord syndrome.

A, B 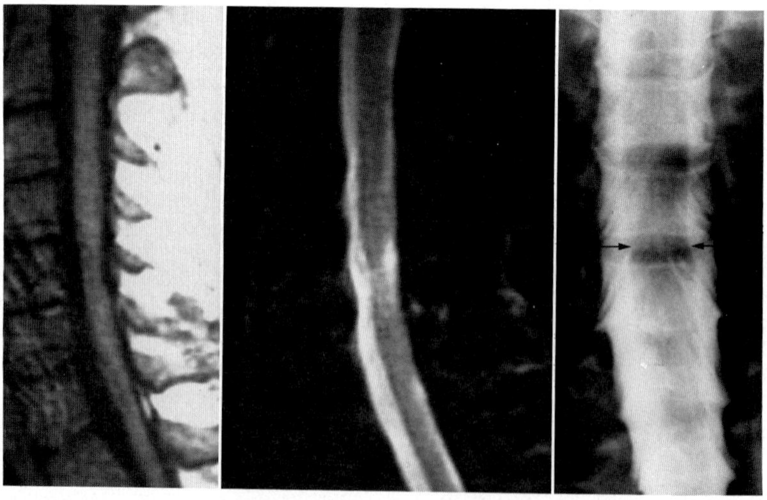 C

FIGURE 6-16. Posttraumatic cord atrophy. **A,** Sagittal T1W scan (SE 800/20) shows focal narrowing of cord at C_5 without obvious abnormal cord signal intensity on T1W image. **B,** Sagittal T2W scan (SE, gated, 2000/100) confirms focal narrowing of cord at C_5 and shows abnormal high signal at this narrowing that indicates damaged cord tissue and probable gliosis. No cyst formation is evident. **C,** Anteroposterior (AP) view of water-soluble myelogram confirms focal cord narrowing at C_5-C_6 level *(arrows)*.

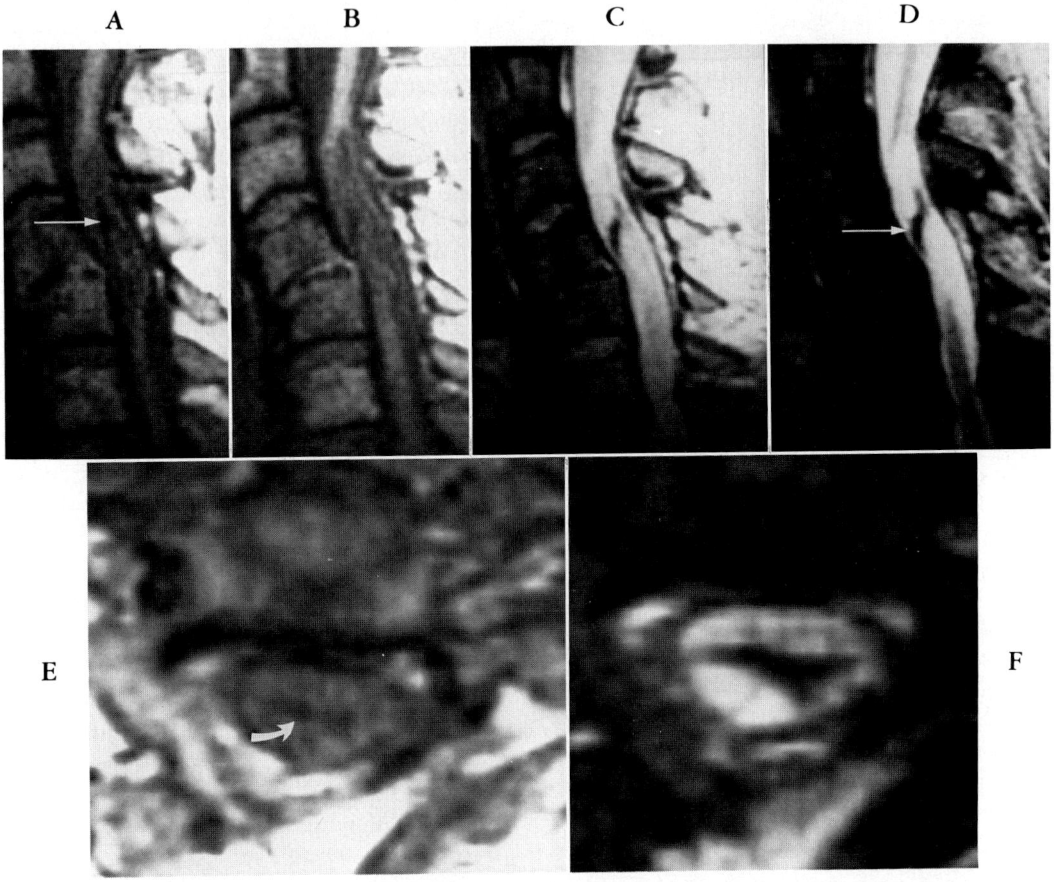

FIGURE 6-17. Old posttraumatic myelomalacia and hematomyelia. **A** and **B**, Sagittal T1W scans (SE 800/20) shows atrophy of upper cervical cord and prominent area of myelomalacia extending from C_3 to C_5. Area is lower signal intensity than normal cord (**A** and **B**) and contains linear area of even lower signal intensity *(arrow)*. Narrowed C_4-C_5 disc space shows partial fusion of C_4-C_5 vertebrae (**A**). **C**, Sagittal T2W scan (SE gated 2200/80) confirms cord atrophy and abnormal signal intensity of cord extending from C_3-C_5. Abnormal high signal of cord is indistinguishable from adjacent CSF. **D**, At C_4 level, linear area of marked low signal intensity suggests magnetic susceptibility effect characteristic of hemosiderin, residua of a previous hemorrhage *(arrow)*. **E**, Axial T1W scan (SE 800/20) through midportion of myelomalacic cord shows that cord tissue is difficult to differentiate from adjacent CSF because of similar signal intensity. Low signal intensity area indicative of hemosiderin deposition can also be seen on T1W scan (*arrow*, **E**). **F**, Axial T2W scan (SE, gated 2200/80) shows triangular-shaped area of marked low signal intensity indicative of hemosiderin deposition.

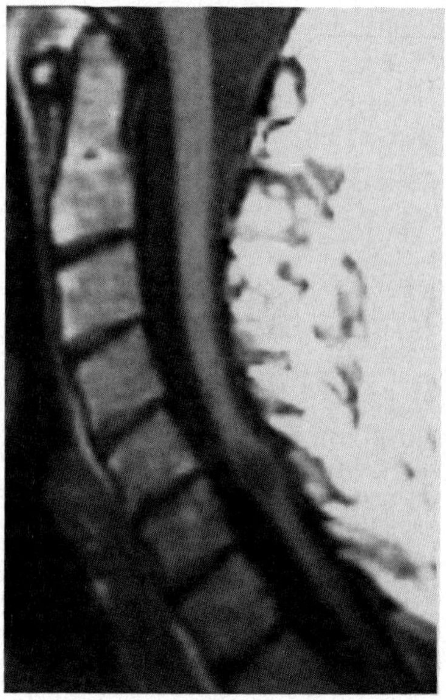

FIGURE 6-18. Posttraumatic myelomalacia: syrinx. Quadraparetic patient with seven-year postinjury. Sagittal T1W scan (SE 600/20) shows focal expansion of cervical cord at C_6 level. Focal area of relative enlargement has low signal intensity at its center with more normal cord signal intensity around periphery of apparent cyst. Overall size of cervical cord is reduced indicating diffuse atrophy. Whether this lesion represents one large cyst or focal area of microcystic change cannot be determined. Probably represents early stage of posttraumatic syrinx. A T2W image could help clarify this. (Courtesy of Dr. David Norman.)

within a normal-sized cord, or the cyst may appear as a focal expansion in an atrophic cord (Figure 6-18). The cyst may appear expansive, but this is relative because the cord is small (see Figure 6-18): the cyst may be similar to or less than the normal cord diameter. The factors resulting in arrested myelomalacia or small cyst formation instead of continued enlargement and extension of cavitation to form a syrinx are not known. Posttraumatic syrinx is a complication that can result in further neurologic deterioration years after the injury. The pathogenesis of posttraumatic syrinx is not well understood but the diagnosis is usually straightforward on T1W images. If the syrinx is small, it may be mistaken for a focal area of myelomalacia. Differentiation usually can be made on T2W images where myelomalacia has intermediate to high signal intensity on the first echo or "balanced image," whereas a fluid-filled syrinx has low signal intensity on the balanced image. If the fluid is pulsating, it is low signal on both echoes with marked signal loss on the second echo (see Chapter 12).

Progressive myelopathy after trauma may occur with lesions that are not syrinx. Two cases of progressive myelopathy occurring years after incomplete cervical spinal cord injury have been described.[10] In both patients, clinical features, as well as the "bull's eye" appearance on a delayed (CT) myelogram and circumscribed low density on the MR scan, suggested posttraumatic syringomyelia. Surgical exploration, however, including intraoperative spinal sonography, failed to reveal a syrinx. Although arachnoiditis was present in both patients, the striking abnormality found at surgery was cord softening with microcystic degeneration of the cord. Microcystic spinal cord degeneration in these cases represents a previously undescribed cause of late deterioration after spinal cord injury that may mimic the clinical, CT-myelographic, and MR features of posttraumatic syringomyelia. The method of differentiation using the first and second echo of a T2W sequence should, however, be accurate. A similar finding has been reported in a short-time interval (4½ months) after injury in which intense gliosis was responsible for clinical neurologic deterioration.[5] T1W images were suggestive of syrinx formation, although this would be too soon for a posttraumatic syrinx. The first echo of the T2W scan shows high signal, which is against the diagnosis of syrinx, and strongly suggests myelomalacia.[5]

There are other posttraumatic conditions that may result in neurologic deterioration besides that caused by the acute injury itself. Subarachnoid adhesions can form after trauma and cause cord tethering or result in loculated subarachnoid cysts,[14] which enlarge and result in cord compression (see Figure 12-10). Such subarachnoid cysts are usually identified easily on T1W scans because of their localized nature, low signal intensity, and impression on the adjacent cord. A late finding of cord trauma is cord atrophy.[14] It may be focal or extensive and may be seen above and below the site of trauma (see above).

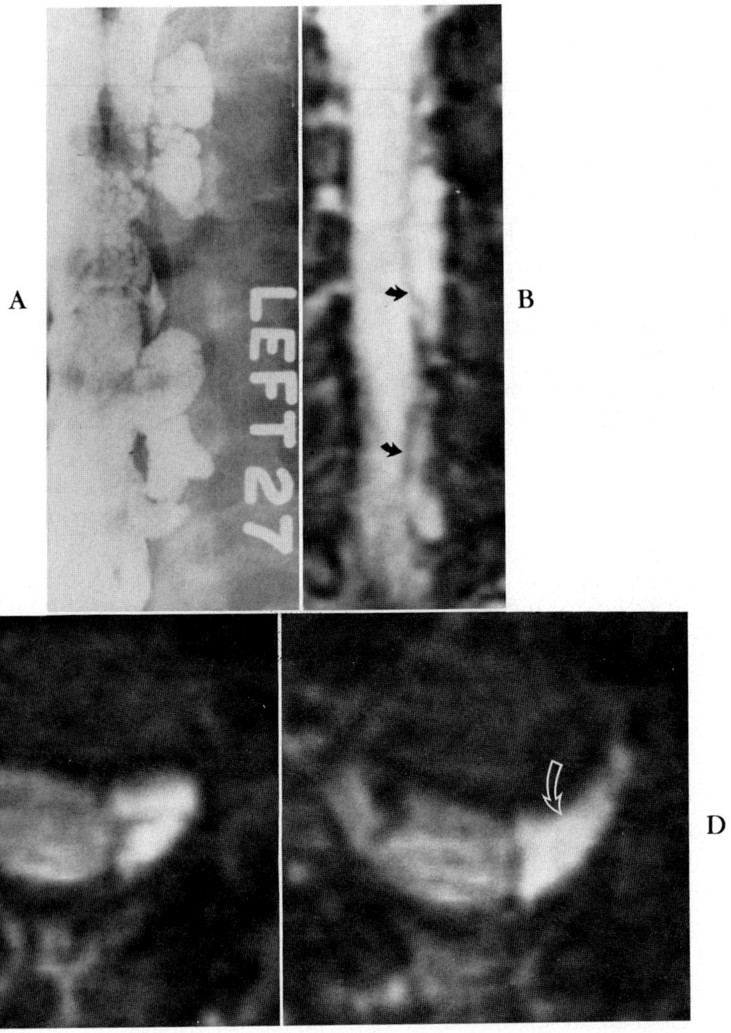

FIGURE 6-19. Cervical nerve root avulsion in 21-year-old male. **A,** Anterorposterior (AP) view of myelogram shows collections of contrast within CSF outpouchings that represent either meningoceles or pseudomeningoceles typical of avulsed nerve root sleeves. **B,** Coronal T2W scan (SE 2500/80) shows close correlation between pouches on myelogram and extradural collections of fluid on coronal MR scan. Note signal intensity of extradural fluid collection is higher than that within dural sac. Thin low signal intensity line representing dura separates intrathecal CSF from that in extradural pouches *(arrows)*. **C** and **D,** Axial T2W images (SE 2500/80) shows difference in signal intensity of CSF on left side of canal compared to right side. Higher signal intensity CSF on left side is trapped within extradural pouches and is higher signal because it is less mobile than CSF within thecal sac. Note characteristic extension of extradural pouch into neural foramen *(arrow)*.

NERVE ROOT AVULSION

Depending on the position of the arm at the time of injury, avulsed nerve roots usually occur in the upper or lower portion of C_5 through T_1. Lesions consist of tearing individual nerve rootlets and the formation of a meningocele or a pseudomeningocele at the root sleeve. Most often roots rupture completely and are not identifiable in the CSF outpouching.[17] A meningocele suggests expansion of the subarachnoid space through a dural tear with the arachnoid membrane remaining intact, whereas a pseudomeningocele would be a more appropriate term when the arachnoid is also disrupted and does not line the outpouching. In any case, the CSF collection can extend through the neural foramen and may extend superiorly or inferiorly within the spinal canal in an extradural location.[17]

MR Findings

MR findings reflect changes similar to those described for CT myelography and are also consonant with typical plain film myelographic findings.[17] The outpouchings—meningoceles or pseudomeningoceles—fill with contrast material on myelographic studies. With CT myelography, dura can be identified between normal subarachnoid space and CSF outpouching. This displaced dura can also be seen on T2W images but not on T1W scans. The retracted individual nerve roots are often not identified on imaging studies. CSF-filled outpouchings may be difficult to identify on T1W images but are easily seen on nonmotion-compensated axial T2W images (Figure 6-19). Because CSF in the outpouchings exhibits less motion than CSF within the subarachnoid space it has relatively higher signal intensity on that basis (see Figure 6-19).[4] Axial T2*W images used for the study of disc disease may miss this diagnosis because parameters used in these pulse sequences are usually chosen because of their insensitivity to CSF motion. Such a sequence therefore may not discriminate between moving and nonmoving CSF, a feature which is an aid to the diagnosis.[4] Diagnosis relies on the anatomic deformity of the thecal sac or nerve roots. The size and extent of the outpouchings may increase over time.

CHRONIC ATLANTOAXIAL SUBLUXATION

A benign fibrous mass can form at the C_1 to C_2 junction secondary to chronic atlantoaxial subluxation without rheumatoid arthritis.[22] The masses at C_1 to C_2 are composed of fibrous and granulation tissue and are presumed secondary to chronic mechanical irritation. The inciting cause may be degenerative disease or congenital dysplasia of the dens. Findings are similar to those seen in rheumatoid arthritis (see Chapter 7). Mass lesions can reach a size sufficient to cause impingement on the spinal canal and result in cord compression.[22] On T1W images the masses are intermediate signal intensity similar to that of bone marrow. Findings on T2W images may show heterogeneous signal intensity, but large portions of the mass are low signal because of the prominent fibrous tissue component. MR bone findings may be similar to those seen in rheumatoid arthritis where pannus has formed at C_1 to C_2.[1]

REFERENCES

1. Aisen AM, Martel W, Ellis JH, et al. Cervical spine involvement in rheumatoid arthritis: MR imaging. Radiology 1987; 165:159.
2. Chakeres DW, Flickinger F, Bresnahan JC, et al. MR imaging of acute spinal cord trauma. AJNR 1987; 8:5.
3. Edeiken-Monroe B, Wagner LK, Harris JH Jr. Hyperextension dislocation of the cervical spine. AJNR 1986; 7:135.
4. Enzmann DR, Rubin JB, DeLaPaz R, et al. Cerebrospinal fluid pulsation: benefits and pitfalls in MR imaging. Radiology 1986: 161:773.
5. Fox JL, Wener L, Drennan DC, et al. Central spinal cord injury: magnetic resonance imaging confirmation and operative considerations. Neurosurgery 1988; 22:340.
6. Hackney DB, Asato R, Joseph PM, et al. Hemorrhage and edema in acute spinal cord compression: demonstration by MR imaging. Radiology 1986; 161:387.
7. Hadley MN, Zabramski JM, Browner CM, et al. Pediatric spinal trauma: review of 122 cases of spinal cord and vertebral column injuries. J Neurosurg 1988; 68:18.
8. Kadoya S, Nakamura T, Kobayashi S, et al. Magnetic resonance image of acute spinal cord injury. Report of three cases. Neuroradiology 1987; 29:252.
9. Kulkarni MV, McArdle CB, Kopanicky D, et al. Acute spinal cord injury: MR imaging at 1.5 T. Radiology 1987; 164:837.
10. MacDonald RL, Findlay JM, Tator CH. Microcystic spinal cord degeneration causing post-traumatic myelopathy. Report of two cases. J Neurosurg 1988; 68:466.
11. McArdle CB, Crofford MJ, Mirfakhraee M, et al. Surface coil MR of spinal trauma: preliminary experience. AJNR 1986; 7:885.
12. Nakstad P. Myelographic findings in cervical spines without degenerative changes. Neuroradiology 1987; 29:256.

13. Nelson E, Gertz SD, Rennels ML, et al. Spinal cord injury: the role of vascular damage in the pathogenesis of central hemorrhagic necrosis. Arch Neurol 1977; 32:332.
14. Osborne DRS, Vavoulis G, Nashold BS, et al. Late sequelae of spinal cord trauma: myelographic and surgical correlation. J Neurosurg 1982; 57:18.
15. Pang D, Wilberger JE. Spinal cord injury without radiographic abnormalities in children. J Neurosurg 1982; 57:114.
16. Penning L. Preveretebral hematoma in cervical spine injury: incidence and etiologic significance. AJNR 1980; 1:557.
17. Petras AF, Sobel DF, Mani JR, et al. CT myelography in cervical nerve root avulsion. J Comput Assist Tomogr 1985; 9:275.
18. Pollack IF, et al. Recurrent spinal cord injury without radiographic abnormalities in children. J Neurosurg 1988; 69:177.
19. Ruge JR, Sinson GP, McLone DG, et al. Pediatric spinal injury: the very young. J Neurosurg 1988; 68:25.
20. Scher AT. Unilateral locked facet in cervical spine injuries. Am J Roentgenol 1977; 129:45.
21. Sherman JL, Barkovich AJ, Citrin CA. The MR appearance of syringomyelia. New observations. AJNR 1986; 7:985.
22. Sze G, Brant-Zawadzki MN, Wilson CR, et al. Pseudotumor of the craniovertebral junction associated with chronic subluxation: MR imaging studies. Radiology 1986; 161:391.
23. Tarr RW, Drolshage LF, Kerner TC, et al. MR imaging of recent spinal trauma. J Comput Assist Tomogr 1987; 11:412.

7

Infection and Inflammation

Dieter R. Enzmann

INFECTIOUS SPONDYLITIS

Infections of the spine involve the vertebral body (osteomyelitis) or the disc space (discitis). In most instances, both regions are involved and therefore *infectious spondylitis*, a more accurate term,[25] is used in this chapter. The term *discitis* is reserved for special circumstances and described later.

In general, the axial skeleton is more frequently involved by infection in adults than in children. Spread of the infectious agent to the spine is believed to occur by three mechanisms[32]:

1. Hematogenous spread through the arterial system
2. Spread through the venous system via Batson's venous plexus
3. Direct inoculation via a diagnostic procedure or surgery

Hematogenous spread is seen in drug abusers who have a high incidence of infectious spondylitis. Batson's venous plexus is believed to be an important route from pelvic sources of infection,[11] which include urinary tract infections, enteric fistulae, surgery, and the postpartum state. Although the exact mechanism is not understood, the extensive, valveless venous plexus connecting the pelvic organs to the lumbar spine is believed to be a potential route of infection. Direct inoculation is usually secondary to surgery or some type of needle puncture for a diagnostic procedure or anesthesia.

Pyogenic spondylitis is commonly caused by *Staphylococcus aureus;* other organisms include streptococcus and gram-negative organisms.[24, 33] The latter, especially pseudomonas, are particularly common in intravenous drug abusers. The common cause of the nonpyogenic spondylitis is tuberculosis, although brucella and various fungi (coccidioidomycosis) can also be causes.[25] The causative organism may be identified by means of a blood culture, but this is the exception. Direct aspiration may be necessary. In nonpyogenic spondylitis, the organism can usually be identified only by tissue biopsy or aspiration.

Clinical symptoms for infectious spondylitis vary greatly and depend on the site, extent, and type of organism. In general, pyogenic spondylitis moves at a more rapid pace than the nonpyogenic type, although the time course is still measured in weeks. Pain is a common symptom, but its presentation varies from being intermittent to constant with a wide spectrum of severity. The patient may be febrile. Paraparesis is a late and rare finding. Nonpyogenic spondylitis is usually more insidious with a slower tempo, although the symptoms may be similar. With tuberculous spondylitis a pulmonary tuberculosis (TB) infection may be present.

Pathogenesis

In the first four weeks of infectious spondylitis the following events may take place. The infecting organism settles in the anterior subchondral space of the vertebral body where the

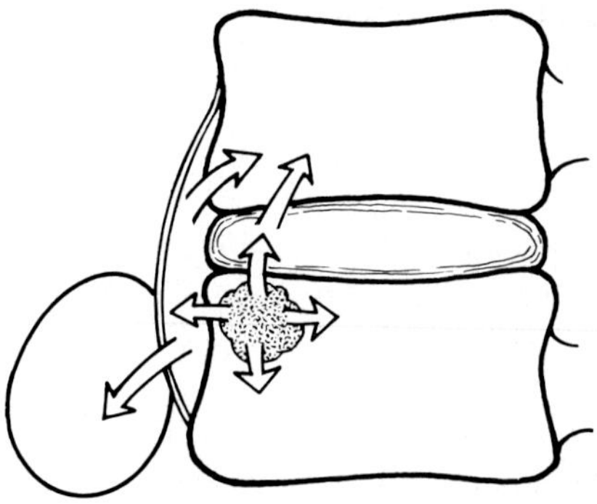

FIGURE 7-1. Schematic diagram of different routes of infection spread from presumed initial subchondral location. From this site, infection can spread to remainder of vertebral body into adjacent disc space or into anterior subligamentous space. From disc it can spread to adjacent vertebral body, obviously resulting in disc space abnormalities. From subligamentous space, spread can be to adjacent vertebra, sparing disc space. Disc space abnormalities may therefore not be evident. From subligamentous space infection can easily spread to paravertebral soft tissue.

infection gains a strong base (Figure 7-1). As it spreads contiguously, the infection may enter the disc space, causing both an osteomyelitis and a discitis.[18] From the disc space the infection then spreads through it to the adjacent vertebrae (Figure 7-1). The infection may, however, bypass the disc space, spread anteriorly into the subligamentous space, and from there track to an adjacent vertebra, thus sparing the disc space. This lack of disc space narrowing is often seen with, and characteristic of, tuberculous and fungal infections. From the subligamentous space the infection may penetrate through the ligament and infect the adjacent soft tissue.[18] In both pyogenic and nonpyogenic spondylitis it is unusual for one vertebra to be involved alone; this occurs in less than 1% of patients[26] (see Figure 7-12). Most often two adjacent vertebrae and the intervening disc show evidence of infection. It is uncommon for the infection to spread posteriorly within bone to involve the pedicles, transverse processes, or the spinous process. When present, this should suggest tuberculosis.

As the host responds to the infection or proper treatment is instituted, various degrees of regenerative processes occur over several weeks to months. The major response is that of bone sclerosis, which can be variable in degree and is present in both pyogenic and nonpyogenic spondylitis. The narrowed disc space may undergo partial or complete bony ankylosis. The degree of vertebral body preservation depends on when and if appropriate treatment is instituted; the earler the treatment, the greater the preservation. With lack of or inappropriate treatment, extensive bony lysis may take place causing significant, if not complete, collapse of the vertebrae. In tuberculous spondylitis, anterior wedging of the vertebral body causing a gibbus deformity is not uncommon.

The pathogenesis of nonpyogenic spondylitis is believed to be similar to the above sequence of events and routes of spread. The site of infection for tuberculous spondylitis, however, centers around L_1 with the frequency dropping off in either direction, becoming extremely rare in the cervical and sacral regions.[19] Although routes of spread through the disc space and the subligamentous regions are the same, the rapidity of spread is slower compared to pyogenic infections. Tuberculous spondylitis also appears to have a greater propensity for soft tissue invasion, especially in an anterolateral location,[30,43] causing the infection to extend to the psoas muscle and resulting in paravertebral abscess that has a strong tendency to calcify. Similar to pyogenic spondylitis, tuberculous spondylitis involves more than one vertebrae, usually in a contiguous fashion. Because the tempo of the infection is slower than pyogenic spondylitis, disc space narrowing is seen later in the course of the disease. Except for this difference in time course, the propensity for paravertebral abscess formation, and posterior element involvement, it can be difficult to differentiate tuberculous from pyogenic spondylitis on gross pathologic features alone (see Figure 7-8). MR may allow earlier diagnosis and thus the presentation of tuberculous spondylitis may be primarily soft tissue abnormality with minimal bony and disc space changes. The inflammatory tissue may be primarily in the spinal canal. Findings can therefore simulate metastatic disease of the spine. Involvement of the posterior bony elements appears to be more common with TB than with other infectious agents. Clinical history is an important consideration in correct diagnosis.

Discitis

As mentioned previously, pyogenic and nonpyogenic spondylitis often involve both the vertebral body and the adjacent disc space. The disc space is usually involved secondarily by extension from the adjacent vertebral body except in rare instances where the infection is caused by direct inoculation of the organism into the disc space. In such instances the infection starts as a discitis. Although there is some controversy regarding the entity of discitis, it may be appropriate to use this term in children, in whom because of the nature of the blood supply a direct hematogenous route to the disc space exists.[14,28] Because of this anatomic feature, an organism may gain direct access to the disc causing infection without first causing osteomyelitis in the adjacent vertebrae. This circumstance is limited to the pediatric age group.[42] In patients where this is suspected, an upper respiratory infection or ear infection is sometimes an antecedent event. The organism, however, is usually not isolated but is presumed to be bacterial. The sites of disc involvement in descending order are lumbar, thoracic, and cervical.[40] X-ray changes typically are subtle and not detectable until late in the disease process. When they become detectable, the hallmark is disc space narrowing, which at first is subtle and then becomes more obvious as the bony end-plates are eroded.[36] Because of the limited bone response, the end stage is similar to other forms of infectious spondylitis, which are also characterized by bone sclerosis and partial or complete bony fusion of the disc space.

Postoperative Discitis

Although the infection is not limited to the disc space, it begins and is most severe there. The route of spread is probably similar to that described for infectious spondylitis (Figures 7-2 and 7-3). Postoperative disc space infections

A, B

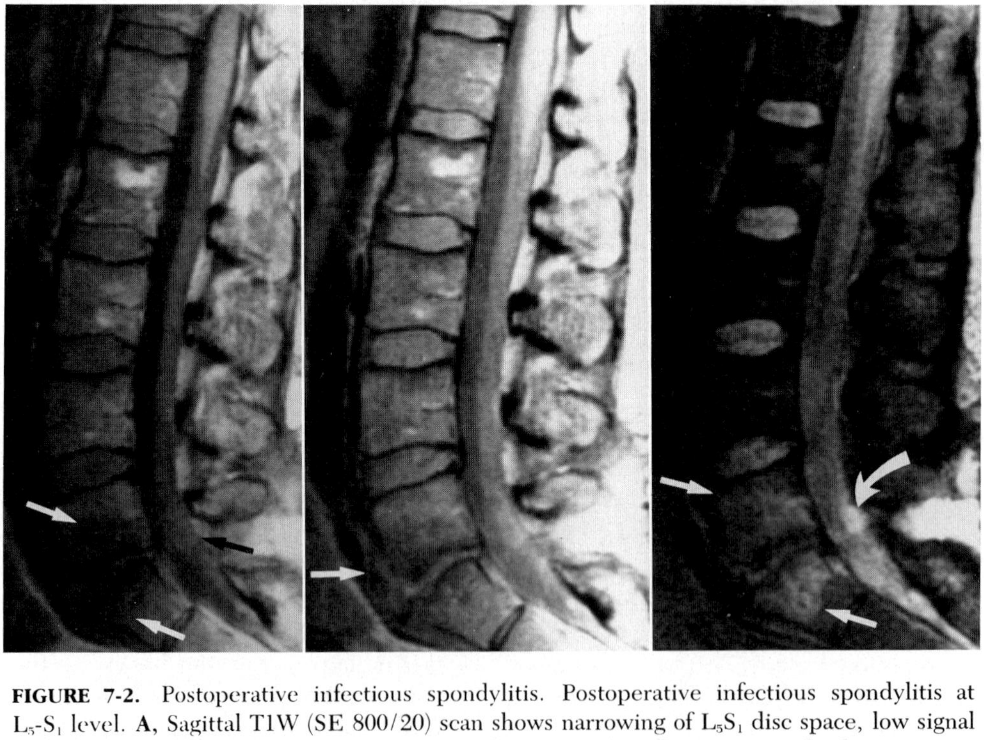

C

FIGURE 7-2. Postoperative infectious spondylitis. Postoperative infectious spondylitis at L_5-S_1 level. **A,** Sagittal T1W (SE 800/20) scan shows narrowing of L_5S_1 disc space, low signal intensity in L_5 and S_1 adjacent to disc space *(white arrows),* and suggestion of soft tissue mass *(black arrow)* in posterior spinal canal. Sagittal T2W scans show (**B,** SE 2000/20) soft tissue extension of inflammation under anterior spinal ligament *(arrow)* and (**C,** SE 2000/80) abnormal high signal in L_5 and S_1 vertebral bodies *(straight arrows)*. Focal area of high signal *(curved arrow)* in dorsal spinal canal at L_5-S_1 corresponds to suspected soft tissue abnormality on T1W scan (**A**). High signal intensity at postoperative site near spinous processes on T1W (**A**) and T2W (**C**) scans indicates hemorrhagic component. L_5-S_1 disc space signal intensity is similar to other disc spaces on T2W scan (**C**).

are not common, .2% to 3.0% of operations. The clinical setting and presentation are obviously a key to the diagnosis. One to four weeks after surgery, patients usually develop severe back pain, which can radiate into the legs, testes, perineum, and abdomen.[31] The pain is accompanied by paravertebral muscle spasm. Laboratory tests may show an elevated erythrocyte sedimentation rate (ESR) and usually a minimal increase in the white blood cell count.[31] The most common isolated organism is staphylococcus.

Conventional x-ray imaging is relatively insensitive to this type of infection but eventually shows changes such as end-plate erosion several weeks after clinical onset.[9] MR findings typical of infectious spondylitis with the changes in disc space and adjacent vertebral bodies present earlier. Evaluation of the bony end-plates may require phase and frequency axes swapping (see phase axes in Chapter 2) so that the frequency axis is perpendicular to the spine. Another approach is a water image that has fat signal suppressed. Bone is well seen in such an image, since there is no chemical-shift artifact.

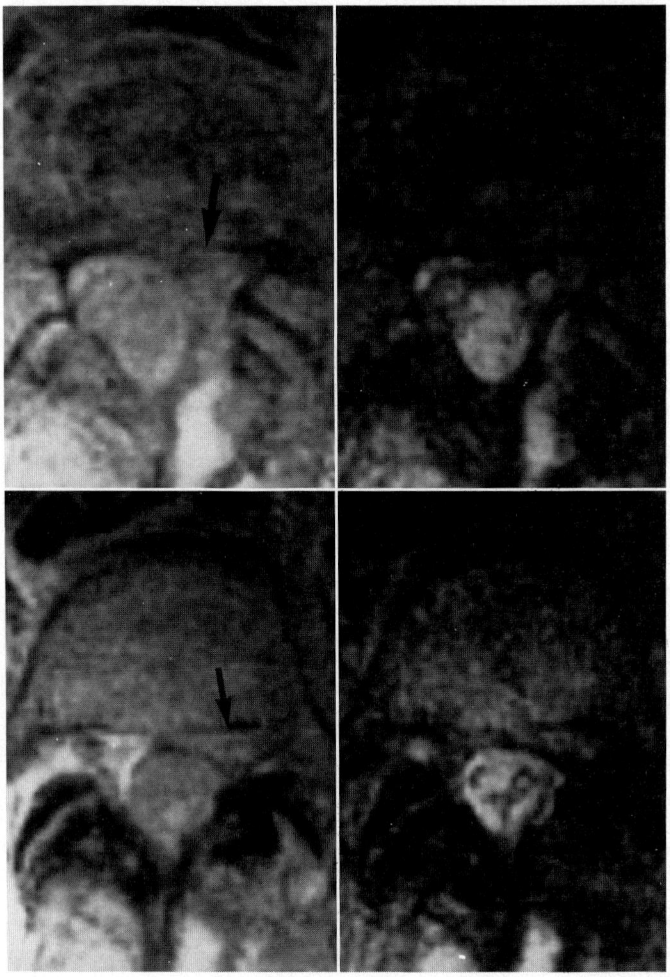

D E F G

FIGURE 7-2, cont'd. Axial T2W scans (SE 2000/20 (**D** and **F**) and T2W SE 2000/80 (**E** and **G**) show replacement of epidural fat in anterolateral recess on left (*arrow*, **D**) and at operative site (*arrow*, **F**). Second echos (**E** and **G**) show no significant impingement on dural sac. Only minimal arachnoiditis is detected as evidenced by adhesion of some of the nerve roots (**G**). Soft tissue postoperative changes may be difficult to differentiate from superimposed infection. Changes in vertebral bodies are pivotal to correct diagnosis and best seen on sagittal scans.

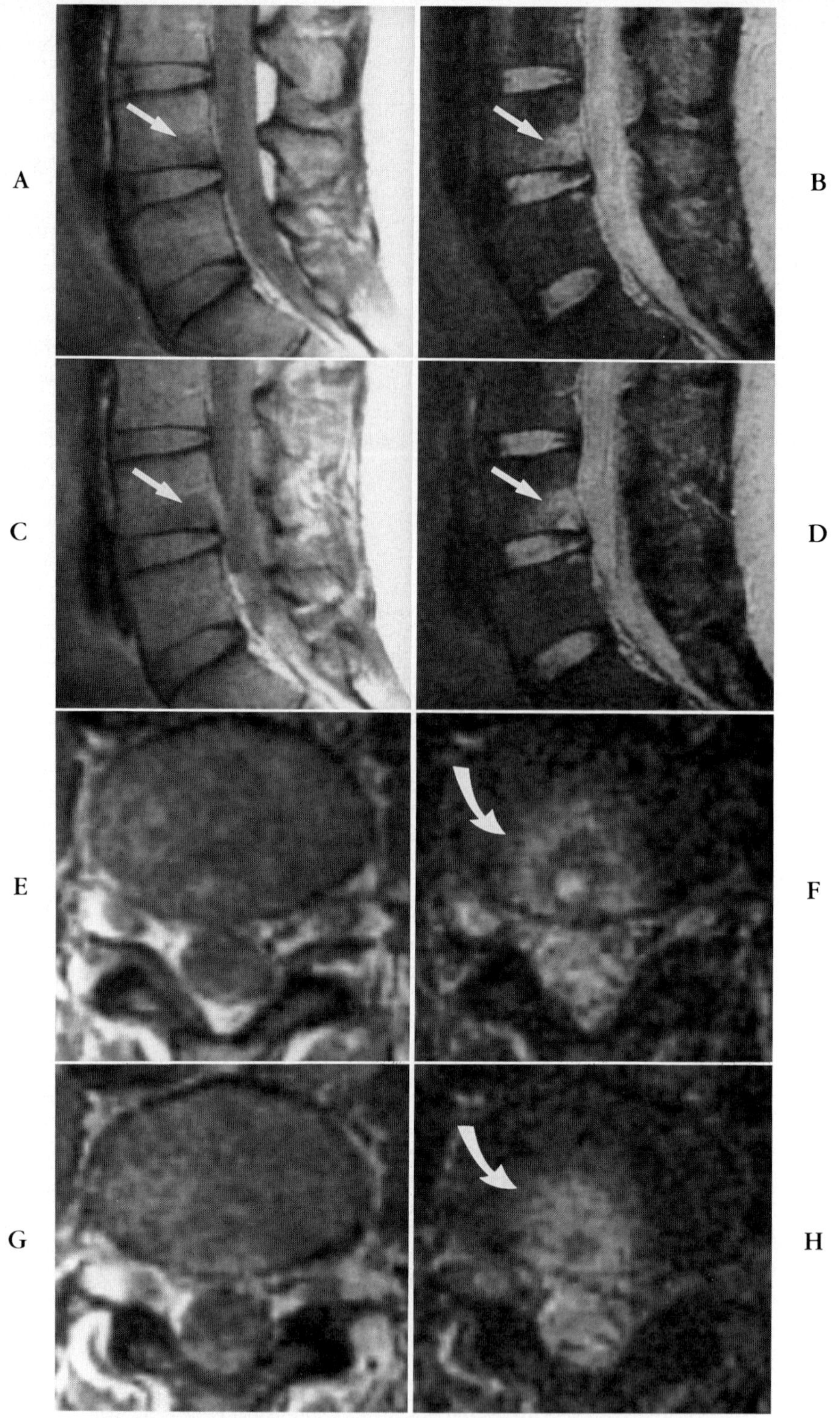

FIGURE 7-3. Infectious spondylitis, secondary to discography. Most abnormal findings appear in vertebral body rather than disc space. Sagittal T1W images (SE 800/20) show low signal in posterior-inferior portion of L_4 (*arrows*, **A** and **C**). Disc space is only minimally narrowed posteriorly. Note no abnormality is seen in L_5. T2W scan (SE gated 2500, 80) shows abnormal high signal intensity in same posterior-inferior portion of L_4 (*arrows*, **B** and **D**). It also shows a small focal area of increased signal in the supero-posterior aspect of L_5 (**B** and **D**). This is an important finding (i.e., two adjacent vertebrae) because it is strong evidence for infection. Axial T2W scans (SE 2500/20, 80) show minimal abnormality on first echo (**E** and **G**) but distinct area of abnormal high signal in vertebral body on second echo (*arrows*, **F** and **H**). Small focal area of marked increased signal intensity corresponds to same area seen on sagittal scan adjacent to disc space (**D**).

MR Findings

MR findings reflect two major characteristics of this disease process: replacement of bone marrow by inflammatory tissue and associated structural changes, i.e., narrowing of the disc space. The relative signal intensity on T1W scans of the inflammatory tissue depends on the intensity of the vertebral body marrow signal, which varies with age. The displacement of marrow by inflammatory tissue is usually seen as abnormal low signal intensity within the vertebral body on T1W images (Figures 7-4 to 7-7; see Figures 7-2 and 7-3). In young children the axial skeleton has a low signal intensity of marrow compared to adults and replacement by inflammatory tissue is more difficult to detect on T1W images. In elderly patients the infection may be of relatively higher signal than the marrow signal (Figure 7-8). This finding should also suggest tuberculosis. A finding highly suggestive of infectious spondylitis is that of vertebral body signal abnormality in adjacent vertebrae even if the intervening disc space is normal. Less characteristic but still suggestive is involvement of only one vertebral body but associated soft tissue swelling (Figure 7-12). Disc space involvement is seen as a physical narrowing of the disc space and as a loss of signal of the nucleus pulposus on T1W images (see Figures 7-2, 7-4, and 7-6). It may show complete obliteration (see Figure 7-5).

The disc space narrowing can also be identified on T2W images. The disc on T2W images may show normal, decreased, or increased signal, higher than normally seen (see Figure 7-4).[29] On T2W images, abnormal increased signal is seen within the vertebral body in regions where one would expect little signal if normal marrow were present (see Figure 7-5). These alterations in signal intensities within the vertebral bodies are accentuated and highlighted by pulse sequences that show only fat signal or water signal (see Figures 7-6, 7-8 and 7-12). Water or fat pulse sequences (including STIR sequences) are used to show abnormal signal intensity within vertebral bodies representing abnormal water content caused by the inflammatory tissue[4] (see Figure 7-6). STIR sequences may have a role in detection of infectious spondylitis. Use of a contrast medium, such as GdDTPA, may have limited application because it can obscure findings (see Figure 7-6). In unusual circumstances there may be multiple sites of involvement. Even more unusual is involvement of the posterior elements without vertebral body involvement (see Figure 7-7). In most patients, bone and disc abnormalities are accompanied by adjacent inflammatory tissue—anterior subligamentous or epidural in the spinal canal (see Figure 7-5). This soft tissue may be granulation tissue or a true abscess and can cause cord compression (see Figure 7-5).

In some instances the vertebral body osteomyelitis is not associated with significant abnormal soft tissue beyond the confines of the vertebral body. In fact, a T1W scan may not show an abnormality, whereas a T2W scan will (Figures 7-3 and 7-9). With significant disc space involvement, however, abnormal soft tissue adjacent to the vertebral body becomes more prominent. Normal fat-water tissue planes are obscured. Although bone is not well seen on MR scans, the low signal intensity from cortical margins becomes difficult to delineate or is lost altogether. This is seen only with extensive disease and marked bony destruction. Cortical margins are well seen on a balanced image, i.e., first echo of a T2W sequence (see Figure 7-5). A water image (i.e., no fat signal) also shows cortical margins well. It is important to be sure that the lack of cortical margin is not caused by a chemical-shift artifact where fat signal is superimposed on the cortical margin. This can be determined by knowing the direction of the phase and frequency encoding axes and by comparing the findings with other vertebral bodies that should experience the same chemical shift artifact.

The end-stage of infectious spondylitis shows narrowing of the disc space or partial-to-complete obliteration by fusion of the vertebral bodies (Figure 7-10), which develop one to two years after the acute infection. Acute inflammatory changes in the vertebral bodies and surrounding soft tissue will have regressed. Often marrow fat destroyed or replaced by the infection is not restored. In nonpyogenic spondylitis anterior wedging is a common finding resulting in a gibbus deformity (Figures 7-11 and 7-12).

Although clinical experience is limited, MR appears to be as sensitive and specific as radionuclide scans (bone, Gallium, white cell) in detecting infectious spondylitis.[29] With use of a contrast agent, MR will likely replace the role of CT in the workup of this disease process. In combination with a high index of clinical suspicion, MR findings will allow accurate diagnosis of this entity.

Text continued on p. 278.

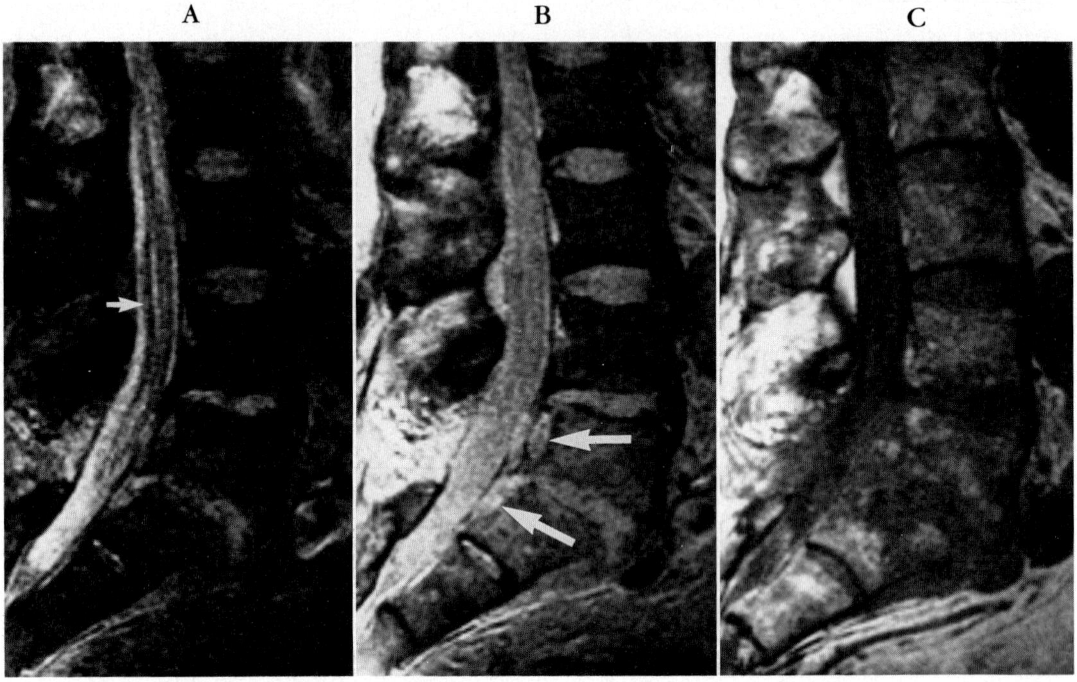

FIGURE 7-4. Staphylococcal infectious spondylitis. Patient with staphylococcal sepsis developed infectious spondylitis involving L_5 and S_1 and, in addition, epidural abscess formed at L_5-S_1 in spinal canal. **A,** T1W scan (SE 800/20) shows extensive destruction of L_4-L_5 and L_5-S_1 disc spaces, L_5 vertebral body, and superior portion of S_1 vertebral body. Abnormal soft tissue in prevertebral space at level of L_5-S_1. **B,** Sagittal first echo, balanced image of T2W sequence (SE gated 2100/30, 80), shows similar findings and bony margins of vertebral bodies are better delineated than on T1W sequence (**A**). Although T1W scan (**A**) showed abnormal soft tissue in spinal canal, epidural location of inflammatory tissue of high signal intensity is better appreciated on "balanced image" (**B,** *arrows*). **C,** More heavily T2W second echo image shows abnormal high signal in L_5 and S_1 vertebral bodies and also in narrowed L_4-L_5 and L_5-S_1 disc spaces. Abnormal epidural inflammatory tissue behind L_5 and S_1 seen as areas of high signal intensity and represent epidural extension of infection. Mild clumping of nerve roots suggests mild arachnoiditis *(arrow)*. Axial T2W scan (SE gated 2100/80) at level of L_5 and S_1 shows abnormal high signal soft tissue in anterior epidural space, representing infection-abscess (*arrows,* **D, F,** and **G**). Extradural defect mass effect deforming dural sac can be appreciated at all levels **D-G**). Right L_5 root sleeve is obliterated by this process (**E**). Infection not limited to bone, disc space, and epidural space but also involves psoas muscles and large portion of posterior paraspinous musculature, seen as high signal behind lamina on all axial images **D-G**). Postcontrast CT scans (**H** and **I**) show marked contrast enhancement in epidural space paraspinous musculature with low density areas suggesting abscess formation (*arrow,* **I**).

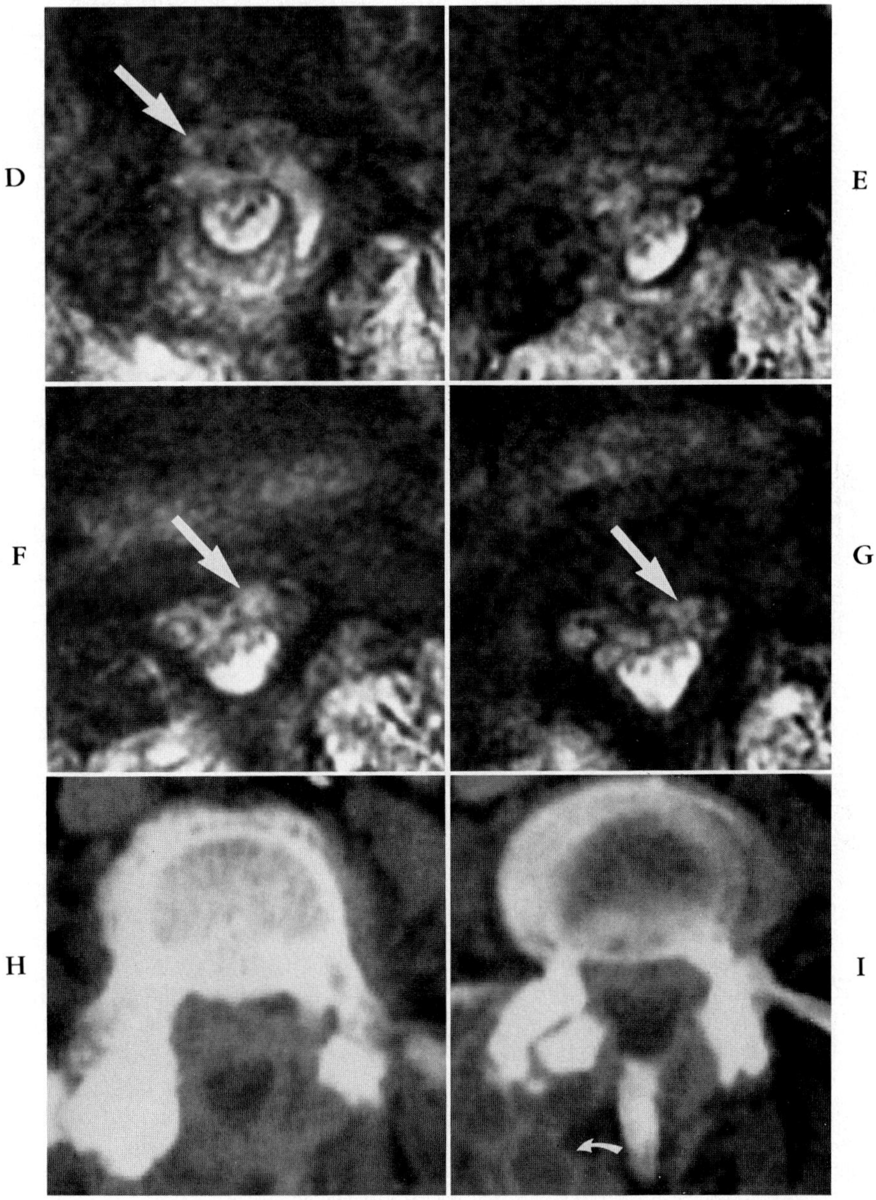
D
E
F
G
H
I

A, B

C

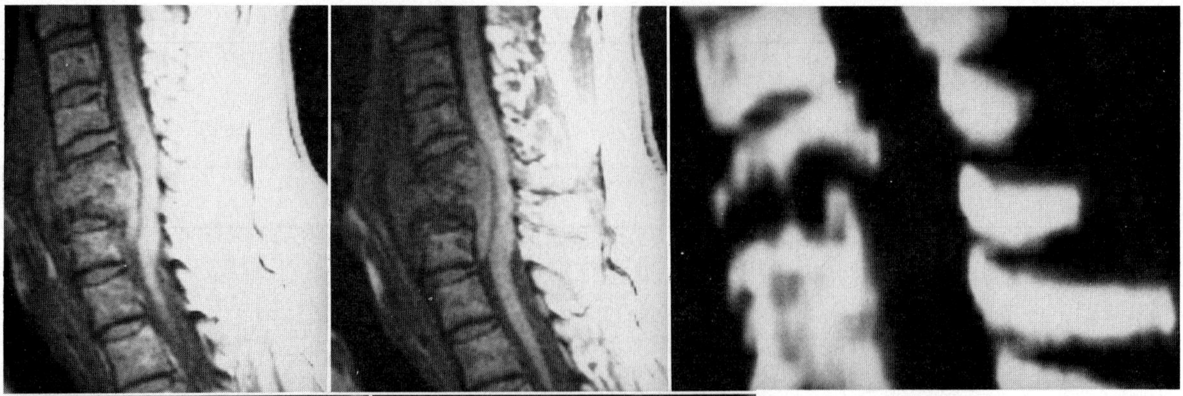

D, E

F, G

H, I

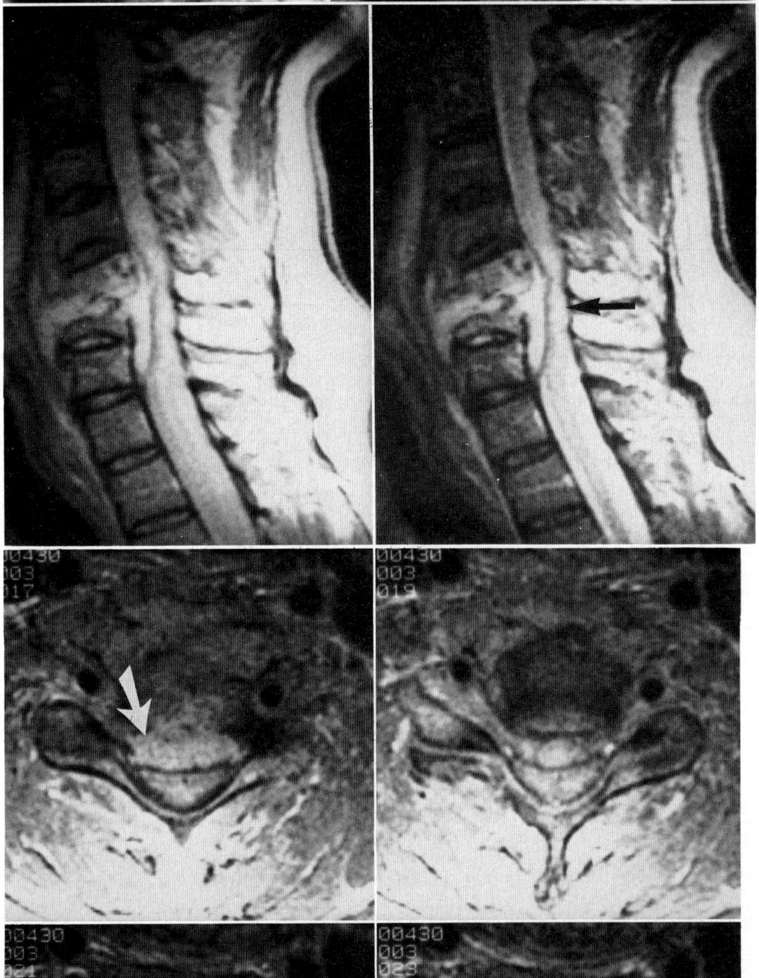

FIGURE 7-5. Staphylococcal infectious spondylitis. Typical findings of aggressive infectious spondylitis caused by staphylococcus. In addition to vertebral body and disc space involvement, large epidural abscess also present. **A** and **B,** T1W scans (SE 600/20) show marked destruction of C_5 and C_6 vertebral bodies with complete obliteration of intervening disc space. Significant abnormal soft tissue is both anterior and posterior to vertebral bodies with posterior component causing significant cord compression. **C,** Reformatted CT scan shows extensive destruction of bony vertebrae and disc space. Sagittal T2W sequence (SE gated 2200/35/70) shows destruction of C_5 and C_6 vertebrae. Note that **D,** first echo of pulse sequence shows bone margins to good advantage and therefore destruction of cortical margins is well seen. **E,** Second echo shows abnormal signal intensity within destroyed vertebral bodies and marked high signal in associated soft tissue, especially in intraspinal component. High signal suggests fluid content indicative of epidural abscess with purulent center. Note also increased signal intensity of compressed cord indicating tissue damage *(arrow)*. **F-I,** Set of four axial images of first echo T2W sequence shows large, well-circumscribed epidural abscess in spinal canal causing cord compression *(arrows)*. Abnormal soft tissue infiltrating neural foramina and surrounding vertebral arteries bilaterally. (Courtesy of Dr. Brant-Zawadski.)

A B

C, D

E, F

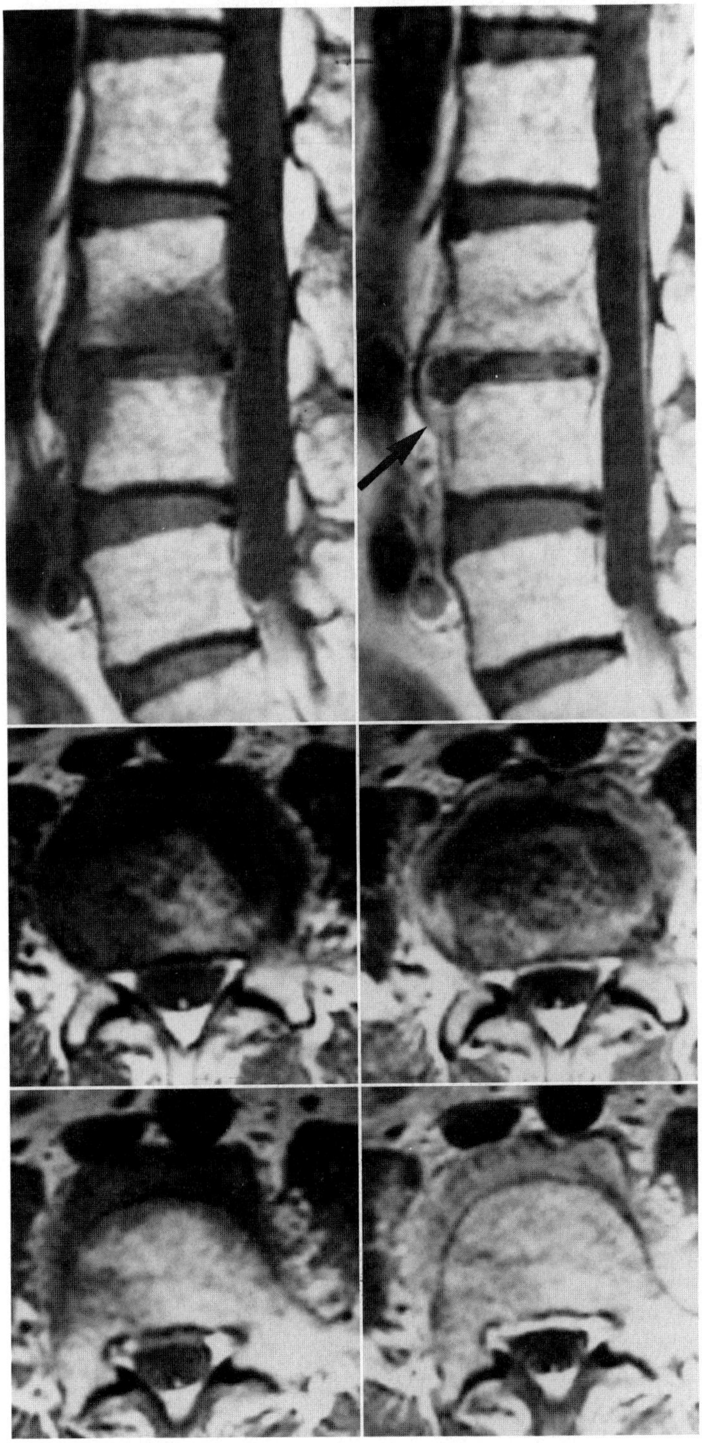

FIGURE 7-6. Aspergillus infectious spondylitis. The use of GdDTPA can obscure MR findings in infectious spondylitis. **A,** Noncontrast T1W scan (SE 800/20) shows typical findings of infectious spondylitis with low signal intensity in adjacent vertebral bodies (L_3 and L_4) associated with disc space narrowing. The disc is of near normal intensity. An anterior subligamentous mass is also present at the L_3-L_4 disc space level. **B,** Post-GdDTPA T1W scan (SE 800/20) shows contrast enhancement of these low signal areas, bringing the signal intensity up to equivalent of that of adjacent normal marrow, thus decreasing their contrast and conspicuity. There is no significant enhancement of the disc space, although inflammatory tissue in the anterior subligamentous space does show enhancement *(arrow)*. Contrast medium such as GdDTPA, therefore, can obscure the delineation of infectious spondylitis. **C-F,** Similar findings are seen on axial precontrast (**C** and **E**) and postcontrast (**D** and **F**) T1W scans (SE 800/20) of the L_3-L_4 disc space. The noncontrast scans (**C** and **E**) show a mottled appearance of the end-plate and abnormal soft tissue mass in the anterior subligamentous space. The post contrast scans (**D** and **F**) show enhancement within marrow space (**D**) and within subligamentous inflammatory tissue (**D** and **F**). Although the findings remain, they are less conspicuous. Postcontrast scans alone, therefore, are not recommended for the investigation of infectious spondylitis.

Continued.

G H I J

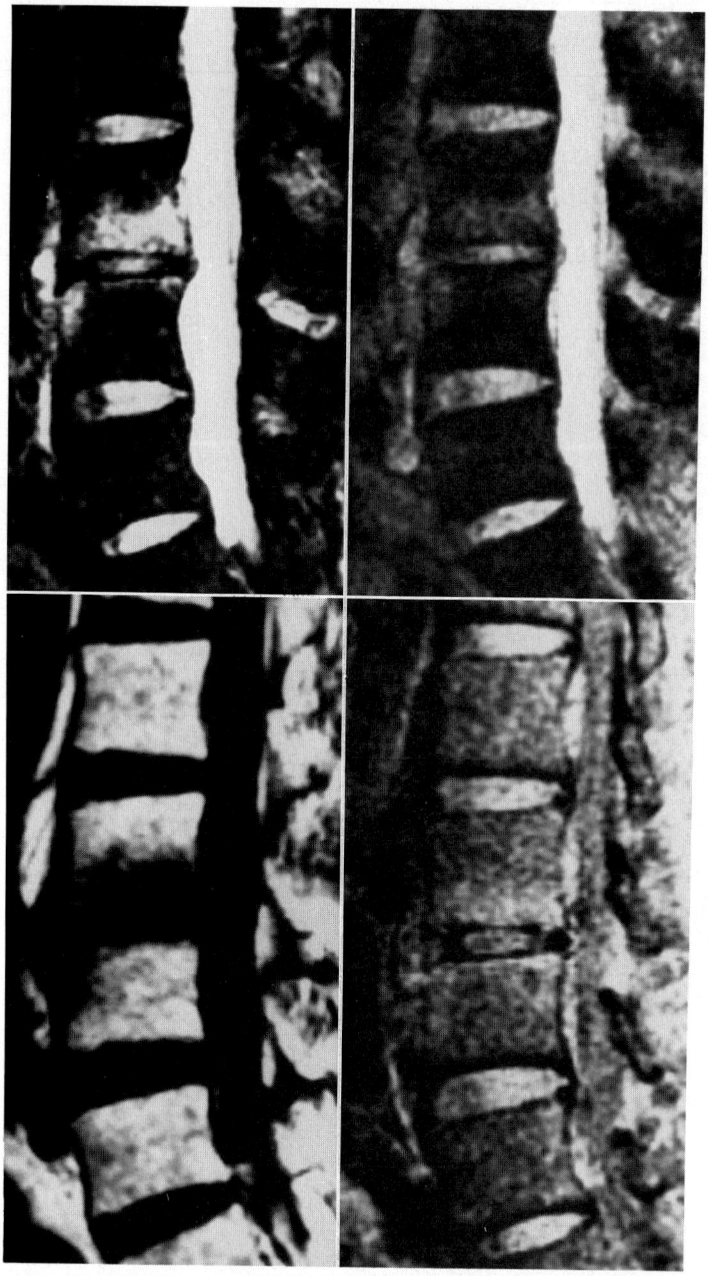

FIGURE 7-6, cont'd. **G,** Sagittal STIR image (IR 1500/40, T1 160) exhibits prominent high signal intensity in adjacent vertebral bodies and in inflammatory tissue in the anterior subligamentous space. High signal corresponds to low signal areas on the T1W image, (**A**). Disc space narrowing is evident, as is some decrease in signal in the disc space. **H,** Sagittal variable flip angle scan (GRASS 40/20, 5°) shows similar findings as the STIR image but signal intensity abnormalities are lower, resulting in lower contrast. Nevertheless the inflammatory tissue in the vertebral body and anterior subligamentous space is seen as high signal. **I,** "Fat" T1W image (SE 800/30) shows displacement of marrow fat by imflammatory tissue in the vertebral bodies in a distribution similar to the low signal on a T1W image (**A**) and the high signal on the STIR (**G**) and variable flip angle (**H**) scans. This represents replacement of fatty marrow by inflammatory infiltrate. **J,** "Water" image (SE 800/30) shows some increased signal in the vertebral bodies adjacent to the narrowed and low signal intensity L_3-L_4 disc space. Abnormal signal intensity is not as high as seen on the STIR image. This image suggests that cortical bone destruction is not yet extensive because the thin black lines outlining the vertebral bodies are only minimally disrupted.

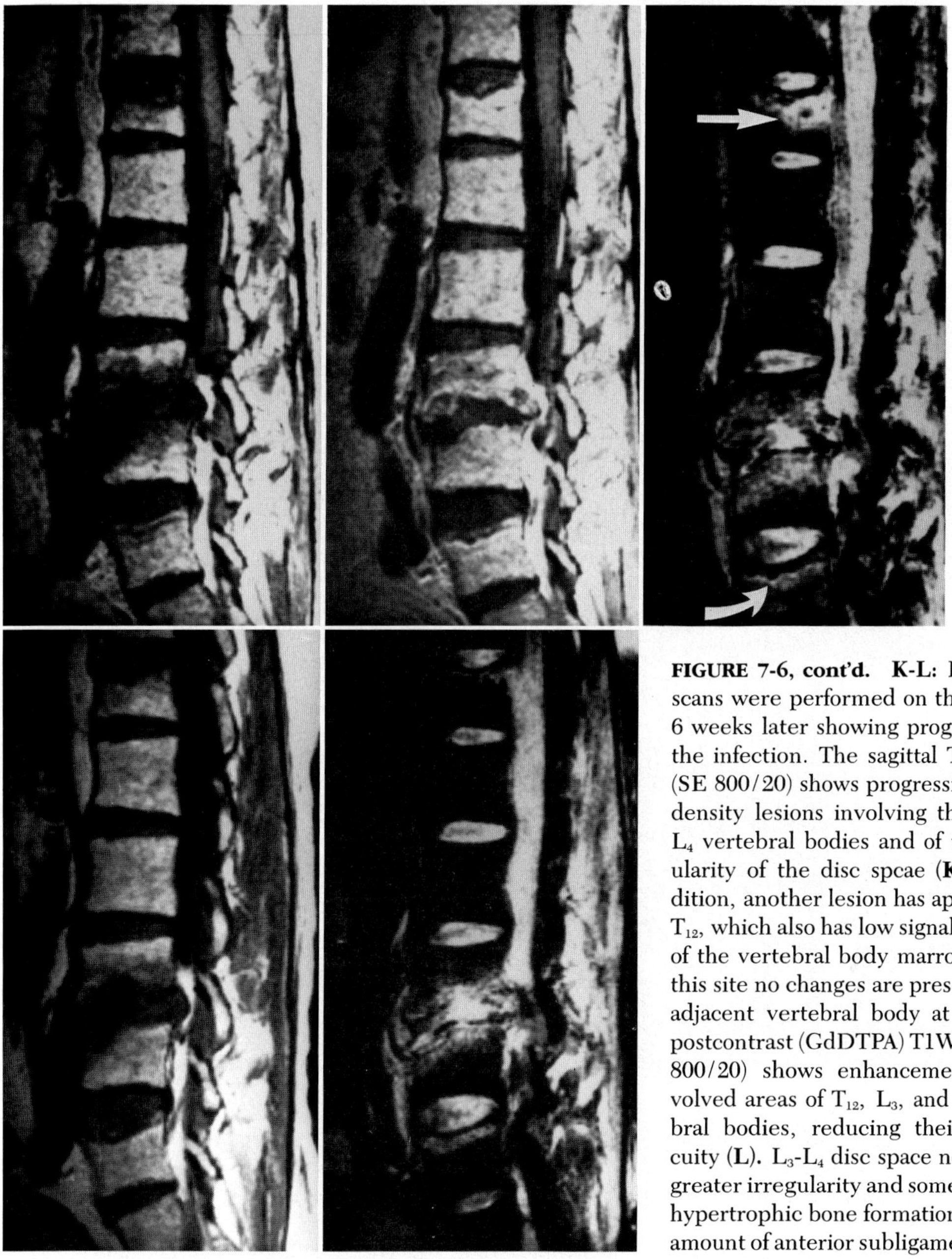

K

L, M

O

FIGURE 7-6, cont'd. K-L: Follow-up scans were performed on this patient 6 weeks later showing progression of the infection. The sagittal T1W scan (SE 800/20) shows progression of low density lesions involving the L_3 and L_4 vertebral bodies and of the irregularity of the disc spcae (**K**). In addition, another lesion has appeared at T_{12}, which also has low signal intensity of the vertebral body marrow, but at this site no changes are present in the adjacent vertebral body at T_{11}. The postcontrast (GdDTPA) T1W scan (SE 800/20) shows enhancement of involved areas of T_{12}, L_3, and L_4 vertebral bodies, reducing their conspicuity (**L**). L_3-L_4 disc space now shows greater irregularity and some adjacent hypertrophic bone formation (**L**). The amount of anterior subligamentous infection has not increased compared to the earlier scan (compared with Figures **A** and **B**). **M:** A sagittal STIR scan (1800/40, TI 150) better illustrates progression of the infection at T_{12} and L_3-L_4 sites. This scan shows additional involvement of L_5 as evidenced by high signal intensity within the marrow, a finding not detectable on the T1W scan (**K**). The STIR scan was most sensitive to the extent of disease and its progression (compared with **G**). **N:** Sagittal noncontrast T1W scan (SE 800/20) obtained 8 weeks after the initial scan *(A-J)* now shows some healing of the lesions at L_3-L_4 and T_{12}. The extent of low signal abnormality is decreased in all of the involved vertebrae. Involvement of L_5 is not evident on the T1W scan. **O:** A STIR scan (1400/40, TI 150) concurrent with the T1W scan (**N**) shows residual high signal intensity in T_{12}, L_3, L_4, and L_5. The degree and extent of high signal abnormality, however, is less compared to the previous STIR (**M**) scan obtained 2 weeks earlier. This *aspergillus* infection is now in the healing stage and the STIR scan shows well the regression of abnormal high signal intensity within the vertebral bodies and disc spaces.

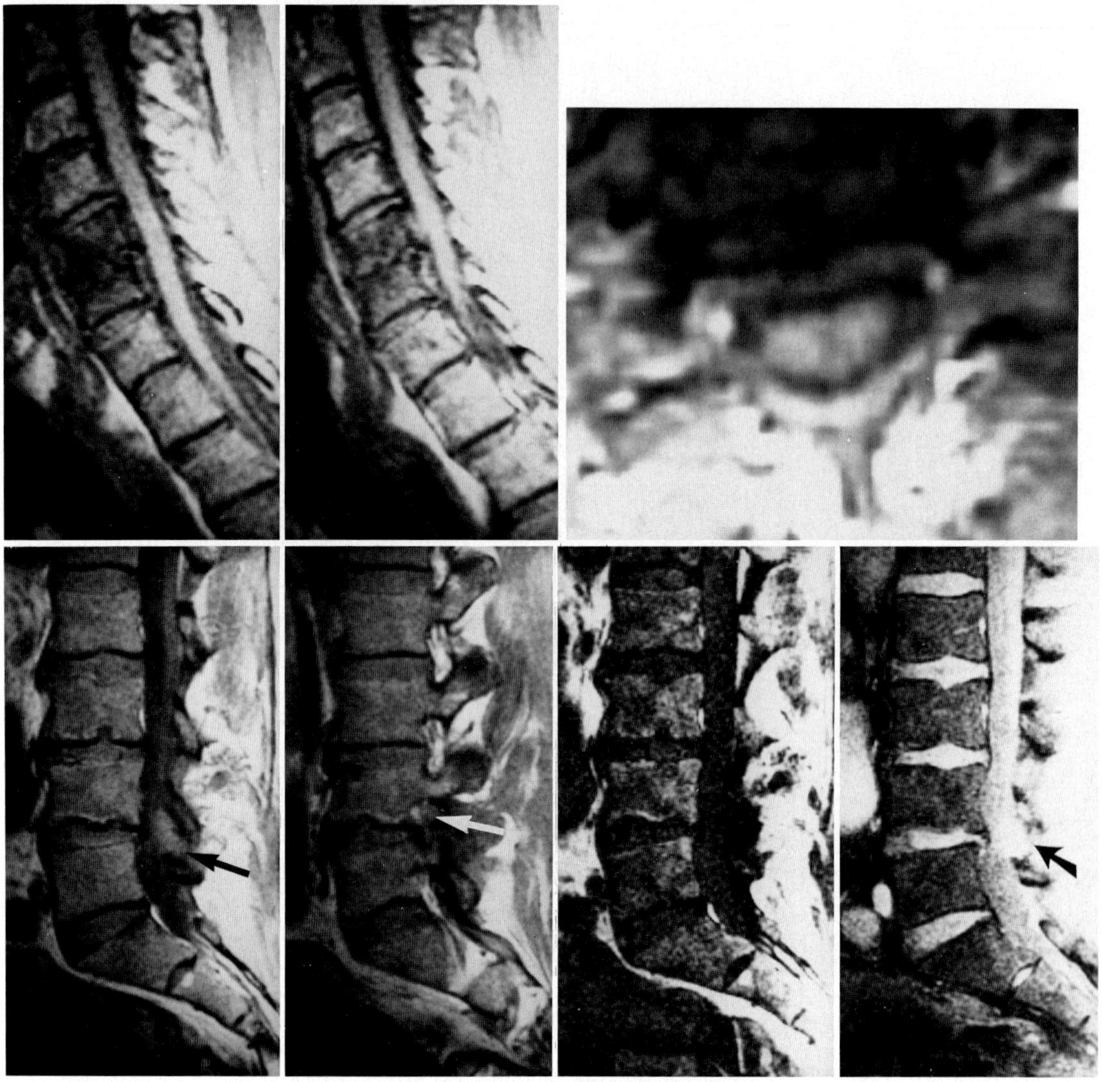

FIGURE 7-7. Streptococcal infectious spondylitis. Infectious spondylitis secondary to beta-streptococcal bacteremia in 70-year-old male with diabetes mellitus. Patient exhibited two simultaneous sites of involvement, in cervical and lumbar spine. Approximately 1 week before MR scans, bone scan was interpreted as equivocal. **A** and **B**, In cervical region, sagittal T1W scans (SE 800/20) show expected changes of abnormal low signal in vertebral bodies, destruction of C_5-C_6 disc space, and abnormal soft tissue posterior to vertebral bodies causing mild posterior displacement of cervical cord. **C**, Axial T1W scan (SE, 1000/20) shows rind of abnormal soft tissue in epidural space at this level. In lumbar spine, manifestation of infectious spondylitis was more unusual in that it involved posterior elements, i.e., lamina and ligamentum flavum, to greater extent than vertebral body and disc space. **D**, Sagittal T1W scan (SE 800/20) shows abnormal soft tissue in dorsal lumbar canal at L_4-L_5 level *(arrow)*. **E**, More lateral slice shows extension of soft tissue mass into intervertebral foramen *(arrow)*. **F**, Corresponding "fat" image and **G**, "water" image show no involvement of vertebral body or disc space. There is abnormal high water signal in posterior spinal canal in soft tissue mass *(arrow)*. **H-K,** Axial T1W scans (SE 1000/20) show unusual nature of inflammatory tissue because it involves right lamina (*arrow,* **I**), apophyseal joint and ligamentum flavum (*arrow,* **K**). Corresponding T2W images (SE, gated 2200/80) show abnormal high signal intensity in inflammatory mass (*arrow,* **M**) and extradural defect caused by involvement of ligamentum flavum (*arrows,* **N** and **O**).

H I J K L M N O

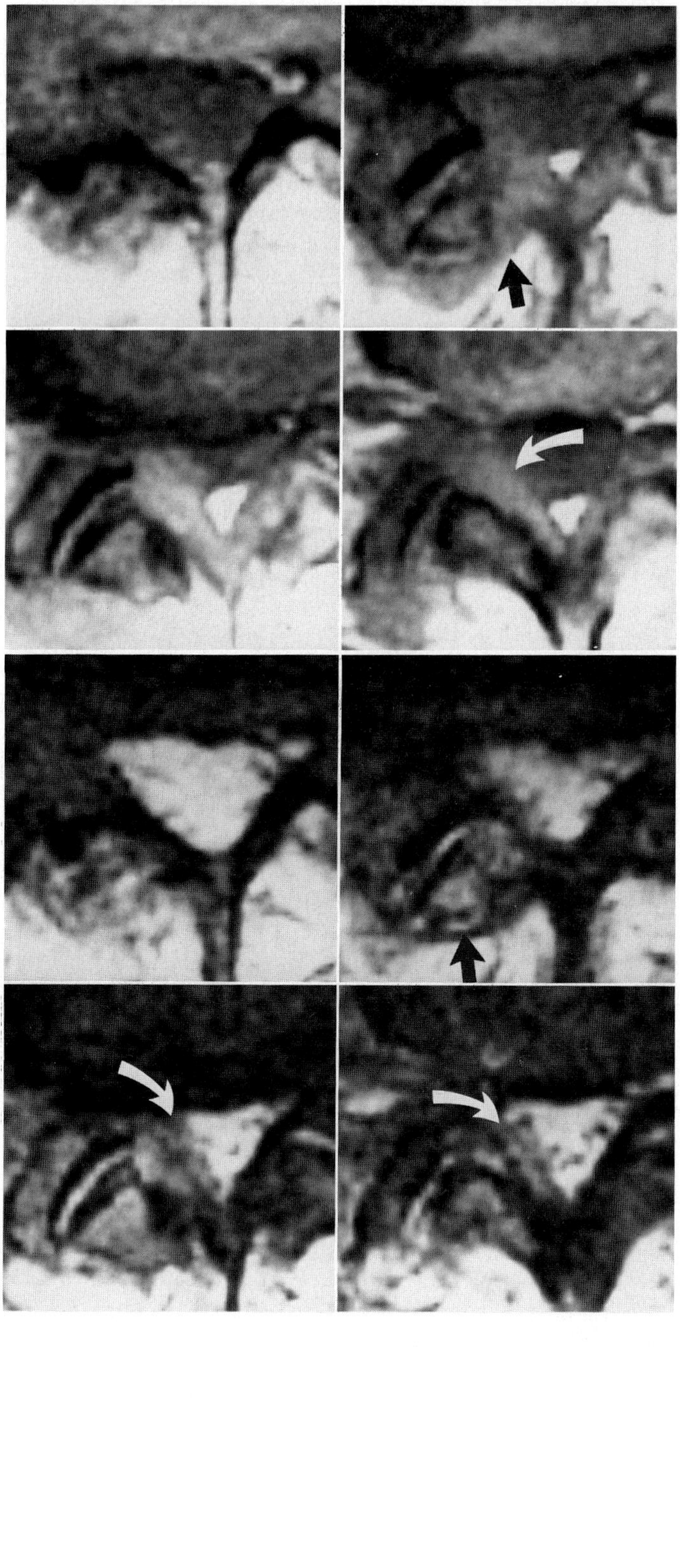

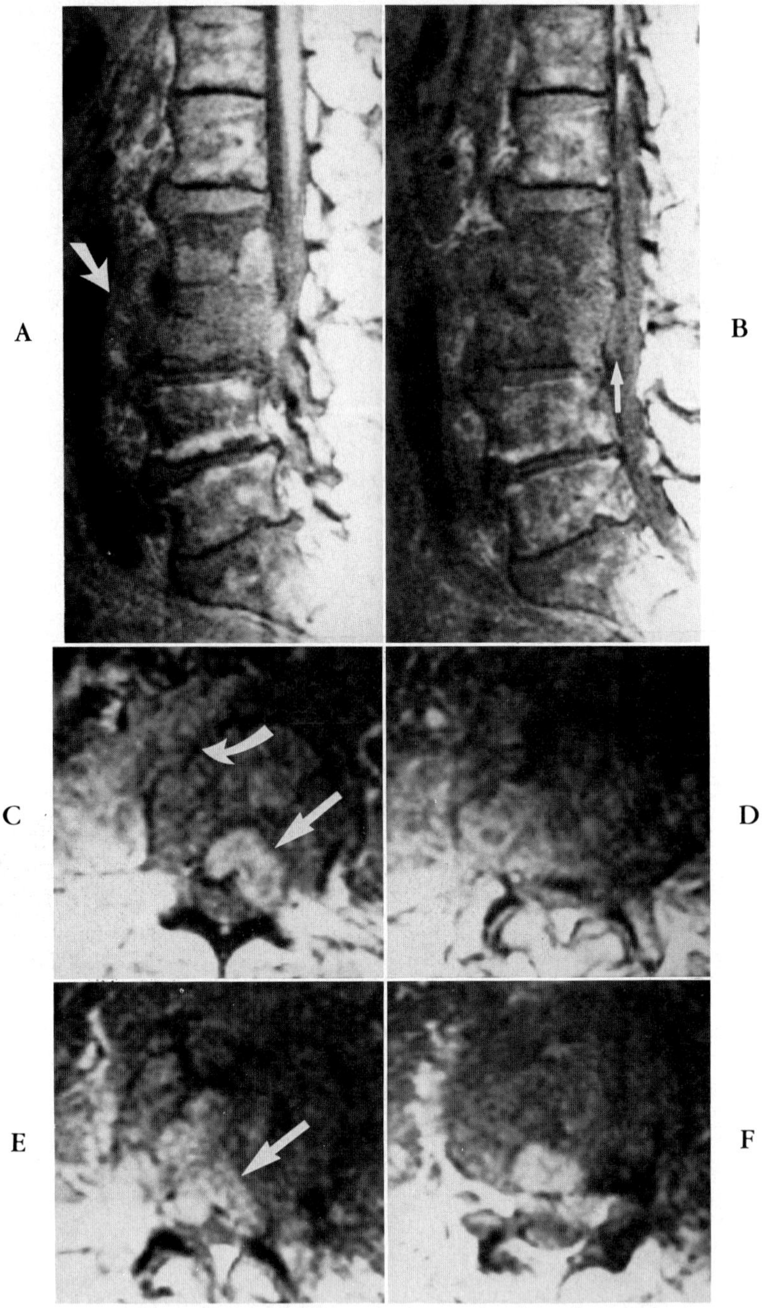

FIGURE 7-8. Tuberculous infectious spondylitis. Typical vertebral body destruction, disc space narrowing, and adjacent soft tissue masses in prevertebral location and within the spinal canal of patient with tuberculous spondylitis. **A** and **B**, Sagittal T1W scans (SE 800/20) show marked destruction of L_2-L_3 disc space and markedly abnormal signal in L_2 and L_3 vertebral body. Vertebral body cortical margins poorly visualized in inferior portion of L_2 and most of L_3. Inflammatory tissue is slightly higher signal intensity compared to upper half of L_2 and inhomogenous signal intensity of L_4 and L_5. Inflammatory tissue extends into prevertebral space (*arrow*, **A**) and spinal canal, compressing cauda equina (*arrow*, **B**). Axial T1W scans (SE 1000/20) show significant intraspinal component of inflammatory tissue (*arrow*, **C** and **E**), which causes spinal stenosis (**D** and **E**). Extension of inflammatory mass through the disrupted cortical margin is visualized on right (*curved arrow*, **C**).

G H I J

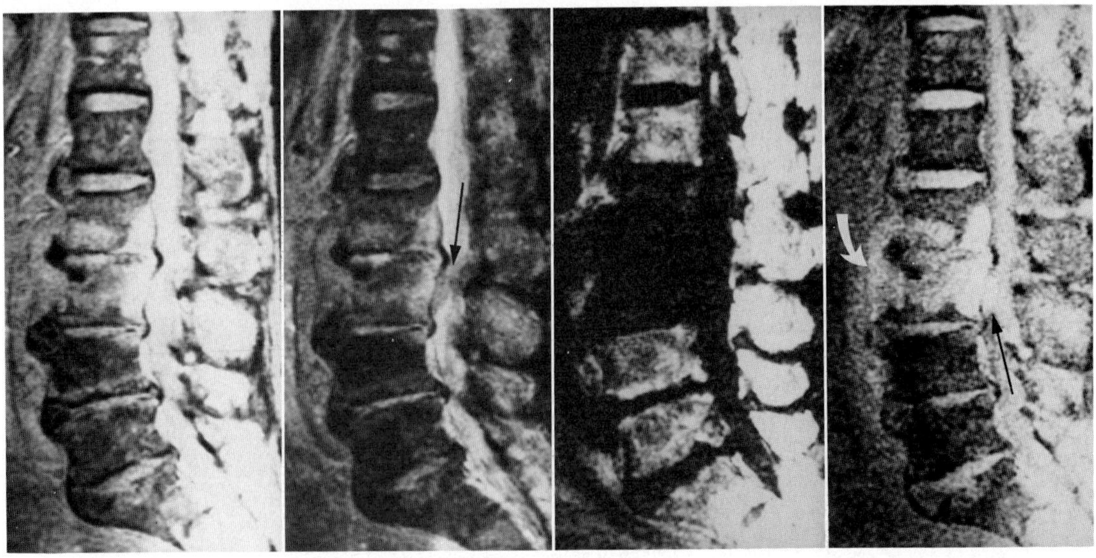

FIGURE 7-8, cont'd. **G** and **H,** Sagittal T2W scan (gated SE 2000/20, 80) at same level as image **A** shows inflammatory tissue of high signal intensity on both echoes. First echo image (**G**) shows disruption of cortical margins, especially anterior margins of L_2 and L_3. Disc spaces appear relatively spared. Epidural mass in spinal canal best visualized on second echo (*arrow,* **H**). Most severely involved disc space (L_2-L_3) shows abnormal high signal intensity on second echo image (**H**). Note T1W images show low signal intensity in some regions and T2W images show abnormal high signal intensity throughout vertebrae. **I,** "Water-suppressed," i.e., fat, image shows complete replacement of marrow fat in L_2-L_3 vertebral body. **J,** "Fat-suppressed," i.e., water, image shows abnormal high signal in L_2 and L_3 in similar configuration as relative high signal seen on T2W images. "Fat-suppressed" image also shows high signal in prevertebral extension *(curved arrow)* and in epidural component *(straight arrow)*. Even in low signal portion of L_2 on T1W image (**A**), water content is slightly increased and fat has been completely replaced, showing total involvement of vertebral body by this infection.

A

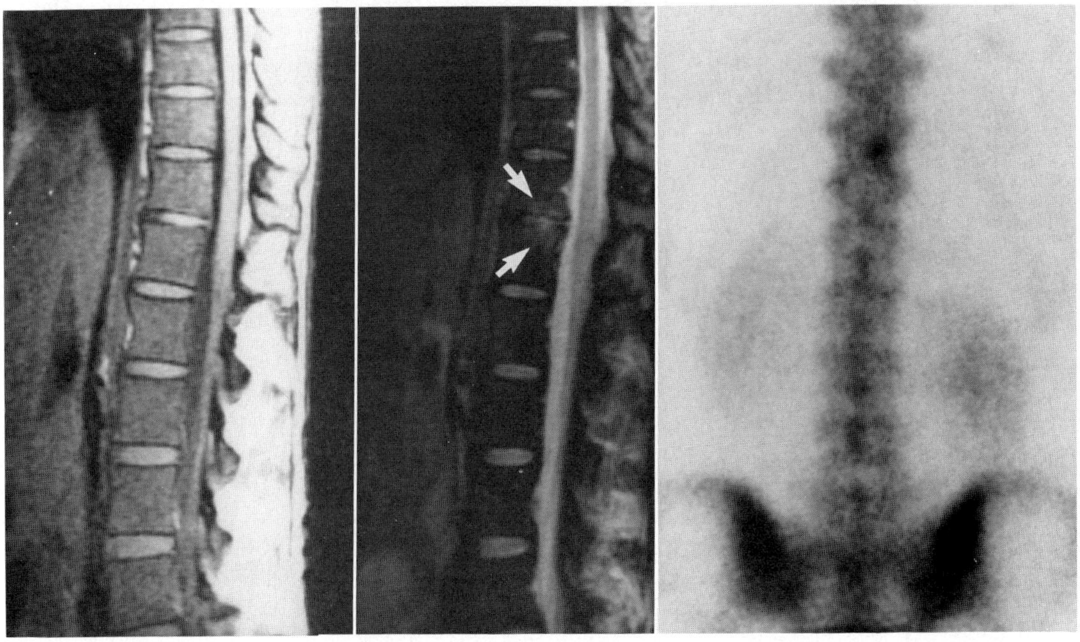

B, C

FIGURE 7-9. Infectious sypondylitis. Subtle form of infectious spondylitis involved T_{11}-T_{12} in febrile patient with mitral valve prolapse. **A,** T1W scan (SE 800/20) shows no significant abnormality except for minimal disc space narrowing at T_{11}-T_{12}. There is no evidence of abnormal signal within vertebral body or disc. **B,** T2W scan (SE gated 1900/80) confirms disc space narrowing at this level and shows abnormal high signal intensity in adjacent vertebral bodies *(arrows)*. **C,** Bone scan positive at this level.

A 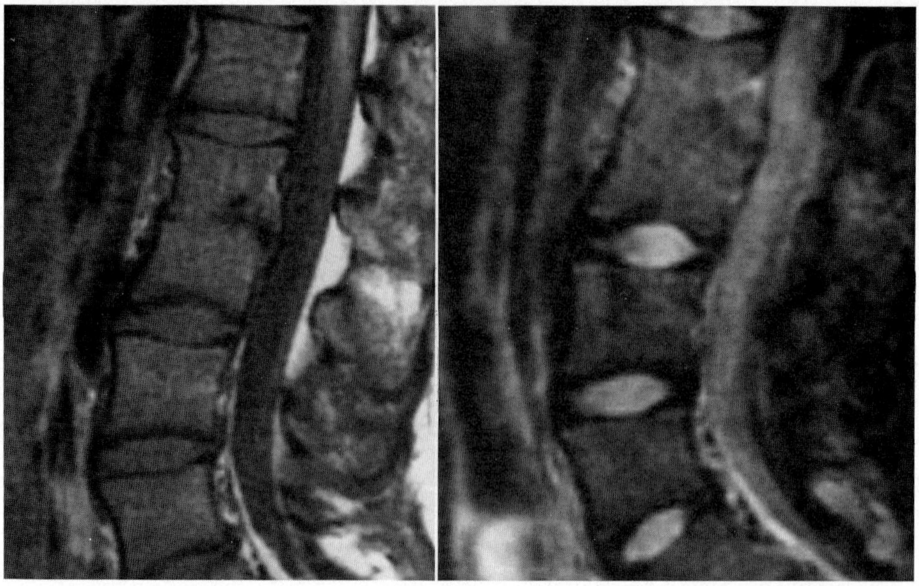 B

FIGURE 7-10. End stage infectious spondylitis. **A,** Sagittal T1W scan (SE 800/20) of 15-year-old female shows end stage of infectious spondylitis with nearly complete obliteration of L_2-L_3 disc space. Note despite marked loss of disc space, vertebral bodies are relatively intact. This is not uncommon in child age group where more pure form of "discitis" is thought to occur. **B,** T2W image (SE 1500/70) confirms near total obliteration of disc space and fusion of L_2-L_3 vertebral bodies. Abnormal high signal intensity still seen throughout both vertebral bodies.

A, B 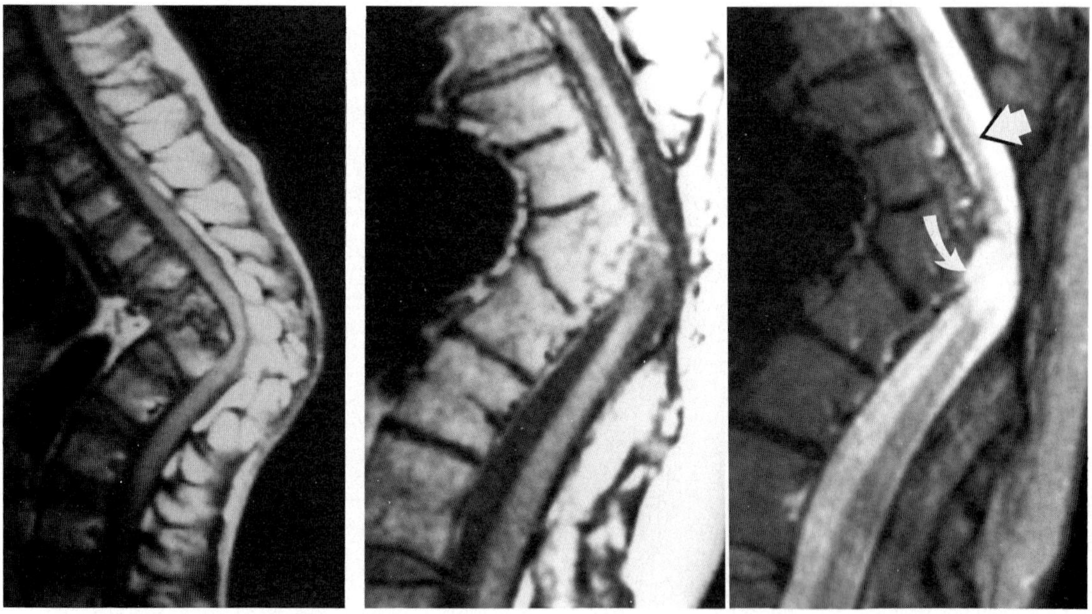 C

FIGURE 7-11. End stage tuberculous spondylitis. **A,** Sagittal T1W scan (SE 600/20) of end stage of tuberculous spondylitis. Note severe gibbus deformity and marked destruction of vertebral bodies and disc spaces. Cord is compressed and deformed at apex of deformity. **B,** T1W scan (400/25) of different patient with gibbus deformity secondary to tuberculous spondylitis. End stage of disease process with affected vertebrae showing increased fat deposition, obvious wedging, and fusion. Spinal cord is normal caliber above and below lesion but of abnormal low signal intensity at apex of gibbus deformity. Cord appears slightly widened and low signal on T1W scan. **C,** On T2W image (SE 2000/80), cord is abnormal high signal intensity indicating myelomalacia *(curved arrow)*. Abnormal cord intensity extends centrally in cord in rostral direction *(straight arrow)*. (**A,** Courtesy of Dr. D. Norman.)

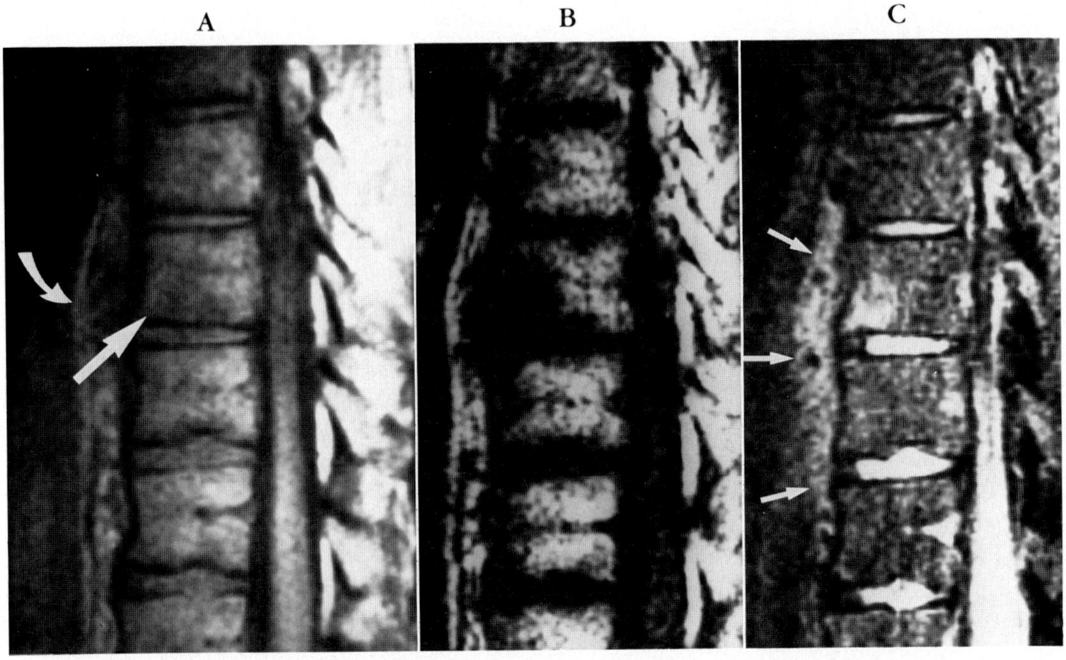

FIGURE 7-12. MR scans of a 29-year-old male with history of drug abuse and acute onset of back pain. Patient was diagnosed as having infectious spondylitis although a specific infectious agent was not cultured. This patient shows only subtle features of infectious spondylitis. The findings on "fat" (**B**) and "water" (**C**) images were clearer than on the conventional T1W scan (**A**). The combination of the vertebral body signal abnormality and associated prevertebral soft tissue swelling is highly suggestive of infectious spondylitis. The more characteristic finding of two adjacent vertebral bodies having signal abnormalities was not present in this patient. **A,** T1W scan (SE 800/20) showed only minimal low signal abnormality in anterior inferior portion of T_9 vertebral body *(straight arrow)*. There was minimal swelling of prevertebral soft tissues, causing slight anterior convexity of the fat planes at the T_9 level *(curved arrows)*. Disc space was within normal limits. **B,** Sagittal "fat" scan (SE 800/20) showed loss of marrow fat signal in anterior-inferior portion of T_9. This low signal area was more prominent than the conventional T1W scan and appeared more extensive. Anterior displacement of the prevertebral fat plane was also evident on this image. **C,** Concurrent sagittal "water" scan (SE 800/20) demonstrated abnormal high signal within the anterior inferior portion of the T_9 vertebral body consistent with presence of inflammatory tissue. Prevertebral soft tissue also showed increased signal intensity extending for length of approximately three vertebral bodies *(arrows)*. This increased soft tissue explains the anterior displacement of the prevertebral fat plane.

EPIDURAL ABSCESS

Spinal epidural abscess is uncommon, but since early diagnosis greatly improves outcome, it is important to be aware of this disease process because MR appears to greatly facilitate the diagnosis.[2] Subdural empyema is even rarer.[21] MR may be positive before a radionuclide bone scan or white cell scan.[2] The epidural abscess may be an extension of an adjacent infectious spondylitis or it may appear separately. In fact, epidural abscess is a misnomer because often the infection can be primarily a cellulitis without an obvious pus-filled abscess cavity. Although this chapter uses the term *abscess*, this includes the cellulitis stage of the disease as well. The source of the organism may be another infection site with spread occurring hematogenously. Drug abusers are at risk for this type of infection.[22] Contiguous spread occurs in the cervical spine from tonsillar and nasopharyngeal infections. All of the organisms causing infectious spondylitis are also etiologic agents for epidural abscess with *Staphylococcus aureus* the most common.[3,22,44] Gram-negative organisms are also important. Tuberculosis can present in a similar manner with most of the abnormality occurring in soft tissue rather than in bone and disc.

Spinal epidural abscess appears in acute and chronic form. Symptoms include spine pain and radicular pain that progress to weakness and eventual paralysis. Stiffness and cramping are often the earliest symptoms.[22] Radicular pain and paresthesia, usually of the lower extremities, develop later.[22] Weakness and paralysis appear last and are clearly the most serious sequellae, which usually are not entirely reversible.[22] The acute form can progress over an interval of 24 hours to a few days, whereas the chronic form may show progression over weeks to months.[3,22] Rapid diagnosis is obviously important in the acute form because timely treatment and decompression can save neurologic function. An experimental model of epidural abscess shows that direct compression of neural tissue is the major cause of damage.[16] Microscopically, white matter is more involved than gray matter, showing vacuolization, myelin loss, and axonal swelling.[16] Interestingly, vessel thrombosis or inflammation is not a prominent pathologic feature.[16] The pathogenesis of neural damage is similar to that of epidural tumor.

Treatment usually consists of antibiotics and surgical decompression. Successful conservative treatment with antibiotics alone is possible.[6] MR may help determine the mode of treatment. If no significant epidural mass is detected and the patient does not have motor weakness, antibiotic treatment alone may be attempted first with close interval follow-up by MR. MR evidence of epidural abscess causing cord compression will likely lead to emergency decompressive surgery.

MR Findings

MR findings are site dependent. Epidural infections in the high cervical spine insinuate into the foramina and around vertebral bodies causing loss of normal water-fat interfaces and replacement of normal epidural fat. On T1W images the inflammatory tissue is abnormal, isointense (with muscle) tissue, obliterating normal landmarks within foramina and in the epidural space (Figures 7-13 and 7-14). The areolar tissue around and above the odontoid process may be

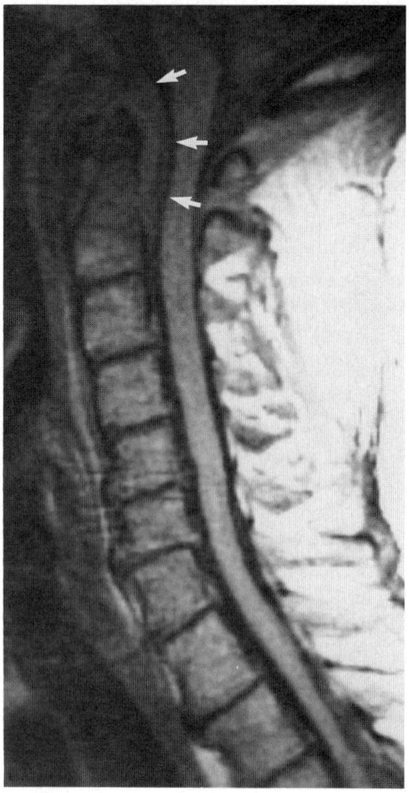

A

FIGURE 7-13, A. For legend see next page.

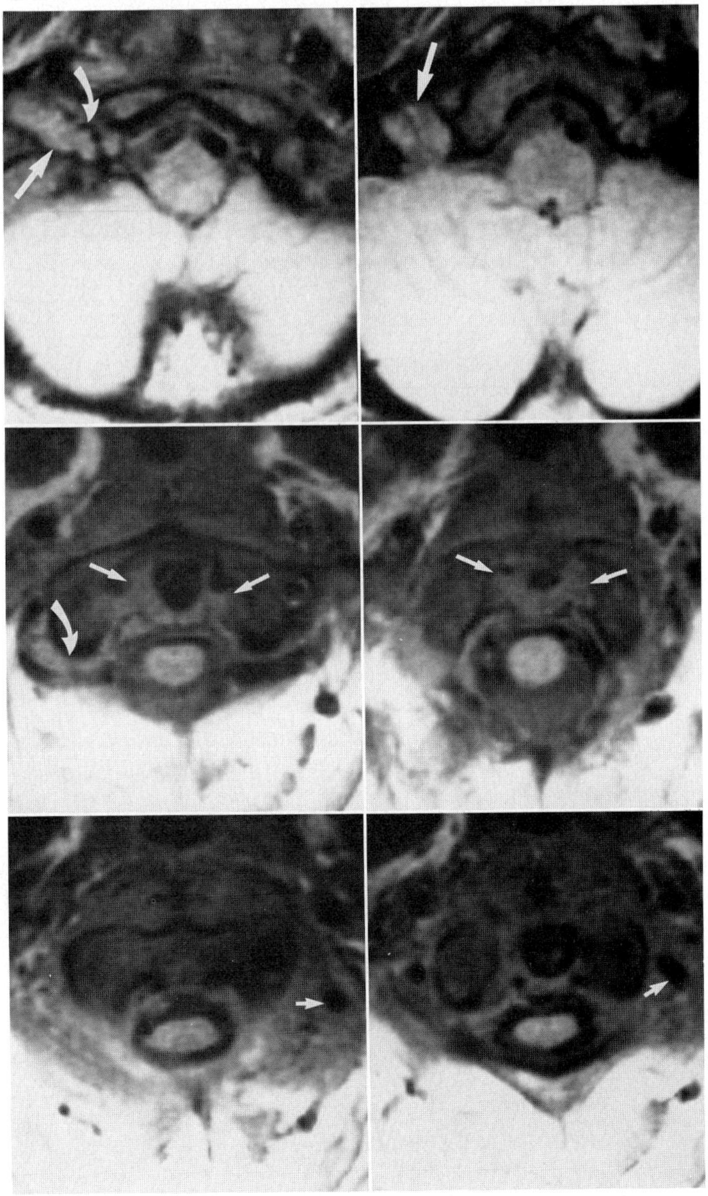

FIGURE 7-13, cont'd. Epidural Abscess. Sagittal and axial MR scans of patient with epidural abscess (cellulitis) causing cord compression at cervicomedullary junction. **A,** Sagittal T1W scan (SE 800/20) exhibits abnormal soft tissue around the craniocervical junction with epidural component *(arrows)* causing cord compression. Normal fat between tip of odontoid and basion not seen because it is replaced by inflammatory tissue. Area of interest is somewhat difficult to see because it lies at edge of sensitive volume of this small posterior surface coil. **B-G,** Axial T1W scans (SE 1000/20) extending from posterior fossa to body of C_2 show abnormal soft tissue in right jugular fossa (*straight arrows*, **B** and **C**), pharyngeal mucosal space, retropharyngeal space, and prevertebral space (**D** and **E**). Right jugular vein is markedly compressed (*curved arrow*, **B**). Soft tissue effaces normal muscle–fat fascial planes and insinuates itself around odontoid process (*straight arrows*, **D** and **E**) and in soft tissue adjacent to vertebral arteries (*curved arrow*, **D** and *small arrows*, **F** and **G**).

Continued.

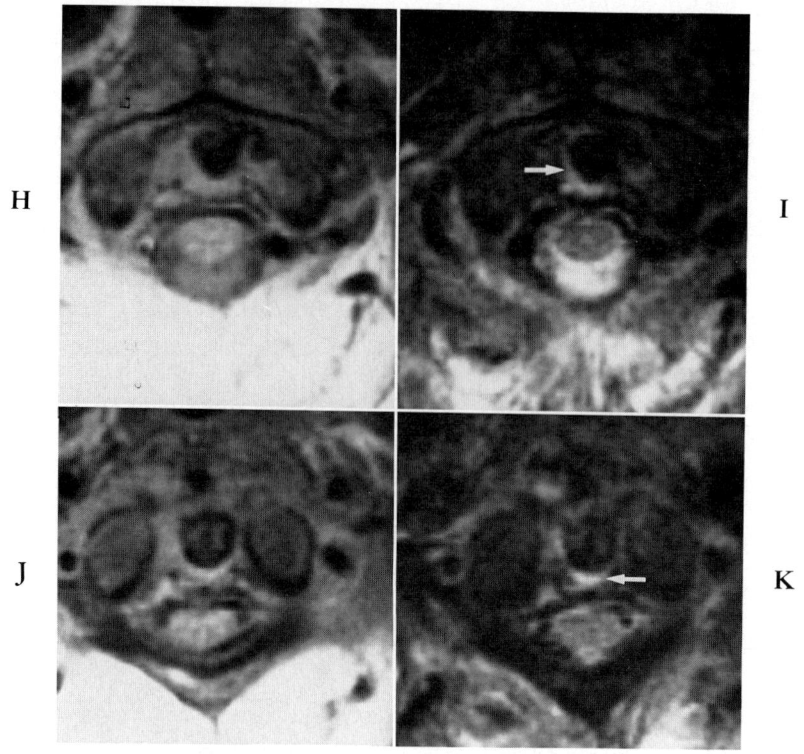

FIGURE 13 cont'd. **H-K**, T2W scans (ungated SE 2000/20, 80) confirm abnormal soft tissue in prevertebral and retropharyngeal spaces and show abnormal high signal intensity in immediate area around odontoid process *(arrows)*.

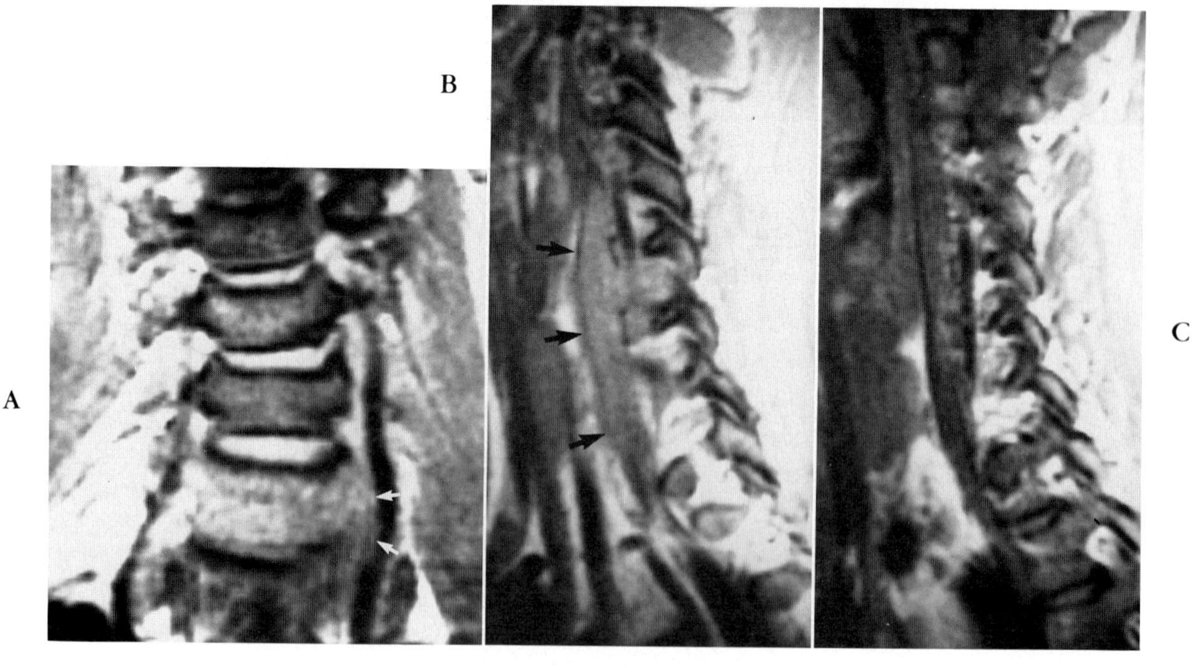

FIGURE 7-14. For legend see next page.

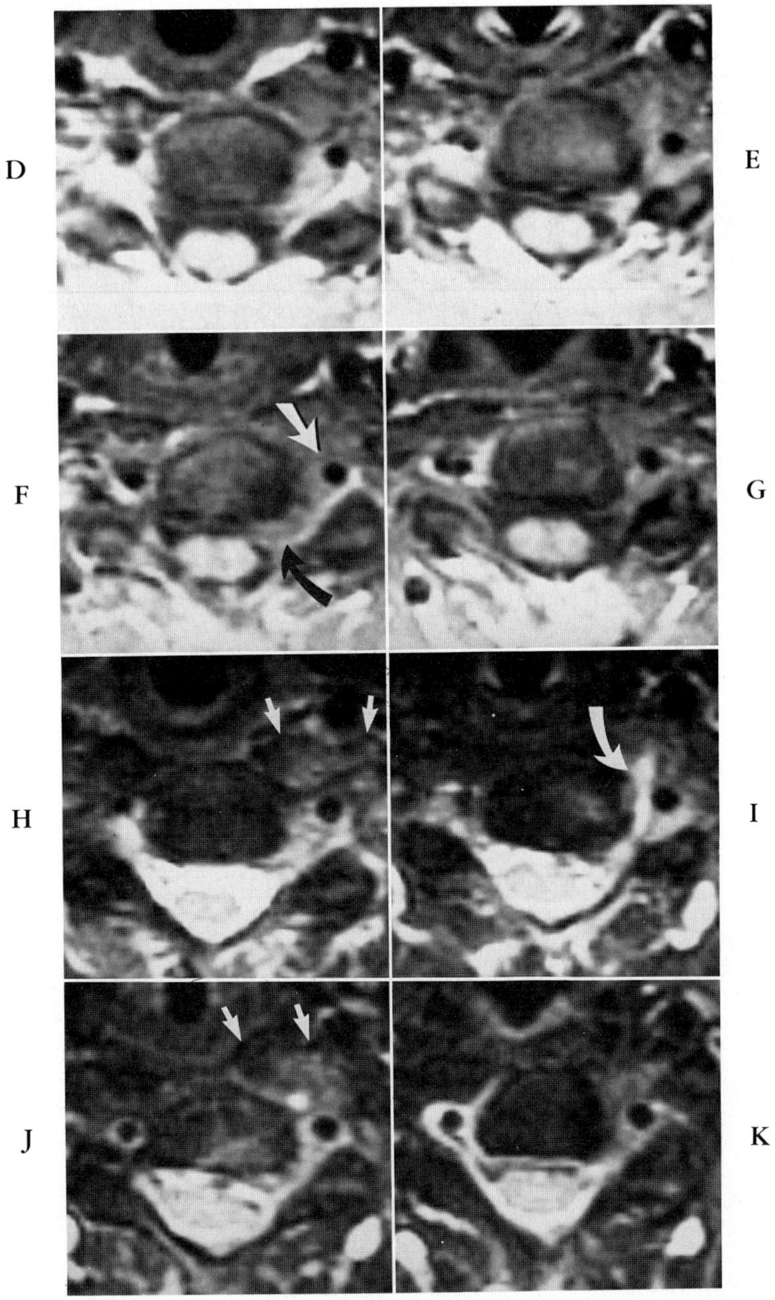

FIGURE 7-14. Cellulitis. Coronal, sagittal, and axial scans accurately depict extent of cellulitis caused by prolonged placement of acupuncture needles in neck. **A,** Coronal T1W scan (SE 800/20) shows abnormal soft tissue adjacent to left vertebral artery causing slight lateral displacement *(arrows)*. Sagittal off-midline T1W scans (SE 800/20) show extent of prevertebral soft tissue abnormality on left side (**B**) compared to normal right side (**C**). **D-G,** Set of four axial scans (SE 1000/20) show cellulitis located in prevertebral space on left with extensions through neural foramina at three different disc levels (**E**, **F**, and **G**). Cellulitis replaced epidural fat around left vertebral artery *(straight arrow)* and within neural foramina *(curved arrow)*. Some inflammatory tissue causes small extradural defect in left anterolateral recess at two different cervical levels (**E;** *curved arrow*, **F**). **H-K,** Set of four axial T2W scans (flow-compensated and gated 2300/80) at same levels as axial T1W scans (**D-G**) show abnormal high signal intensity tissue in prevertebral space and around left vertebral artery (*arrow*, **I**). High signal around right vertebral artery (**J**) represents venous sinus continuous with sinus in intervertebral foramen (**K**). Entire area of cellulitis has inhomogeneous signal intensity ranging from intermediate to high signal (*arrows*, **H** and **J**).

Continued.

L 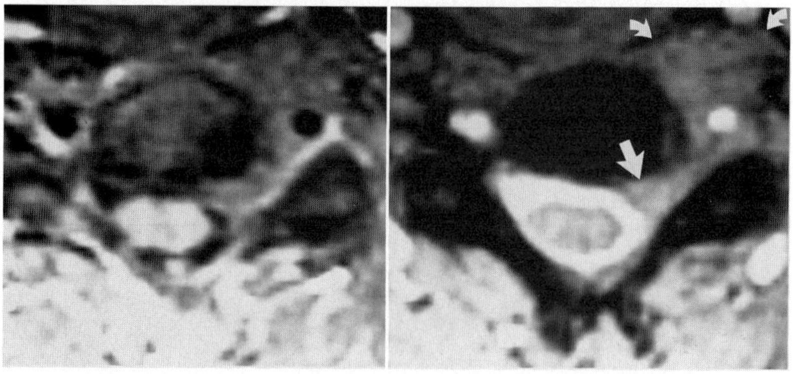 M

FIGURE 7-14, cont'd. Comparison of **L**, axial T1W scan (SE 1000/20) with **M**, variable flip angle scan (GRASS 25/13, 7°) at same level shows T1W scan superior in delineating cellulitis, especially at interfaces with fat, such as in left intervertebral foramen. Although mass effect of cellulitis is evident on variable flip angle scan *(small arrows)*, distinction between inflammation and normal fat planes is less clear, but extension of cellulitis into spinal canal is well visualized *(large arrow)*. Inflammatory mass on variable flip angle sequence has similar signal intensity as epidural fat. One might therefore suspect extension of inflammatory mass into dorsal spinal canal (**M**); this would be in error because T1W scan (**L**) shows this to be normal epidural fat.

A 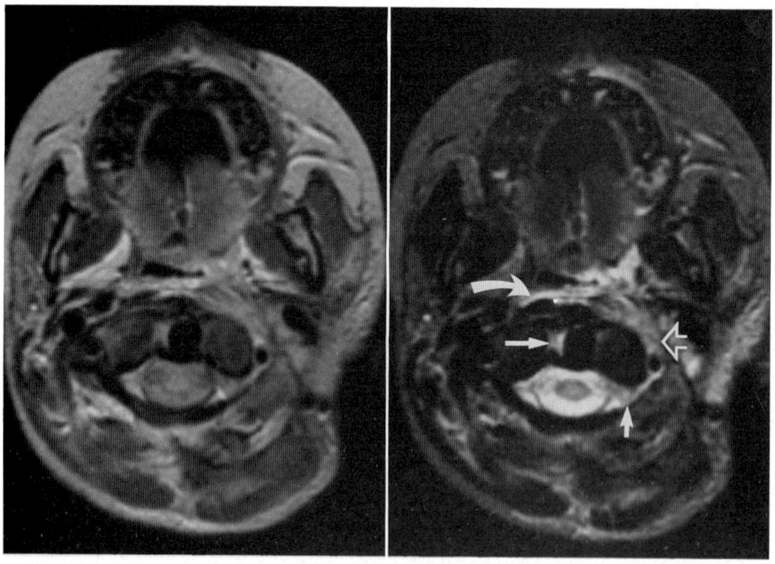 B

FIGURE 7-15. Cellulitis. **A** and **B**, Axial T2W scans (SE 2000/20, 80) of patient with postoperative nasopharyngeal infection involving pharyngeal mucosal space, left parapharyngeal space, retropharyngeal space (*curved arrow*, **B**), prevertebral space on left, and soft tissue adjacent to odontoid process on right *(medium straight arrow)*. One route of infection spread to spine occurs laterally around C_2 (on left), involving tissue around vertebral artery *(open arrow)* to spinal canal behind lateral mass *(vertical arrow)*. In high cervical region, route of spread following course of vertebral artery is one route of access to spinal canal.

replaced by this intermediate signal intensity (see Figure 7-13). When frank abscess (i.e., purulent center) is present, it will appear as an epidural soft tissue mass on T1W images (see Figure 7-5), may not have an obvious low signal center, and may be quite extensive, involving several vertebral body levels and their respective foramina (see Figure 7-14). On T2W images, inflammatory tissue exhibits high signal intensity in these same regions (Figure 7-15; see Figures 7-13 and 7-14). This is particularly striking in the areas where epidural fat that is low signal intensity is normally expected. The high signal may be marked where a purulent fluid collection is present. A frank abscess exhibits high signal in a mass that is convex toward the cord (see Figure 7-5). A compressed cord may show abnormal high signal on a T2W scan indicating tissue damage (see Figure 7-5).

Epidural abscesses can be extensive, especially in the thoracic region because of the large potential epidural space (Figures 7-16 and 7-17). In the thoracic region, the most common site of involvement, epidural abscess is usually located dorsally, whereas in the cervical and lumbar regions infection is usually located ventrally (see Figures 7-16 and 7-17). The soft tissue inflammatory component in paravertebral tissues is less in the thoracic region compared to cervical and lumbar regions. Also in the thoracic region, although this may occur elsewhere, the infection may have a significant hemorrhagic component (see Figures 7-16 and 7-17), presumably secondary to rupture of epidural veins caused by the expanding inflammatory mass. This means on T1W images the infection may have the appearance of a subdural or epidural hematoma, i.e., high signal intensity on the T1W image (see Figures 7-16 and 7-17). This could even be mistaken for epidural fat in the dorsal spinal canal, although the hemorrhage will be seen as continuous, whereas normal epidural fat should have a segmental distribution. A T2W image will make the differentiation and avoid a MR mis-

A

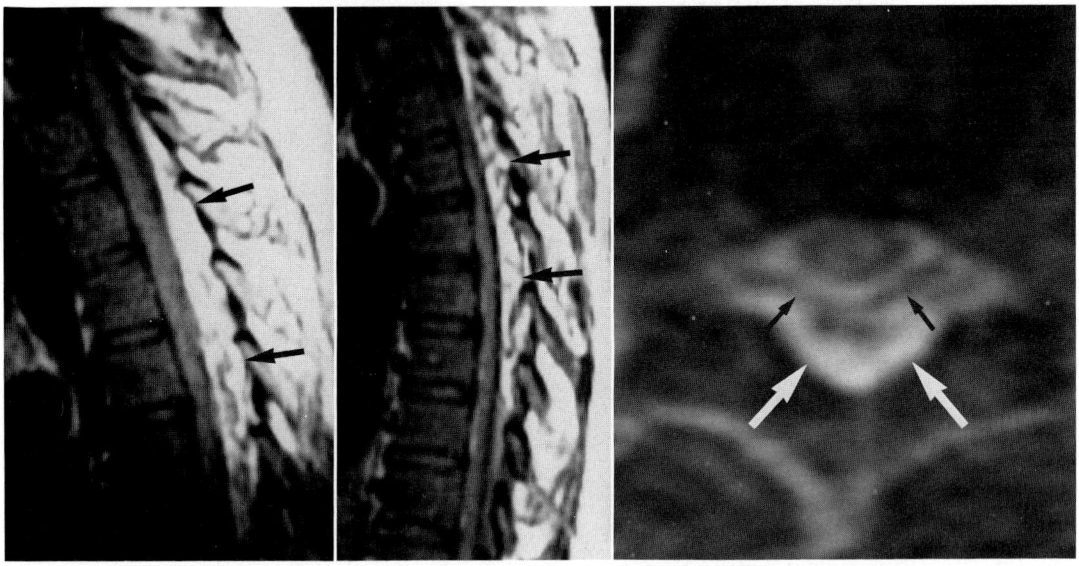

B, C

FIGURE 7-16. Staphylococcal epidural abscess. MR scans show hemorrhagic characteristics of epidural abscess in 24-year-old male. T1W sagittal images (SE 600/20) of **A**, upper and **B**, lower thoracic spine show prominent long area of high signal intensity in dorsal spinal canal causing cord compression *(arrows)*. High signal area is not uniform but shows significant heterogeneity with multiple, irregular, and linear areas of low signal intensity. **C**, Axial T2W (flow-compensated 2500/80) image demonstrates abnormal high signal intensity in dorsal canal *(white arrows)* causing forward displacement of dura *(black arrows)*. Dorsal area of high signal also demonstrates inhomogeneous low signal within it on T2W images. Cord is compressed anteriorly and surrounded by uniform high signal CSF. There is suggestion of abnormal high signal intensity within cord itself. (Courtesy of Dr. Robert Jahnke.)

interpretation. On T2W images high signal intensity consistent with chronic hemorrhage and inflammatory tissue can be seen in the epidural space (see Figures 7-16 and 7-17). T2W image findings rule out increased fat deposition. Normal thoracic epidural fat should not compromise the spinal canal and compress the cord. A rare entity, epidural lipomatosis, could be mistaken for epidural abscess in the thoracic region both clinically and by MR if only T1W images are obtained. Clinically the symptoms may be similar in the chronic presentation and this entity is seen in the setting of chronic low-dose corticosteroid therapy (see Chapter 8).

In the thoracic region the infection may be circumferential around the dural sac causing the dural sac to be constricted around the cord and causing high signal around the dura. The dura is seen as a thin low signal intensity circle that, in turn, surrounds a high signal ring, which is the narrowed subarachnoid space (see Figure 7-16). In the center of all this is the intermediate signal cord. It appears that the dura is more easily stripped from bone and compressed by epidural disease processes in the thoracic region compared to either the cervical or lumbar regions. The same phenomenon is seen with epidural metastatic tumors, which have the same tendency in the thoracic region. Epidural metastatic tumor has not shown any features sug-

A 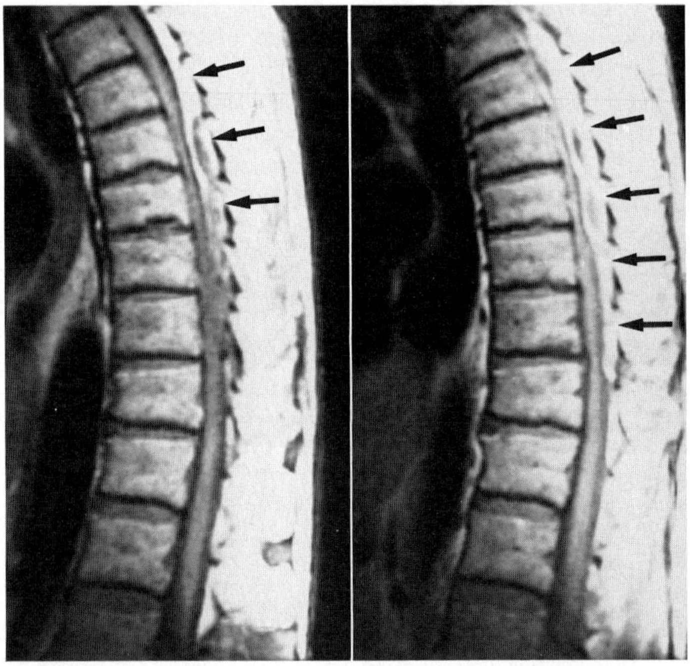 B

FIGURE 7-17. Thoracic epidural abscess. **A** and **B**, Adjacent sagittal T1W scans (SE 800/20) show long segment of increased signal intensity dorsal to cord *(arrows)* causing significant cord compression in upper thoracic spine. Area of increased signal intensity shows some inhomogeneity with interspersed areas of low signal intensity and has similar signal intensity to epidural fat but does not have segmental distribution. **C** and **D**, Axial T1W scans (SE 800/20) through upper thoracic region confirm prominent area of high signal intensity in dorsal spinal canal *(black arrows)*. Inhomogeneity of signal is confirmed on axial scans (**D** and **F**) where areas of low signal intensity are seen dorsal to compressed cord *(white arrows)*. **G-J**, Axial T2W scans (SE 2000/80) at same levels as axial T1W images show complex mixture of signal intensities, major portion of which is high signal dorsal to cord. On T1W images high signal intensity areas remain high signal on T2W images indicative of hemorrhage (**G** and **I**). Areas of low signal on T1W images (**D** and **F**) appear as high signal on T2W images (**H** and **J**), indicating fluid. It is evident from all views that mass in dorsal spinal canal causes severe compression of thoracic spinal cord **C-J**).

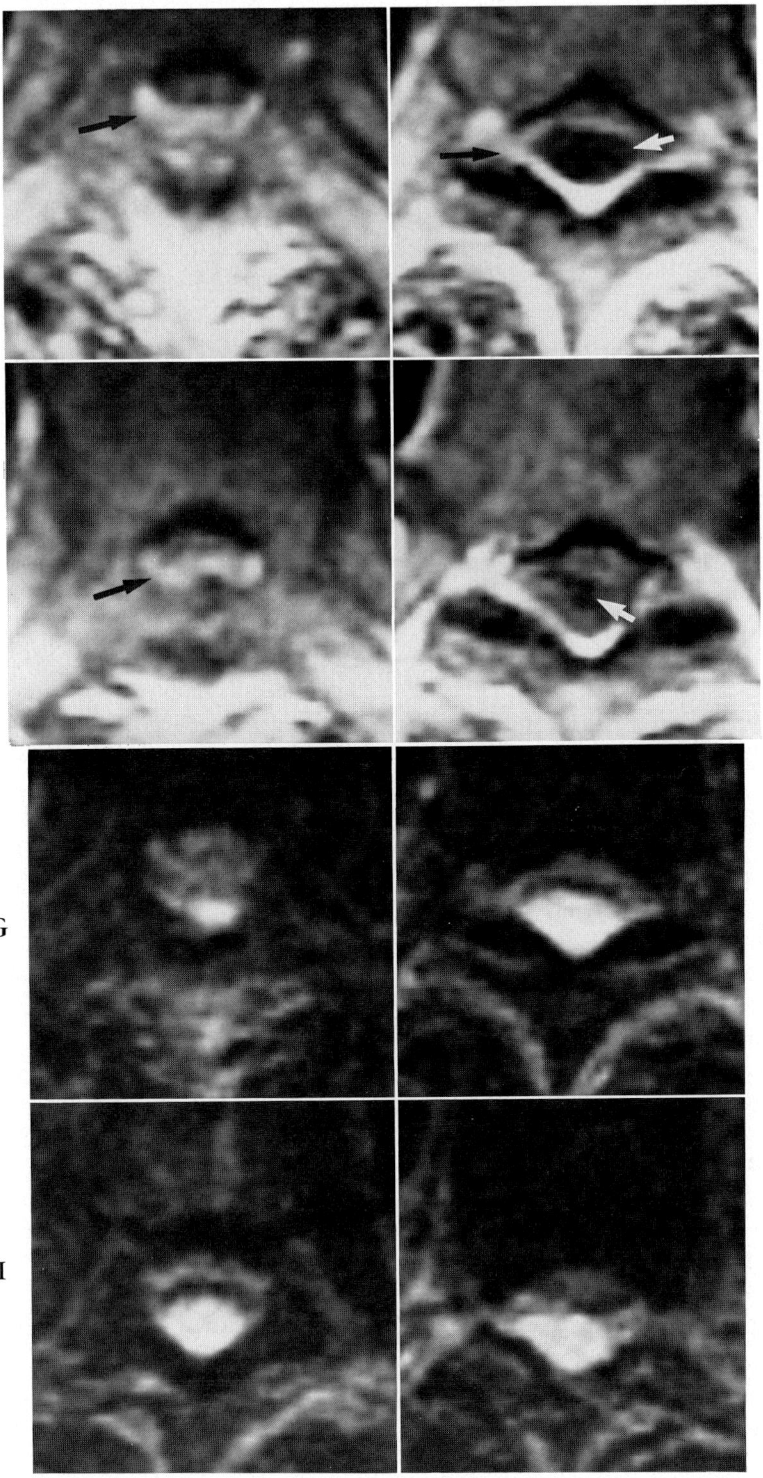

C D E F G H I J

gesting hemorrhagic components as seen with these infections.

The epidural abscess often extends for several segments and sometimes involves the entire thoracic region. This differs from metastatic tumor, which is more localized and associated with local and focal bone invasion and destruction. Hematopoietic tumors are exceptions and can have extensive multilevel involvement. The epidural abscess is often remarkable for the lack of associated bony changes.[44] Involvement of adjacent bone anywhere in the spine is seen as increased signal in the vertebrae replacing the low signal marrow on T2W images. This is as sensitive of bone involvement as detecting bone erosion on CT.

The major differential point from metastatic disease is disc space narrowing, which is the most reliable sign but may not yet be detectable early in the disease. The widespread obscuration of fat-water interfaces helps differentiate infection from tumor. The presence of multiple fluid collections in soft tissue masses favors infection.

CORD INFECTIONS

Considering the rather limited blood supply to the cord, bacterial infections of the cord are quite rare, making generalizations difficult.[5] An important feature, however, is the rapid progression of a mass lesion in the confined space in the spinal canal.[5] With MR's ability to image the spinal cord, the same problems encountered in the diagnosis of brain infections can be expected in spinal cord infections. Unfortunately noncontrast and even postcontrast MR scan findings are also nonspecific. With accurate visualization of the cord, many infectious organisms will be found to infect it. Mycobacteria and even unusual infections such as cysticercosis already have been imaged.[17]

In general, most infections will show a focal mass effect and low signal intensity on T1W images. On T2W images high signal is seen in the inflammatory region and in the surrounding edema. If a contrast agent, such as gadolinium diethylenetriamine penta-acetic acid (GdDTPA) is used, ring or nodular areas of high signal enhancement are seen on T1W images. GdDTPA helps localize the abscess, granuloma, etc. in the cord, which may be difficult on noncontrast T1W and T2W images because of the similarity of signal with surrounding edema (Figure 7-18).

High quality T2W images reveal lesions in the spinal cord that could not previously be imaged or diagnosed, such as in patients with AIDS (Figure 7-19). Multiple areas of abnormal high signal intensity within the cord on T2W images are as nonspecific as they often are in the brain (see Figure 7-19). Because aggressive surgical intervention is rarely undertaken in the cord, the specific etiology of these lesions has not been determined, although in all likelihood they represent the same spectra of lesions seen in the brain in patients with AIDS.

Transverse Myelitis

Transverse myelitis is a heterogeneous clinical diagnosis that presents in a variety of different clinical settings: allergic reaction related to previous infection or vaccination, direct infection by a virus, a paraneoplastic type process (also allergic), vascular insufficiency, and multiple sclerosis. A preceding viral illness is a common associated infectious illness. A minority of patients diagnosed as having transverse myelitis eventually develop multiple sclerosis.[34] Clinically, an important diagnostic goal is to exclude treatable entities such as extraaxial tumor, spinal vascular malformation, or epidural abscess.

Most patients present with ascending paresthesia (numbness, tingling, "pins and needles") or leg weakness that evolve over one to eleven days.[37] Findings are ascending because cord damage masks any neurologic deficits at a lower spinal level. Caudal progression that is seen neuropathologically is usually not expressed clinically. Some patients have a very acute onset, i.e., evolving over a few hours. Symptoms include pain, leg weakness, and paresthesia. The primary symptom is pain, which is usually interscapular in location. There is also a longer, stuttering onset that evolves over 10 to 30 days.[37] The prognosis is reasonably good except for patients with acute onset; in these cases prognosis is poor.[37]

Pathologically, tissue damage is characterized by necrosis,[37] which involves both gray and white matter, and by demyelination. Long segments of cord are usually diffusely involved. The midthoracic cord is commonly involved but this predilection has not been explained.[37]

MR scan may be normal on both T1W and T2W images[27] performed early in the course of the disease. After the initial phase, the MR scan

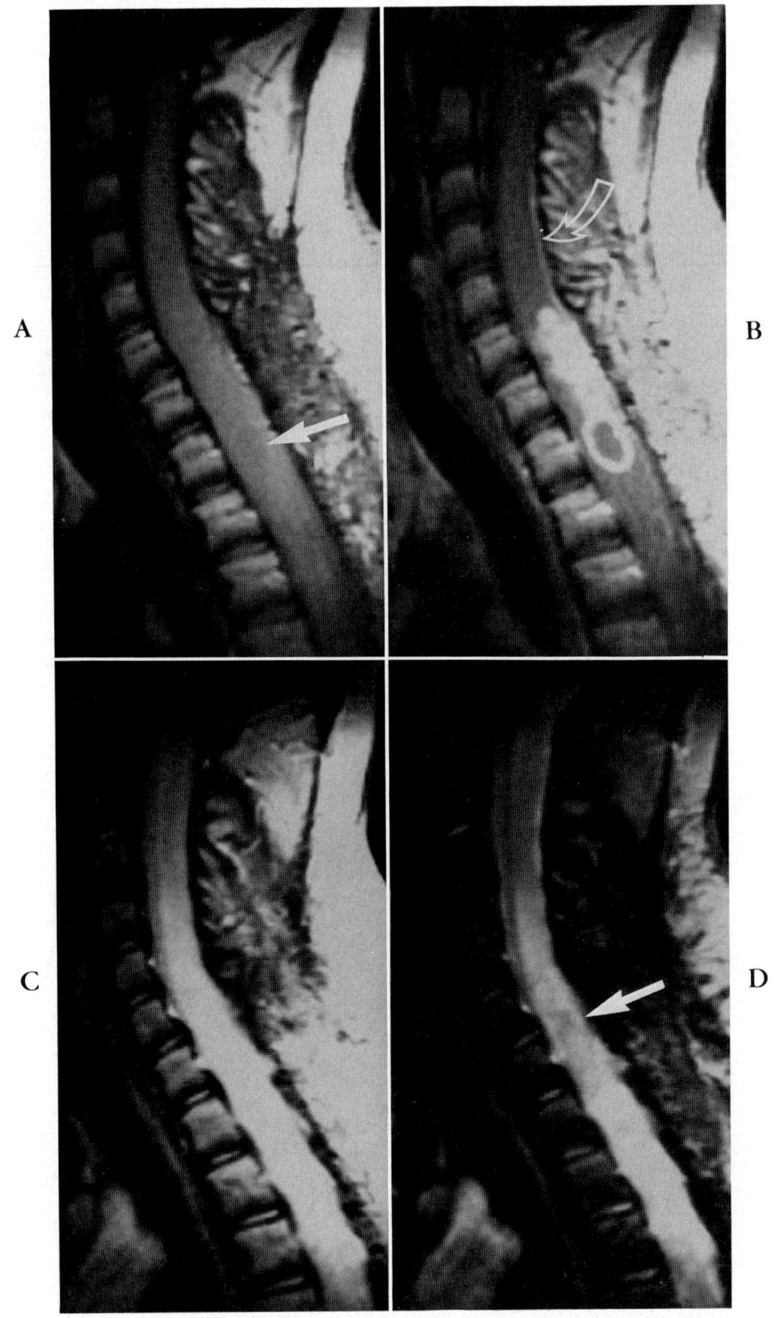

FIGURE 7-18. Spinal cord tuberculosis. Both intramedullary and leptomeningeal tuberculosis in the spine of this 14-year-old female. **A,** Sagittal precontrast T1W scan (SE 800/20) shows marked enlargement of the mid- and low cervical cord, which is of relatively homogeneous signal intensity. Close inspection shows subtle areas of lower signal intensity suggesting cystic components *(arrow)*. **B,** Postcontrast GdDTPA T1W scan shows a prominent area of contrast enchancement in the low cervical cord characterized by numerous areas of ring enhancement representing multiple granulomas. Meningeal enhancement is also present dorsal to the cord *(arrow)*. **C** and **D,** Sagittal T2W scans (SE 2000/20, 80) show abnormal cord enlargement throughout, with the major area of infection seen as abnormal high signal extending from C_6 to T_2 on both echoes. Second echo image shows signal heterogeneity in region of actual granulomas *(arrow)*, as shown by the area of contrast enchancement (**B**). Note high signal edema extends cranially up to level of the medulla. *Continued.*

E F G H I J

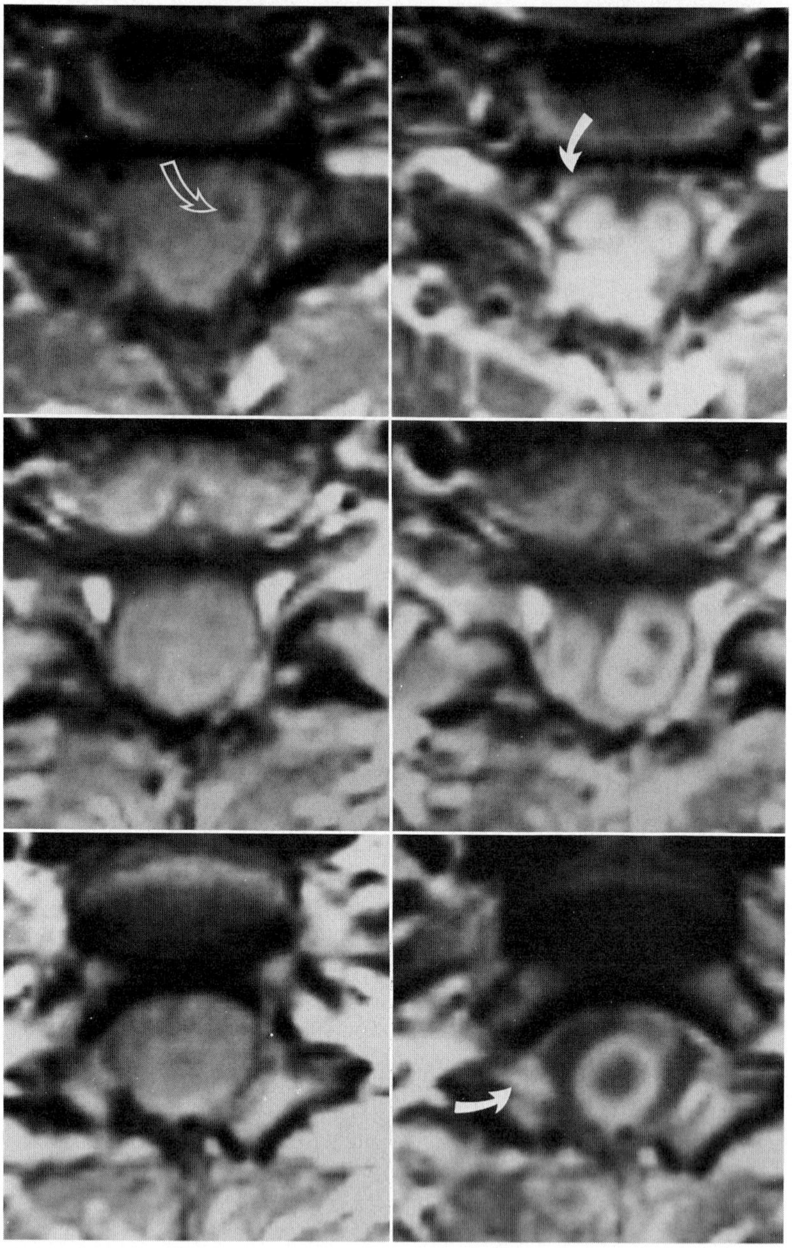

FIGURE 7-18, cont'd. E-J, Axial precontrast (**E**, **G**, **I**) and postcontrast (**F**, **H**, **J**) T1W scans (SE 800/20) show marked cord enlargement and an aggregate of nodular granulomas. The precontrast T1W scans (**C** and **E**) show only a few areas of decreased signal intensity within the enlarged cord suggesting cystic components to the lesion (*arrow*, **E**). Postcontrast GdDTPA scans (**F**, **H**, **J**) show multiple, contiguous areas of ring enhancement. Findings are typical of infectious disease with the ring lesions representing multiple granulomas. In addition to the parenchymal lesions, abnormal contrast enhancement is noted in the subarachnoid space indicating leptomeningeal involvement by this tuberculous infection (*arrows*, **F** and **J**).

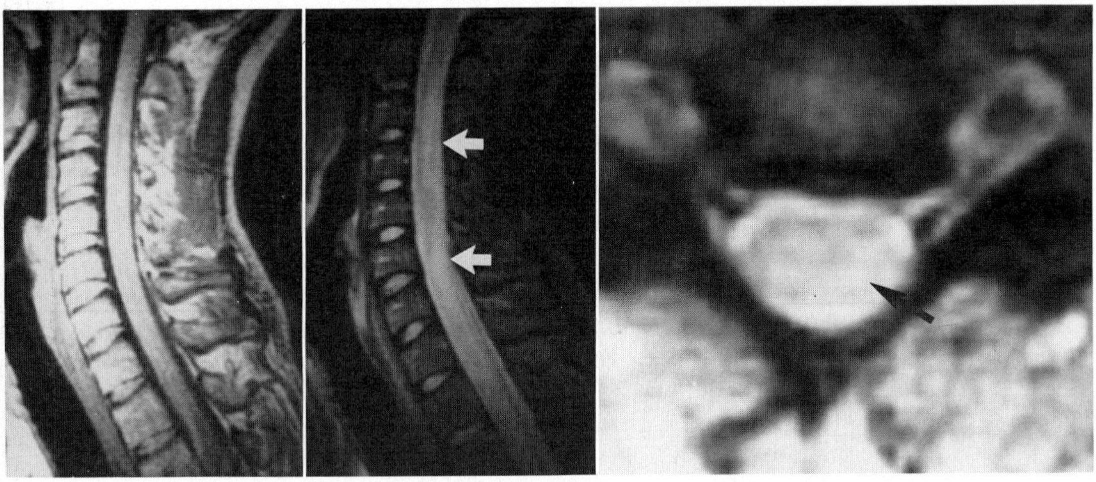

B, C

FIGURE 7-19. AIDS myelopathy. Cervical cord lesion of unknown etiology in patient with AIDS related complex (ARC) and bowel and bladder symptoms plus bilateral lower extremity dysesthesia. **A,** T1W (SE 800/20) scan of cervical cord is essentially normal although minimal enlargement may be suspected at C_4-C_5 level. **B,** T2W scan (SE gated 1600/80) shows marked abnormal signal within cord extending from C_3 to C_7 *(arrows)*. **C,** Axial variable flip angle scan (GRASS 40/12, 7°) shows cord enlargement and diffuse abnormal high signal within cord *(arrow)*. Unfortunately, abnormal high signal on T2W scans in spinal cord is as nonspecific as it is in the brain of patients with ARC. It is clear that CNS infections are not limited to the brain; this could represent an HIV infection of the cervical cord.

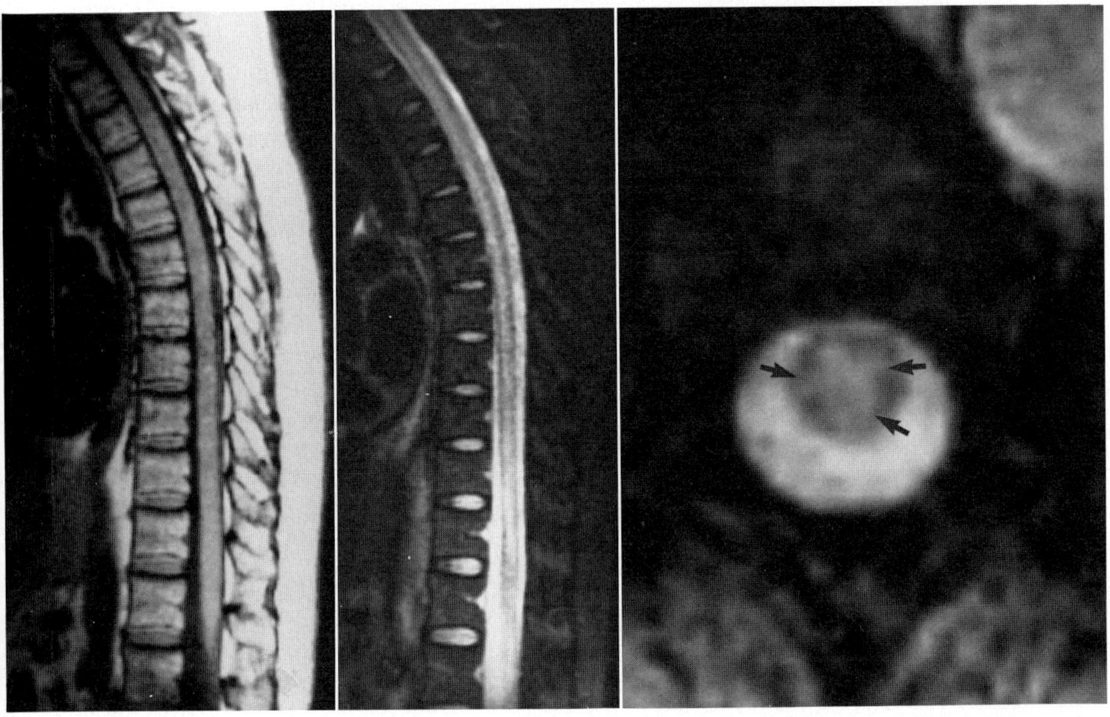

B, C

FIGURE 7-20. Transverse myelitis. MR scans of a 38-year-old female with clinical history most consistent with transverse myelitis. **A,** T1W (SE 800/20) scan shows mild enlargement of entire thoracic cord—a subtle finding but should be considered in view of the fact that the entire cord is nearly same size as conus medullaris. **B,** T2W scan (SE 2300/80) shows abnormal signal intensity extending through entire thoracic cord, primarily central in location and relatively homogeneous in signal intensity. This is not a Gibb's artifact as matrix size is 256 × 256. **C,** Abnormal cord signal intensity confirmed by axial, variable flip angle scan (GRASS 40/20, 7°) that demonstrates its central location and somewhat irregular border *(arrows)*.

may show cord enlargement over several segments.[27] The MR scan reflects the full pathologic extent by showing more extensive cord involvement than might be suspected clinically from the identifiable sensory level. Part of the MR spectrum includes abnormal high signal intensity involving long segments of the thoracic cord (Figure 7-20), but cord enlargment may not be evident despite this extensive abnormal signal. Cord swelling is likely to change over time as the disease evolves and may only be evident in the subacute stage. Although there is little experience with this disease entity, the nonMS form of the disease appears to be more extensive in the cord compared to multiple sclerosis (MS) of the cord, which shows abnormal high signal and appears to have a more limited and scattered distribution (see Chapter 9).

LEPTOMENINGEAL INFECTIONS

Leptomeningeal infections of the spinal canal are not usually discussed as a separate entity because they often accompany cranial leptomeningeal infections. The disease entities of interest are those that cause chronic meningitis intracranially. The main organisms are *Mycobacterium tuberculosis*, *Coccidioides immitis*, and cysticercosis *(Taenia Solium)*. These organisms cause a granulomatous inflammation involving the basal cisterns, can extend into the spinal canal, and incite fibrotic reactions that can be quite severe. The spinal manifestation of the disease therefore is simply an extension of the inflammation and arachnoiditis seen in the basal cisterns. Because cranial symptoms predominate, patients are initially studied for intracranial problems. In rare instances, spinal manifestations are the presenting symptoms and spine MR scan is the key to the correct diagnosis.

A rare and obscure disease entity, pachymeningitis cervicalis hypertrophica, presents as a severe arachnoiditis by MR imaging (Figure 7-21). The etiology of this entity is unknown although a variety of organisms have been implicated.[38] Pathologically, it is characterized by chronic but nonspecific inflammation and hyaline fibrosis. The inflammation is not granulomatous. The dura is typically involved (thus pachymeningitis), but the inflammation often extends to the leptomeninges.[38] Stains and culture for microorganisms are often negative.[38] This disease entity seems to represent a final common pathway of severe spinal pachymeningitis when the inciting factor cannot be definitively identified.

MR Findings

Major MR findings are severe arachnoiditis that in most instances not only involves the spinal canal but extends to involve the basal cisterns and the region around the foramen magnum. On T1W scans, normal CSF spaces and cisterns are obscured or completely obliterated by soft tissue. This may be particularly evident around the foramen magnum. On a T1W sequence, the spinal cord may appear enlarged and have an irregular margin. This increase in size and irregular border is more easily detected on axial scans compared to sagittal scans. The axial scan may show a thin halo of signal intensity surrounding the cord circumferentially. On T2W images some of these findings are obscured in that cord enlargement and irregular cord margin may be less obvious. What may be evident on T2W images, however, is abnormal signal within the cord related to the leptomeningeal infection, which may be more prominent in the acute stages of the meningitis and could represent either underlying edema or myelitis. In the late, chronic, fibrotic stage this abnormal signal in the cord may be less evident and, if present, represents scattered areas of myelomalacia caused by an inflammatory vasculitis. Clumping of nerve roots are a residua of the arachnoiditis (Figure 7-22). Depending on the severity of the arachnoiditis, small, potentially multiple, subarachnoid cysts may form that can be seen as low signal areas on T1W scans (see Chapter 12, Figure 12-10) and can be identified by their deformation of the adjacent cord and by their high signal intensity on T2W scans. If these cysts do not cause cord deformity they are difficult to detect, but they are also of little clinical significance.

There is currently no extensive experience with the contrast agent GdDTPA but it is apparent that various forms of spinal arachnoiditis exhibit enhancement with this contrast agent. If spinal arachnoiditis, infectious or noninfectious, is suspected, GdDTPA can demonstate abnormal enhancement of the leptomeninges and thus make the correct diagnosis (Figure 7-23) (see Chapter 12). The enhancement may be exten-

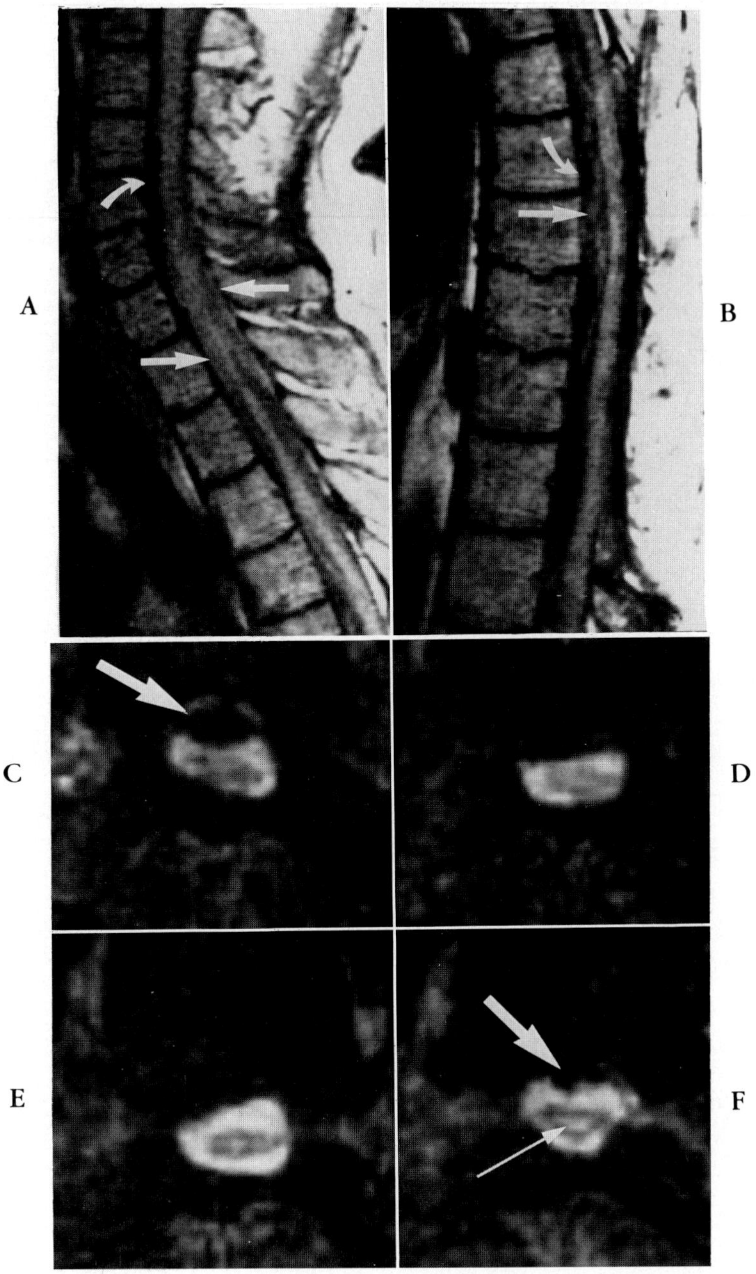

FIGURE 7-21. Pachymeningitis cervicalis hypertrophica. MR scans of 51-year-old male with progressive lower extremity dysfunction and biopsy proven diagnosis of pachymeningitis cervicalis hypertrophica. MR scan findings appear to be combination of severe arachnoiditis and ossification of posterior longitudinal ligament (see Figure 10-55). Sagittal T1W images (SE 800/20) of **A,** cervical and **B,** upper thoracic spine show irregular, shaggy outline of cord with abnormal signal in subarachnoid space *(arrows)*. In addition, irregular areas of low signal intensity in anterior spinal canal represent thickened and calcified (ossified?) posterior longitudinal ligament (*curved arrow,* **A**). **C-F,** Set of four axial, variable flip angle/gradient echo scans (GRASS 22/12, 7°) in upper thoracic region show impingement on spinal canal by ligament–dural hypertrophy in anterior spinal canal, seen as marked low signal *(wide arrows)*. Cord markedly atrophic and exhibits abnormal signal intensity centrally *(thin arrow)*.

A, B

C

D, E

F

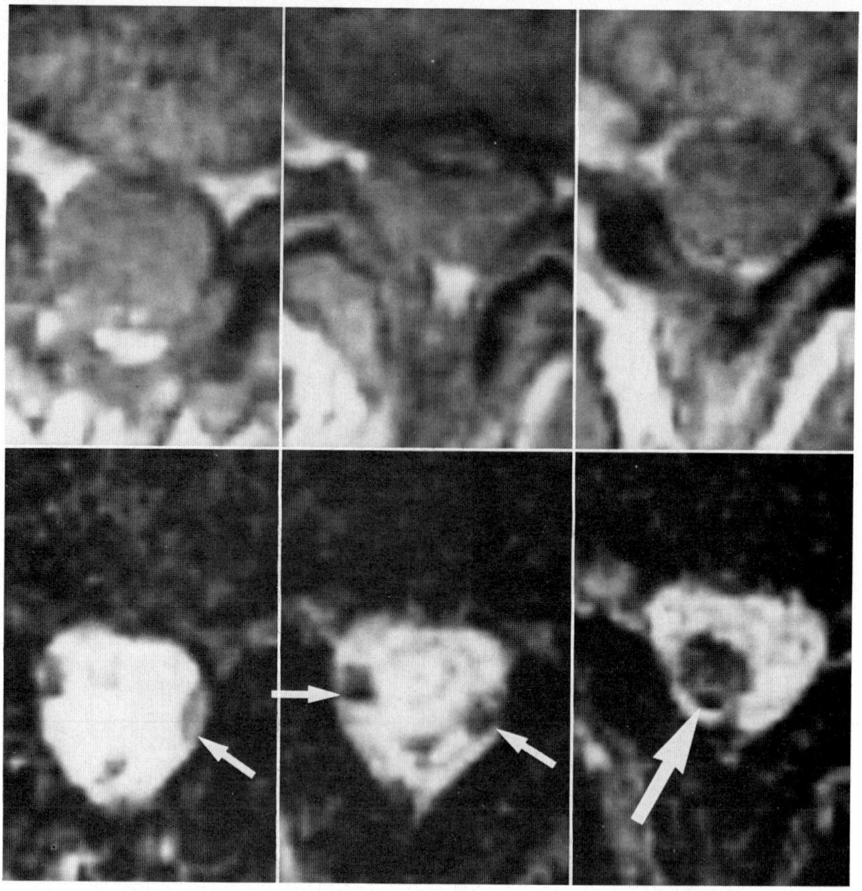

FIGURE 7-22. Tuberculous arachnoiditis. Axial T2W scans (SE gated 2000/20, 80) of lumbar spinal canal in patient with moderate arachnoiditis secondary to tuberculous meningitis. **A-C,** First echo images (TE 20) do not yield sufficient information about structures within dural sac. **D-F,** Second echo images (TE 80) show marked clumping of nerve roots (*arrows,* **D, E,** and **F**). In lower canal, nerve roots are located peripherally in dural sac and form three distinct groups (**D** and **E**), as they progress rostrally these three groups merge into single large mass of adhered nerve roots (*arrow,* **F**).

A

B

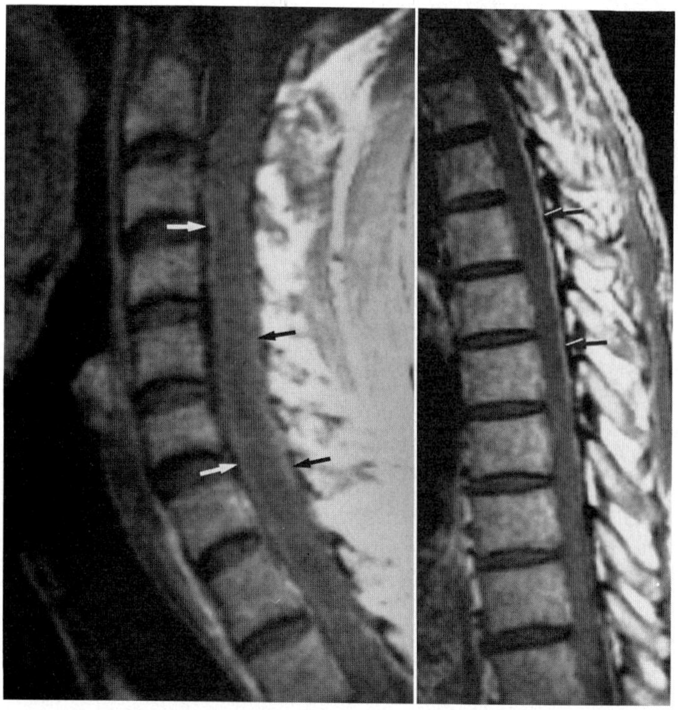

FIGURE 7-23, **A** and **B,** For legend see next page.

C D

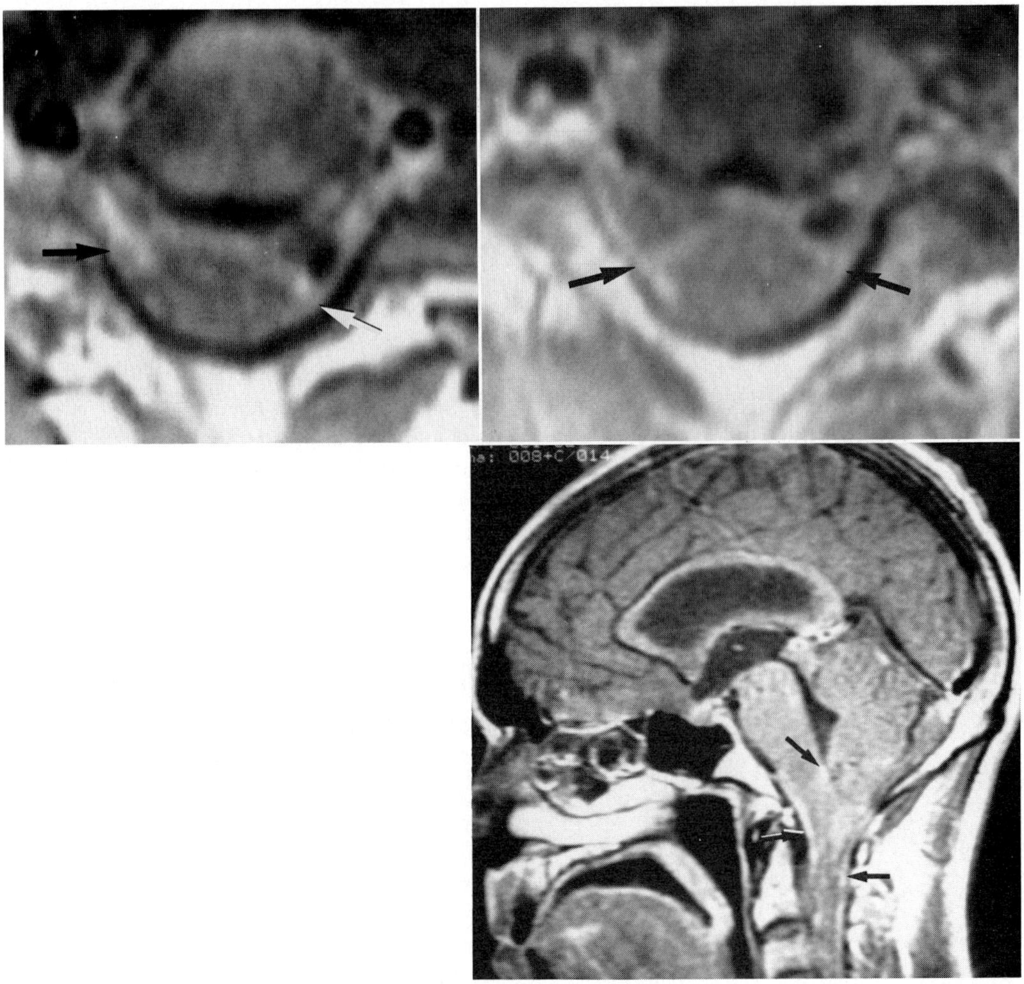

E

FIGURE 7-23. Coccidioidal meningitis. Series of MR scans shows contrast enhancement of leptomeninges after intravenous administration of GdDTPA in patient with coccidioidal meningitis. **A,** Postcontrast sagittal T1W scan (SE 600/20) shows apparently widened cervical spinal cord. Note thin line of contrast enhancement dorsal-ventral to cord *(arrows)* indicating abnormal enhancement of leptomeninges. **B,** Sagittal T1W scan (SE 800/20) of thoracic spine shows similar findings, although thin line of contrast enhancement *(arrows)* is most evident on dorsal aspect of cord. **C** and **D,** Postcontrast axial T1W scans (SE 800/20) show enhancement of leptomeninges in subarachnoid space *(arrows)* and obliteration of an area of signal void normally seen in the right anterolateral recess, indicating soft tissue replacement of normal subarachnoid space and disruption of normal CSF flow patterns. **E,** Sagittal T1W scan (SE 600/20) of brain and cranio-cervical junction shows marked abnormal contrast enhancement around foramen magnum obliterating normal margins of medulla, vallecula, and inferior vermis. Abnormal contrast enhancement in subarachnoid space well delineated by high signal produced by GdDTPA *(arrows)*. *(Courtesy of Dr. Michael Brant-Zawadski.)*

be subarachnoid space (see Figure 7-23). Cord enhancement may be visualized if a myelitis or cord infarction accompanies the leptomeningeal infection.

CYSTICERCOSIS

Central nervous system (CNS) cysticercosis develops when a person accidentally becomes the intermediate host, rather than the definitive host, for *T. solium*. The intracranial manifestations of the disease in its various stages have been well described. The spinal manifestations of neurocysticercosis are more uncommon and assume one of two forms: (1) intramedullary cyst and (2) subarachnoid cyst and arachnoiditis. Spinal cord intramedullary cysticercosis is rare.[12] Just as in the brain, intramedullary lesions are believed to be secondary to hematogenous spread and their distribution is related to the amount of blood flow—because blood flow to the spinal cord is much less than to the brain, parenchymal lesions in the cord are less frequent. Although not documented by imaging tests, presumably the intramedullary lesions of the cord progress through the same cyst, granuloma, and calcified nodule stages typical of brain parenchymal cysticercosis.

Spinal involvement by cysticercosis is uncommon, and the subarachnoid form of the disease, consisting of cysts and arachnoiditis, is more frequent than the intramedullary form. Increasing use of MR scans may provide more accurate data. The pathogenesis of spinal subarachnoid cysticercosis is thought to be the spread from the intracranial space into the spinal subarachnoid space via the posterior fossa.[45] The cervical, thoracic, and lumbar regions are affected equally.[10,15] Because of the difficulty in diagnosis, it is likely that estimates of the spinal forms of cysticercosis are low. In subarachnoid cysticercosis, cysts in the subarachnoid space can be and are typically mobile. Associated with the cysts is an arachnoiditis of variable severity[41] that can be severe enough to cause a complete block. For unknown reasons, the arachnoiditis is more severe in females than in males.

Few intramedullary cysticercosis generalizations can be made with regard to clinical presentation; it will be a function of the lesion site. Both extremity weakness and pain have been reported.[12] In spinal subarachnoid cysticercosis, patients experience lower extremity weakness, paresthesia, and bowel and bladder symptoms. It is common for cranial signs and symptoms of the disease to dominate the spinal findings. The initial clinical presentation may therefore relate primarily to hydrocephalus,[45] and it may be several months before spinal symptoms appear, whether or not the hydrocephalus is treated.[45]

MR Findings

Focal cord enlargement caused by single or multiple cysts within the cord is seen on T1W scans of intramedullary cysticercosis. The granuloma stage of the disease in the spinal cord has not been reported. The differential diagnosis of the cyst on T1W scans includes cystic cord tumors and small localized syrinxs. On T2W scans, the cystic form of the disease shows high signal intensity within the cyst at the site of cord enlargement.[12] Again, the granulomatous form of the disease has not been described in the spinal cord but presumably is similar to the intracranial presentation.[23] Granuloma is characterized by the high signal center, a low signal rim of capsule, and surrounding high signal caused by adjacent edema on T2W images. On T2W scans the differential diagnosis includes syrinx, which often contains signal loss caused by fluid motion, something not expected in a cysticercosis cyst.[12] Cord tumors show abnormal signal within an enlarged cord separate from the cyst, another finding not expected with a cysticercosis cyst. A degenerative cyst with a granulomatous capsule could show adjacent edema but the low signal within the capsule will help differentiate it from cord tumor.

There are two major findings in the subarachnoid form of cysticercosis. Individual cysts may be identified, although their mobility may be more difficult to demonstrate by MR than by myelography.[39] On T1W scans, subarachnoid cysts appear as well circumscribed, low signal intensity, intradural and extramedullary masses or may be identifiable only by their deformity of the adjacent spinal cord. On T2W scans such cysts will show high signal intensity similar to that of adjacent CSF if gating and flow compensation techniques are used. In ungated scans the cyst may stand out because of adjacent low signal produced by pulsating CSF. The other major finding is general to all forms of severe arachnoiditis: diffuse enlargement of the cord associated with an ill-defined margin. This irregular, "shaggy" margin to the cord is most visible on axial T1W scans. A T2W scan shows abnormal signal intensity within the cord representing secondary damage. On T1W and T2W scans, findings in subarachnoid cysticercosis may be similar to those seen in arachnoiditis of other etiologies. Secondary arachnoid cysts appear similar to the primary cysts of cysticercosis. In most instances, the subarachnoid form of cysticercosis will not be a diagnostic problem because the cranial manifestations have already been diagnosed. If spinal cysticercosis, intramedullary or subarachnoid, is suspected a brain scan and complement fixation titers are probably useful confirmatory diagnostic tests.

RHEUMATOID ARTHRITIS

The cervical spine has some manifestations of rheumatoid arthritis in up to 60% to 70% of patients,[34] occurring in synovial and cartilaginous articulations, as well as in tendonous and ligamentous insertions. Many of these changes are visible by plain film radiography. Of major concern in rheumatoid arthritis patients is the involvement of the occipital to C_2 area because this poses a threat to the patient's cervical spinal cord. All important features in this area are best seen with MR.[8,35] Because suspected atlantoaxial subluxation may trigger a myelogram, it is therefore one of the major reasons for obtaining an MR scan. The atlantoaxial joint is involved in up to 20% to 25% of rheumatoid arthritis patients.[13,35]

Subluxation and impaction, two major abnormalities of the atlantoaxial joint, can result in compressive myelopathy. Most often subluxation is anterior, although posterior and lateral subluxations occur. Impaction results in "settling" of the cranium and a relative cephalad position of the odontoid that encroaches on the foramen magnum and the structures within it.

Atlantoaxial joint involvement can result in pain that is localized in the neck or referred to the temporooccipital or orbital regions. Impingement on the cervical cord may result in paraparesis, quadraparesis, and paresthesia. A compressive myelopathy is fortunately uncommon. In rare instances, vertebrobasilar insufficiency can occur if there is compromise of one or both of the vertebral arteries; this can cause a variety of brainstem symptoms. Because the odontoid process is weakened, minimal trauma can fracture it, resulting in neurologic symptoms on that basis. With atlantoaxial impaction, the odontoid process may sublux in a cranial direction through the foramen magnum causing brainstem symptoms by direct compression.[26]

Changes in rheumatoid arthritis are caused primarily by effects secondary to synovial inflammation and the effects of hyperemia. Pannus formation results, which causes destruction of cartilage and bone seen as erosion. Ligamentous structures are also involved; they may be weakened or they may be thickened by fibrosis. Atlantooccipital subluxation (>2.5 mm gap between the arch of C_1 and the odontoid, i.e., the atlantodental distance)[8] and odontoid erosion can be visualized on plain x-rays. Subluxation is the result of laxity or disruption of the transverse ligament secondary to local synovial inflammation. Other ligaments, cruciate, alar, apical, etc. are also involved. As the disease progresses, erosion becomes more evident at the base of the odontoid process anteriorly and posteriorly and can become quite severe, causing significant osteolysis of the odontoid process. The presence of these erosions at the odontoid base increases the risk of odontoid fracture even with minimal trauma.

MR Findings

The odontoid process is well visualized in the normal adult cervical spine because of its marrow content. The signal intensity of the marrow in the odontoid is equivalent to that of other cervical vertebral bodies. A thin black, cortical line can be visualized around the entire odontoid process in sagittal and axial views. Fat can normally be identified between the odontoid process and the basion. Structures such as the anterior longitudinal ligament, the anterior atlantooccipital membrane, apical ligament (outlined by fat), and transverse ligament are routinely visualized.[8] On T2W images in axial and sagittal views, signal intensity of the odontoid process decreases because of the fat content in the marrow. No significant signal is detected in the region of the normal synovial joints.

With rheumatoid involvement of the odontoid process, the signal intensity on T1W images re-

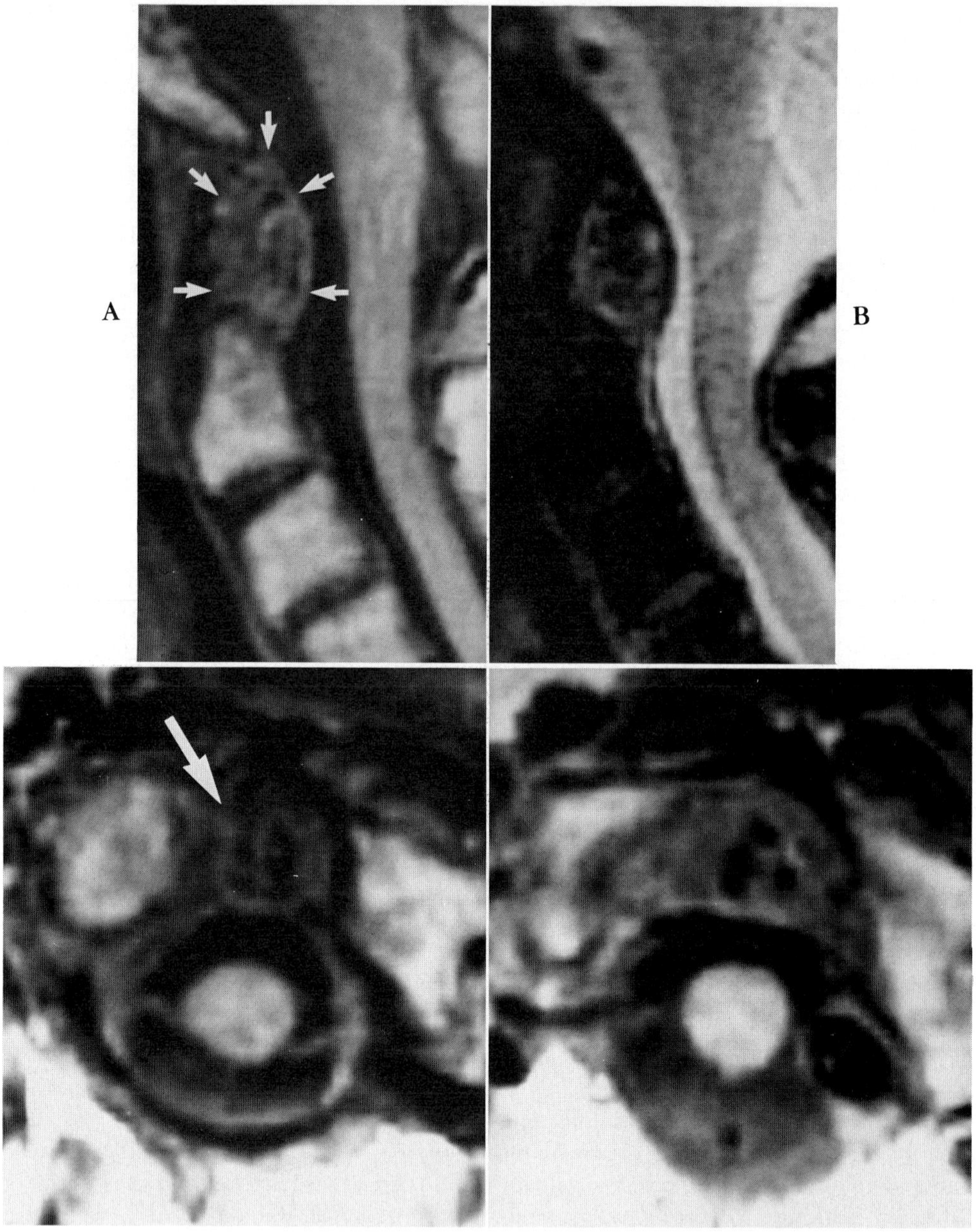

FIGURE 7-24. Rheumatoid arthritis. MR scan of 77-year-old female with rheumatoid arthritis shows inflammatory mass (pannus) replacing odontoid process. **A**, Sagittal T1W (SE 800/20) scan shows soft tissue mass *(arrows)* of intermediate and inhomogeneous signal intensity replacing superior portion of odontoid process. Soft tissue mass represents predental, retrodental, and supradental pannus that replaces normal fat between odontoid process and basion, narrowing atlantooccipital distance. **B**, Sagittal variable flip angle scan (GRASS 40/20, 5°) at same level shows only minimal impingement on spinal canal. Pannus itself consists of inhomogeneous areas of low signal and high signal intensity. Sagittal variable flip angle scan could be used for obtaining dynamic information at C_1-C_2 junction by scanning in flexed position to assess atlantodental distance. Axial T1W scan (SE 1000/20) shows pannus of intermediate inhomogeneous signal intensity replacing normal marrow in odontoid process (*arrow*, **C**) and extending into body of C_2 (**D**). No significant impingement into spinal canal is seen.

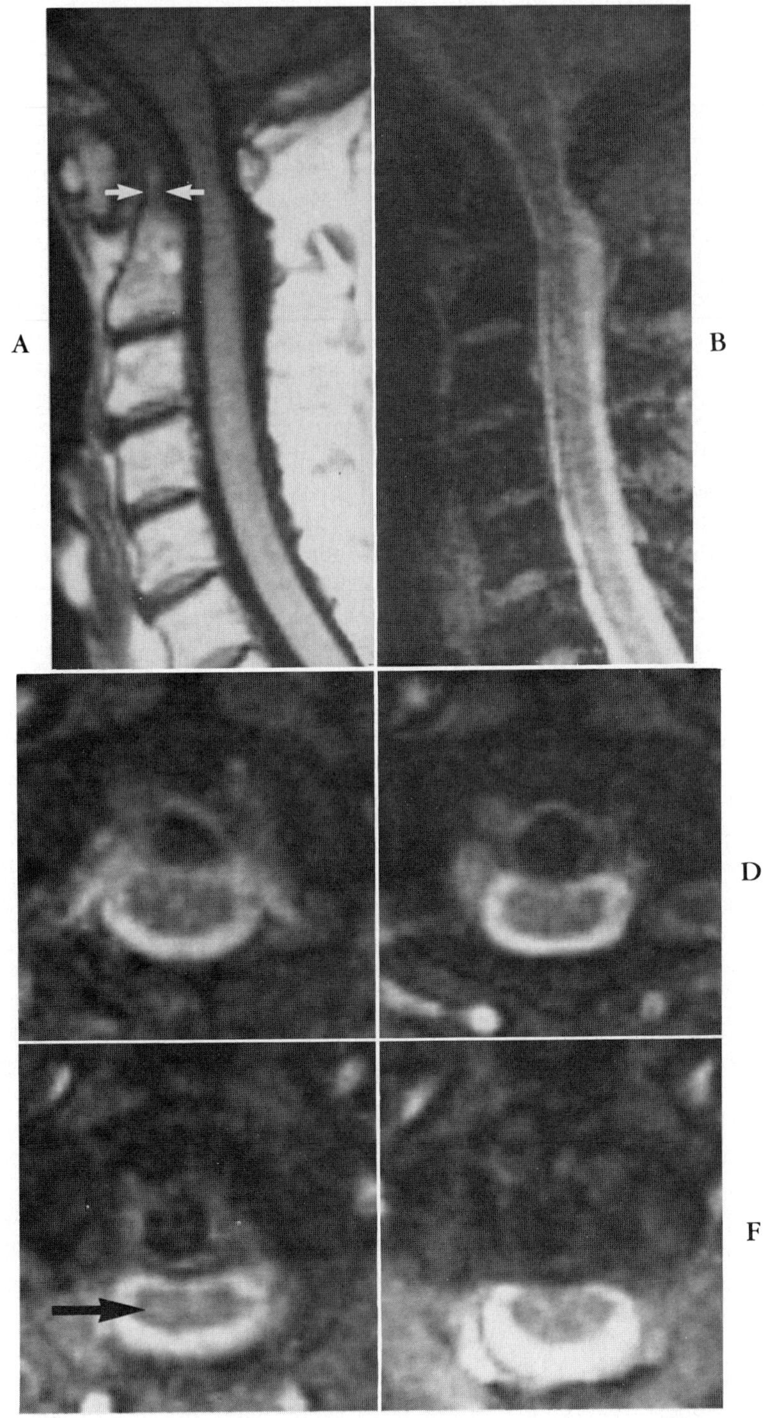

FIGURE 7-25. Rheumatoid arthritis. Subluxation of C_1 on C_2 causing compression of upper cervical cord in 69-year-old female with rheumatoid arthritis. **A,** T1W image (SE 800/20) shows marked anterior subluxation of C_1 on C_2 associated with predental pannus formation around anterior arch of C_1 and partial erosion of odontoid process *(paired arrows)*. Marrow-containing space is thinned *(arrow)*. Apical fat between odontoid and basion has been replaced. **B,** Sagittal variable flip angle/gradient echo scan (GRASS 25/13, 5°) better depicts narrowing of spinal canal, which is somewhat underestimated on T1W scan because some tissue posterior to odontoid process is of same low signal intensity as CSF (**A**). **C-F,** Set of four axial variable flip angle scans (GRASS 25/13, 7°) at level of odontoid process shows constriction of spinal canal and compression deformity of cord. At area of maximum narrowing, abnormal signal can be detected within cord (*arrow,* **E**). Area around odontoid process on axial images shows intermediate signal intensity indicative of pannus in this region.

mains intermediate signal intensity although more heterogeneous in nature (Figure 7-24). Characteristic of the disease process is pannus formation in a predental and retrodental location. Fat that is normally present between the odontoid and basion is replaced by this inflammatory tissue (Figure 7-25; see Figure 7-24). Pannus is of intermediate signal intensity on both T1W and T2W (or T2*W) images. T2W or T2*W images show heterogeneous signal in the region of the odontoid process with some areas of high signal indicating an abnormally high water content (see Figure 7-24). The odontoid cortical margin is partially eroded or totally absent with severe involvement. The odontoid process may be eroded and appear thinned (see Figure 7-25).[8] Odontoid erosion can be better visualized by MR compared to plain films.[1] The size of the odontoid process may appear enlarged because of the increased amount of pannus within and around it, and may extend more caphalad than normal decreasing the basion-dental interval. This also occurs with impaction. Retrodental pannus causes a convex posterior border, which can impinge upon the upper cervical canal.

The degree of impingement upon the cervical canal and the upper cervical cord is a clinical concern. Atlantoaxial subluxation and those below C_2 are well detected by MR,[7] and can be detected by a sagittal view in a neutral position or accentuated in a flexed position. Impingement into the spinal canal is best evaluated by a pulse sequence that yields a "myelogram" effect; a sagittal variable flip angle/gradient echo scan or T2W images generated with some form of motion compensation, CSF gating or gradient moment nulling, or both (see Figures 7-24 and 7-25). The time it takes to perform the latter scans makes them less practical for a flexion view. Sagittal variable flip angle/gradient echo scans can be used to produce fast "myelographic" images in flexion and extension, less than a minute in a single-slice mode. The variable flip angle scan is a useful alternative to myelography for studying atlantoaxial dynamics.

If patients have neurologic deficits MR scans show cord and brainstem indentation. In one study where patients had two objective signs of a compressive myelopathy, all had MR evidence of cord impingement.[7] In another study not only did all patients show cord indentation but five of seven patients also showed abnormal high signal within the cord on T2W image.[1] MR is therefore an important study in the investigation and possibly in the screening of RA patients. Subluxation as determined from plain radiographs correlates poorly with the presence of compressive myelopathy.[7]

PSORIATIC ARTHRITIS

Two to six percent of psoriatic patients have manifestations of psoriatic arthritis, a form of arthritis that has widespread skeletal manifestations involving the appendicular skeleton. In many respects, psoriatic arthritis is similar to rheumatoid arthritis but is seronegative. The similarity is present because both disease processes share a significant component of synovial inflammation. Conversely psoriatic arthritis involves cartilagenous joints which is uncommon with rheumatoid arthritis. Patients with prominent involvement of the axial skeleton with spondylitis have evidence of the human lymphocyte B7 antigen. Spine changes are characterized by erosive changes similar to rheumatoid arthritis and prominent bony proliferation in a paravertebral distribution. These areas of ossification vary from quite thick to thin and resemble syndesmophytes of ankylosing spondylitis. Another feature shared with rheumatoid arthritis is the erosive change around the odontoid process resulting in atlantoaxial subluxation. This is relatively common with psoriatic spondylitis.[20]

MR Findings

MR findings in the atlantoaxial region may be similar to those found in rheumatoid arthritis (Figure 7-26). The T1W image can show erosion of the odontoid process and subluxation of C_1 of C_2. The gap between the arch of C_1 and the odontoid process is filled with abnormal soft tissue, which is of intermediate signal intensity on a T1W image and intermediate signal intensity on a variable flip angle/gradient echo scan (Figure 7-26). Because the basic pathogenesis of synovial inflammation in this location is the same, findings are also similar in psoriatic and rheumatoid arthritis. Abnormalities of the vertebral bodies and disc spaces of psoriatic arthritis are similar to that seen with severe degenerative osteoarthritis. The low signal intensity extend-

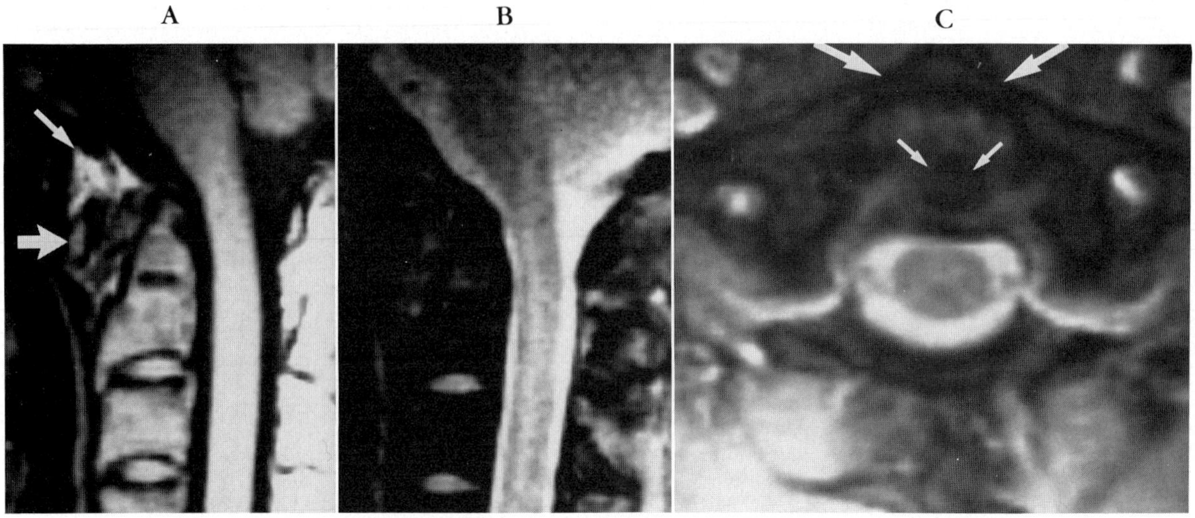

FIGURE 7-26. Psoriatic arthritis. Atlantoaxial subluxation in psoariatic arthritis is similar to that in rheumatoid arthritis. **A,** T1W scan (SE 800/20) shows abnormal separation of odontoid process and arch of C_1 by intervening soft tissue *(large arrow)*. Fat tissue between arch of C_1 and basion remains intact *(small arrow)*. **B,** Sagittal variable flip angle/gradient echo scan (GRASS 40/20, 5°) shows some compromise on spinal canal but no cord compression. **C,** Axial variable flip angle scan (GRASS 22/12, 7°) shows separation between arch of C_1 *(large arrows)* and odontoid process *(small arrows)*. Abnormal intervening soft tissue surrounding odontoid process is intermediate signal intensity. There is mild anterior extradural impingement into the spinal canal.

ing into the vertebral body from the involved disc space may suggest the possibility of metastatic disease (see Chapter 8, Figure 8-86). Although the paravertebral ossification may be difficult to identify by MR, this hypertrophic bone formation can be identified by the extensive area of low signal caused by the ossified masses.

REFERENCES

1. Aisen AM, Martel W, Ellis JH, et al. Cervical spine involvement in rheumatoid arthritis: MR imaging. Radiology 1987;165:159.
2. Angtuaco EJC, McConnell JR, Chadduck WM, et al. MR imaging of spinal epidural sepsis. AJNR 1987;8:879.
3. Baker AS, Ojemann RG, Swartz MN, et al. Spinal epidural absess. N Engl J Med 1975;293:463.
4. Bertino RE, Porter BA, Stimac GK, et al. Imaging spinal osteomyelitis and epidural abscess with short T1 inversion recovery (STIR). AJNR 1988;9:563.
5. Blacklock JB, Hood TW, Maxwell RE. Intramedullary cervical spinal cord abscess. J Neurosurg 1982;57:270.
6. Bouchez B, Arnott G, Delfosse JM. Acute spinal epidural abscess. J Neurol 1985;231:343.
7. Breedveld FC, Algra PR, Vielvoye CJ, et al. Magnetic resonance imaging in the evaluation of patients with rheumatoid arthritis and subluxations of the cervical spine. Arthritis Rheum 1987;30:624.
8. Bundschuh C, Modic MT, Kearney F, et al. Rheumatoid arthritis of the cervical spine: surface-coil MR imaging. AJNR 1988;9:565.
9. Burke DR, Brant-Zawadzki. CT of pyogenic spine infection. Neuroradiology 1985;27:131.
10. Cabieses F, Vallenas M, Landa R. Cysticercosis of the spinal canal. J Neurosurg 1959;16:337.
11. Carson HW: Acute osteomyelitis of the spine. Br J Surg 1930;18:400.
12. Castillo M, Quencer RM, Post MJD. MR of intramedullary spinal cysticercosis. AJNR 1988;9:393.
13. Conlon PW, Isdale IC, Rose BS. Rheumatoid arthritis of the cervical spine. An analysis of 333 cases. Ann Rheum Dis 1966;25:120.
14. Coventry MB, Ghormley RK, Kernohan JW. The intervertebral disc: its microscopic anatomy and pathology. J Bone Joint Surg 1945;27A:105.
15. Dorfsman J. Radiological aspects of spinal cysticercosis. Acta Radiol 1966;6:1003.
16. Feldenzer JA, McKeever PE, Schaberg DR, et al. Experimental spinal epidural abscess: a pathophysiological model in the rabbit. Neurosurgery 1987; 20:859.
17. Gokalp HZ, Ozkal E. Intradural tuberculomas of the spinal cord. J Neurosurg 1981;55:289.
18. Goldman AB, Freiberger RH. Localized infectious and neuropathic diseases. Semin Roentgenol 1979;14:19.
19. Hodgson AR. Infectious disease of the spine. In: Rothman RH, Simeone FA, eds. The spine. Philadelphia: W.B. Saunders Co., 1982.
20. Killebrew, Gold RH, Sholkoff SD. Psoriatic spondylitis. Radiology 1973;108:9.
21. Knudsen LL, Voldby B, Stagaard M. Computed tomographic myelography in spinal subdural empyema. Neuroradiology 1987;29:99.
22. Lasker BR, Harter DH. Cervical epidural abscess. Neurology 1987;37:1747.

23. Lotz J, Hewlett R, Alheit B, et al. Neurocysticercosis: correlative pathomorphology and MR imaging. Neuroradiology 1988;30:35.
24. Mallowaski SK. Pyogenic infection of the spine. Int Orthop (SICOT) 1977;1:125.
25. McGahan JP, Graves DS, Palmer PES. Coccidioidal spondylitis. Radiology 1980;136:5.
26. Menezes AH, VanGilder JC, Clark CR, et al. Odontoid upward migration in rheumatoid arthritis. J Neurosurg 1985;63:500.
27. Merine D, Wang H, Kumar AJ, et al. CT myelography and MR imaging of acute transverse myelitis. J Comput Assist Tomogr 1987;11:606.
28. Mineiro JD. Coluna vertebral humana: alguns aspectos da sua estrutura e vascularizacao. Lisboa 1: Dissertacao de Doctoramento, 1965.
29. Modic MT, Feiglin DH, Piraino DW, et al. Vertebral osteomyelitis: assessment using MR. Radiology 1985;157:157.
30. Postacchini F, Montanaro A. Tuberculous epidural granuloma simulating a herniated lumbar disk: a report of a case. Clin Orthop 1980;148:182.
31. Rawlings CE, Wilkins RH, Gallis HA, et al. Postoperative intervertebral disc space infection. Neurosurgery 1983;13:371.
32. Resnick D, Niwayama G. Osteomyelitis, septic arthritis, and soft tissue infection: the axial skeleton. In: Resnick D, Niwayama G, eds. Diagnosis of bone and joint disorders. Philadelphia: W.B. Saunders Co., 1981.
33. Resnick D, Niwayama G. Osteomyelitis, septic arthritis, and soft tissue infection: the organisms. In: Resnick D. Niwayama G, eds. Diagnosis of bone and joint disorders. Philadelphia: W. B. Saunders Co., 1981.
34. Resnick D, Niwayama G. Rheumatoid arthritis. In: Resnick D, Niwayama G. eds. Diagnosis of bone and joint disorders. W. B. Saunders Co., 1981.
35. Reynolds H, Carter SW, Murtagh FR, et al. Cervical rheumatoid arthritis: value of flexion and extension views in imaging. Radiology 1987;164:215.
36. Rocco HD, Eyring EJ. Intervertebral disk infections in children. Amer J Dis Child 1972;123:448.
37. Ropper AH, Poskanzer DC. The prognosis of acute and subacute transverse myelopathy based on early signs and symptoms. Ann Neurol 1978;4:51.
38. Rosenfeld JV, Kaye AH, Davis S, et al. Pachymeningitis cervicalis hypertrophica. J Neurosurg 1987;66:137.
39. Savoiardo M, Cimino C, Passerina A, et al. Mobile myelographic filling defects: spinal cysticercosis. Neuroradiology 1986;28:166.
40. Smith RF, Taylor TKF. Inflammatory lesions of intervertebral discs in children. J Bone Joint Surgery 1967;49:1508.
41. Sotelo J, Marin C. Hydrocephalus secondary to cysticercotic arachnoiditis. J Neurosurg 1987;66:686.
42. Wenger DR, Bobechko WP. Spectrum of intervertebral disc-space infection in children. J Bone Joint Surgery 1978;60:100.
43. Whelan MA, Naidich DP, Post JD, et al. Computed tomography of spinal tuberculosis. J Comput Assist Tomogr 1983;7:25.
44. Whelan MA, Schonfeld S, Post JD, et al. Computed tomography of nontuberculous spinal infection. J Comput Assist Tomogr 1985;9:280.
45. Zee C-S, Segall HD, Ahmadi J, et al. CT myelography in spinal cysticercosis. J Comput Assist Tomogr 1986;10:195.

8
Tumor

Dieter R. Enzmann
Robert L. DeLaPaz

SPINAL CORD TUMORS

Astrocytoma

Astrocytomas represent approximately 40% of spinal cord tumors. Generally, astrocytomas in the cord are less malignant than those in the brain. In one series of 86 spinal cord astrocytomas, 52% were grade I, 24% were grade II, 18% were grade III, and 6% were grade IV.[67] Approximately 90% of brain astrocytomas are grade III or IV in adults.[67] The distribution of astrocytomas is fairly uniform in the spinal cord regardless of tumor grade.[67] Approximately 75% of lesions occur at the thoracic and cervical levels, 20% occur in the distal cord, and 5% occur in the filum terminale. The longitudinal extent of most symptomatic tumors is two to three vertebral segments, but some lesions involve ten or more vertebral levels. Generally, more malignant tumors are not more extensive than low-grade astrocytomas.[67]

Most patients with spinal cord astrocytomas present in their thirties and forties, with a slight tendency for more malignant lesions to become symptomatic earlier.[67] They vary in age from 16 months to 63 years with a mean of 35 years for grade I, 39 years for grade II, 30 years for grade III, and 23 years for grade IV tumors. The usual presentation (50% to 75% of patients) is pain in the back, neck, or legs. Motor disturbances of spasticity and stiffness occur frequently in the legs, are the presenting signs in 20% to 30% of patients, and are more frequent than pain in higher grade tumors. Sensory changes (numbness or tingling), constipation, and urinary incontinence may also be present.

The survival period for patients with spinal cord astrocytomas varies and depends primarily on the grade of the tumor. Low-grade tumors tend to survive approximately eight times longer than high-grade astrocytomas; 8 years vs. 1 year in an older series.[67] The survival period was equal to approximately 2 to 3 times the pretreatment symptom time interval. The prognosis and possibility of cure is changing. More aggressive surgical resection, previously attempted primarily with ependymomas, appears to improve survival statistics with astrocytomas[11] but necessitates accurate tumor localization. MR, especially with intravenous contrast gadolinium diethylenetriamine penta-acetic acid

A

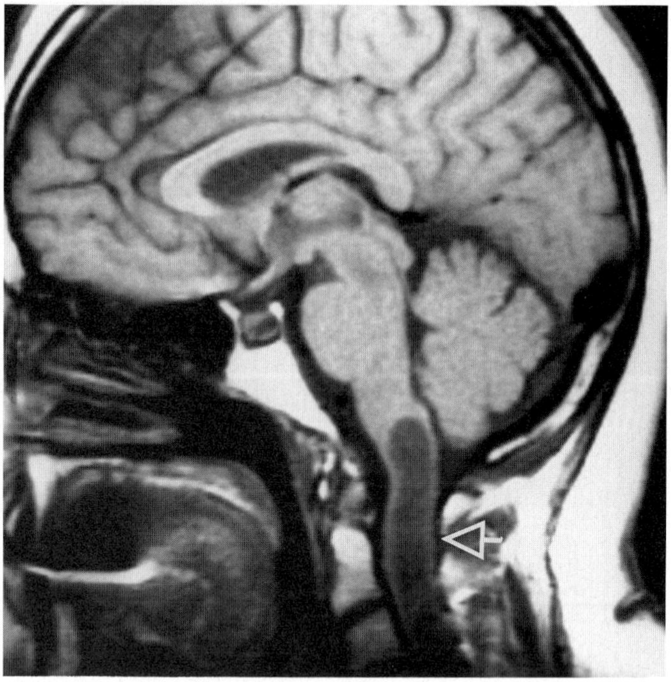

FIGURE 8-1. Astrocytoma of the cervical and thoracic spinal cord with an adjacent cyst in 56-year-old female. Sagittal T1W (SE 800/20) images of spinal cervicomedullary function (**A**), cervical cord (**B**) and thoracic cord (**C**) show extensive intramedullary lesion extending from foramen magnum to T_{10}. Heterogeneous signal intensities are seen within cord and most homogeneous portion of involved cord, from C_6 to T_2 (**B**, *solid straight arrow*). Above and below is irregular low and intermediate signal intensity (**B** and **C**, *curved arrows*). Low signal within areas is indistinctly marginated and reflects variation in water content rather than cyst formation. An intramedullary low signal cyst with sharp margins is present superiorly (**A** and **B**, *open arrows*), enlarging cord and lower medulla. **D**, Axial T1W image (SE1000/20) at C_4-C_5 through midcervical solid portion of tumor shows enlargement of cord with loss of normal internal architecture. Signal within enlarged cord is intermediate intensity, similar to normal cord, with small areas of low signal, high water content tissue *(arrow)*. **E**, Axial T2W image (SE 2000/80) at C_4-C_5 also shows enlarged cord and loss of normal internal architecture. Foci of high signal indicate areas of higher water content tissue and correspond to low signal on T1W image. Two small regions of low signal *(arrow)* are present in dorsal cord that correspond to isointense signal areas on T1W and probably represent small amounts of hemosiderin from petechial hemorrhage within tumor. **F**, Axial T1W image (SE 1000/20) at C_2 level through cyst shows sharply defined region within cord with very low signal, similar to CSF. Thin rim of intermediate signal cord tissue surrounds cyst *(arrow)*. Low signal within cyst is typical of most tumor-associated cysts. Some cysts have signal isointense with cord because of high protein content or hemorrhage in cyst fluid (see Figure 8-3). **G**, Axial T2W image (SE 2000/80) at C_2 shows sharply defined region in central cord with homogeneous, high signal that is higher than CSF. Relative lower signal in CSF is due to its oscillatory motion in subarachnoid space. Thin rim of normal low signal cord surrounds cyst *(arrow)*. Region of high signal is slightly larger than corresponding low signal of cyst seen on T1W image because high signal is produced by free water in cyst fluid and by high water content of cord tissue at cyst margin. Both cysts and solid tumor show high signal on T2W images. The key to differentiating cyst from tumor is usually the signal on first echo of the T2W sequence. Cysts have low signal compared to cord (similar to CSF), whereas tumor has relatively high signal to cord.

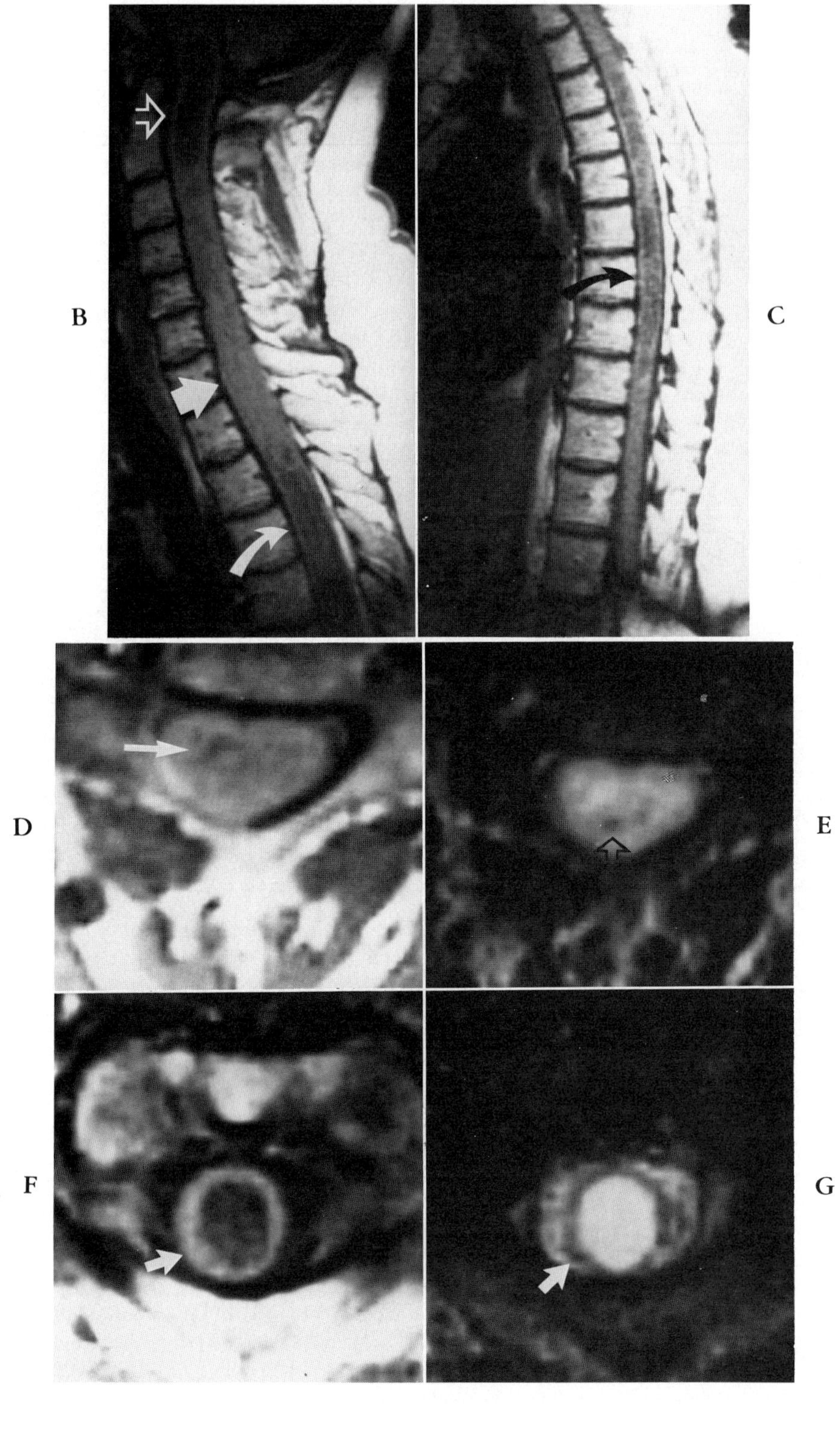
B
C
D
E
F
G

sive and occupy portions of what normally would (GdDTPA), provides important information for the newer surgical techniques used in treating spinal cord astrocytoma.

MR Imaging

MR is very sensitive in the detection of primary spinal cord tumors. It is relatively nonspecific, however, with regard to histology in nonvascular primary tumors of the cord. MR signal intensity does not distinguish cord astrocytomas from other tumors. MR scans in one series of 32 patients with surgically confirmed primary cord tumors (11 astrocytomas, 10 ependymomas, 5 vascular lesions and 6 gliomas)[65] showed all lesions to have high signal on T2W images and low signal on T1W images. Although no specific morphologic or signal patterns were found that differentiated the two types of tumor (astrocytoma and ependymoma) some characteristics were more common in one or the other. A tumor involving the full diameter of the cord with homogeneous high signal on T2W images is most likely an astrocytoma. A smaller, well-defined nodule associated with extensive cysts is most likely an ependymoma.

Typical cord astrocytomas are relatively large and involve multiple levels, with the tumor of lower signal intensity than cord on T1W images (Figures 8-1 to 8-4). The heterogeneity of low signal intensity depends on the size of the tu-

A, B

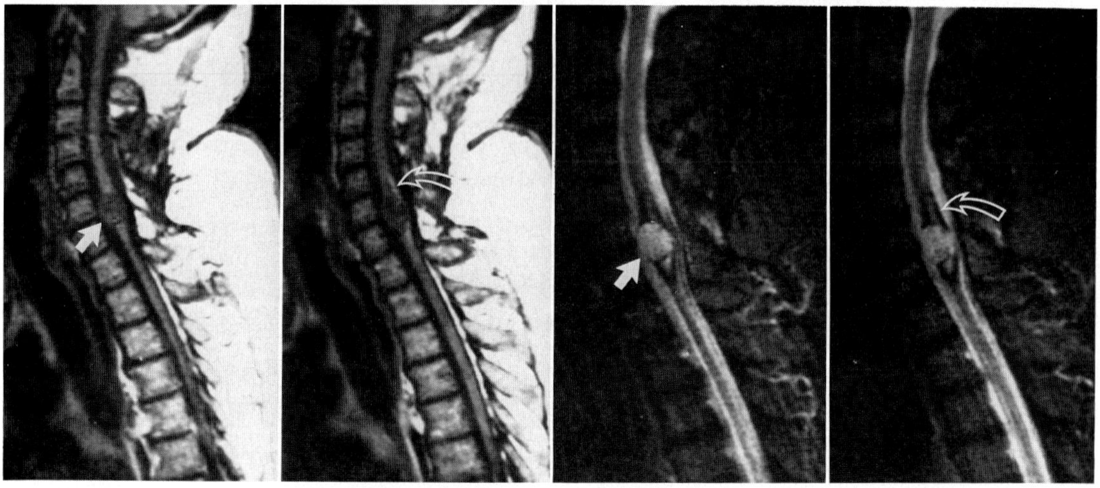

C, D

FIGURE 8-2. Cervical spinal cord astrocytoma in 62-year-old male. Sagittal T1W images (SE 800/20) show well-circumscribed intermediate signal, fusiform mass (*arrow*, **A**) in cervical spinal cord at C_6-C_7 level. Region of low signal in central cord tapers superiorly and inferiorly from mass (*arrow*, **B**) that corresponds to high signal on T2W images and probably represents edema rather than cyst formation. Sagittal T2W images (SE 2000/100) show mass as high signal (**C**, *arrow*). Fusiform enlargement of cord is present with central high signal tapering superiorly (*arrow*, **D**) and inferiorly from mass. Indistinct margins and tapering of region are more consistent with edema or myelomalacia than cyst. Marked low signal outlines these regions above and below mass and probably represents hemosiderin staining from previous hemorrhage. Presence of magnetic susceptibility effects suggests possibility of slow flow (cryptic) AVM. Low signal is not around main mass as it would be around a chronic hematoma. Axial T2W images (SE 2000/20, **E**; 80, **F**) at C_6-C_7 level show enlarged cord filling most of thecal sac. Cord is nearly completely replaced by tumor. Slightly exophytic portion of tumor projects to right posterolaterally *(arrows)*. Signal in mass is intermediate and similar to cord on first echo image, **E**, and higher and less homogeneous than cord on second echo image, **F**. Hemosiderin staining is not seen at this level. **G**, Axial CT image with intrathecal contrast (iopamidol) at C_6-C_7 shows enlarged cord with small exophytic component on right outlined by thin rim of opacified CSF *(arrow)*. **H**, Anteroposterior (AP) view of cervical myelogram shows marked focal widening of cord caused by tumor *(arrow)*. Although consistent with intramedullary tumor, appearance is nonspecific.

E, F

G

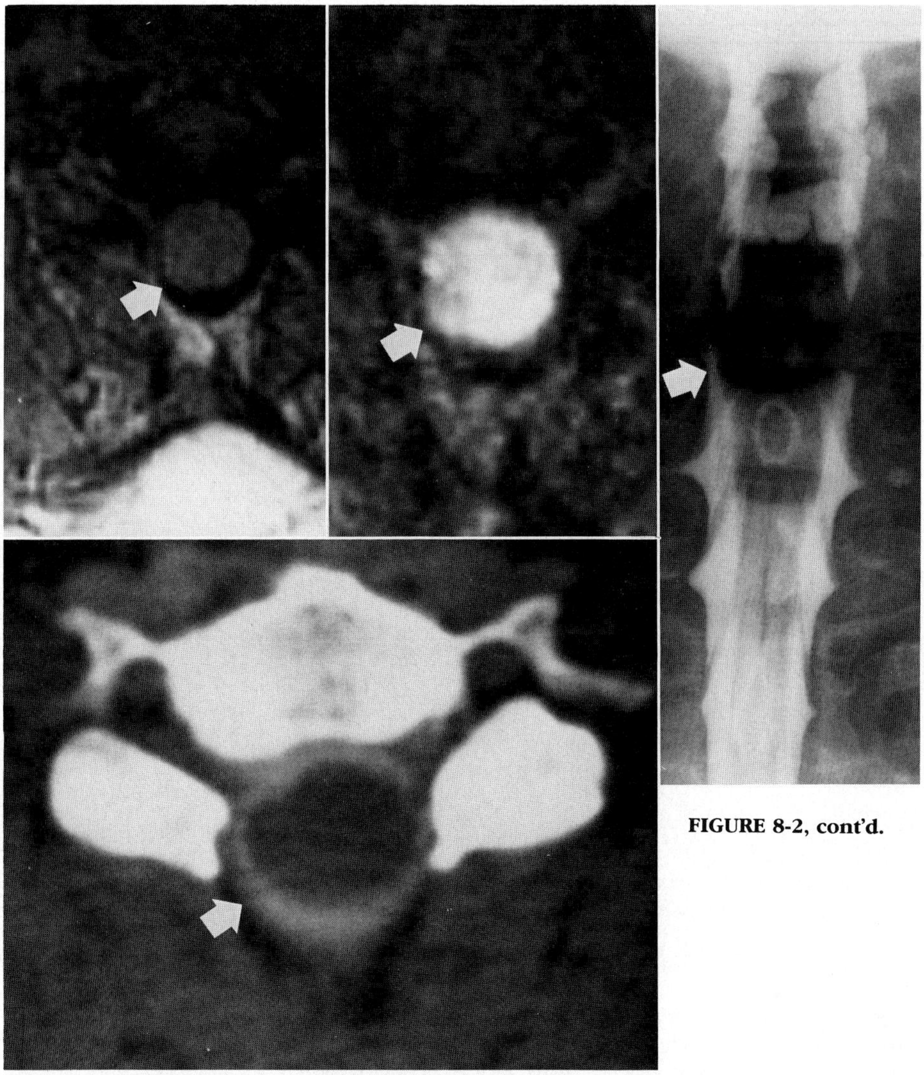

H

FIGURE 8-2, cont'd.

A

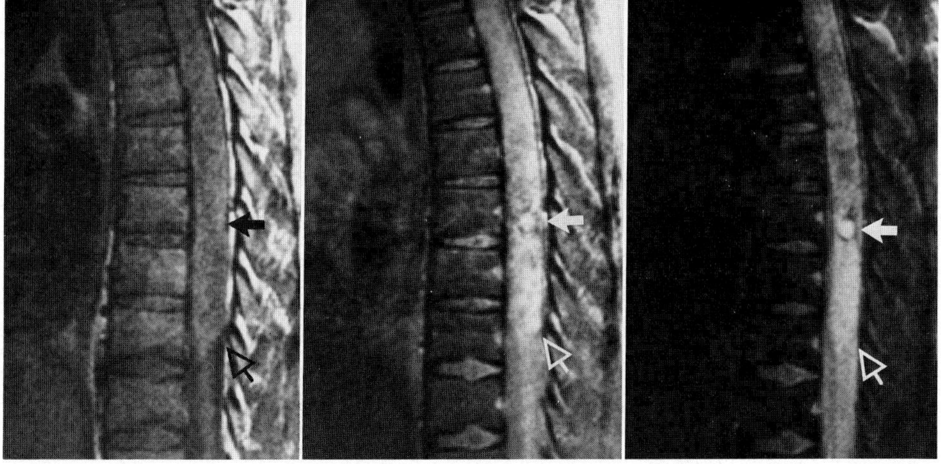

B, C

FIGURE 8-3, A-C. For legend see p. 306.

D E

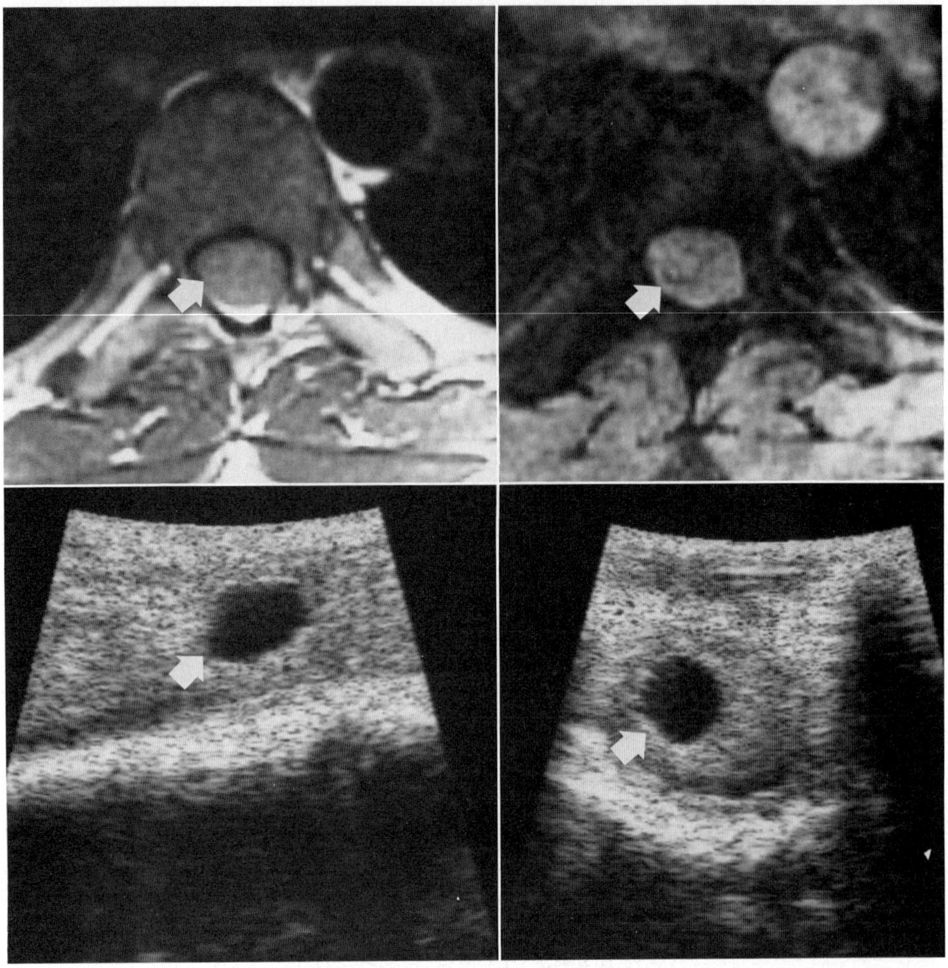

F G

FIGURE 8-3, cont'd. Surgically confirmed thoracic cord astrocytoma in 22-year-old male. **A,** Sagittal T1W image (SE 800/20) shows marked enlargement of thoracic spinal cord extending inferiorly to T_9 level *(open arrow)*. Mottled pattern of intermediate and low signal is typical of astrocytoma on T1W images. No evidence for typical, sharply defined, low signal cyst is seen, but an ill-defined focus of signal *(closed arrow)* corresponds to cyst seen on T2W images and intraoperative ultrasound. Relatively high signal in cyst (equal to cord) is probably result of high protein content of cyst fluid. Sagittal T2W images (SE 2022/30, **B;** 80, **C**) show diffuse enlargement of thoracic spinal cord by tumor with abnormal high signal. Inferior margins of cord are less well defined than on T1W image *(open arrows)* because elevated signal is nearly isointense with CSF. Mottled signal is seen in enlarged cord on T2W images. Mottled signal on T1W image is result of intrinsic variation within cord tumor. Pattern on T2W images is primarily result of motion artifact along phase-encoding gradient from cardiac motion (phase ghosting). Small, well-defined high signal focus at T_7 (**C,** *closed arrow*) represents proteinaceous cyst corresponding to isointense lesion on T1W image *(closed arrow,* **A**). **D,** Axial T1W image (SE 1000/20) through level of cyst at T_7 shows enlarged spinal cord *(arrow)* without visualization of cystic portion of lesion. Homogeneous intermediate signal of enlarged cord fills entire thecal sac. **E,** Axial variable flip angle/gradient echo image (GRASS 25/13, 7°) through cyst at T_7 shows area on right side in enlarged cord that is isointense with cord but outlined by thin low signal margin *(arrow)*. This corresponds to cyst on sagittal T2W images and axial intraoperative ultrasound, **G.** Thin margin of low signal probably represents hemosiderin. **F,** Sagittal and **G,** axial intraoperative ultrasound images with 10 MHz transducer show round anechoic region *(arrows)* representing cyst within cord tumor at T_7 level.

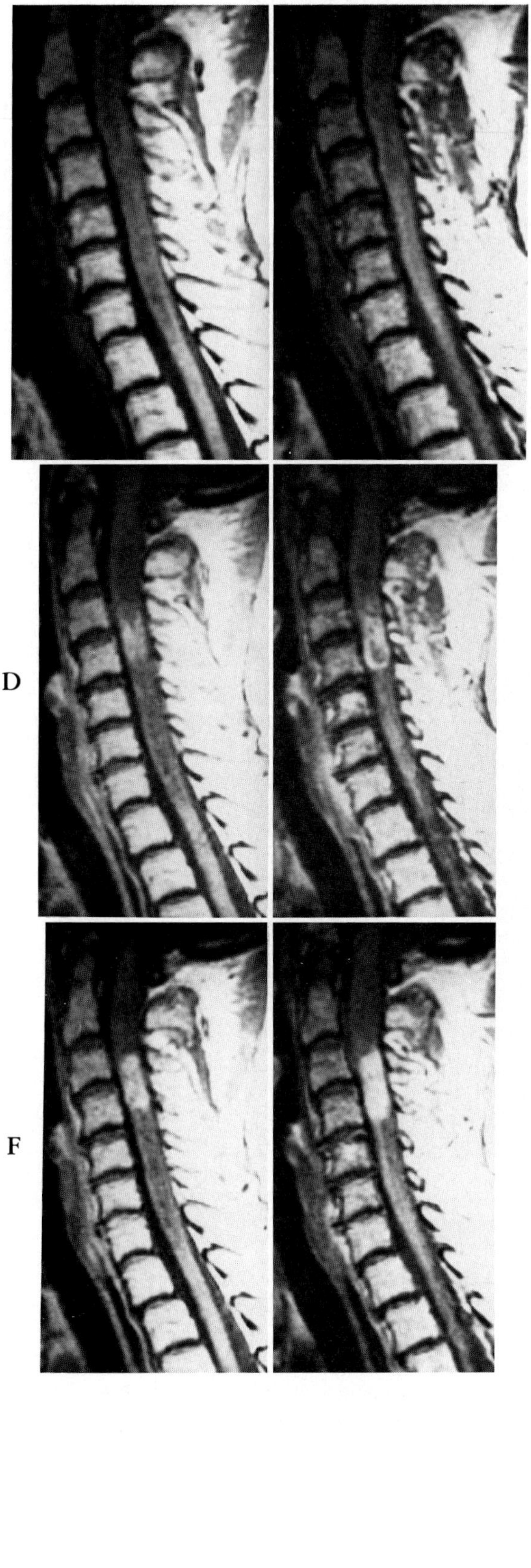

A B

C, D

E, F

FIGURE 8-4. Astrocytoma. Use of GdDTPA and T2W images illustrates evaluation of tumor extent and growth in patient with cervical glioma. **A** and **B,** Sagittal T1W scans (SE 800/20) show diffuse low signal in enlarged cervical cord. Low signal is somewhat inhomogeneous at C_3-C_4 level. Differentiation of tumor from adjacent edema on T1W images is difficult. **C** and **D,** Post-GdDTPA scan (SE 800/20) shows enhancement of cord at C_3-C_4 level. **E** and **F,** Delayed postcontrast scan (45 minutes) shows increased enhancement of tumor with more homogeneous pattern, although area of enhancement is similar.

G H

I J

K L

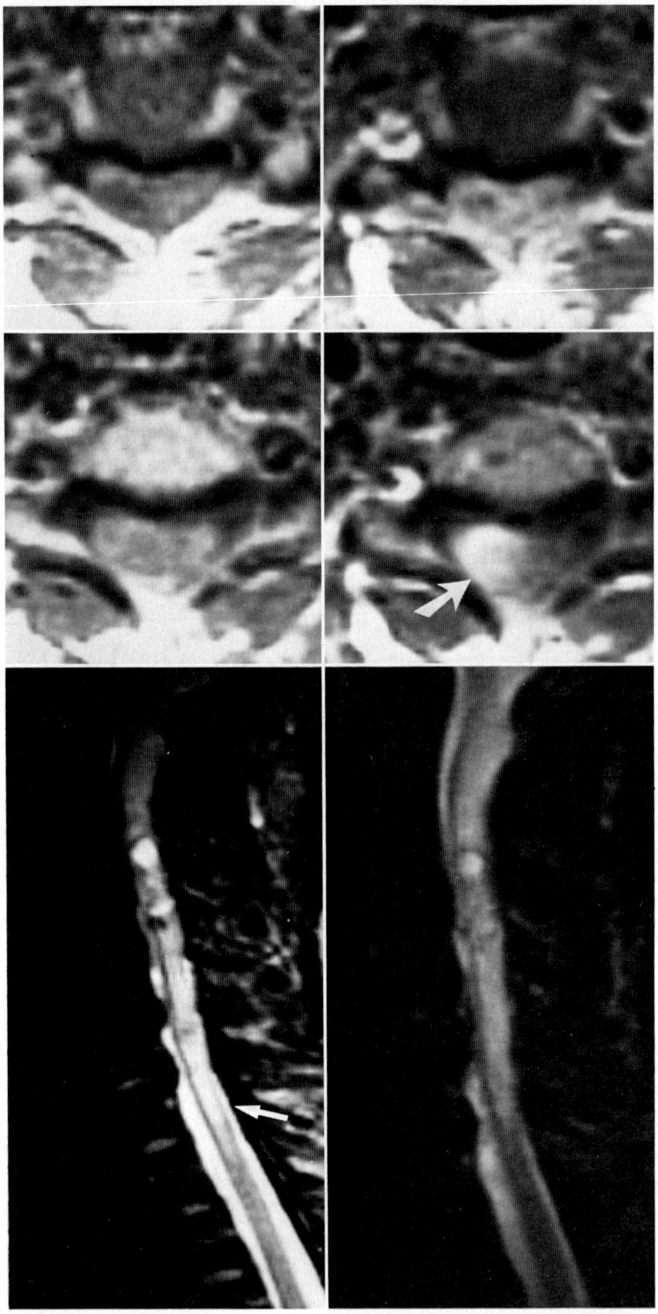

FIGURE 8-4, cont'd. G and **J**, Axial T1W scans (SE 1000/20) show heterogeneity of signal in cord (**G**), enhancement involving entire cord at some levels (**H** and **I**), and partial cord enhancement at another level (*arrow*, **J**). **K** and **L**, T2W sagittal scan (SE 2500/80) at same time shows abnormal high signal in enlarged cord in similar distribution as low signal area (**A** and **B**). Inhomogeneous signal was present at C_3-C_4, the site of enhancement (**K**). Tumor and edema are difficult to determine. Contrast enhancing area may not be the only tumor present (**C-F**). Extensive high signal within cord (**K**) could be tumor or edema. T1W images (**A** and **B**) show no appreciable difference from a year earlier. T2W sagittal scan, however, showed further caudal extension of intramedullary high signal (*arrow*, **K**) compared to year earlier (**L**).

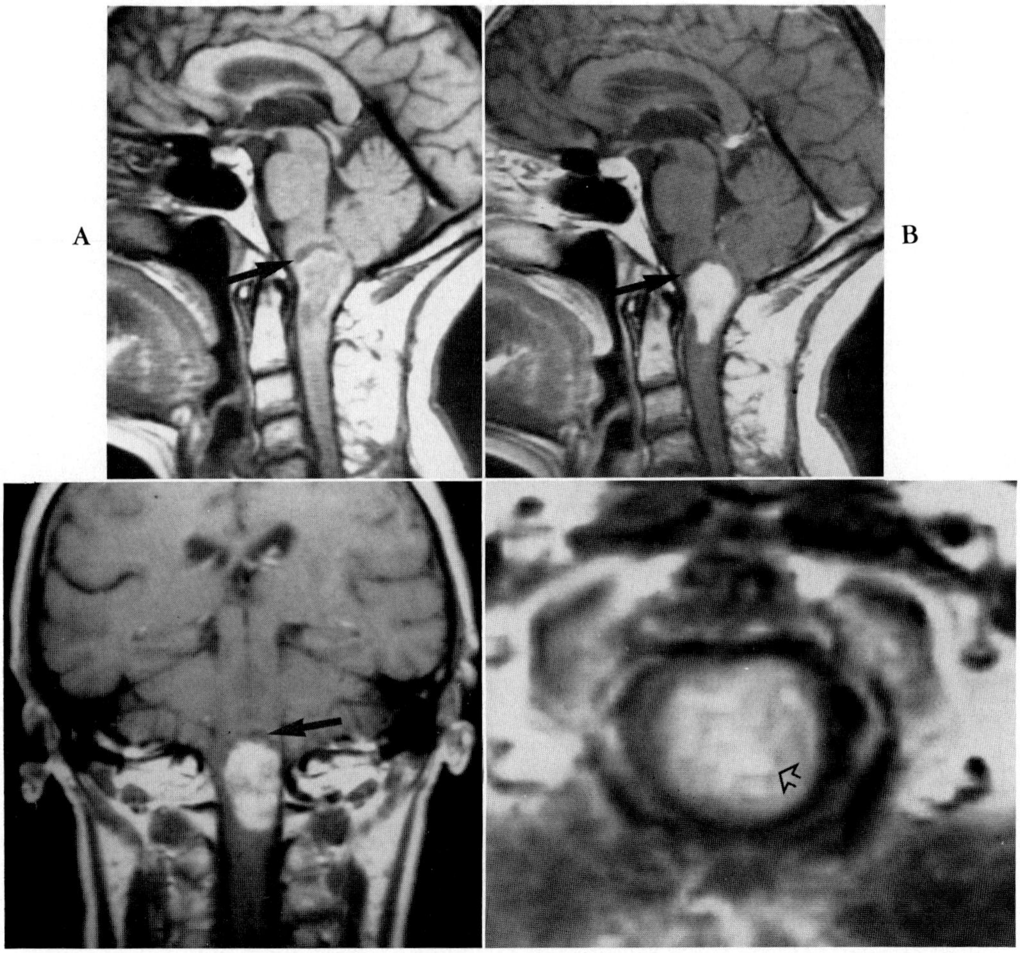

FIGURE 8-5. Before intravenous gadopentetate (GdDTPA) and postGdDTPA in cervicomedullary junction astrocytoma of 62-year-old female. **A,** Sagittal T1W image (SE 600/20) obtained before intravenous injection of GdDTPA shows intermediate signal astrocytoma at cervicomedullary junction. Central region of mass shows mottled signal with two well-defined low signal regions superior (**A-C,** *arrows*) and inferior to mass that represent cyst formation at margins of astrocytoma. **B** and **C,** Sagittal and coronal T1W images (SE 600/20) obtained at approximately 5 minutes and 10 minutes after injection of 0.1 mmol/kg GdDTPA show intense contrast enhancement of tumor. There is marked increase in signal centrally in mass. No enhancement is in low signal cystic areas superior *(arrows)* and inferior to tumor. **D,** Axial T1W image (SE 600/20) obtained approximately 15 minutes after GdDTPA administration shows enlarged cord with irregular high signal enhancement centrally *(arrow)*. *(Courtesy of Dr. Doyon.)*

mor. Cysts and areas of hemorrhage identified within tumor add to the heterogeneity (see Figures 8-2, 8-3, and 8-6).[28] Edema is difficult to distinguish from tumor on conventional T1W or T2W images (see Figure 8-4) because both have low signal on T1W images and high signal intensity on T2W images (see Figure 8-4).

With a contrast agent such as GdDTPA, astrocytomas exhibit enhancement seen as high signal on T1W images (Figures 8-5 to 8-7; see Figure 8-4), which distinguishes between tumor and adjacent edema. GdDTPA is a marker for an abnormal blood-brain barrier (blood-cord) and may not show enhancement in areas of tumor (i.e., low grade) with an intact barrier (see Figures 8-4 to 8-7). Delayed MR scans (30 to 60 minutes) may show a larger area of enhancement and an increase in signal intensity (see Figure 8-4). Therefore the same dilemma that occurs with iodinated contrast media and CT in brain

A B C D

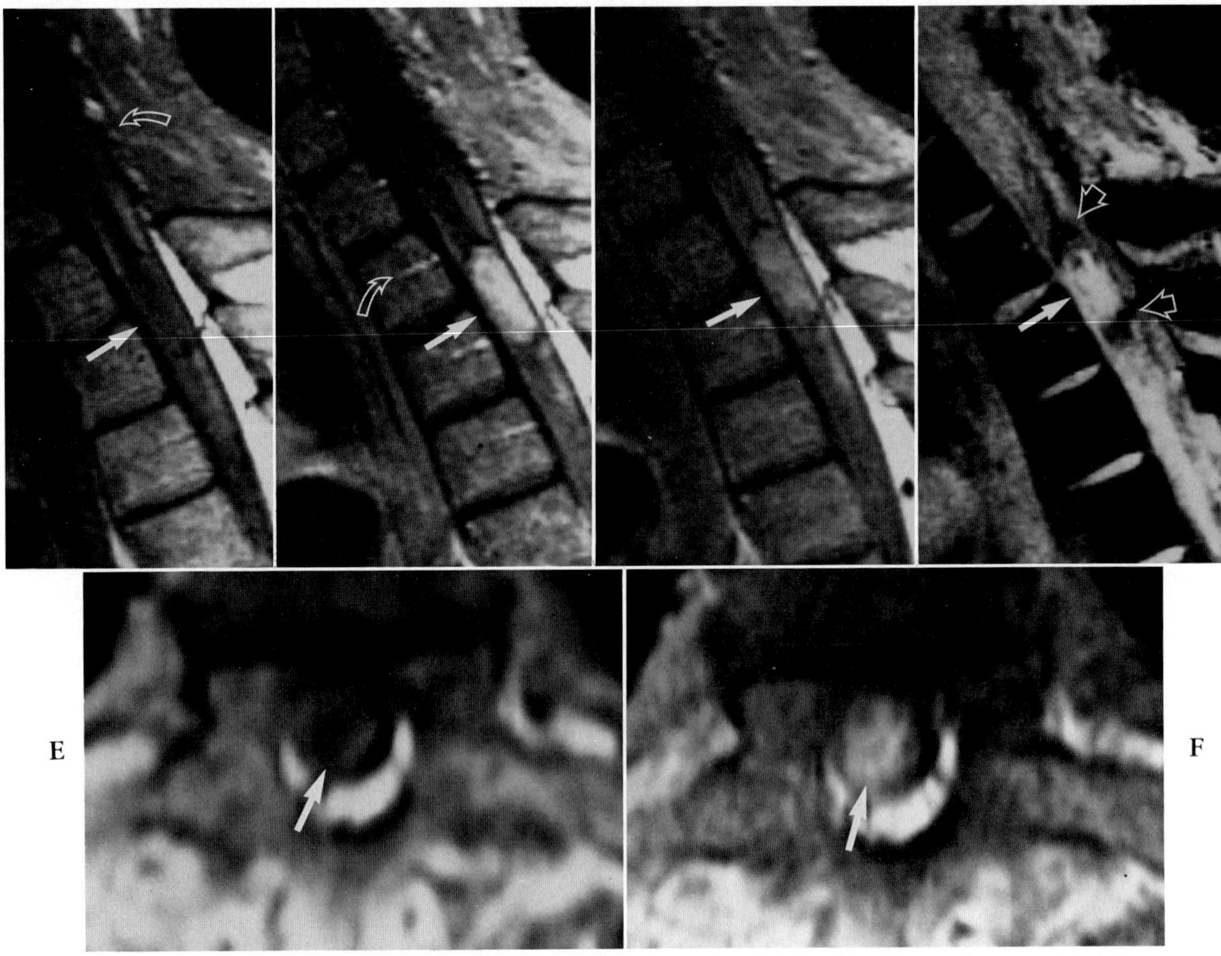

E F

FIGURE 8-6. Astrocytoma of cervical spinal cord in 60-year-old female. **A,** Sagittal T1W image (SE 600/20) shows well-circumscribed mass within spinal cord at C_7-T_1 *(straight arrow)*. Curvilinear low signal at superior margin of mass is consistent with deposition of hemosiderin from previous hemorrhage (see GRASS image, **D**). Cord tapers to normal diameter below tumor mass but appears widened superior to it. Indistinctly marginated central low signal in cord through this enlarged region is consistent with edema or "gliosis". In this case it may represent residual of cyst that was present preoperatively. Indistinct posterior margin of cord at laminectomy site is result of postsurgical pia-arachnoid adhesions and extradural fibrotic changes *(curved arrow)*. **B** and **C,** Sagittal T1W images (SE 600/20) after intravenous GdDTPA (0.1 mmol/kg) show maximal enhancement of tumor nodule at 5 minutes (*straight arrow,* **B**) and reduced enhancement at 60 minutes (*arrow,* **C**). Enhancement is uniform in tumor, suggesting absence of central necrosis. No enhancement in cord outside tumor nodule is seen. Note increased signal in basivertebral veins (*curved arrow,* **B**) on 5 minute image. Curvilinear low signal at tumor margins are consistent with hemosiderin deposition from previous hemorrhage (see GRASS image, **D**). **D,** Sagittal variable flip angle/gradient echo image (GRASS 400/15, 10°) at 15 minutes after GdDTPA injection shows high signal in central nodule *(solid arrow)*. Broad areas of low signal with indistinct margins are present at superior and inferior borders of tumor mass *(open arrows)*. These low signal regions are wider than corresponding thin dark lines on T1W images because of greater sensitivity of GRASS image to magnetic susceptibility effect of hemosiderin deposits. Dense fibrotic capsule would appear as thin line of low signal on both images (result of low proton density) and would not "bloom" on GRASS images. Linear extension of low signal from superior margin is also seen. **E** and **F,** Axial T1W images (SE 600/20) pre-GdDTPA (**E**) and post-GdDTPA (**F**) through middle of tumor mass. Precontrast image shows tumor mass as central low signal in cord (*arrow,* **E**) with three zones of intermediate signal cord surrounding it. Postcontrast image shows signal enhancement through most of central cord (*arrow,* **F**). (**A-F,** Courtesy of William Dillon, M.D..)

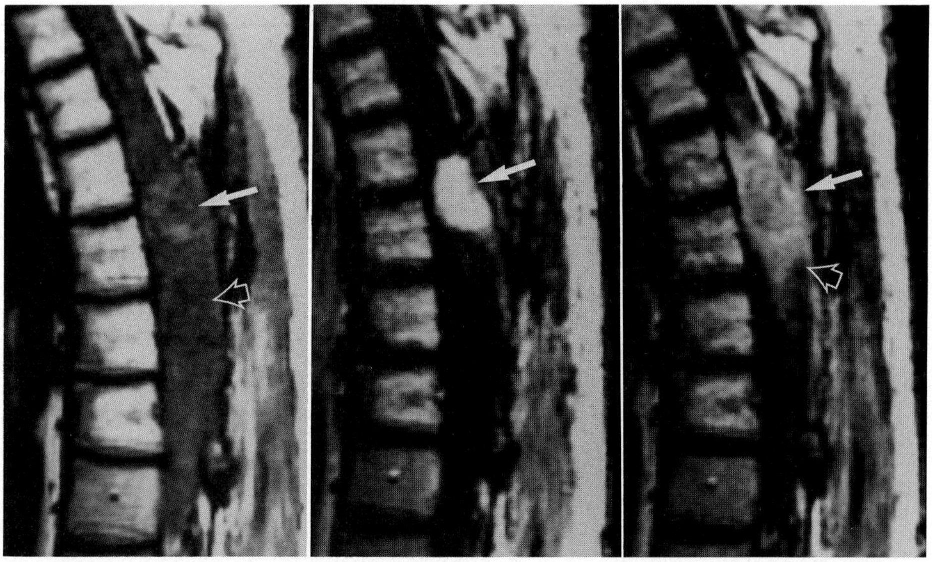

FIGURE 8-7. Astrocytoma in thoracic spinal cord with GdDTPA after surgery and radiation therapy in 34-year-old male. **A,** Sagittal T1W image (SE 600/20) taken before contrast injection shows fusiform enlargement of cord through upper thoracic region adjacent to large laminectomy. Ovoid area of irregular slightly higher signal *(closed arrow)* represents central tumor nodule. Enlarged cord adjacent to apparent nodule is lower in signal than normal cord *(open arrow)*. This area is ambiguous on this image and may represent infiltrative tumor or postsurgical or postradiation changes. Cystic change is less likely. High signal in vertebral bone marrow is result of fatty infiltration in response to radiation exposure. **B,** Sagittal T1W image (SE 600/20) immediately (5 minutes) after intravenous infusion of 0.1 mmol/kg GdDTPA shows marked enhancement of tumor nodule *(arrow)*. Uniformity of enhancement suggests absence of central necrosis in lesion. No enhancement in adjacent cord or at laminectomy site at this time. **C,** Sagittal T1W image (SE 600/20) 90 minutes after contrast injection shows persistent but low intensity enhancement of tumor nodule compared to early postcontrast image (**B**). New enhancement at laminectomy site posterior to nodule (*closed arrow,* **C**) and in spinal cord superior and inferior (*open arrow,* **C**) to main nodule. Enhancement at laminectomy site indicates presence of fibrosis and granulation tissue. Delayed enhancement in cord probably represents additional, infiltrative tumor. Edema and "gliosis" are associated with intact blood-brain barrier (blood-cord barrier) and do not show contrast enhancement. (**A-C,** From Dillon WP, et al.: Radiology 1989; 170:229.)

tumors occurs in MR and GdDTPA cord tumors. Although enhancement localizes the main portion of the tumor, it does not necessarily depict its microscopic boundaries. A T2W image shows the tumor to be of greater extent than a postcontrast T1W scan because tumor with or without edema is detected (see Figure 8-4). In an untreated tumor a T2W scan could be more sensitive to tumor progression than a contrast enhanced T1W scan, if progression is primarily in the form of increased edema rather than increased tumor size (see Figure 8-4).

GdDTPA (or other contrast medium) is essential to detect residual or recurrent tumor after surgery because the usual morphologic-anatomic landmarks no longer serve as diagnostic criteria; abnormal enhancement is the key to this diagnosis (see Figure 8-7). Abnormal high signal on T2W images is less helpful because it could represent tumor, edema, or postsurgical change (myelomalacia) (see Figure 8-7). Postsurgical T2W scans show heterogeneous signal that can have a hemorrhagic (hemosiderin) component from the surgery itself (Figure 8-8). Cord enlargement after treatment may not represent tumor (Figure 8-9). Serial studies showing cord

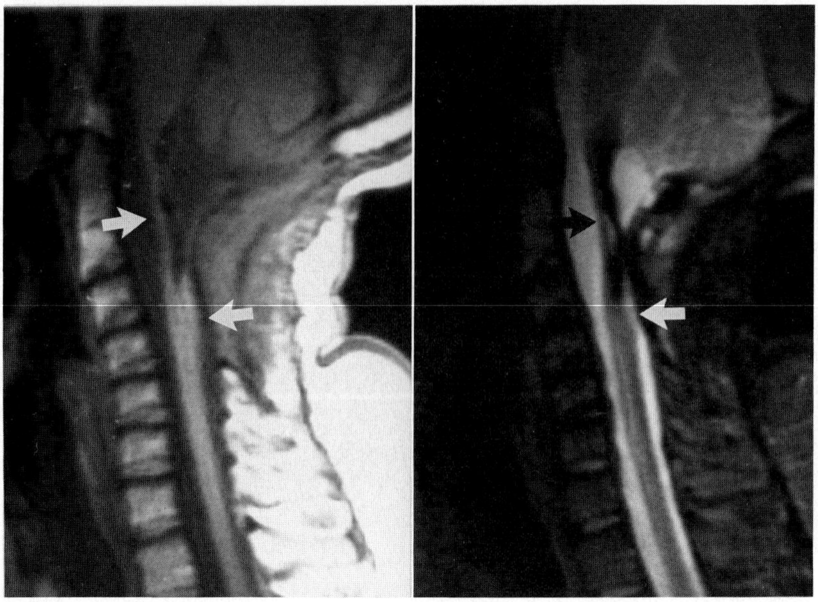

FIGURE 8-8. Postoperative changes after resection of cervicomedullary junction astrocytoma in 26-year-old male. **A,** Sagittal T1W image (SE 1000/20) shows thinning of spinal cord from cervicomedullary junction to C_3 *(upper arrow)*. Immediately posterior to thinned cord is strip of very low signal, which represents dense hemosiderin staining, seen with this pulse sequence because of some T2-weighting imparted by relatively long TR time. At C_3-C_4 level, cord appears relatively widened *(lower arrow)*. **B,** Sagittal T2W image (SE 2000/80) shows atrophy of upper cervical spinal cord *(black arrow)*. Low signal in cord represents hemosiderin staining and is more extensive on this image as a result of greater sensitivity to shortened T2* caused by hemosiderin deposits. At C_3-C_4 level, where T1W image shows relative cord widening, intermediate signal is present in posterior cord on T2W image (*white arrow*), which probably represents myelomalacia in posterior cord.

enlargement or increasing contrast enhancement are the current criteria for tumor recurrence.

An important differential diagnostic consideration in a cord lesion with mass effect and abnormal signal intensity is multiple sclerosis (MS) (or transverse myelitis of other causes). Acute MS lesions may show focal enlargement of the cord, be indistinguishable from astrocytoma, and be extensive enough to enlarge the entire cervical cord (see Chapter 9). MS plaques are usually more homogenous in signal intensity than astrocytomas, even in large lesions, and may involve the cord asymmetrically when viewed on axial images, whereas cord tumors tend to have more symmetrical diffuse involvement. On sagittal T2W scans, large MS lesions usually show a peripheral rim of normal cord intensity that is less common with astrocytomas. An acute MS plaque can exhibit contrast enhancement. MS lesions often show resolution of the mass effect in 3 to 6 months whereas high signal on T2W images persists beyond 6 months. Cord atrophy can accompany high signal intensity in the late stage. Clinical history may not allow differentiation between new-onset acute MS and early signs of primary cord tumor. For these reasons, caution should be exercised in recommending surgery for atypical cord lesions; serial MR studies may be a more prudent approach.

Ependymoma

Spinal ependymomas are slow-growing benign tumors that arise from ependymal cells in the central canal or in ependymal rests that are present in filum terminale or sacral locations. It is rare for the cells to be cytologically malignant. These tumors are normally well circumscribed, although not usually encapsulated. This has important implications because many if not most

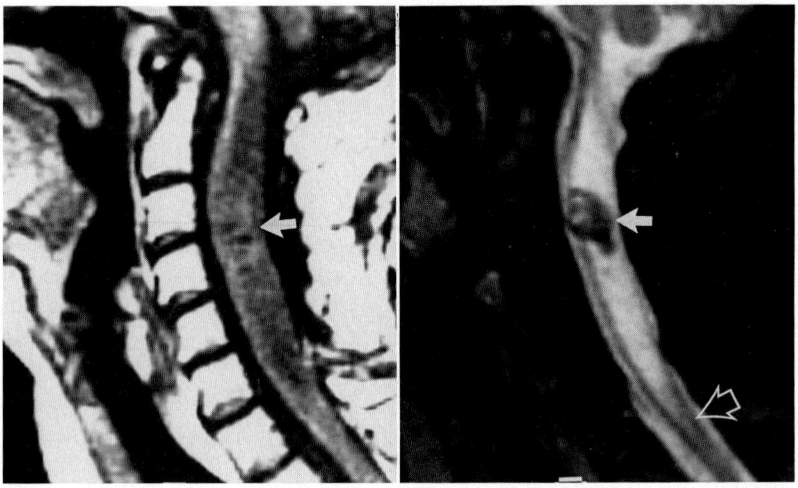

FIGURE 8-9. Cervical spinal cord grade II astrocytoma in 59-year-old female, 2 years after radiation therapy. Biopsy 3 months after MR study showed "gliosis" without evidence of recurrent tumor. **A,** Sagittal T1W image (SE 400/25) shows increased anteroposterior (AP) diameter of entire cervical cord with low signal centrally and posteriorly (sparing thin anterior margin of normal cord signal). Low signal tapers superiorly to cervicomedullary junction and inferiorly to C_7. Finding is nonspecific and may represent delayed radiation change (demyelination and edema), vasogenic edema reaction to tumor recurrence, or recurrent tumor itself. Irregular area of relatively increased signal at site of original tumor nidus at C_2-C_3 represents gliotic remnant *(arrow)*. High signal in vertebral bone marrow is consistent with radiation-induced fatty change. **B,** Sagittal T2W image (SE 2000/50) shows similar enlargement of cord with high signal extending over same region as low signal on T1W image. This represents tissue with high water content and has signal similar to CSF intensity. Characteristics that distinguish area from typical tumor cyst are signal on T1W image (higher than CSF) and indistinct margins with "flame shaped" tapering *(open arrow)* into central cord at superior and inferior extents. Complex focus of low signal at C_2-C_3 corresponds to focus of higher signal on T1W image *(closed arrow)*. Gliotic remnant of treated tumor may contain small amount of hemosiderin from previous hemorrhage, as suggested by low signal focus at inferior part of nidus (*open arrow,* **B**).

of these tumors can be enucleated surgically, effecting a cure.[11,61] Ependymomas occur predominately in the third to sixth decades of life, and they are less common in children. Ependymomas represent 60% to 70% of spinal cord tumors and can be associated with neurofibromatosis.

Although ependymomas can occur anywhere in the spinal cord, 60% typically occur in the conus medullaris region and in the cauda equina or filum terminale. Ependymomas in the filum terminale are usually of the myxopapillary type, which has a prominent collagenous stroma characterized by a central core of hyalin (acellular material) around a small vessel.[61] This tumor may undergo a mucinous change also characteristic of filum terminale sites. Microscopically, ependymomas may show hemorrhage and can rarely be the cause of subarachnoid hemorrhage. Similar to other intramedullary cord tumors, these tumors may undergo cystic degeneration and be associated with spinal cord cysts in or adjacent to the tumor. The cysts vary in size.

The most common site for extradural and extraspinal ependymomas[46,64] is the sacral region, either presacral in location or posterior to the sacrum. Besides location, these ependymomas differ from others in that they have an increased propensity for systemic metastases.

As mentioned previously, because these tumors are benign and well circumscribed an aggressive surgical approach is usually taken to effect a cure.[11] This approach works well for patients who do not have severe motor deficits of the lower extremities[11] and is aided by the more accurate localization allowed by modern imaging techniques: CT with intrathecal contrast and intraoperative ultrasound.[11] The improved ability of MR to detect and localize spinal cord tumors improves localization by demonstrating internal cord anatomy and allowing the total resection approach for ependymomas, as well as astrocytomas.[11] When ependymoma tumors recur the recurrence is often local with tumor remaining cytologically benign. Recurrence rarely shows dedifferentiation of cells.[61]

MR Findings

Intramedullary ependymomas are relatively easy to detect on T1W images by focal cord enlargement (Figure 8-10). Cord enlargement can be extensive, but when it is focal and limited to a few spinal levels an ependymoma is favored over astrocytoma (Figure 8-11; see Figure 8-10). Cord enlargement is usually obvious but more subtle presentations can be expected if MR scans are obtained early in the natural history of these tumors. On the T1W sequence, the cord may show homogeneous or heterogeneous areas of low signal intensity that can represent tumor, cystic degeneration within tumor, or tumor with adjacent cysts.[28] Localization is more problematic in the conus region (Figure 8-12) where it may be difficult to determine whether the tumor involves the cauda equina or the filum terminale. In addition, on a T1W sequence the signal intensity of an ependymoma may be similar to that of CSF distal to the tumor (see Figure 8-12). Signal intensity of CSF in the lumbar sac distal to the tumor may be increased for two reasons: (1) increased protein content and (2) dampening of CSF pulsation resulting in increased signal intensity characteristic of stationary fluid (see Figure 8-12). Failure to see a well-defined conus to cauda equina transition should be viewed with suspicion; axial views are necessary to clarify findings.

On T2W images, intramedullary ependymoma exhibits increased signal intensity compared to cord (see Figures 8-10 to 8-12). This

A, B

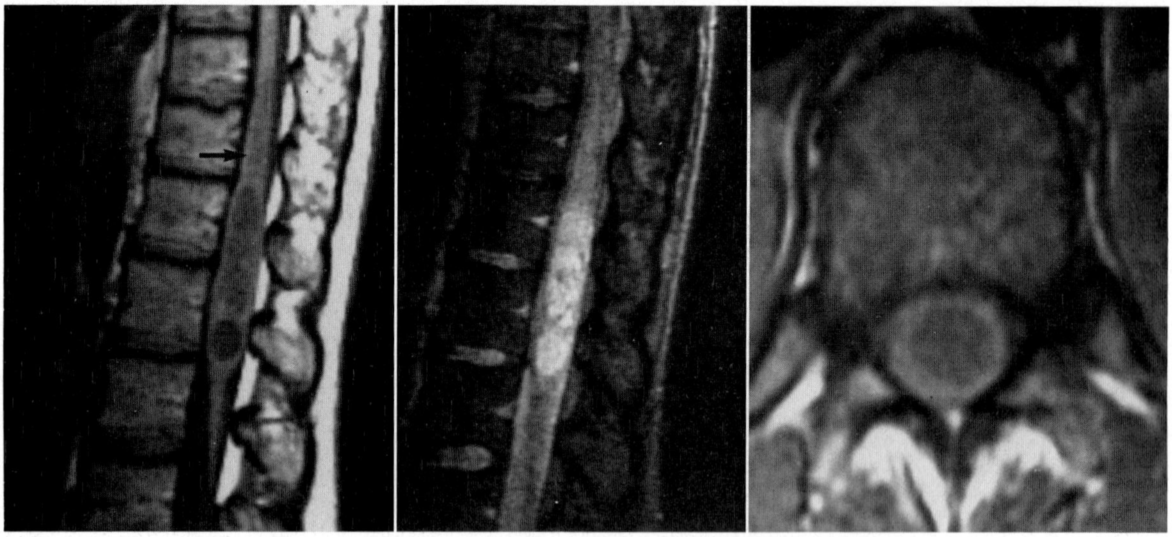

C

FIGURE 8-10. Ependymoma of conus medullaris in 31-year-old female with neurofibromatosis. **A**, On sagittal T1W image (SE 600/25) tumor shows focal enlargement of distal cord and conus extending for approximately three vertebral segments. Low signal intensity tumor has multiloculated appearance and is well circumscribed. Tapered area of low signal at rostral end is consistent with adjacent edema *(arrow)*. **C**, On T1W axial view (SE 1000/25) cord shows symmetric enlargement with low signal tumor situated centrally. **B**, Sagittal T2W scan (SE ungated, 2500/80) shows area of increased signal in conus and distal cord corresponding to area of low signal intensity in T1W image. Tumor appears well circumscribed but shows some internal inhomogeneity similar to apparent "septations" on T1W image (**A**). Suspected area of edema (*arrow*, **A**) is lower signal intensity than tumor on T2W image (**C**). Surgery confirmed localized and circumscribed nature of this ependymoma.

area of high signal intensity is well circumscribed with smaller ependymomas. The circumscribed nature of the tumor may not be apparent on T1W images. A T2W sequence is more useful than a noncontrast T1W sequence in delineating tumor margins (see Figures 8-10 and 8-11), which nevertheless can be obscured on T2W images by adjacent edema, which is also high signal. Tumor localization in the cauda equina and filum terminale can be as difficult on T2W images as it is with T1W images (see Figure 8-12). Because these tumors show high signal intensity on T2W images, there may be little contrast between tumor and adjacent static CSF, especially with tumors in the conus and cauda equina location, which often cause complete block of CSF flow (see Figure 8-12).[32] Because these tumors have some propensity to hemorrhage, areas of marked low signal intensity in and around the tumor indicative of the magnetic susceptibility effect caused by hemosiderin may be visualized (see Figures 8-11 and 8-12). Although evident on T1W images, such hemorrhagic findings are accentuated on T2W images. A variable flip angle/gradient echo scan can further accentuate this magnetic susceptibility effect.

Contrast-enhanced T1W MR scans are superior to T2W scans in detecting and delineating ependymomas because they generally have a permeable blood-brain barrier and are well circumscribed. GdDTPA can be used to delineate tumor margins and distinguish tumor from edema or associated cysts (Figure 8-13).[15] Ependymomas typically show well-circumscribed, homogeneous areas of high signal enhancement on T1W images. The histologic subcategories of ependymoma, subependymoma, and myxopapillary types cannot be differentiated by signal characteristics.

The purpose of surgical intervention for ependymomas is to achieve a complete removal and thus a cure. Tumor localization is crucial and best results are obtained with an intravenous contrast agent such as GdDTPA. Because tumor recurrence is local it is recommended that T1W and T2W images be obtained after surgery to establish a new baseline for the tumor site. Tu-

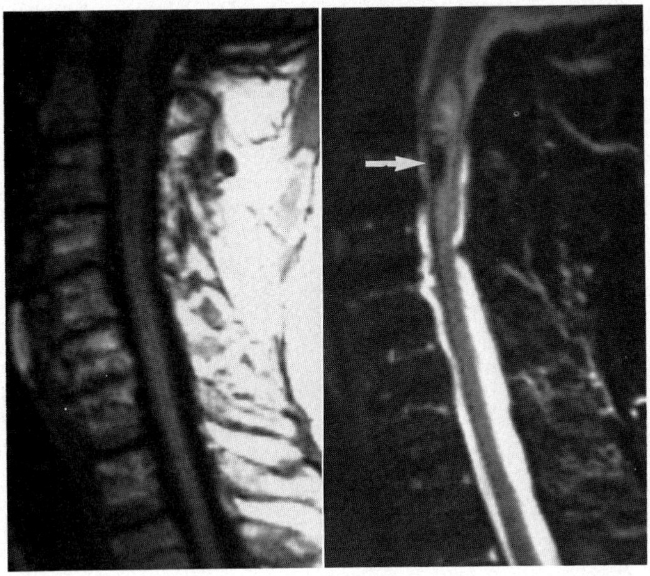

FIGURE 8-11. Ependymoma. Preoperative and postoperative T1W and T2W scans of 72-year-old male with myxopapillary ependymoma of upper cervical cord. **A**, Preoperative sagittal T1W scan (SE 800/20) shows focal enlargement of cervical cord of C_2-C_4 levels. Central cord shows low signal intensity surrounded by rim of cord tissue with relatively normal signal intensity. **B**, Preoperative T2W scan (SE gated, 2100/100) shows tumor of high signal intensity and relatively well circumscribed. Tumor extent is well seen because of contrast with normal surrounding cord. Circumscribed nature of ependymoma was confirmed at surgery. Area of marked low signal within tumor at level of C_3 suggests magnetic susceptibility effect seen with hemosiderin deposition *(arrow)*.

Continued.

C D

E F

G H

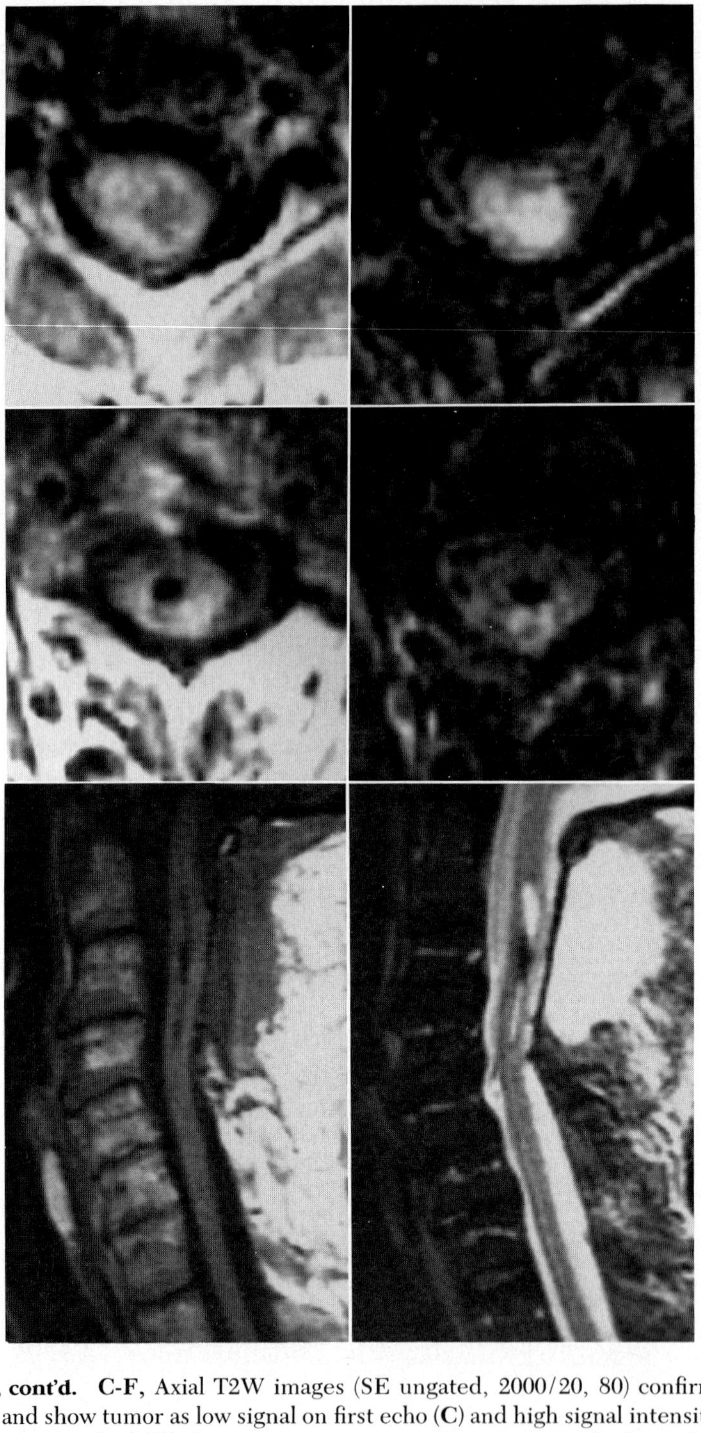

FIGURE 8-11, cont'd. **C-F**, Axial T2W images (SE ungated, 2000/20, 80) confirm focal cord enlargement and show tumor as low signal on first echo (**C**) and high signal intensity on second echo (**D**), suggesting fluid-filled cyst. Tumor is somewhat eccentrically located in cord. At another level, area of marked low signal intensity in central cord is consistent with magnetic susceptibility effect of hemosiderin on the first (**E**) and second (**F**) echos. After complete surgical removal of ependymoma this patient shows only residual postoperative changes. **G,** Postoperative T1W scan (SE 800/20) shows long area of low signal intensity at site of tumor bed. **H,** T2W scan shows persistent low signal in previous area of hemosiderin deposition and new focal linear areas of high signal intensity in tumor bed. A baseline, postoperative scan is important because ependymomas recur locally and the scan can be used for future comparisons.

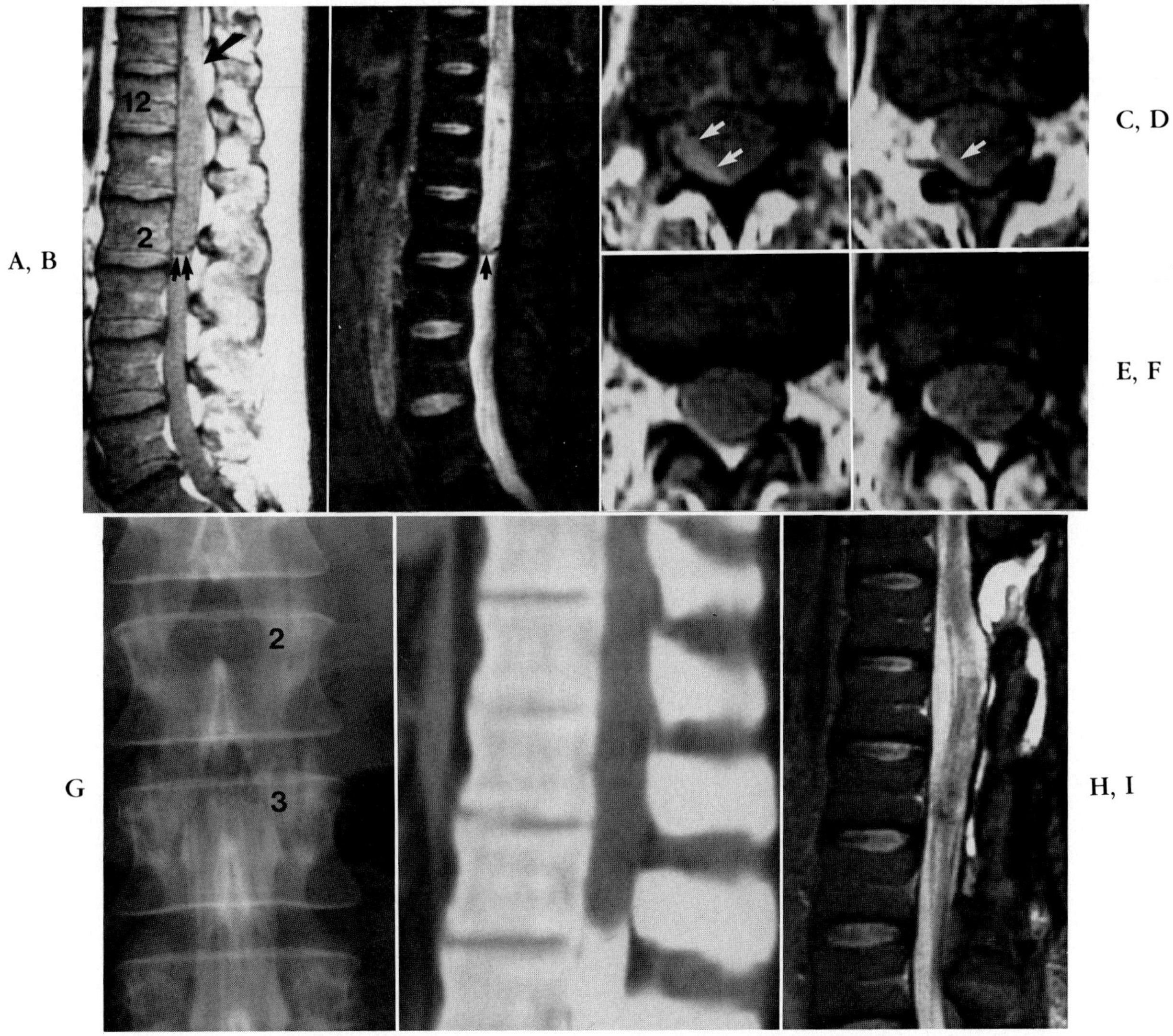

FIGURE 8-12. Ependymoma of cauda equina in 36-year-old male. **A,** T1W sagittal scan (SE 800/20) shows subtle lesion extending from T_{12} to L_2. Spinal canal has lower signal intensity than conus above it and CSF below it. Conus *(large arrow)* is displaced posteriorly by ependymoma. Thin black line delineates lower extent of ependymoma and CSF below it at level of L_2-L_3 *(small arrows)*. **B,** Corresponding T2W image (SE gated, 2200/80) shows ependymoma to be of high signal intensity but still difficult to detect because of lack of contrast with high signal CSF. Thin black line at L_2-L_3 represents border between ependymoma and stationary CSF below it *(arrow)*. Low signal suggests hemosiderin effect indicative of hemorrhage. CSF is high signal because of CSF gating and complete block caused by ependymoma (see myelogram [**G**] and CT scan [**H**]). Note posterior deviation of conus at T_{12}. Tumor shows minimal inhomogeneity within it. **C-F,** Four axial T1W images (SE 1000/20) starting rostrally and going caudally show posterolateral displacement of conus *(arrows)*, which is relatively high signal compared to tumor. Below level of conus, tumor occupies entire spinal canal and is difficult to differentiate from normal dural sac (**E** and **F**). **G,** Water soluble myelogram shows complete block at L_2-L_3 corresponding to caudal tumor margin seen as thin low-intensity line on sagittal MR scans (**A** and **B**). It did not characterize the tumor further. Reformatted post-metrizamide CT scan confirmed the complete block, lower end of mass, and failure of any contrast material to pass by the ependymoma. The MR scan yielded superior information compared to CT or myelogram. **I,** T2W postoperative scan (SE gated 2400/80) shows soft tissue postoperative changes and adhesion of cauda equina to posterior dural sac within small pseudomeningocele. Cauda equina shows adhesion of nerve roots indicating arachnoiditis. Because ependymomas recur locally a baseline postoperative scan is recommended for future follow-up.

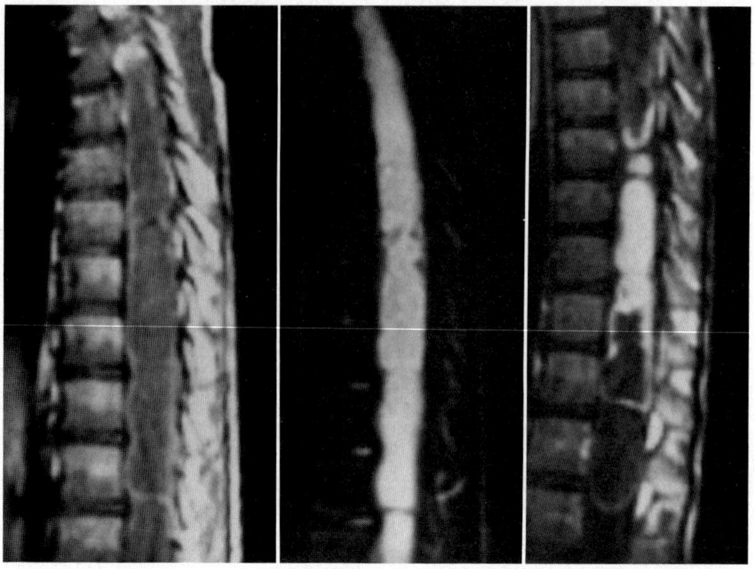

A, B C

FIGURE 8-13. Ependymoma. Sagittal T1W and T2W scans of child with ependymoma that has prominent cystic components. **A,** Sagittal T1W scan (SE 600/20) shows diffuse enlargement of thoracic cord with major portion of cord of low signal intensity (**A**). **B,** Sagittal T2W scan (gated, flow-compensated SE 1700/100) shows diffuse high signal within cord in same region as area of low signal intensity on T1W image (**A**). Tumor nodule and cystic portions of tumor cannot be distinguished when cysts are this extensive. **C,** Postcontrast GdDTPA scan (SE 600/20) differentiates between enhancing tumor, which is high signal intensity, and cyst that remains low signal intensity on this T1W image. Neither T1W precontrast scan (**A**) nor T2W image (**B**) clearly localizes main body of the tumor, which is an important consideration with ependymoma considering surgical successes in completely removing this type of tumor. (Courtesy of William Dillon, M.D.. From Dillon WP, et al.: Radiology 1989; 170:229). Reprinted by permission of *Radiology*.)

mor recurrence can then be determined by any changes in cord morphology or signal intensity, although these changes can be subtle on noncontrast scans. GdDTPA scans are probably most sensitive to the presence of residual and recurrent tumor by showing abnormal enhancement within the cord (see Figure 8-14). The postsurgical site can show residual low signal in the cord on T1W images and high signal on T2W images, representing postsurgical myelomalacia. Contrast enhancement secondary to surgical changes should resolve over 2 to 3 months. Evidence for hemorrhage may persist in the tumor bed on T2W images. After surgery, marked deformity of the conus and cauda equina and fixation to the dura usually occurs secondary to postsurgical adhesions (see Figure 8-11). The appropriate follow-up interval for postsurgical patients remains to be determined.

Hemangioblastoma

Hemangioblastoma is a benign tumor whose cell of origin is believed to be the endothelial cell. This tumor is composed of a dense network of capillary and sinus channels.[61] Between the capillaries lies a stroma, which may contain fat and hemosiderin.[61] Hemangioblastoma is found primarily in the posterior fossa (brain stem and cerebellum), in the spinal cord (uncommon), and in the supratentorial space (rare). It is usually intramedullary in the spine, although it can be intradural extramedullary when it involves the posterior roots or the cauda equina. It may even involve the filum terminale. Hemangioblastoma may be present as a solitary lesion or as a multicentric tumor; in the latter case, it is usually associated with von Hippel-Lindau disease, which is a familial disorder. Such patients have angiomatosis retinae and numerous renal and

A

B

C, D

E

F

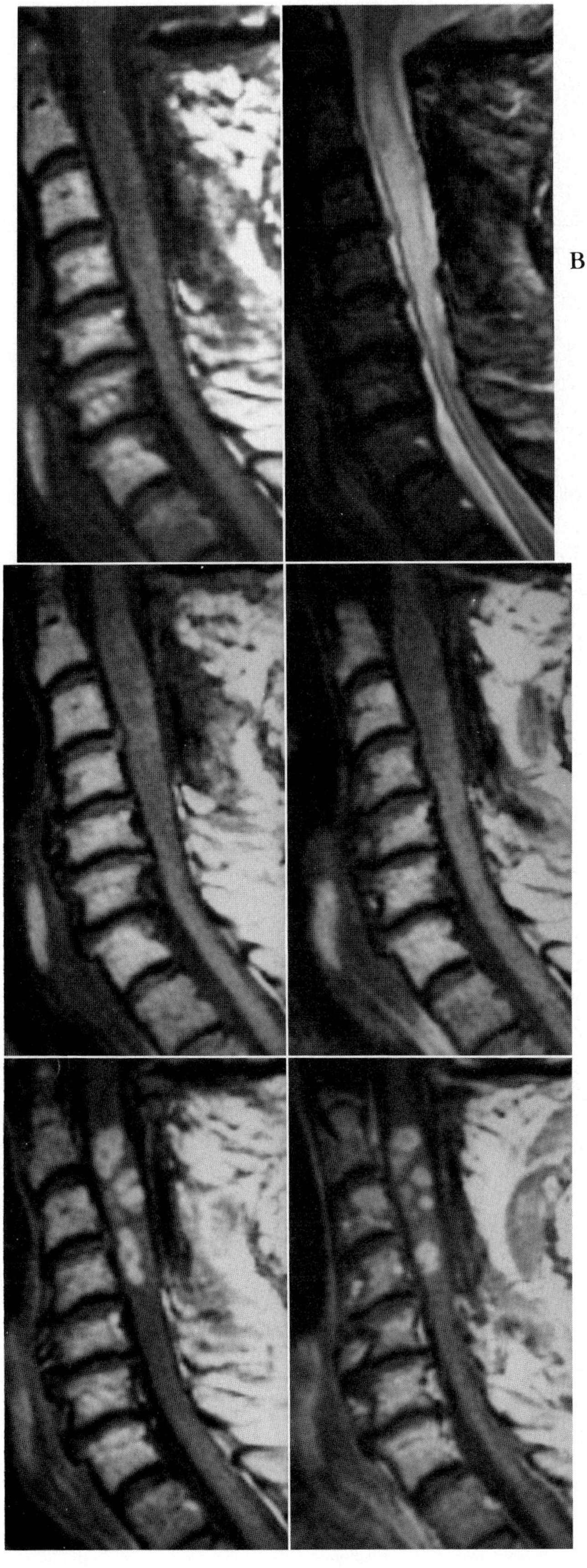

FIGURE 8-14. Ependymoma. MR scans of 65-year-old male with recurrent ependymoma. **A,** Sagittal T1W scan (SE 800/20) of patient 1 year after surgical removal of an ependymoma. T1W scan shows low signal inhomogeneity of enlarged upper cord. Residual/recurrent tumor is suspected because of the mass effect. Note radiation change in marrow signal. **B,** Sagittal T2W scan (SE gated 2000/80) confirms cord enlargement and shows diffuse central area of high signal intensity. There is some heterogeneity of cord signal. These findings are consistent with presence of tumor, but it cannot be delineated or separated from edema. **C** and **D,** Follow-up MR scans 1 year later. Precontrast T1W scan (SE 800/20) shows diffuse cord enlargement with abnormal low signal intensity in upper half of cervical cord and minimal increase in cord size in the year interval. Compare to **A.** A C_3-C_4 disc herniation is incidentally noted. Tumor cannot be differentiated from adjacent edema. **E** and **F,** Postcontrast GdDTPA T1W scans (SE 800/20) show multiple enhancing tumor nodules within low signal area of cord enlargement. *Continued.*

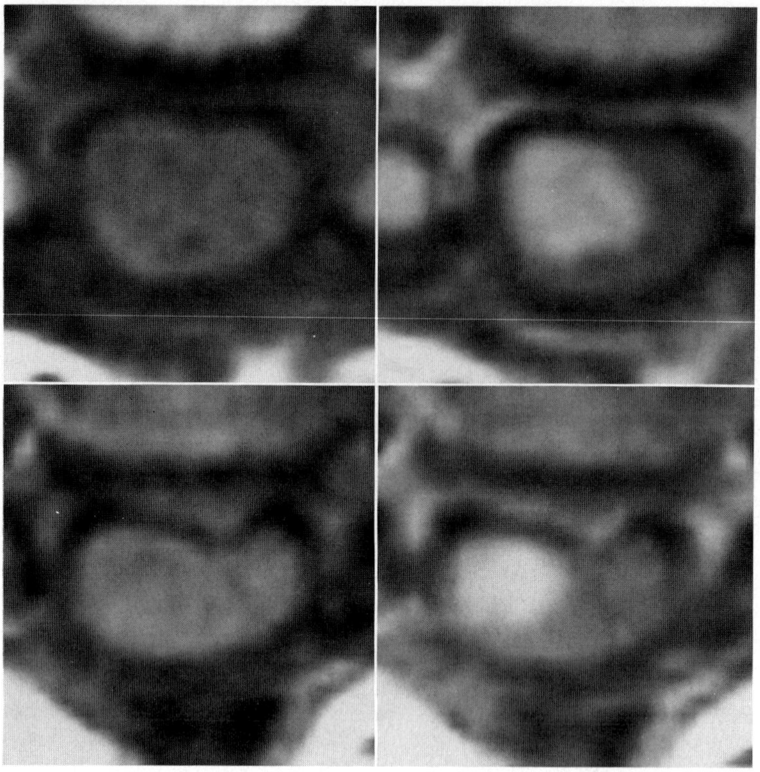

FIGURE 8-14, cont'd. **G** and **J**, Axial precontrast (**G** and **I**) and post GdDTPA scans (**H** and **J**) in upper cervical cord confirm findings on the sagittal scan. Precontrast scans show cord enlargement and diffuse low signal intensity within the cord (**G**). Disc herniation is also seen (**I**). Areas of contrast enhancement representing recurrent tumor (**H** and **J**) could not be differentiated on precontrast scan. Tumor nodules are well circumscribed, whereas low density adjacent to nodules presumably represents edema.

pancreatic cysts. Later in life these patients develop renal cell carcinoma. An important feature of hemangioblastoma is the presence of an associated cyst that usually extends beyond the tumor, or it may be entirely separate from it. Characteristically, the tumor nodule is a "mural" nodule in the cyst. The cyst is lined by fibrillary astroglia, not tumor tissue[61] and it may contain hemorrhage. In addition, its wall may contain hemosiderin.[61] Hemorrhagic components may also be identified within the tumor nodule.

Cerebellar tumors become symptomatic earlier in patients with both cerebellar and spinal hemangioblastomas. In the spinal cord, the tumor is more often in the thoracic than in the cervical cord.[7] Some patients have only spinal hemangioblastoma. These spinal tumors become symptomatic at a median age of approximately 30 years.[7] The well-known polycythemia seen with hemangioblastoma occurs only when cerebellar tumors are present. The clinical presentation depends on the location of the tumor, but spastic paraparesis and posterior column sensory loss are common findings. Radicular pain may be present if the tumor involves the posterior roots.

MR Findings

On T1W images, hemangioblastomas characteristically present with a long area of diffuse and extensive enlargement of the spinal cord (Figures 8-15 and 8-16) in which mutliple inhomogeneous areas of low signal intensity can be seen. Some of these low signal intensities are well circumscribed and suggest cyst formation (see Figure 8-15). Others are often limited to the central cord region where the peripheral rim of the cord has normal signal intensity (Figures 8-17 to 8-19; see Figure 8-15). A major feature and an important clue to the diagnosis is the presence of focal abnormal prominent vasculature in the cord and on its dorsal surface (see Figures 8-15 and 8-16). The areas of signal void representing vasculature may be punctate or serpigenous depending on whether they are seen in cross section or within the plane of the scan. These tumors can have prominent, dilated draining veins that can be well seen on the dorsal surface of the cord on the MR scan. Visualization of this abnormal vasculature is important because it localizes the site of the tumor nodule (see Figures 8-15 and 8-16), which helps direct the spinal arteriogram that is necessary to confirm the diagnosis. A spinal atriovenous malformation (AVM) may have a similar appearance, although associated cyst formation, as well as extensive cord enlargement, would be unusual. AVMs tend to be more focal. Conversely, hemangioblastoma can appear similar to a cryptic AVM, although the cyst formation distinguishes the two entities (see Figure 8-17). Specialized pulse sequences such as variable flip angle/gradient echo scans can be used to highlight the abnormal vasculature (see Figure 8-15). Using the appropriate flip angle, arterial or venous blood flow can be highlighted as high signal on such scans when they are used in a single-slice mode. These scans can distinguish areas of low signal caused by flowing blood from areas of low signal caused by the magnetic susceptibility effect of hemosiderin.

On T2W scans, hemangioblastoma shows extensive areas of high signal within the cord extending for long distances (see Figures 8-15 and 8-16). These areas are relatively homogeneous and represent edematous and cystic cord. Cysts may be conspicuous as areas of even higher signal, but often they blend in with the edema. The tumor nodule itself cannot be distinguished on T2W scans other than by the presence of abnormal vasculature, seen as signal voids on T2W scans (see Figures 8-15 and 8-16). T2W images effectively show the unusual characteristic of hemangioblastoma: a small tumor nodule with extensive cyst formation and edema seem-

A

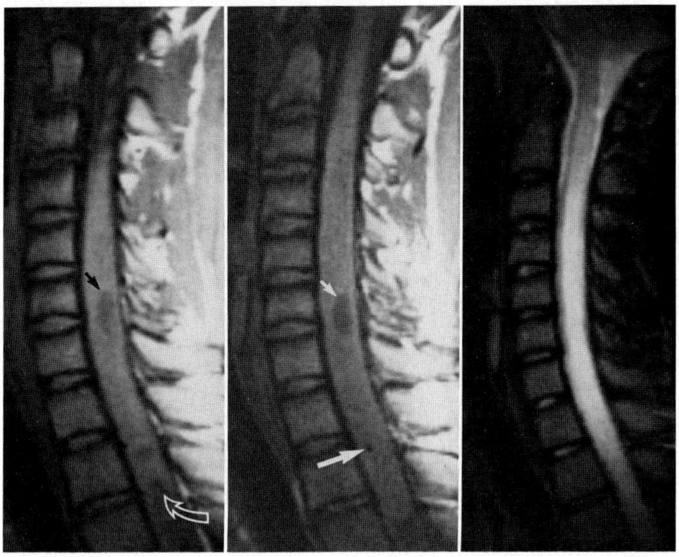

B, C

FIGURE 8-15. Hemangioblastoma. MR scans of cervical hemangioblastoma in 13-year-old male with von Hippel-Lindau disease. Spinal lesion was the only CNS hemangioblastoma. **A** and **B**, T1W sagittal views (SE 800/20) show diffuse enlargement of cervical cord with well-defined area of low signal at C_6, suggesting well-circumscribed cyst *(small arrows)*. Two small subtle areas of very low signal suggesting vascular signal voids are seen at level of T_2 *(curved arrows)*. Small hemangioblastoma nodule is not well visualized on T1W scan and is detected primarily by presence of abnormal vasculature. **C**, T2W scan (SE gated, 2300/80) shows diffuse enlargement of cord and relatively homogeneous high signal intensity throughout central cervical cord. Relatively homogeneous appearance of high signal suggests cord edema.

Continued.

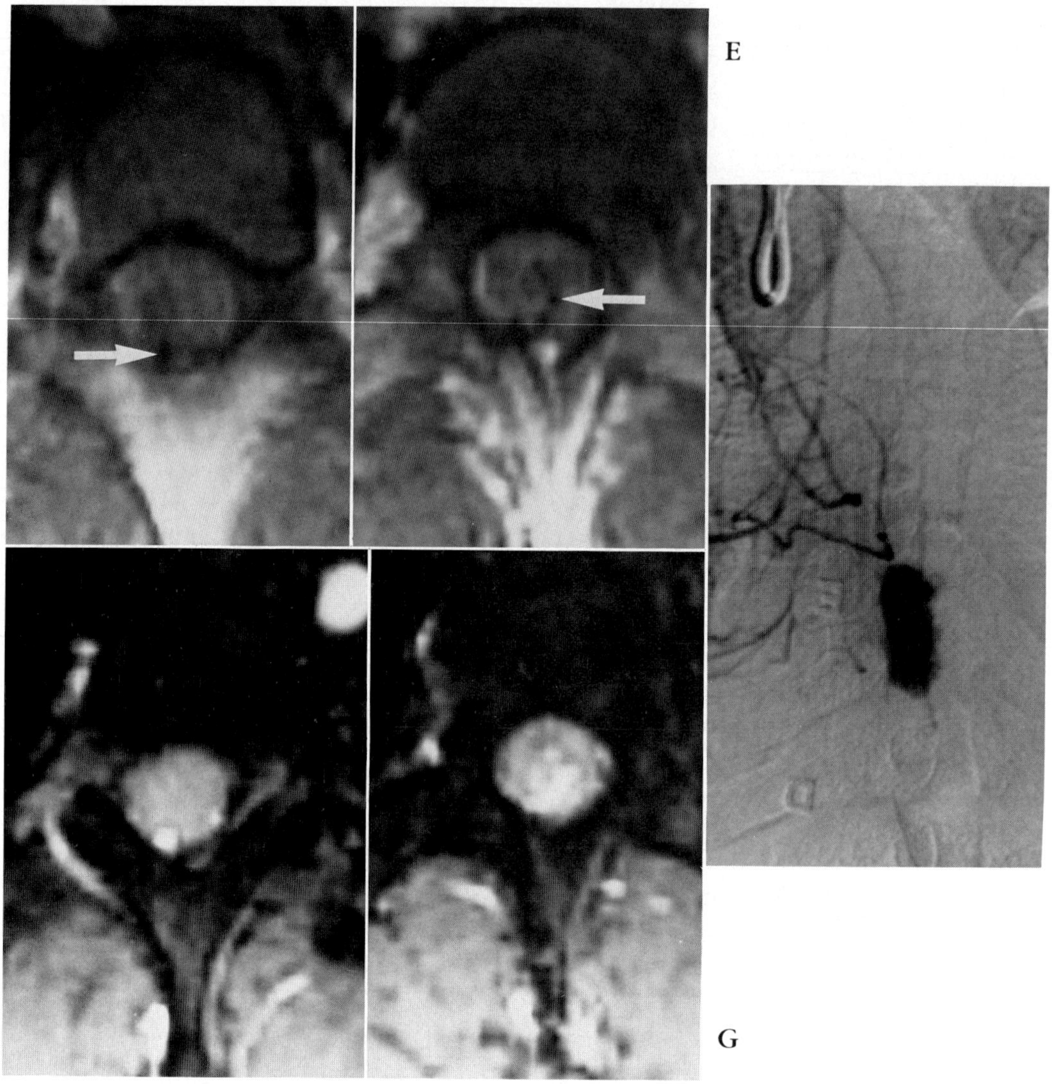

FIGURE 8-15, cont'd. D and **E,** Axial T1W scans (SE 1000/20) show diffuse cord enlargement and definite areas of signal void representing abnormal vasculature *(arrows)*. Small round and serpiginous areas of low signal are well seen dorsal to cord (**D**) and penetrating cord (**E**). **F** and **G,** Axial variable flip angle scans with 33° flip angle, which makes sequence sensitive to blood flow, show high signal intensity in same regions of previous signal void, indicating relatively rapid blood flow. **H,** Spinal arteriogram confirms presence of localized hemangioblastoma tumor nodule at T_2 level.

ingly out of proportion to the tumor size (see Figures 8-15 and 8-16).

A contrast agent such as GdDTPA makes the diagnosis of hemangioblastoma considerably easier compared to conventional, noncontrast MR (see Figures 8-17 to 8-19). Tumor nodules show intense contrast enhancement, as they do with CT; they vary in size and number but are well circumscribed (see Figures 8-18 and 8-19); and they may be in the wall of a cyst or separated from it in the cord parenchyma (see Figures 8-18 and 8-19). The cyst wall does not enhance with contrast because it does not contain neoplastic tissue. GdDTPA scans show a high sensitivity to these tumors, revealing multiple tumors that might otherwise be difficult to detect (see Figure 8-19).

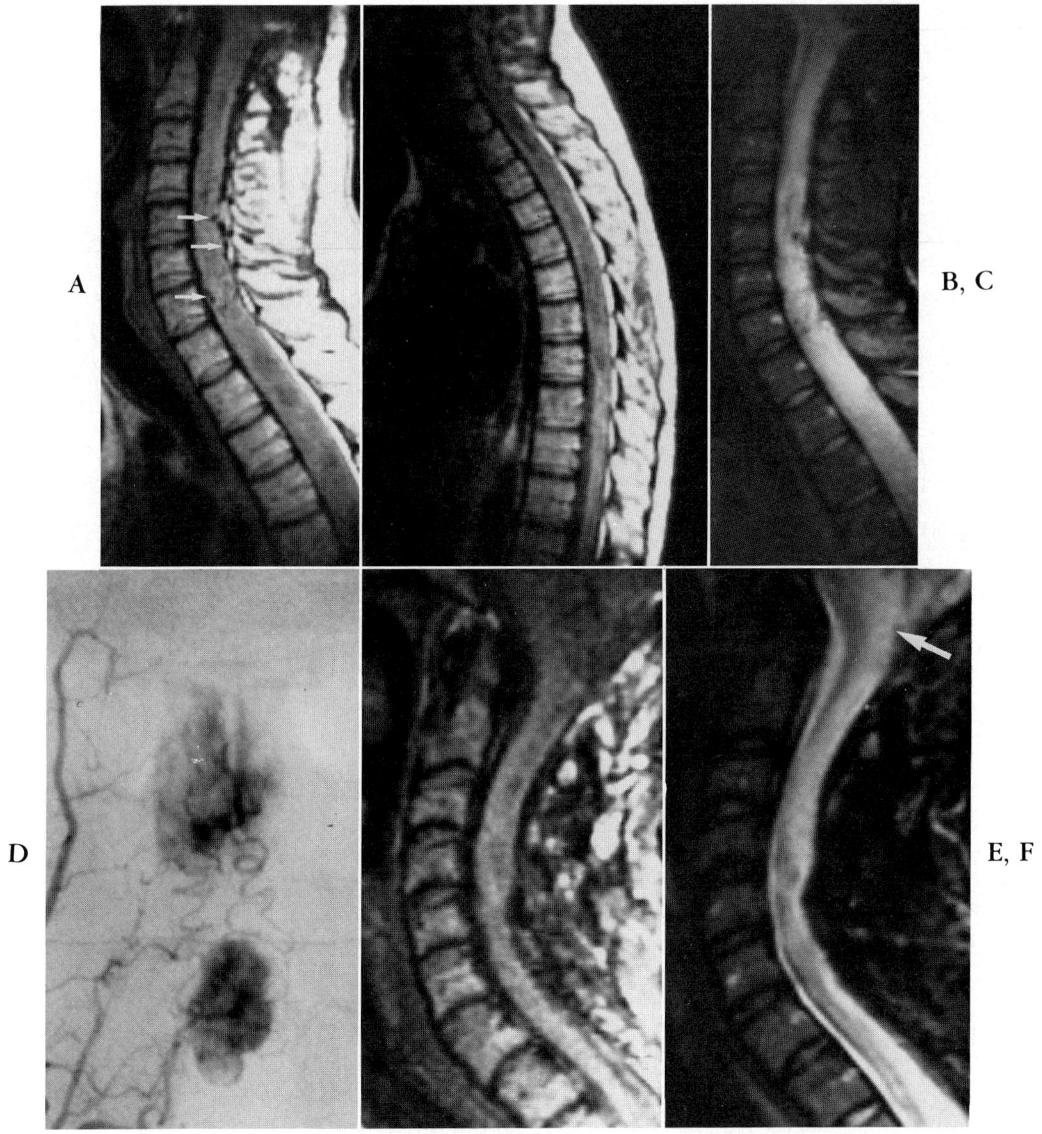

FIGURE 8-16. Multiple hemangioblastomas of cervical cord in patient with concomitant multiple hemangioblastomas in posterior fossa. T1W scans (SE 800/20) of **A**, cervical and **B**, thoracic cord show diffuse marked enlargement of spinal cord to midthoracic level. Signal intensity of cord is inhomogeneous, showing multiple irregular areas of low signal intensity. Prominent serpiginous areas of low signal intensity at C_5-C_7 levels (*arrows*, **A**) are located on ventral and dorsal aspect of cord and indicate abnormal vascularity. No signal voids are seen in thoracic cord (**B**). **C**, T2W scan (SE gated 1900/75) shows diffuse abnormal high signal throughout entire cervical cord. Areas of signal void in cervical region are again well seen. Abnormal vasculature indicates site(s) of actual tumor nodules, whereas extensive and marked cord enlargement elsewhere in cord represents secondary effect of hemangioblastoma. **D**, Spinal arteriogram anteroposterior (AP) view shows two separate tumor nodules in C_5-C_7 cord region. **E**, Postsurgical scan shows incomplete resolution of cord mass effect and signal abnormality in cervical region, but normal or atrophic cord in thoracic region. T1W scan (SE 800/20) shows persistent, although less severe, cord enlargement and persistent normal low signal intensity in upper cervical cord. **F**, Postsurgical T2W scan (SE gated 2050/80) shows abnormal high signal in remaining areas of cord enlargement; note that mass effect and abnormal signal extends into medulla *(arrow)*.

A, B

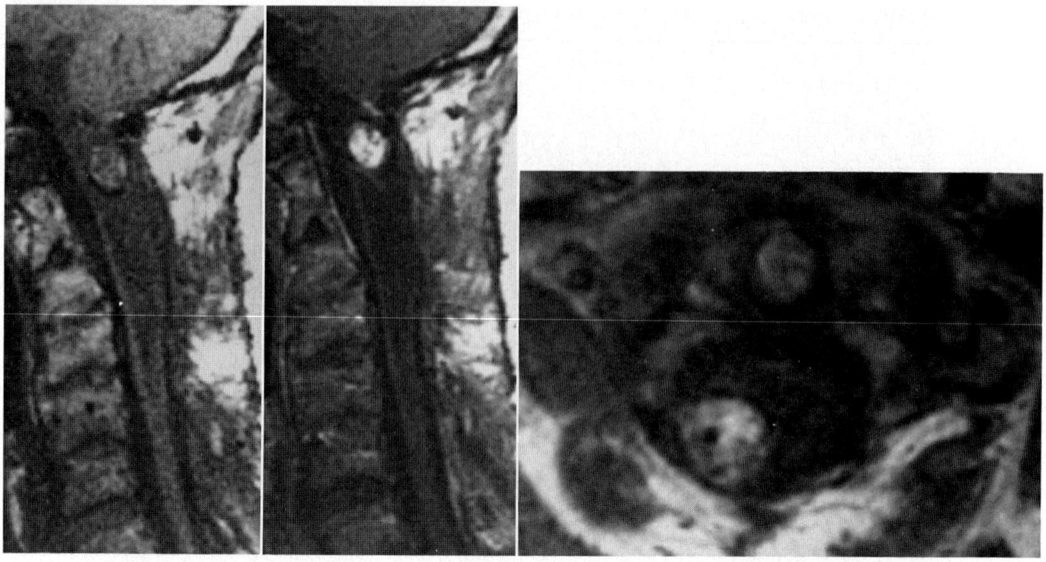

C

FIGURE 8-17. Hemangioblastoma. Precontrast and postcontrast scans (GdDTPA injection) in patient with hemangioblastoma at C_1 level. **A,** Precontrast T1W (SE 600/20) scan shows large area of low signal indicative of cyst extending from medulla to C_4. Within cyst is tumor nodule that can be easily identified and has increased signal within it compared to cord. It has low signal rim around nodule. This combination of findings suggests previous hemorrhage, although part of the low signal rim may represent signal void in enlarged vessels. Tumor has superficial resemblance to low flow AVM. Tumor nodule is inhomogeneous and has stippled areas of low signal intensity within it, suggesting signal voids in vascular channels. **B,** Postcontrast T1W scan (SE 600/20) shows intense enhancement of tumor nodule but not of areas of low signal around and within tumor nodule. **C,** Axial postcontrast scan shows distinct small round signal voids indicative of vasculature with high velocity flow. The GdDTPA scan shows areas of increased blood-brain barrier permeability, but with conventional SE images arteries are characterized by typical signal voids because of rapid blood flow while venous structures are enhanced by GdDTPA. (Courtesy of William Dillon, M.D.)

Cyst formation and extensive cord enlargement are often reversed simply by removal of the small tumor nodule (see Figure 8-16). The cysts require no separate surgical attention. After tumor removal, cord enlargement regresses and may return to normal size or even to a small or atrophic state. The cause of the extensive cord enlargement is not understood but is characteristic of spinal hemangioblastomas. It is doubtful that merely high arterial blood flow and increased venous pressure is responsible because similar extensive findings are not seen with spinal AVM of any type (see Chapter 11). The tumor, however, may secrete a substance that increases vascular permeability, as has been demonstrated with some meningiomas. This could explain cord enlargement as extensive edema that is reversible only by tumor removal.

Intradural Lipoma

Lipomas are benign neoplasms composed of mature fat cells. The three main types of spinal lipomas are lipoma of the filum terminale, intradural lipoma, and lipomyelomeningocele. Filum lipoma (Figure 8-20) and lipomyelomeningocele are discussed in detail in Chapter 5. Intradural lipomas are usually intramedullary with some subpial extension and confined to the spinal canal, which may be normal, widened, or bifid. The overlying skin is normal. The lipoma may involve several segments of the cord. There is usually no clear demarcation between cord tissue and lipoma because the two tissues are merged (Figures 8-21 and 8-22). Lipomas may be partially encapsulated but there is usually no clear demarcation between lipoma and cord tissue around its entirety. Neural tissue can be found mixed with fat cells. The fat titssue may

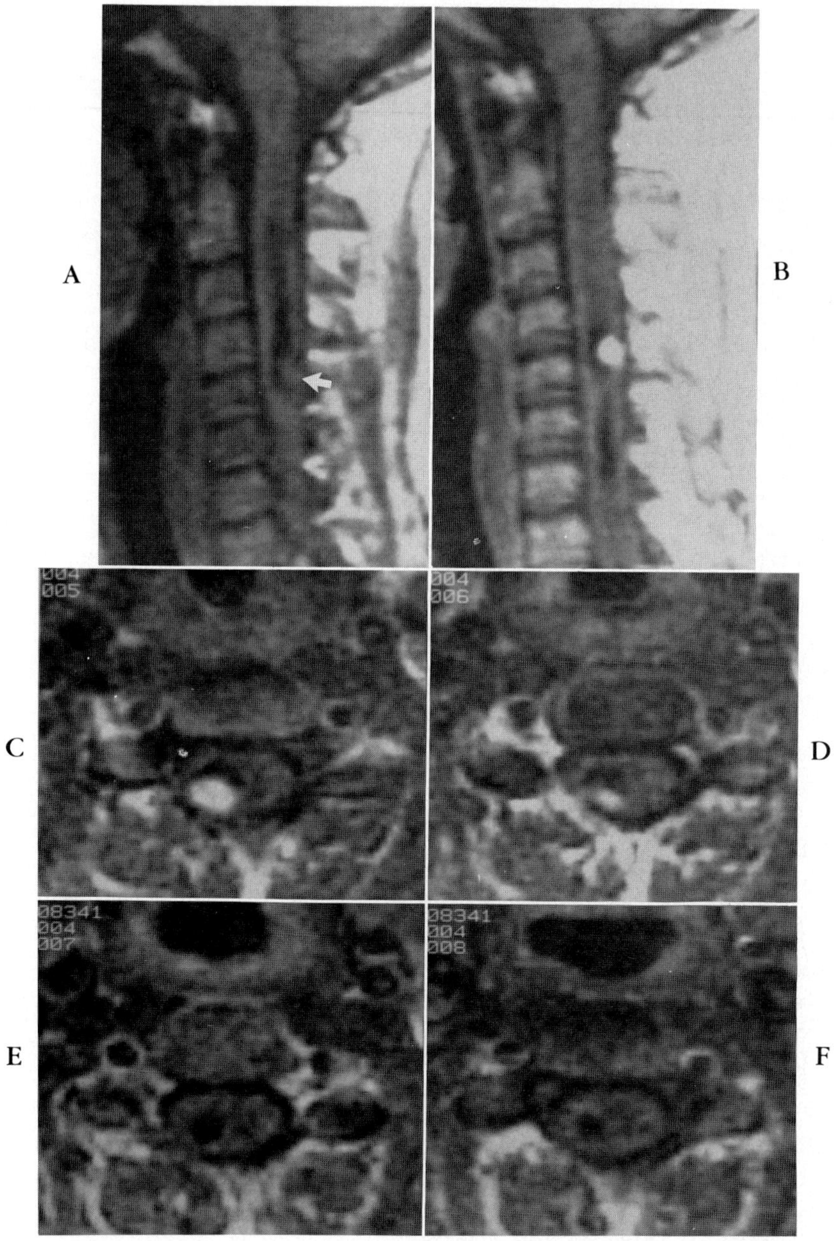

FIGURE 8-18. Precontrast and postcontrast T1W scans of single hemangioblastoma associated with cyst in the cervical cord. **A,** Precontrast scan shows tumor isointense with cord *(arrow)*. **B,** Post-GdDTPA scan demonstrates intense contrast enhancement of the hemangioblastoma. **C-F,** Axial postcontrast T1W scans show tumor nodule in one portion of cyst wall (**C**); cyst wall itself does not enhance with contrast (**D-F**). (Courtesy of Professor Doyon.)

A, B

C, D

E

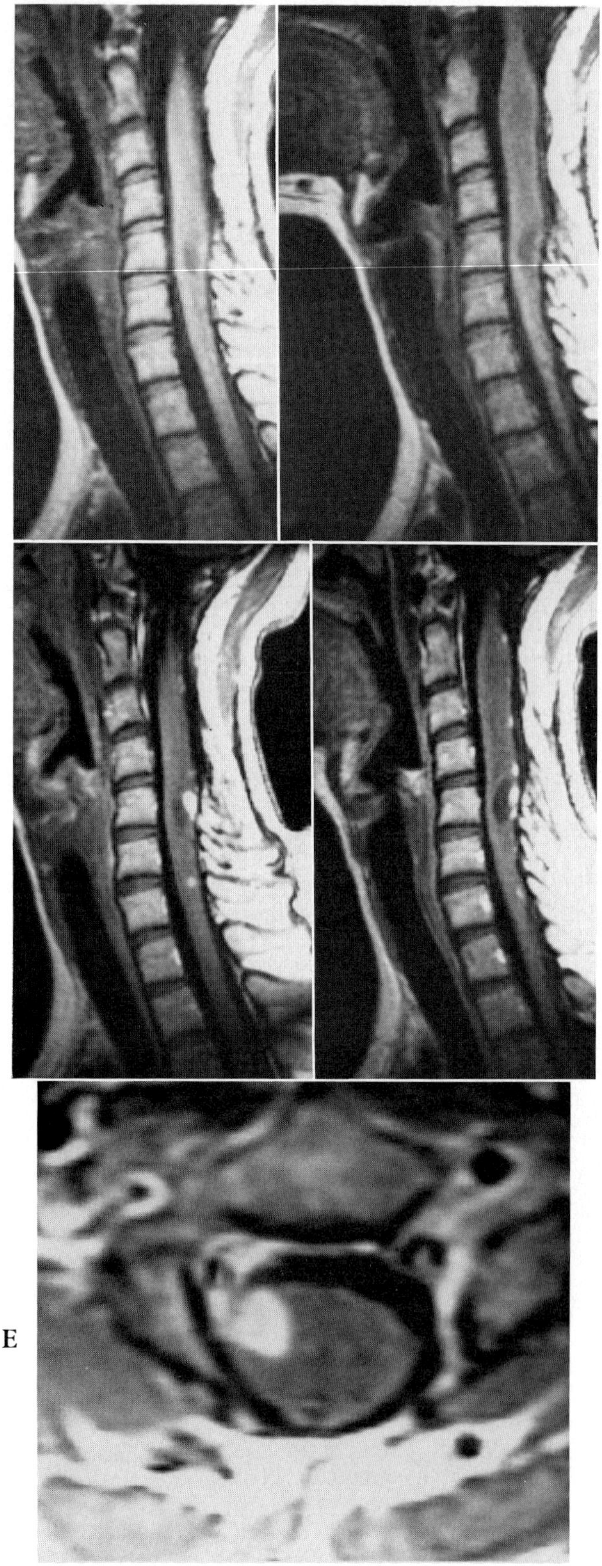

FIGURE 8-19. Hemangioblastoma. Value of contrast medium, GdDTPA, in detecting multifocal tumors is demonstrated in patient with multiple spinal hemangioblastomas. **A** and **B,** Precontrast T1W scans (SE 800/20) show cord enlargement in upper cervical region with diffuse low density in central cord and focal area of low signal intensity, suggesting cyst at C_5 level (**B**). Hemangioblastomas are isointense with cord. **C** and **D,** Postcontrast GdDTPA sagittal T1W scans (SE 800/20) show multiple nodular areas of intense contrast enhancement (high signal intensity) indicative of hemangioblastoma. Several nodules of enhancement are adjacent to cyst at C_5 level. Low signal intensity area in upper cervical cord most likely represents diffuse cord edema. **E,** Axial postcontrast T1W (SE 800/20) shows focal, well-defined area of contrast enhancement in enlarged upper cervical cord. Cord shows abnormal low signal intensity consistent with diffuse cord edema. (Courtesy of Dr. Michael Brant-Zawadzki.)

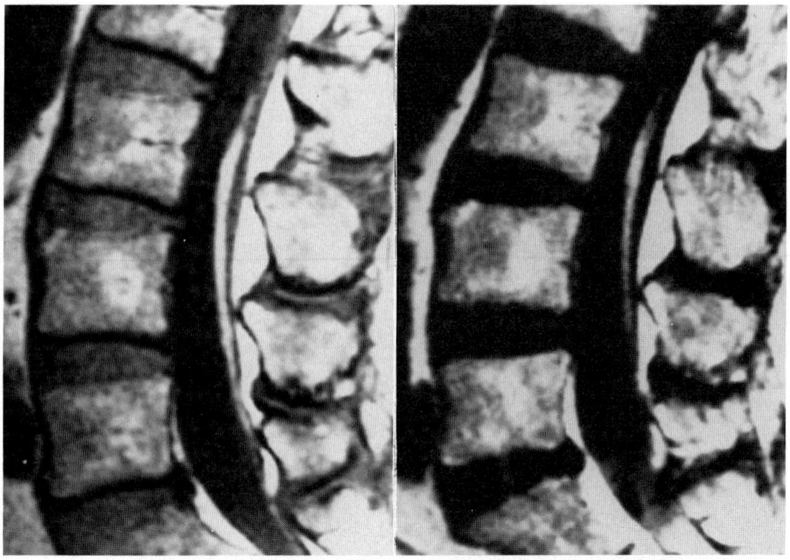

FIGURE 8-20. Lipoma of filum terminale. **A,** Sagittal T1W scan (SE 800/20) in 70-year-old male presenting with signs and symptoms compatible with cord tethering shows lipoma of filum terminale. **B,** "Fat" image shows high signal in filum indicating presence of adipose tissue.

contain collagen and occasionally areas of calcification. Lipomas involve primarily the thoracic cord, extending from T_1 to L_1, and males are more commonly affected than females (see Figure 8-22).

Symptoms develop between the second and fourth decades and consist of paraparesis, sensory changes, urinary incontinence, and, sometimes, pain localized to the level of the lipoma.[3] The pain is rarely radicular, although this does occur. The time course over which these symptoms appear can be quite variable, extending from a few weeks to many years.[74] Operative intervention with attempts to remove these lipomas has met with limited success and aggressive resection is not warranted.[74] Decompression of the spinal canal and biopsy often yield results as good as or better than attempted resection.[74]

MR Findings

Lipomas are normally easy to diagnose because of their prominent high signal intensity on T1W images. The only time they are subtle is when they are small in size. With small lipomas, both sagittal and axial views may be necessary to detect the lesion. The lipoma can be seen in both an intramedullary and extramedullary location (see Figure 8-21). In a few circumstances, in which high signal intensity in the T1W image could be mistaken for hemorrhage, a T2W scan can be used because fat exhibits lower signal intensity than hemorrhage. Acute hemorrhages may exhibit low signal on T2W images because of the dephasing effect of deoxyhemoglobin. The T2W scan can be indeterminate. The chemical shift artifact at the fat-cord interface may be helpful in discriminating fat from hemorrhage. A better method for demonstrating fat is the use of "fat" and "water" images (see Figures 8-21 and 8-22). Water suppression images (fat only) show prominent high signal intensity wherever lipoma is located (see Figures 8-20, 8-21 and 8-22). On a fat suppression image (i.e., water only), large areas of absent signal show where the lipoma is located (see Figure 8-22). This method clearly differentiates fat from hemorrhage.

Intramedullary Spinal Cord Metastases

True intramedullary metastases of the spinal cord are uncommon and are probably seen in only 1% to 3% of tumor patients.[12] The source

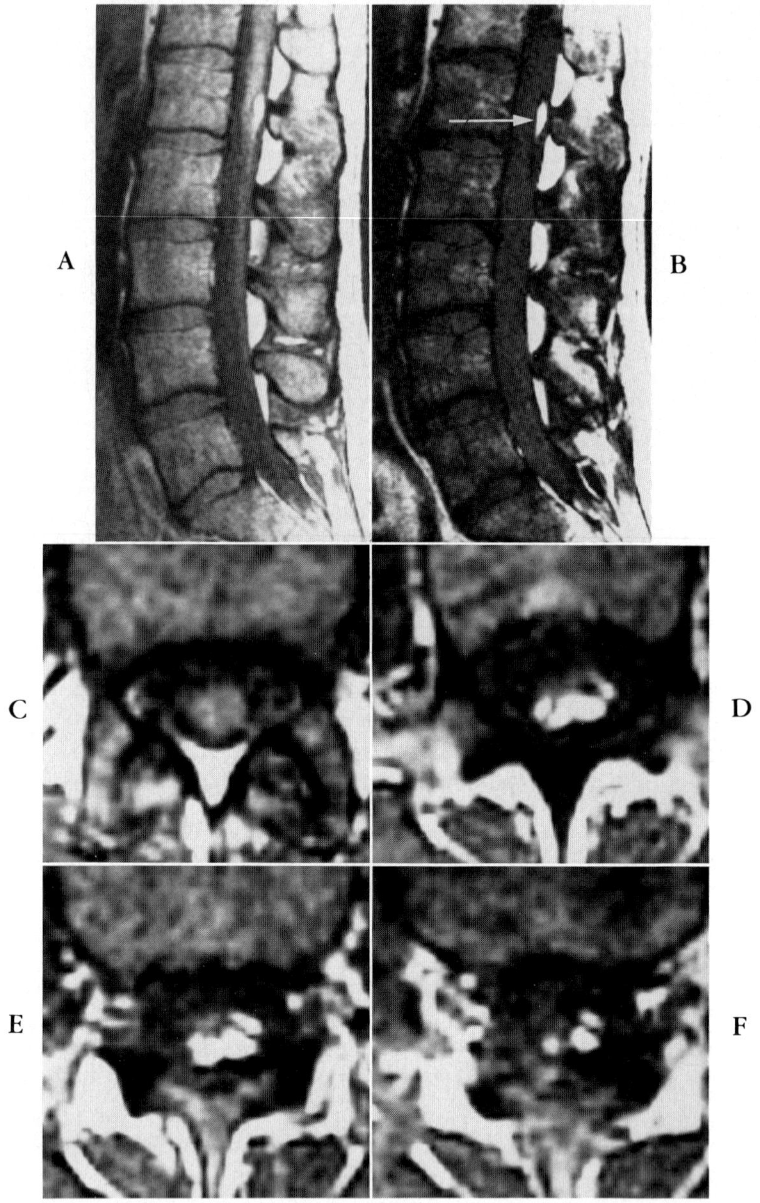

FIGURE 8-21. Lipoma. Incidental lipoma of conus and cauda equina detected in workup for acute back pain. **A,** Sagittal T1W scan (SE 800/20) shows focal elliptic area of high signal intensity at junction of conus and cauda equina. Focal hemorrhage could be a consideration. **B,** Water-suppressed image shows focal area of high signal to be fat tissue *(arrow)*. **C-F,** Set of four axial T1W scans (SE 1000/20) shows irregular mass of fat tissue extending from tip of conus (**C** and **D**) into cauda equina (**E** and **F**). Roots of cauda equina are interspersed within lipoma (**E** and **F**), which appears to have intramedullary and extramedullary components.

of intramedullary metastases are from neoplasms outside the central nervous system (CNS) and from primary CNS tumors.[12,56] Common non-CNS tumors are lung and breast carcinoma (Figure 8-23).[12,47] Melanoma is a tumor that can metastasize to the cord. Lymphoma and leukemia are two other neoplasms that may show cord involvement. Non-CNS tumors spread to the spinal cord via two proposed mechanisms: hematogenous spread and cord penetration from leptomeningeal tumor.[12] In a few patients (2%) with spinal cord metastases, this represents the first manifestation of non-CNS tumor in which the primary site may never be identified.[12]

The second major source of spinal cord metastases is a primary CNS tumor, most commonly glioblastoma, ependymoma, and medulloblastoma (Figures 8-24 and 8-25). Medulloblastoma exhibits this type of metastatic spread more than other tumors[14] (see Figure 8-25). The mechanism of spread is via the subarachnoid space; thus intramedullary and leptomeningeal tumors may coexist.

Intramedullary metastatic sites may be single or multiple and are more common in the thoracic cord than in the cervical cord.[12] With the hematogenous type of spread, metastatic nodules in the cord may partially or completely replace cord tissue. The metastasis is often well demarcated (see Figure 8-23). The metastatic tumor may be small enough that it does not enlarge the cord.[12] With hematogenous spread, leptomeningeal involvement is not a pathologic feature. The exception is if the metastatic nodule completely replaces the cord tissue and spreads into the adjacent meninges. Even then this is usually not accompanied by diffuse subarachnoid spread. Metastatic tumor resulting from hematogenous spread causes focal irregular cord enlargement, whereas contiguous spread from

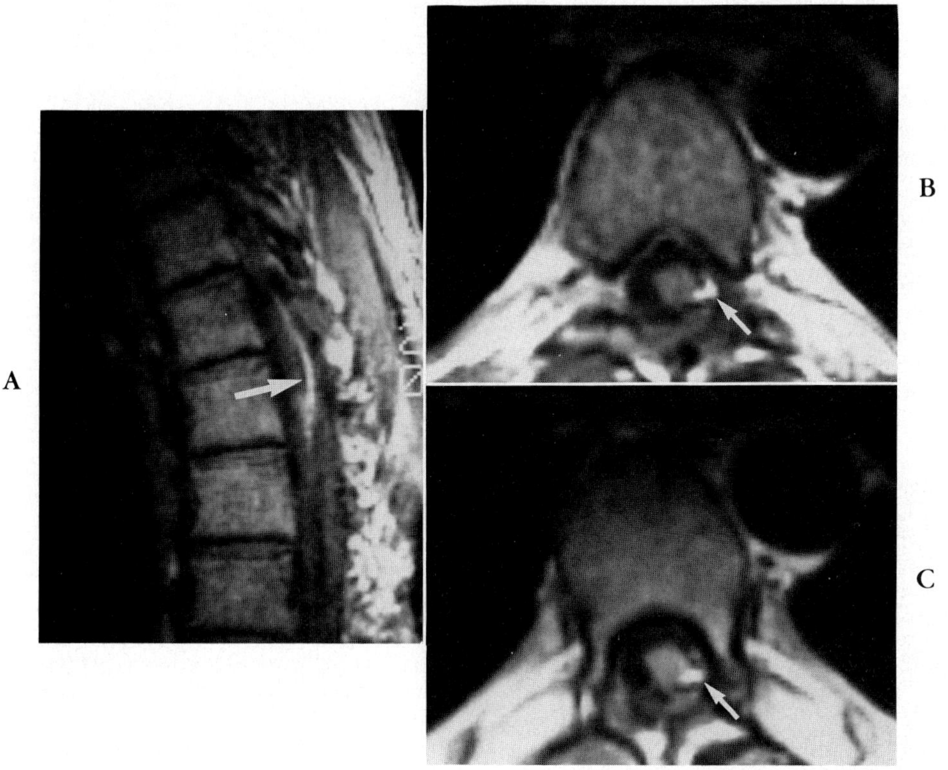

FIGURE 8-22. Intradural lipoma in 32-year-old male 1 year after biopsy. **A,** Sagittal T1W image (SE 800/20) of midthoracic spine shows curvilinear high signal structure *(arrow)* in spinal canal. Differential diagnosis for high signal on T1W images includes fat and subacute or chronic hemorrhage. In this case, lesion is a lipoma. **B** and **C,** Axial T1W images (SE 1000/20) through lipoma show small focus of high signal *(arrows)* lying posterior and lateral to spinal cord. Intermediate signal tissue posterior to cord in midline represents postoperative fibrosis.
Continued.

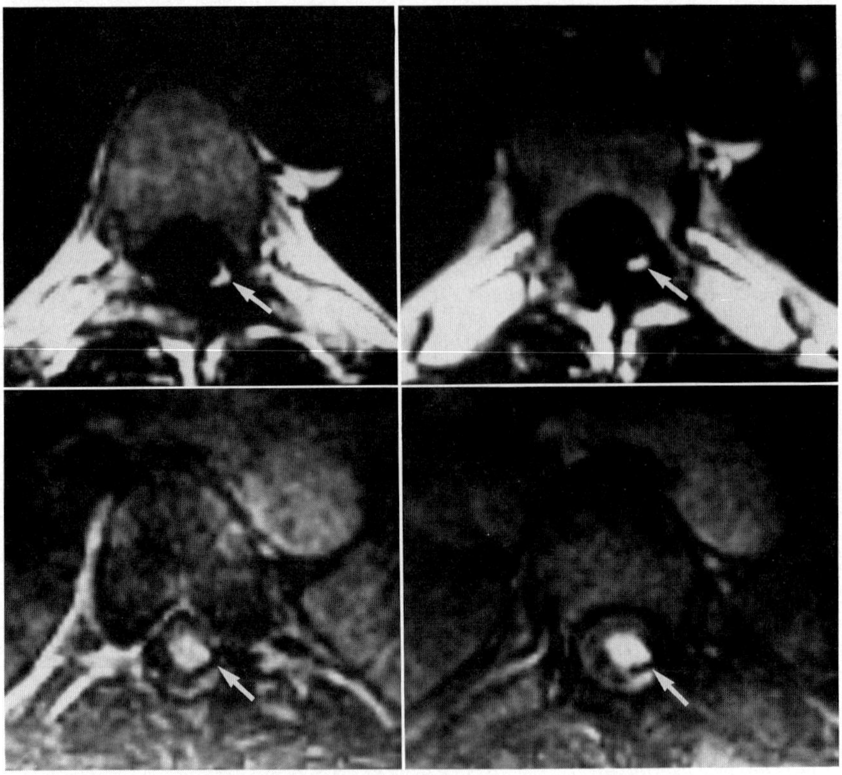

FIGURE 8-22, cont'd. **D** and **E**, Axial "water-suppressed" images (signal is from fat protons only) clearly show that high signal focus adjacent to cord *(arrows)* is composed of fat. This positively confirms presence of lipoma and excludes hemorrhage (signal from hemorrhage is generated from water protons). Spinal cord is not seen because signal from water protons in cord and CSF are equally suppressed. **F** and **G**, Axial "fat-suppressed" images (signal is from water protons only) also confirm presence of fat as low signal *(arrows)* adjacent to high signal spinal cord. Findings are less striking than with "water-suppressed" images. Presence of low signal is less specific than on "water-suppressed" images because low signal may be produced by proton relaxation effects such as short T2 or low proton density (e.g., acute hemorrhage or hemosiderin with short T2 or cortical bone with low proton density). Cord appears as high signal relative to CSF because oscillatory motion decreases signal of CSF.

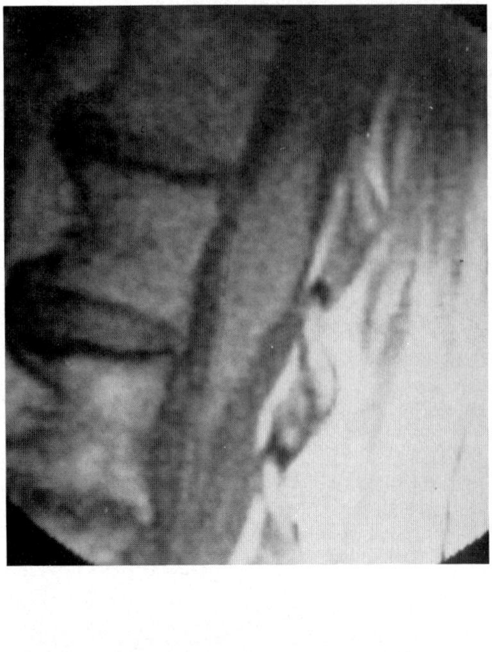

FIGURE 8-23. Intramedullary breast metastasis. T1W scan (SE 1016/26) of breast carcinoma diagnosed 7 years previously in female who now complains of back pain and had no known metastases before this time. Magnified view shows marked enlargement of conus caused by breast metastasis. Subsequent CT scan showed multiple intracranial metastases. Focal nature of metastasis suggests spread by hematogenous route. (Courtesy of Dr. Michael Brant-Zawadzki.)

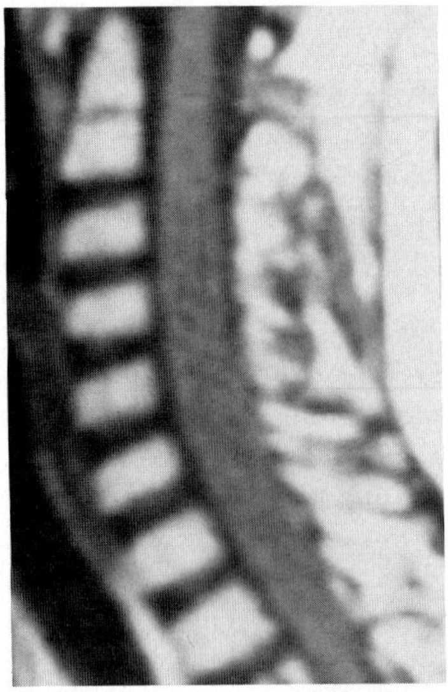

FIGURE 8-24. Intramedullary metastases from intracranial astrocytoma in child. Enlarged cervical cord shows diffuse, abnormal low signal intensity on T1W image (SE 400/25). Cord enlargement extends throughout entire cervical and upper thoracic cord. Note increased signal intensity in vertebral bodies indicative of previous radiation therapy. Appearance is similar to primary cord tumor, although history makes differentiation clear.

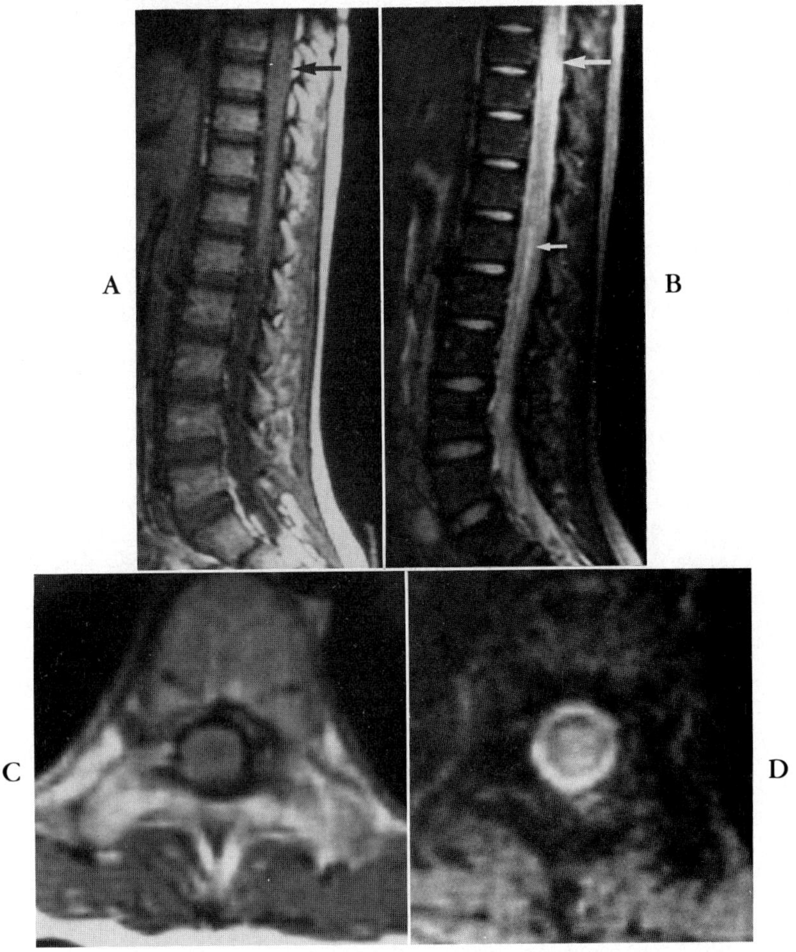

FIGURE 8-25. Intramedullary metastasis from medulloblastoma in 7-year-old female. **A,** T1W sagittal scan (SE 800/20) shows focal enlargement of distal thoracic cord above conus *(arrow)*. **B,** Sagittal T2W scan (SE gated 1900/80) shows focal area of high signal within cord in same region of cord expansion *(large arrow)*. Cord below metastatic site is of normal signal intensity. **C,** Axial T1W scan (SE 1000/20) confirms focal enlargement of cord and area of low signal intensity in its center. **D,** Variable flip angle/gradient echo scan (SE 40/20, 7°) shows area of increased signal intensity in central cord corresponding to area of low signal intensity on T1W axial scan (**C**). Cord signal around metastasis appears normal.

leptomeningeal tumor results in long segments of cord enlargement. Cord invasion secondary to leptomeningeal tumor occurs by direct extension, usually by tracking into the cord via the Virchow-Robin (perivascular) spaces and then penetrating the pia.

Clinical presentation depends on the site of the metastases. Progression of symptoms is usually rapid, ranging from days to a few weeks.[12,17] Typical progression occurs over 1 to 5 weeks. Patients experience progressive pain and weakness leading to paraplegia or tetraplegia; they may complain of numbness, and may develop bowel and bladder dysfunction. Typically the prognosis is poor, patients respond poorly to any form of treatment, and death usually ensues within a few months.

Diagnosis of spinal cord metastases was difficult before MR. Metastatic disease may be suspected clinically, although the differential diagnosis usually includes epidural tumor, a paraneoplastic syndrome, and transverse myelitis. CSF cytology studies are characteristically negative in intramedullary metastases without a leptomeningeal component. Spinal metastases may be the first presentation of tumor; sometimes the initial tumor diagnosis was made so long ago (up to 20 years) that tumor is not strongly considered, as may be the case with breast carcinoma. In patients with no known tumor the differential diagnosis includes the previous named entities, as well as MS. Although spinal cord metastases are unusual, they need to be included in the differential diagnosis of acute and subacute myelopathy. In such patients, a chest x-ray and a CT or MR brain scan may be indicated to locate a primary tumor.[12]

MR Findings

T1W scans show cord enlargement at the site of the metastases (see Figures 8-23 to 8-25). With the hematogenous type of spread the enlargement is focal (see Figure 8-23), whereas metastases secondary to leptomeningeal spread show longer segments of enlargement. In the latter type of tumor spread, nodules can be seen in an intradural extramedullary distribution (see leptomeningeal tumor spread). The intramedullary mass may be associated with osseous metastatic disease but usually is not associated with epidural tumor. The area of cord enlargement shows decreased signal intensity with minimal inhomogeneity on T1W images (see Figures 8-23 to 8-25). T2W images show abnormal increased signal intensity within the cord parenchyma at the site of cord enlargement and extending somewhat beyond. In some instances the extent of abnormal signal may involve long segments of the cord, or the entire cord (Figure 8-26). Cord size may be normal. Abnormal signal can extend into the brainstem (see Figure 8-26). The major portion of this high signal intensity represents edema spreading from the metastatic site. Depending on the size of the metastasis, normal cord tissue may surround the metastatic nodule and edema on axial views. The central location of the lesion and edema suggests this diagnosis, although a small focal cord tumor such as ependymoma may have a similar appearance (see Figure 8-25). Diseases such as lymphoma and leukemia usually show more extensive involvement than is seen with other non-CNS tumors (Figure 8-27). Lymphoma may show extensive areas of increased signal intensity within the cord without significant cord enlargement (see Figure 8-27).

It may be difficult to differentiate tumor from surrounding edema, transverse myelitis, or a paraneoplastic syndrome by conventional noncontrast MR images. A contrast agent such as GdDTPA will help detect and differentiate metastases that enhance, and most will enhance just as in the brain.[73] Because metastatic tumors characteristically have an abnormal blood-brain barrier, marked contrast enhancement would be expected in tumor nodules (Figure 8-28). The enhancement may be only moderate (Figure 8-29). On T1W scans contrast enhancement may be the only abnormality (see Figure 8-29) and is unlikely to be present in transverse myelitis or a paraneoplastic syndrome (autoimmune processes). When MS is a consideration, however, an acute MS plaque may show contrast enhancement. The clinical history allows the distinction. With extensive edema, localization can be difficult without a contrast agent (see Figure 8-26).

EXTRAMEDULLARY TUMORS

Meningioma

Meningiomas account for approximately 25% of intraspinal tumors, second only to neurinomas (29%)[67] and generally occur in adults between 20 and 60 years of age with a peak incidence at 45 years. A strong female predominance (F:M

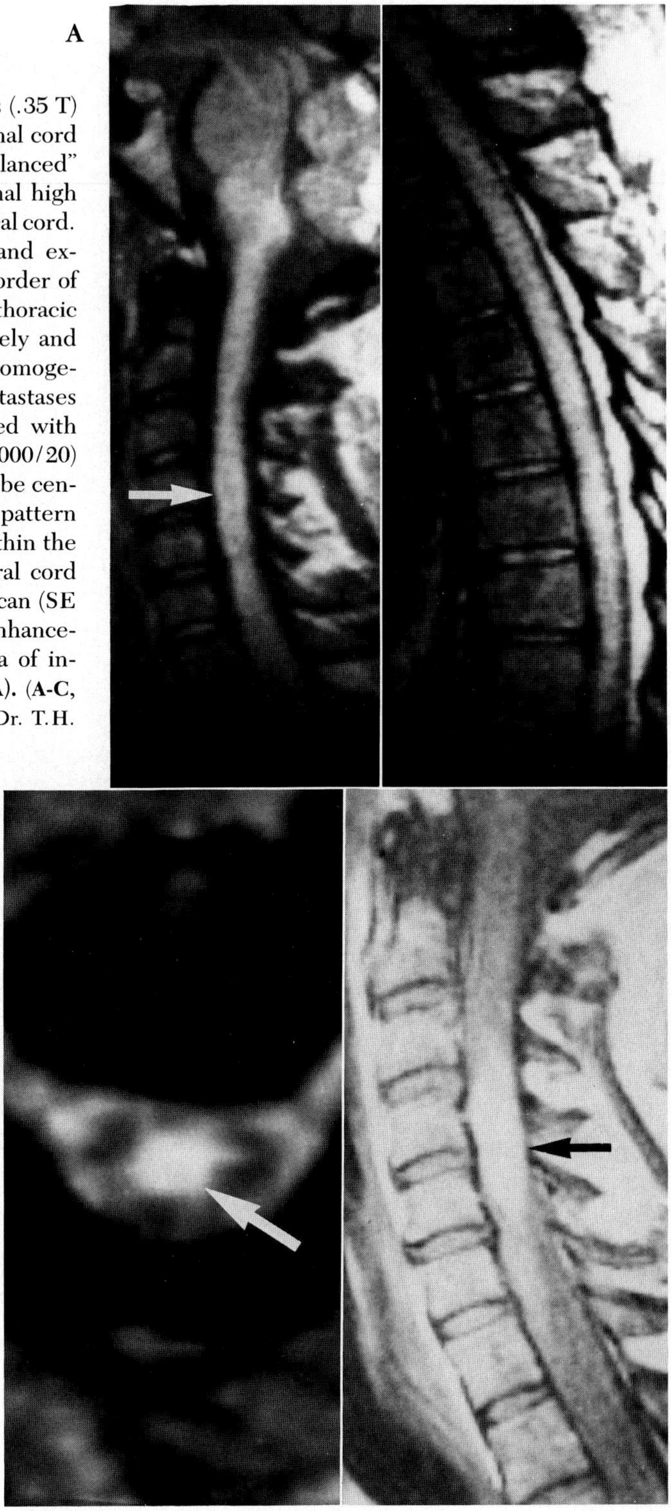

FIGURE 8-26. Cord metastases. MR scans (.35 T) of 36-year-old male with metastases to spinal cord from lung carcinoma. **A** and **B**, Sagittal "balanced" images (SE 1500/40) show diffuse abnormal high signal throughout entire thoracic and cervical cord. This abnormal signal represents edema and extends into the medulla up to the caudal border of the pons. Cervical cord is normal size but thoracic cord starting at approximately T_1 is diffusely and mildly enlarged. Subtle area of cord inhomogeneity at C_4-C_5 level was site of actual metastases shown on subsequent MR scan performed with GdDTPA (**D**). **C**, Axial .35T scan (SE 1000/20) shows abnormal high signal within cord to be centrally located. This appears to be a common pattern seen with longitudinal spread of edema within the cord *(arrow)*. Signal intensity of peripheral cord is within normal limits. **D**, Sagittal T1W scan (SE 600/20) after GdDTPA shows marked enhancement of metastasis, corresponding to area of inhomogeneity noted on noncontrast scan (**A**). (**A-C**, Courtesy of Dr. Bruce Nixon; **D**, Courtesy of Dr. T.H. Newton. Submitted for publication to AJNR.)

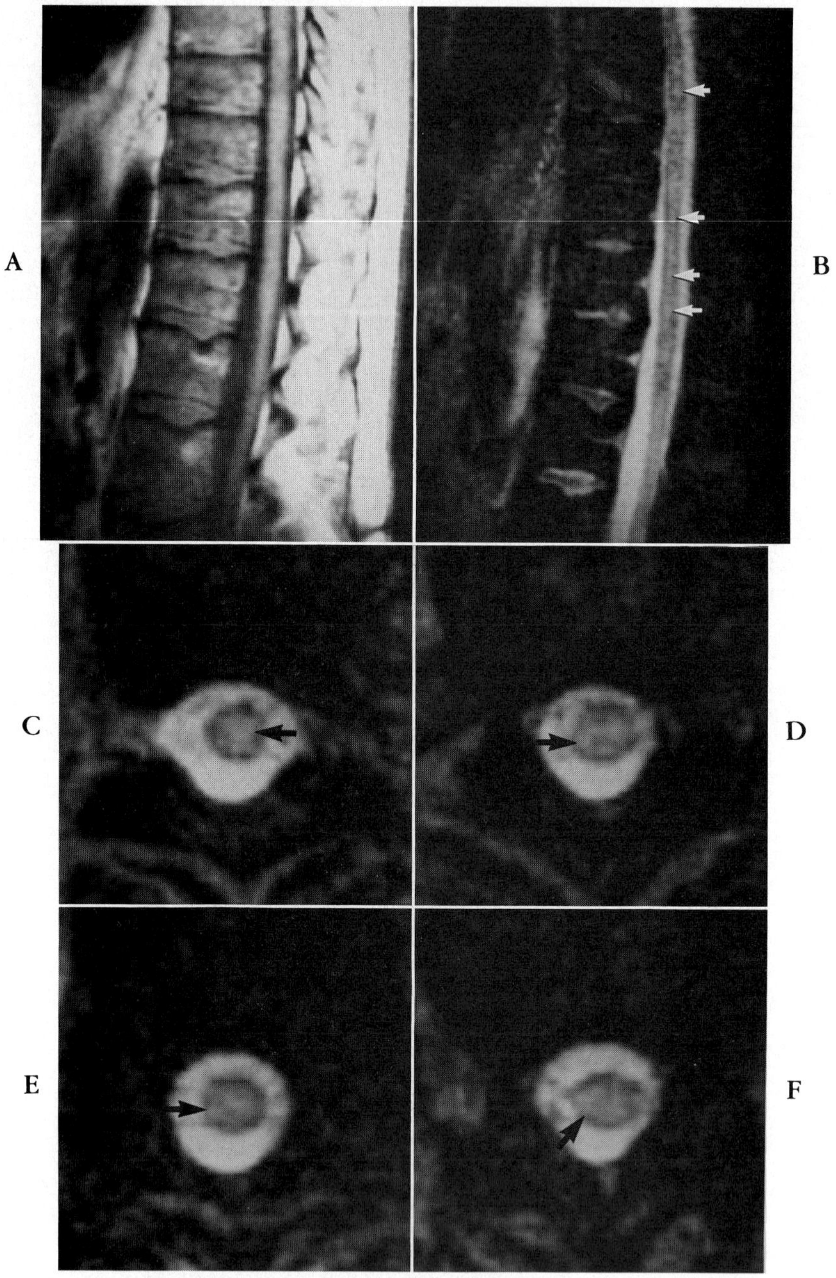

FIGURE 8-27. Lymphoma. MR scans of patient with clinical diagnosis of lymphomatous infiltration of cord, although this was not pathologically proven. **A,** T1W (SE 800/20) scan shows normal size of cord. **B,** T2W scan (gated SE 2000/80) shows thin line of abnormal tissue in central cord *(arrows)* extending throughout entire thoracic region without focal enlargement of cord. This is not a Gibbs (truncation) artifact. **C-F,** Set of four axial T2W scans (SE gated, 2100/80) confirm abnormal high signal in central cord throughout thoracic region *(arrows)*.

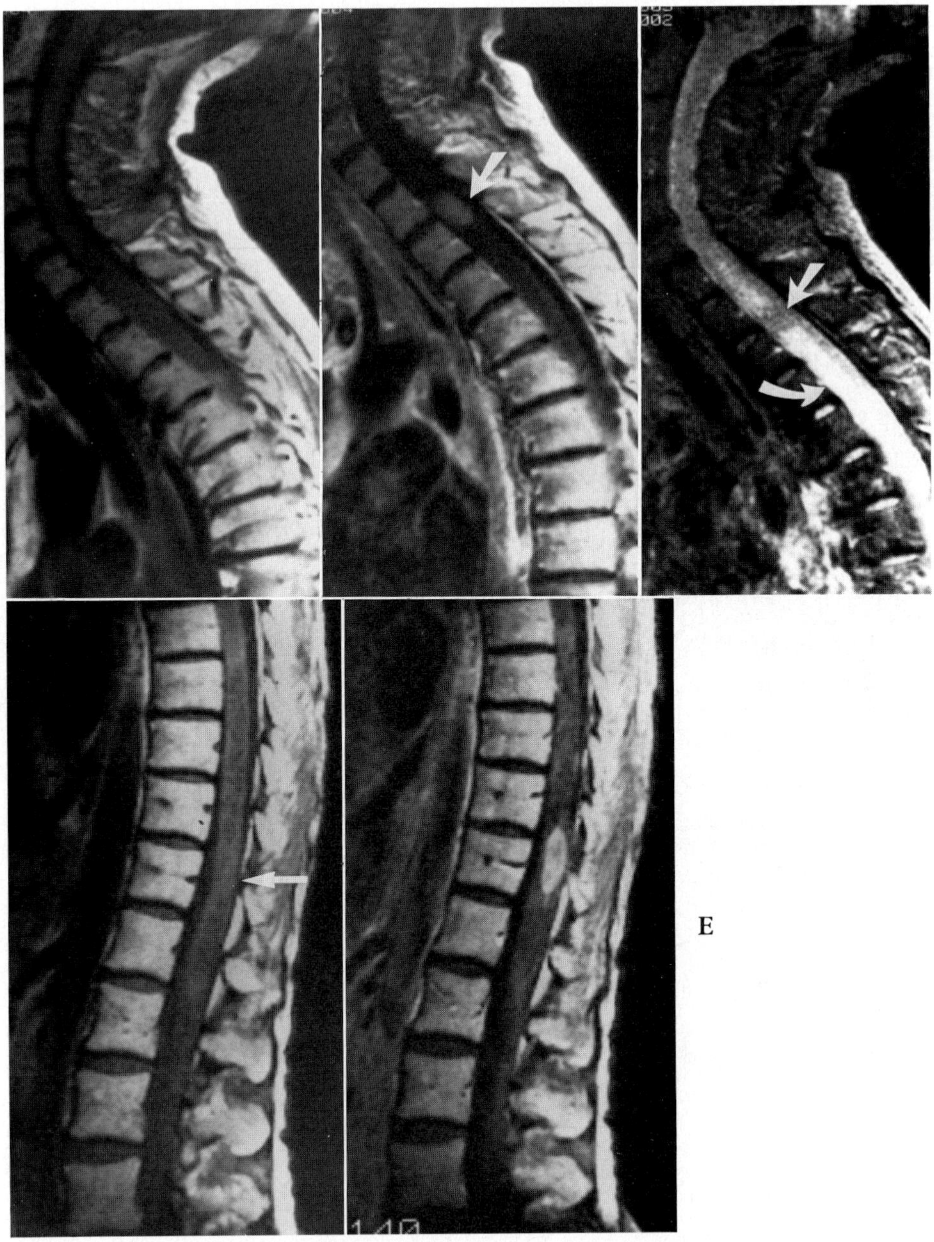

FIGURE 8-28. Cord metastases: breast. MR scan of 45-year-old female with lower extremity weakness and paresthesias had two intramedullary breast metastases: in the cervical cord and in the thoracic cord. **A,** Sagittal precontrast T1W scan (SE 600/20) shows lower cervical and upper thoracic cord enlargement. **B,** Postcontrast (GdDTPA) scan shows well-marginated oval area of enhancement within cord that was not detectable on precontrast scan. **C,** Sagittal T2W scan shows cervical metastasis to be isointense with cord *(straight arrow)*, but is flanked by high signal edema minimally above and markedly below it *(curved arrow)*. **D,** Sagittal precontrast T1W scan (SE 600/20) of lower thoracic cord shows diffuse enlargement and extensive long areas of low signal within cord. Metastasis is isointense with cord *(arrow)*. **E,** Sagittal postcontrast (GdDTPA) T1W scan (SE 600/20) shows focal nature of intramedullary metastases. Area of contrast enhancement is well marginated and degree of contrast enhancement is intense. Cord swelling above and below metastases is secondary to adjacent edema. (Courtesy of Dr. Gordon Sze. From Sze G, Drol G, Zimmerman RD, et al. AJNR 1988; 9:847.

A, B

C

D

E

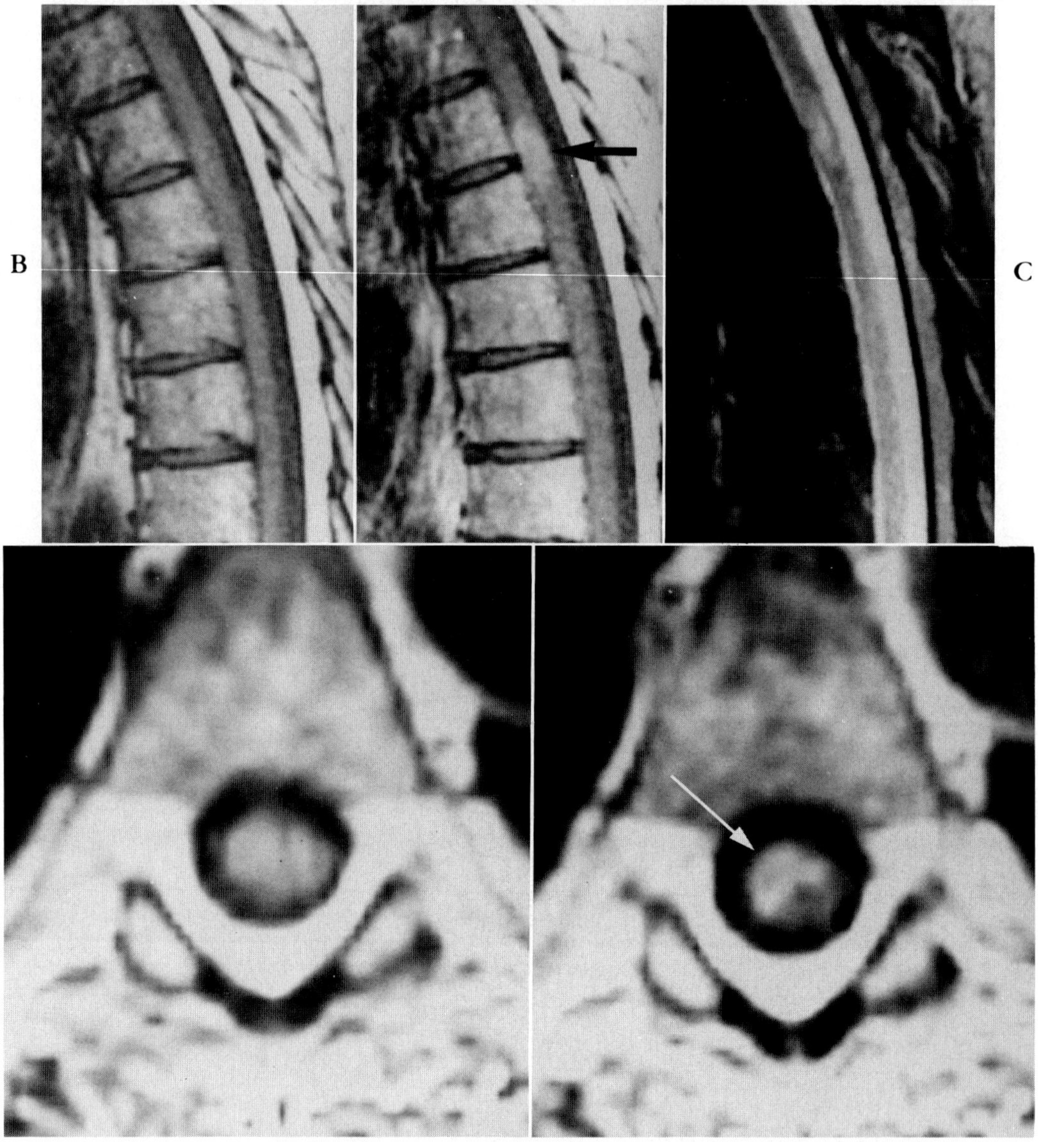

FIGURE 8-29. Spinal cord metastasis. MR scans of 45-year-old female with oat cell metastasis to the spinal cord. **A** and **B**, Pre- and post-sagittal GdDTPA T1W scans (SE 800/20) show contrast enhancing lesion at level of T_5 (**B**). Precontrast scan shows minimal cord swelling at this site and no significant signal inhomogeneity within cord (**A**). Postcontrast scan shows well circumscribed area of moderate enhancement within cord consistent with metastasis (*arrow*, **B**). **C**, Sagittal T2W scan (SE gated 2600/80) shows focal area of high signal intensity within cord at same site as contrast-enhancing lesion. Area of high signal extends slightly further caudad than area of enhancement, suggesting adjacent edema. Both T2W scan (**C**) and post-contrast T1W scan (**B**) show this relatively small intramedullary metastasis. **D** and **E**, Pre- and post-GdDTPA axial T1W scans (SE 800/20) confirm the findings on the sagittal scans. Precontrast scan shows minimal cord enlargement on the right (**D**). A well-circumscribed area of enhancement is noted at this site of enlargement that involves the right and anterior portion of the spinal cord *(arrow)*.

4:1) of intraspinal meningiomas is even more pronounced than in intracranial lesions.[61] Intraspinal meningiomas are usually solitary but may be multiple in neurofibromatosis where they may be associated with multiple other intraspinal tumors, including neurinomas, neurofibromas, and intramedullary gliomas and ependymomas.[61]

Intraspinal meningiomas arise primarily from arachnoid cells at sites of arachnoid villi, accounting for their predominance at the exits of spinal nerves from their dural sleeves. This location also corresponds to the most frequent site of neurinomas and neurofibromas of the spine. Meningiomas project from the dura into the subdural space of the thecal sac (85%), half of the remainder are extradural, and the rest are both intradural and extradural.[67] Meningiomas are most common in the thoracic spine.[61] The rare en plaque meningioma may produce a circumferential ring of tissue that compresses the cord.[68]

Microscopic psammomatous calcification is a common histologic feature of meningiomas, but dense grossly visible calcification is uncommon in spinal meningiomas, reported in 1% to 5% of cases.[67,68] Almost all meningiomas are histologically benign, slow growing, and compress but do not directly invade spinal nerves or cord. Rare malignant meningiomas probably arise from the angioblastic histologic type (hemangiopericytoma of the meninges) and tend to invade neural tissue.[61]

Typical clinical signs of intraspinal meningiomas are slow, progressive nerve root and cord compression, lasting from 6 months to 2 years.[63] Findings, depending on location of the lesion, include focal sensorimotor disturbances, transverse myelitis, hemiparesis, paraparesis, and loss of sphincter control.

A

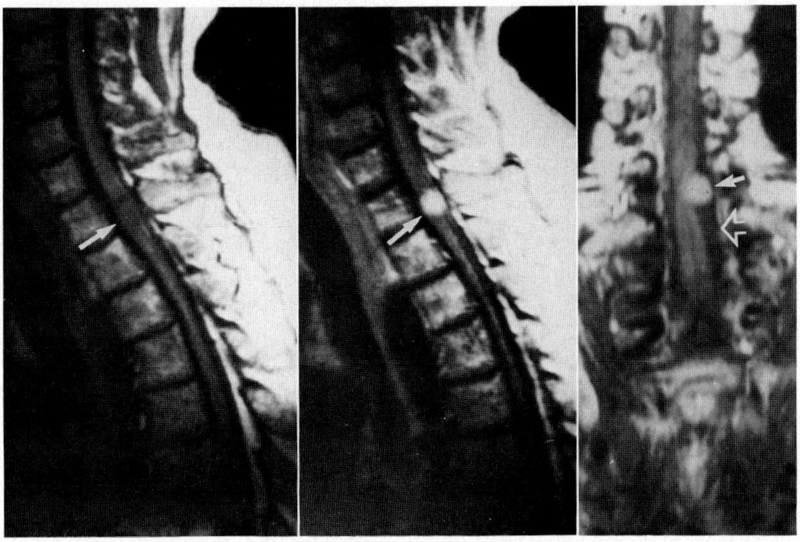

B, C

FIGURE 8-30. Meningioma. GdDTPA contrast enhancement of intraspinal meningioma. **A**, Sagittal T1W image (SE 800/20) shows subtle widening of spinal cord at C_7-T_1 level with slightly lower signal than normal cord *(arrow)*. Finding is ambiguous and may be caused by intramedullary mass or extrinsic mass compressing cord laterally. In this case, cord is compressed by right-sided intraspinal meningioma. Orthogonal axial or coronal images are needed to clarify relationship of cord to mass. **B**, Sagittal T1W image (SE 800/20) immediately after intravenous administration of 0.1 mmol/kg GdDTPA shows markedly increased signal and sharp margination of lesion *(arrow)*. Image remains ambiguous and does not discriminate between enhancing intrinsic or extrinsic cord lesion. **C**, Coronal T1W image (SE 800/20) after GdDTPA clearly shows relationship of extraaxial enhancing meningioma to cord *(closed arrow)*. Mass impinges on spinal cord and deviates it to left. Widening of low signal subarachnoid space above and below lesion *(open arrow)* is analogous to widening of contrast column seen on myelography with extramedullary lesions. (Courtesy of Dr. David Norman.)

A B C, D E

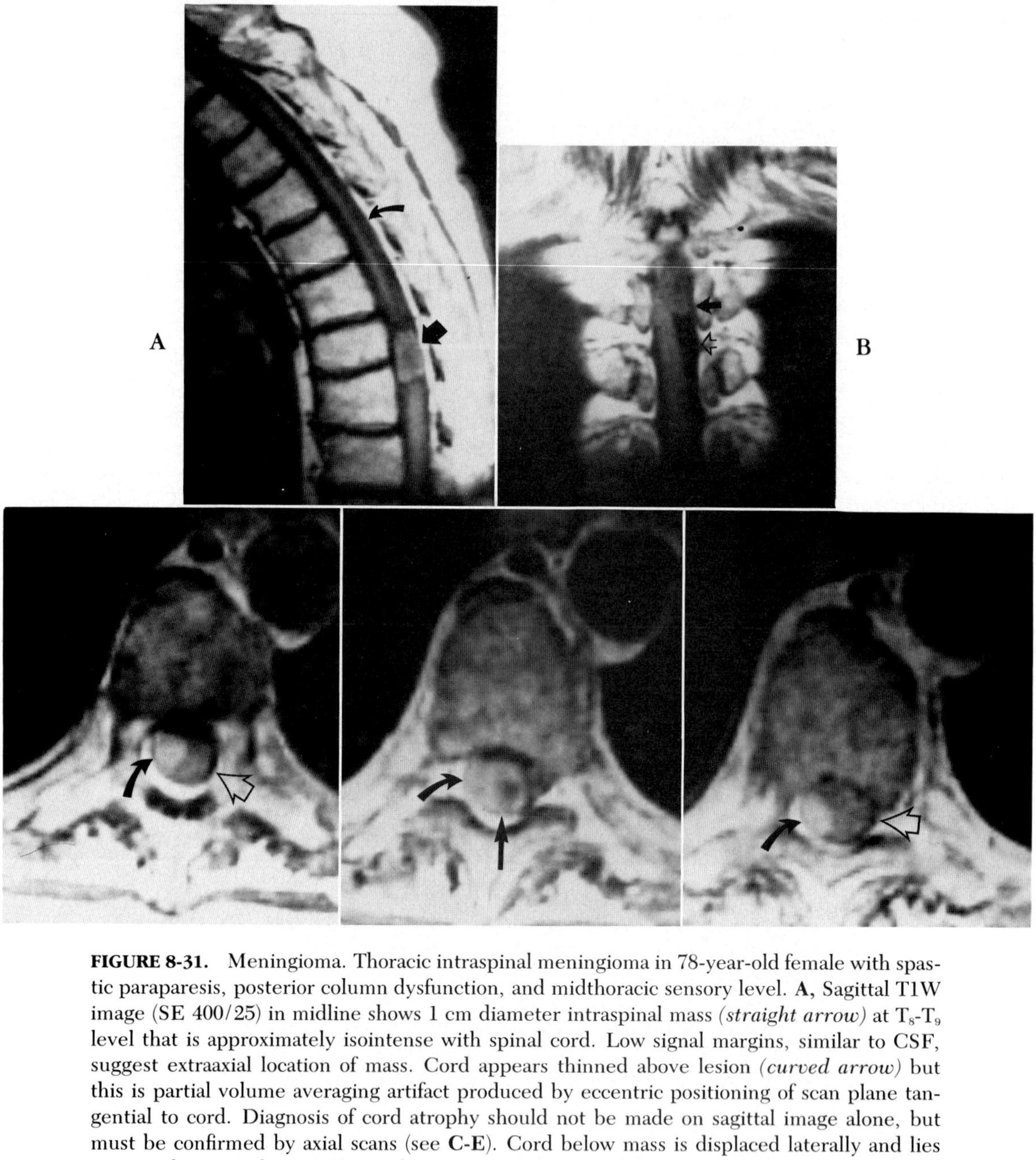

FIGURE 8-31. Meningioma. Thoracic intraspinal meningioma in 78-year-old female with spastic paraparesis, posterior column dysfunction, and midthoracic sensory level. **A,** Sagittal T1W image (SE 400/25) in midline shows 1 cm diameter intraspinal mass *(straight arrow)* at T_8-T_9 level that is approximately isointense with spinal cord. Low signal margins, similar to CSF, suggest extraaxial location of mass. Cord appears thinned above lesion *(curved arrow)* but this is partial volume averaging artifact produced by eccentric positioning of scan plane tangential to cord. Diagnosis of cord atrophy should not be made on sagittal image alone, but must be confirmed by axial scans (see **C-E**). Cord below mass is displaced laterally and lies more within scan plane. **B,** Coronal T1W image (SE 400/25) shows meningioma *(closed arrow),* projecting from left side of spinal canal, producing marked deviation and distortion of spinal cord. Diameter of cord below lesion is normal and deviation to right produces widening of left subarachnoid space *(open arrow)* analogous to widening of contrast column seen on myelography with extramedullary lesions. Axial T2W images (SE 2500/40) **C,** above, **D,** at, and **E,** below level of meningioma show compression and deviation of spinal cord adjacent to extraaxial mass. **D,** Mass *(straight arrow)* is isointense with compressed cord *(curved arrow)* and fills most of spinal canal cross section. Cord above (**C,** *curved arrow*) and below (**E,** *curved arrow*) lesion is normal in diameter. Deviation of cord to right produces widening of subarachnoid space on left (**C** and **E,** *open arrows*).

MR Findings

Meningiomas appear as discrete mass lesions with signal similar to the spinal cord on T1W and T2W images. Cord compression by meningiomas can be clearly seen in sagittal and axial images. Intradural extramedullary meningiomas deviate the cord and produce widening of the adjacent subarachnoid space, similar to the effect seen on myelography (Figures 8-30 and 8-31). Occasionally, meningiomas may invaginate severely into the cord and appear to be intramedullary lesions in some views. Additional orthogonal images usually allow better discrimination between cord and meningioma. Slight differences in signal intensity on T1W and T2W images may also allow differentiation of invaginating extramedullary lesions from intramedullary tumors. Intravenous contrast enhancement with GdDTPA is the best means for detection of meningiomas and for clarification of their extramedullary location. Meningiomas enhance densely and consistently with GdDTPA, appearing as sharply defined high-signal masses on T1W images.[63]

Intraspinal meningiomas have a similar appearance to intradural neurinomas and neurofibromas on MR images. All tend to have signal similar to the spinal cord on T1W and T2W images, enhance with GdDTPA,[32,63] and often present as intradural extramedullary mass lesions. Differentiation may be difficult in some cases and may depend on anatomic considerations. The tendency for neurinomas and neurofibromas to grow through and expand neural foramina helps to distinguish these tumors from meningiomas. Lesions that are not in contact with the thecal sac, such as isolated masses on nerve roots of the cauda equina, are more likely to be neurinomas than meningiomas or neurofibromas (Figure 8-33).

MR imaging has a safety advantage over myelographic evaluation of large intraspinal masses causing spinal cord compression in that it is noninvasive and precludes the 14% to 26% risk of acute worsening of symptoms from "spinal coning" that exists with myelography in masses producing subarachnoid block.[34] In cases of severe block, lumbar myelography may demonstrate only the caudal end of the lesion and a second puncture at C_1-C_2 may be required to demonstrate the cephalad extent of the mass. The noninvasive nature of MR spinal imaging is an advantage over CT scanning of spinal meningiomas. Complete characterization of lesions with CT usually requires lumbar puncture for instillation of intrathecal contrast material with the attendant risks and limitations similar to myelography. CT may be advantageous in unusual cases of densely calcified meningiomas or those that produce significant reactive bony hypertrophy, less common in spinal meningiomas than intracranial lesions. MR should be the initial imaging technique in cases of suspected spinal meningioma.

Neurinoma

Neurinomas are benign tumors composed of Schwann cells that are also known as neuromas, Schwannomas, neurilemomas, and peripheral fibroblastomas.[62] Schwann cells form the axonal myelin sheaths in the peripheral nervous system. Neurinomas—the most frequent type of extramedullary spinal tumor (29% of cases) with meningiomas second most common—almost always originate from sensory nerve roots, with rare reports of lesion in ventral motor roots, and usually occur in the cervical and thoracic regions but are found in the lumbar region in 40% of cases. The peak incidence is in the fifth decade of life and, in contrast to intracranial neurinomas, are seen predominantly in males.[61]

Neurinomas are generally single solitary lesions, except when associated with von Recklinghausen's neurofibromatosis. With neurofibromatosis, spinal neurinomas are often multiple and frequently associated with intracranial neurinomas (acoustic nerve lesions), multiple intracranial and spinal meningiomas, and gliomas.[61] Neurinomas are well-encapsulated, firm, mass lesions that compress adjacent tissues. Large lesions may be lobulated (Figure 8-32) with occasional internal hemorrhage and cyst formation. Intraspinal neurinomas are more frequently cystic than intracranial neurinomas.[61] Intraspinal neurinomas are usually located in the subdural space of the thecal sac but may also extend through neural foramina, resulting in "hour glass-" or "dumbbell-" shaped lesions that may produce large masses outside the spinal canal and considerable erosion of the neural foramen. Rare intramedullary lesions have been reported, probably originating from peripheral nerve elements accompanying branches of the

A, B

C, D

E

F

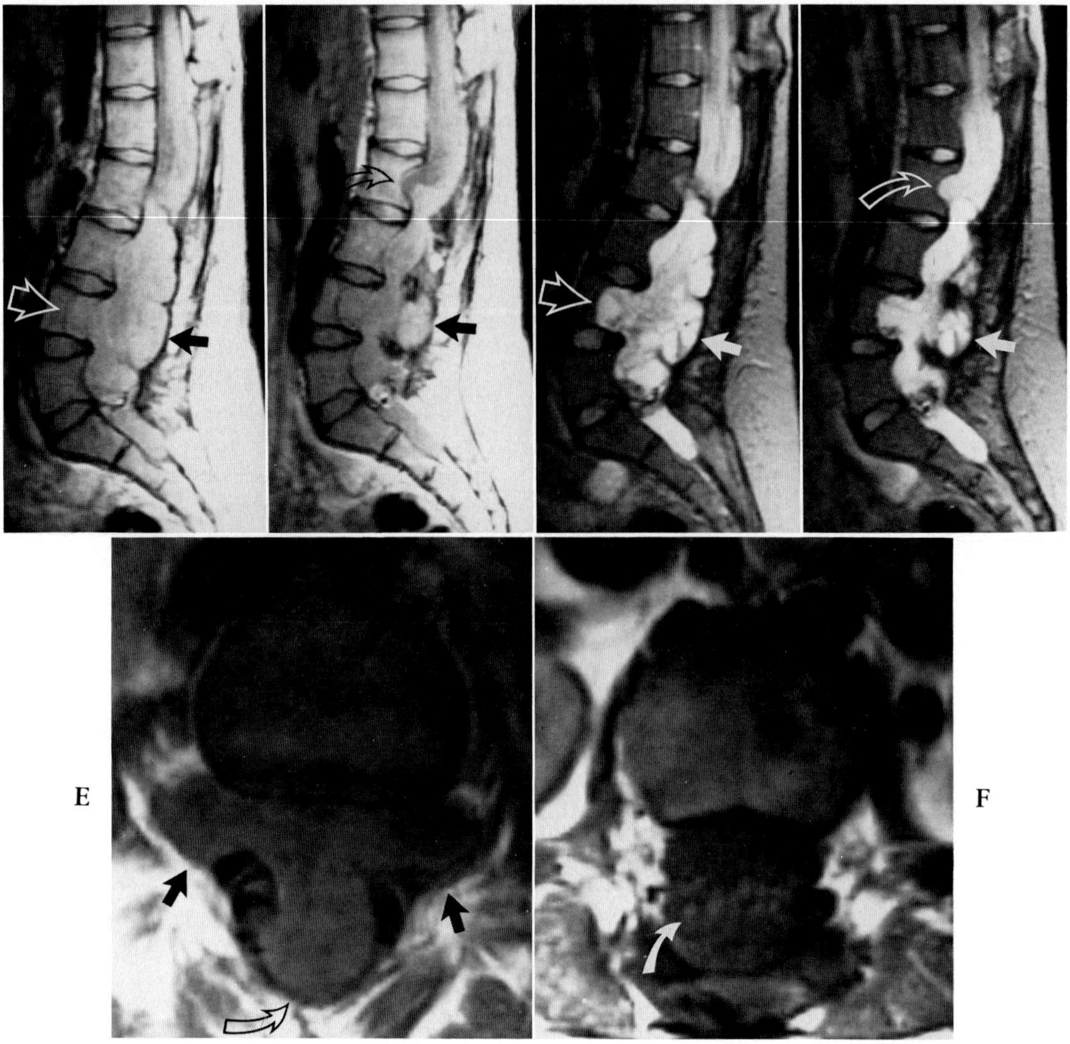

FIGURE 8-32. Schwannoma in 32-year-old female. Sagittal T2W images (2000/20, **A** and **B**; 80, **C** and **D**) show extensive, complex mass in lumbar spinal canal. Lesion appears homogeneous intermediate signal below L_2 on first echo images (**A** and **B**, *closed arrows*) and complex high signal with lobulated architecture on second echo images (**C** and **D**, *closed arrows*). Widening of lumbar spinal canal apparent with focal penetration of tumor into posterior body of L_4 (**A** and **C**, *open arrows*). Lesion extends caudally to level of S_2. Immediately superior to mass is area of dural ectasia with extension into posterior body of L_2 that appears as region of low signal on first echo image, as a result of CSF motion, and as intermediate to high signal on second echo image (**B** and **D**, *curved arrows*). Surgical changes posteriorly are from previous partial resection. Axial T1W images (1000/20) through midportion of mass at L_3-L_4 (**E**) and L_2 (**F**) levels show uniform signal in mass with extension bilaterally through neural foramina (**E**, *straight arrows*) and posteriorly through surgical defect (**E**, *curved arrow*). Superiorly at L_2 level, anterior sac is moderately enlarged with normal intermediate signal roots arrayed in posterior sac (**F**, *arrow*).

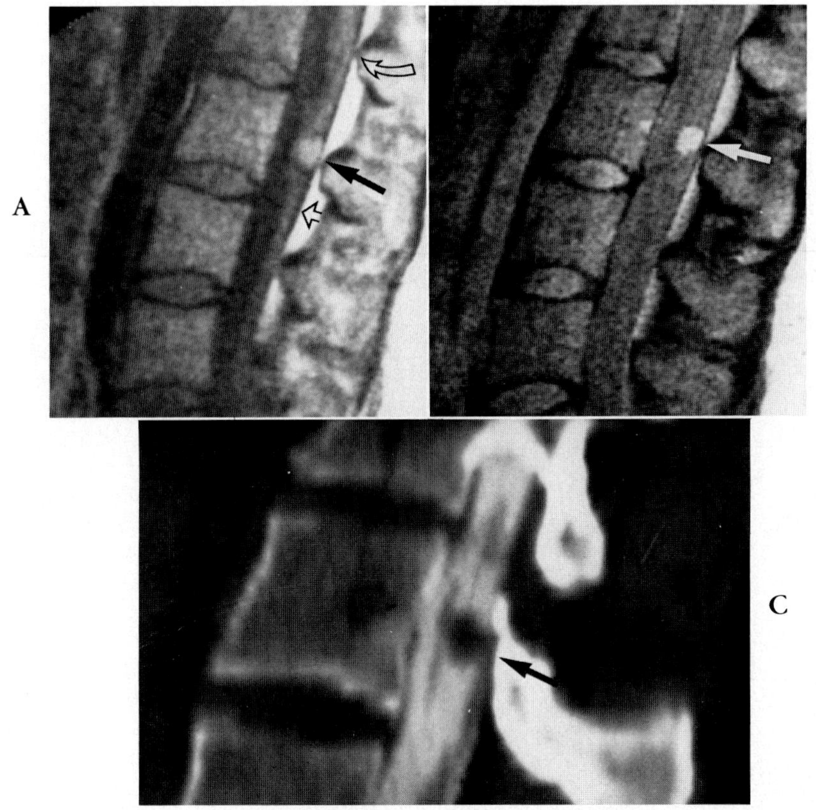

FIGURE 8-33. Confirmed neurinoma of cauda equina in 29-year-old female. Scans performed on .5T machine. **A,** Sagittal T1W image (SE 750/26) shows 1 cm diameter moderately high signal mass in cauda equina at L_2 level *(black arrow)*. Signal in neurinoma is slightly higher than cauda equina *(open straight arrow)* and conus medullaris *(open curved arrow)*. **B,** Sagittal T2W image (SE 1500/60) shows neurinoma as very high signal *(arrow)* contrasted against lower signal CSF. Conus and cauda equina are isointense with CSF. **C,** Sagittal reformation of intrathecal contrast-enhanced CT scan shows neurinoma as negative defect in contrast column posterior to L_2 *(arrow)*. (Courtesy of Dr. Michael Brant-Zawadzki.)

anterior spinal artery into the spinal cord or the result of developmental inclusion of neural crest cells within the cord.[61,67]

Neurinomas are histologically benign lesions, and although peripheral nerve lesions may undergo malignant transformation, intraspinal lesions probably do not become malignant.[61] Neurinomas are distinguished from neurofibromas by their extrinsic location relative to the nerve root of origin and their largely homogeneous histology. Neurofibromas are less clearly demarcated than neuromas and enlarge within the nerve, resulting in a mixture of proliferating Schwann cells, fibroblasts, and myelinated and unmyelinated nerve fibers. Grossly, neurinomas and neurofibromas may have very similar appearances, including predominantly intrathecal location and extension through neural foramina (Figure 8-32).

Clinical presentation of intraspinal neurinomas is usually that of focal nerve root compression with related sensory deficits.[61] Large intraspinal masses cause progressive deficits from cord compression. Cauda equina lesions (Figure 8-33) usually produce specific distal nerve root deficits, often chronic sciatica. Neurofibromatosis symptoms as a result of neurinoma may be inseparable from those resulting from nerve root and cord compression by neurofibromas or meningiomas.

MR Imaging

Neurinomas appear as discrete mass lesions with signal similar to or lower than that of spinal

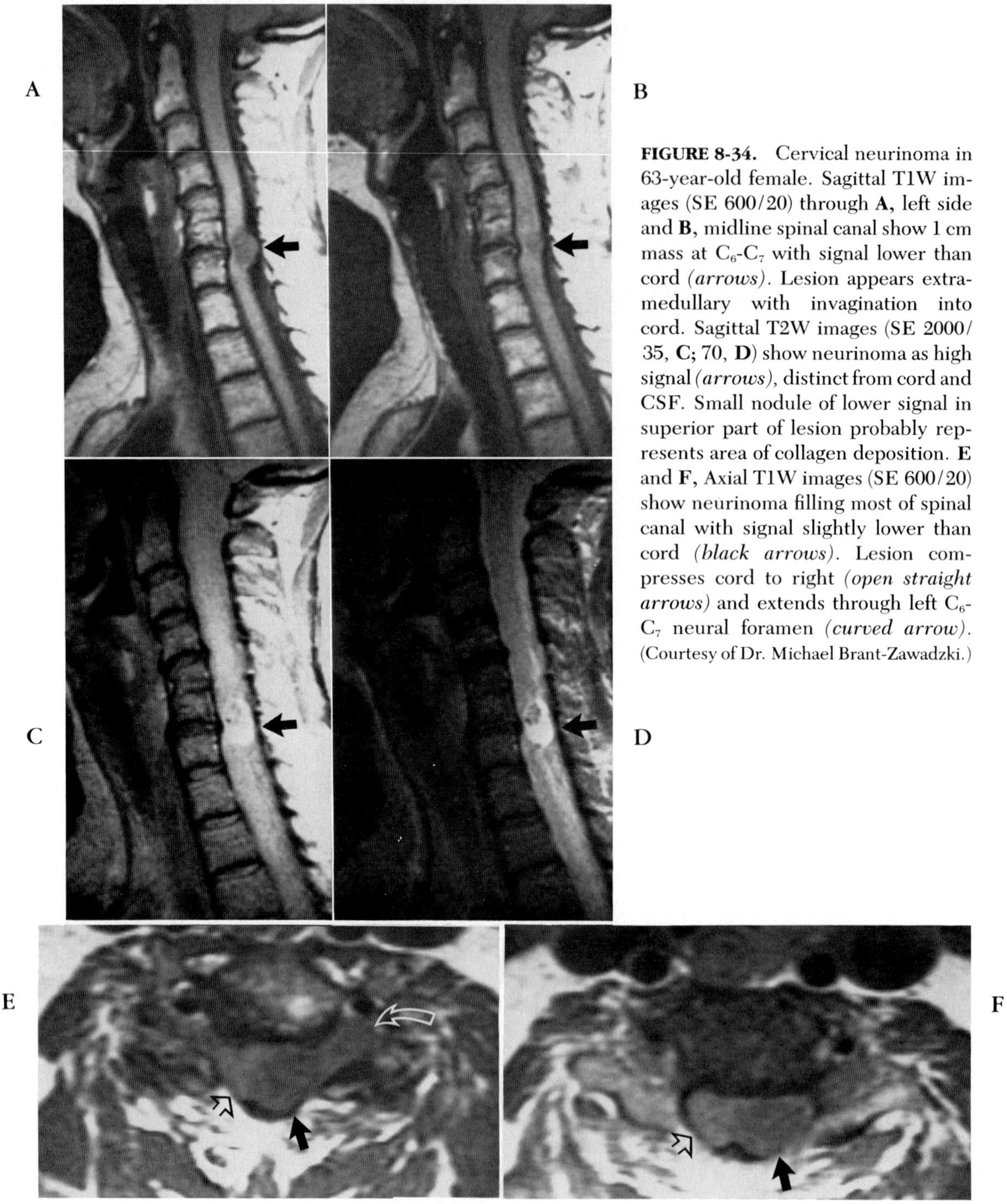

FIGURE 8-34. Cervical neurinoma in 63-year-old female. Sagittal T1W images (SE 600/20) through **A,** left side and **B,** midline spinal canal show 1 cm mass at C_6-C_7 with signal lower than cord *(arrows)*. Lesion appears extramedullary with invagination into cord. Sagittal T2W images (SE 2000/35, **C;** 70, **D**) show neurinoma as high signal *(arrows)*, distinct from cord and CSF. Small nodule of lower signal in superior part of lesion probably represents area of collagen deposition. **E** and **F,** Axial T1W images (SE 600/20) show neurinoma filling most of spinal canal with signal slightly lower than cord *(black arrows)*. Lesion compresses cord to right *(open straight arrows)* and extends through left C_6-C_7 neural foramen *(curved arrow)*. (Courtesy of Dr. Michael Brant-Zawadzki.)

cord on T1W images. Cord compression by neurinomas can be clearly seen in sagittal and axial images despite their isointensity. Intradural neurinomas deviate the cord with widening of the adjacent subarachnoid space, similar to the effect seen with intradural extramedullary masses on myelography. Occasionally, the neurinoma may invaginate into the cord with severe compression and appear to be intramedullary in some images (Figure 8-34). Orthogonal images are used to discriminate between cord and neurinoma. Neurinomas extending through the neural foramina can usually be seen best on axial images (see Figure 8-27). Sagittal images may show lesions in the neural foramina on laterally positioned images. Foraminal lesions appear as intermediate signal, replacing high signal fat on T1W images and heterogeneous high signal venous structures and intermediate signal fat on T2W images.

Intravenous contrast enhancement with GdDTPA allows easy detection of neurinomas and differentiation of extramedullary from intramedullary masses. Neurinomas consistently enhance with GdDTPA, appearing as sharply defined high signal masses on T1W images.[63]

Differential diagnosis of neurinoma includes meningioma and neurofibroma. All of these lesions may have similar signal intensities on T1W and T2W images and enhance with GdDTPA so that differentiation may be difficult in some cases and may depend on anatomic considerations. For example, a lesion within the thecal sac isolated on a nerve root in the cauda equina is more likely to be a neurinoma than meningioma or neurofibroma. Extension through a neural foramen is unusual for meningioma; a solitary lesion favors neurinoma, while multiplicity favors neurofibroma.

Neurofibromatosis

Neurofibromatosis (von Recklinghausen's disease) can be divided into three forms that usually present the following distinctive clinical and pathologic features[60,61]:

1. Central form consists of multiple intracranial and intraspinal tumors that arise from the parenchyma of the CNS, meninges, and cranial and spinal nerves.
2. Peripheral form is characterized by large numbers of peripheral and subcutaneous nerve sheath tumors associated with multiple cutaneous cafe-au-lait patches.
3. Visceral form has ganglioneuromas and nerve sheath tumors involving the viscera and autonomic nervous system. It may be associated with other visceral neoplasms derived from the neural crest such as peripheral neuroblastomas, adrenal ganglioneuromas, and pheochromocytomas.

The three forms of neurofibromatosis tend to overlap slightly, and it is typical that the peripheral form seldom shows central manifestations, whereas, the central form shows few of the peripheral manifestations. Patients with the central form tend to manifest symptoms at a younger age than those with the peripheral form. All forms may be present within the same family.[61]

Central Neurofibromatosis

Tumors associated with central neurofibromatosis are Schwannomas (neurinomas) that usually involve cranial and spinal nerve roots. Multiple meningiomas are also found intracranially and within the spinal canal.[59,60,61] Intraparenchymal tumors of glial origin are common and of two basic types: pilocytic astrocytomas and ependymomas. Astrocytomas are typically located adjacent to the third ventricle and ependymomas are frequently multiple and situated in the spinal cord. Diffuse gliomas of the spinal cord may occasionally be present.[60,61]

Neurofibromas are tumors of the cranial and spinal nerves that are almost unknown in the absence of von Recklinghausen's neurofibromatosis[10,61] and are histologically less sharply marginated than Schwannomas.[61] These tumors are derived from and composed of Schwann cells and fibroblasts; they often include collagen and nerve fibers, which may or may not be myelinated.[61] Fusiform masses are present in the nerves that consist of endoneural myxoid matrix (acid mucopolysaccharides) and large amounts of fluid that spread axons apart. Condensations of relatively cellular fibrous tissue may occur at the center of these fusiform masses.[31,61] A variant of these lesions, aggressive fibromatosis, is a relatively acellular lesion consisting of dense collagen.[2] Unlike Schwannomas, neurofibromas in nerve roots may progress from malignant degeneration to neurofibrosarcoma.[61]

Intramedullary lesions associated with neurofibromatosis include astrocytomas, ependymomas, central neurinomas (central schwannosis[61]) and harmartomas.[4] A peculiar association of central neurofibromatosis producing both intramedullary lesions and bilateral acoustic neuromas occurs in neurofibromatosis and is believed to be a distinct genetic disorder.[18] Most cases thought to be intramedullary schwannoma associated with neurofibromatosis are, in fact, pilocytic gliomas.[61] Rare true intramedullary schwannomas have been reported that presumably grow in from peripheral nerve sheath elements that accompany the intraspinal branches of the anterior spinal artery.[61]

MR Findings

Spinal manifestations of neurofibromatosis can be evaluated using conventional radiography, myelography, and CT scanning. Abnormalities include bony dysplasias, extradural masses, dural ectasia, lateral meningocele, and peripheral nerve tumors outside the spinal canal. MR has several advantages over these techniques because of its ability to visualize intramedullary and extramedullary lesions without intrathecal contrast; this is important in view of the multiplicity of tumors.

The MR appearance of neurofibromas is complex and probably related directly to topographic variation. Spinal nerve lesions (Figures 8-35 to 8-41) show slightly greater signal intensity than muscle on T1W images, increased signal on T2W images,[8] and correspond to low density lesions on CT scans.[8] Low signal on T1W images and high signal on T2W images is probably the result of the high water content of the endoneural myxoid matrix, which is complex with large acid mucopolysaccharide molecules interacting with water, resulting in relaxation times dominated by high water content but shorter than those of free water such as CSF.[8] Central areas of low signal in neurofibromas are frequently seen on T2W images. These low signal areas are well defined and extend longitudinally through the center of the neurofibroma.[8] Pathologically, central areas of low signal correspond to areas of Schwann cell proliferation within regions of dense collagen surrounded by myxoid tissue and may be explained by the presence of collagen, which has fewer mobile protons and a very short T2 relaxation time.[8] Larger neurofibromas (3 to 5 cm diameter) may exhibit several distinct rings of low signal.[8] Some very large neurofibromas may show less well-defined central areas of variable signal instead of the typical low signal changes; these correspond pathologically to necrosis.[8]

Large neurofibromas can be difficult to distinguish from anterior meningoceles (see Figure 5-33) (see Chapter 5). In general, meningoceles are filled with fluid that is similar to CSF, tend to be lower signal than muscle on T1W images, and homogenous high signal on T2W images. In some large meningoceles, however, motion of fluid within the meningeal sac may produce inhomogenous signal on T2W images, mimicking necrosis in larger neurofibromas. Images may be further complicated by variation of signal across the meningocele as a result of signal falloff from the posteriorly placed surface coil (higher signal near the coil falling off distally on T2W images) (see Figure 5-33). Two potential solutions to the dilemma are available. The first least invasive and least expensive method is an ultrasound study, which will clearly demonstrate the difference between solid and cystic masses. However, this solution is limited to lesions not surrounded by bone or with no bone or bowel gas lying between the lesion and the skin surface. The second alternative is an intravenous (IV) contrast-enhanced CT study. Although most neurofibromas do not clearly enhance, when they do the pattern of double density is characteristic.[77] Insufficient experience is available with IV paramagnetic contrast enhancement (GdDTPA) with MR to assess whether this will be a useful means for distinguishing large neurofibromas from cystic meningoceles, but it is likely that it will.

Malignant neurofibrosarcoma may occur within an area of extensive plexiform neurofibromatosis. These lesions are distinguished from smaller benign neurofibromas by the absence of a well-defined central area of low signal on T2W images. Heterogenous, irregularly marginated central signal within these lesions on T2W images corresponds pathologically to areas of necrosis. Unfortunately, the appearance may be similar to and indistinguishable from the internal appearance of some large, benign neurofibromas—those without the typical ring pattern of central low signal.[8]

Plexiform "dumbbell" neurofibromas in the neural foramina often enlarge sufficiently within the spinal canal to produce spinal cord compression (Figure 8-36). These lesions are typically transdural so that the intraspinal portion com-

A

B

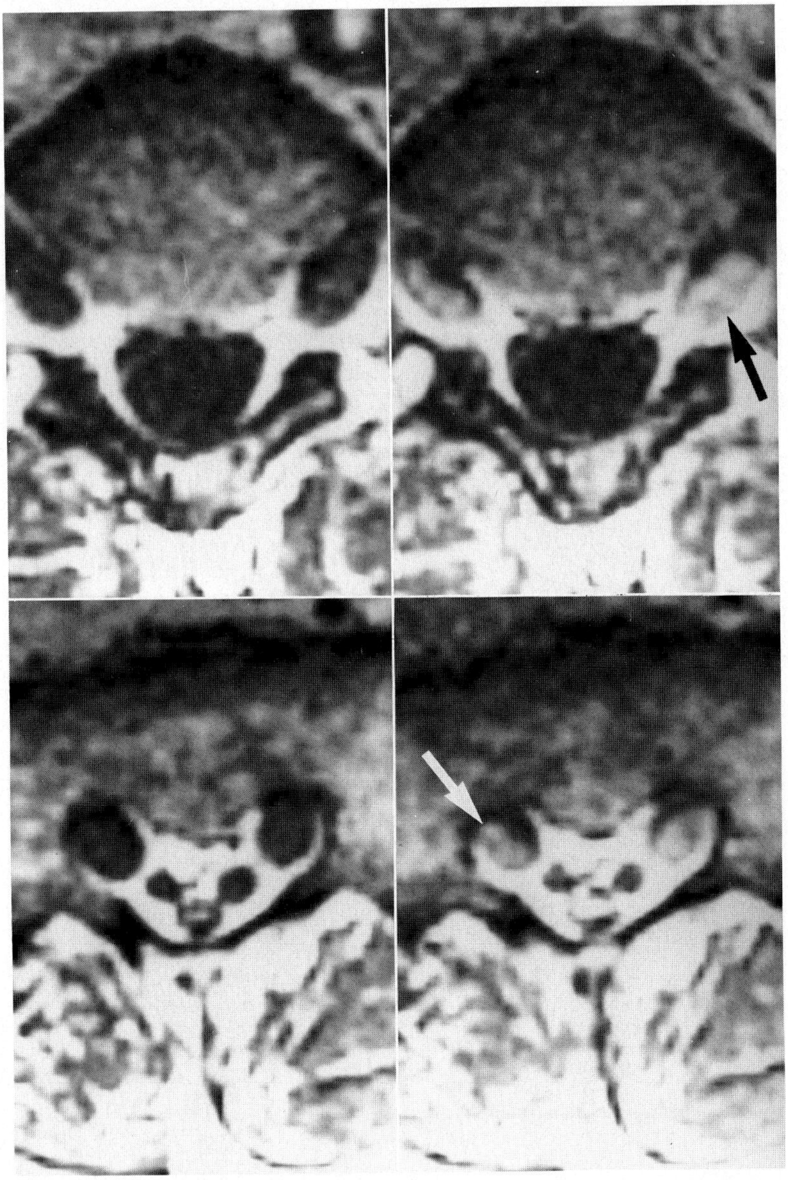

C

D

FIGURE 8-35. Lumbar root lesions in 41-year-old male with neurofibromatosis. **A** and **C**, Precontrast T1W scans (SE 1000/20) show bilaterally symmetrical enlarged nerve root sleeves suggestive of perineural cysts (Tarlov's cysts). **B** and **D**, Postcontrast (GdDTPA) T1W scans (SE 1000/20) demonstrate contrast enhancement within nerve root sleeves *(arrows)*. This increased signal represents enhancement of neurofibromata. Note area of low signal intensity around the tumors within nerve root sleeves that may represent a thickened perineureum or dilated subarachnoid space.

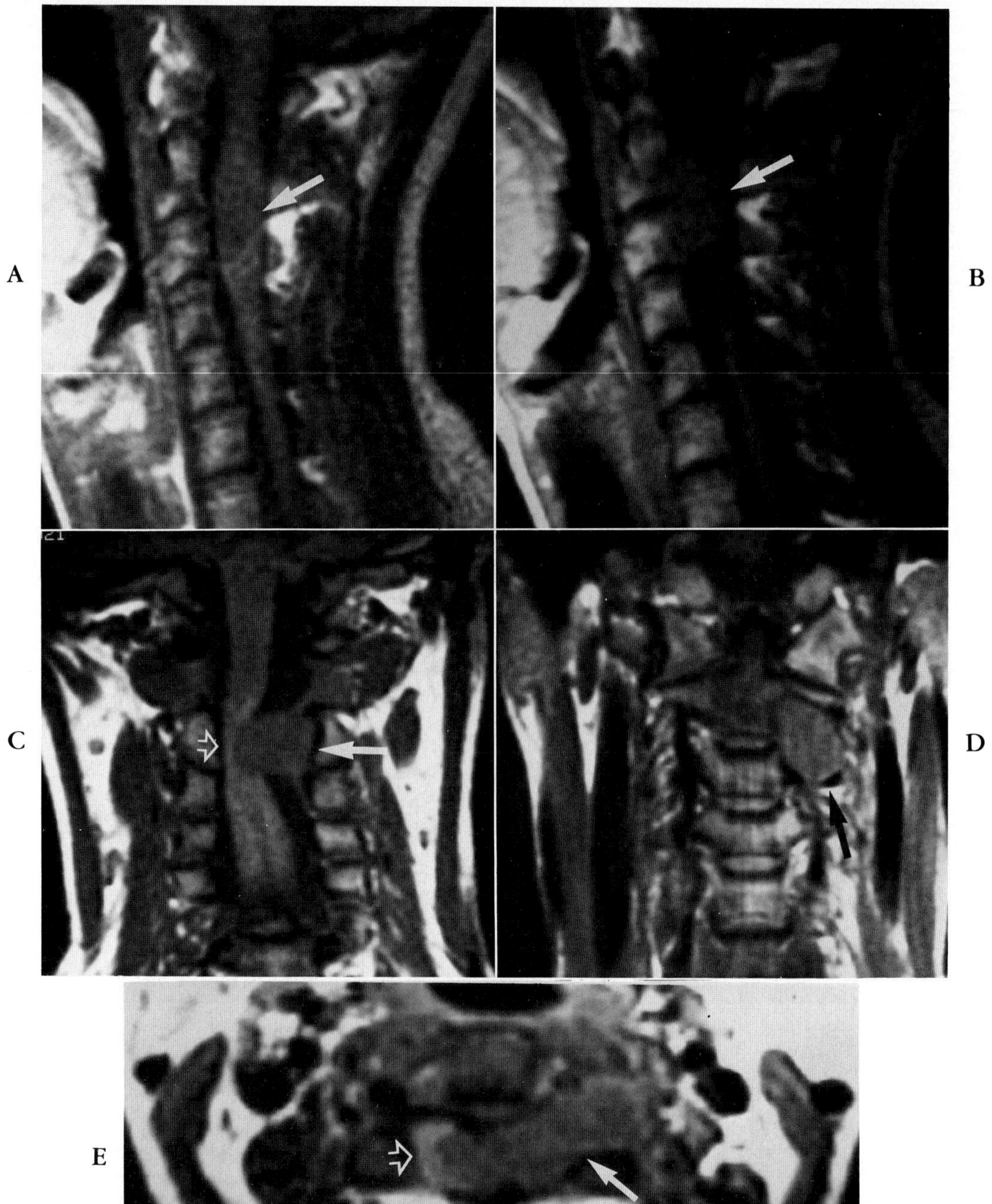

FIGURE 8-36. Cervical neurofibroma in 38-year-old female with neurofibromatosis. **A** and **B**, Sagittal T1W images (SE 800/20) of upper cervical spine show widening of cervical spinal cord at C_2-C_3 in midline image (**A**). Slightly lower signal is seen at widest point *(arrow)*. This image alone is ambiguous and may represent either an intramedullary mass or invagination of a lateral extramedullary mass partially averaged with the cord. Image to left of midline (**B**) shows that mass is, in fact, extramedullary *(arrow)*, which is confirmed on orthogonal coronal and axial images. **C** and **D**, Coronal T1W images (SE 800/20) show extramedullary mass (**C**, *closed arrow*), with signal slightly lower than cord, filling the left spinal canal and compressing the cord to right *(open arrow)*. Lesion extends through left C_2-C_3 neural foramen and forms a mass adjacent to the vertebral bodies on the more anterior coronal image (**D**, *arrow*). **E**, Axial T1W image (SE 800/20) shows neurofibroma filling most of the spinal canal and compressing the higher signal spinal cord to right *(open arrow)*. Lesion extends from the spinal canal through enlarged C_2-C_3 neural foramen *(arrow)* into the paraspinous region.

A B

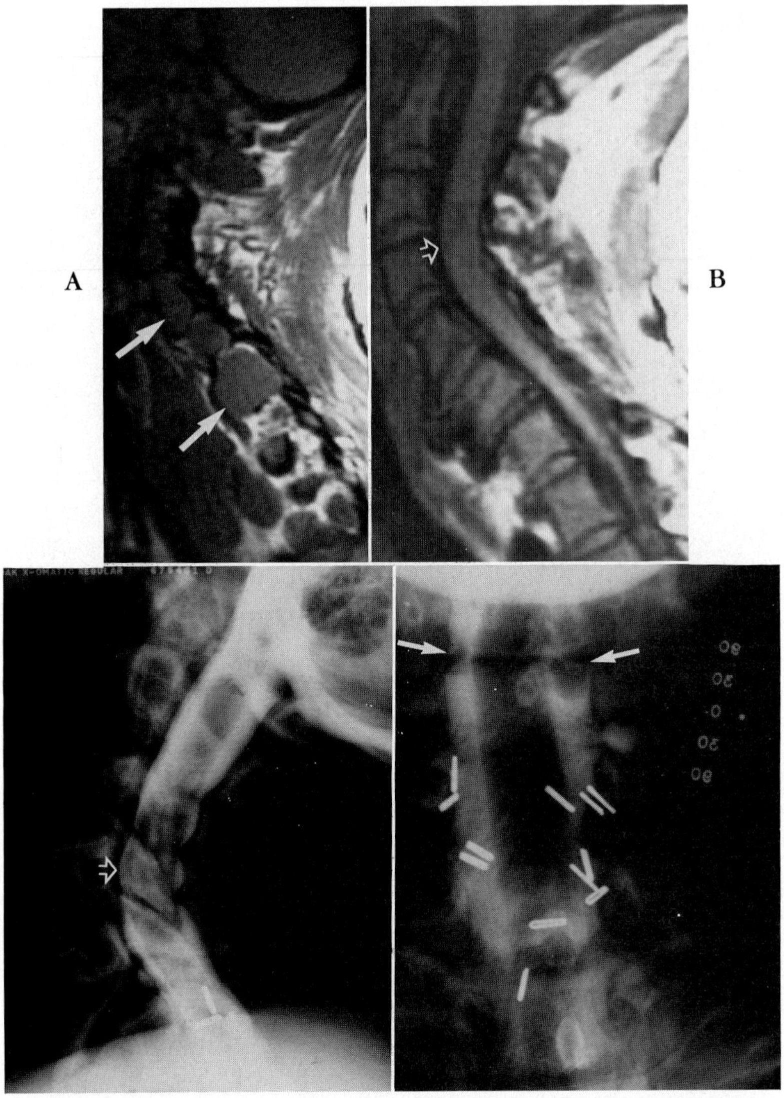

C D

FIGURE 8-37. Cervical neurofibromatosis in 35-year-old female. Sagittal T1W image (SE 800/20) shows multiple intraforaminal neurofibromata (**A**, *arrows*) with widening of neural foramina. **B**, Midline sagittal image shows widening of anteroposterior (AP) dimension of cord *(arrow)* as result of lateral compression from intraspinal neurofibromata. Appearance of cord cannot be differentiated from intrinsic enlargement on sagittal images alone. Axial images are needed to clarify size and shape of cord and demonstrate intraspinal components of foraminal neurofibromata. **C**, Lateral and **D**, AP films from metrizamide cervical myelogram show widening of spinal cord in lateral view *(open arrow)* that appears similar to midline sagittal T1W MR image (**B**). AP view shows bilateral intradural extramedullary masses, left larger than right, with deviation of cord to right at C_3-C_4 level (**D**, *arrows*). Multiple surgical clips overlie mid- and lower cervical spine from previous laminectomy for partial resection of intraspinal neurofibromata. Axial GRASS images (TR 22 ms, TE 12 ms, flip angle 7°, contiguous 5 mm thick) at C_3-C_4 (**E**) and C_6-C_7 (**F**) levels. **E**, Four images at C_3-C_4 show foraminal neurofibromata *(closed arrows)* with extension into spinal canal and compression and deviation of spinal cord *(open arrow)*. Interface between neurofibromata and cord is indistinct and the two tissues are nearly isointense. High signal anterior to cord is produced by oscillatory motion of CSF through plane of image. **F**, Images at C_6-C_7 level show large foraminal neurofibromata *(closed straight arrows)* that do not enter spinal canal and show wider variation in signal than those at C_3-C_4. Very low signal areas posterior to spinal canal represent magnetic artifacts from surgical clips *(curved arrows)* (see myelogram and CT images).

Continued.

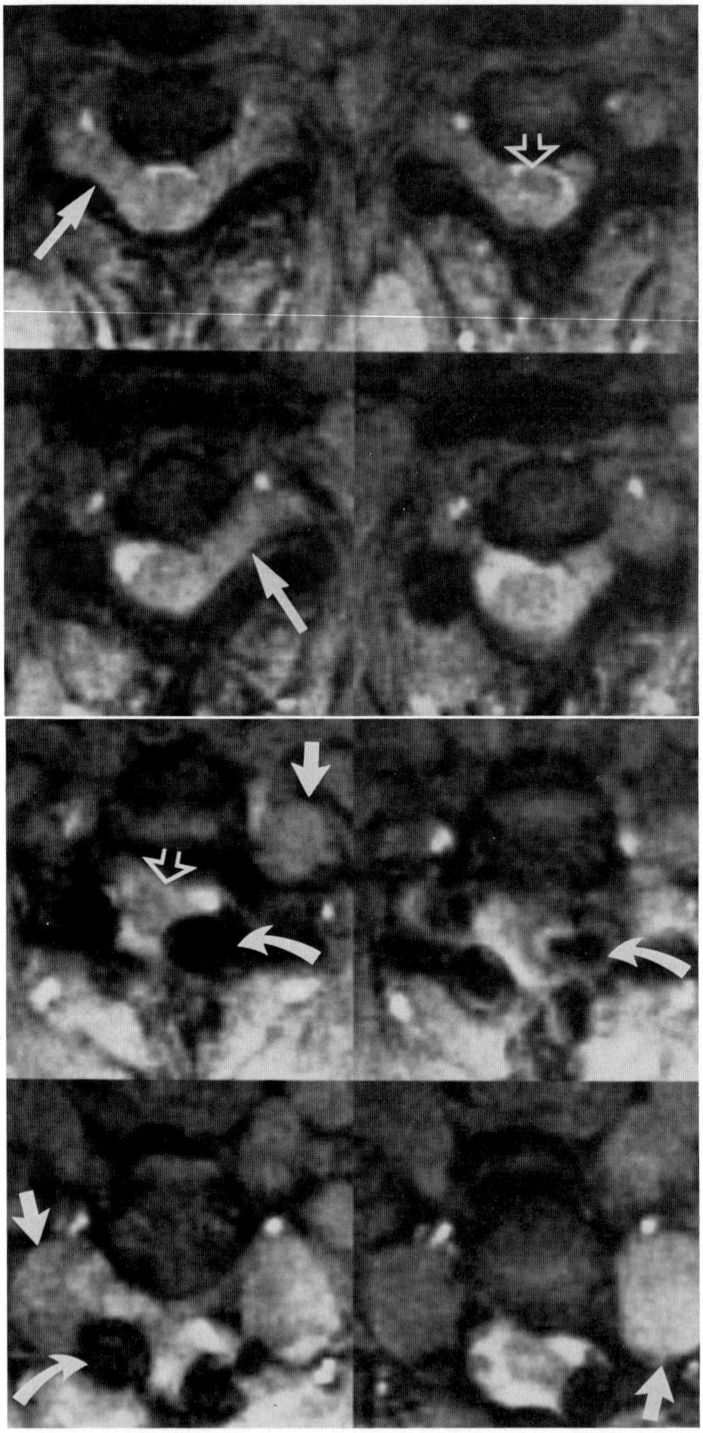

E

F

FIGURE 8-37, cont'd. Spinal cord *(open arrow)* is partially obscured by these artifacts and, in fact, is not compressed by mass lesions. Axial T1W images (SE 1000/20) at C_5-C_6 (**G**) and C_6-C_7 (**H**) levels show large foraminal neurofibromata (**G,** *closed arrow*) that do not extend into spinal canal. Spinal cord *(open arrow)* lies in central spinal canal after resection of intraspinal components of foraminal neurofibromata. **H,** Low signal regions posterior to spinal canal represent artifact from surgical clips *(curved arrow)* that are less pronounced than those seen on more GRASS images. **I-L,** Axial CT scans with intrathecal metrizamide at C_3-C_4 and C_6-C_7 levels.

G

H

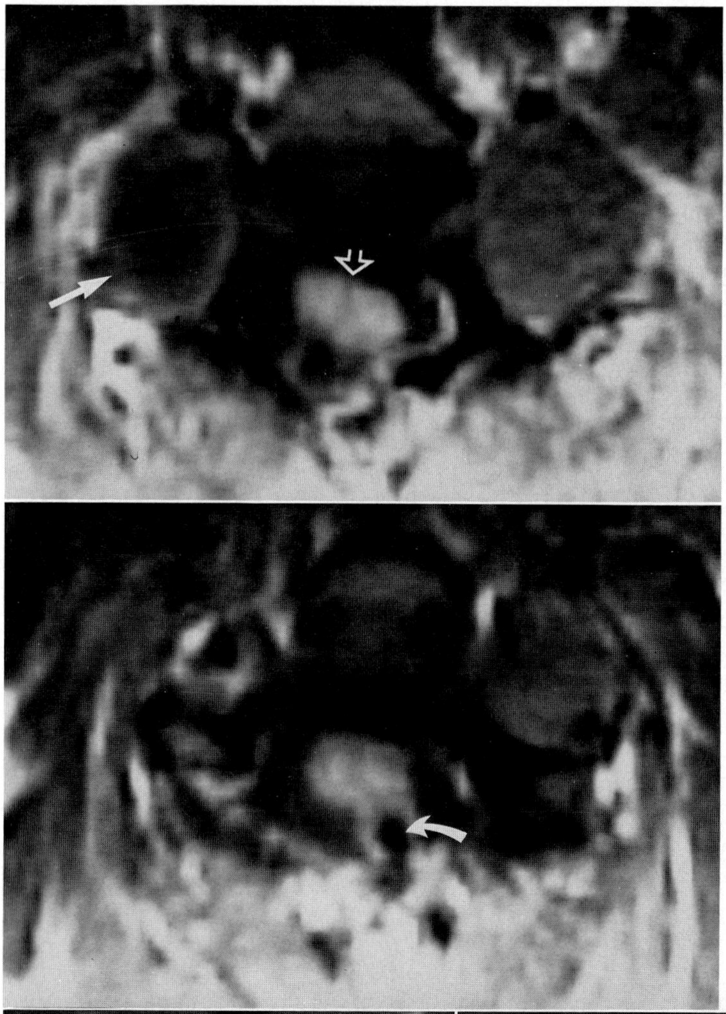

FIGURE 8-37, cont'd. **I** and **J**, At C_3-C_4, masses in neural foramina *(black arrows)* enter spinal canal and produce distortion of spinal cord (**J**, *open arrow*). CT shows better discrimination between neurofibromata extending into spinal canal and spinal cord. **K** and **L**, At C_6-C_7, foraminal masses on MR images are not well seen. Enlargement of lateral bony foramina *(straight arrows)* is secondary sign of large neurofibromata. Streak artifacts, formed by dense surgical clips *(curved arrows)* obscure central canal and prevent clear visualization of spinal cord.

I

J

K

L

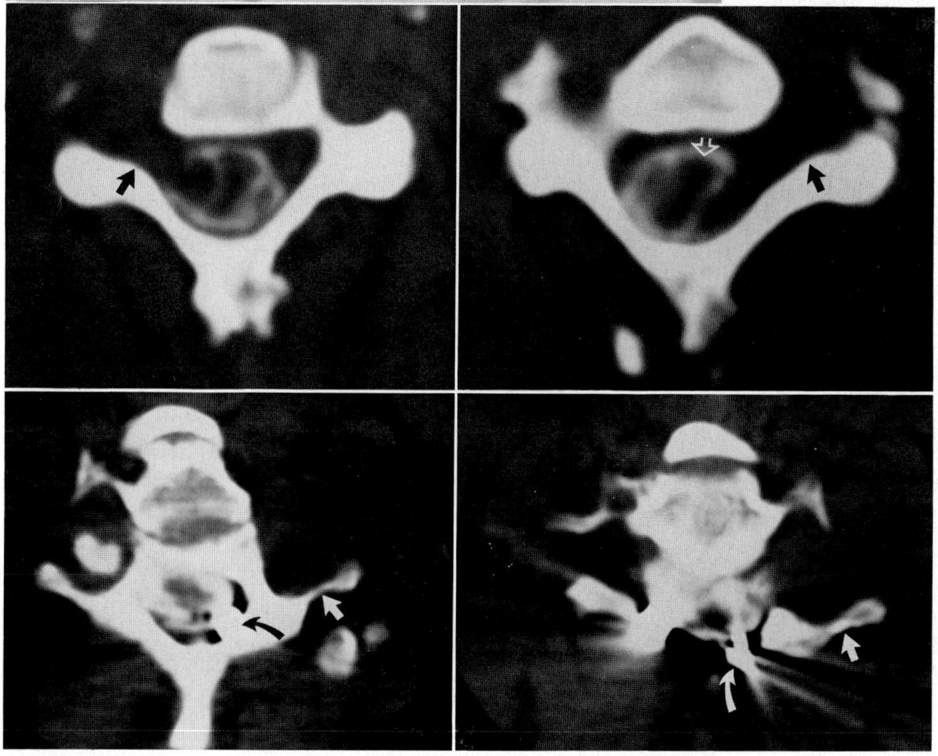

A B

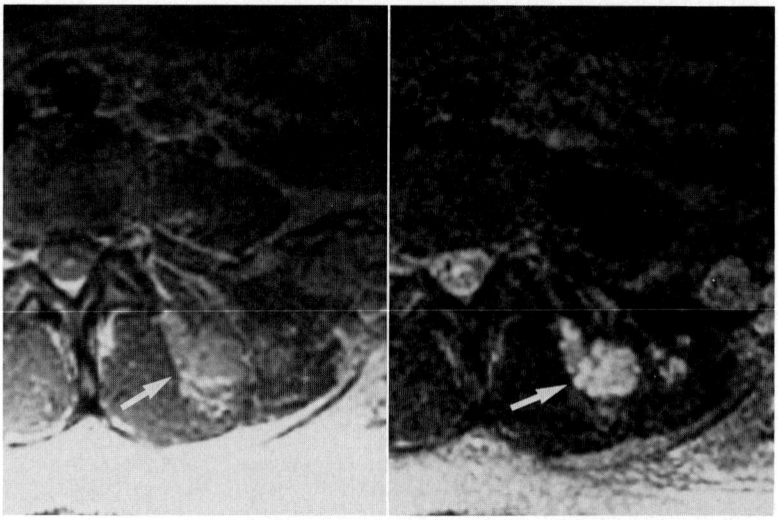

FIGURE 8-38. Plexiform neurofibroma in 30-year-old female. Axial T2W images (SE 2400/20, **A**; 80, **B**) through lumbar spine show plexiform neurofibroma in left paraspinous muscle *(arrows)*. Lesion is complex and multilobular without signs of central fibrosis that may be seen in large simple neurofibromata. A smaller lateral component is also present.

A, B C

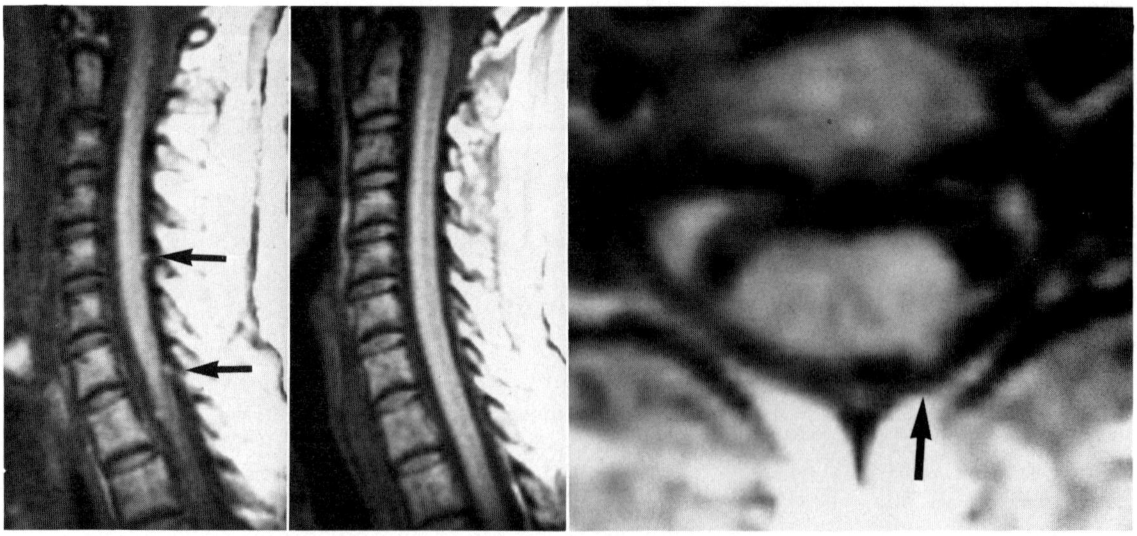

FIGURE 8-39. Central neurofibromatosis in 37-year-old female. Sagittal T1W images (SE 800/20) show **A,** multiple, small, intrathecal extramedullary masses in cervical spinal canal *(arrows)*. **B,** Small neurofibromata clustered to left not seen in midline slice. **C,** Axial T1W image (SE 1000/20) at C_5-C_6 shows one of small neurofibromata on left posterolateral surface of spinal cord *(arrow)*.

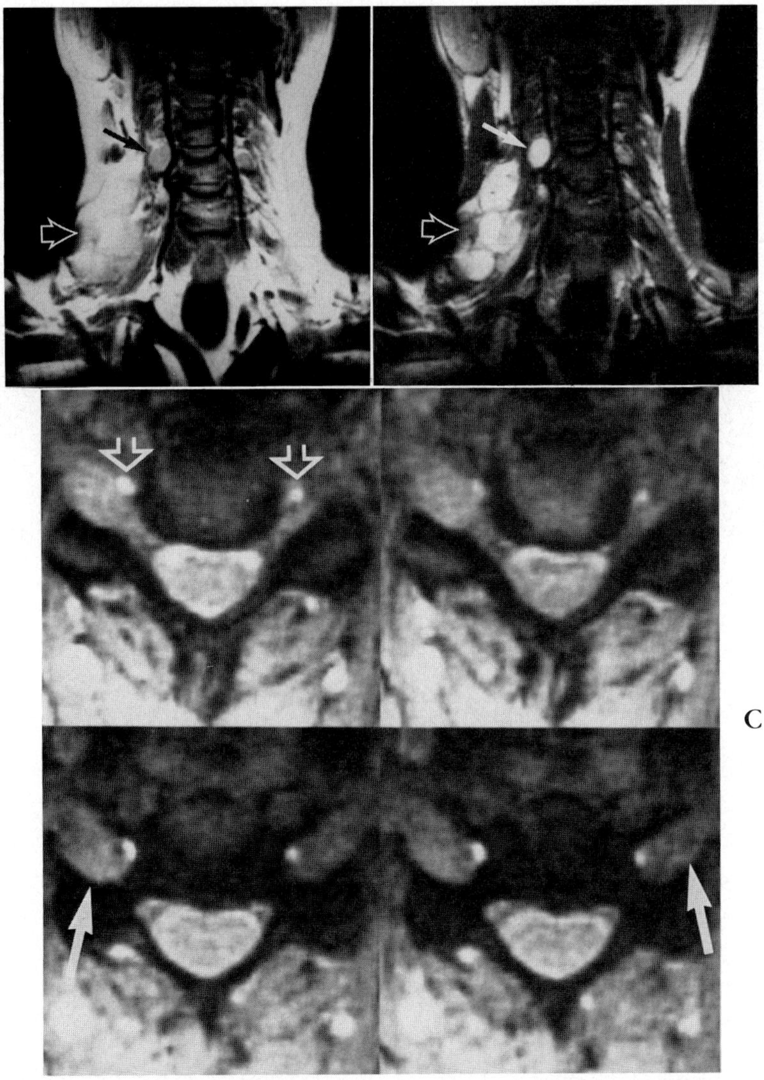

FIGURE 8-40. Brachial plexus neurofibromata in 41-year-old female. Coronal T2W images (SE 1500/20, **A,** and 70, **B**) show multiple 1 cm to 2 cm diameter, well-circumscribed masses in right C_4-C_5 neural foramen *(closed arrows)* and brachial plexus *(open arrows)*, representing multiple neurofibromata and appearing as intermediate signal on first echo image and as high signal on second echo image. Vertebral artery seen as curvilinear signal void appears deviated medially by C_4-C_5 mass. **C,** Axial GRASS images (TR 22, TE 12, Flip angle 7°, contiguous 5 mm thick) at C_4-C_5 show bilateral intermediate signal neurofibromata in neural foramina *(closed arrows)* without intraspinal extension. Vertebral arteries seen as high signal foci (flow effect) adjacent to neurofibromata *(open arrows)*.

pressing the cord is an intradural, extramedullary mass. The advantage of MR over myelography is clear in cases with multiple large masses producing cord compression at different levels. The most caudad or cephalad lesion may produce a complete block to intrathecal contrast introduced via lumbar or upper cervical routes, respectively. Consequently, other lesions may not be visualized by myelography or CT when the degree of obstruction to contrast flow is severe (usually the case). Intraspinal neurofibromatosis may be sufficiently extensive to completely obstruct the subarachnoid space over long segments of the canal (Figure 8-41). Demonstration of these lesions noninvasively by MR is a simple, direct procedure that allows positive

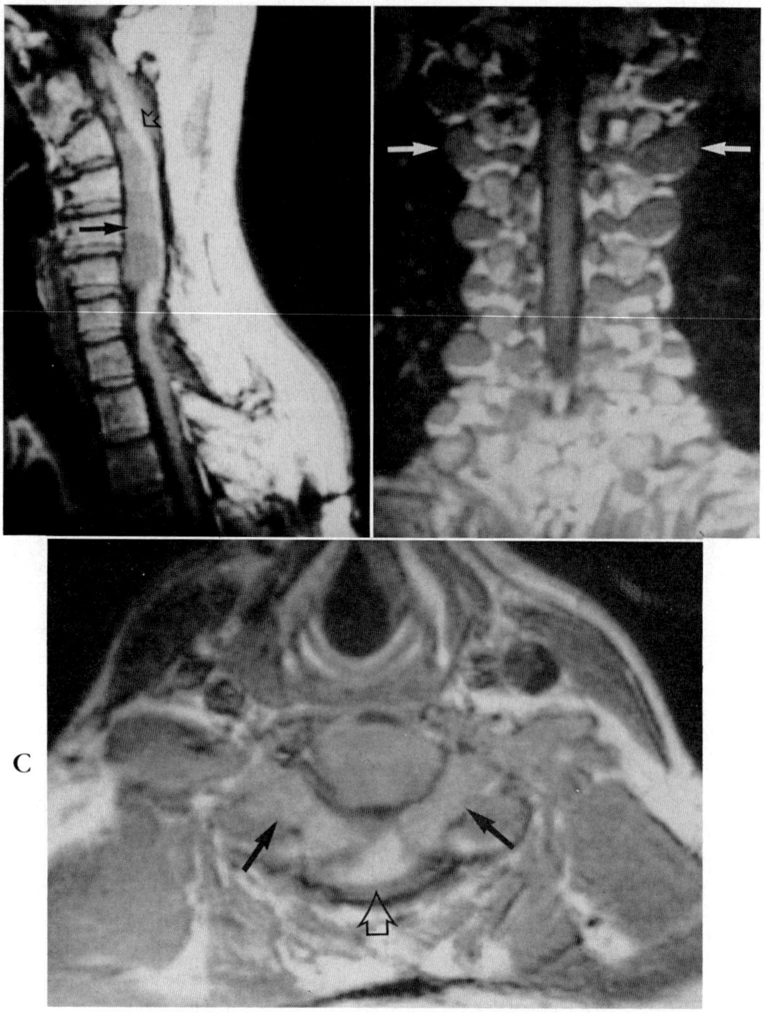

FIGURE 8-41. Extensive cervical central neurofibromatosis with cord compression in 30-year-old male. **A**, Sagittal T1W image (SE 600/20) shows large intraspinous neurofibroma *(black arrow)* displacing and compressing spinal cord posteriorly through most of cervical spinal canal. Neurofibroma is slightly lower signal than cord, which appears as thin high signal structure draped over mass *(open arrow)*. **B**, Coronal T1W image (SE 600/20) demonstrates presence of numerous neurofibromata in all neural foramina in cervical spine *(arrows)*. **C**, Axial T1W image (SE 600/20) shows neurofibromata in neural foramina bilaterally *(black arrows)* with extension into spinal canal and distortion of higher signal spinal cord *(open arrow)*.

identification of the neurofibromas and their relationship to the neural foramina, canal, thecal sac, and spinal cord. In patients with multiple intraspinal lesions, surgical resection of individual mass lesion is often followed by new cord compression by another lesion; a "losing battle" in these unfortunate patients that eventually results in unrelenting progressive paraparesis or quadriparesis.

CONGENITAL TUMORS

Teratomas are frequently cystic neoplasms that contain disarrayed tissues belonging to all three germ cell layers in locations where they do not normally occur.[25] The term *teratoid* is used to describe closely related tumors that do not clearly contain tissue from all three germ cell layers. The embryogenesis of teratomas is complex and not precisely understood. They

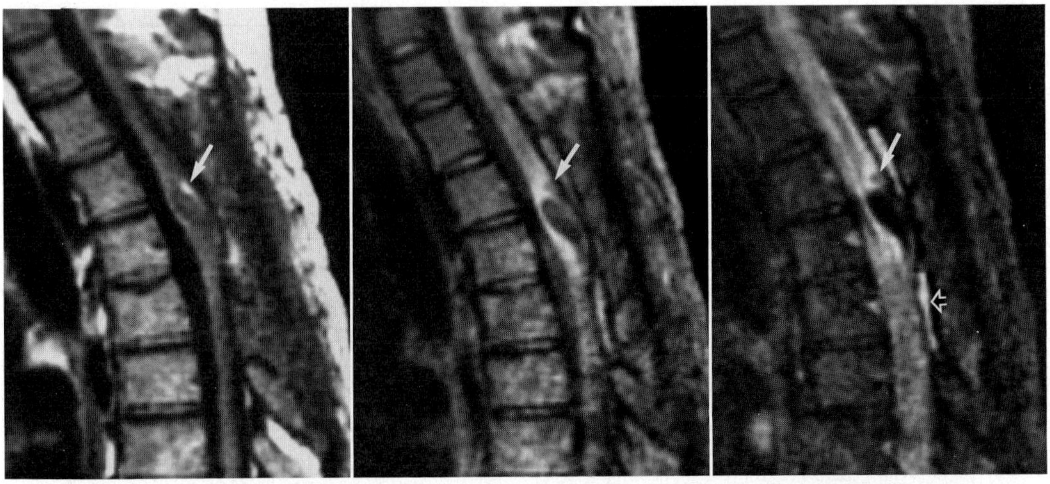

FIGURE 8-42. Intramedullary teratoid tumor 1 year after biopsy in 42-year-old female. **A**, Sagittal T1W image (SE 400/25) shows focal enlargement of upper thoracic spinal cord adjacent to laminectomy site. Central area of enlargement is low signal with border of intermediate signal anterior and small focus of high signal posterior *(arrow)*. Central area represents dense fibrotic nodule with border of normal cord anterior and fat present posteriorly at high signal focus. Posterior position of cord within spinal canal is result of arachnoid adhesions fixing it to laminectomy site. Sagittal T2W images (SE 2000/50, **B**, and 100, **C**) show area of spinal cord enlargement predominantly low signal surrounded by high signal cord tissue. Dense, fibrotic center of cord lesion is low signal on first and second echo images. Cord anterior to mass is higher signal than cord distal to mass and probably represents gliotic change and, possibly, some edema. Area of low signal posterior to mass *(closed arrows)* corresponds to high signal focus of fat on T1W image. Small amount of fluid accumulation at laminectomy site is immediately posterior to thecal sac *(open arrow)*.

may arise parthenogenetically by proliferation of displaced germ cells or of pluripotential cells left behind during migration of Hensen's node.[50] The presence of Barr bodies in 50% of tumors in males suggests that haploid germ cells may fuse and induce organization of adjacent cells.[50] Teratomas may arise from tissue rests that escape control of inducers early in embryogenesis, thus growing freely and chaotically.[50]

Intraspinal Teratoma

Intraspinal teratomas are unusual lesions, constituting approximately 0.15% of all intraspinal tumors.[67] Male and female incidence is equal and all ages are affected (32% below age 6; 26% ages 6 to 19; 42% over age 20).[67] These tumors may be found at any level of spinal canal but frequently involve the dorsal aspect of the thoracolumbar cord and are usually focal, extending over 1 to 2 vertebral segments[25,27,58] (Figures 8-42 to 8-44). Clinical presentation is usually that of intermittent pain and cord compression with occasionally striking periods of spontaneous relief.[25,50]

Teratomas may be solid, partially cystic, or completely cystic (unilocular or multilocular). The cysts may be thick- or thin-walled and contain clear, milky, or dark fluid with amorphous debris.[27,50,58] Bone and cartilage elements may also be present, sometimes in the form of a tooth. Intraspinal teratomas rarely show malignant recurrence of dissemination.[50] Teratomas may be intramedullary, intraarachnoid, or intradural in location. True intramedullary lesions are unusual. Intramedullary solid lesions may replace the cord diffusely, whereas cystic lesions tend to expand the cord into a thin shell surrounding the cyst,[27,50] (see Figures 8-43 and 8-44), and tumors are usually large at clinical presentation and compress and displace the spinal cord anteriorly (see Figure 8-42). The cord often shows histologic signs of pressure degeneration and may be hemorrhagic.[50] Syringomye-

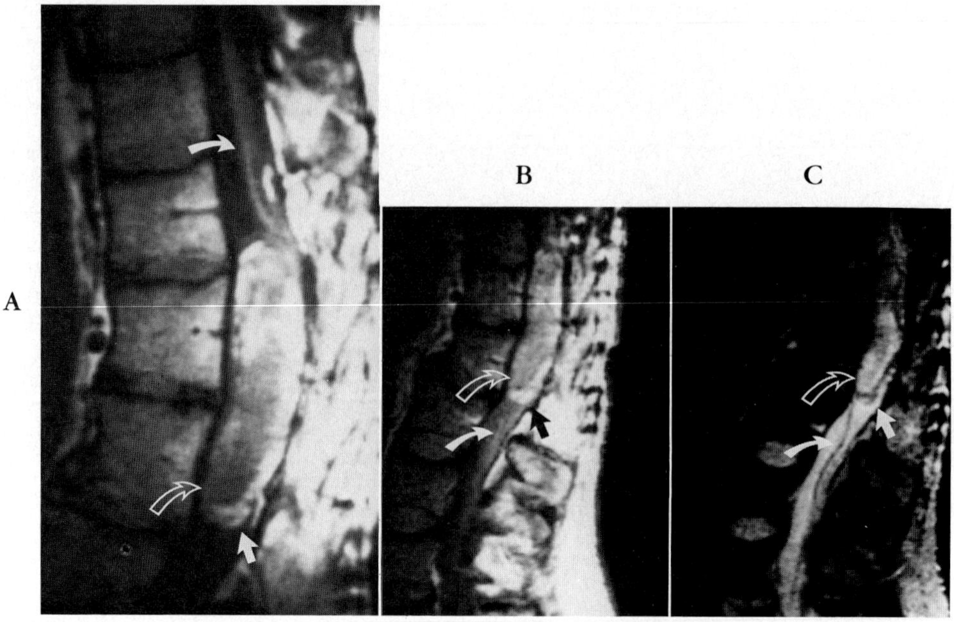

FIGURE 8-43. Large thoracolumbar intraspinal teratoma in 21-year-old male. **A**, Sagittal T1W image (SE 800/20) shows large intraspinal mass filling spinal canal at T_{12}-L_1 level that produced posterior displacement of distal conus medullaris *(curved closed arrow)* and proximal cauda equina. Central area of lesion inferiorly *(curved open arrow)* is lower signal than margins *(straight arrow)* of mass but not as low as CSF. Unclear from this image alone whether low signal area represents cystic or solid tissue. High signal marginal areas represent fatty components of lesion. Sagittal T2W images (SE 2500/20, **B**, and 80, **C**) through lumbosacral teratoma show mass displacing cauda equina posteriorly *(curved closed arrows)*. Area of low signal on T1W image in inferior part of mass corresponds to relatively low signal on first echo image and high signal on second echo image *(curved open arrows)*. Region remains ambiguous and may be solid tissue or cyst filled with highly proteinaceous fluid or cellular debris. Fatty, marginal components of lesion are high signal on first echo image and low signal on second echo image *(straight arrows)*.

lia may be present above or below the point of compression. The teratoma is usually adherent to the cord with a poorly defined interface formed by tumor connective tissue and spinal cord reactive gliosis.[50,58] Less frequently, cystic lesions may be attached only by a short pedicle to the pia of the spinal cord, the dura, or to the roots of the cauda equina.[50,58] In the lumbar region, the roots of the cauda equina are frequently adherent to the walls of the lesion and draped around it dorsally or ventrally[50,58] (see Figure 8-42).

Intraspinal teratomas are usually not associated with other congenital spinal anomalies. The skin overlying intraspinal teratomas is usually intact with rare occurrence of superficial cyst, skin dimple, or nevus.[50] The spinal canal is usually developmentally normal with only rare occurrences of spina bifida, block vertebrae, Klippel-Feil syndrome, spurs of diastematomyelia, or anomalously long spinous processes.[50] With large lesions, the spinal canal may be enlarged with signs of pressure erosion, including thinned pedicles, widened interpedicular distance, thinned laminae, and posterior scalloping of vertebral bodies.[50] Scoliosis and reversal of the normal cervical or lumbar lordosis may also be present.[50]

Sacrococcygeal Teratoma

Sacrococcygeal teratomas are a different clinical entity from intraspinal teratomas and have a strong tendency to undergo malignant transformation. Lesions that are diagnosed between 4 months and 5 years have a 50% to 60% chance

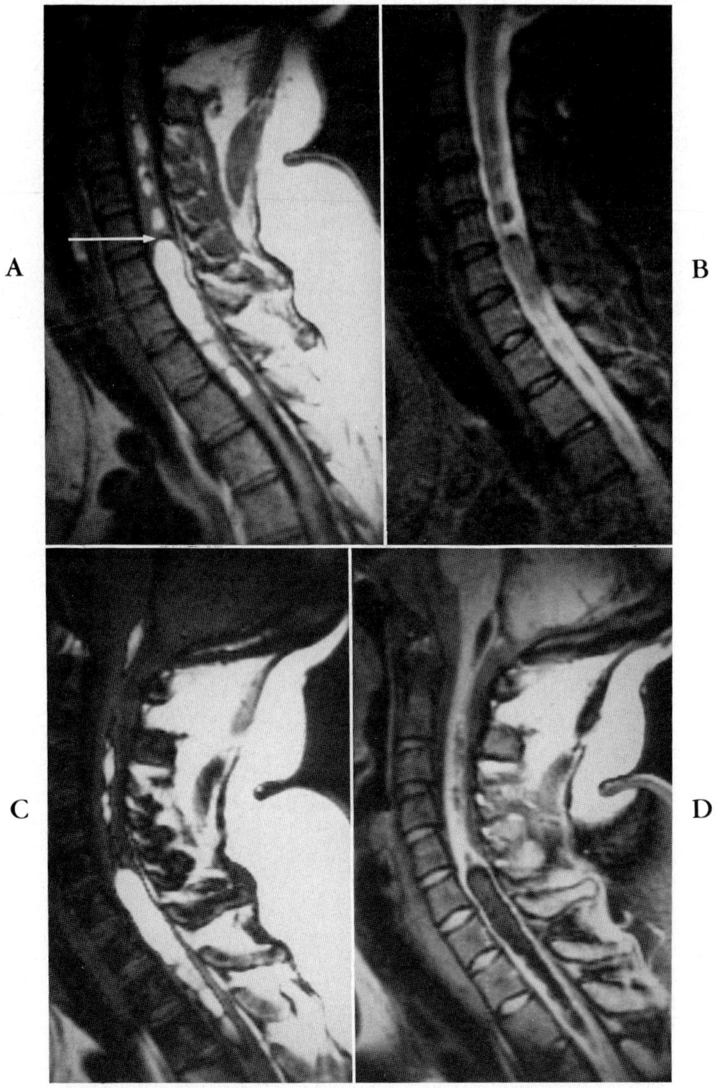

FIGURE 8-44. Teratoma. MR scans of 45-year-old female with extensive intramedullary teratoma. **A,** T1W sagittal scan (SE 800/20) shows several discontinuous nodular areas of increased signal intensity within cervical cord. Largest, at C_6-C_7, causes cord enlargement. Signal intensity is similar to that of subcutaneous fat. **B,** Sagittal T2W scan (gated SE 2300/80) shows decreased signal intensity in intramedullary masses that is consistent with lipid and not hemorrhage. **C,** Sagittal "fat" image (water-suppressed) shows high signal intensity from each fatty mass within cord. Note little signal is derived from water protons. **D,** On "water" image (fat-suppressed, SE 800/20) lesions show very low signal intensity. These images are a definitive way of separating lipid from water signal when lesions have large amounts of fat, although one must be aware of the chemical shift artifact. Close inspection shows curvilinear areas of signal loss on the superior aspect of each discrete lesion in the cervical cord on the sagittal image (*arrow*, **A**), representing chemical shift artifact where fat signal is displaced caudally because this is the frequency encoding direction. Thin rim of absent signal is artifact and should not be confused with magnetic susceptibility effect of hemosiderin deposition. The latter would be circumferential if this were hemorrhage. Differentiation can identify fat or hemorrhage on T1W scan. *Continued.*

E

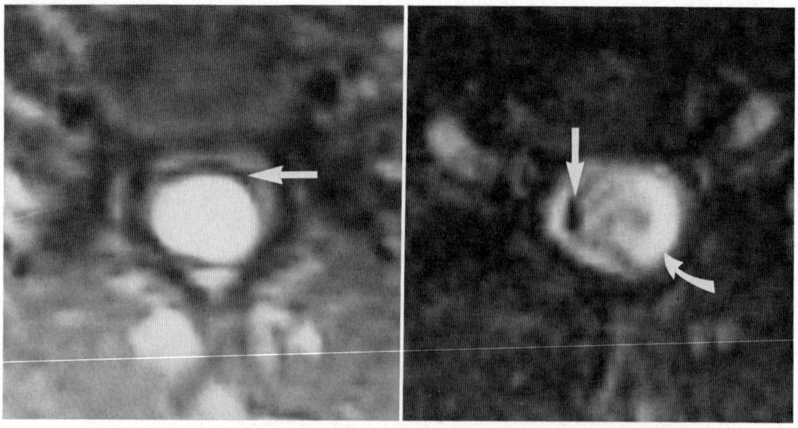

F

FIGURE 8-44, cont'd. **E,** On axial T1W scan (SE 1000/20) thin curvilinear area of signal loss outlines anterior margin of lipoma, and also represents chemical shift artifact *(arrow)*, and not magnetic susceptibility effect, because frequency encoding axis is anteroposterior direction. **F,** On T2W image (gated SE 2300/80) at same level as **E,** although fat signal has decreased in intensity. Chemical shift artifact is still identified but area of signal loss is on right side of cord *(straight arrow)* and area of summated fat and water signal is on left side *(curved arrow)*. In this image frequency axis is oriented right to left. This change in orientation of the curvilinear area of low signal is definitive for chemical shift artifact and differentiates it from low signal intensity related to magnetic susceptibility effects.

A

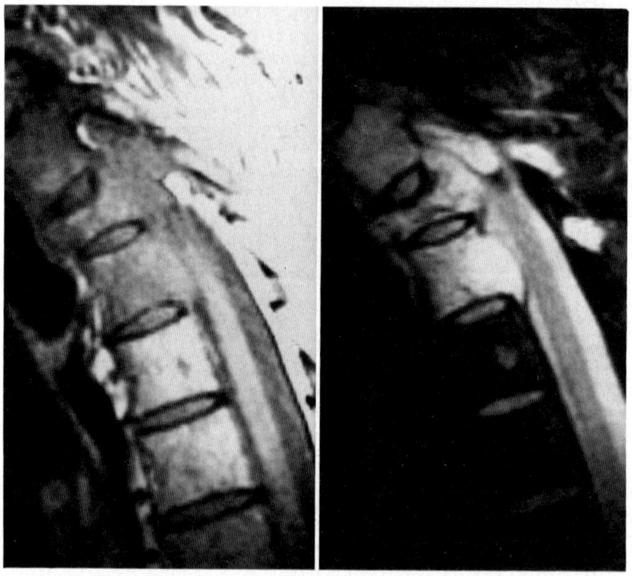

B

FIGURE 8-45. Lymphoma: comparison of T1W and STIR images in patient with complete spinal block caused by lymphoma. **A,** Sagittal T1W scan (SE 800/20) shows involvement of three upper thoracic vertebrae with replacement of bone marrow by intermediate signal intensity tumor, extension of tumor into spinal canal, and a compression fracture of the middle vertebrae. Tumor signal intensity is somewhat lower than normal marrow signal intensity. **B,** Sagittal STIR image (IR 1400/40, TI 150) shows tumor involvement as marked increased signal with the vertebrae. Contrast between tumor and bone marrow is much greater than on the T1W image. Extent of tumor, spinal canal mass, and compression fracture are well seen. Bone erosion is well seen on this STIR image. The "myelogram effect" on this sagittal STIR scan is of high quality because the tumor has caused a complete block and thus has damped the normal CSF pulsation. This results in high signal CSF without artifact. STIR images normally have poor delineation of the intraspinal contents and poor cord-CSF contrast because they lack motion compensation characteristics, which prevent the CSF pulsation artifacts. High quality "myelogram" effect on the STIR scan, therefore, is indicative of high grade CSF block.

of being malignant, whereas those diagnosed before or after this period have only a 5% to 6.5% chance.[35] The occurrence of lesions is usually sporadic, with rare reports of familial cases. There is a clear female predominance (F:M 4:1).[62]

Tumor mass in the sacral region may project externally from the perineum between the buttocks or may be completely internal, presenting as a retroperitoneal mass[62] that may be solid, partially cystic, or wholly cystic. Wholly or partially cystic lesions are less likely to be malignant than solid lesions.[62] The sacrum is often intact and when destruction of the bony sacrum occurs it is usually minimal, involving only the distal segments. The diagnosis of sacral teratoma is unlikely if more than two sacral segments are involved.[16] Sacrococcygeal teratomas may be associated with other congenital anomalies in the "Currarino triad." Malformations forming this triad are (1) anorectal anomalies (especially anorectal stenosis), (2) a curved sacrococcygeal bony defect (scimitar sacrum), and (3) a presacral tumor (anterior meningocele, dermoid cyst, neurenteric cyst, teratoma, or combination of these).[33]

MR Imaging

MR imaging is useful for defining the pathologic anatomy of spinal teratomas, especially in relation to the spinal cord, and for differentiating these lesions from other types of tumors. As with other mass lesions, depiction of the anatomic relationships to the spine and spinal cord is best achieved with sagittal and axial (occasionally coronal) T1W images (see Figures 8-42 to 8-44). The presence of spinal cord distortion and compression with extramedullary lesions and enlargement of the cord by intramedullary lesions is usually clearly seen. The relationship of the sacrococcygeal teratoma to the sacrum and to the retroperitoneal and pelvic organs is also well defined on T1W images.

Characterization of the type of tissue within spinal teratomas requires both spin echo (SE) T1W and T2W images and, in some cases, specialized pulse sequences. Differentiating cystic lesions from solid lesions may be fairly clear on T1W and T2W images with cystic areas behaving more like CSF with very low signal on T1W images and high signal on T2W images. However, teratoma cysts are often filled with highly proteinaceous or cellular debris and the fluid may take on relaxation characteristics resembling solid tissue (see Figure 8-42). In some cases, fluid motion effects (on T2W images or specialized motion-sensitive sequences) may help identify cysts, whereas in others, only intraoperative ultrasonography may be able to positively identify a cyst. Irregularity of the cyst wall, often seen with teratomas, may also create a confusing picture and make identification of cysts difficult.

Fat content is the other major characteristic component of teratomas that may be identified with MR. Fat, combined with a solid or cystic mass, strongly favors the diagnosis of teratoma over that of another spinal tumor or simple lipoma. The presence of fat is usually first suggested by high signal on the T1W image with low signal in the same region on the heavily T2W image. However, subacute hemorrhage (e.g., 3 to 7 days) may have a similar appearance and differentiating between the two can be critical to patient management. The presence of a chemical shift artifact at the fat-water interface is a useful diagnostic sign on the T2W image. It is a sharply defined, crescentic or semicircular low signal band (signal void) at the margin of the fatty tissue that is paired with a similar high signal band at the opposite margin. These two bands should be oriented perpendicular to the frequency encoding gradient (the chemical shift is along the frequency encoding gradient). The low signal band should not be confused with hemosiderin staining at the margin of the lesion, which is usually less well-defined, often surrounds the lesion, is not in a fixed orientation to the frequency-encoding gradient, and is not paired with a high signal band (see Figure 8-43). When the chemical-shift artifact is not present, more direct identification of fat can be obtained using specialized pulse sequences that display only signal from fat protons (water-suppressed images) (see Figure 8-43).

Dermoid and Epidermoid Tumors

Dermoid and epidermoid tumors are discussed in Chapter 5.

Neuroblastoma and Ganglioneuroblastoma

Neuroblastomas are unusual tumors of infancy and childhood that are composed of primitive

A, B

C

D

E

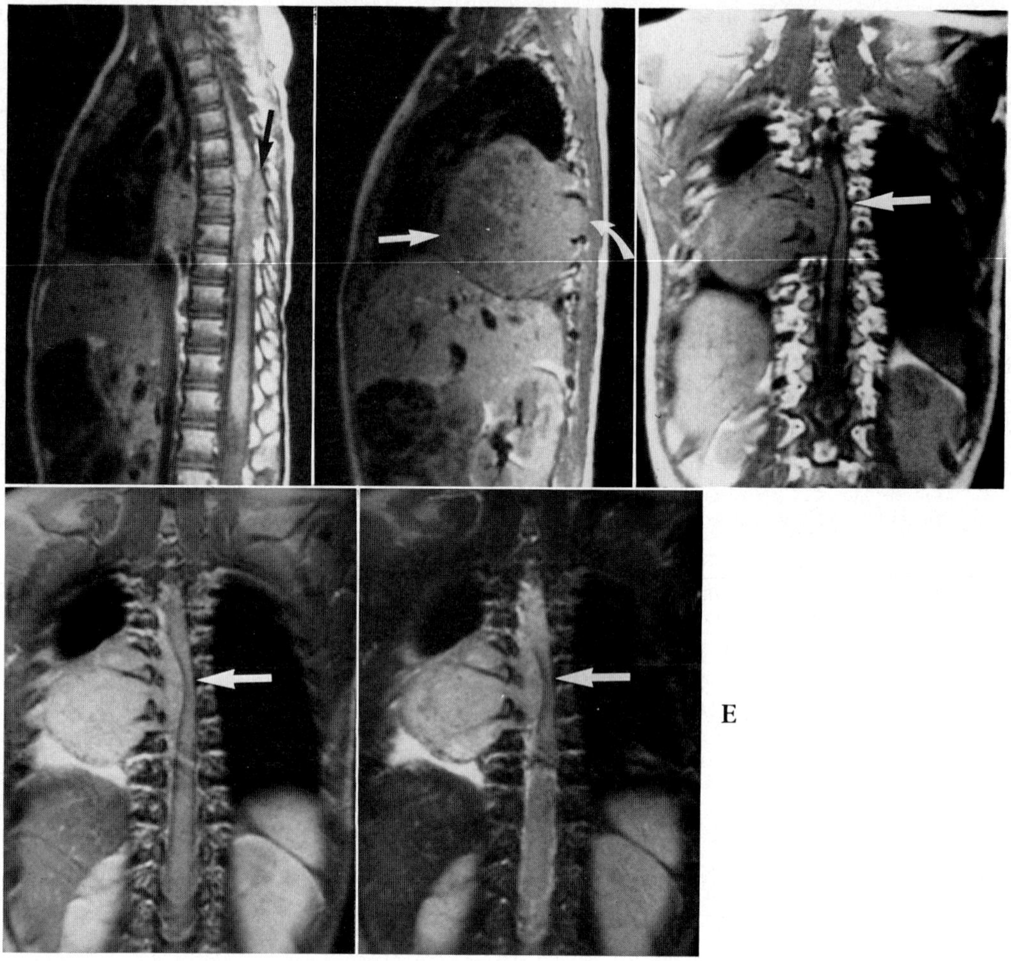

FIGURE 8-46. Ganglioneuroblastoma in 2-year-old female with mild paraparesis. Sagittal T1W images (SE 8000/20) in **A,** midline and **B,** right of midline show large right mediastinal tumor mass with intraspinal epidural tumor tissue. Tumor within spinal canal (**A,** *arrow*) is intermediate in signal and appears to compress and displace spinal cord. Confirmation of cord compression needs to be obtained from axial images (see **F** and **G**). **B,** Tumor mass extends from posterior mediastinum to form large posterior thoracic mass with mixed internal signal *(straight arrow)* and posterior extension causing rib spreading *(curved arrow)*. Calcification in tumor mass on CT scan is not apparent on these MR images. Coronal T1W (SE 800/20, **C**) and T2W images (SE 2000/30, **D** and 80, **E**) show large right chest mass with direct extension through three midthoracic neural foramina forming large intraspinal epidural tumor mass. Deviation of spinal cord to left is apparent *(arrows)*. Compression of cord may be present, but needs to be confirmed with axial images. Signal from cord on second echo images (heavily T2W images) is normal, suggesting no significant edema or gliosis in segments adjacent to tumor mass. Axial images T1W (SE 800/20, **F**) and GRASS (TR 22, TE 12, flip angle 7°, **G**) show large posterior mediastinal mass on right with direct extension into spinal canal producing cord and thecal sac deviation to right *(arrows)*. This is point of maximal deviation of cord and does not confirm cord compression suggested by sagittal and coronal images. Extension of tumor through neural foramina without destruction of vertebral bodies is typical of ganglioneuroblastoma.

F

G

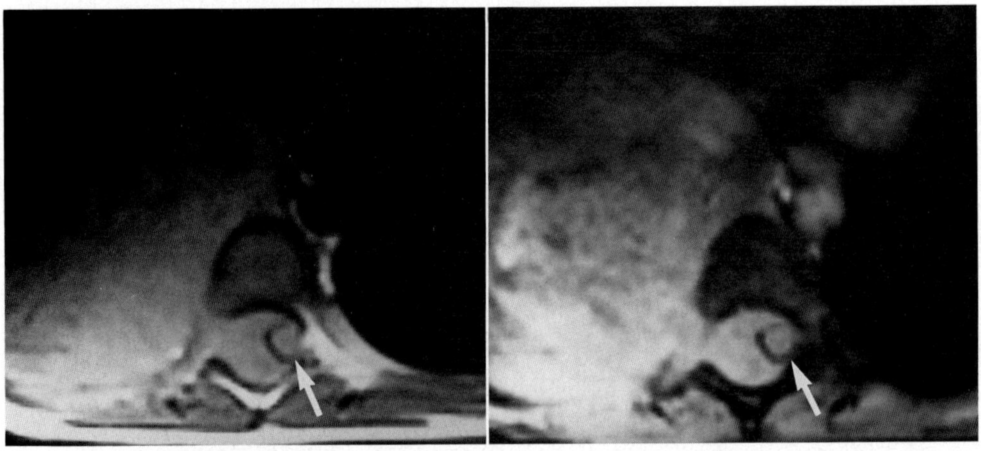

FIGURE 8-46, cont'd. For legend see previous page.

cells identical to fetal neuroblasts, occurring in 1 in 10,000 live births.[16] They arise in the sympathetic nervous system with the most frequent site of origin being the adrenal gland (65%). Other typical sites include the paraspinous sympathetic chain (especially upper lumbar), the carotid ganglia, the aortic bodies, and the organs of Zuckerkandl.[55] Metastases are common, especially in patients over 2 years old, and are present in 74% of cases at the time of presentation.[55] Metastases are most frequently adjacent to lymph nodes, but are also common in the spine and appendicular skeleton. Adjacent pinal involvement is common (see Figures 8-48 and 8-49), but spinal cord compression is usually seen only in the late stages of disease (only 1% to 4% present with cord compression).[16] Calcification is common in these masses and may be detected on plain radiographs in as many as 30%.[16]

Ganglioneuroblastomas and ganglioneuromas are also tumors of the sympathetic nervous system and may represent stages in maturation of neuroblastomas. Ganglioneuroblastomas show histologic and biologic behavioral features intermediate to the aggressive neuroblastoma and the relatively benign ganglioneuroma.[1,16] The age of presentation is similar to neuroblastoma for ganglioneuroblastomas but is delayed until adolescence or adulthood for ganglioneuromas.[16] The posterior mediastinum is the frequent site for ganglioneuromas and ganlioneuroblastomas (40%), followed by the abdomen (30%) and other sites (30%, pelvis and neck).[55] Intraspinal extension through neural foramina, rather than destructive invasion of the adjacent spine, is relatively frequent (Figure 8-46). A "dumbbell" extension of the mass into the spinal canal eventually produces spinal cord compression. The intraspinal component tends to produce superior and inferior tapered extensions, which helps to differentiate it from rounded intraspinal neuromas or neurofibromas that might also occur in this age group.[16] Ganglioneuromas and ganglioneuroblastomas are frequently calcified.

MR Imaging

MR imaging is useful for studying the anatomic relationships of neuroblastomas, ganglioneuroblastomas, and ganglioneuromas to the spine and spinal cord (Figures 8-46 to 8-48). This is especially true when there is local invasion of the spine by neuroblastoma or "dumbbell" extension through neural foramina by ganglioneuroblastoma or ganglioneuroma. Definition of the relationship of intraspinal extension of these tumors to the spinal cord requires lumbar puncture and instillation of intrathecal contrast with conventional imaging, whereas MR can directly demonstrate cord involvement noninvasively. In general T1W sagittal and axial images are sufficient for showing anatomic relationships (see Figure 8-47). T2W images may be useful for assessing the status of the spinal cord to rule out compressive edematous changes. Characterization of the tumor is not a major function of MR

A

B, C

D

E

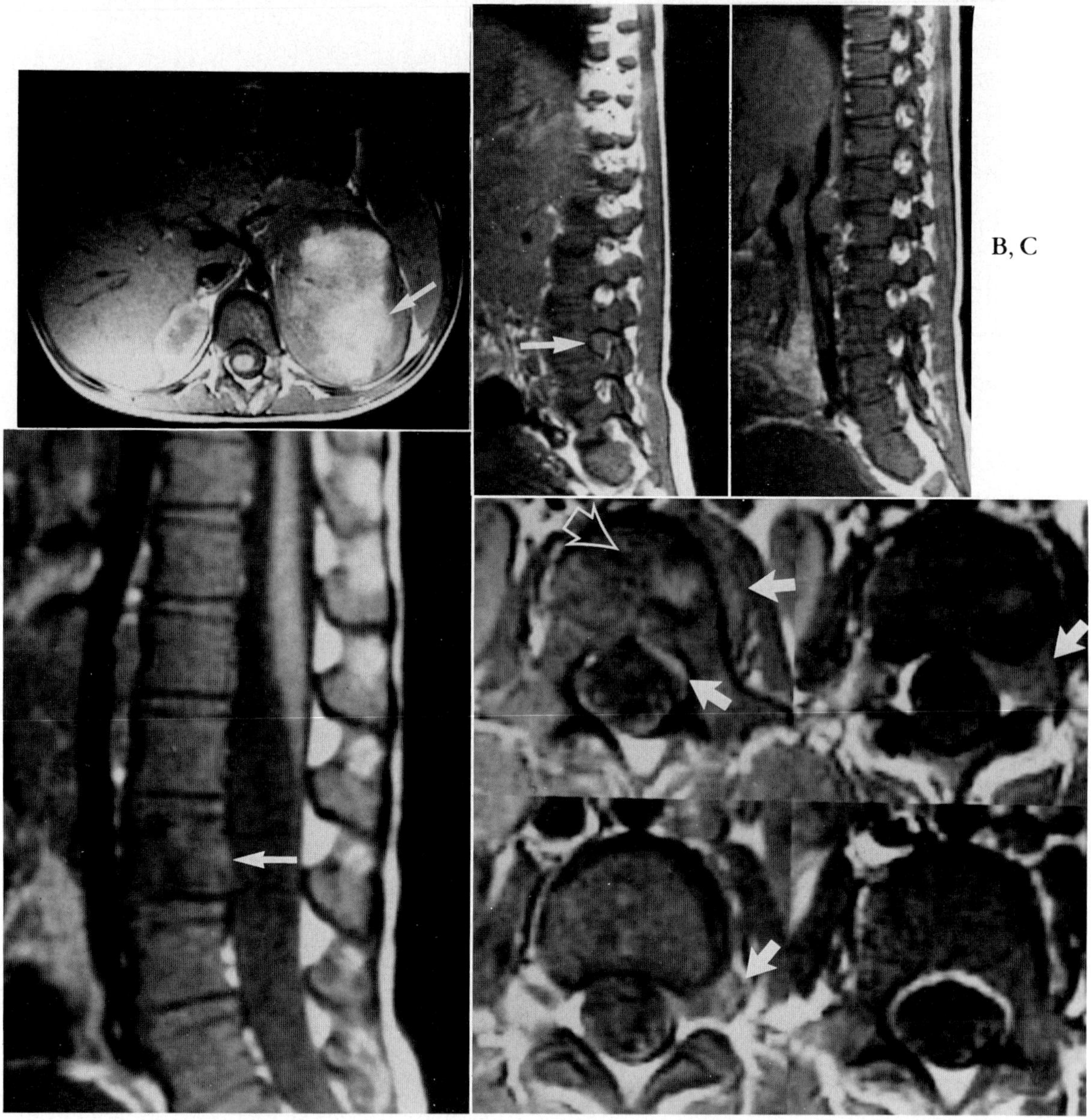

FIGURE 8-47. Retroperitoneal neuroblastoma with noncontiguous metastases to lumbar spine in 3-year-old female. **A,** Axial T1W image (SE 800/20) at T_{12} shows large left retroperitoneal mass with central hemorrhage *(arrow)*. Vertebra, spinal canal, and cord appear normal with no evidence of direct invasion by tumor. **B-D,** Sagittal T1W images (SE 800/20) through lumbar spine show irregular low and intermediate signal in L_3 vertebral body on midline sagittal image (**D**). Intermediate signal tissue appears to extend through posterior L_3 cortex and replace epidural fat anterior to thecal sac *(arrow)*. Left lateral sagittal images show replacement of normal fat in L_3-L_4 neural foramen by intermediate signal tissue (**B,** *arrow*). Changes are not contiguous with large retroperitoneal tumor mass and represent either thin pedicle of tumor spread or distant metastasis to L_3 with local epidural extension. **E,** Axial T1W images (SE 1000/20, contiguous 5 mm thick) through L_3-L_4 level show irregular signal in inferior L_3 vertebral body *(open arrow)* with paraspinous and epidural tumor replacing fat adjacent to thecal sac and pedicle with extension into left neural foramen *(closed arrows)*.

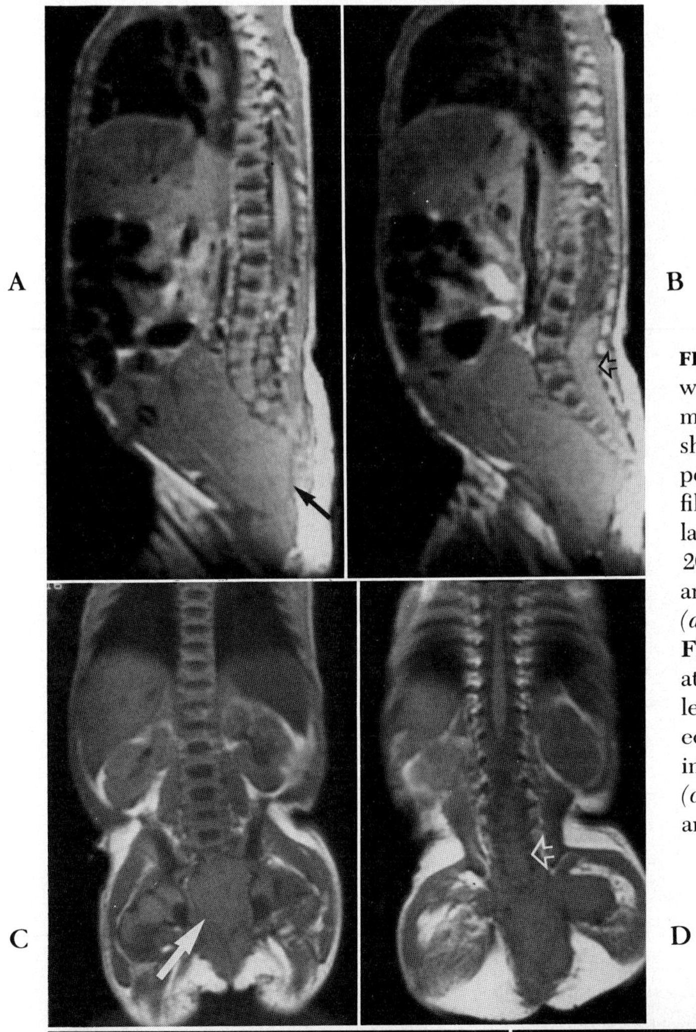

FIGURE 8-48. Pelvic neuroblastoma mass with intraspinal extension in 2-month-old female. Sagittal T1W images (SE 800/20) show **A,** large, intermediate signal mass in pelvis *(arrow)* with **B,** intraspinal extension filling distal spinal canal *(arrow)*. Sacrum is largely intact. Coronal T1W images (SE 800/20) also show **C,** central pelvic mass *(arrow)* and **D,** extension of tumor into spinal canal *(arrow)*. Axial T2W images (2000/20, **E** and **F**; 80, **G** and **H**) show pelvic mass *(arrows)* at midsacral (**E** and **G**) and L_5-S_1 (**F** and **H**) levels. Mass is intermediate signal on first echo image and high signal on second echo image. Tumor extension into spinal canal *(open arrows)* shows similar signal pattern and is seen best at L_5-S_1 level.

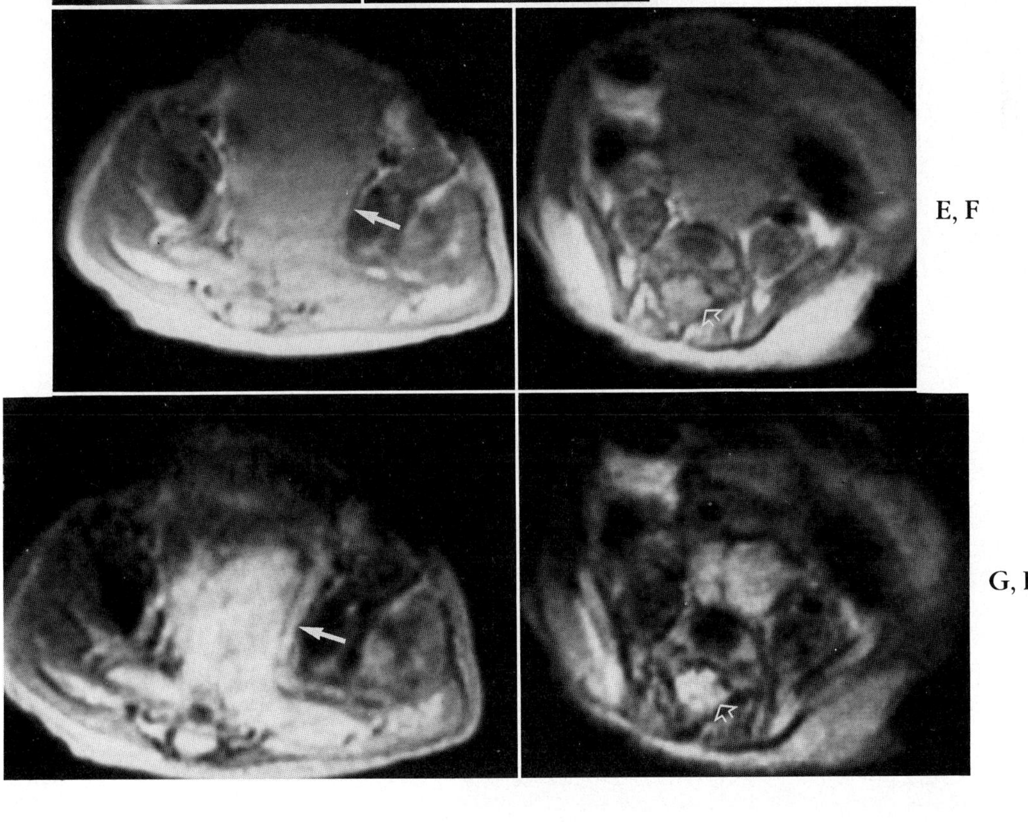

A, B

C

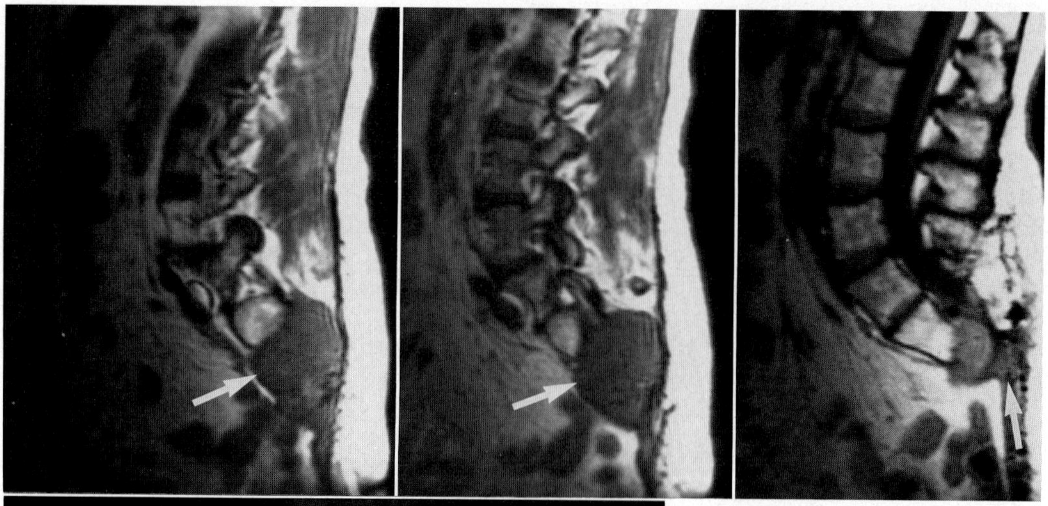

D

E

F

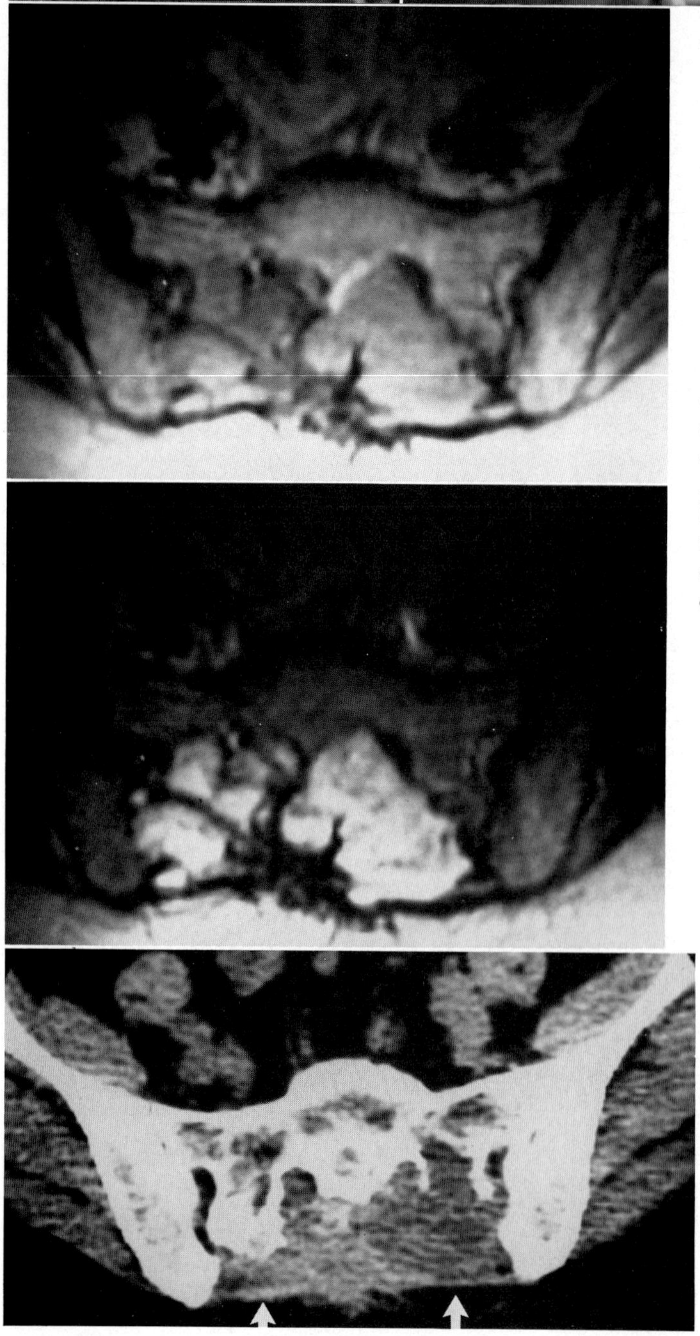

FIGURE 8-49. Sacral chordoma in 64-year-old female. **A-C,** Sagittal T1W images (SE 800/20) to left and in midline show large soft tissue mass *(arrows)* replacing distal sacrum. Destructive changes apparent in midline (**C**) with loss of cortical bone at interface between mass and upper sacrum. Axial T2W images (SE 2500/20, **D**; 80, **E**) show tumor mass lying posterior to S_1 vertebral body *(arrows)* with intermediate signal on first echo image and high signal on second echo image. Posterior spinal elements are distorted and replaced by tumor. **F,** Axial CT image through S_1 vertebral body shows soft tissue mass in posterior sacrum *(arrows)* with direct demonstration of destructive bone changes.

primarily because a major indication of these lesions is calcification, which is often poorly detected on T1W and T2W SE images. Gradient echo techniques may be useful for identification of calcification, but there is currently insufficient experience to assess their reliability and discrimination between calcification and small hemorrhages.

Epidural Lipomatosis

Lipomas associated with spinal dysraphism are discussed in Chapter 5. Abnormal amounts of normal adipose tissue can be found in the epidural space in some patients with endogenous obesity but in clinical situations are most commonly seen in patients receiving exogenous corticosteroids.[40] Patients with epidural lipomatosis often have the clinical stigmata of Cushing's syndrome and are on relatively high-dose steroids, taking more than 40 mg of Prednisone per day. When associated with corticosteroid treatment, clinical signs and symptoms of cord compression appear approximately 4 years after initiation of drug therapy.[30] Although symptoms may be delayed for several years, they can occur as early as a few months after drug initiation.[9] This syndrome can be seen in transplant patients and also in patients with rheumatoid arthritis,[30] who are treated with relatively low doses of corticosteroids. The appropriate treatment is to discontinue the corticosteroid.

One location of abnormal increased accumulations of fat is within the epidural space in the spinal canal, often the thoracic and lumbar regions (Figures 8-50 and 8-51). The epidural fat is mature benign fat tissue, which in some patients can be seen in the epidural space or elsewhere in the spinal canal with no specific inciting cause identifiable. The adipose tissue can be intermixed with prominent vasculature, prompting the term *angiolipoma*[41] and may cause nonspecific clinical symptoms that range from sensory changes and dysesthesia to spastic

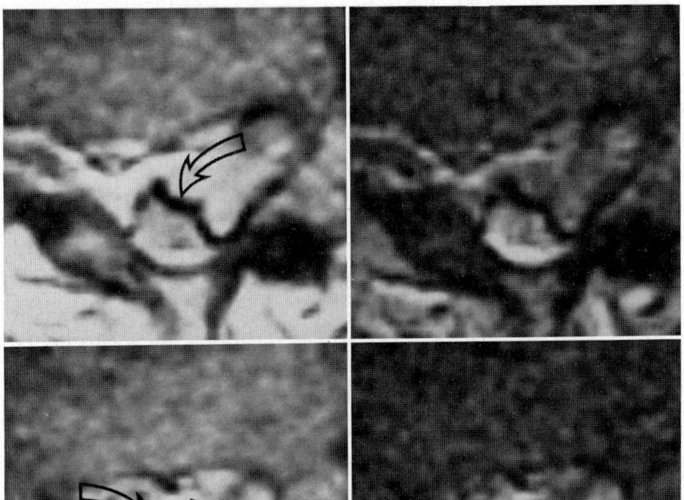

FIGURE 8-50. Epidural lipomatosis. Patient has epidural lipomatosis in upper lumbar spine with asymmetrical distribution. Axial T2W images (SE gated 2100/20, 80) show scalloped appearance to dural sac resulting from increased epidural fat. **A** and **C**, On first echo images, dural sac is displaced posteriorly and fat surrounds exiting nerve root, which appears stretched *(straight arrow)*. Note prominent chemical shift artifact as thick black line on anterior margin of dural sac *(curved arrows)*. Second echo images (**B** and **D**), confirm findings and show a decrease in signal typical of fat tissue.

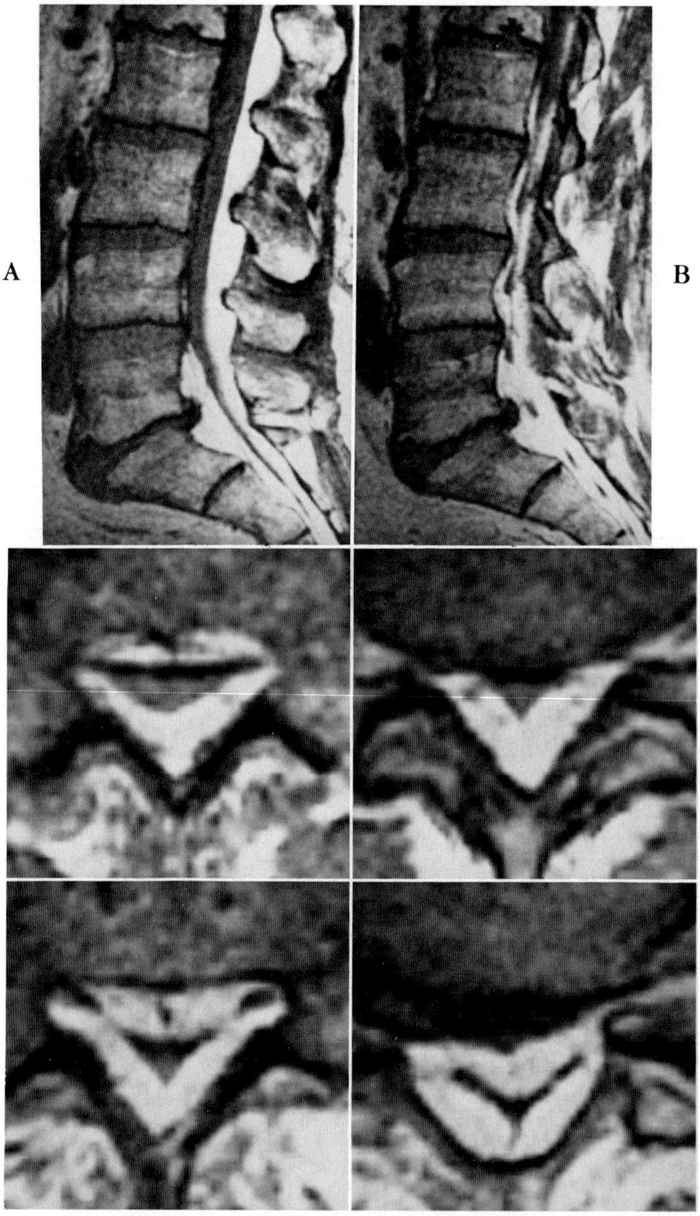

FIGURE 8-51. Epidural lipomatosis. **A** and **B**, Sagittal T1W images (SE 800/20) show large amount of epidural fat in lumbar spinal canal causing marked compression of dural sac. Lipomatous tissue is primarily dorsal except at level of L_5 and below where there is significant ventral deposition. **C-E**, Axial balanced images (SE gated, 2100/20) in lower lumbar region (images rostral to caudal) show marked lipomatous tissue deposition dorsally in midlumbar region (**C** and **D**) and more symmetrically around dural sac in lower lumbar region (**E** and **F**) resulting in inverse "Mercedes sign" at level of L_5 (**F**). Dural sac and root sleeves are symmetrically compressed but not displaced. Findings are typical of lumbar epidural lipomatosis.

paraparesis. There is some question whether such fat deposition represents a true disease entity. CT and MR have clearly shown significant mass effect on the cord and dural sac caused by such fat deposition. If the clinical status does not require urgent action, cessation of corticosteroid treatment may be sufficient. If clinical progression is severe and rapid, laminectomy may be necessary to decompress the spinal canal. In patients with long-term corticosteroid therapy, other considerations for spinal cord symptoms are epidural abscess, as a result of chronic immunosuppression; compression fractures, as a result of steroid induced osteoporosis; myopathy; and peripheral neuropathy.[30] The MR scan can therefore be useful in the diagnostic workup of such patients.

MR Findings

The T1W image is the key to the diagnosis of epidural lipomatosis by showing abnormally large amounts of epidural fat in the spinal canal, most commonly in the thoracic and sometimes in the lumbar region (see Figure 8-51). In the thoracic region, abnormal epidural fat is usually dorsal in location, whereas in the lumbar region it may be both dorsal and ventral. It can be focal and asymmetric (see Figure 8-50). In severe cases it may be circumferential around the dural sac, causing compression and resulting in a trefoil appearance of the lumbar sac and an inverted "Mercedes star" sign in the low lumbar and sacral regions (see Figure 8-51). Abnormal fat distribution is usually characteristic in the lumbar region. In the thoracic region, a T2W confirmation scan is recommended to ensure that the high signal intensity dorsal to the cord represents fat and not the hemorrhagic component of an epidural abscess or hematoma (see Chapter 7).[30] A selective "fat" image would yield similar information.

SPINE METASTASES

Epidural and paraspinous metastases are closely related to vertebral body metastases in location and incidence and usually coexist with vertebral lesions. It is usually not possible to determine whether the origin of these combined lesions is epidural or vertebral.[16,75] Breast and lung carcinomas are the most frequent sources of epidural and paraspinous metastases, followed by carcinomas of the prostate and kidney. In contrast to carcinomas, lymphomas are frequently located in epidural and paraspinous tissues without involvement of adjacent vertebral bodies.[16,20,24] Ewing's sarcoma, although less common, is one of the primary neoplasms that may metastasize to the epidural space without involvement of the vertebral body.[16] The muscle groups in the paraspinous region are often involved and the fatty tissue planes between muscle groups provide the route for spread up and down the spine from the initial implantation site.[16]

Lymphoma and Leukemia

Malignant lymphomas (e.g., lymphosarcoma and reticulum cell sarcoma) frequently infiltrate the spinal canal, especially the epidural space and dura. The typical route of metastasis for lymphoma is by direct, contiguous spread from the retroperitoneum to the paraspinous and epidural spaces via the neural foramina (Figures 8-52 to 8-56). Leukemic involvement of the epidural space is uncommon, except with the occasional occurrence of mass lesions.[16] Neurologic symptoms are usually the result of spinal cord compression (Figure 8-45), but direct infiltration of the spinal cord and nerve roots may also occur. The route of direct parenchymal infiltration is probably along perivascular spaces. Extensive nerve root infiltration can produce massive enlargement of the cauda equina, filling the thecal sac and lumbar canal.[61] Infiltration of the subarachnoid space may also be significant, producing a coating of the spinal cord, individual nerve roots, and cauda equina by a pannus of tumor[61] (see Multiple myeloma) (see Figure 8-92). Hodgkin's lymphoma may infiltrate the epidural space and meninges, similar to the more malignant lymphomas, but it rarely extends to direct infiltration of the spinal cord or nerve roots.[61] Occasionally, dural invasion may disrupt meningeal veins and capillaries, resulting in a spinal subdural hematoma.[61]

MR Findings

Metastases to the spine usually show vertebral body involvement accompanying the paraspinous soft tissue mass (Figures 8-52, 8-53, 8-56,

Text continued on p. 372.

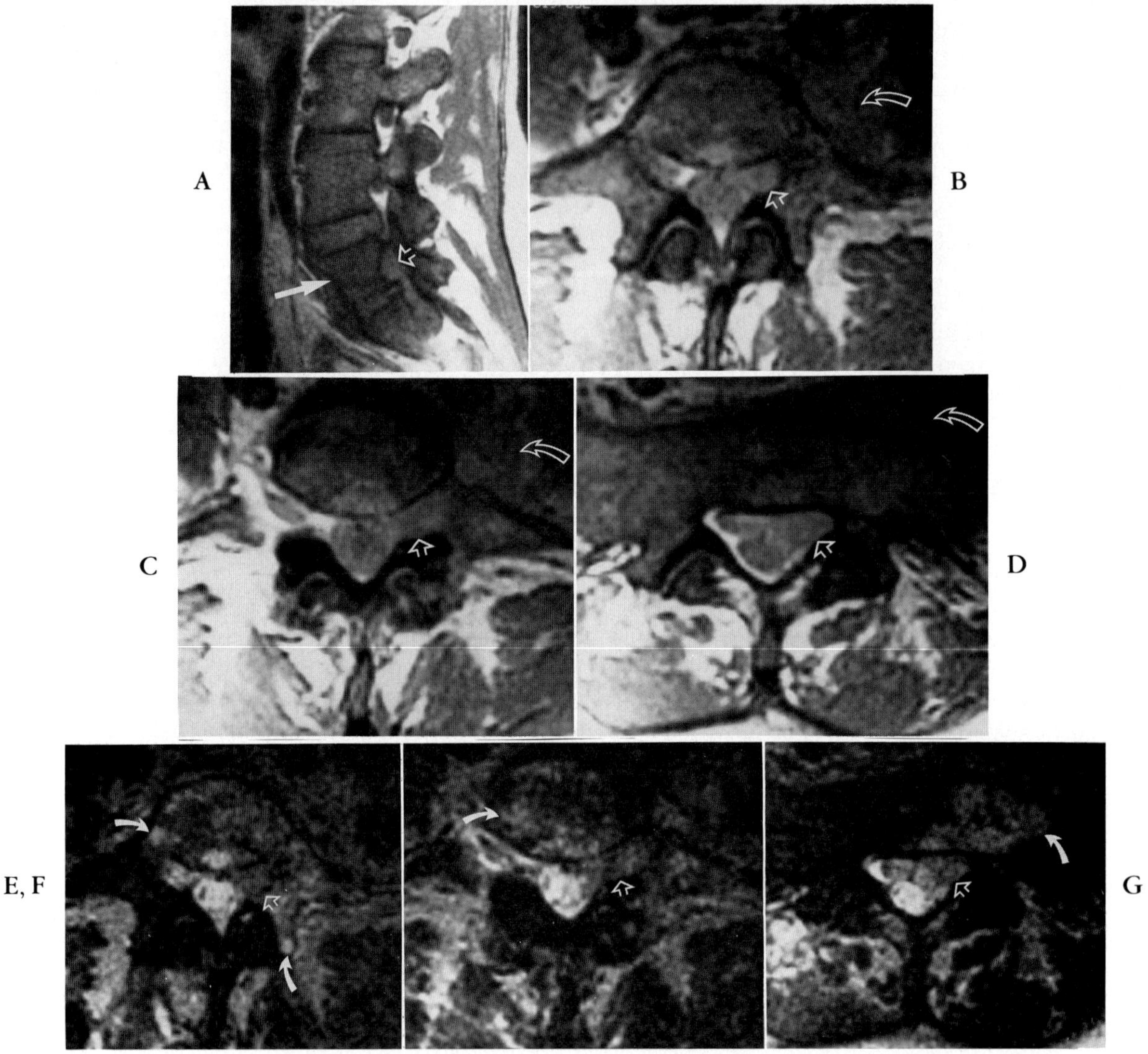

FIGURE 8-52. Lymphoma metastases to vertebral body and epidural space in 41-year-old female. **A,** Sagittal T1W image (SE 800/20) throughout lumbosacral junction shows slightly low signal in L_5 vertebral body *(closed arrow)* consistent with metastatic tumor involvement. Intermediate signal tissue, metastatic lymphoma, fills adjacent neural foramen and lateral recess of spinal canal *(open arrow)*. Axial T2W images (SE 2222/20, **B-D** and 80, **E-G**) show extensive paraspinous *(open curved arrows)* and epidural *(open arrows)* tumor tissue filling neural foramen and lateral recess of spinal canal. Margins of thecal sac and nerve root sleeves, normally seen with high contrast against epidural fat, are obscured by isointense tumor tissue. Identification of metastatic tumor in vertebral bodies is difficult on first echo images but is seen clearly as high signal within marrow spaces on second echo images *(closed curved arrows)*.

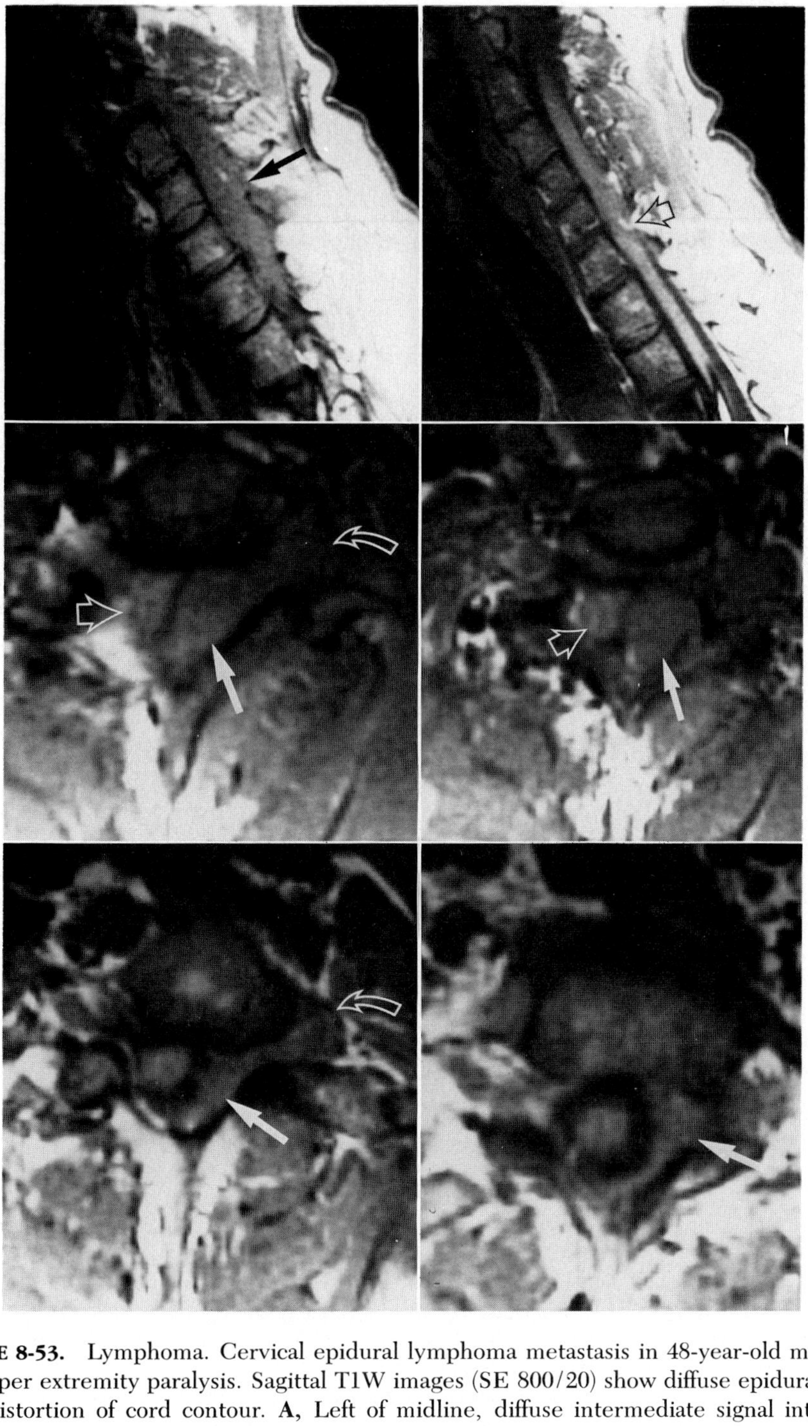

A B C D E F

FIGURE 8-53. Lymphoma. Cervical epidural lymphoma metastasis in 48-year-old male with left upper extremity paralysis. Sagittal T1W images (SE 800/20) show diffuse epidural tumor with distortion of cord contour. **A,** Left of midline, diffuse intermediate signal intraspinal tumor extends from C_4-C_7 levels *(arrow)*. **B,** In midline, distortion and widening of spinal cord is at C_6-C_7 levels *(arrow)*. Whether metastatic tumor is epidural, intradural, or intramedullary in these sagittal views cannot be determined without additional axial images. **C-F,** Axial T1W images (SE 1000/20) through intraspinal tumor, from superior to inferior, show that tumor is epidural in location and produces extrinsic spinal cord compression. **C** and **D,** At C_6-C_7 level, tumor fills most of spinal canal *(closed arrows)*, compressing and distorting thecal sac and spinal cord *(open arrows)*. As tumor tapers inferiorly (**E** and **F,** *straight arrows*) it wraps partially around thecal sac, shifting it and the spinal cord to right at C_7-T_1 level. Tumor extends through left neural foramina and into paraspinous fat at both levels (**C** and **E,** *curved arrows*).

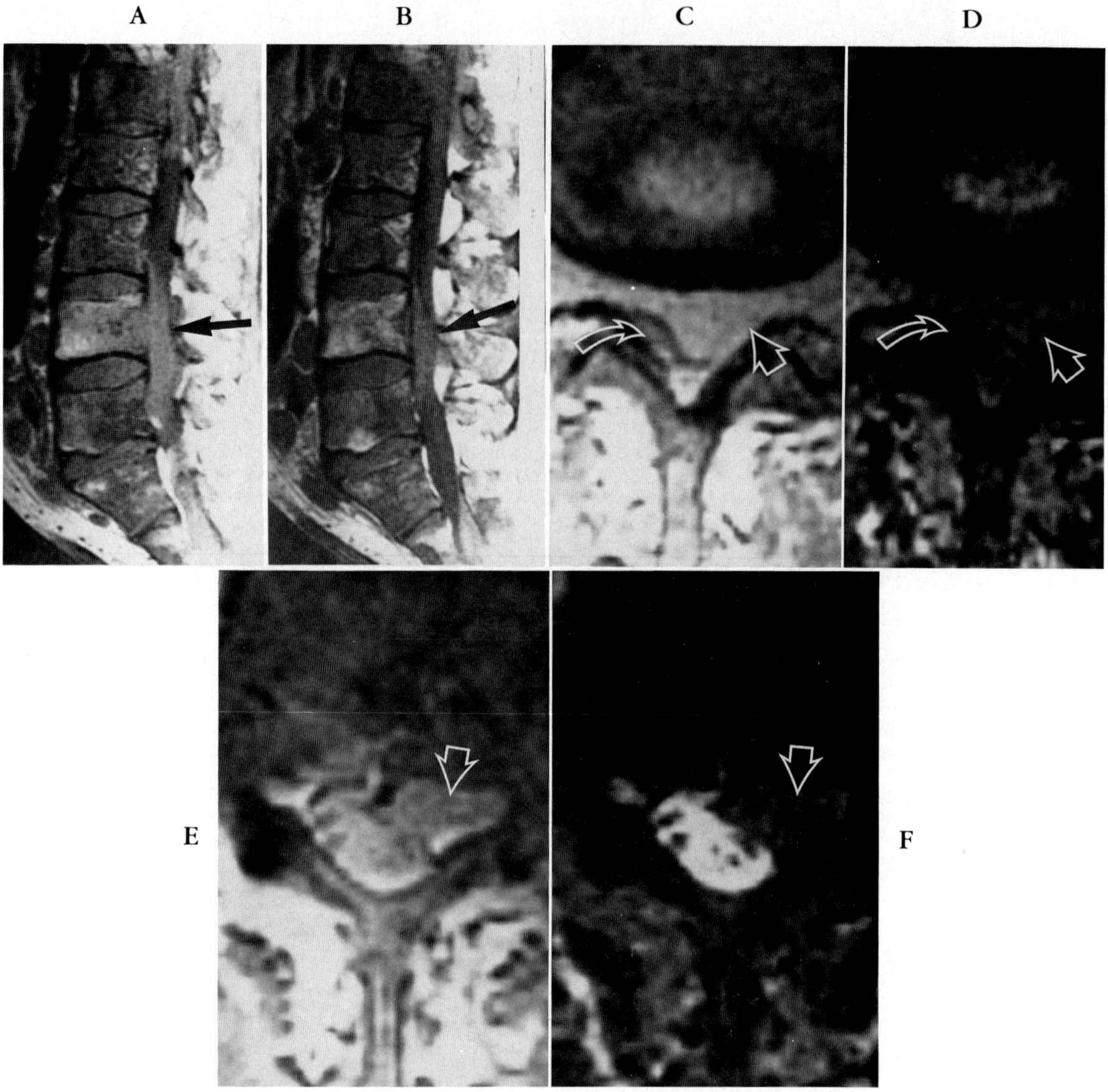

FIGURE 8-54. Extensive vertebral and epidural lymphoma metastases in 30-year-old male. Sagittal T1W images (SE 800/20) of lumbar spine to **A,** left and **B,** in midline show generalized patchy low signal (lower than disc) caused by tumor infiltration of vertebral marrow. Posterior to L_4 and L_5, intermediate signal tumor *(arrows)* replaces normal low signal of thecal sac and high signal of epidural fat. Destruction of posterior cortical margin of L_4 by tumor invasion along course of basivertebral vein is also seen (**A**). Axial T2W images (3158/20, 80) at L_4-L_5 disc (**C** and **D**) and at mid-L_5 (**E** and **F**) show relationship of epidural tumor to thecal sac and neural foramina. At disc level, tumor fills neural foramina bilaterally and most of spinal canal *(straight open arrows)*, markedly compressing thecal sac displacing it to right *(open curved arrows)*. Contents of compressed thecal sac are isointense with tumor tissue because little free CSF is present. At L_5 level, tumor mass is smaller and fills only lateral recess of spinal canal (*arrows*, **E** and **F**). Mass effect distorts thecal sac, giving lesion appearance similar to "free" disc fragment. Relationship to thecal sac is seen best on second echo image (**F**) where CSF is high signal.

A B C D

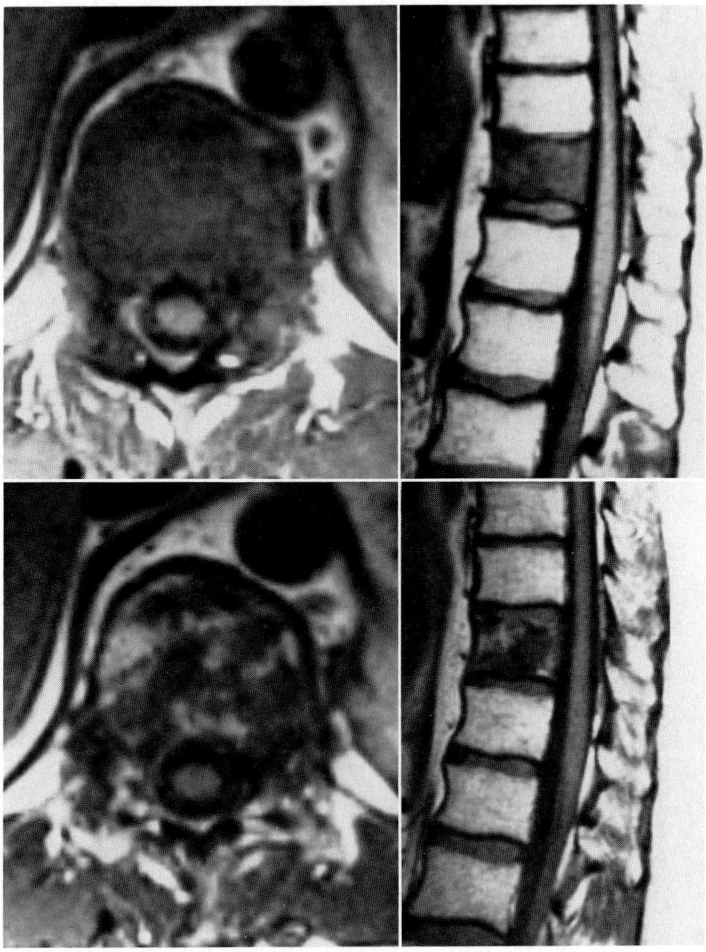

FIGURE 8-55. **A-D,** Scans done 1 year apart show partial response of metastatic lymphoma to treatment as evidenced by increased fat deposition in affected vertebral body. Initial T1W scans in **A,** axial (SE 1000/20) and **B,** sagittal (SE 800/20) projections show low signal intensity throughout T_{11} vertebra. Axial scan (**A**) shows diffuse involvement with vertebral body and some infiltration into immediate adjacent soft tissue and epidural space. On sagittal view (**B**) it is apparent that adjacent vertebrae have increased signal secondary to increased fat deposition as a result of previous irradiation. MR scans obtained one year after further treatment show infiltration of fat into affected vertebral body causing inhomogeneous signal pattern on axial (SE 1000/20, **C**) and sagittal (SE 800/20, **D**) scans. **E,** "Fat" image (SE 800/30) confirms inhomogeneous high signal is caused by fat. **F,** "Water" image (SE 800/30) shows increased signal in posterior portion of vertebral body corresponding to low signal intensity area on conventional T1W image (**D**). **G,** Sagittal T2W scan (SE gated 2000/80) shows increased signal intensity throughout vertebrae but is most prominent posteriorly in same area as high signal on "water" image (**F**). Although increased fat deposition suggests some response to treatment, abnormal high signal on "water" image (**F**) and T2W image (**G**) suggests residual tumor. Whether sterilized tumor with residual fibrosis also exhibits such abnormal high signal on "water" or heavily T2W images has not been determined at this time.

E, F

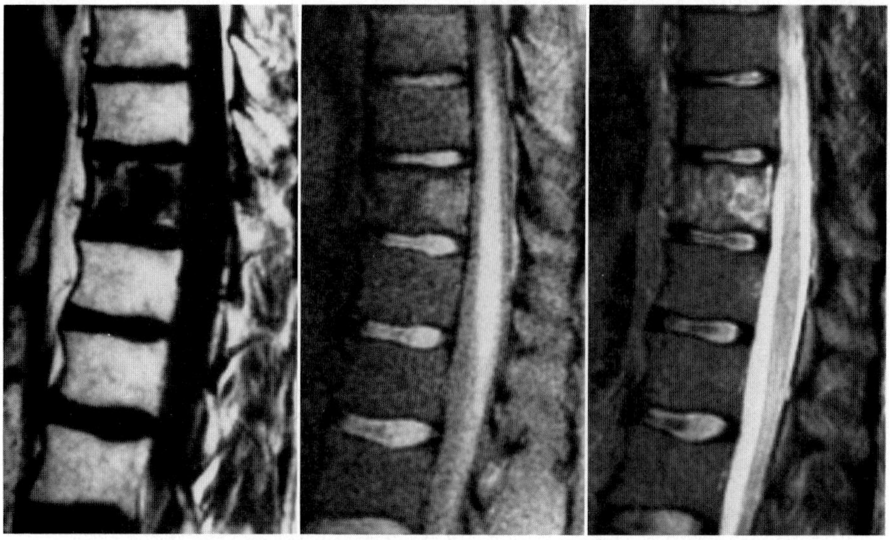

G

FIGURE 8-55, cont'd. For legend see previous page.

A

B

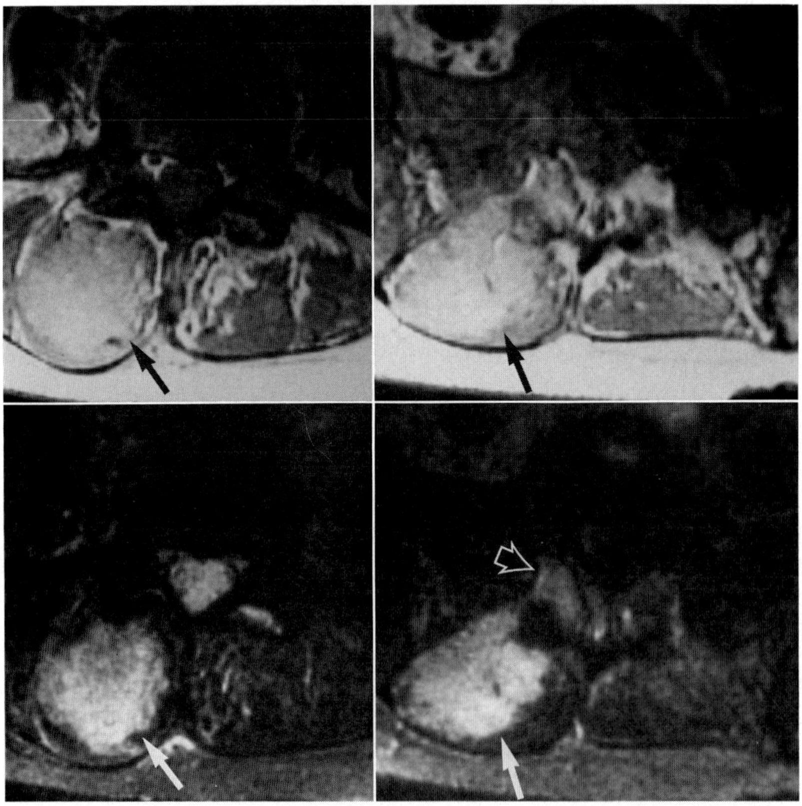

C

D

FIGURE 8-56. Acute myelogenous leukemia (AML) chloroma in 65-year-old female. Axial T2W images (SE 2143/20, **A** and **B**; 80, **C** and **D**) at L_5-S_1 show large, high signal right paraspinous chloroma *(closed arrows)* partially replacing erector muscle of the spine. Tumor also extends medially through the neural foramen to form an epidural mass *(open arrow)* in sacral canal.

A

B, C

D

E, F

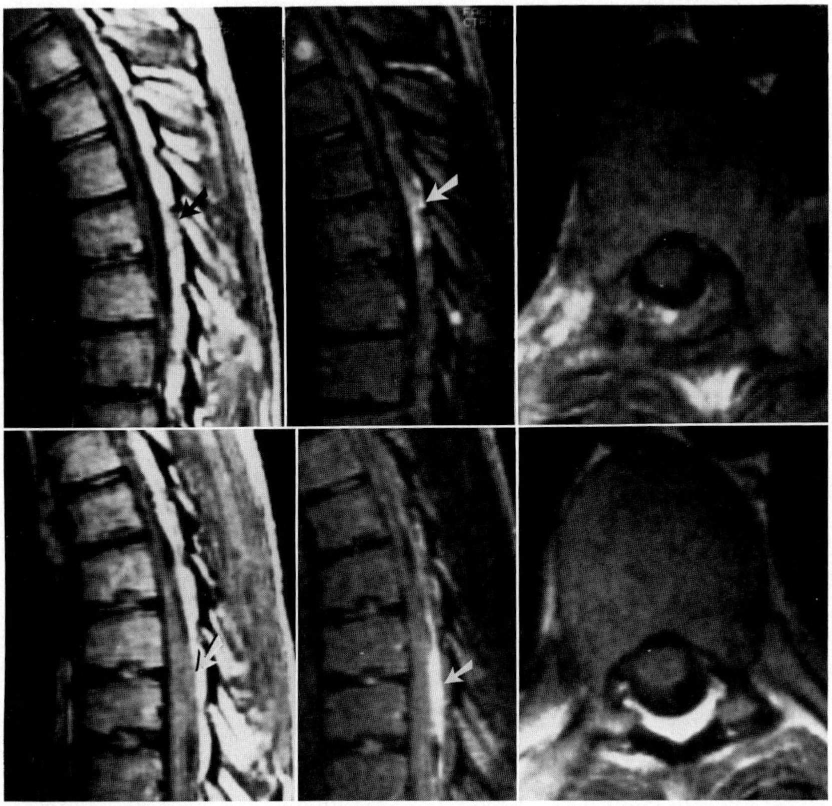

FIGURE 8-57. Ewing's sarcoma. Scans show potential for false positive interpretation of metastatic tumor on T2W scans in thoracic region caused by stationary CSF dorsal to cord. Sagittal first echo T2W scans (SE 2500/20) show subtle area of signal change in dorsal epidural fat (*arrow*, **A**) and irregular area of intermediate signal intensity occupying space between cord and epidural fat (*arrow*, **D**). Second echo (SE 2500/80) at same location shows abnormal high signal within dorsal epidural fat (*arrow*, **B**); note another metastatic site in high thoracic vertebral body (**B**). Increased signal intensity is identified between thoracic cord and epidural fat (see *arrow*, **E**). Tumor infiltration of dorsal epidural fat is confirmed at this level on axial T1W scan (SE 800/25, **C**) by its replacement of fat with lower signal intensity tissue. The area of increased signal in (**D**) represents static CSF and the axial T1W scan (**F**) shows epidural fat to be normal. T1W scans are sufficient to make correct diagnosis because normal high signal of dorsal epidural fat provides adequate contrast for tumor infiltration.

and 8-58). The verbetral body lesion is usually of relative lower signal than marrow on T1W images (see Figure 8-52, 8-54, and 8-55). This low signal abnormality may be subtle in children and can also be difficult to detect in older patients who have heterogeneous marrow signal. In leukemia, T1W changes in marrow signal have been related to relapse.[44,45]

Hematopoietic malignancies infiltrate epidural tissue around the dural sac and in the neural foramen (Figure 8-56). Neoplasm is detected where it replaces normal epidural fat, i.e., low-signal intensity replacing high signal, or by morphologic change where abnormal tissue contour is present. Lymphoma often dissects dura off bone, causing circumferential narrowing around the cord; the dura is seen as an irregular dark ring (see Figure 8-98). Contributing to the dark ring is signal-loss from pulsating CSF. Because the subarachnoid space is narrowed, velocity and amplitude of pulsation increase, making flow effects more evident in T1W images. T2W images are usually not needed for diagnosis but hematopoietic tumors exhibit high signal on T2W images (see Figure 8-55). Epidural disease can be mistaken for static CSF trapped in arachnoid septations in the dorsal thoracic region[19] (Figure 8-52).

The differential diagnosis for paraspinous lesions include primary soft tissue tumors and sarcomas of muscle and connective tissue. Inflammatory and infectious disease may be difficult to differentiate from these neoplasms, especially when typical vertebral end-plates and disc space changes are absent. Epidural replacement of normal fat and formation of mass lesions in the epidural space and paraspinous muscles may occur with granulomatous inflammatory processes. Asymmetry of the paraspinous muscles due to unilateral atrophy should not be misinterpreted as neoplastic enlargement of the normal side. The distinction from neoplasm can usually be based on the exaggerated contour of the atrophied muscle with relatively greater fat at its margin and fat interposed between the muscle and the spine and, in some cases, the elevated signal of severely atrophied muscle.

Multiple Myeloma

Myeloma is a malignant proliferation of plasma cells, usually within bone marrow of the spine, which may also form localized mass lesions, and is spread throughout the body in its later stages. Myeloma comprises approximately 34% of cases of malignant bone tumors and shows a peak incidence at 50 to 70 years of age (60% of cases).[51] The predominant sites of diffuse spinal marrow involvement are the thoracic, especially midthoracic and lower-thoracic (66%), lumbar (18%), cervical (11%), and sacrum (5%).[51] Solitary spinal myelomas (plasmacytomas) are paraspinous mass lesions that occur in the same age range and anatomic distribution as the disseminated variety but may have a slightly better prognosis with a tendency to proliferate later in the disease process.[51] The major systemic effects of multiple myeloma are anemia and cachexia with Bence Jones protein and renal failure. Rarefaction of vertebral bodies by disseminated disease or local destruction by plasmacytoma produce bone pain and pathologic fractures with consequent involvement of neural structures. Early identification of vertebral disease may allow prevention of many neurologic sequelae by early institution of radiation or chemotherapy.[26]

A, B

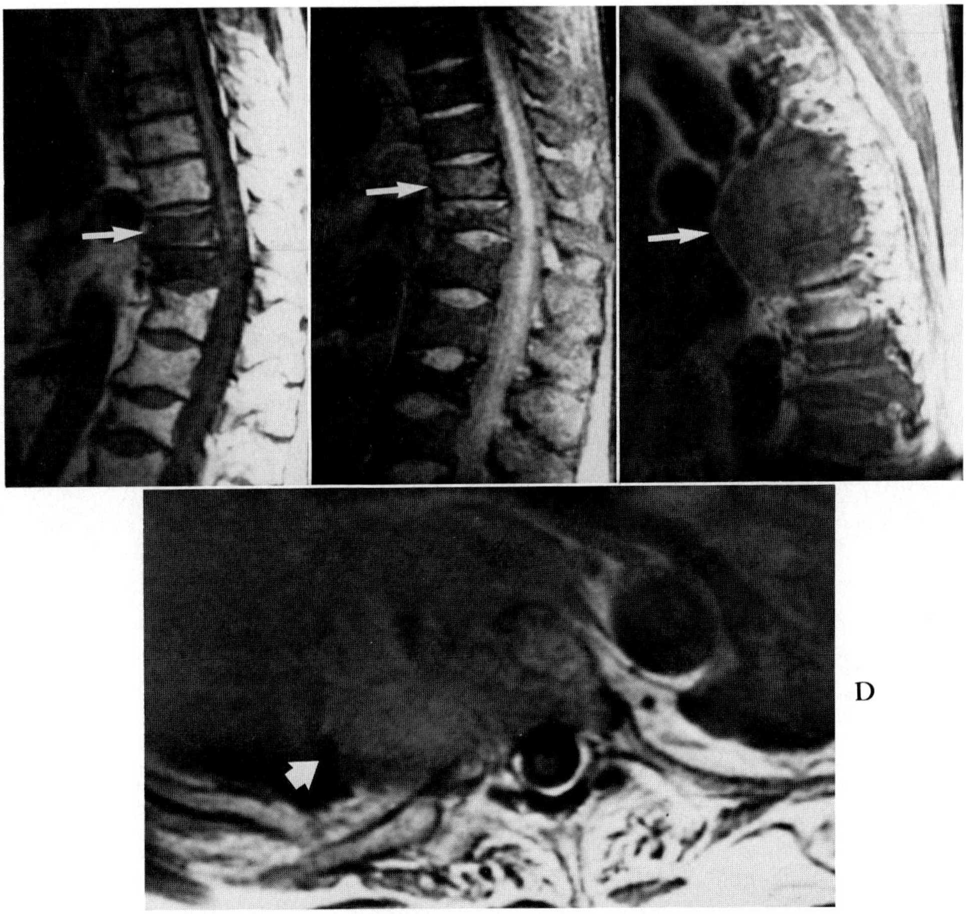

C

D

FIGURE 8-58. Multiple myeloma. Paraspinous plasmacytoma in 65-year-old male after radiation therapy. **A**, Sagittal T1W image (SE 800/20) shows uniform low signal in T_{10} *(arrow)* and T_{11} vertebral bodies indicating replacement by myeloma. Signal intensity is lower than radiation-induced high signal of other vertebral bodies and lower than adjacent discs. Partial collapse of vertebral bodies is also present. Pattern of uniform involvement of individual vertebral bodies is typical of metastases from other types of tumors, but is within spectrum of multiple myeloma. **B**, Sagittal "water" image (fat-suppressed) corresponding to **A** shows high signal in T_{10} *(arrow)* and T_{11} vertebral bodies representing replacement of normal marrow by high water content tumor cells. Signal intensity in involved vertebral bodies is lower than discs and higher than fatty marrow in irradiated vertebrae. Spinal cord is higher signal than CSF because of motion-induced signal loss in CSF. **C**, Sagittal T1W image (SE 800/20) right of midline shows large paraspinous plasmacytoma at T_5-T_7 levels *(arrow)*. Replacement of bone marrow is adjacent to mass not seen on midline sagittal images (**A** and **B**). **D**, Axial T1W image (SE 1000/20) through T_5 shows large right paraspinous mass with local invasion of vertebral body.

A B C

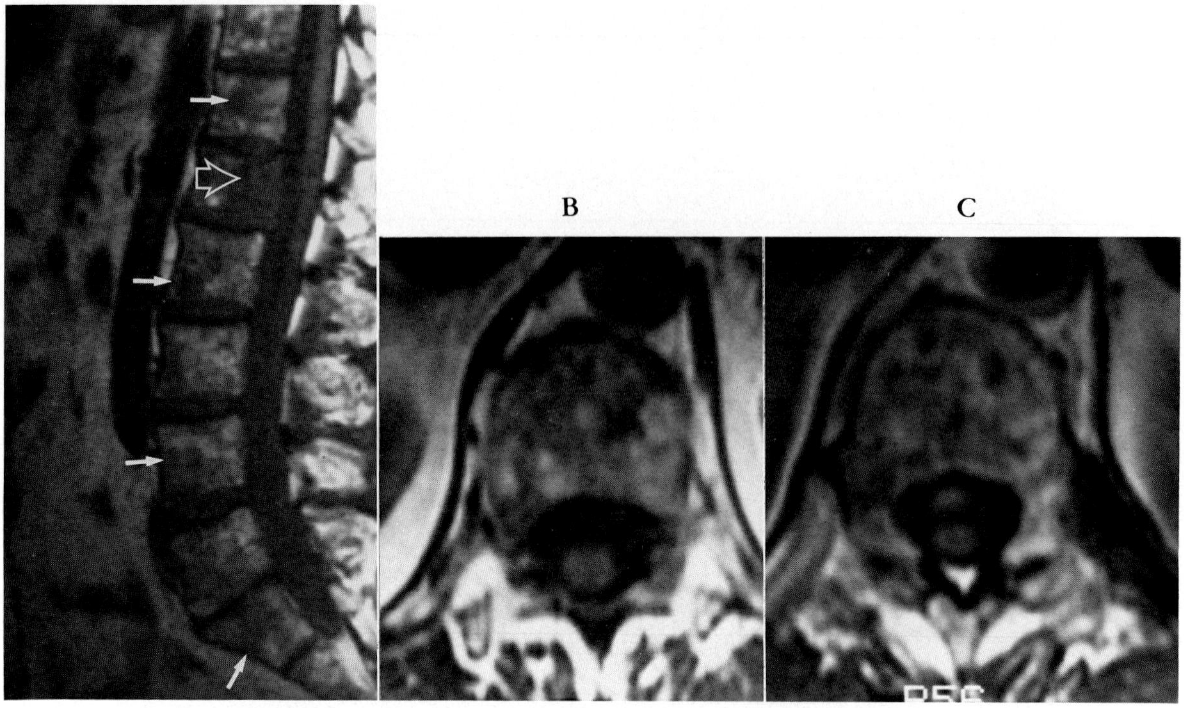

FIGURE 8-59. Multiple myeloma. Diffuse lumbar spine involvement in 49-year-old female. **A,** Sagittal T1W image (SE 800/20) of lumbar spine shows multiple low signal areas *(small arrows)* caused by replacement of marrow by high water content tumor. Confluent low signal with partial vertebral body collapse is present at L_1 *(open arrow)*. Pattern is typical of multiple myeloma but also is seen with carcinoma and lymphoma metastases. No epidural tumor is seen. Axial T1W images (SE 1000/20) through T_{11} (**B**) and T_{12} (**C**) also show mottled signal pattern with low signal representing replacement of marrow by tumor. No epidural tumor is seen; high signal immediately anterior to cord at T_{12} (**B**) represents in-flow enhancement of CSF.

MR Imaging

The typical appearance of untreated multiple myeloma on MR images is similar to that of other metastatic lesions that replace fatty bone marrow. Compared to normal marrow, lesions are low signal on T1W images and high signal on T2W images (Figures 8-58 and 8-59). The usual pattern of involvement is diffuse marrow replacement in multiple vertebral bodies, often as multiple well-circumscribed lesions (see Figure 8-59). Diffuse replacement of marrow in individual vertebral bodies may be seen, especially adjacent to a paraspinous plasmacytoma (see Figure 8-58). In the late stages of disseminated disease, all normal marrow may be replaced. In general, myeloma involves the central vertebral body and may include the pedicles. In cases where only the pedicles are involved, diagnosis of another metastatic tumor type may be more likely, although this does not exclude myeloma.[51] After radiation therapy, vertebral myeloma lesions may show low signal relative to marrow on both T1W and T2W images.[26] In general, sagittal and axial T1W images are sufficient for detection of multiple myeloma and demonstration of destructive vertebral changes or paraspinous masses. Pathologic collapse of vertebral bodies is easily identified on sagittal T1W images, and axial images can further delineate relationships to cord and nerve roots. Occasionally, collapsed vertebral bodies may not show abnormally low signal within the marrow.[26] MRI is much more sensitive for detection of vertebral myeloma lesions than plain radiography or radionuclide bone scan. In a recent series, lesions seen on MRI in 42 vertebral bodies were detected in 11 (27%) with plain radiographs and in only 2 (5%) with radionuclide bone scanning.[26]

A B C D

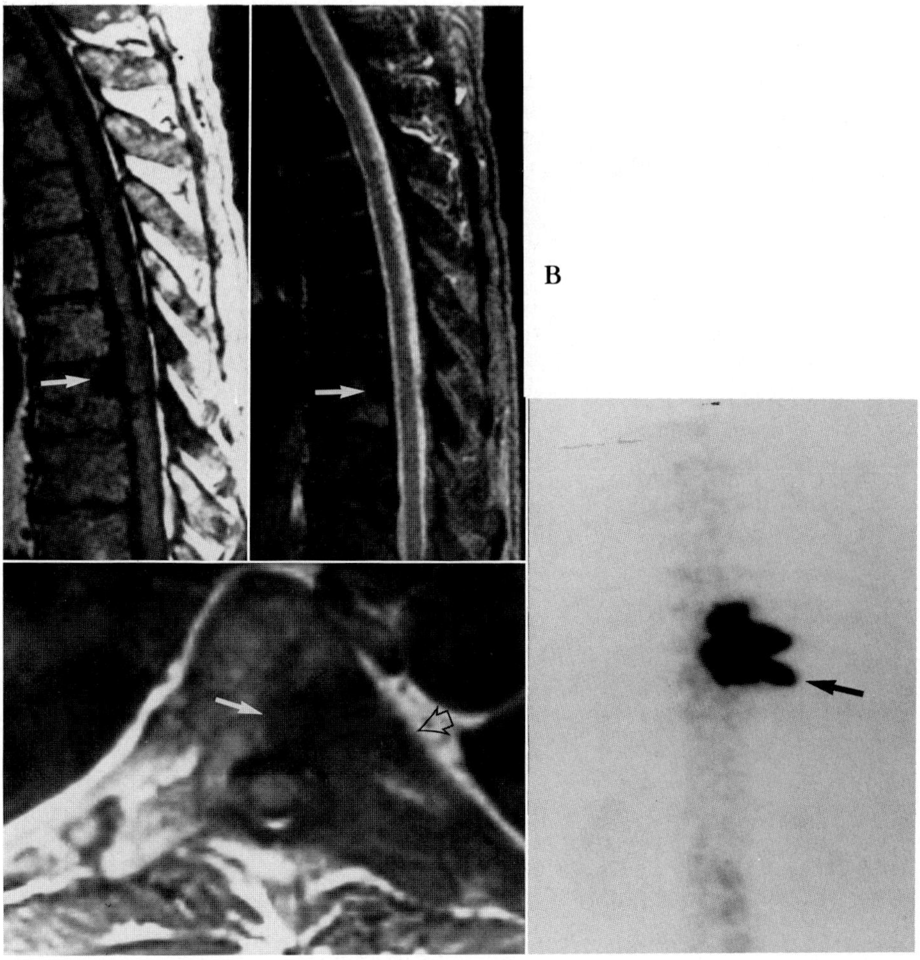

FIGURE 8-60. Metastases. Prostate carcinoma in 75-year-old male. **A,** Sagittal image T1W (SE 800/20) shows low signal in posterosuperior T_8 vertebral body *(arrow)* consistent with metastatic disease from carcinoma. Epidural disease is not apparent on this image. **B,** Sagittal T2W image (SE 2400/80) shows region of low signal *(arrow)* (i.e., low proton density) that is also relatively low signal on the T1W image, suggesting a region of bone sclerosis commonly found with prostate carcinoma metastases. Area of high signal around low signal region has normal signal intensity on T1W image; this represents metastatic tumor replacing normal marrow. **C,** Axial T1W image (SE 800/20) shows abnormal low signal tumor in left T_8 vertebral body *(white arrow)* with extension into pedicle, lamina, and adjacent proximal rib *(open arrow)*. Destruction of cortical bone is present where tumor has invaded posterior elements and rib. **D,** Bone scan (99mTc MDP) shows very high activity in region of left T_7-T_9 vertebral bodies with extension into adjacent ribs *(arrow)*.

Vertebral Metastases

The primary tumor that is frequently metastatic to the spine is breast tumor, followed by prostate, lung, and renal cell carcinomas. Other neoplasms that metastasize to the spine include sarcomas, Ewing's sarcoma, neuroblastoma, and melanoma.[21] Diffuse neoplasm such as lymphoma, leukemia, and multiple myeloma also involve the vertebral column. Metastases show a strong predilection for bone marrow as a result of its high vascularity and, in the case of pelvic neoplasm, the transport of tumor cells through the venous system (Batson's plexus) to the thoracolumbar vertebral bodies.

The initial change in marrow with metastatic disease is the replacement of normal fatty bone marrow with nonfatty tumor cells. At a later stage, destruction of trabeculae occurs, usually without a periosteal response, but in breast and prostate carcinoma a reactive bone response may occur that generates an osteoblastic or sclerotic reaction at the sites of metastatic involvement. Most metastases are osteolytic; breast and prostate carcinomas are the exception.

MR has advantages over plain films in the detection of metastatic disease because it shows more subtle signs of tumor invasion, i.e., replacement of normal fatty marrow when presumably little change in the trabecular bone pattern has occurred. Plain films are abnormal at a clinically determined level in 60% to 85% of patients with signs of spinal cord compression. Myelography, the gold standard, is virtually 100% sensitive to symptomatic complete or partial block in such patients.[22,75] The major advantage of MR, of course, is that it allows noninvasive direct visualization of the cord and the mass lesion that may be compressing it.

Most metastases are osteolytic. Bone changes are more important to the diagnosis of metastases with procedures such as plain films and CT that show bone changes directly. More relevant to MR imaging is the replacement of bone marrow (normally 50% to 70% fat) by nonfatty tumor cells, which produces a marked change in MR signal of vertebral bodies as a result of the higher water and lower fat content of neoplasm. These changes can be seen separately on "fat" and "water" images. Metastases show a lack of signal on "fat" images compared to normal marrow and increased signal intensity on "water" images in the same areas that show signal loss on the "fat" image. This change in composition causes lower signal on T1W (or T2*W) images and higher signal on T2W images regardless of bone changes. Marked sclerosis, however, can cause low signal on both T1W and T2W images. MR imaging appears to be more sensitive to early bone marrow metastases than plain radiography and 99mTc MDP bone scanning, before bone destruction or reactive bone formation.[26,29] Plain radiographs depend on relative marked bone destruction for tumor detection, and 99mTc MDP bone scans, although more sensitive, depend on reactive bone formation after bone destruction and detect marrow involvement only by indirect signs of metaphyseal expansion.[29]

MR Findings

The appearance of the vertebral body metastatic lesion is relative on T1W images. Because signal intensity of vertebral bodies can vary, relative intensity of the metastatic lesion also varies. Most often tumor of low signal is compared to the adjacent vertebral body (Figures 8-60 to 8-73). This is always the case after radiation where normal marrow has been replaced by fat (see Figures 8-62, 8-66, 8-67, and 8-69). The metastatic tumor can also be of higher signal intensity than the adjacent, uninvolved vertebral body (see Figures 8-70 and 8-71). In some instances the tumor and remainder of the vertebral body are similar signal intensity, making detection difficult (Figures 8-74 and 8-75). Such relative increased tumor signal intensity is also seen if there is significant bone sclerosis that produces a low signal background. Because of the difficulty in identifying a normal vertebra the extent of bony metastases may be difficult to assess in some patients. Other pulse sequences such as STIR or "water" images provide a more absolute high signal abnormality for vertebral metastases and rely less on relative differences (Figures 8-76 to 8-80). STIR scans may detect diffuse metastatic disease that may be undetectable on a conventional T1W scan (see Figure 8-80).

Metastatic tumor may be difficult to detect by signal intensity changes on T1W images (see Figures 8-74 and 8-75). This is especially true in older patients with heterogenous marrow sig-

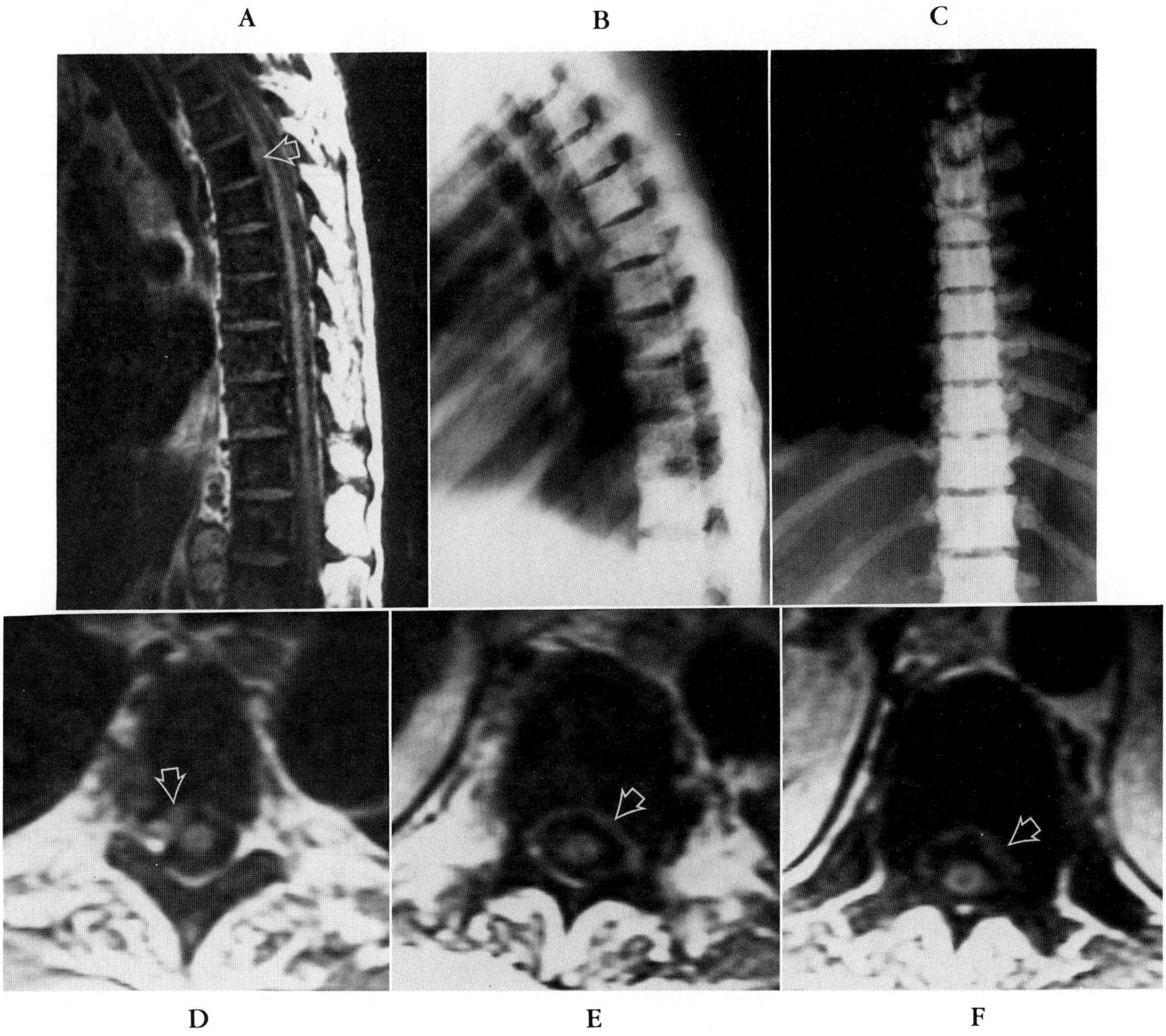

FIGURE 8-61. Prostate carcinoma metastases throughout thoracic spine in 75-year-old male. **A,** Sagittal T1W image (SE 800/20) shows unusually low signal (lower than disc) in vertebral bodies at all levels as a result of dense vertebral sclerosis (see **B** and **C**). Small intermediate signal area (higher than vertebral body and similar to disc) behind T_6 vertebral body *(arrow)* represents metastatic prostate carcinoma extension into epidural fat. At other levels epidural fat between vertebral bodies and thecal sac appears approximately normal in signal, although smaller areas of epidural tumor cannot be completely excluded. **B** and **C,** Plain radiographs of thoracic spine show dense sclerosis of vertebral bodies throughout, secondary to diffuse prostate metastases. **D-F,** Axial T1W images (SE 800/20) at T_6 (**B**), T_{11} (**C**), and T_{12} (**C**) show consistent diffuse low signal in vertebral bodies as seen on sagittal images. Intermediate signal epidural tumor is clearly present at T_6 level on right with local mass effect (**D,** *open arrow*). Epidural space at T_{11} and T_{12} is intermediate signal anteriorly (**C** and **D,** *open arrows*), rather than high signal seen in paraspinous fat, indicating presence of epidural tumor at these levels as well. Pattern of "reverse contrast," where vertebral body is lower signal than epidural spread of tumor, is common with prostate carcinoma, or any tumor that produces dense vertebral sclerosis.

Continued.

G, H 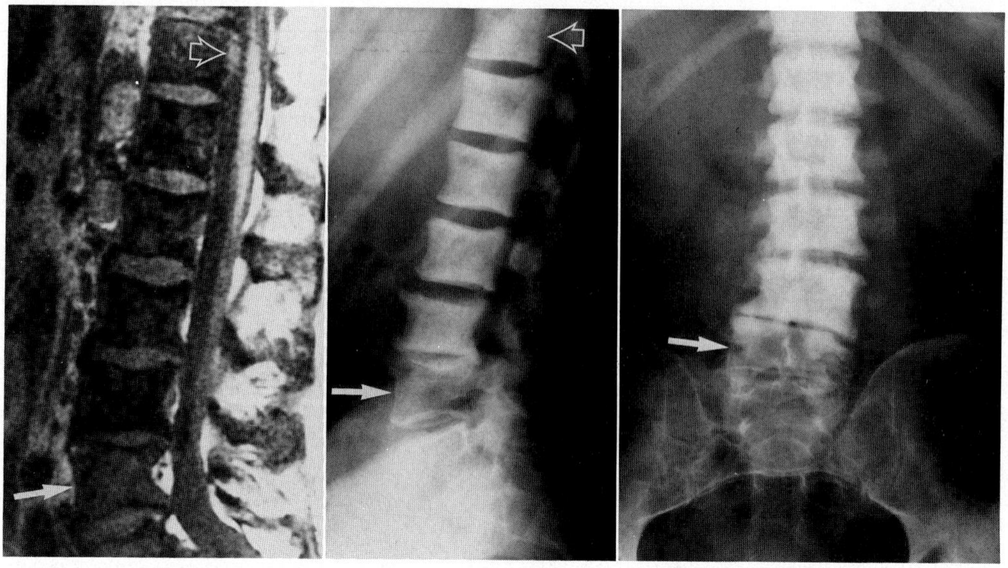 I

FIGURE 8-61, cont'd. **G,** Sagittal T1W image (SE 800/20) of lumbar spine shows low signal in vertebral bodies, except L_5 *(closed arrow)* and S_1, which show signal closer to normal marrow. Low signal vertebrae correspond to dense sclerosis on plain radiographs (**H** and **I**), whereas L_5 and S_1 correspond to nonsclerotic vertebrae. As in upper thoracic spine, small amount of epidural tumor replaces fat at posterior vertebral margins, most notably at T_{12} *(open arrow)*. **H** and **I,** Plain radiographs of lumbar spine show dense sclerosis in T_{12}-L_4 vertebral bodies with sparing of L_5 *(closed arrows)* and S_1 vertebrae. Posterior margin of T_{12} is indistinct *(open arrow)*, consistent with tumor extension from vertebral body into epidural space, but this finding is not specific.

nal that yields poor contrast. "Water" and "fat" images can help decipher changes in signal caused by metastases (see Figures 8-74 and 8-75). Metastatic involvement usually results in total displacement of marrow tissue at the tumor site, resulting in lower signal on T1W images and absent signal on "fat" images (see Figures 8-73 to 8-75). "Water" images show increased signal because of higher water content, i.e., higher than normal marrow signal on T1W and "water" images (see Figures 8-73 to 8-75). It is possible for these effects to nearly offset each other; in which case the metastatic tumor may be difficult to visualize on a T1W image that reflects both components (see Figures 8-73 and 8-74). In detecting vertebral body metastases "fat" and "water" images can be useful because these effects are separated. Another pulse sequence useful in this regard is the STIR sequence, which can summate the effects of long T1 and long T2 relaxation times of tumor tissue while suppressing fat signal, making it more sensitive than a conventional T1W image (see Figures 8-76 to 8-79). It is probably similar in sensitivity to a "fat" and "water" image combination, which takes approximately the same amount of scanning time (see Figures 8-76 to 8-79).

When bone destruction occurs, it is best seen on proton density or "water" images. The thin, low signal of bone cortex can be seen as thinned or interrupted by soft tissue signal. In evaluating bone destruction the direction of the frequency encoding axis and its chemical shift must be kept in mind. Although an IV contrast agent such as GdDTPA is necessary for the diagnosis of leptomeningeal tumor (see leptomeningeal tumor), its use may obscure vertebral body metastases[69] (Figures 8-81 to 8-83) because tumor enhancement may raise the signal intensity of the vertebral body so that the low signal tumor on T1W images increases to match that of adjacent normal marrow, reducing or eliminating contrast between tumor and marrow and decreasing lesion detectability. Such obscuration of metastases can occur when adjacent vertebrae have high signal as a result of radiation-induced fat replacement of normal marrow (see Figure 8-83).

Text continued on p. 398.

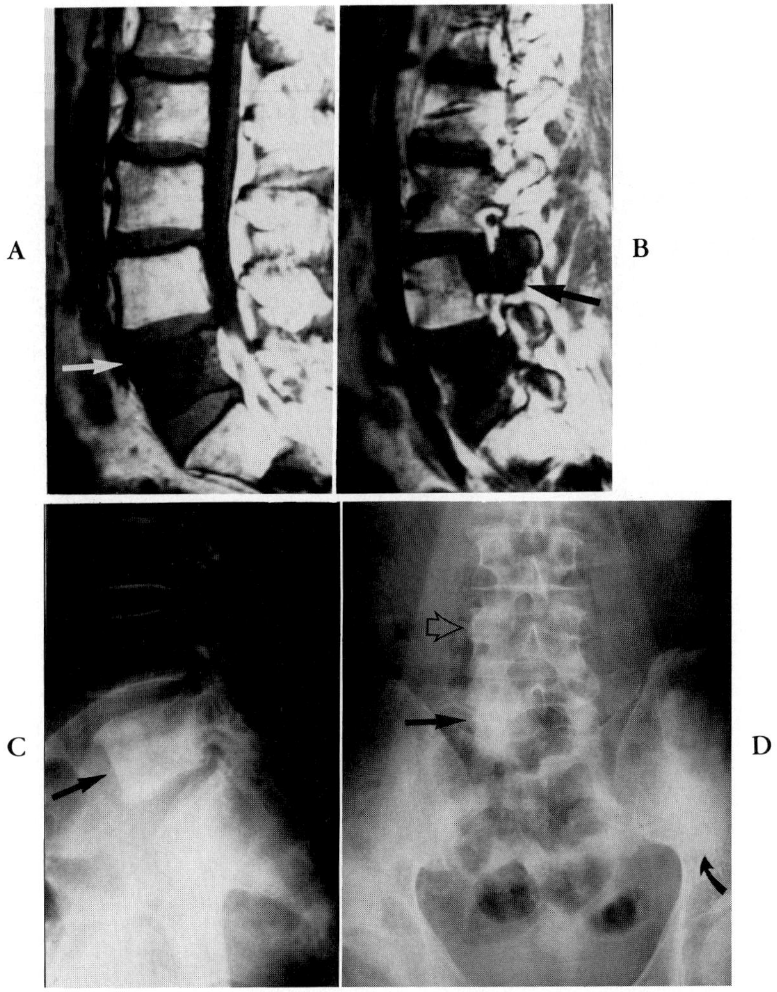

FIGURE 8-62. Prostate carcinoma metastases in 64-year-old male after radiation therapy to pelvis and lumbar spine. **A** and **B**, Sagittal T1W images (SE 800/20) of lumbar spine. High signal in vertebral bodies at most levels represent fatty degeneration of normal bone marrow in response to radiation exposure. Low signal replaces most of marrow in L_5 vertebral body (**A**, *arrow*) consistent with metastatic disease. In addition, there is well-circumscribed low signal abnormality in right pedicle at L_4 level (**B**, *arrow*) and S_2 vertebral body. **C**, Lateral and **D**, anteroposterior (AP) plain radiographs of lumbar spine show dense sclerosis of right L_5 vertebral body *(straight black arrows)* corresponding to low signal on sagittal T1W image. AP film shows poor definition of cortical margins of right L_4 pedicle (**D**, *open arrow*) consistent with lytic metastatic tumor involvement. Dense sclerosis in left medial ilium is adjacent to sacroiliac joint *(curved arrow)*.

Continued.

E

F

G

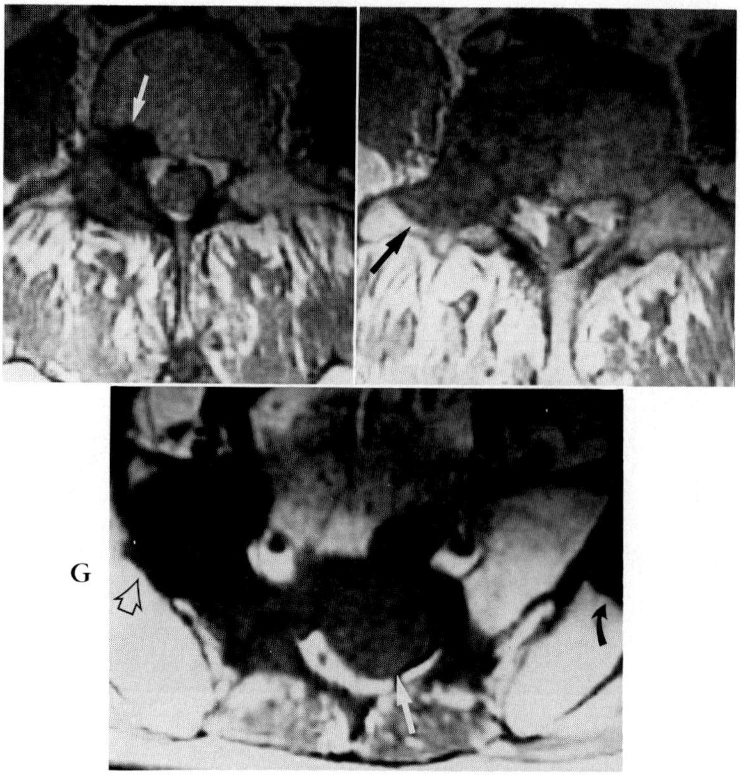

FIGURE 8-62, cont'd. Axial T2W images (SE 2500/20) through L_4 (**E**) and L_5 (**F**) show well-circumscribed low signal lesion in right L_4 pedicle (**E**, *arrow*). Cortical margins of pedicle are not clearly seen, corresponding to indistinct appearance on plain film (**D**). Small amount of epidural tumor is present medial to pedicle. At L_5 right half of vertebral body and transverse process are low signal (**F**, *arrow*), which corresponds to dense sclerosis on plain films. **G**, Axial T1W image (SE 800/20) through S_1 level shows extensive low signal in lateral sacrum representing metastatic prostate carcinoma with extension through cortical bone, invasion of sacroiliac joint *(open arrow)*, and formation of large intraspinal mass *(white arrow)*. Very low signal in left medial ilium *(curved arrow)* corresponds to dense sclerosis in plain films.

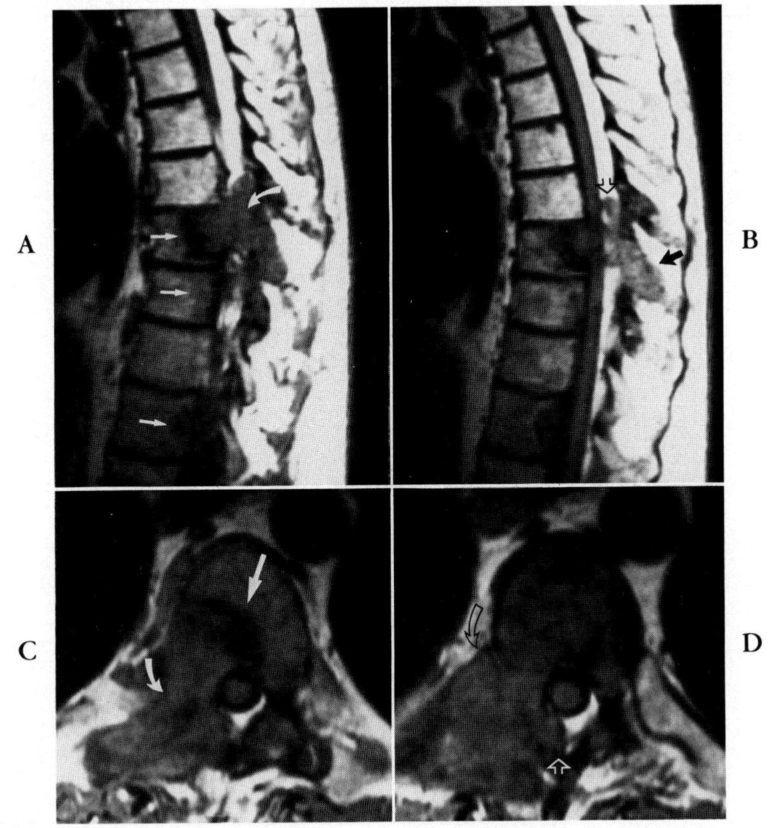

FIGURE 8-63. Lung carcinoma metastases in 36-year-old male. Sagittal T1W images (SE 800/20) show abnormal low signal in posterior T_8, T_9, and T_{11} vertebral bodies (**A,** *straight arrows*). Very low signal in T_8 lesion is result of sclerotic vertebral reaction. Abnormal signal on right posteriorly at T_8 (**A,** *curved arrow*) is result of extension of tumor into lateral spinal canal from pedicle. **B,** Replacement of normal high signal in posterior epidural fat *(open arrow)* represents tumor infiltration. Tumor signal also replaces marrow signal in pedicle adjacent to epidural tumor *(solid arrow)*. High signal in T_3-T_7 vertebral bodies is secondary to previous radiation therapy. Axial T1W images (SE 1000/20) show abnormal low signal in right posterolateral T_8 vertebral body (**C,** *straight arrow*) where metastatic tumor and bony sclerosis have replaced normal marrow. Intermediate signal tissue (similar to marrow signal with this pulse sequence) replaces right pedicle (**C,** *curved arrow*), causes destruction of cortical bone and proximal rib (**D,** *curved arrow*), and infiltrates epidural fat (**D,** *open arrow*).

A 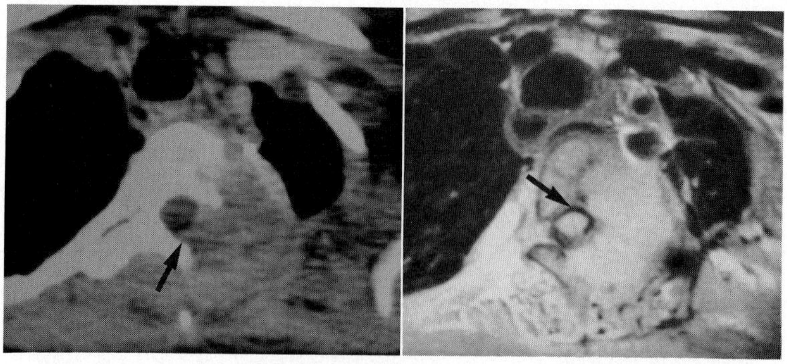 B

FIGURE 8-64. Metastasis. Apical lung carcinoma in 55-year-old male. **A,** Axial noncontrast CT scan shows contiguous spread of left apical lung tumor causing destruction of adjacent vertebral body and posterior vertebral elements. Invasion of spinal canal is shown *(arrow)* but relationship of tumor mass to spinal cord is unclear and cord compression cannot be excluded without intrathecal contrast injection. **B,** Axial T1W image (SE 400/25) shows left apical lung tumor as relatively high signal, spreading medially and causing destruction of vertebral body and posterior elements, similar to findings on CT scan. Invasion of spinal canal is shown but relationship between tumor and cord is better delineated than on CT. Cord cross section is clearly seen surrounded by semicircle of low signal anteriorly *(arrow),* which represents pulsating CSF through constricted subarachnoid space. Posteriorly, CSF is relatively static and appears higher signal than anteriorly but lower signal than cord. Findings separate cord from tumor and exclude cord compression. Direct visualization of bone destruction is better with CT but determination of status of spinal cord is better shown by MR study.

A, B 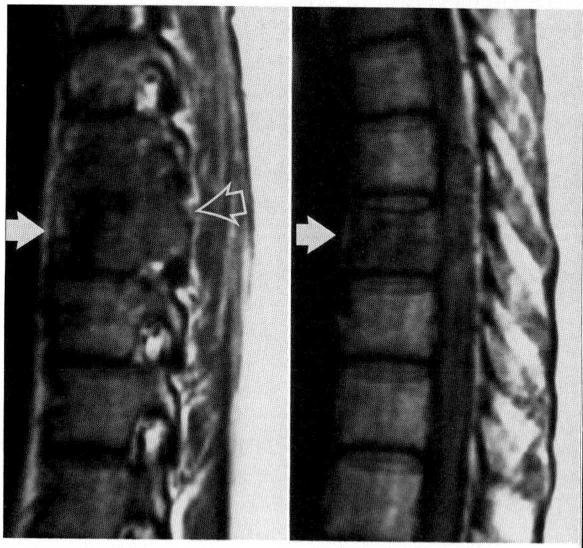

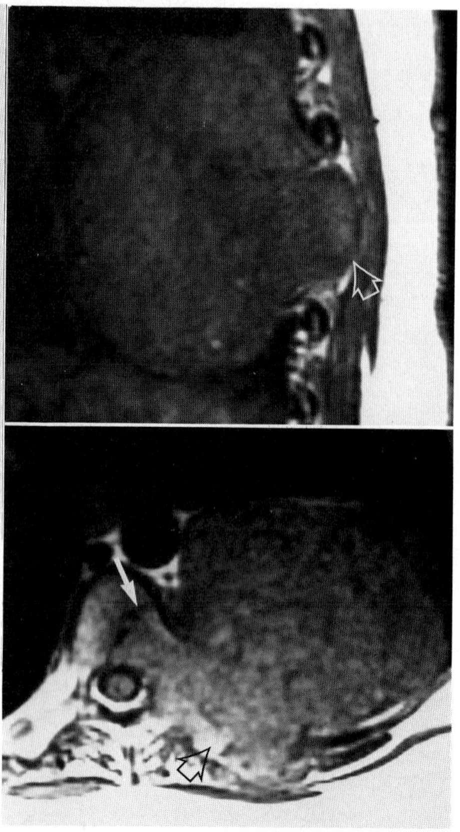 C

D

FIGURE 8-65. Malignant fibrous histiocytoma with local invasion of thoracic spine in 29-year-old female. Sagittal T1W images (SE 800/20) through left neural foramina (**A**) and midline (**B**) show subtle signal reduction in T_7 and T_8 vertebral bodies *(closed arrows).* Abnormal signal is posterior, replacing normal high signal of fat in neural foramina and obscuring pedicle of T_8 *(open arrow).* **C,** Sagittal T1W image (SE 800/20) left of thoracic spine shows large thoracic mass (malignant fibrous histiocytoma) with posterior extension destroying and replacing eighth rib *(arrow).* **D,** Axial T1W image (SE 1000/20) through T_8 shows large left thoracic mass with local invasion of vertebral body *(closed arrow)* and posterior extension destroying proximal eighth rib *(open arrow).* Spinal cord is not compressed.

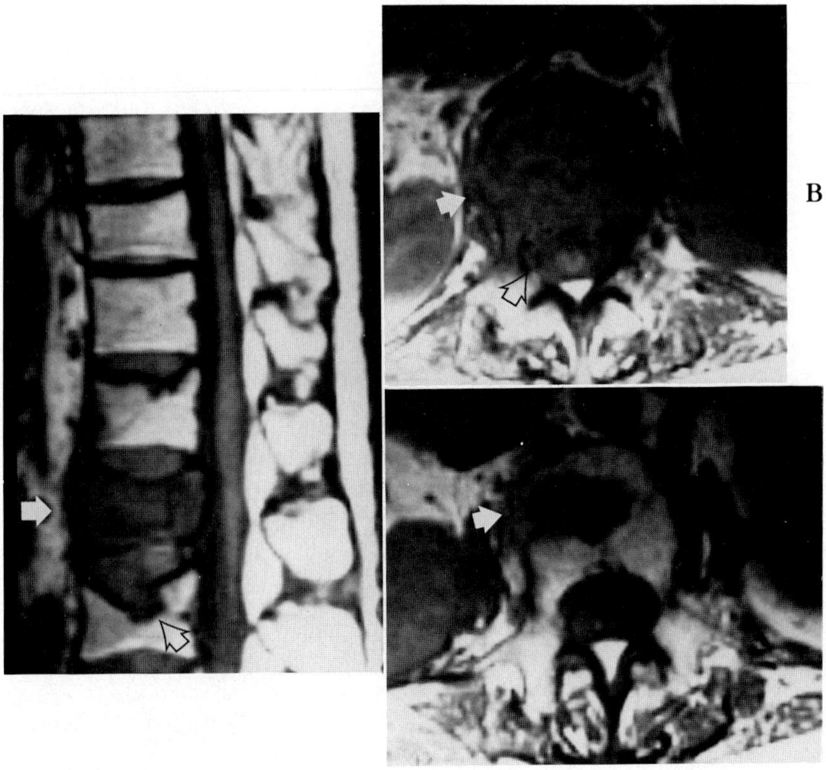

FIGURE 8-66. Breast metastasis to T_{12} after radiation therapy in 58-year-old female. **A,** Sagittal T1W image (SE 800/20) shows diffuse, uniform high signal in bone marrow of T_8-T_{11} and L_1 representing fatty infiltration of marrow in response to radiation exposure. Low signal in T_{12} indicates replacement of marrow by tumor metastasis *(solid arrow)*. Partial collapse of T_{12} is present with posterior expansion but no impingement of conus medullaris. Apparent Schmorl's indentation in superior end-plate of L_1 has some unusual features suggesting that it may actually represent metastatic tumor. Signal in anterior portion of T_{12}-L_1 disc is lower than that posteriorly and this tissue appears to extend into central L_1 vertebral body *(open arrow)*. In addition, low signal adjacent to disc at superior margin of L_1 (end-plate plus chemical shift artifact at disc-marrow interface) is less prominent centrally, suggesting penetration of tissue through end-plate. Destruction of vertebral cortex adjacent to this area on axial T1W images (**B** and **C**) supports hypothesis. **B,** Axial T1W image (SE 800/20) through midbody of T_{12} shows diffuse low signal representing complete replacement of marrow by metastatic tumor. Destruction of cortical bone with extravertebral tumor *(solid arrow)* and epidural extension of tumor *(open arrow)* medial to right pedicle are also present. Direct impingement on conus medullaris is not detected. **C,** Axial T1W image (SE 800/20) through midbody of L_1 shows low signal centrally with extension to right anterior vertebral body margin. Destruction of vertebral cortex *(arrow)* confirms presence of metastatic tumor suggested on sagittal image (**A**).

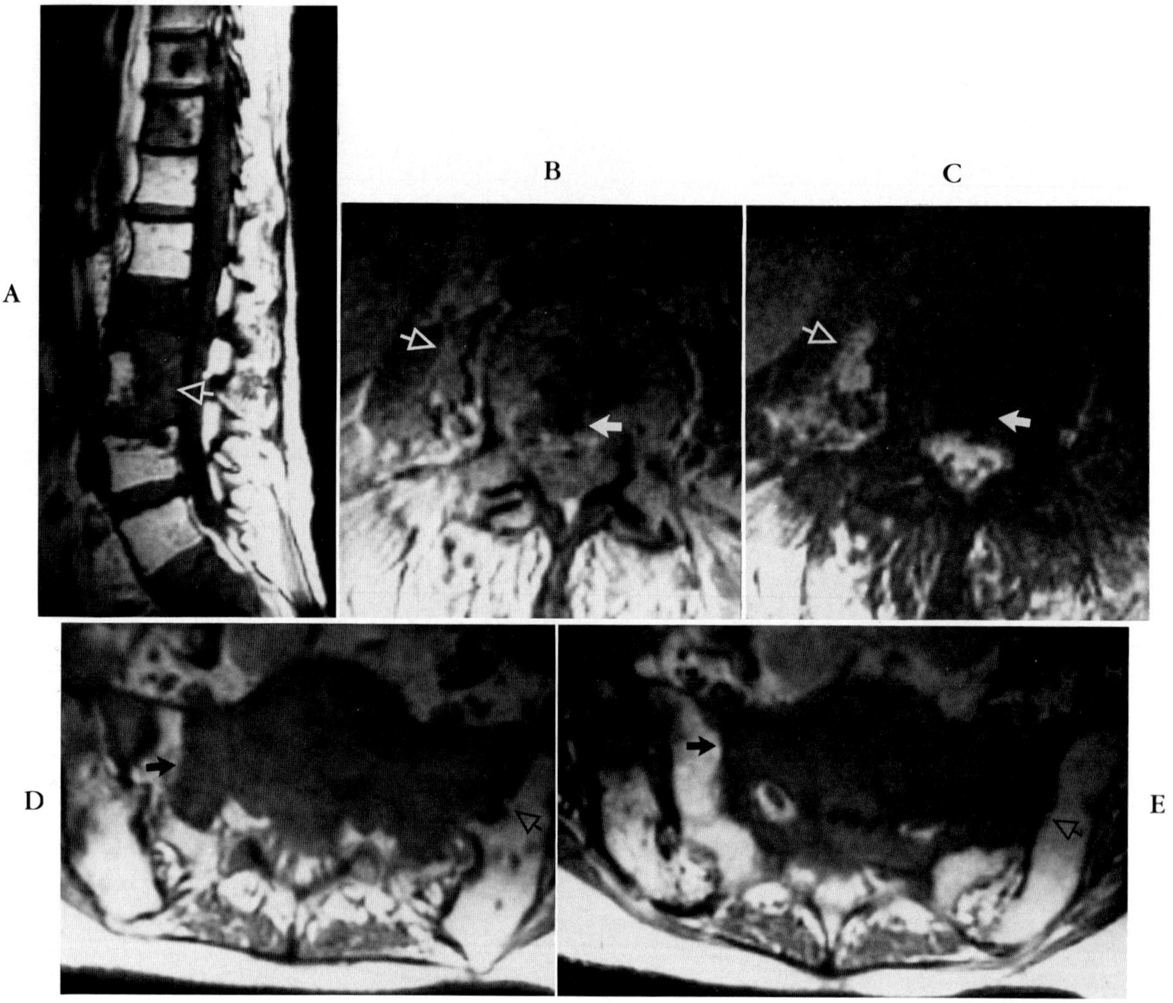

FIGURE 8-67. Breast metastases to lumbar and thoracic spine after radiation therapy in 49-year-old female. **A,** Sagittal T1W image (SE 800/20) shows well-circumscribed lesions in T_{10}, T_{11}, L_2-L_4 (small focus superiorly), and S_1. Tumor in posterior half of L_3 is isointense with adjacent discs *(arrow)*. High signal in uninvolved marrow is result of fatty infiltration of marrow in response to radiation exposure. Note lesion in L_4 is lower signal intensity than L_3 lesion. Axial T2W images (SE 2400/20, **B**; 80, **C**) through lesion in superior part of L_4 vertebral body. First echo image (**B**) shows low signal in mid- and posterior vertebral body *(solid arrow)* corresponding to low signal lesion on sagittal T1W image (**A**). Signal on second echo image (**C**) is isointense with adjacent bone marrow *(solid arrow)*. Signal in lesion, low on first echo image and isointense on second echo image, suggests partially sclerotic metastasis. Mixed water (long T1) and bone (low proton density) in each pixel produces low signal relative to fat on first echo image. Same combination limits elevation of signal in lesion on second echo image to isointensity with fat because of "dilution" of water signal by low proton density bone and T2* shortening secondary to bone magnetic susceptibility effects. Paraspinous spread of metastatic tumor to right psoas muscle is also present, as intermediate signal intensity, slightly higher than muscle, on first echo image (**B**, *open arrow*) and high signal on second echo image (**C**, *open arrow*). **D** and **E**, Axial T1W images (SE 1000/20) through S_1 level show extensive low signal metastatic tumor through most of sacrum with sharply defined margins *(black arrows)* and extending to sacroiliac joint on left *(open arrows)*.

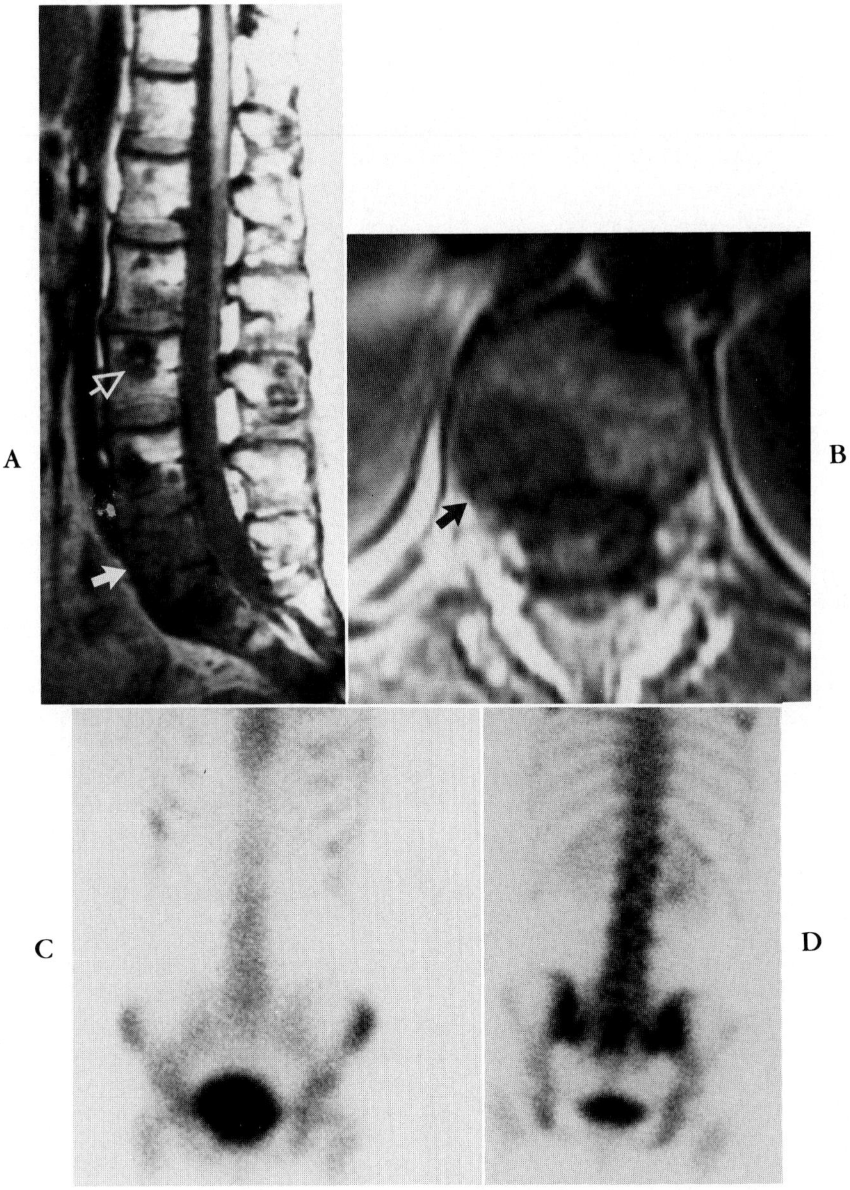

FIGURE 8-68. Breast metastases to thoracolumbar spine in 49-year-old female with normal bone scan. **A,** Sagittal T1W image (SE 800/20) shows multiple low signal lesions in lumbar spine, including inferior body of L_2, round lesions in L_3 and L_4, and complete replacement of normal marrow signal in L_5 *(solid arrow)* and S_1. Very low signal in L_3 and L_4 vertebral bodies represents sclerotic lesions *(open arrow)*. **B,** Axial T1W image (SE 1000/20) through T_{12} vertebral body shows low signal, well-circumscribed metastatic lesion on right *(arrow)*. **C,** Anterior and **D,** posterior views of bone scan (99mTc MDP) show no abnormal radionuclide uptake in thoracolumbar vertebral bodies. No evidence of multiple lesions on MR images.

A 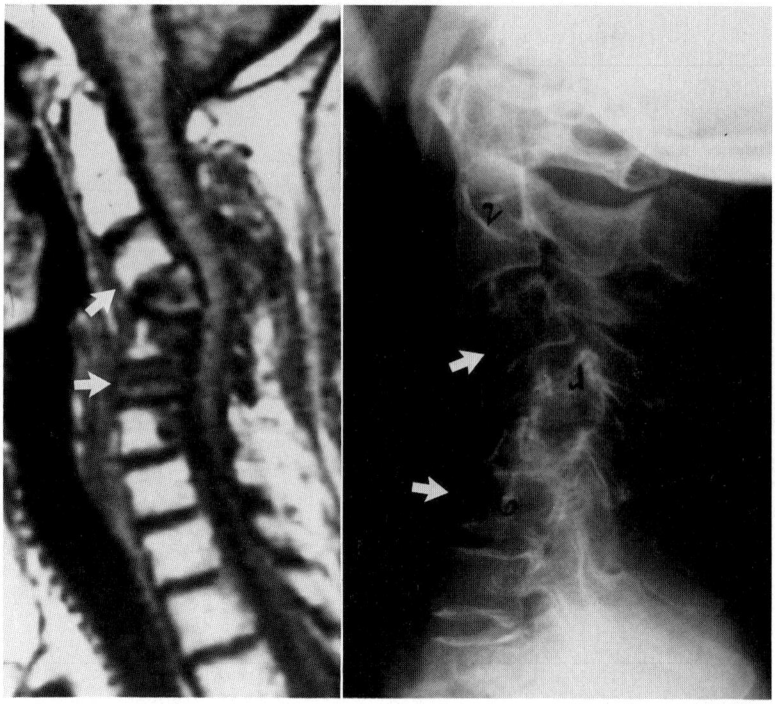 B

FIGURE 8-69. Breast metastases to cervical spine in 61-year-old female. **A,** Sagittal T1W image (SE 20/400) shows abnormal low signal in C_4-C_6 and C_7 vertebral bodies with pathologic fracture and anterior wedging of C_4. Sharp posterior angulation of cervical vertebral column at C_4 produces marked deviation of spinal cord. Posterior laminectomy defect is present at level of angulation. Note marked difference in signal in anterior C_3 and C_6 vertebral bodies *(arrows)*. C_3 shows high signal from fatty marrow, whereas C_6 is low signal, consistent with metastatic tumor involvement. **B,** Lateral plain film of cervical spine shows pathologic anterior wedging of C_4 and posterior angulation of vertebral column. Appearance of anterior vertebral bodies at C_3 and C_6 *(arrows)* is similar on this plain film, but clearly different on MR image.

A, B 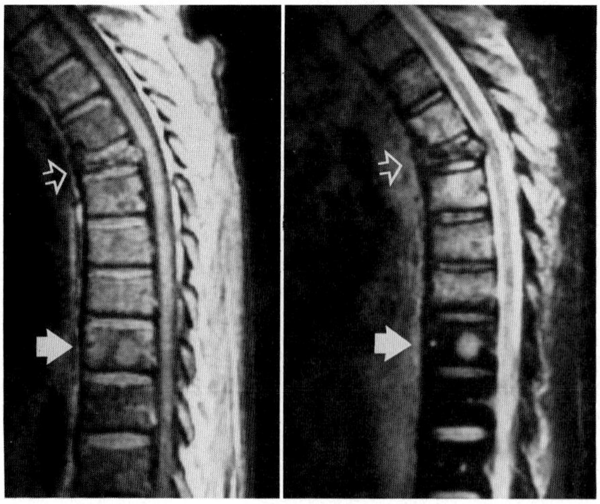

FIGURE 8-70. Breast metastases to thoracic spine in 61-year-old female. **A,** Sagittal T1W image (SE 800/20) shows high signal in upper thoracic vertebral bodies and lower intermediate signal in lower bodies. At T_{10}, anterior part of vertebral body is high signal *(solid arrow)* as is focal round area in center of vertebral body. Collapse of T_6 vertebral body (**A** and **B,** *open arrows*) with posterior protrusion and impingement on thoracic spinal cord is also seen. Marrow within collapsed body is high signal. Unclear from this image whether high or low signal marrow, or both, represent metastatic disease. T2W or fat-suppressed image is needed to assess whether signal in vertebral bodies is produced by water or fat protons. **B,** Sagittal T2W image (SE 2400/80) shows persistence of high signal in upper thoracic vertebrae and further reduction in signal in lower thoracic region. High signal on both T1W and T2W images in upper thoracic vertebrae is result of high water content (with prolonged T2) and therefore represents metastatic tumor infiltration rather than normal bone marrow. Signal fall-off between T1W and T2W images in lower thoracic vertebrae is typical of normal bone marrow with high fat content (i.e., shorter T2 than metastatic tumor). Contrast between these regions is shown clearly in T_{10} (**A** and **B,** *solid arrows*), where anterior body and round lesion have equally high signal on T1W image. On T2W image anterior body is low signal (fatty marrow) and round lesion remains high signal (metastasis). Marrow in collapsed T_6 vertebral body (**A** and **B,** *open arrows*) shows persistent high signal on T2W image, indicating metastatic tumor involvement and pathologic fracture.

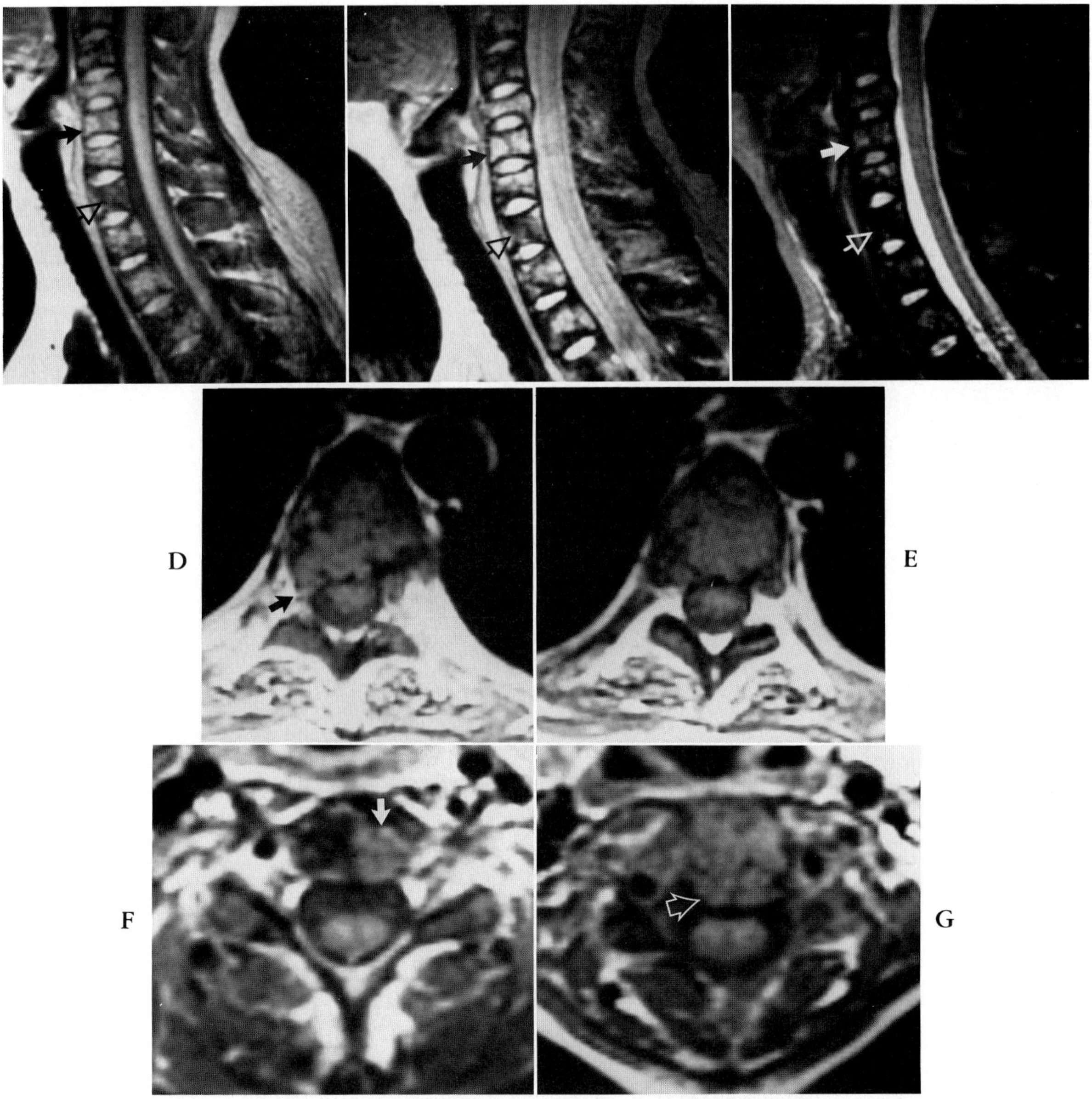

FIGURE 8-71. Breast metastasis to cervicothoracic spine in 31-year-old female. **A,** Sagittal T1W image (SE 800/20) shows unusual high signal vertebral metastases at multiple cervical and thoracic levels (C_3-C_6 and T_1-T_3). Findings are most prominent in partially collapsed body of C_4 and in anterior C_5 body *(solid arrow)*. Signal is higher in these lesions than in uninvolved marrow, such as in C_7 vertebral body *(open arrow)*. Persistence of high signal in lesions on T2W images (**C** and **D**) differentiates them from fat in normal marrow. Explanation for this atypical appearance is unclear. It may be result of very high water content and unusually prolonged T2 relaxation times (high signal can be result of "T2-contrast" in this nominally "T1-weighted" SE pulse sequence). If metastatic involvement of bone marrow is sufficiently extensive, compensatory hematopoiesis in normal marrow may shift it toward lower fat content, resulting in lower signal on T1W images. Sagittal T2W images (SE 2200/30, **B**; 80, **C**) show persistent high signal in multiple lesions on T1W image, especially in partially collapsed C_4 vertebral body and anterior body of C_5 *(solid arrows)*. Lower signal is seen in normal marrow in C_7 vertebral body *(open arrows)*. **D** and **E,** Axial T1W images (SE 1000/20) through T_6 vertebral body show relatively high signal metastatic tumor (higher than marrow) replacing central vertebral body with exophytic posterior extension into epidural space (**D,** *arrow*). Axial T1W images (SE 1000/20) through C_6 (**F**) and C_4 (**G**) show high signal tumor replacing normal marrow in left half of C_6 (**F,** *arrow*) and throughout C_4. In addition, partial collapse of C_4 results in posterior protrusion of vertebral body (**G,** *arrow*) and narrowing of spinal canal (without cord compression).

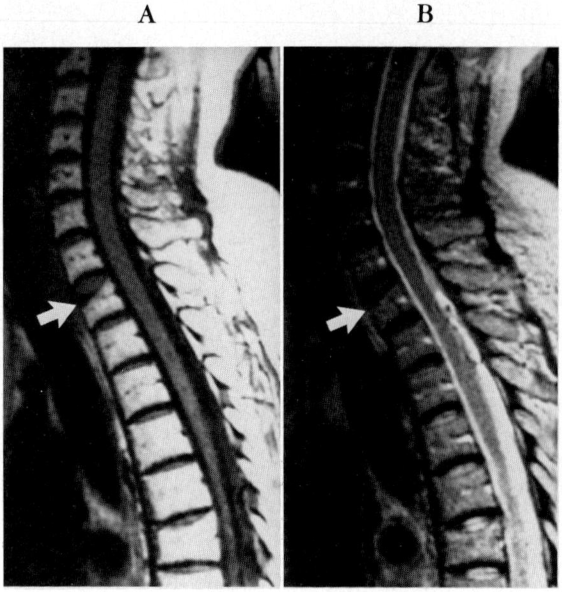

FIGURE 8-72. Breast metastasis to T_1 in 56-year-old female. Sagittal T1W images (**A,** SE 800/20) and T2W (**B,** SE 1905/80) through cervicothoracic spine show subtle low signal lesion at anterior-superior margin of T_1 on T1W image (**A,** *arrow*). Not completely clear whether this represents lesion in vertebral body or is inferior extension of adjacent disc anulus. Question is answered on T2W image where disc is seen as normal configuration (**B**). Overall signal in normal bone marrow is elevated on T1W image because of fatty change induced by previous radiation therapy. Metastasis is seen because of fat replacement. On T2W image increased signal of increased fat matches lesion signal, which has a higher water content. In this situation the T2W image clarifies nature of the lesion but provides poorer contrast for detection. Distance from surface coil contributes to low SNR and poor contrast.

A 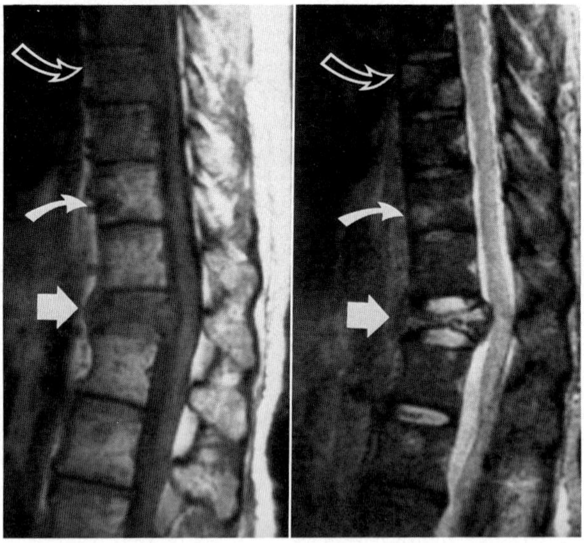 B

FIGURE 8-73. Breast carcinoma metastases with pathologic fracture of T_{12} in 46-year-old female. Sagittal T1W (**A,** SE 800/20) and T2W (**B,** SE 2000/80) images through thoracolumbar spine show collapsed T_{12} vertebral body *(straight arrows)*. Posterior protrusion of body impinges on distal spinal cord at conus medullaris (**B**). Signal within collapsed body is lower on T1W image and higher on T2W image relative to marrow in adjacent vertebral bodies. Signal characteristics are typical of metastatic tumor involvement that replaces normal fatty marrow with high water content tumor cells. Other areas of metastatic involvement are present. At T_{10}, there is region of typical signal change with low signal on T1W image and high signal on T2W image *(solid curved arrows)*. At T_7, there are two regions of high signal on T2W image that appear isointense with neighboring normal marrow on T1W image *(open curved arrows)*.

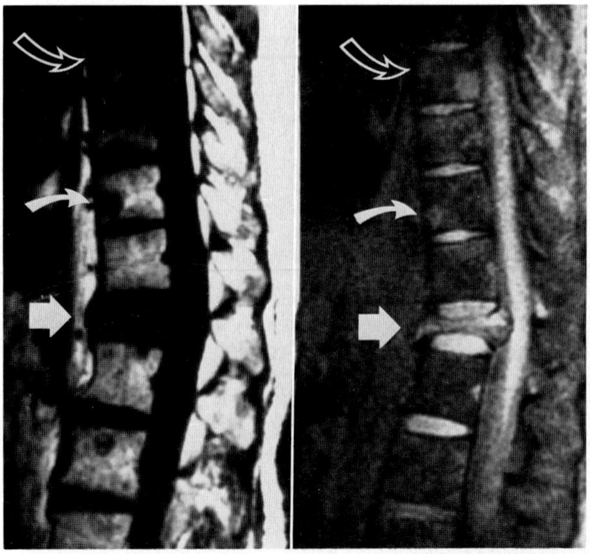

C, D

FIGURE 8-73, cont'd. Lesions appear to represent tumor replacement of normal marrow (see **C**) but with less prolongation of T1 than lesion in T_{10}. Sagittal "fat" image (water-suppressed, **C**) and "water" image (fat-suppressed, **D**) of metastatic lesions. Collapsed T_{12} vertebral body shows absence of signal on "fat" image (**C**) and high signal on "water" image (**D**) *(straight arrows)* indicating complete replacement of normal marrow by metastatic tumor. Note parallel signal changes in adjacent high water content discs. Other sites of metastatic tumor also show signal changes indicating replacement of marrow by high water content tumor cells. At T_{10}, lesion is low signal on "fat" image and high signal on "water" image (*solid curved arrows,* **C** and **D**). Lesions at T_7 *(open curved arrows),* which are isointense with marrow on T1W image (see **A**), show same signal pattern, indicating replacement of marrow fat by metastatic tumor cells rather than mix of tumor and fat cells.

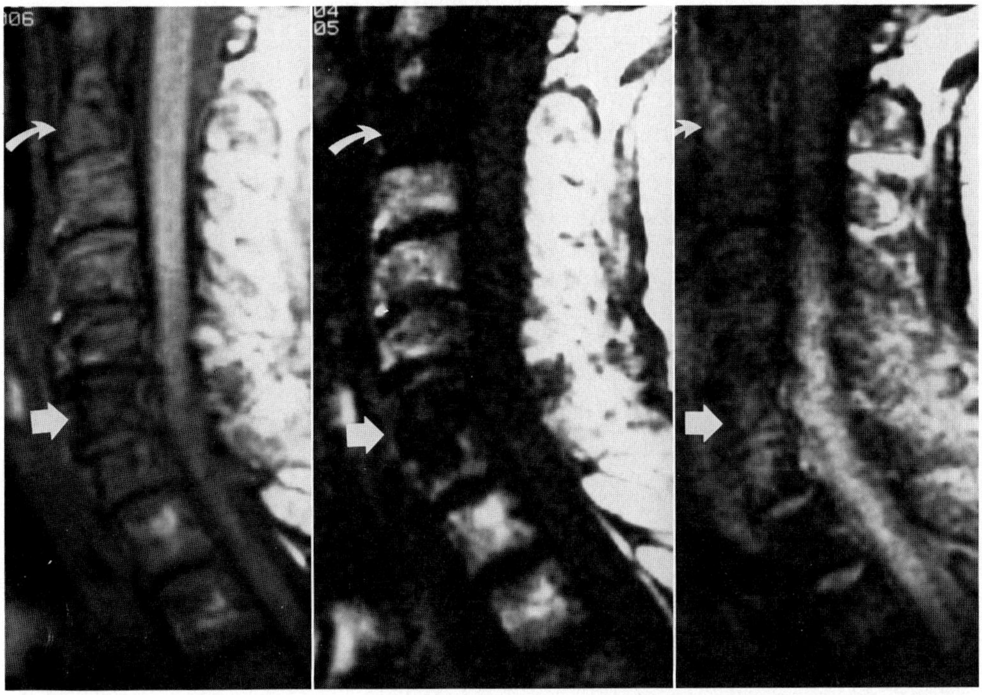

A

B, C

FIGURE 8-74. Breast carcinoma metastases in 65-year-old female. **A,** Sagittal T1W image (SE 800/20) shows slightly lower signal in C_6 and C_7 vertebral bodies *(straight arrow).* Finding is consistent with but not diagnostic of metastatic disease by itself. Signal in body of C_2 is within normal limits *(curved arrow).* Irregular high signal in C_3-C_5 and T_1-T_2 vertebral bodies is typical of patchy fatty degeneration of normal marrow seen in patients of this age. **B,** Sagittal water-suppressed image (low signal represents water protons; high signal is from fat protons) matching T1W image in **A** shows marked loss of signal in C_6 and C_7 vertebral bodies *(straight arrow),* indicating that source of signal on T1W image is water and not fat. Focal absence of fat indicates presence of metastatic neoplasm. Patchy high signal in C_3-C_5 and T_1-T_2 vertebral bodies is result of normal fatty infiltration of marrow. Low signal in body of C_2 *(curved arrow)* also indicates metastatic disease, which was not evident on T1W image. **C,** Sagittal "water" image (fat-suppressed) shows areas of metastatic tumor involvement as high signal (representing water protons) in C_6 and C_7 vertebrae *(straight arrow)* and C_2 *(curved arrow).* Combination of low signal on "fat" image and "high" signal in corresponding area of "water" image appears sensitive for metastatic tumor.

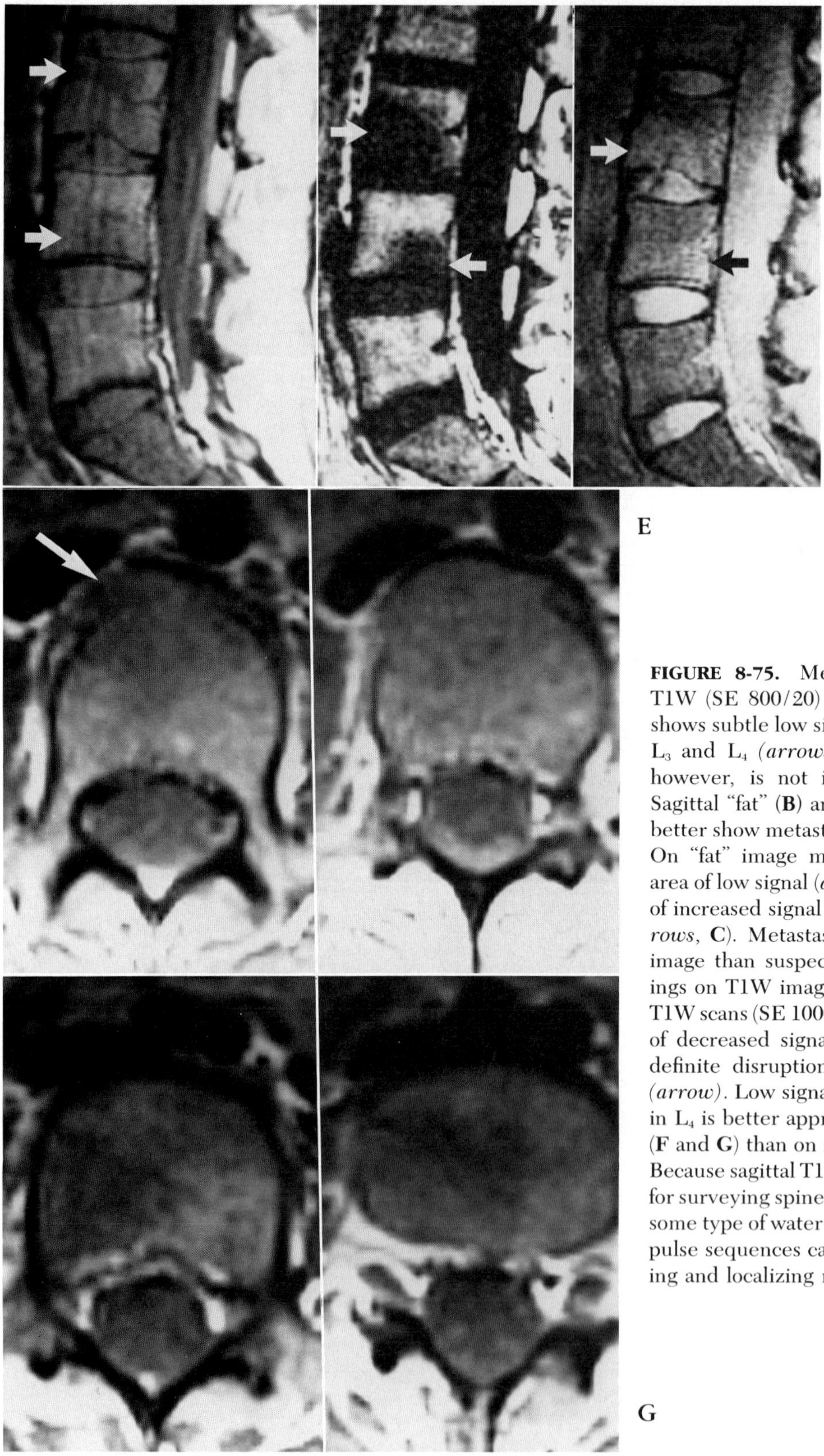

A B, C D E F G

FIGURE 8-75. Metastases. **A,** Sagittal T1W (SE 800/20) scan of lumbar spine shows subtle low signal intensity areas in L_3 and L_4 *(arrows)*. Metastatic tumor, however, is not immediately obvious. Sagittal "fat" (**B**) and "water" (**C**) images better show metastatic sites in L_3 and L_4. On "fat" image metastatic sites are an area of low signal (*arrows*, **B**) and an area of increased signal on "water" image (*arrows*, **C**). Metastases are larger on "fat" image than suspected from subtle findings on T1W image (**A**). **D** and **E,** Axial T1W scans (SE 1000/20) show subtle area of decreased signal intensity in L_3 and definite disruption of cortex anteriorly *(arrow)*. Low signal intensity metastases in L_4 is better appreciated on axial scans (**F** and **G**) than on sagittal T1W scan (**A**). Because sagittal T1W scan is usually used for surveying spine for metastatic lesions, some type of water and fat discrimination pulse sequences can be useful in detecting and localizing metastatic tumor.

A

B, C

D

E, F

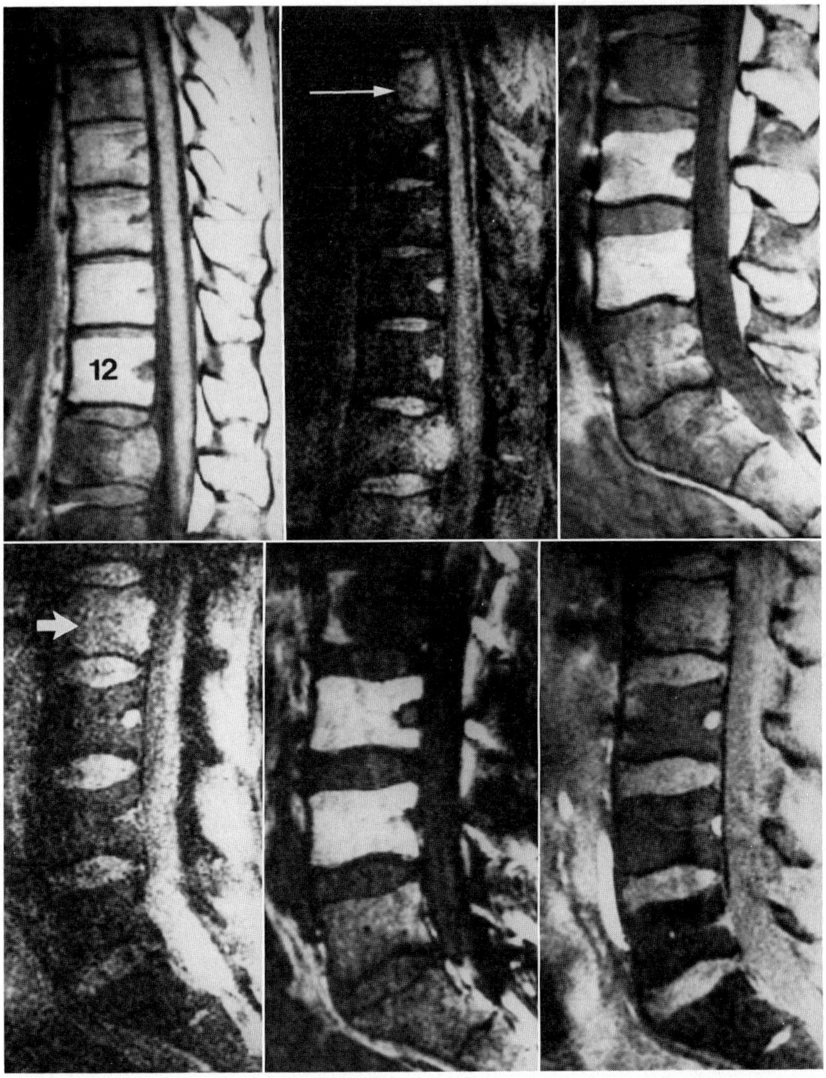

FIGURE 8-76. Metastatic renal cell carcinoma. T1W images (SE 800/20, **A** and **C**) compared with STIR images (IR 1400/40, TI 100, **B** and **D**) and "fat" (**E**) and "water" (**F**) images. In thoracic spine T1W scan (**A**) shows several degrees of signal abnormality in vertebral bodies. T_{11} and T_{12} show increased signal intensity secondary to fat replacement of normal marrow. T_8, L_1, and L_2 show abnormal low signal intensity on T1W image (**A**) that corresponds to abnormal high signal intensity on STIR image (**B**). No abnormal signal is noted on STIR images in postradiation fat replaced vertebra (**B**). Note that on T1W image (**A**) metastatic deposit in T_8 is difficult to visualize, whereas on STIR sequence (*arrow*, **B**) metastatic site is easily detectable. In lumbar spine T1W scan (**C**) shows increased marrow signal in L_3 and L_4 indicative of postradiation effect. L_2 shows marked abnormal low signal intensity indicative of metastatic disease. L_5 and S_1 show heterogeneous intermediate signal intensity higher than that of metastatic disease but lower than postradiation vertebra. Tumor involvement of vertebrae is problematic because of unusual signal intensities of adjacent comparative vertebrae. STIR sequence shows abnormal signal intensity of L_2 (*arrow*, **D**) but normal signal intensities of L_3-L_5. "Fat" (**E**) and "water" (**F**) images confirm lack of metastatic involvement of L_3-L_5. "Fat" image shows marked increased signal intensity of postradiation vertebrae L_3 and L_4. L_5 is uninvolved, showing intermediate signal intensity. "Water" image (**F**) shows abnormal increased signal intensity of L_2 but normal signal intensities of L_3-L_5. Postradiation vertebrae, L_3 and L_4, show slight increase in signal intensity compared to L_5, indicating minimal degree of increased water content.

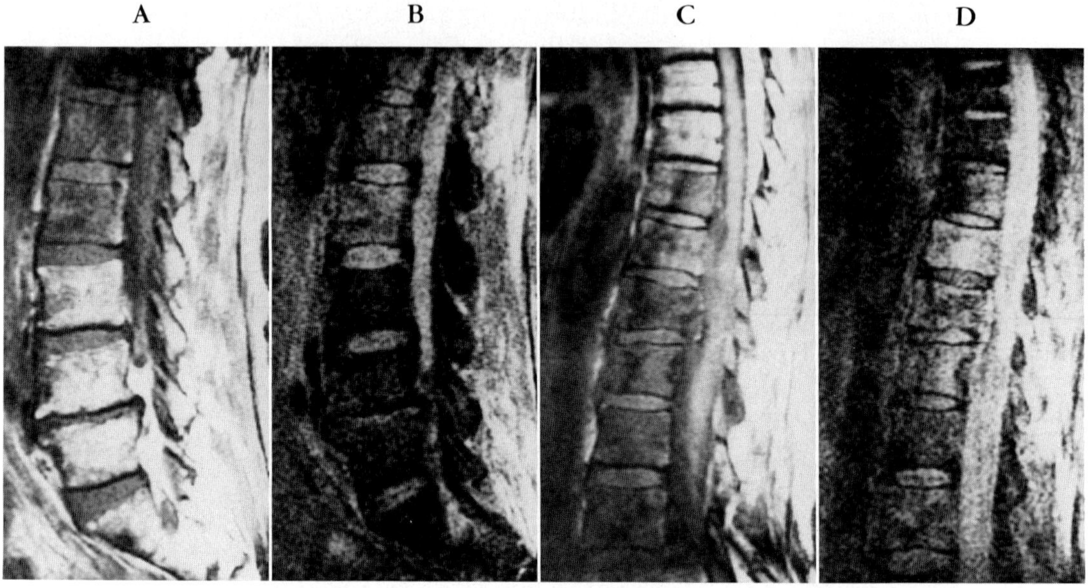

FIGURE 8-77. Metastasis: breast carcinoma. Comparison of T1W scans (SE 800/20) with STIR scans (IR 1400/40, T1 100) in patient with metastatic breast carcinoma. **A,** In lumbar spine sagittal T1W scan shows abnormal low signal intensity of L_1 and L_2 indicative of metastatic disease. **B,** On STIR image the two vertebrae show abnormal high signal compared to more normal signal seen in L_3-L_5 with this pulse sequence. **C,** In thoracic spine vertebra body signal intensity is inhomogeneous on the T1W scan. Many vertebrae show abnormal low signal intensity. Upper vertebra show increased signal intensity because of marrow replacement by fat as a result of radiation therapy. **D,** STIR image shows abnormal high signal in areas corresponding to low signal in T1W image (**C**). Abnormal soft tissue within spinal canal is better appreciated on T1W scan (**C**) compared to STIR scan (**D**). STIR images, despite lower SNR, have high contrast between abnormal neoplastic tissue in vertebra compared to normal marrow. Contents of spinal canal are better appreciated on T1W scan in part because STIR sequence is susceptible to flow effects, which are more detectable when CSF has relative high signal.

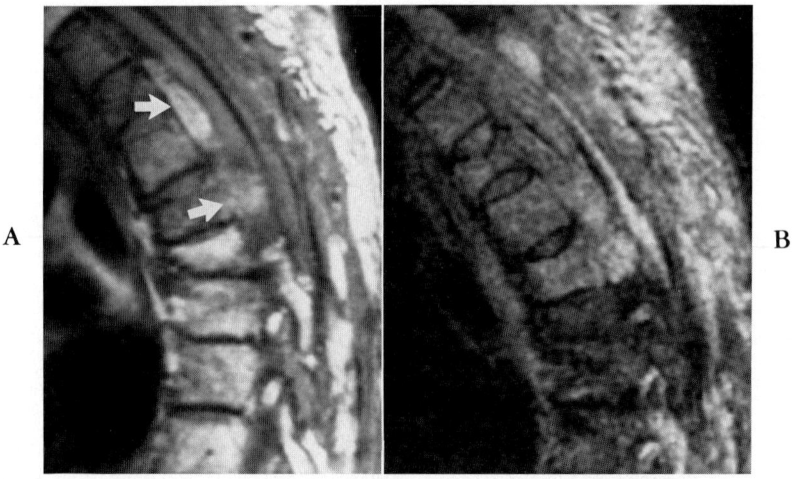

FIGURE 8-78. Metastasis: liposarcoma. Scans of a patient with metastatic liposarcoma compare findings on T1W scan (SE 800/20, **A**) with those on STIR scan (IR 1400/40, TI 100, **B**). T1W scan shows midthoracic vertebral bodies involved by metastases to be lower signal intensity than unaffected vertebral bodies. STIR sequence shows involved vertebrae of increased signal intensity. T1W scan has advantage of better delineating epidural tumor, which can cause cord compression (*arrows*, **A**), whereas STIR sequence does not adequately differentiate between epidural tumor, cord, and CSF (**B**). Pulse sequences can yield complementary information in patients with metastatic disease of spine.

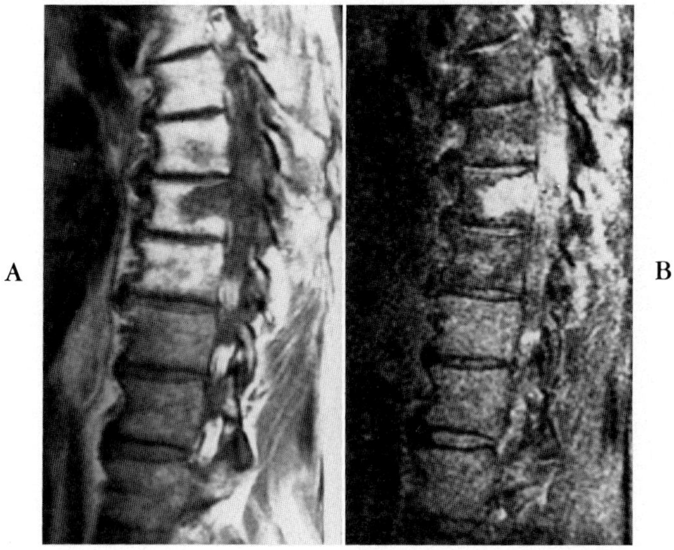

FIGURE 8-79. Metastases: lung. Scans of 65-year-old male with lung carcinoma show comparison of T1W scan (SE 800/20, **A**) and concomitant STIR scan (IR 1400/40, TI 100, **B**). Metastatic site is low signal intensity on T1W scan (**A**), whereas comparable area is high signal on STIR scan (**B**). Fat replacement of marrow causes high signal of vertebrae in radiation field (**A**). Fat-replaced vertebrae are lower signal intensity on STIR sequence than normal uninvolved lower thoracic vertebrae. Although STIR sequences are low signal to noise ratio when TI is chosen to suppress fat, some residual signal is detected in normal vertebrae.

A 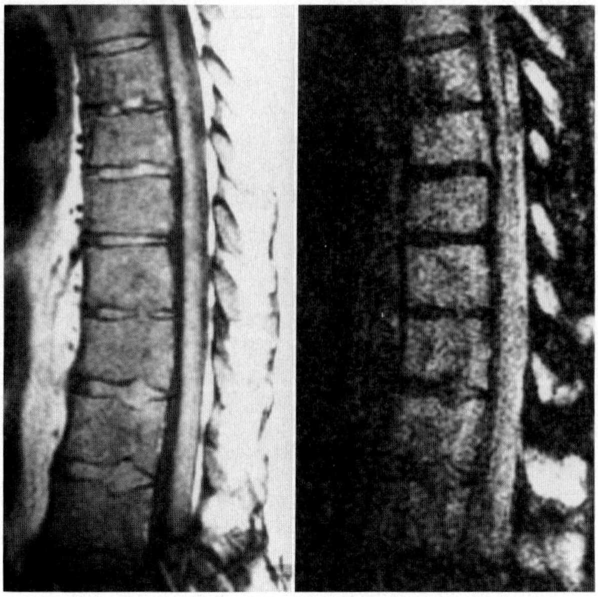 B

FIGURE 8-80. Lung metastases. Diffuse metastatic disease to the vertebrae is not detected on conventional T1W scan but is well seen on a STIR scan. **A,** Sagittal T1W scan (SE 800/20) shows minimal inhomogeneity of signal intensity of vertebral bodies that is not unusual for a 61-year-old male. Mineral degenerative changes are noted. **B,** Sagittal STIR scan (SE 1400/40, TI 150) shows diffuse abnormal high signal indicative of diffuse metastatic disease throughout all of the vertebrae (biopsy proven). Detection of vertebral metastatic disease is dramatically more evident on STIR sequence compared to conventional T1W scan.

A 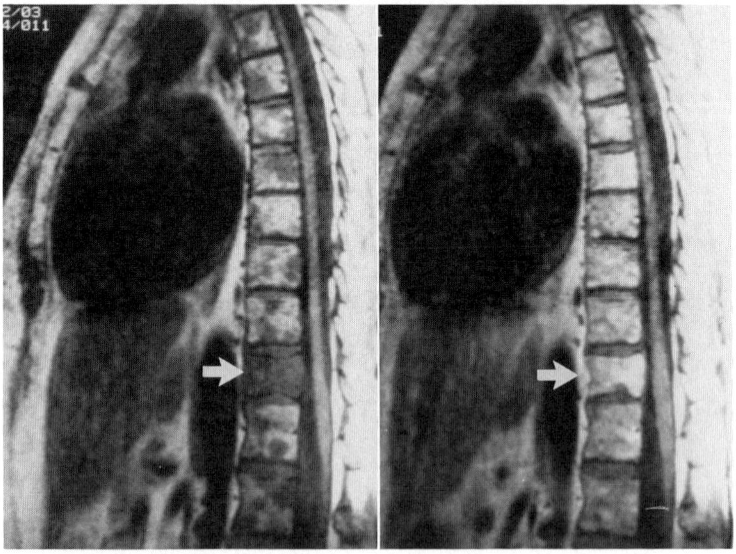 B

FIGURE 8-81. Metastases. Sagittal T1W scans show potential of contrast agent GdDTPA to obscure metastatic disease in vertebral bodies. **A,** Precontrast T1W scan shows obvious heterogeneous low signal lesions throughout thoracic and upper lumbar spine. **B,** After infusion of GdDTPA signal intensity of vertebral bodies is more homogeneous and diagnosis of metastases to vertebral bodies is more difficult. Note prominent enhancement of low thoracic vertebrae that is converted from grossly abnormal (*arrow*, **A**) to nearly normal (*arrow*, **B**). GdDTPA therefore is not recommended in routine investigation of metastases to spine. (Courtesy of Dr. David Norman.)

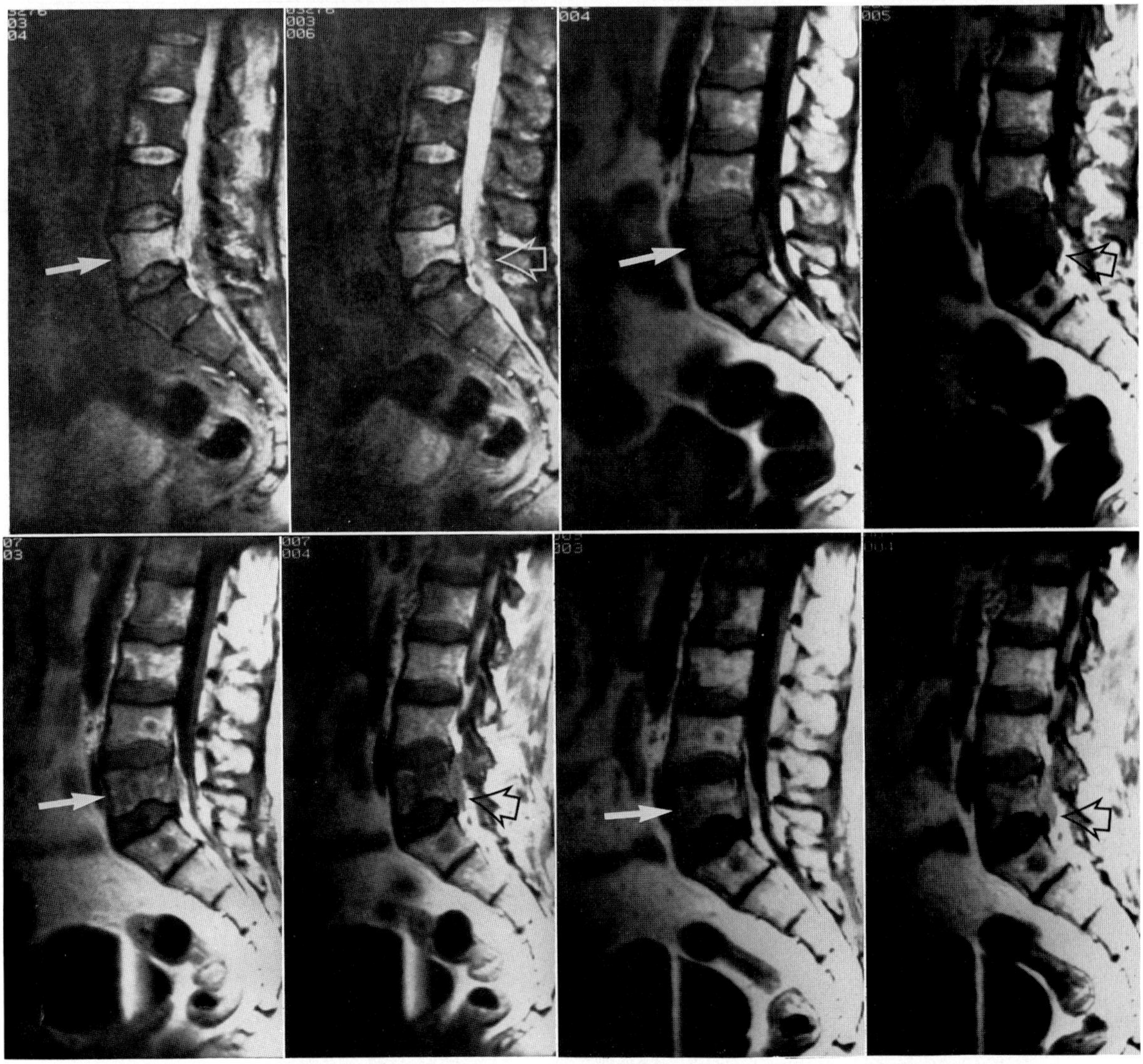

, B C, D

, F G, H

FIGURE 8-82. Colon carcinoma metastases with GdDTPA contrast enhancement in 59-year-old male. **A** and **B,** Sagittal T2W images (SE 2000/70) show marked high signal from metastatic tumor throughout L_5 vertebral body *(solid arrow)* and anterior portions of L_2 and L_3 bodies. Epidural tumor posterior to L_5 vertebral body is also present as area of mixed signal *(open arrow).* **C** and **D,** Sagittal T1W images (SE 600/20) show low signal (similar to disc and lower than normal marrow) metastases corresponding to high signal on T2W images in L_2, L_3, and L_5 *(solid arrow).* Epidural tumor posterior to L_5 appears as intermediate signal tissue replacing fat *(open arrow).* Round areas of low signal in L_4 and S_1 vertebral bodies are isointense on T2W images and probably represent sclerotic focus. **E** and **F,** Sagittal T1W images (SE 600/20) immediately after intravenous administration of 0.1 mmoles/kg GdDTPA show partial enhancement of signal throughout L_5 vertebral body, bringing signal up to level similar to normal marrow in adjacent vertebral bodies *(solid arrow).* Lesions in anterior portions of L_2 and L_3 show reduced contrast against adjacent marrow signal. Epidural tumor posterior to L_5 shows enhancement and slightly reduced contrast against epidural fat *(open arrow).* **G** and **H,** Sagittal T1W images (SE 600/20) obtained 1 hour after GdDTPA administration show further enhancement of signal in L_5 vertebral body *(solid arrow)* that is nearly isointense with normal marrow. Contrast between epidural tumor *(open arrow)* and fat posterior to L_5 is also reduced. Little change seen in other metastatic foci. (Courtesy of Dr. Gordon Sze.)

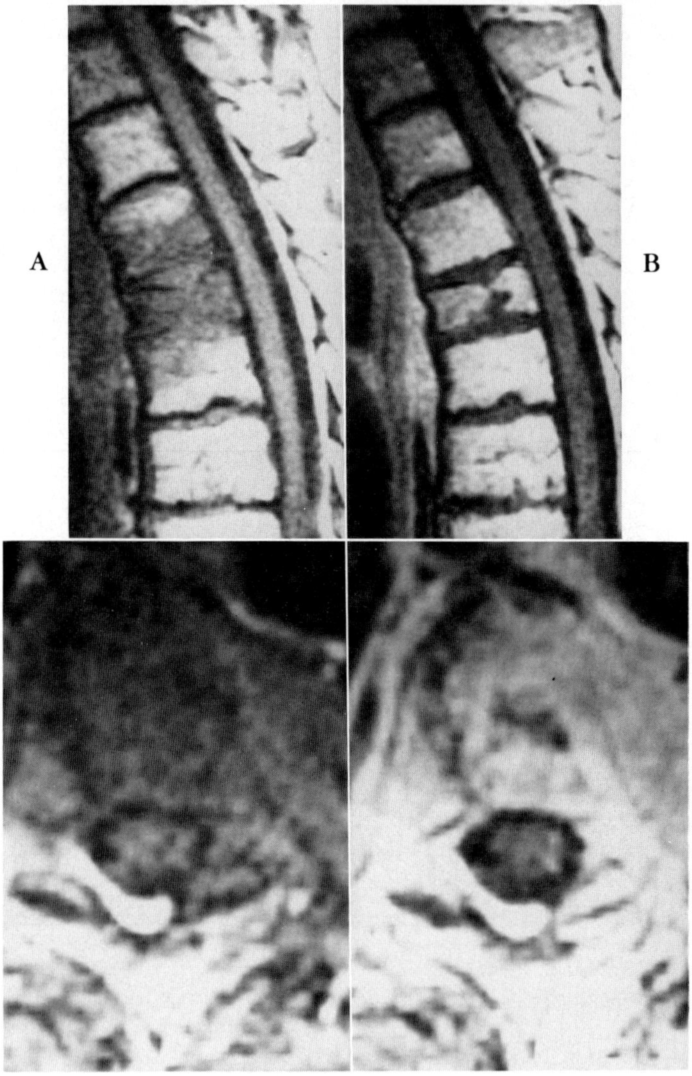

FIGURE 8-83. Lymphoma. Pre-GdDTPA (**A**) and post-GdDTPA (**B**) sagittal T1W scans (SE 800/20) of patient with lymphoma in which contrast enhancement of tumor diminishes its detectability. Contrast enhancement within thoracic vertebrae causes signal intensity of involved vertebrae to become similar to high signal intensity of adjacent vertebrae that exhibit typical radiation change. Compression fracture remains evident. Axial precontrast (**C**) and postcontrast (**D**) shows enhancement of vertebral body tumor, as well as soft tissue and epidural components (**D**).

A B C D E F

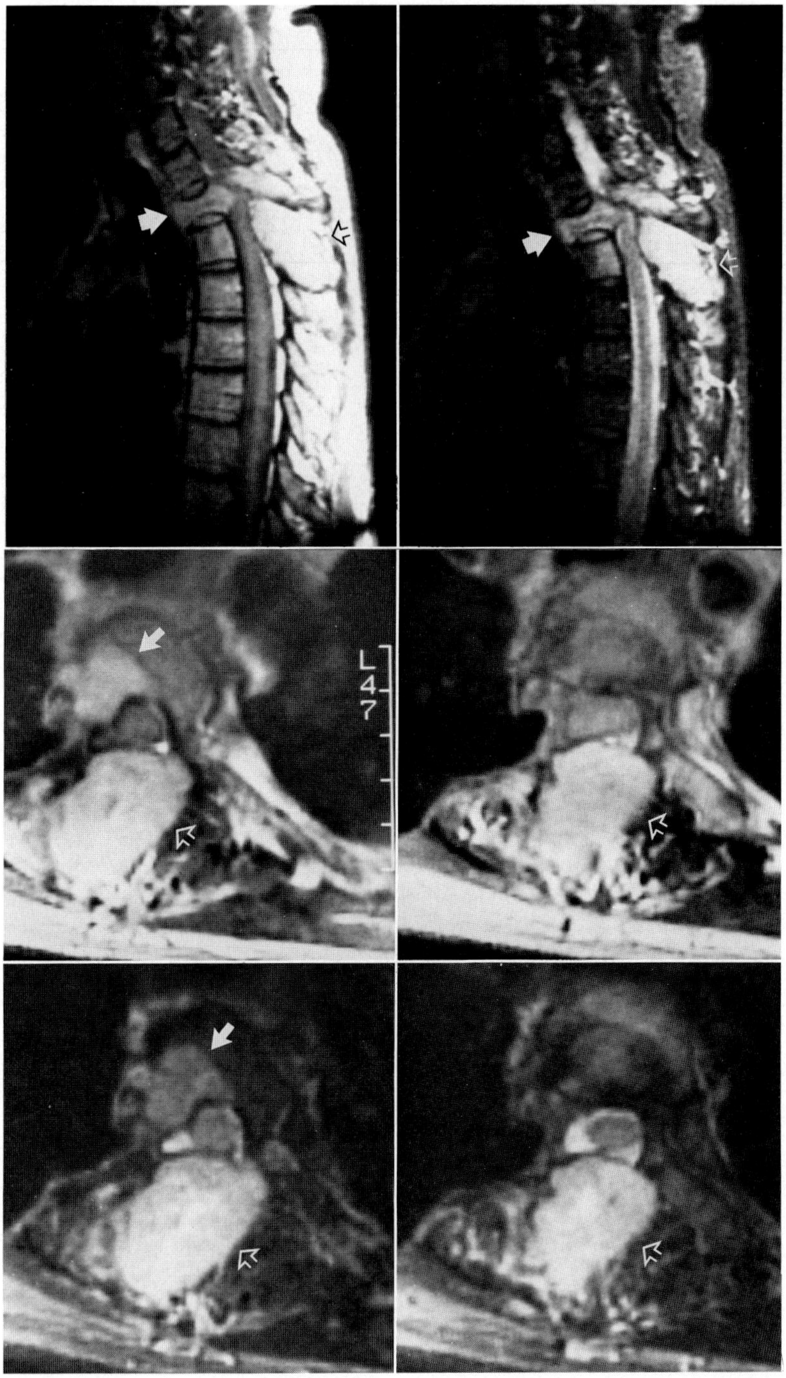

FIGURE 8-84. Metastasis. Thyroid carcinoma in 48-year-old male. **A** and **B**, Sagittal T2W images (SE 2500/25, 80) show collapse of T_2 with high signal metastasis *(solid arrows)* in marrow causing posterior protrusion of vertebral body. Large posterior metastatic mass is also present *(open arrows)*. Spinal cord, seen best on second echo image (**B**), appears to be compressed between collapsed vertebral body and posterior mass. **C-F**, Axial T2W images (SE 2500/25, 80) at T_3 show moderately high signal metastasis in right side of vertebral body (**C** and **E**, *solid arrows*). Large mass (**C** and **E**, *open arrows*) with same signal characteristics is present posteriorly and replaces posterior vertebral elements. Distinction between spinal cord and CSF is unclear on first echo images (**C** and **D**) but is clarified on second echo images (**E** and **F**), which show cord displacement but not compression suggested by sagittal images. Tumor impingement on spinal canal is severe enough to dampen CSF pulsation (**B**). CSF is seen without motion artifact in these scans, which have no motion compensation attributes.

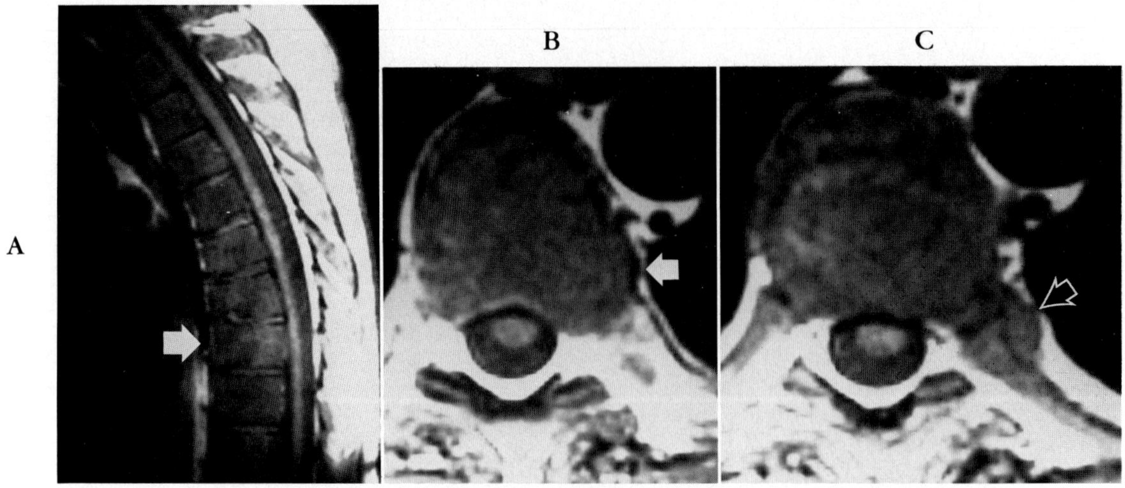

FIGURE 8-85. Lung carcinoma metastases with subtle thoracic spine findings in 38-year-old male. **A,** Sagittal T1W image (SE 800/20) shows subtle mottled pattern of high and low signal throughout thoracic spine. Some areas have more sharply circumscribed, geographic appearance suggestive of metastatic disease (i.e., low signal in anterior T_{10} vertebral body *(arrow)*, but it is difficult to make a definite diagnosis. Posterior margin of T_{10} is indistinct, raising question of whether relative high signal metastasis is present and causing destruction of cortical bone. Axial images through T_{10} are needed to clarify these ambiguities. **B** and **C,** Axial T1W images (SE 1000/20) through T_{10} show enlargement of left posterolateral vertebral body (**B,** *arrow*). Enlargement represents destructive enlargement of metastatic disease and is slightly lower signal than normal marrow on right side of vertebral body. Extension of metastasis laterally, adjacent to proximal rib is also seen on right (**C,** *arrow*). High signal in posterior part of T_{10} on sagittal image (**A**) appears to represent normal marrow slightly to right of midline (cord is included by partial volume averaging in this 5 mm thick, off-midline sagittal slice).

Metastatic disease in some patients may be obvious but interpretation of findings requires thought and two perpendicular views (Figure 8-84). The question of cord compression requires axial views for confirmation (see Figure 8-84), and perpendicular views are recommended for any suspicious area because axial views may provide crucial diagnostic information (Figure 8-85). This is certainly true for degenerative disease that could mimic metastatic disease. Partial volume averaging of normal high-signal marrow on T1W images with adjacent lower signal intensity disc material should not be confused with metastatic deposits. This problem occurs frequently in the axial plane when an oblique axial slice includes normal disc tangentially, or when a large Schmorl's node indentation into the vertebral body end-plate is present and partially imaged. Orthogonal sagittal or coronal images will usually clarify the anatomy and alleviate any confusion between partial volume averaging artifacts and metastatic deposits. A similar problem may be seen on sagittal images at lateral margins of the vertebral bodies where low signal cortical bone may be partially averaged with higher signal marrow on T1W images. This becomes a problem with severe degenerative changes of the spine, especially with subchondral sclerosis (Figure 8-86). With such artifacts, reference to an orthogonal image plane will usually clarify the anatomy and exlude or confirm the presence of metastatic disease. Infection of vertebral bodies results in signal changes similar to those caused by replacement of marrow by neoplastic cells. However, the distribution of these changes differs (see Chapter 7) and the adjacent disc space usually exhibits some signal changes. T2W images are helpful in delineating disc space and epidural tissue signal abnormalities. Obviously the clinical history is important in the differentiation. (Figures 8-86 and 8-87).

A B

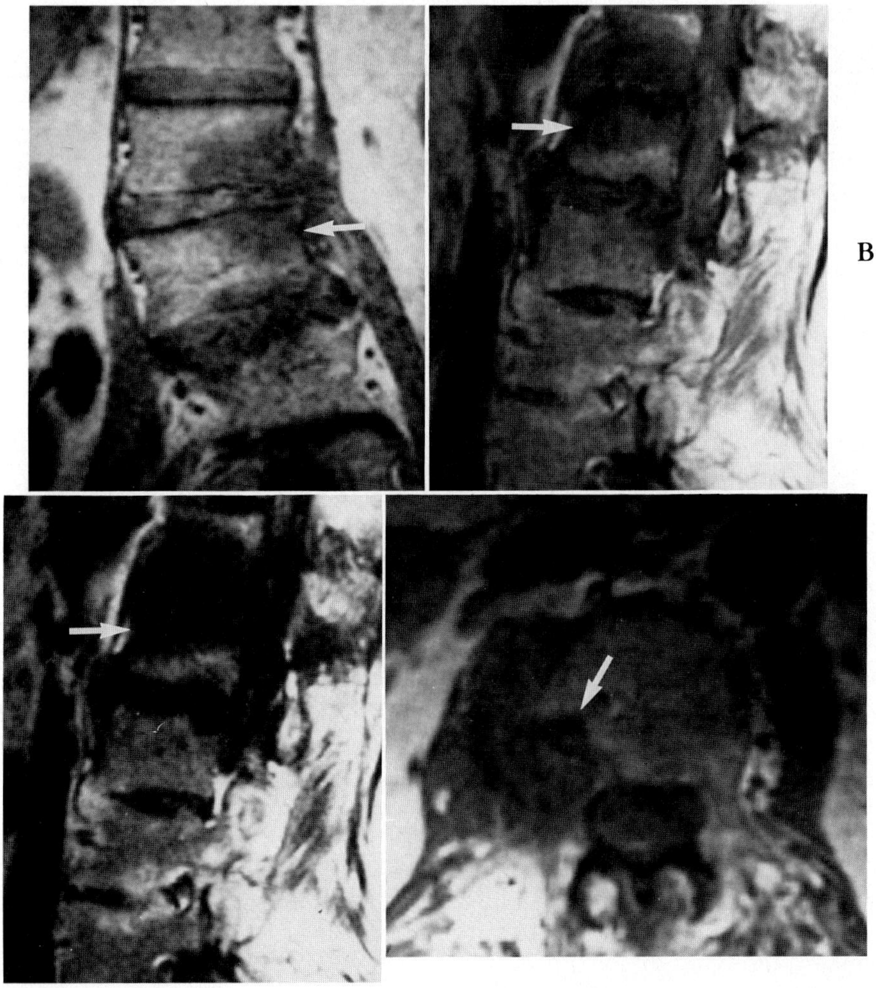

C D

FIGURE 8-86. Psoriatic arthritis mimicking metastatic disease in 75-year-old male. **A,** Coronal T1W image (SE 800/20) through thoracolumbar spine shows low signal replacing normal marrow on left at T_{12} and L_1 *(arrow)*. Disc is asymmetrically narrowed. Changes are caused by sclerosis and inflammatory changes rather than metastatic disease. However, in patient of this age, metastatic disease is always a prime consideration. **B,** Sagittal T1W image (SE 800/20) shows low signal areas in T_{12} and L_1 *(arrow)* adjacent to narrowed disc. **C,** Sagittal "water-suppressed" image (signal from fat only) shows that areas of low signal on T1W image correspond to nonfatty regions of marrow, probably combined effect of sclerosis and inflammation replacing normal marrow. **D,** Axial T1W image (SE 600/20) through L_3 vertebral body shows changes in pedicle and posterior vertebral body *(arrow)* very suggestive of metastatic diseases that were, in fact, result of patient's psoriatic arthritis.

A 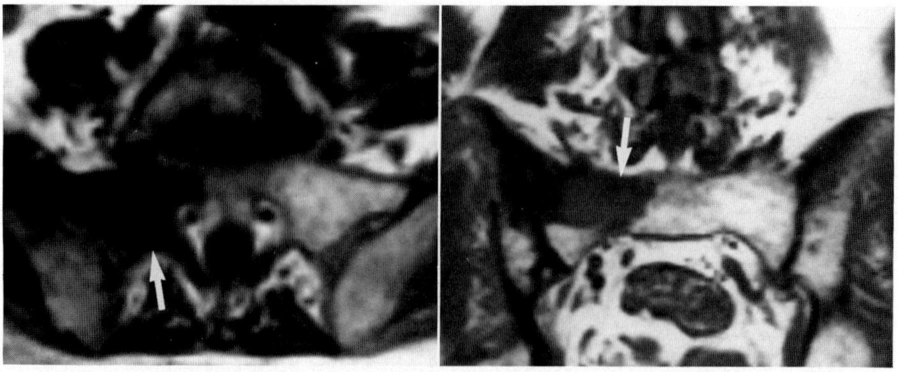 B

FIGURE 8-87. Paget's disease mimicking metastatic disease in 73-year-old male. **A,** Axial and **B,** coronal T1W images (SE 800/20) show uniform low signal with sharp margins replacing normal marrow signal in S_1 on the right *(arrows)*. These changes correspond to sclerotic lesions of Paget's disease. Patient's history and the presence of other characteristics of Paget's disease may be the only way to distinguish these abnormalities from sclerotic metastases.

Leptomeningeal Tumor

Leptomeningeal tumor spread occurs with primary non-CNS and CNS tumors. Non-CNS tumors include lung carcinoma, breast carcinoma, and melanoma. Non-Hodgkin's lymphoma is a relatively common cause of leptomeningeal tumor spread. In rare instances, leptomeningeal tumor from a non-CNS source is the primary manifestation of tumor and the primary tumor is never identified (Figure 8-88). Leptomeningeal tumor spread from primary CNS tumors occurs with glioblastoma, ependymoma, medulloblastoma, and pineal tumors (primary pineal and germinal cell tumors).[14]

Meningeal infiltration occurs with acute leukemia. Leukemic infiltration of the dura appears in 70% of patients with acute lymphocytic leukemia and 59% of patients with acute myelocytic leukemia. Arachnoid infiltration occurs in 30% of cases, more frequently with lymphocytic leukemia, and more commonly in children than adults. As with malignant lymphomas, infiltration may extend along the perivascular spaces to invade the parenchyma of the spinal cord and nerve roots.[43] Meningeal infiltration may produce presenting symptoms in as many as 15% of cases of leukemia.[66]

Leptomeningeal tumor is characterized pathologically by sheets of tumor cells coating the leptomeninges. In such instances, even gross examination of the meninges may not reveal tumor. As the amount of tumor increases the leptomeninges become thickened and opalescent. In addition to the thin layer of tumor cells, the subarachnoid spread of tumor may result in the formation of large nodules. The term *carcinomatous meningitis* is used to reflect an inflammatory component that can be seen in some patients.

The clinical presentation of leptomeningeal tumor is often nonspecific.[36,52,54] A common presentation is that of simple back pain that is not well localized. Some patients may show evidence of meningeal irritation. In more severe cases, if cord invasion is also present, the patient may present with a myelopathy. Diagnosis can be difficult, especially in patients with no known primary tumor. Intracranial leptomeningeal spread may accompany the spinal form of the disease. These patients may show intracranial symptoms: headache, change in mental status, and cranial nerve deficits.

A definitive diagnosis is made when cerebrospinal fluid (CSF) cytology is positive. Imaging studies can be helpful in the diagnosis. Myelography and intrathecally enhanced CT are useful in showing findings indicative of tumor spread: nodular filling defects in the subarachnoid space, adhesion of nerve roots, and irregularity of nerve roots. MR without benefit of an intravenous contrast agent has low sensitivity to this disease process, having a false negative rate around 40%.[37] The use of GdDTPA greatly improves sensitivity and reduces false negatives.[5,72]

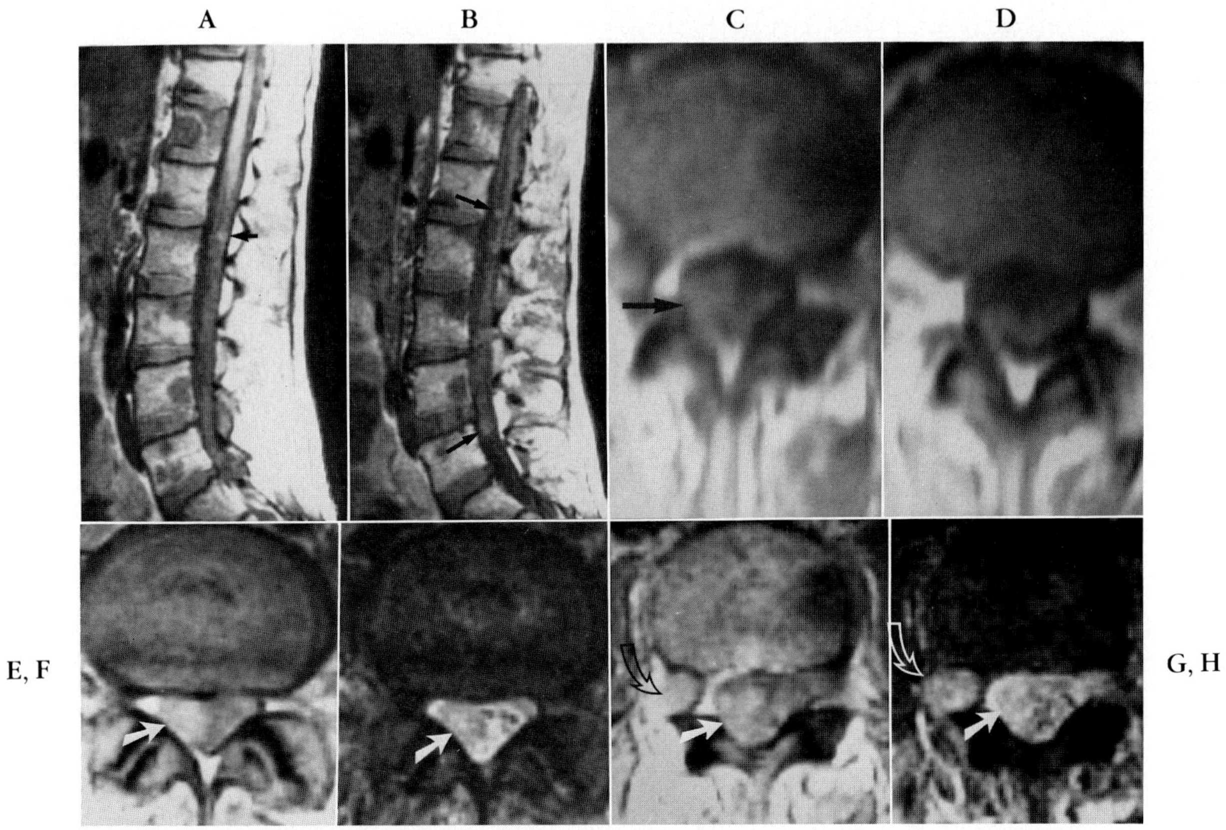

FIGURE 8-88. Leptomeningeal carcinomatosis. **A** and **B,** T1W sagittal scans (SE 800/20) show diffuse metastatic lesions in vertebrae and nodular lesions in cauda equina *(arrows)*. Cauda equina normally has smooth tapering appearance with homogeneous signal intensity; in this patient it is irregular with inhomogeneous signal intensity. In addition, intermediate signal intensity structure is seen as low as L_4-L_5, a location where normal cauda signal is not seen. **C** and **D,** Axial T1W scans (SE 1000/20) show abnormal soft tissue signal intensity within dural sac (**C,** *arrow*). Axial T2W scans (SE gated, 2100/20, 80) show some areas of increased signal intensity on first echo (*solid arrows,* **E** and **G**) and intermediate to high signal nodules on second echo (*solid arrows,* **F** and **H**). Second echo T2W images demonstrate individual nerve roots that can only be identified individually in left half of spinal canal because they are obscured on right side by tumor and adhesions. Significant finding and clue to diagnosis of leptomeningeal carcinomatosis is enlarged ganglion on right side, seen on both first and second echo images (**G** and **H,** *curved arrows*). Spread of leptomeningeal tumor to ganglion causing enlargement is important indirect finding in diagnosing disease processes that involve subarachnoid space.

A

B

C

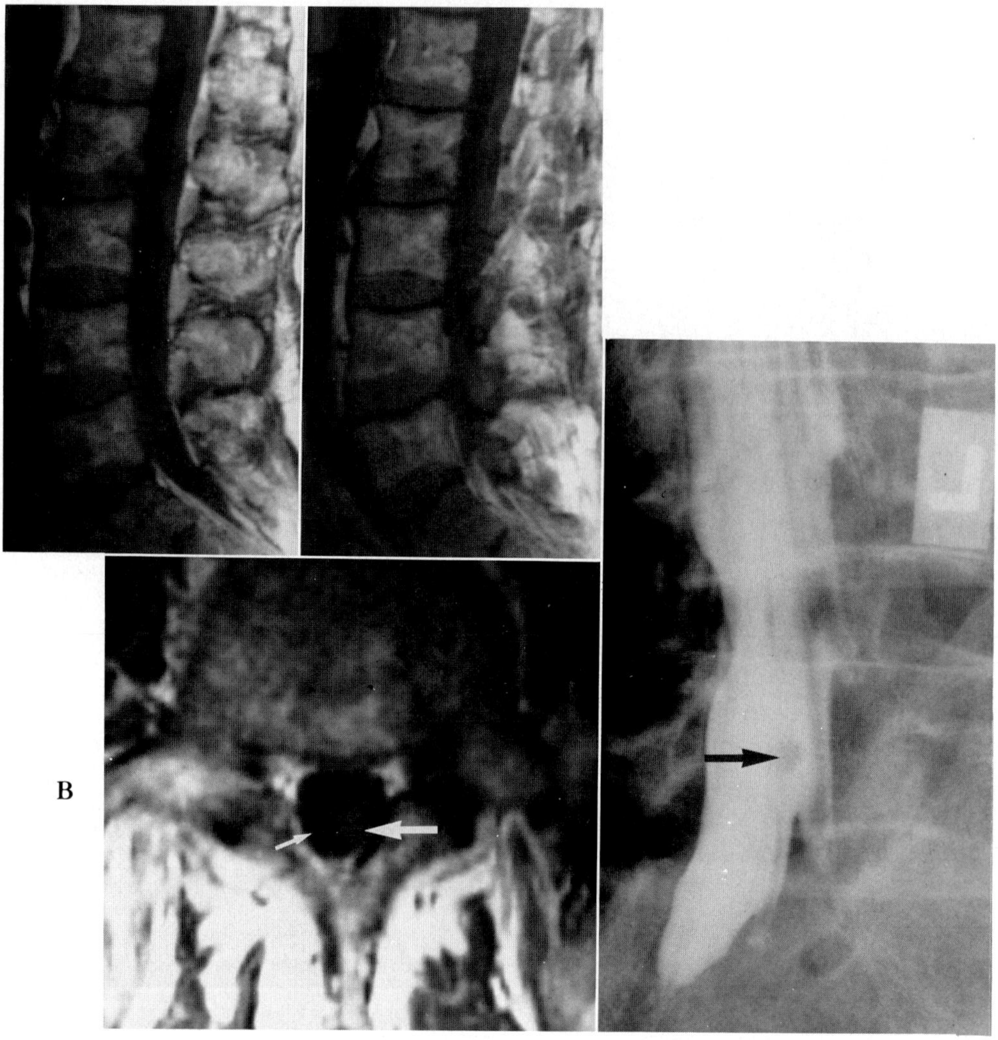

FIGURE 8-89. Subarachnoid seeding from cervical ependymoma (see Figure 8-11) is not well seen on sagittal T1W image (SE 800/20) but visualized on axial T1W scan (SE 1000/20). **A** and **B,** On sagittal scan, tumor nodule is difficult to detect posterior to L_5 vertebrae. **C,** Tumor nodule is clearly seen on the axial scan at this level *(large arrow)*. Individual lumbar and sacral nerve roots can be seen as punctate areas of increased signal compared to surrounding CSF (*small arrow,* **C**). **D,** Water soluble myelogram confirms presence of tumor nodule at L_5 level *(arrow)*.

MR Findings

T1W images may be negative or demonstrate only subtle findings in leptomeningeal tumor. Diagnostic criteria are similar to those used in myelography and CT. The important diagnostic finding is one of identifying small nodules on the surface of the cord or attached to nerve roots of the cauda equina (Figure 8-89; see Figure 8-88). Although nodules can appear anywhere in the spinal canal (Figure 8-90), they are most easily visualized in the cauda equina or lower in the lumbar sac where one does not expect to see significant soft tissue signal intensity. The T1W manifestation of leptomeningeal tumor may resemble that of arachnoiditis, i.e., adherence or matting of nerve roots (Figures 8-91 and 8-92). This is especially prominent in the cauda equina, which normally has a uniform signal intensity and a gradual tapering shape.[42] Leptomeningeal carcinomatosis may cause the cauda equina to appear irregular and have areas of inhomogeneous signal intensity without obvious tumor nodules. Both sagittal and axial images are important in confirming areas of suspected abnormal soft tissue signal intensity. T1W images may show little or no evidence of leptomeningeal tumor (see Figures 8-94 to 8-96). Axial T1W images could produce false positive images in which clumping of nerve roots could be simulated by the end-slice in-flow phenomenon (Figure 8-93).

T2W images are of limited value because tumor nodules may have high signal intensity similar to that of normal CSF, reducing contrast between tumor and CSF and making detection difficult (see Figures 8-88 and 8-96). In the axial view they may be useful in an indirect way because individual nerve roots in the cauda normally can be identified. Roots that are matted together, obscured, or asymmetrically distributed in the spinal canal indicate adhesion that may be secondary to leptomeningeal tumor, infection, or to arachnoiditis of various etiologies (see Figure 8-88). An important finding on T2W images that may also be seen on T1W and T2W images is that of enlargement of the spinal ganglia (see Figure 8-88). In leptomeningeal carcinomatosis the spinal ganglia may be enlarged and show abnormal high signal intensity on T2W images. This is not seen in simple arachnoiditis.

It is clear from the previous discussion that subtle areas of leptomeningeal tumor, especially when it forms thin sheets in the subarachnoid space, can be missed on conventional T1W and T2 weighted images (Figure 8-94; see Figure 8-96). Therefore, contrast material such as GdDTPA is necessary to make the correct diagnosis.[5,79] A difficult diagnosis with conventional MR images becomes relatively simple with the use of GdDTPA (Figures 8-95 and 8-96; see Figures 8-92 and 8-94), which shows enhancement of tumor in the subarachnoid space on T1W images. The enhancement can be intense and virtually fill the subarachnoid space (see Figure 8-96) or it may be subtle, causing only a thin line of enhancement along the margin of the cord (Figure 8-97). This enhancement reflects increased permeability of the blood-brain (cord) barrier similar to that seen in the intracranial cavity with contrast enhancement of leptomeningeal tumor. The fact that leptomeningeal tumor may have an inflammatory component probably increases the blood-brain barrier permeability that, in turn, increases the usefulness of contrast media. Whereas noncontrast MR has low sensitivity, GdDTPA MR scans have high sensitivity to leptomeningeal tumor spread[72] and is the examination of choice.

Radiation Changes

In children and adults the vertebral bodies contain red marrow, hematopoietic marrow, which contains reticulum cells and other hematopoietic precursors. It is characterized by extensive sinosoidal vascular space. Sinosoidal system characteristics are associated with increased deposition of metastases. Whereas the vertebral body has red marrow, the pedicles and posterior elements have yellow marrow characterized by fat-laden reticulum cells and a paucity of hematopoietic elements. Instead of a sinosoidal system, the vascular channels have characteristics of capillaries and venules. Yellow marrow typically is a rare site for metastatic implants. The exception is the vertebral pedicle that in spite of having yellow marrow still has significant vascularity, causing it to be a relatively common site for metastases. In the more peripheral portions of the skeleton, bone marrow converts to yellow marrow with increasing age. If there is stress to the hematopoietic system, yellow marrow can reconvert to red marrow.

Marrow space, as well as red and yellow marrow, may undergo fatty infiltration that is localized to adipose tissue rather than fat-laden reticulum cells. This is considered a normal aging process, noted in the spine, and causes increased heterogenity of marrow tissue with increasing age.

Radiation of red marrow in the spine causes a loss of reticulum cells and the hematopoietic cursors. Red marrow is replaced by adipose tissue. This tissue does not reconvert to red marrow because it basically differs from yellow marrow. If neoplastic tissue is present in the marrow and it replaces red marrow, radiation may result in the neoplastic tissue being replaced by adipose tissue or the neoplastic tissue being replaced by fibrotic tissue. In either case, normal marrow does not reoccupy metastatic sites. These basic concepts help to understand the MR appearance of the spine after radiation therapy.

Continued on p. 413.

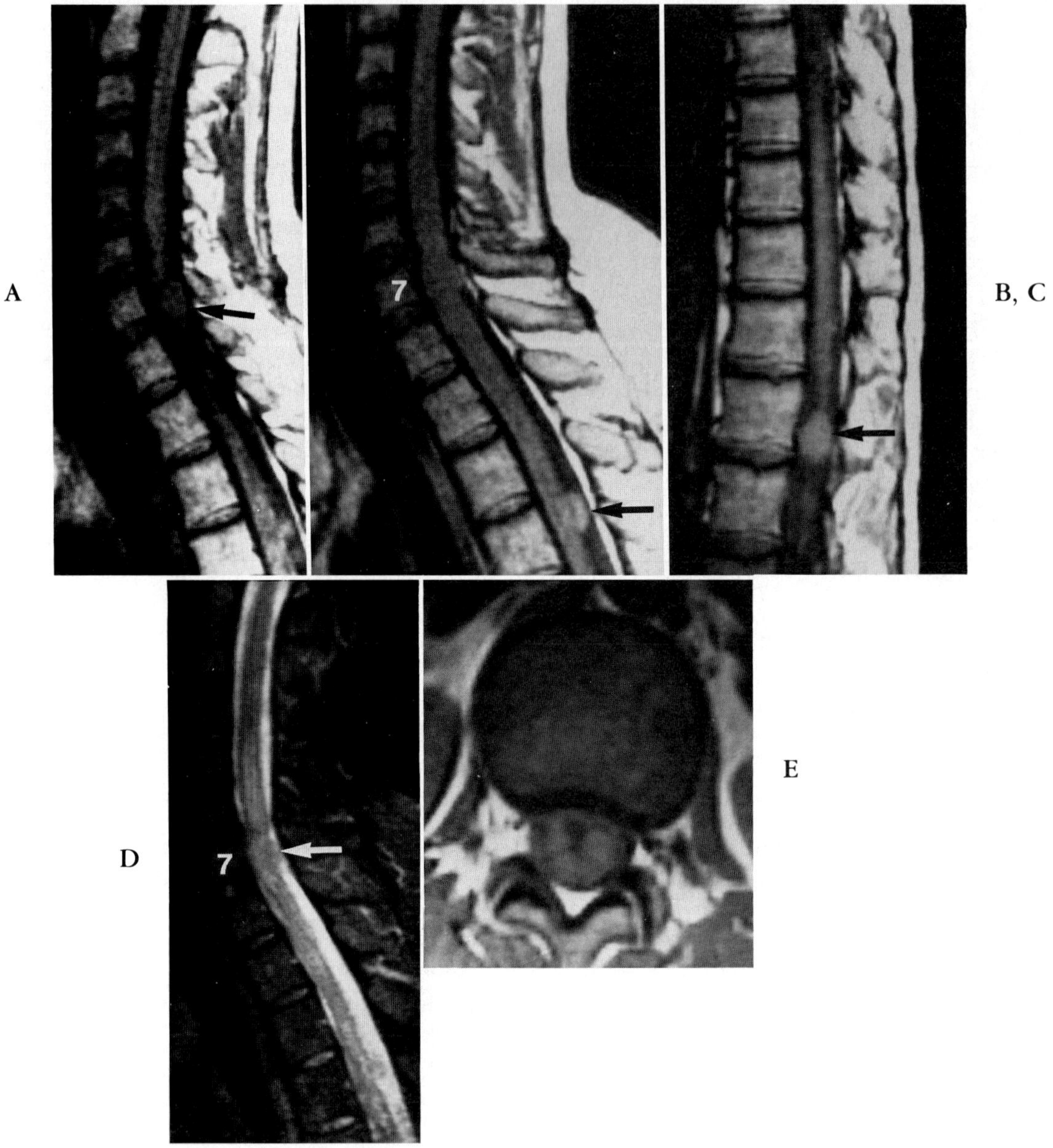

FIGURE 8-90. Leptomeningeal tumor spread of glioblastoma. MR images of 30-year-old female with leptomeningeal metastases from intracranial glioblastoma. Multiple extramedullary, intradural nodular masses are identified on sagittal T1W scan (SE 800/20) throughout spinal canal in cervical (*arrows*, **A** and **B**) and thoracic region (*arrow*, **C**). In midcervical region cord is diffusely enlarged secondary to compression from subarachnoid mass dorsolateral to cord (*arrow*, **A**). Cord signal intensity is low, suggesting edema within cord secondary to compression by extramedullary mass at C_7 level (**A**). **D**, T2W sagittal scan (gated SE 2300/80) of cervical cord shows abnormal signal intensity in midcervical region (C_5-C_7) of cord enlargement *(arrow)*. This most likely represents edema in anteriorly displaced cord *(arrow)*. **E**, Metastatic site was also present in cauda equina (**C**). Multiple nodules present in this location were identified on axial T1W image (SE 1000/20) just distal to conus (**E**).

A, B

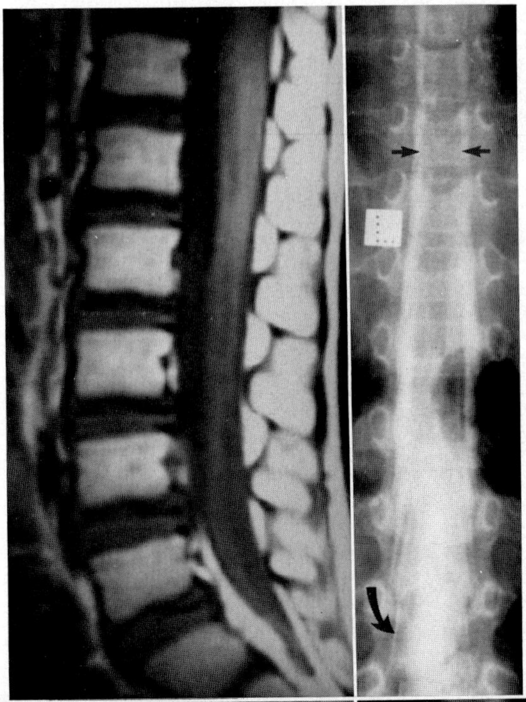

FIGURE 8-91. Leptomeningeal medulloblastoma. Series of T1W images shows marked extensive leptomeningeal spread from posterior fossa medulloblastoma. **A,** Sagittal view (SE 800/20) shows prominent, irregular, and inhomogeneous cauda equina. Fine striations normally seen in cauda are lost because of nerve root adhesions caused by leptomeningeal tumor (**A**). **B,** Myelogram anteroposterior (AP) view shows apparently widened cord and conus *(paired arrows)*. Adhesion of nerve roots causes them to clump laterally in subarachnoid space *(curved arrow)*. **C-F,** set of T1W images (SE 1000/20) through midthoracic cord shows prominent circumferential abnormal signal intensity around thoracic cord indicative of leptomeningeal tumor *(arrows)*.

C D

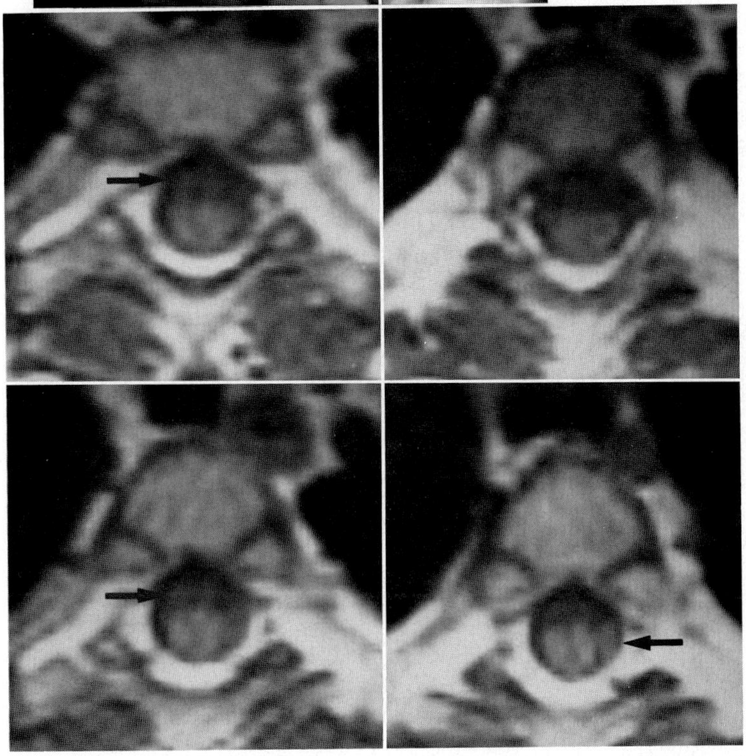

E F

Continued.

G, H

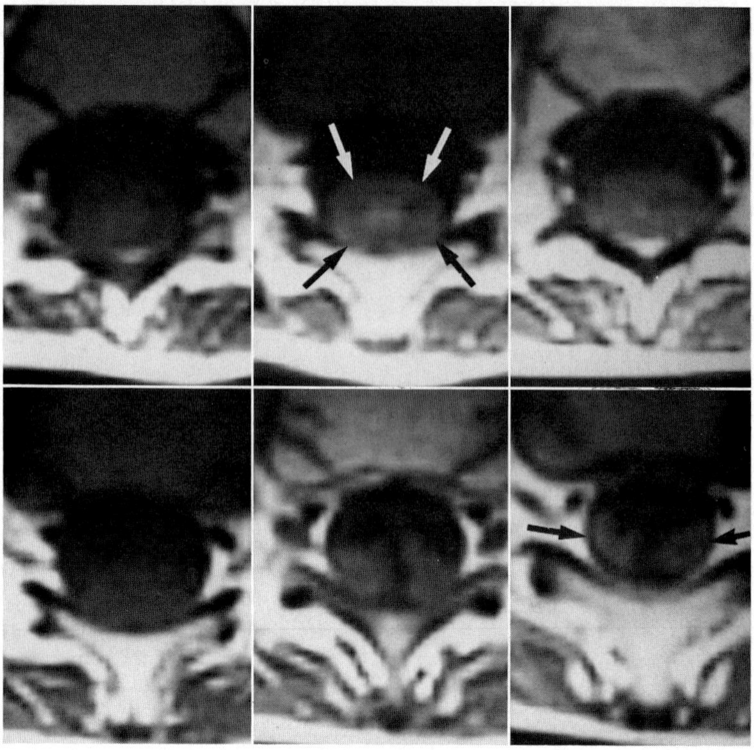

I

J, K

L

FIGURE 8-91, cont'd. **G-L**, Series of six axial T1W scans (SE 800/20) through cauda equina beginning at lower conus (**G**) shows thick "halo" of tumor coating of conus (**H**, *arrows*). Cauda equina instead of showing normal "wing-shaped" roots shows posteriorly situated mass (**I** and **J**) that eventually splits into two large columns of clumped roots (**K**; and **L**, *arrows*).

A

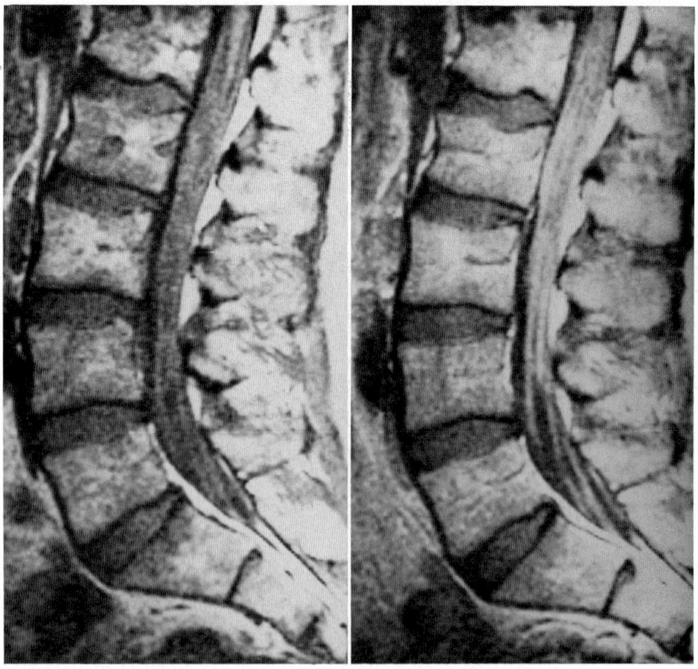

B

FIGURE 8-92. For legend see next page.

C

D, E

F

G, H

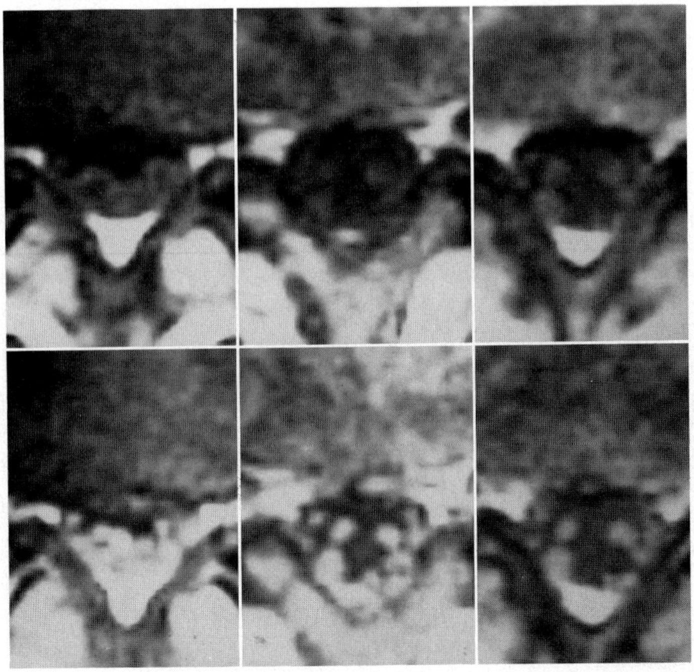

FIGURE 8-92, cont'd. Leptomeningeal lymphoma. **A**, Precontrast GdDTPA sagittal T1W scan (SE 800/20) shows increased signal intensity of entire cauda equina. **B**, Postcontrast GdDTPA scan shows diffuse enhancement of cauda equina and individual nerve roots lower in lumbar canal. **C-H**, Axial T1W scans (SE 1000/20) show enlarged lumbar roots even on precontrast scan (**C-E**). Roots enhance markedly on postcontrast scan (**F-H**) obtained at same anatomic levels.

A

B

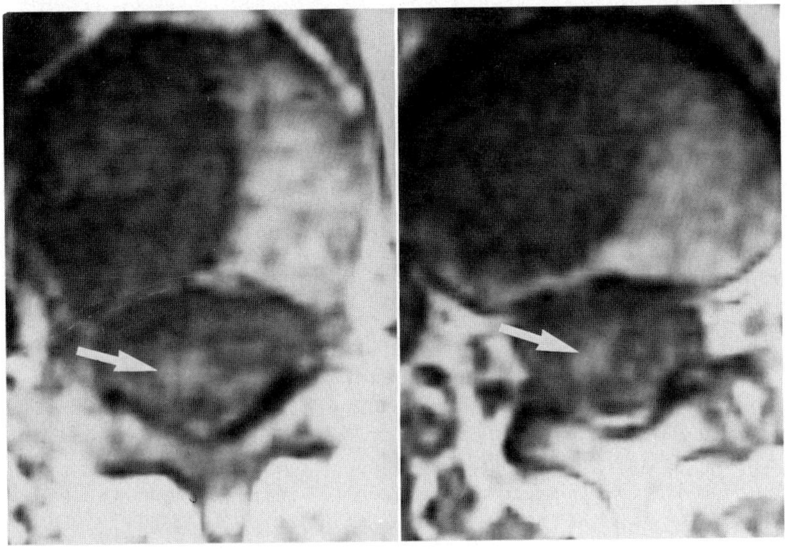

FIGURE 8-93. False positive leptomeningeal tumor. **A** and **B**, Axial T1W scans (SE 1000/20) show obvious low signal metastatic lesion in vertebral body. Within dural sac irregular area of increased signal suggests thickening or clumping of nerve roots in cauda equina *(arrows)*. These two slices were end-slices; finding was not confirmed by sagittal images or another set of axial views.

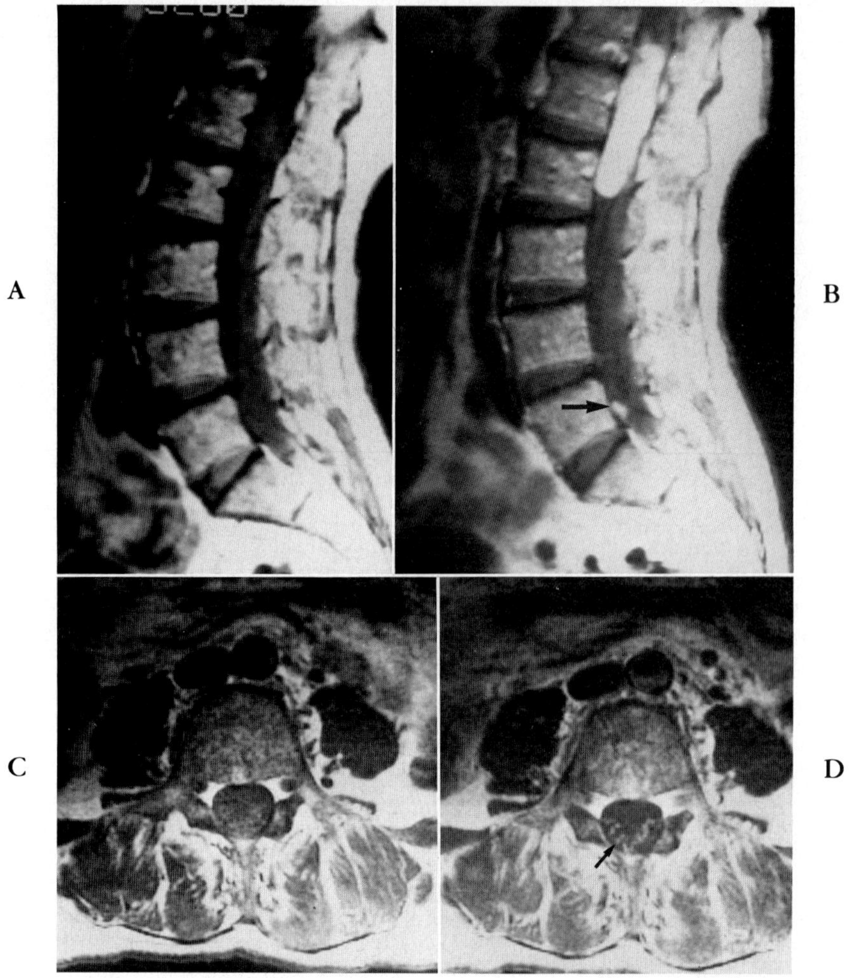

FIGURE 8-94. Leptomeningeal ependymoma. GdDTPA T1W scans in 71-year-old male with back pain show value of contrast agent in detecting leptomeningeal tumor; seeding from ependymoma. **A,** Precontrast T1W (SE 600/20) sagittal scan does not definitely show tumor, although conus and cauda equina are not well seen. **B,** Postcontrast T1W scan (SE 600/20) clearly shows contrast-enhanced high signal intensity ependymoma at T_{12}-L_2. Note small metastatic deposits at level of L_5 *(arrow)*. **C,** Precontrast axial T1W scan (SE 600/20) of cauda equina shows no definite abnormality because roots are individually visualized. **D,** Postcontrast scan (SE 600/20) shows definite enhancement of cauda equina indicating presence of leptomeningeal tumor *(arrow)*. At surgery tumor was found to be ependymoma with leptomeningeal spread distal to it. (Courtesy of Dr. Gordon Sze.)

A B C D E F

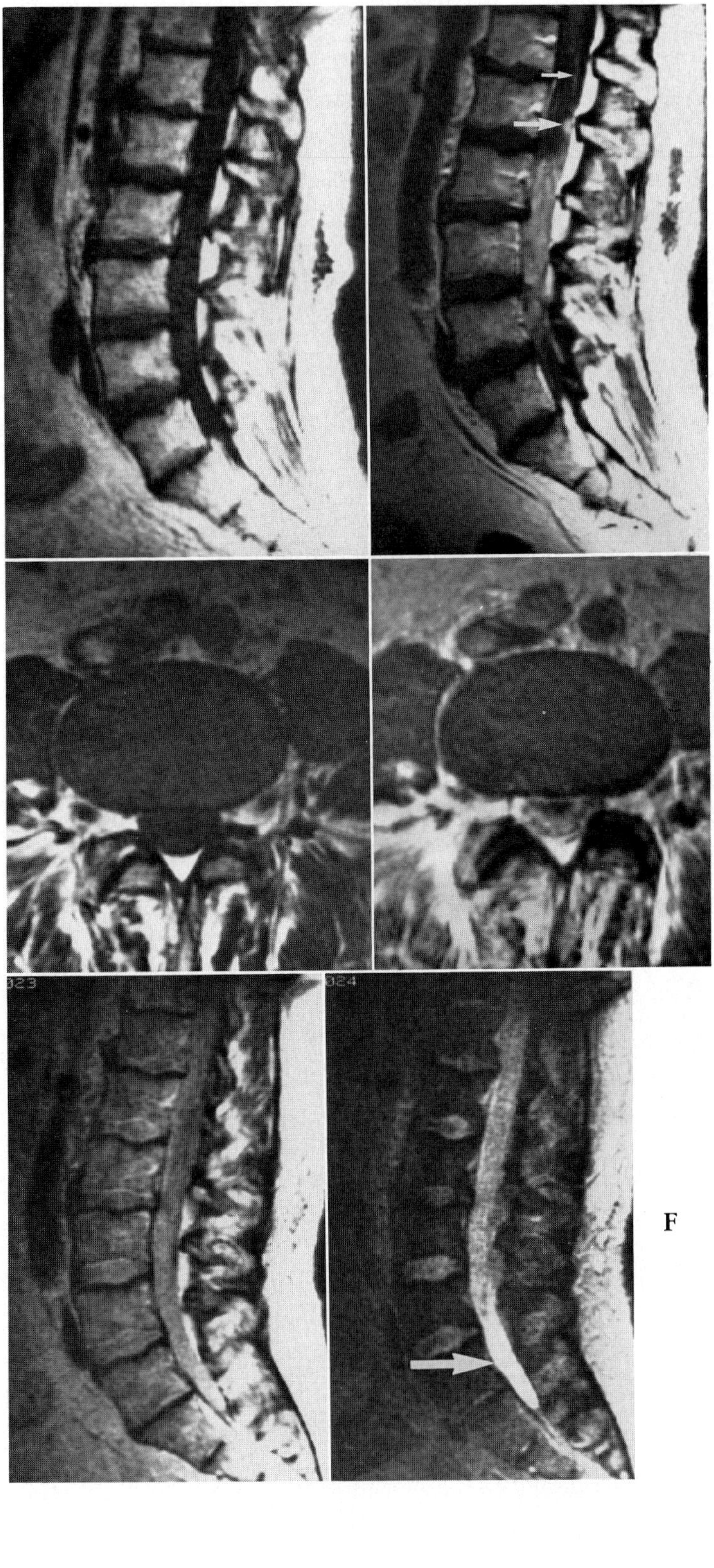

FIGURE 8-95. Leptomeningeal spread of glioblastoma. Series of T1W (SE 600/20) and T2W (SE 2000/35, 70) scans of patient with known glioblastoma who developed back pain and leg weakness. Precontrast T1W scans in sagittal (**A**) and axial (**C**) views show no definite abnormality. Postcontrast GdDTPA sagittal (**B**) and axial (**D**) scans show marked enhancement of intradural leptomeningeal spread of tumor extending at least from L_1 to L_4 (**B**). Although metastatic tumor is relatively confluent (L_2-L_3), individual nodules (**B**, *large arrow*) and individual nodular nerve roots *(small arrow)* can be visualized. **D,** Postcontrast axial scan shows enhancement of aggregate of adherent nerve roots. T2W scans (TE 35, **E**; TE 70, **F**) show no definitive finding for leptomeningeal tumor. High signal intensity (**F,** *arrow*) of CSF in distal lumbar sac suggests pocket of stationery CSF indicating possible obstruction above this level. (Courtesy of Dr. Gordon Sze.)

A 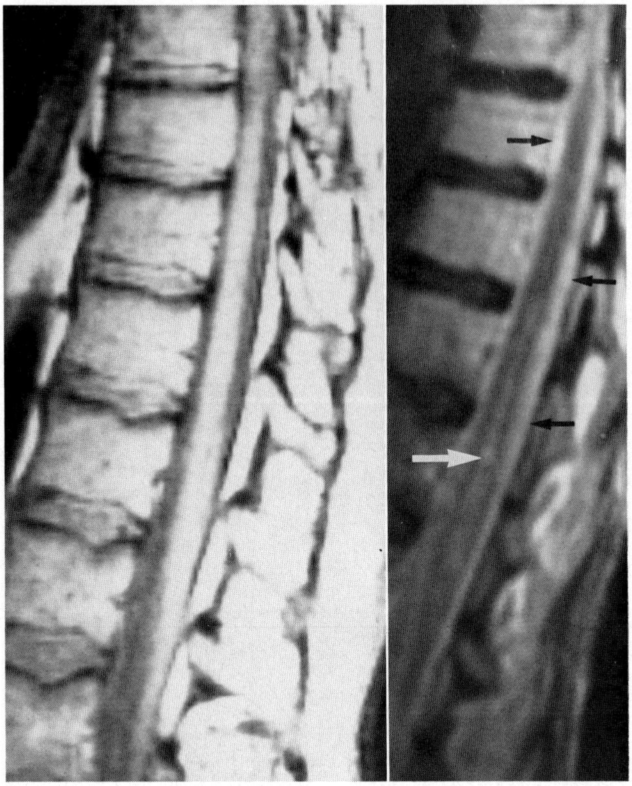 B

FIGURE 8-96. Leptomeningeal ependymoma. **A,** Sagittal T1W scan (SE 800/20) does not show clear evidence of diffuse leptomeningeal metastases from ependymoma. **B,** Post-GdDTPA T1W scan (SE 800/20) shows contrast enhancement, seen as increased signal in subarachnoid space, diffusely filming subarachnoid space around lower thoracic cord and conus *(black arrows)*. In addition, abnormal enhancement in central cord suggests cord invasion by metastatic ependymoma *(white arrow)*. (Courtesy of Dr. Michael Brant-Zawadzki.)

A, B 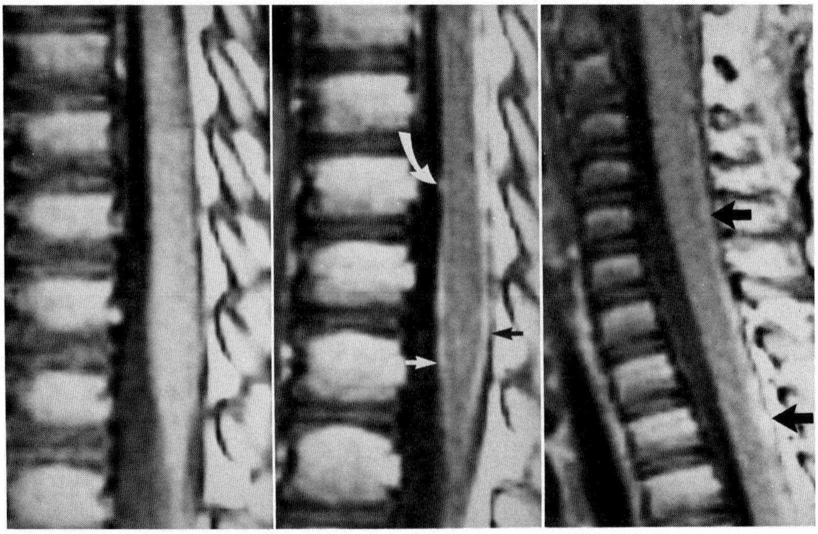 C

FIGURE 8-97, A-C. For legend see next page.

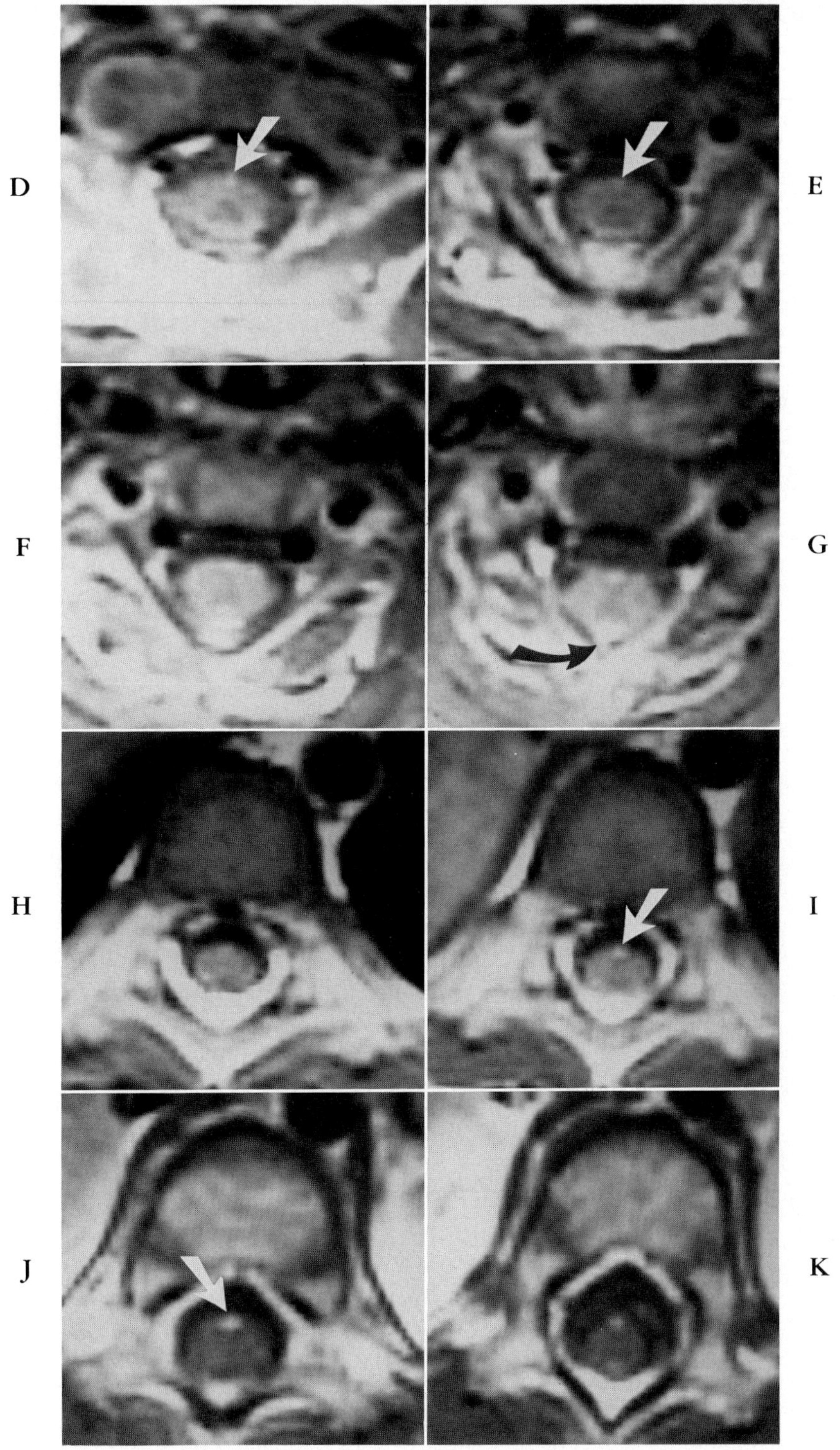

FIGURE 8-97, cont'd. Leptomeningeal spread of medulloblastoma. **A,** Precontrast T1W scan (SE 800/20) shows normal distal cord and conus with no evidence of leptomeningeal tumor. **B,** Post-GdDTPA T1W scan (SE 800/20) shows thin layer of abnormal enhancement outlining surface of distal thoracic cord and conus *(straight arrows)*. Small nodular lesions are also noted *(curved arrow)*. **C,** Postcontrast T1W scan (SE 800/20) in cervical region shows abnormal contrast enhancement on surface of cord, primarily in dorsal location *(arrows)*. Abnormal enhancement is confirmed on axial T1W images (SE 1000/20) in cervical region where abnormal nodular enhancement is noted on anterior and posterior surfaces of cord (*arrows*, **D-G**). Abnormal enhancement is also noted in distal thoracic cord and conus region (*arrows*, **H-K**).

A

B

C

D

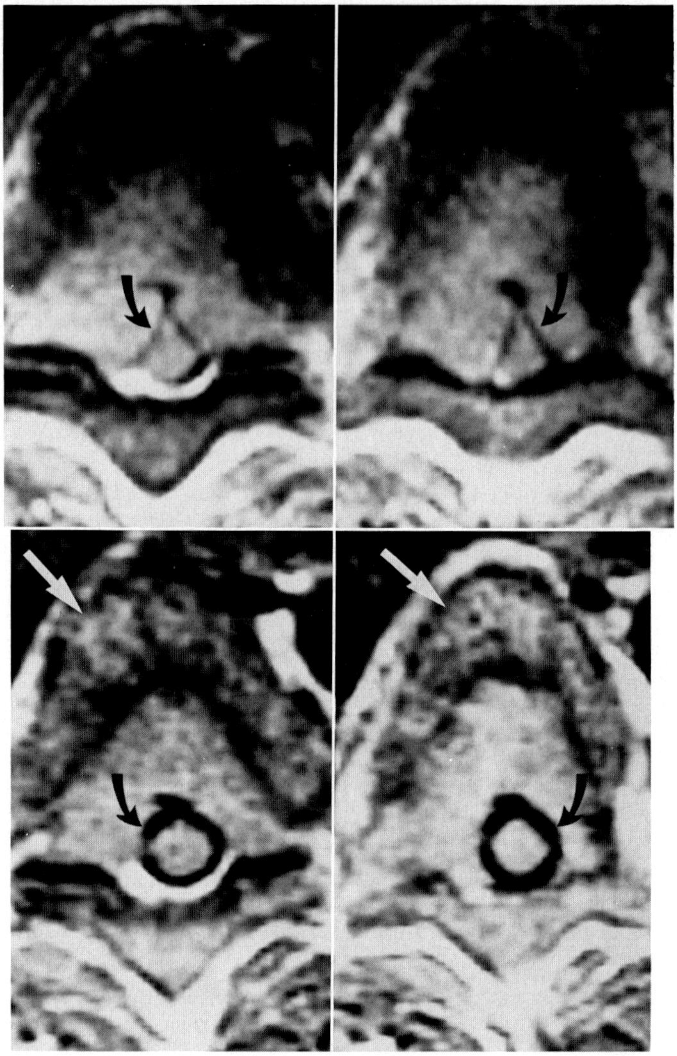

FIGURE 8-98. Renal cell metastasis. Axial T1W scans (SE 1000/20) show response of vertebral body marrow and metastatic renal cell carcinoma to radiation therapy. Initial scan (**A** and **B**) shows metastatic tumor involvement of posterior vertebral body with extension into epidural space and spinal canal, causing marked cord compression. Signal intensity of metastatic tumor is higher than vertebral body marrow. Thin black line separating tumor from cord represents combination of dura and thin layer of pulsating CSF *(arrows)*. **C** and **D**, T1W scan performed 2 months after radiation therapy shows interval increase in signal intensity of vertebral body marrow indicating fat replacement of normal red marrow *(white arrows)*. In addition, cord is no longer compressed and size of subarachnoid space around cord has increased *(curved arrows)*. Images show two responses to radiation therapy: increased signal in marrow indicating fat replacement and some regression of tumor size in spinal canal and at junction of normal marrow and tumor. Junction between tumor and marrow shows clearer demarcation (**C** and **D**) compared to pretreatment scans (**A** and **B**).

MR Findings

Marrow in vertebral bodies has the characteristics of red marrow, that is, lower signal intensity on T1W images compared to marrow in peripheral bones, yellow marrow, which has high signal intensity on T1W images. Signal intensity is homogeneous in children and young adults but becomes increasingly heterogeneous with age. The heterogeneity reflects increased fatty infiltration seen in normal aging, which may manifest as large spherical infiltrations or multiple small round infiltrations that are more difficult to define discretely but result in a mottled appearance in the vertebral body. Heterogeneity can make the diagnosis of a diffuse infiltrative disorder in older age groups difficult on T1W images. When fat and water components are separated using "fat" and "water" sequences, one can find moderate amounts of fat in normal marrow as indicated by the signal intensity seen in the vertebral bodies on "fat" images. "Water" images, however, show a moderate amount of such protons in normal vertebral bodies.

Radiation-induced fatty infiltration results in a marked increase in signal intensity of vertebral bodies on T1W images (see Figure 8-73). "Water" images of postirradiation vertebral bodies show a reduced amount of water protons. The evolution from normal red marrow to a stable level of fatty infiltration after radiation occurs over an approximate 3-month period. If metastases are present in the vertebral bodies, the residual normal red marrow undergoes fatty infiltration, whereas the metastatic site often does not (Figure 8-98). In some diffuse neoplastic infiltrations such as lymphoma, fatty infiltration may be seen within the metastatic focus. "Fat" images are very sensitive to displacement of fat components in red marrow or fatty infiltration and are highly sensitive to metastatic sites. Untreated metastases show increased signal intensity on "water" images. After treatment, the signal intensity of metastatic foci decreases, but it does not disappear on "water" images. It is not known at this time whether this represents residual tumor or fibrotic tissue of a sterilized metastatic site. The postirradiation vertebral body provides high contrast for assessing any increase in size of new or old metastatic deposits. Further growth of neoplastic tissue encroaches and replaces adipose tissue, making such increases in size readily detectable.

Radiation therapy does not significantly change the signal intensity of the metastatic focus in the short term (see Figure 8-98). The use of radiation for metastases causing spinal block seems to result in enough tumor regression to allow opening up of some subarachnoid space (see Figure 8-98).

BONE TUMORS

Hemangioma

Hemangioma, a benign vascular neoplasm that commonly involves vertebral bodies, consists of cavernous, capillary, and venous vascular channels intermixed between thickened osseous trabeculae. Spinal angiography shows these tumors to be extremely vascular. Trabeculae form vertical striations commonly seen on plain x-ray films and the honeycombed appearance seen on plain films and CT. The tumor may have cystic spaces within it.

Bone hemangiomas are more common in females than in males and are often single instead of multiple, although they can occur in multiple locations. The vertebral body is a common location and the thoracic spine is the common spinal level. Hemangioma rarely extends beyond the vertebral body to involve the posterior elements. It, however, can reach considerable size and extend beyond the confines of the bony margins of the vertebral body. In such instances it can result in cord compression. When hemangiomas reach a large size, they normally involve the entire vertebral body and can extend into the neural arch, i.e., the pedicles. The soft tissue mass can expand beyond the bony margins, which already exhibit expansion.[38]

Hemangiomas are usually asymptomatic, but if they become symptomatic it is usually after the second decade of life and the common clinical presentation is that of pain, often a painful compression fracture. In rare instances, patients may present with progressive paraparesis over a period of weeks to months. Progression may be more rapid during pregnancy. The cause of cord compression is usually an extension of the soft tissue mass beyond the confines of the vertebral body. This complication commonly occurs at the T_3 to T_9 level.[38]

MR Findings

Hemangiomas exhibit high signal intensity within the vertebral body on T1W images. The extent may vary from a small round sphere to involvement of the entire vertebral body (Figures 8-99 and 8-100). Signal intensity of the hemangioma is high and relatively homogeneous as a result of an increased amount of fat within the hemangioma. When selective "water" and "fat" images are obtained, most of the high signal on a T1W image can be attributed to an increased fat content (see Figure 8-100). Very little is related to an increase in the water content of the vertebral body. Nevertheless, portions of the hemangioma can show increased water compared to normal marrow (see Figure 8-100) and may correspond to the more vascular regions in the tumor. On the late echo of the T2W sequence, signal from fat is low and the hemangioma shows little signal. The high signal appears unrelated to thrombosis or methemoglobin. In rare instances of cord compression, the soft tissue mass extending beyond the confines of the vertebral body is clearly shown by a T1W scan.

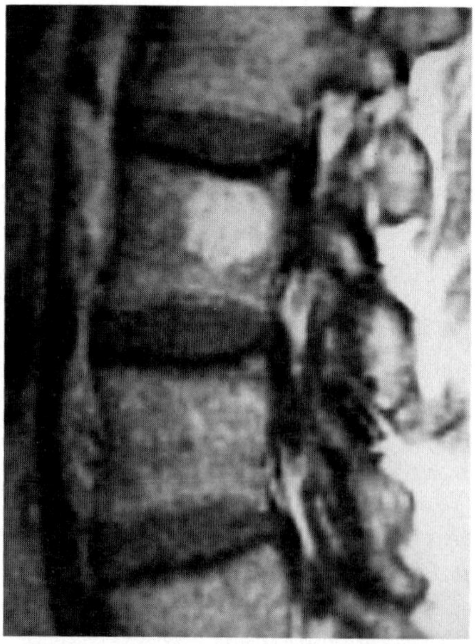

FIGURE 8-99. Hemangioma. T1W scan (SE 800/20) shows typical hemangioma as well-circumscribed circular lesion of high signal intensity compared to normal marrow signal intensity. High signal intensity is result of increased fat deposition in lesions.

Osteochrondroma (Exostosis)

These bone tumors have both cartilaginous and bony elements. A cartilagenous cap has bony trabecullae underneath it. The cortex of the osteochondroma is continuous with the cortex of the underlying bone and the same is true for the spongiosa. In most cases these tumors are considered spontaneous, although they have been reported after radiation, especially if this occurred before the age of two.[48] Osteochondromas also present in a multiple form that is associated with a hereditary syndrome expressed as an autosomal dominant and is most likely to involve the vertebrae. Vertebral involvement may cause cord compression.[39,76] Osteochondromas can grow in childhood and compress adjacent structures such as vessels, nerves, and tendons. These benign bone tumors can undergo malignant degeneration, especially in the hip and shoulder. The primary manifestation is a rapid increase in tumor size (see Chondrosarcoma).

MR Findings

MR scans show a surprising amount of soft tissue in tumors that with x-ray imaging techniques are seen because of their bone and calcium content (Figure 8-101). Areas of calcification and ossification appear on MR as low signal intensity on all pulse sequences, but the findings are less dominant than with x-ray studies (see Figure 8-101). Even in areas with marked calcification or ossification as determined by CT, significant amounts of soft tissue are still visualized on MR scans (see Figure 8-101). The major importance of imaging in the spine is to assess potential spinal cord compression. The MR scan accurately delineates cord deviation and compression by such a lesion.

Chondrosarcoma

Chondrosarcoma is a bone tumor composed of a sarcomatous stroma that produces cartilage, calcification, and sometimes ossification.[57] It may have a large soft tissue component and calcification within the tumor increases with time[49] It is considered primary when it arises de novo and secondary when it arises in a chondroma, osteochondroma, or parosteal chondroma (the latter type is less common). This tumor is slow growing, has low metastatic potential, a ten-

A 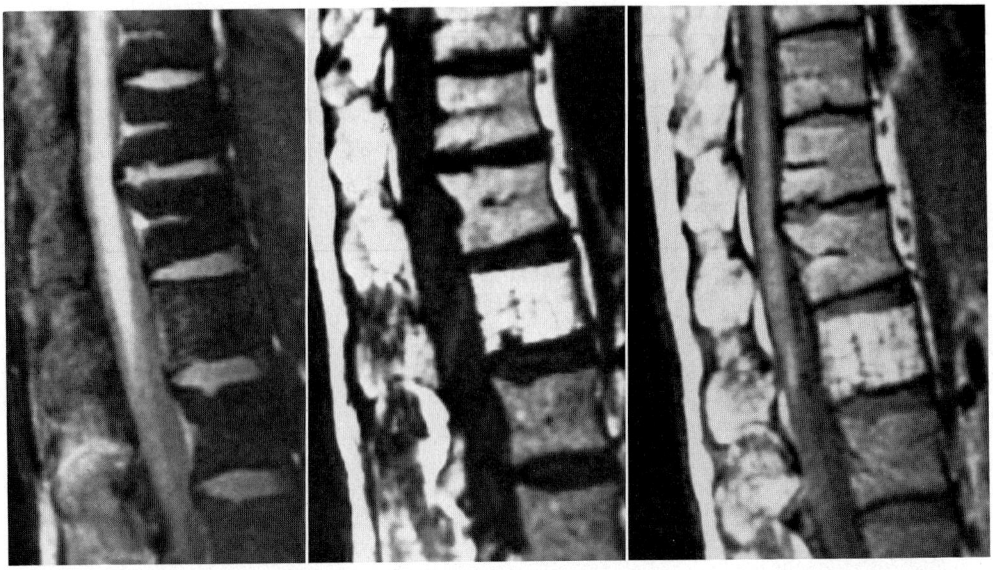 B, C

FIGURE 8-100. Vertebral body hemangioma. Analysis of hemangioma signal intensity with use of "water" and "fat" images. T1W (SE 800/20, **A**), fat (SE 800/20, **B**), and water (SE 800/20, **C**) images of vertebral body hemangioma in 39-year-old male. **A,** Routine T1W image shows diffuse increased signal within L_1. Prominent bony trabeculae are seen as irregular linear areas of decreased signal intensity within vertebral body. Hemangioma is confined entirely to vertebral body. It is evident from "fat" image (**B**) that most of increased signal within vertebral body is result of increased lipid within marrow space. **C,** "Water" image shows increased water content in posterior half of vertebra whereas the remainder is normal compared to other normal vertebral bodies.

A 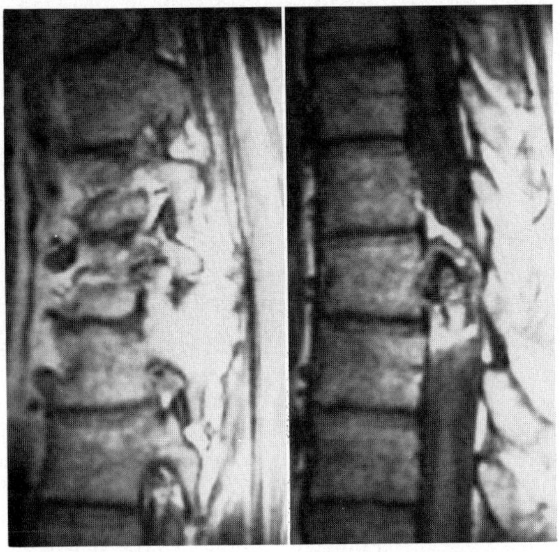 B

FIGURE 8-101. Spinal osteochondroma. Sagittal (**A** and **B**) and axial (**C** and **D**) T1W scans (SE 800/20) of patient with familial multiple exostoses, one of which shows impingement into spinal canal. Sagittal scans show extensive soft tissue abnormality outside of spinal canal and neural foramen (**A**) in addition to component in spinal canal that displaces and compresses spinal cord (**B**). Fat is seen on rostral and caudal ends of osteochondroma, but rather than being part of lesion it represents secondary fat deposition caused by displacement of dura by cartilagenous tumor.

Continued.

C D

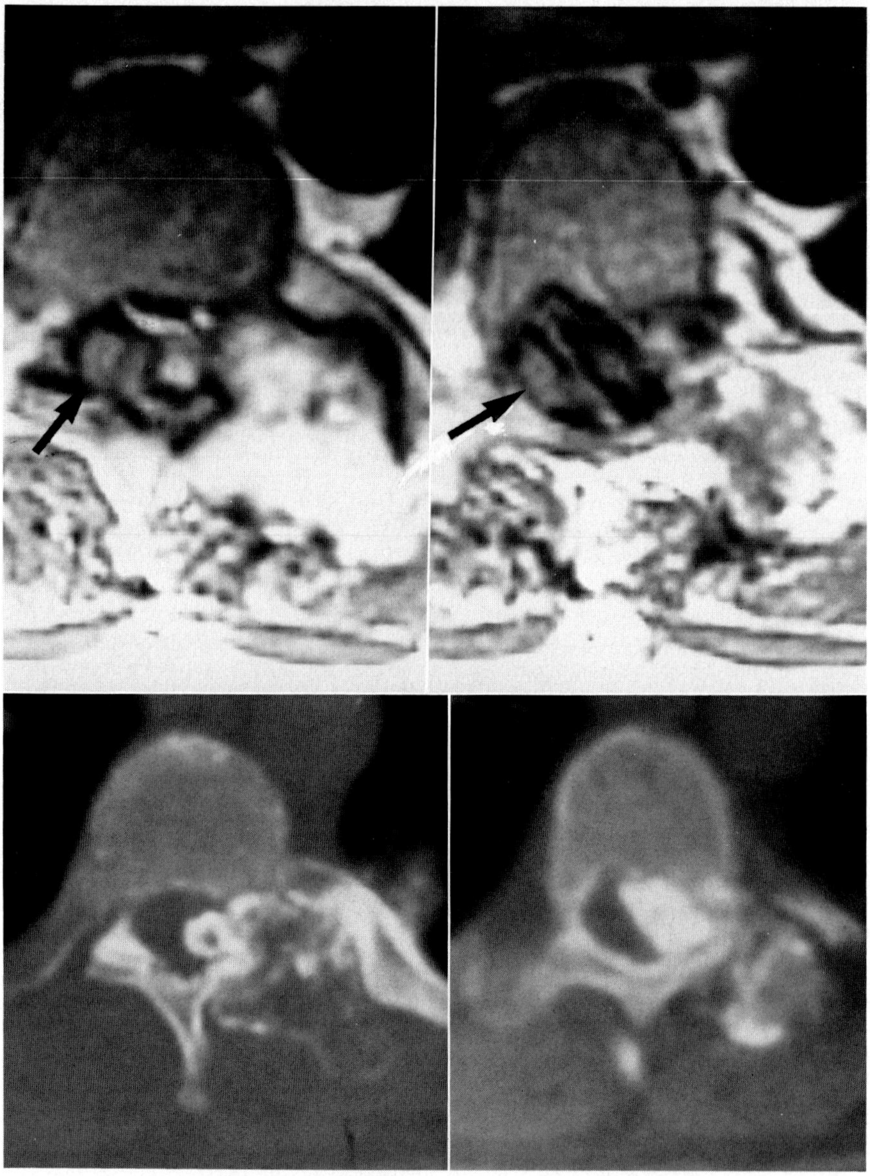

E F

FIGURE 8-101, cont'd. **C** and **D**, Axial scans show marked cord displacement and impingement *(arrows)*; these two levels correspond to the CT scans (**C** to **E** and **D** to **F**). **E** and **F**, On CT scan in areas where no significant ossification or calcification is seen, soft tissue density is apparent on MR scan. Even where dense calcification is seen in canal on CT scan (**F**), significant soft tissue density is still visualized on MR scan (**D**). Dense calcification and ossification on MR scan is circumferential low signal intensity around central soft tissue in this tumor. Note extensive soft tissue abnormality involving left foramina, facet joint, and pedicle (**C**) where bone expansion is visualized on CT scan (**E**). Although both studies yield useful information, MR scanning gives more accurate information about tumor extent and status of spinal cord.

dency for local recurrence, and is most frequent in tubular bones. Vertebral body involvement is less common but may manifest as a destructive lesion resulting in compression fracture.

This tumor spans a wide age range, beginning in childhood and extending to old age, with the highest frequency occurring in the fifth and sixth decade.[49] Clinically, pain and swelling may indicate its presence, although many chondrosarcomas are asymptomatic.

A recognized clinical entity is the *dedifferentiated chondrosarcoma*,[13,23] a poor descriptive term that refers to the appearance of a higher grade sarcoma within the chondrosarcoma. This new highly malignant sarcoma is noncartilagenous and may show histologic features of fibrosarcoma, osteosarcoma, or malignant fibrohistiocytoma. Development of a second high-grade sarcoma occurs in 10% to 20% of chondrosarcomas, but is a rare event in the spine. Its appearance is marked by soft tissue extension with little or no calcification compared to the more benign underlying chondrosarcoma. Metastases are common.

MR Findings

The MR scan is sensitive to the soft tissue component of chondrosarcoma (Figures 8-102 and 8-103). Typically this tumor has character-

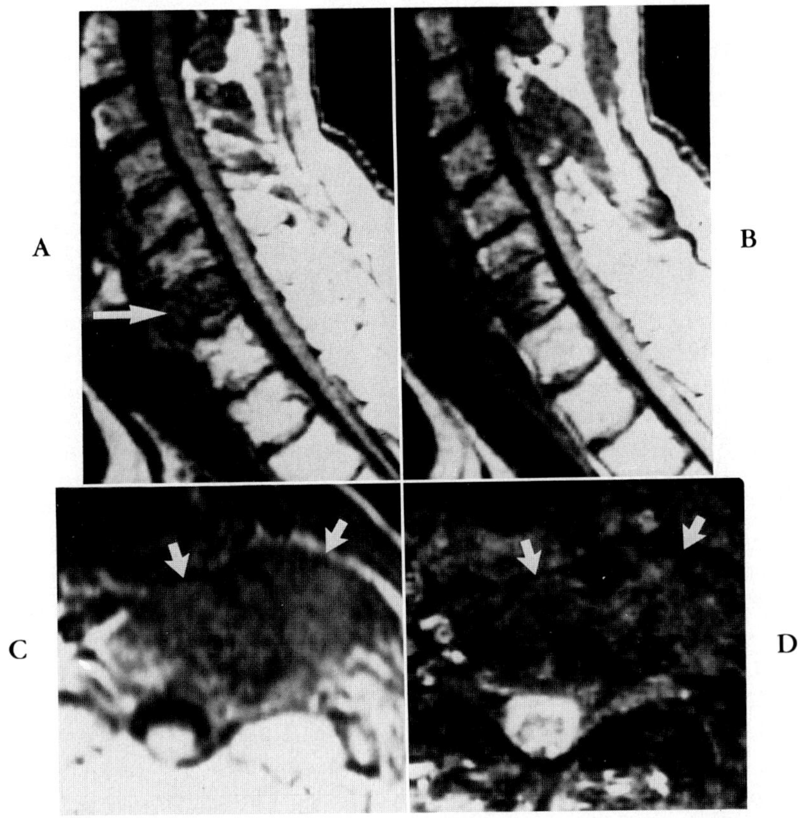

FIGURE 8-102. Chondrosarcoma. In this patient with chondrosarcoma of C_7, tumor and its local extent can be appreciated on T1W scan (SE 600/25, **A** and **B**). Tumor is lower signal intensity than normal vertebral body marrow, which has been nearly entirely replaced in C_7 (*arrow*, **A**). **C**, Adjacent soft tissue invasion is better appreciated on axial T1W scan (SE 1000/25) *(arrows)*. **D**, Gradient echo scan (SE 500/20) shows mild impingement on dural sac in left anterolateral recess, but tumor margins are less well delineated with this pulse sequence because of similarity in signal intensity of tumor and fat. Anterolateral tumor margin is seen because of intravoxel destructive interference effect of water and fat protons yielding artifactual (black) border (*arrows*, **D**).

A

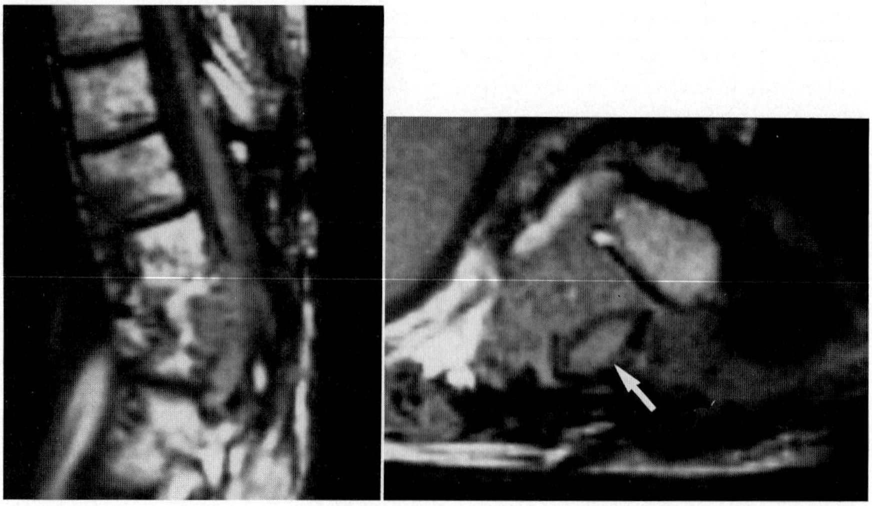

B

FIGURE 8-103. Chondrosarcoma. **A,** Sagittal (SE 600/20) and **B,** axial T1W scans (SE 1000/20) of patient after surgery and radiation for chondrosarcoma. Tumor has caused marked destruction of vertebral body and has significant soft tissue component that impinges on spinal canal, compressing spinal cord (*arrow,* **B**).

istics of long T1 and T2 relaxation times; shows low signal on T1W images; and high signal, often prominent, on T2W images.[53,71] Findings are similar to osteosarcoma in that extension within the vertebrae is seen on T1W images primarily as an area of signal intensity lower than normal marrow (see Figure 8-102). Tumor delineation therefore relies on the depiction of normal marrow fat tissue. Soft tissue expansion beyond the vertebral body is well depicted by MR on both T1W and T2W images (see Figures 8-102 and 8-103). It is delineated by distortion of normal anatomy and by abnormal increased signal on T2W images. T2*W images may not be as informative because the signal intensity of tumor may be similar to that of adjacent muscle or fat tissue on this pulse sequence (see Figure 8-102). Nevertheless, the tumor border can be delineated by the artifactual black rim at the interface of fat and water (muscle) or, in this case, fat and tumor (see Figure 8-102).

Osteosarcoma

Osteosarcoma is a tumor consisting of a spindle cell stroma that produces primarily osteoid and immature bone.[57] The tissue that composes this tumor is varied and includes bone (causing sclerosis), osteoid (causing lytic lesions), cartilage (causing calcification) and fibrous and vascular tissue. It occurs most frequently in the metaphysis of tubular bones; the skull and spine are only rarely involved.

Clinically the tumor presents, similar to other tumors, with local pain and swelling. The peak incidence of this tumor is in the second and third decades, and occurs in males more frequently than in females. A second peak occurs in an older age group when the tumor is related to Paget's disease. Osteogenic sarcoma may appear after radiation therapy as part of a dedifferentiated chondrosarcoma, may arise isolated in soft tissue, or have a multicentric presentation. One unusual association of osteogenic sarcoma is its presentation as a second tumor approximately 10 years after the detection of retinoblastoma.[70] This linkage between retinoblastoma and osteosarcoma occurs in the hereditary form of retinoblastoma (autosomal dominant) and the nonhereditary retinoblastoma. The hereditary form occurs in approximately 40% of patients and is usually associated with bilateral retinoblastoma, whereas the nonhereditary form occurs in approximately 60% of patients and is more often associated with a unilateral retinoblastoma. Both bilateral and unilateral retinoblastoma are linked with osteosarcoma, although this is more frequent with the hereditary form.[70]

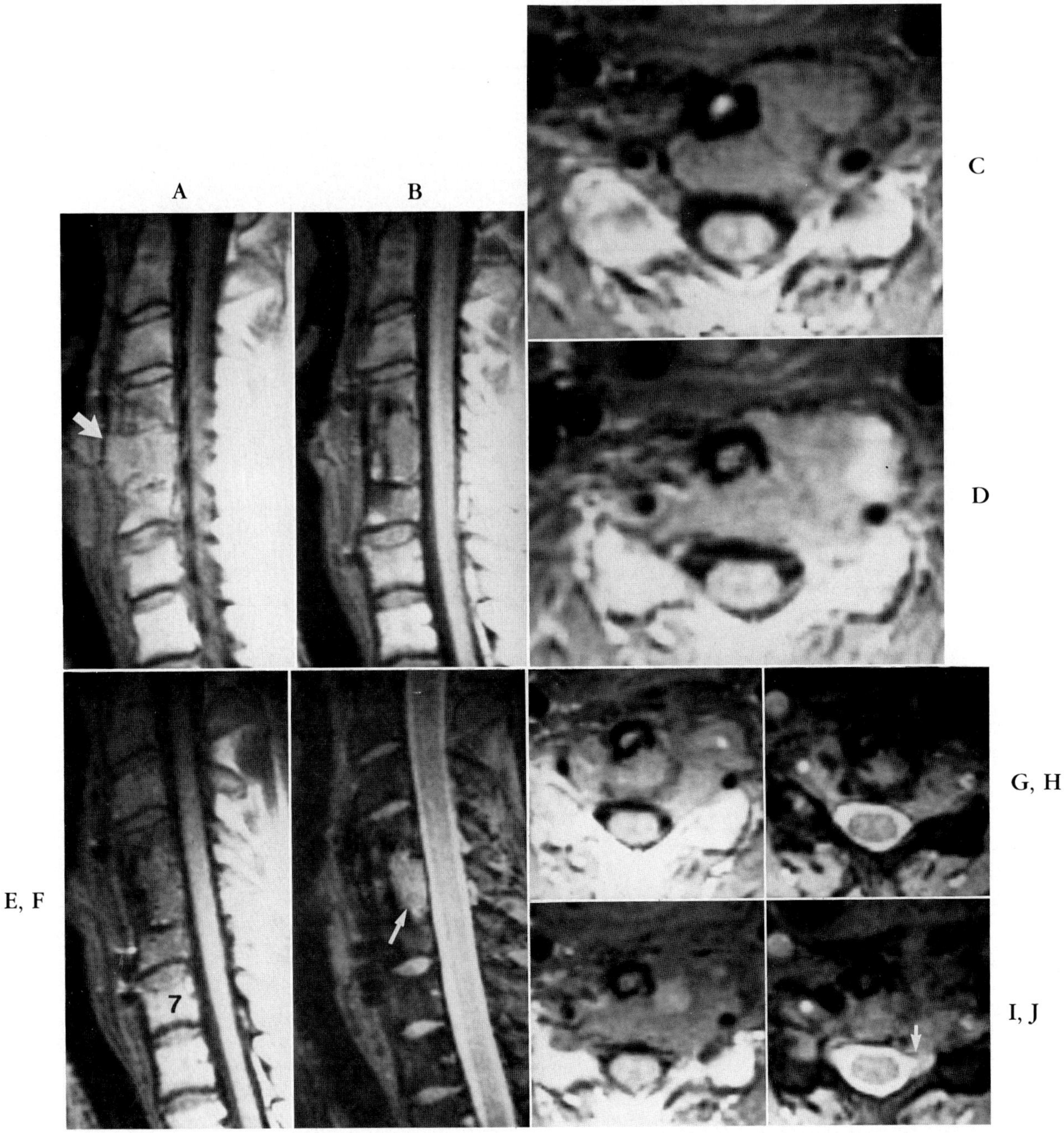

FIGURE 8-104. Osteosarcoma. Sagittal and axial scans of cervical spine osteosarcoma in patient previously treated for retinoblastoma. Osteosarcoma has invaded three contiguous vertebral bodies, C_4-C_6, replacing marrow and expanding C_5 (*arrow*, **A**). **A** and **B,** On sagittal T1W scans (SE 800/20) tumor is intermediate signal intensity similar to normal marrow but lower compared to high signal from radiation-induced fat-replaced marrow of lower cervical vertebrae. **C** and **D,** On axial T1W scans (SE 1000/20), tumor has destroyed cortical margins of C_5 and expanded into prevertebral space and both foramina. Tumor is slightly higher signal intensity than adjacent muscle. Circle of low signal intensity on anterior edge of tumor mass is a fibular strut, which has also been invaded by tumor, i.e., marrow fat is replaced (**D**). **E,** Sagittal T1W scan (SE 800/20) performed 1 month later appears similar (**E** to **B**). **F,** On sagittal T2W scan (SE gated 2110/80) part of tumor exhibits high signal intensity (*arrow*, **F**). Axial T1W scans (SE 1000/20), 1 month later, show progression of tumor as evidenced by further encasement and displacement of both vertebral arteries (**G** and **I**). **H** and **J,** Axial variable flip angle scans (GRASS 25/13, 7°) show tumor to be intermediate signal intensity with tumor margins somewhat harder to delineate compared to comparable T1W scans (**G** and **I**). Impingement on dural sac and left root sleeve (*arrow*, **J**) is well seen.

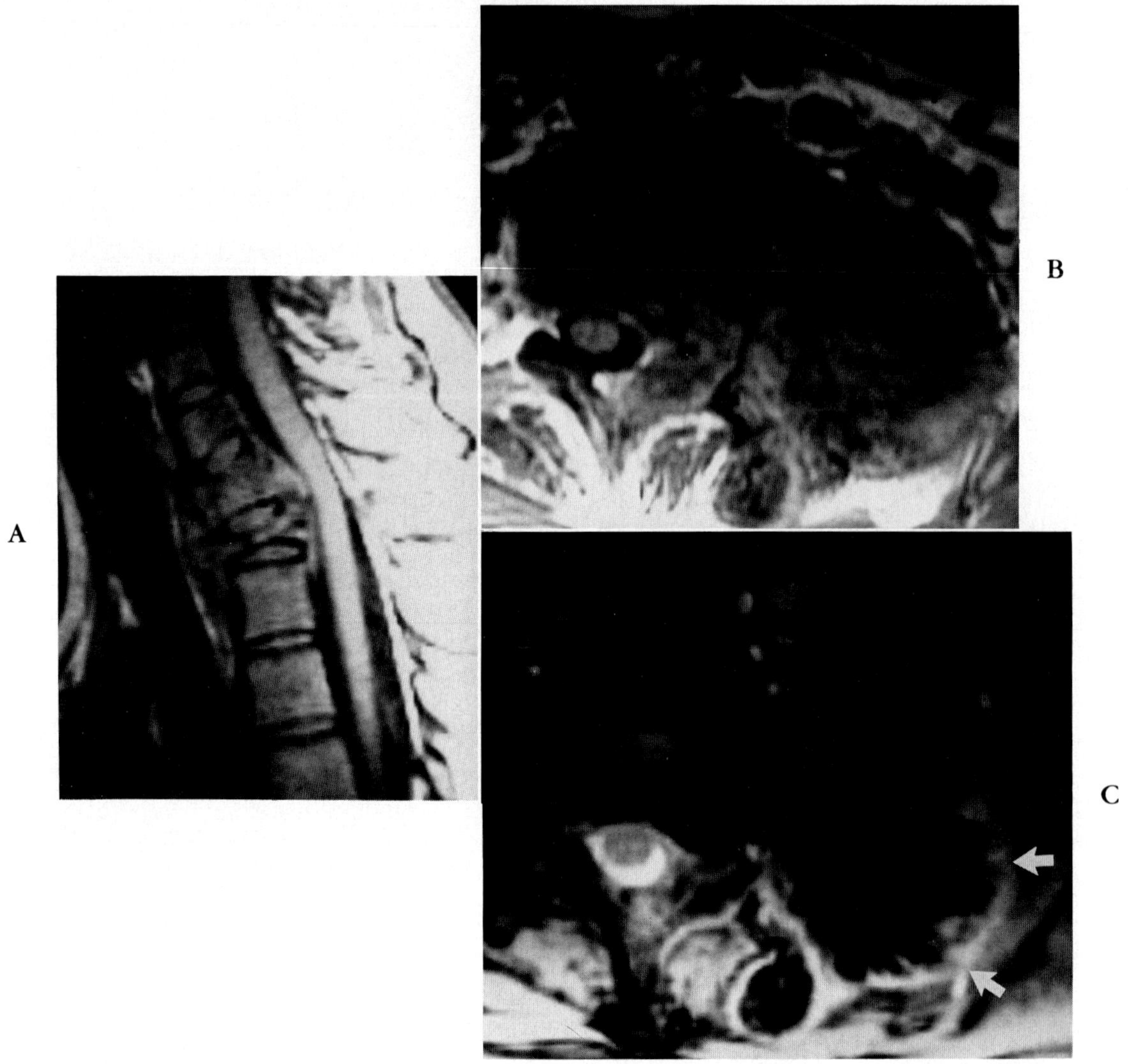

FIGURE 8-105. Osteosarcoma involving spine can cause marked vertebral body destruction, cord compression, and massive soft tissue extension. **A,** T1W scan (SE 800/20) shows tumor extension into C_7, T_1, and T_2 vertebrae with marked loss of height of T_2. Tumor extends beyond vertebral bodies with posterior soft tissue component causing cord compression. **B,** Axial T1W scan (SE 800/20) at level of T_1 shows extension of osteosarcoma from vertebral body into posterior elements and into soft tissue of left lung apex. **C,** Variable flip angle scan (GRASS 22/12, 7°) better shows diffuse areas of calcification and ossification as low signal intensity within vertebral body tumor and within large soft tissue component. Halo of high signal intensity on tumor periphery indicates edema in adjacent soft tissue *(arrows)*. Edema is also noted in paraspinous musculature. Variable flip angle scan is more sensitive to calcification and ossification in this tumor than T1W scan (**B**).

MR Findings

In general, the bony extension of osteosarcoma is best seen on T1W images where intramedullary extension is depicted as relative low signal by the replacement of normal high signal marrow. A very cellular tumor may have similar relative signal intensity (Figure 8-104). If the osteosarcoma has a prominent sclerotic component, very low signal is seen on T1W and T2W images (Figure 8-105). Considering the wide variety of tissue types in this tumor, the degree and pattern of signal intensity can be quite inhomogeneous. Expansion of the tumor through the cortex is seen as a disruption of the thin black line representing cortex on T1W images and as an obvious extraosseous soft tissue mass (see Figures 8-104 and 8-105). T1W and T2W images show extraosseous extension, with the T1W image relying primarily on distortion of normal anatomic structures, whereas the T2W images depict the tumor as abnormal high signal.[6,71] T2*W images may have poor contrast between the tumor and surrounding soft tissue (see Figure 8-105). Because of the magnetic susceptibility effects as a result of ossification and calcification, variable flip angle/gradient echo scans may depict this tumor as low signal intensity (see Figure 8-105). The tumor may progress rapidly (see Figure 8-104). Both sagittal and axial scans are necessary for complete depiction of the tumor.

REFERENCES

1. Adam A, Hocholzer L. Ganglioblastoma of the posterior mediastinum: a clinicopathologic review of 80 cases. CANCER 1981;47:373.
2. Aisen AM, Martel W, Braunstein EM, et al. MRI and CT evaluation of primary bone and soft-tissue tumors. AJR 1986;146:749.
3. Ammerman BJ, Henry JM, DeGirolami U, et al. Intradural lipomas of the spinal cord: a clinicopathological correlation. J Neurosurg 1976;7:331.
4. Barson AJ, Cole FM. Neurofibromatosis with congenital malformation of the spinal cord. J Neurol Neurosurg Psychiatry 1967;30:71.
5. Berns DH, Blaser S, Ross JS, et al. MR imaging with Gd-DTPA in leiptomeningeal spread of lymphoma. J Comput Assist Tomogr 1988;12:499.
6. Boyko OB, Cory DA, Cohen MD, et al. MR imaging of osteogenic and Ewing's sarcoma. AJR 1987;148:317.
7. Browne TR, Adams RD, Roberson GH. Hemangioblastoma of the spinal cord. Arch Neurol 1976;33:435.
8. Burk DL, Brunberg JA, Kanal E, et al. Spinal and paraspinal neurofibromatosis: surface coil MR imaging at 1.5T. Radiology 1987;162:797.
9. Butcher DL, Sahn SA. Epidural lipomatosis: a complication of corticosteroid therapy. Ann Intern Med 1979;90:60.
10. Canale DJ, Bebin J. Von Recklinghausen disease of the nervous system. In: Vinken PJ, Bruyn GW, eds. Handbook of clinical neurology: the phakomatoses. vol. 14. New York: American Elsevier, 1972.
11. Cooper PR, Epstein F. Radical resection of intramedullary spinal cord tumors in adults. J Neurosurg 1985;63:492.
12. Costigan DA, Winkelman MD. Intramedullary spinal cord metastasis. J Neurosurg 1985;62:227.
13. deLange EE, Pope TL, Fechner RE. Dedifferentiated chondrosarcoma: radiographic features. Radiology 1986;161:489.
14. Deutsch M, Reigel DH: The value of myelography in the management of childhood medulloblastoma. Cancer 1980;45:2194.
15. Dillon WP, Bolla K, Mark A, et al. Intradural spinal lesions: GdDTPA-enhanced MR imaging. Radiology 1989; 170:229.
16. Dorwart RH, LaMasters DL, Watanabe TJ. Tumor. In: Newton TH, Potts DG. Computed tomography of the spine and spinal cord. San Anselmo, CA: Calvedel Press, 1983.
17. Edelson RN, Deck MDF, Posner JB. Intramedullary spinal cord metastases. Clinical and radiographic findings in nine cases. Neurology 1972;22:1222.
18. Eldridge R. Central neurofibromatosis with bilateral acoustic neuroma. In: Riccardi VM, Mulvihill JJ, eds. Advances in Neurology, neurofibromatosis (von Recklinghausen disease). vol 29. New York: Raven Press, 1981.
19. Enzmann DR, Rubin JB, DeLaPaz R, et al. Cerebrospinal fluid pulsation: benefits and pitfalls in MR imaging. Radiology 1986;161:773.
20. Epstein BS. The spine: a radiological text and atlas, ed. 4. Philadelphia: Lea & Febiger, 1976.
21. Fisher MS. Lumbar spine metastasis in cervical carcinoma: a characteristic pattern. Radiology 1980;34:631.
22. Fornasier VL, Horne JH. Metastases to the vertebral column. Cancer 1975;36:590.
23. Frassica FJ, Unni KK, Beabout JW, et al. Dedifferentiated chondrosarcoma. J Bone Joint Surg 1986;68:1197.
24. Friedman M, Kim TH, Panahon AM. Spinal cord compression in malignant lymphoma. Cancer 1976; 37:1485.
25. Friede RL. Developmental neuropathology. New York: Springer-Verlag, 1975.
26. Fruehwald FX, Tscholakoff D, Schwaighofer B, et al. Magnetic resonance imaging of the lower vertebral column in patients with multiple myeloma. Invest Radiol 1988;23:193.
27. Garrison JE, Kasdon DL. Intramedullary spinal teratoma: case report and review of the literature. Neurosurgery 1980;7:509.
28. Goy AMC, Pinto RS, Raghavendra BN, et al. Intramedullary spinal cord tumors: MR imaging, with emphasis on associated cysts. Radiology 1986;161:381.
29. Gulenchyn KY, Papoff W. Technetium-99m MDP scintigraphy. An insensitive tool for the detection of bone marrow metastases. Clin Nucl Med 1987;12:45.
30. Haid RW, Kaufman HH, Schochet SS, et al. Epidural lipomatosis simulating an epidural abscess: case report and literature review. Neurosurgery 1987;21:744.
31. Harkin JC, Reed RJ. Tumors of the peripheral nervous system: atlas of tumor pathology, series 2, fascicle 3. Washington, D.C.: Armed Forces Institute of Pathology, 1969.
32. Haughton VM, Rimm AA, Czervionke LF, et al. Sensitivity of Gd-DTPA-enhanced MR imaging of benign extraaxial tumors. Radiology 1988;166:829.
33. Holdthusen W, Birtel T, Brinkmann B, et al. The Currarino triad. An autosomal-dominant inherited complex of the anorectal malformation, sacrococcygeal defect and presacral tumor. Observations of 9 further cases. ROFO 1985;143:83.
34. Hollis PH, Malis LI, Zappulla RA. Neurologic deterioration after lumbar puncture below complete spinal subarachnoid block. J Neurosurg 1986;64:253.
35. Hunt P, Van Leeuwen G, Bingham H, et al. Sacrococcygeal teratomas. A report of three cases and survey of present knowledge. Clin Pediatr 1968;7:165.
36. Kim KW, Ho SU, Weinberg PE, et al. Spinal leptomeningeal infiltration by systemic cancer: myelographic features. AJNR 1982;3:233.
37. Krol G, Sze G, Malkin M, et al. MR of cranial and spinal meningeal carcinomatosis: comparison with CT and myelography. AJNR 1988;9:709.
38. Laredo JD, Reizine D, Bard M, Merland JJ. Vertebral hemangiomas: radiologic evaluation. Radiology 1986; 161:183.

39. Magigan R, Worrall T, McClain EJ: Cervical cord compression in hereditary multiple exostosis. Review of the literature and report of a case. J Bone Joint Surg 1974;56A:401.
40. Maehara T, Tanohata K, Noda M, et al. Medically treated steroid-induced epidural lipomatosis. Neuroradiology 1988;30:281.
41. Matsushima K, Shinohara Y, Yamamoto M, et al. Spinal extradural angiolipoma: MR and CT diagnosis. J Comput Assist Tomogr 1987;11:1104.
42. Monajati A, Wayne WS, Rauschning W, et al. MR of the cauda equina. AJNR 1987;8:893.
43. Moore EW, Thomas LB, Shaw RK, et al. The central nervous system in acute leukemia: a postmortem study of 117 consecutive cases, with particular reference to hemorrhages, leukemic infiltrations and the syndrome of meningeal leukemia. Arch Intern Med 1960;105:451.
44. Moore SG, Gooding CA, Ehman R, et al. Intensity measurement of the marrow in patients with acute lymphocytic leukemia. In press. Magnetic Resonance in Imaging.
45. Moore SG, Gooding CA, Ehman RL, et al. Prolongation of T1 relaxation times in patients with acute lymphocytic leukemia. Radiology 1985;157:216.
46. Morantz RA, Kepes JJ, Batnitsky SB, et al. Extraspinal ependymomas. J Neurosurg 1979;51:383.
47. Murphy KC, Feld R, Evans WK, et al. Intramedullary spinal cord metastases from small cell carcinoma of the lung. J Clin Oncol 1983;1:99.
48. Murphy FD Jr, Blont WP. Cartilaginous exostoses following irratiation. J Bone Joint Surg 1962;44A:662.
49. Murray RO, Jacobson JG: The radiology of skeletal disorders. ed 2. Edinburgh: Churchill Livingstone, Inc., 1977.
50. Naidich TP, McLone DG, Harwood-Nash DC. Spinal dysraphism. In: Newton TH, Potts GD, eds. Computed tomography of the spine and spinal cord. San Anselmo, CA: Clavadel Press, 1983.
51. Onofrio BM, Svien HJ. Solitary and multiple vertebral myelomas. In: Vinken PJ, Bruyn GW. Handbook of clinical neurology, vol 20. Tumors of the spine and spinal cord, New York: North Holland Publishing, 1976.
52. Olson ME, Chernik NL, Posner JB. Infiltration of the leptomeninges by systemic cancer: a clinical and pathological study. Arch Neurol 1974;30:122.
53. Oot RF, Melville GE, New PFJ, et al. The role of MR and CT in evaluating clival chordomas and chondrosarcomas. AJNR 1988;9:715.
54. Parsons M. The spinal form of carcinomatous meningitis. Q J Med 1972;42:509.
55. Pochedly C. Neuroblastoma. Acton, Mass: Publishing Sciences Group, 1976.
56. Post JDM, Quencer RM, Green BA, et al. Intramedullary spinal cord metastases, mainly of nonneurogenic origin. AJR 1987;148:1015.
57. Resnick D, Niwayama G, eds. Diagnosis of bone and joint disorders. vol 3. Philadelphia: W.B. Saunders Company, 1981.
58. Rewcastle NB, Francoeur J. Teratomatous cysts of the spinal canal; with "sex chromatin" studies. Arch Neurol 1964;11:91.
59. Rodriguez HA, Bethrong M. Multiple primary intracranial tumors in von Recklinghausen's neurofibromatosis. Arch Neurol 1966;14:467.
60. Rubinstein LJ. Tumeurs et hamartomatomes dans la neurofibromatose centrale. In: Michaus L, Feld M, eds. Les phakomatoses cerebrales. Paris: S.P.E.I. Editerus, 1963.
61. Rubinstein LJ. Tumors of the central nervous system: atlas of tumor pathology, series 2, fascicle 6. Washington D.C.: Armed Forces Institute of Pathology, 1972.
62. Schey WL, Shkolink A, White H. Clinical and radiographic considerations of sacrococcygeal teratomas: an analysis of 26 new cases of review of the literature. Radiology 1977;125:189.
63. Schroth G, Thron A, Guhl L, et al. Magnetic resonance imaging of spinal meningiomas and neurinomas: improvement of imaging by paramagnetic contrast enhancement. J Neurosurg 1987;66:695.
64. Seigel RS, Williams AG, Mettler FA, et al. Intraspinal, extradural ependymoma. J Comput Assist Tomogr 1982;6:189.
65. Scotti G, Scialfa G, Colombo N, et al. Magnetic resonance diagnosis of intramedullary tumors of the spinal cord. Neuroradiology 1987;29:130.
66. Shaw RK, Moore EW, Freireich EJ, et al. Meningeal leukemia: a syndrome resulting from increased intracranial pressure in patients with acute leukemia. Neurology 1960;10:823.
67. Sloof JL, Kernohan JW, MacCarty CS. Primary intramedullary tumors of the spinal cord and filum terminale. Philadelphia: W.B. Saunders, 1964.
68. Stechison MT, Tasker RR, Wortzman G. Spinal meningioma en plaque: report of two cases. J Neurosurg 1987;67:452.
69. Stimac GK, Porter BA, Olson DO, et al. Gadolinium-DTPA-enhanced MR imaging of spinal neoplasms: preliminary investigation and comparison with unenhanced spin-echo and STIR sequences. AJNR 1988;9:839.
70. Sudanese A, Toni A, Baldina N. Osteosarcoma as a primary second tumor in a patient with nonhereditary retinoblastoma. Tumori 1986;72:535.
71. Sundaram M, McGuire MH, Herbold DR. Magnetic resonance imaging of osteosarcoma. Skeletal Radiol 1987;16:23.
72. Sze G, Abramson A, Krol G, et al. Gadolinium-DTPA in the evaluation of intradural extramedullary spinal disease. AJNR 1988;9:153.
73. Sze G, Drol G, Zimmerman RD, Deck MDF. Intramedullary disease of the spine: diagnosis using gadolinium-DTPA-enhanced MR imaging. AJNR 1988;9:847.
74. Thomas JE, Miller RH: Lipomatous tumors of the spinal canal: a study of their clinical range. Mayo Clin Proc 1973;48:393.
75. Torma T. Malignant tumors of the spine and the spinal extradural space: a study based on 250 histologically verified cases. Acta Chir Scand (suppl) 1957;225:1.
76. Vinstein AL, Franken EA Jr. Hereditary multiple exostoses: report of a case with spinal cord compression. AJR 1971;112:405.
77. Yahgmai I. Spine changes in neurofibromatosis. RadioGraphics 1986;6:261.

9

Demyelinating Disease of the Spinal Cord

Robert L. DeLaPaz

MULTIPLE SCLEROSIS

Multiple sclerosis (MS) is a demyelinating disease of the central nervous system (CNS) characterized by multifocal, fluctuating sensory and motor symptoms, which often runs a chronically progressive course.[12,30] The age of onset is between 10 and 50 years, and there is a clear geographic tendency, with the greatest prevalance of disease in northern Europe, Great Britain, Canada, and the United States. MS affects cerebral and spinal cord white matter with almost equal frequency; plaques in the cord are a common pathologic finding.[1,32] However, cord lesions are rarely demonstrated by myelography or CT scanning. Reports are limited to anecdotal demonstrations of cord atrophy on myelography, focal cord swelling on myelography and CT in acute disease (two cases), and one case of IV contrast enhancement on CT.[9,18,31,35] The ability to image subtle changes in water content and proton relaxation times with MR allows sensitive identification of MS plaques with clear superiority over conventional techniques. The ability of MR to demonstrate multiple lesions in the brain, as well as in the cord, helps to confirm the diagnosis of clinically suspected MS by satisfying the diagnostic criterion of dissemination in space.[2,41] The appearance of individual cord plaques is nonspecific on MR. Their existence in the setting of clinically definite MS and changes from the acute to the chronic phase of disease allow differentiation from other lesions, such as primary or metastatic neoplasm and infection.

History

From the earliest descriptions of MS the spinal cord has been known as a major site of disease. The first detailed clinical and pathologic descriptions of "disseminated sclerosis" were by Cruveilhier in 1835 and Carswell in 1838,[6,10,12] who focused on lesions in the spinal cord and only incidentally noted those in the brain. The earliest illustration of these lesions, by Cruveilhier, emphasized with remarkable accuracy many of the anatomic features of the disease in the spinal cord that are now known to be characteristic (Figure 9-1). Cruveilhier described the abnormalities as "sclérose en taches" (sclerotic spots) or "sclérose en îles" (sclerotic islands) and the tissue within the lesions as

> . . . dense, more dense than the cord, and it exactly replaces [normal tissue], neither plus nor minus, as though it is destined to replace a void . . . some medullary fibers have escaped degeneration, and are contrasted by their white color against the grey color of the degenerated tissue.

The anatomic distribution of these grey areas of degeneration was also consistent with modern experience of predominantly posterior and lateral column locations. In Cruveilheir's case description:

> The anterior columns of the cord contain a very small number of grey tissue islands, which intercept a part of the fibers of the long tracts. . . . The anterior and posterior spinal nerve roots have undergone notable atrophy. As to the more profound areas of degeneration, they were quite variable, according to the region. The cut in Figure 1 [Figure 9-1, *B*], shows this degeneration, which invades the posterior fasciculus

> and lateral fasciculus, not completely superficial, but penetrating nearly to the center of the cord . . . relative to the grey degeneration, the midline was not a limit, . . . the grooves separating the medullary tracts were also not a limit, and . . . the alteration seemed to invade almost indifferently to groups of fasciculi. . .

The correlation between symptoms and lesion location was also accurately deduced by Cruveilhier, according to the then new concepts of functional organization of the spinal cord.

> As for the effects of this grey degeneration of the cord on sensation and movement, they are entirely confirmatory of the modern doctrine on the columns and nerve roots of sensation and on the columns and nerve roots of movement. [In this patient] sensation was much more profoundly injured than movement . . . [and] the alterations of the posterior and lateral columns of the cord were much better appreciated and more profound than the alterations of the anterior cord.

Unfortunately, Cruveilhier's concepts of pathophysiology did not have the benefit of modern biochemistry, neurophysiology, and immunology, and he attributed the etiology of his "sclérose en taches" to

> . . . a suppression of sweat and more often a suppression of insensible perspiration. The suppressions of sweat are those that ordinarily result in acute rheumatism of the joints. . .

Later in the nineteenth century, Charcot published definitive clinical and pathologic accounts of MS, emphasizing cerebral as well as spinal cord involvement.[7] His detailed histologic descriptions of the "sclérose en plaque" have not been significantly improved upon by more modern staining techniques.[12] He clearly demonstrated demyelination, sparing of axons, gliosis, and accumulation of perivascular fat-laden macrophages.[12]

More recent accounts of MS have emphasized cerebral lesions, especially studies using CT scanning. Current research in MS is focused on immune mechanisms of pathogenesis and on the biochemistry of myelin and oligodendroglial cells.[12]

Pathology

Historic evidence suggests that plaques in the spinal cord are an almost universal finding in MS, and they may be the sites of earliest disease.[32] MS is frequently restricted to the spinal cord, often in association with optic neuritis (e.g., Devic's disease, see below).[32] The distribution of MS plaques along the cord is variable. In the late stages of typical MS, plaques may be evenly distributed through the cervical, thoracic, and lumbar cord, but in early disease there is a clear tendency for lesions to appear first in the cervical cord.[32] Cervical cord lesions may predominate in some patients in association with cervical spondylosis, which some authors suggest is a causative factor through mechanical stresses on the cord, pia, and blood vessels via the denticulate ligaments.[5,40]

Grossly, spinal cord plaques are characterized by their elongated configuration and may extend longitudinally in the cord for several centimeters.[10,32] Acute lesions tend to be edematous and can cause significant cord swelling.[27] Plaques enlarge with new activity at their periphery, and those in the cord are more likely than intracerebral lesions to be confluent .[1,32] Lesions in the posterior and anterior columns are often bilaterally symmetric.[32] Plaques occur preferentially in the dorsal and lateral segments of the cord and do not respect boundaries between specific tracts or between grey and white matter.[32] Plaques are often wedge-shaped in cross section with a broad subpial base and apex pointing to the center of the cord.[32] The contours of plaques appear to be more closely related to the venous anatomy of the cord than to white matter tracts or grey matter columns. This characteristic is consistent with the perivenous inflammation seen on microscopic examination.[20,32]

In some lesions in the spinal cord, demyelination may be restricted to specific white matter tracts and may not be caused by local plaque formation. Remote plaques, usually in the brain, can cause axonal injury in major fasciculi, resulting in descending Wallerian degeneration.[8] Cases of extensive demyelination in the lumbar cord, caused by large plaques in the pyramidal motor tracts of the brain stem, have been described pathologically.[32]

Microscopically, MS plaques are defined as perivenous inflammatory lesions that produce "periaxial demyelination," that is, myelin destruction with preservation of axons.[1] In the acute phase of plaque formation, perivenous inflammation with polymorphonuclear neutro-

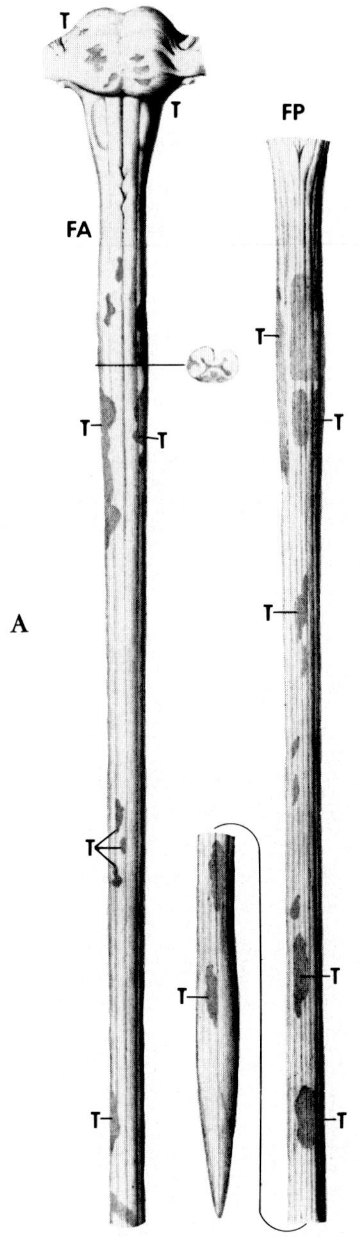

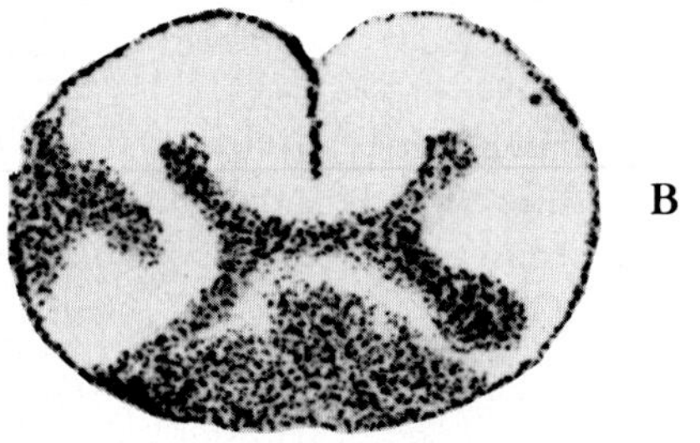

FIGURE 9-1. Cruveilhier's lithograph of *Maladies de la Moelle Epiniere (diseases of the spinal cord)* from the autopsy of 38-year-old female who suffered from bilateral sensory symptoms (reduced pain and light touch), primarily in lower extremities with mild paraparesis. **A,** Gross anatomy of entire spinal cord is viewed from anterior (*FA*, face anterieur) and posterior (*FP*, face posterieur) surfaces. Irregular areas of grey degeneration (degeneration grise) are dark areas labeled with letter *T*, for sclerotic spots (sclérose en taches) that are present throughout length of the cord and are predominant in the posterior and lateral aspects. **B,** Enlarged drawing of cord cross section at midcervical level (line in **A**) shows posterior and lateral areas of grey degeneration with typical wedge shape of spinal cord MS plaques. Lesions lie in major white matter tracts and extend irregularly toward the central cord, without being limited by the midline or to specific fasciculi. Central grey matter is largely spared.

phils predominates and is accompanied by interstitial edema.[1] Demyelination then occurs and myelin disintegration is associated with microglial proliferation and lipid phagocytosis.[1] These changes may be seen in white or grey matter, although white matter is usually more severely involved.[1] At later stages of the disease process, 6 to 12 weeks after onset of clinical symptoms,[32] lymphocytic and plasma cell infiltration is present with extensive gliosis (reactive astrocytosis).[33] As the disease approaches the end stages of its evolution, a thin rim of active myelin breakdown and perivenous lymphocytic cuffing may persist at the edges of the "chronic active plaque."[33] Later in the "chronic inactive plaque," the cellular infiltrate resolves and the central part of the lesion contains intact axons surrounded by extensive astrocytic hyperplasia and hypertrophy (gliosis) with increased perivascular reticulin.[1] Most neurons adjacent to plaques are normal; a few show chromatolysis secondary to axon degeneration.[1] The physiologic effect of demyelination is to reduce the velocity of impulse conduction along the affected axons by removing saltatory conduction.[11] There is only meager evidence that remyelination occurs in MS plaques.[11] Thus, remission of symptoms is usually only partial and may be attributed to factors such as correction of transient interstitial chemical and physiologic disturbances and increases in the numbers of sodium channels in demyelinated axon membranes.[11,48]

MR imaging

Techniques

Magnetic resonance imaging of suspected spinal cord MS produces best results with cardiac-gated and flow-compensated T2W spin echo (SE) images in the sagittal plane. T2W images are very sensitive to the increases in water content that accompany perivenular inflammation and edema in acute lesions. Such areas are seen

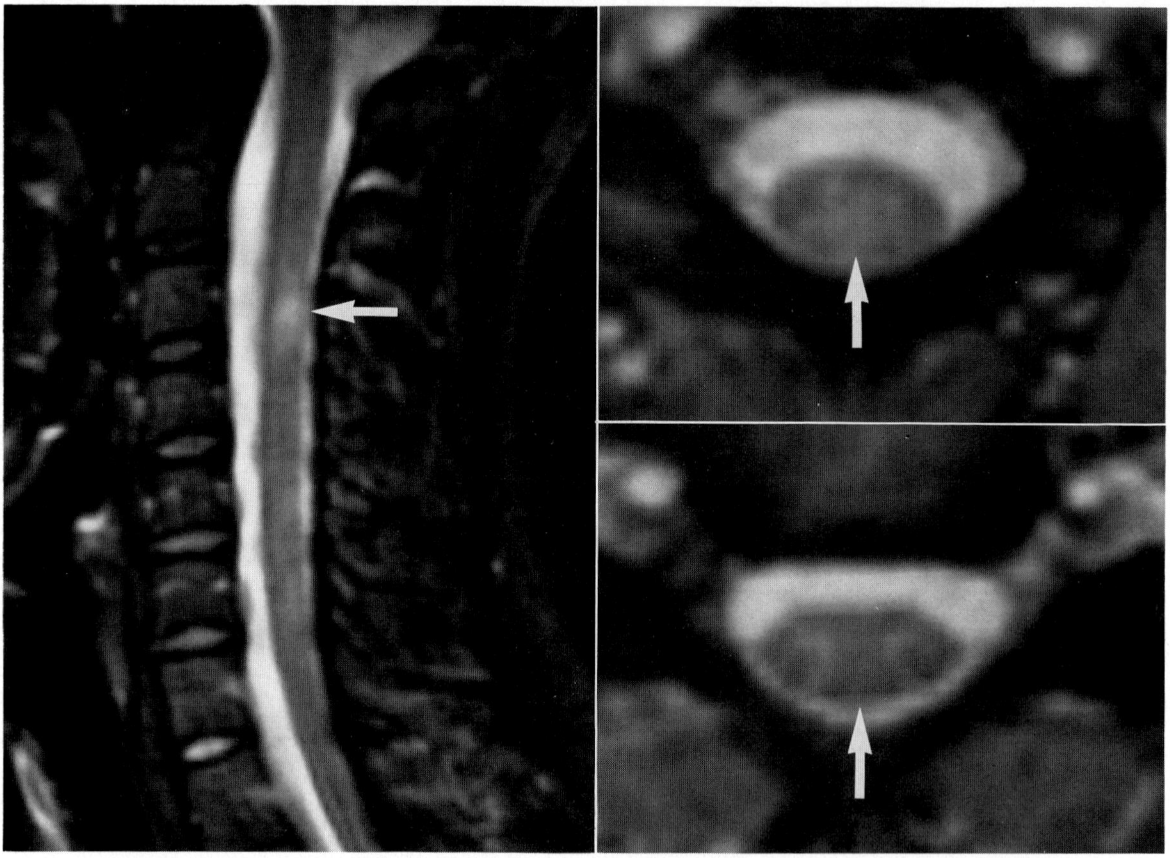

FIGURE 9-2. Typical cervical cord MS plaque in 24-year-old female with history of intermittent myelopathic numbness. **A,** Sagittal T2W image (gated, flow-compensated SE 2500/80) shows high signal focus within cervical cord at C_3 level without mass effect *(arrow)*. Central portion of lesion is higher signal than peripheral areas, which are indistinctly marginated. These differences may represent different stages of evolution of the plaque. **B,** Axial variable flip angle/gradient echo image (TR 40, TE 20, FA 7°) through the lesion at C_3 shows abnormal high signal in central and posterior cord *(arrow)*. Lesion appears to occupy most of the posterior column white matter and cannot be differentiated from central grey matter. Cord swelling is not present. **C,** Axial variable flip angle/gradient echo image (TR 40, TE 20, FA 7°) through cord at C_5 shows normal low signal in white matter of the posterior columns *(arrow)* and symmetric high signal in central grey matter.

as high signal relative to normal cord[24] (Figures 9-2 to 9-4; 9-6 to 9-8). High signal is also seen in chronic lesions at sites of extensive demyelination, gliosis, and atrophy (Figure 9-5). Gated T2W SE sagittal images appear superior to T2*W variable flip angle/gradient echo sagittal images for lesion detection at 1.5T[16] (see Figure 9-3 and Figures 2-19 and 2-34). Long TR variable flip angle/gradient echo images with proton density weighting may be more useful than T2*W variable flip angle/gradient echo images in some circumstances (see Chapter 2). Because T2*W variable flip angle/gradient echo images tend to show significant magnetic susceptibility artifacts, it is recommended that high signal areas within the cord be interpreted with caution and confirmed with sagittal T2W SE images (see Figure 9-3). Axial T2*W variable flip angle/gradient echo images may be used with sagittal T2W SE images to locate plaques within the cross-section of the spinal cord for correlation with clinical symptoms (see Figures 9-2 and 9-6). The best combination in terms of lesion detection and localization with minimum scanning time is a cardiac-gated flow-compensated T2W SE sagittal image set (e.g., TR 1800-2200, TE 20 and 80 msec) followed by axial T2*W variable flip angle/gradient echo images (e.g., TR 40 msec, TE 20 msec, with FAs of 6° to 8°) through suspected lesions. These images are usually sufficient when cord size is not in question. Additional T1W sagittal and axial images may be useful for detecting subtle mass effect with acute lesions or confirming cord atrophy in chronic lesions (see Figures 9-4 to 9-6). The increased water content of acute lesions and demyelination and gliosis in the chronic lesions, are often not appreciated on T1W images. However, loss of landmarks such as the normal low signal in the posterior columns may be a clue to the diagnosis (see Figure 9-6). T1W images are needed if intravenous paramagnetic contrast agents (e.g., GdDTPA) are used (see Figures 9-6 and 9-8).

The specific indications for use of paramagnetic contrast agents with spinal cord MS have not been clearly defined by a comprehensive series of patients. Based on MR experience with cerebral lesions, contrast enhancement may differentiate acute "active" MS plaques from nonenhancing chronic "inactive" lesions. Enhancement in cerebral lesions appears to correlate with active symptoms[23] (see Figure 9-6). Acute

A

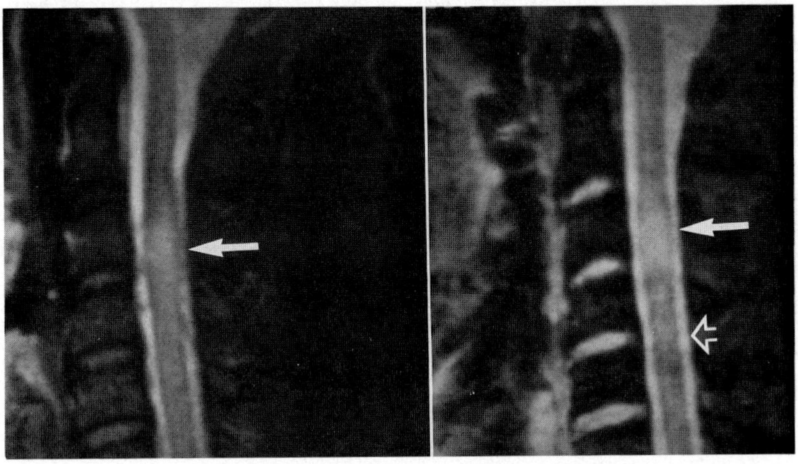

B

FIGURE 9-3. Acute cervical cord MS plaque with swelling in 36-year-old male with recent onset of cord symptoms. **A,** Sagittal T2W (gated, flow-compensated SE 2200/80) shows abnormal high signal at C_3 level with focal swelling of the cord *(arrow)*. Abnormal signal is homogeneous with indistinct superior and inferior margins and occupies most of the diameter of the enlarged cord. No other lesions are identified. **B,** Sagittal variable flip angle/gradient echo image (TR 40, TE 20, FA 7°) also shows lesion at C_3 *(arrow)*. Abnormal high signal area appears slightly larger than on T2W image in **A.** Focal cord swelling is also evident. Area of suspicious high signal in cord at C_4-C_5 *(open arrow)* is artifactual and is not seen on the T2W image in **A.**

A 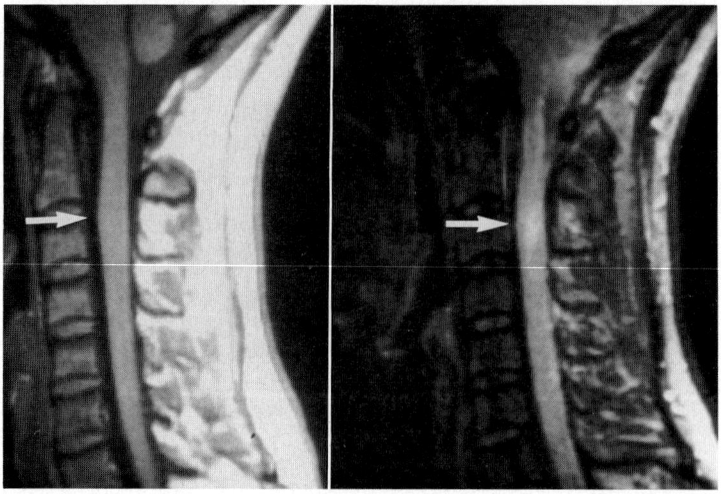 B

FIGURE 9-4. Subtle cord swelling with cervical MS plaque in 28-year-old female with recent onset of cord symptoms. **A,** Sagittal T1W image (SE 800/20) shows fusiform widening of cord contour at C_2-C_3 *(arrow)*. Signal within cord is normal. **B,** Sagittal T2W image (SE 2000/20) shows high signal within cord at C_2-C_3 *(arrow)*. Subtle mass effect seen on T1W image in **A** is not as apparent.

plaques are more likely to enhance than older lesions because of the presence of "leaky" endothelium and blood-brain barrier (blood-cord barrier) breakdown associated with perivascular cellular infiltration and vascular wall complement deposition.[24,44] Contrast enhancement of acute cerebral MS plaques resolves on MR after steroid therapy, probably as a result of steroid-induced repair of the blood-brain barrier.[42] Some acutely enhancing cerebral lesions may resolve completely on follow-up MR after steroid therapy, suggesting that the acute inflammatory phase of the disease may not always progress to permanent demyelination or gliosis.[42] The same repair of the vascular endothelium and blood-brain barrier may occur with the spontaneous resolution of MS plaques. Persistence of active inflammation at the edges of chronic active plaques may account for the marginal enhancement in some lesions on MR (see Figure 9-6). Some areas of apparent plaque (high signal on T2W images) may not enhance, because they represent areas of demyelination secondary to Wallerian degeneration rather than active inflammation.[8] Potential confusion of enhancing MS plaques with neoplastic, infectious, or other inflammatory lesions is subsequently discussed.

Findings

MR (0.35T to 1.5T) is superior to myelography and CT scanning for detecting spinal cord MS plaques[13,19,34,36] and may also be more sensitive to cord lesions than somatosensory evoked potentials, especially in the cervical cord.[36] Spinal cord MR is positive in 75% to 86% of cases with clinically suspected cord MS.[13,36,39] Lesions in the cervical spinal cord were seen in 48% of cases with or without myelopathic symptoms in one series.[34] As mentioned previously, T2-weighted SE images are most sensitive to cord lesions. In one series of 38 patients, T2W SE images were positive in 100% of cases, whereas T1-weighted SE images were positive (low signal or mass effect) in 42% and T2*W variable flip angle/gradient echo images were positive (high signal foci) in 82%.[13] In the various MR series, lesions are seen predominantly in the cervical region. This may reflect early stages of disease, may be a sampling bias in the cases selected, or may be a result of technical factors (such as higher signal to noise images obtained with the smaller or circumferential surface coils used in the cervical region). In one series, 8% of lesions were at the cervicomedullary junction, 86% were in the cervical cord, and 6% were in the thoracic cord.[13] Lesions were seen at multiple levels (usually two

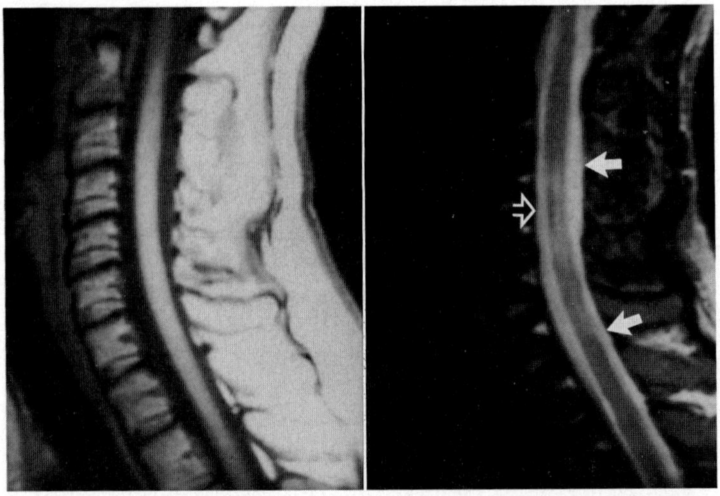

FIGURE 9-5. Chronic cervical cord MS plaques in 43-year-old female with long history of recurrent cord symptoms. **A,** Sagittal T1W image (SE 800/25) shows normal-appearing cervical cord. **B,** Sagittal T2W image (gated SE 2100/80) shows multiple confluent lesions with indistinct irregular margins from C_4-C_7 *(between arrows)*. Appearance of atrophy at C_4-C_5 *(open arrow)* is not supported by the T1W image and may be caused by low contrast between high signal in posterior columns and adjacent CSF, or slight deviation of the cord out of the plane of the scan.

or three) in 12% to 40% of cases in two series[13,34] (see Figure 9-5).

There is a good correlation between location of the plaque in the cord cross section on MR and clinical myelopathic findings (see Figure 9-6). In one series, MR lesions corresponded to focal clinical signs in 77% of cases.[36] Clinical findings typically include the Brown-Sequard syndrome with hemicord lesions, limb deafferentiation and Lhermitte's symptom with posterior lesions, and focal motor deficits with anterior cord lesions. Clinical symptoms may be difficult to correlate directly with specific lesions when widely disseminated cerebral and cord disease is present.[38] This was true in one study where clinical symptoms were not precisely correlated with lesions in 60% of cases (with widely disseminated disease) and appeared to be associated with specific cord lesions in the other 40% of cases.[34] Vertebral spondylosis may be associated with cervical cord lesions, possibly a result of mechanical stress on the cord (see pathology section).[5,40] In one MR series, significant spondylosis was present at the levels of cervical cord lesions in 14% of cases.[13]

Confirmatory laboratory evidence for active MS, such as cerebrospinal fluid (CSF) protein electrophoresis with oligoclonal bands, may not be as helpful with spinal cord MS as with cerebral disease.[17] One MR series showed a strong correlation between the presence of CSF oligoclonal bands and positive brain MR, but exhibited a poor correlation with spinal cord lesions on MR. Oligoclonal bands were frequently absent with extensive cord disease on MR in patients with clinically definite MS.[13,19]

Typical periventricular cerebral lesions of MS are seen in most cases with myelopathic symptoms and positive spinal cord MR, 81% in one series[13] (see Figure 9-6). However, spinal cord lesions may be present with a normal brain MR study, and conversely, brain lesions may be seen with a normal spinal cord study in patients with myelopathy. In one MR series, cord lesions were seen with a normal brain MR in 16% of cases and brain images were positive with a normal cord MR in 19%.[13] In another MR study, 50% of spinal cord lesions were not accompanied by brain lesions.[26] The rate of true negative spinal cord MR studies is not precisely known because pathologic material is not available from most MS patients. There may be undetected lesions in the cord in those patients with myelopathic symptoms and normal cord MR or, in some

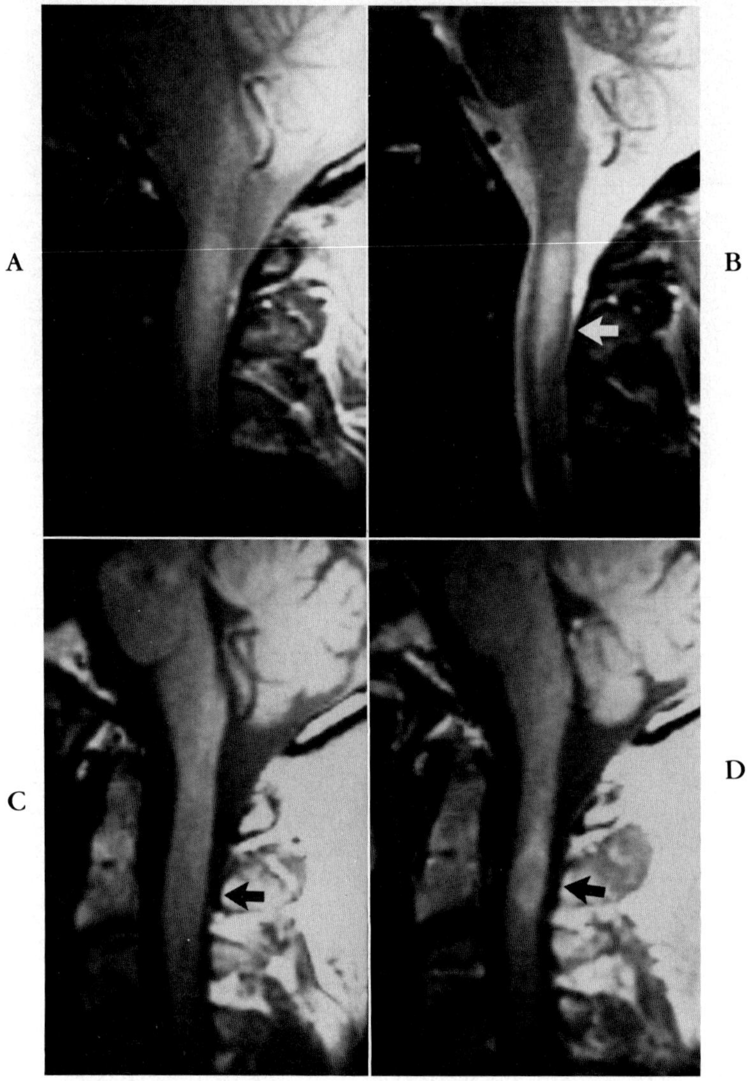

FIGURE 9-6. GdDTPA enhancing upper cervical cord MS plaque in 48-year-old male with episodic left hemiparesis and dysesthesias (numbness and tingling). Sagittal T2W images (gated, flow-compensated SE 2200/20, **A**; 80, **B**) show large, high signal plaque extending from cervicomedullary junction to C_2-C_3 level. Slight cord swelling is present at C_2 level (**B**, *arrow*). **C** and **D**, Sagittal T1W images (SE 800/30) before and immediately after GdDTPA injection. **C,** Precontrast image shows normal cord signal in plaque with mild cord swelling at C_2 level *(arrow)*. **D,** Postcontrast image shows irregular high signal enhancement with greatest degree at margins of the plaque, probably result of greater inflammatory activity at periphery of the plaque. Note that area of enhancement does not correspond precisely to area of high signal on the T2W images (**A** and **B**). Region of greatest enhancement *(arrow)* corresponds only to central and lower region of high signal on the T2W images. Axial variable flip angle/gradient echo images (TR 40, TE 20, FA 7°) through lesion at C_2 (**E**) and through normal cord at C_4 (**F**). Abnormal high signal of plaque occupies most of the central and posterior cord cross section (**E,** *arrow*). Normal bilateral areas of high signal in central grey matter and low signal in posterior columns (**F,** *arrow*) are seen at C_4 level. **G** and **H,** Axial T1W images (SE 1000/20) through lesion before and after GdDTPA injection. **G,** Precontrast image shows slight enlargement of cord with loss of normal landmarks (e.g., absence of low signal in posterior columns).

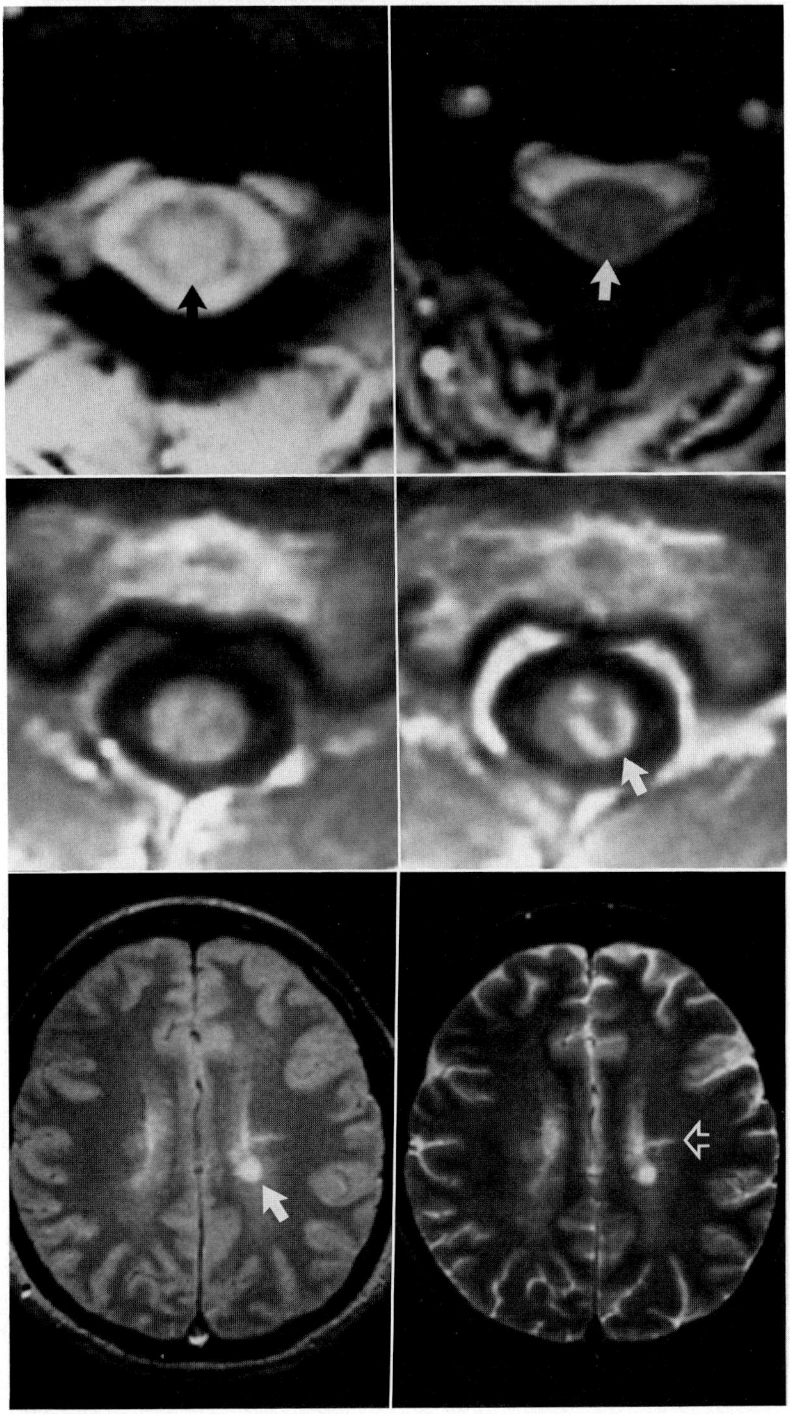

FIGURE 9-6, cont'd. **H,** Postcontrast image shows incomplete ring of enhancement centered to left of midline *(arrow)*, a more pronounced pattern of marginal enhancement of the plaque than that seen in the sagittal image. Enhancement in the left cord corresponds to patient's left-sided symptoms and may represent more "active" areas of the plaque with acute inflammation and demyelination. Axial T2W images (SE 2000/30, **I**; 80, **J**) of the brain show left-sided, round, high signal periventricular lesion typical of MS (**I,** *arrow*) and second linear high signal lesion (**J,** *open arrow*), which probably also represents demyelinating disease.

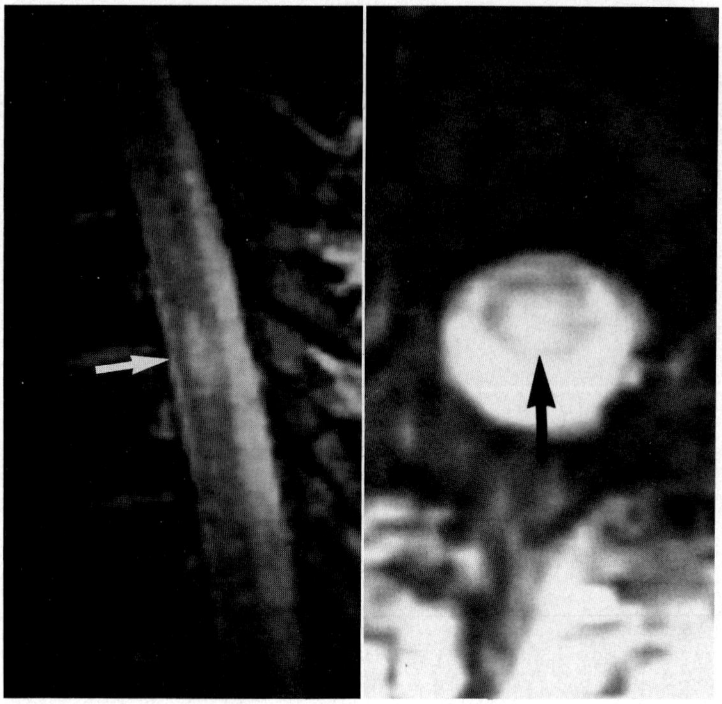

FIGURE 9-7. Thoracic cord MS plaque in 37-year-old male. **A,** Sagittal variable flip angle/gradient echo (TR 40, TE 15, FA 7°) shows high signal abnormality in central midthoracic cord with slight swelling *(arrow)*. **B,** Axial variable flip angle/gradient echo (TR 40, TE 15, FA 7°) shows high signal abnormality in central and posterior cord *(arrow)*. Swelling of cord is not appreciated as well in this axial image.

cases, cerebral lesions may produce symptoms that mimic a spinal cord etiology.[38,43]

Swelling of the spinal cord with acute plaques is well known from pathologic studies (see pathology section) and is seen in 18% to 26% of cases in MR studies.[13,36] The appearance of this swelling on MR is nonspecific and cannot be reliably differentiated from neoplastic, inflammatory, or infectious lesions of the cord on a single examination[13,36] (see Figures 9-3, 9-4, 9-6 and 9-7). Clinical and laboratory findings are needed to differentiate acute MS plaques from other inflammatory or infectious lesions (see Immune-mediated lesions).[36] Serial studies demonstrating spontaneous reduction in mass effect with MS plaques are useful for differentiation from neoplastic disease. In one MR study, focal cord enlargement with high signal on T2W images was seen in five patients during the acute symptomatic phase of MS (2 to 3 weeks after onset of symptoms). Follow-up MR showed perceptible decreases in mass effect after 3 to 4 weeks and a mean time to resolution of swelling of approximately 8 weeks.[13] The reduction in swelling correlated well with spontaneous clinical improvement in these patients, who were not treated with steroids or adrenocorticotrophic hormone (ACTH). A more rapid reduction in mass effect along with symptomatic improvement on corticosteroid therapy should raise the question of an immune-mediated myelitis in the proper clinical setting. Based on this experience, it is recommended that acute cord swelling in suspected MS be followed up with MR at approximately 3 months to confirm significant reduction or resolution of mass effect.[13] Biopsy should be considered with caution at the acute onset of symptoms and, if symptoms stabilize or improve spontaneously, should be avoided until a follow-up MR is performed. Unchanged or increased swelling at the 3 month follow-up may indicate neoplasm, such as astrocytoma, ependymoma, or metastasis, and biopsy should be considered.

Enhancement of MS plaques in the cord may help identify "active" symptomatic lesions

A 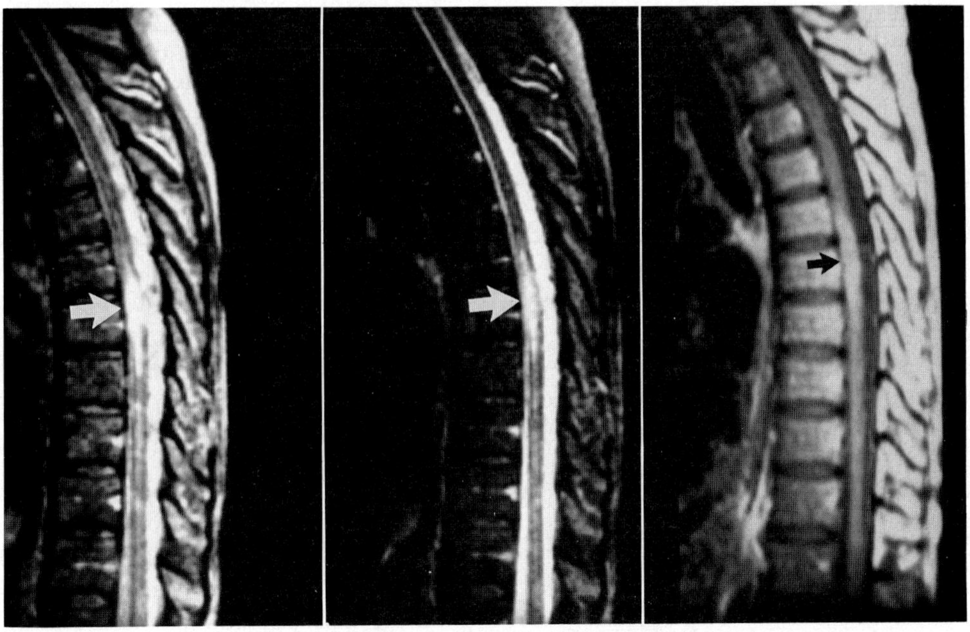 B, C

FIGURE 9-8. Contrast enhancing thoracic cord MS plaque in 30-year-old female. Sagittal T2W images (gated SE 2000/20, **A**; 80, **B**) show high signal fusiform lesion in central midthoracic cord *(arrows)*. Apparent cord swelling is not supported by T1W image in **C** and may be caused by low contrast between anterior cord and CSF. **C**, Sagittal T1W image (SE 600/20) immediately after infusion of intravenous GdDTPA shows uniform high signal from contrast enhancement of the cord lesion *(arrow)*. Contrast enhancement corresponds to high signal on T2W images. Cord swelling is not definitely present. (Courtesy of Dr. Michael Brandt-Zawadzki.)

but can create a diagnostic dilemma (see Figures 9-6 and 9-8). Enhancement may actually decrease diagnostic specificity because an enhancing lesion in the cord may also represent active inflammatory or infectious disease and, especially with cord enlargement, neoplastic involvement. One must rely on the clinical picture to support the diagnosis of acute MS and note changes in the lesions over time to confidently differentiate MS from neoplasia.

Devic's disease

Devic's disease *(neuromyelitis optica)* is a rapidly progressive demyelinating disease restricted to optic nerves and spinal cord. It is probably an especially fulminant form of MS that progresses to severe disability or death before other lesions and the periodicity of the disease can manifest themselves.[33] Massive edema in Devic's disease with acute demyelination can cause secondary circulatory insufficiency that results in cord necrosis.[1] One case of Devic's disease reported in the MR literature is a 20-year-old male with rapid onset of visual blurring and blindness, flaccid paraplegia, urinary retention, and sensory loss below the T_9 level.[46] During the acute disease, MR (0.15T) showed cord swelling and high signal on T2W images from the T_{10} level through the conus, which was unchanged on a repeat scan 1 month later. At 5 months after onset, the patient remained paraplegic with sensory loss below T_{10} and the MR showed severe cord atrophy from T_6 through T_{11}. The MR findings were probably due to inflammatory infiltrate with cord edema, acutely followed by demyelination and, eventually, severe gliosis and atrophy in the chronic stages of the disease. The correlation of MR findings and neurologic symptoms is similar to that for typical MS, with the exception that more severe atrophy occurs and more profound symptoms persist after acute disease.

Other pathologic processes may also produce an association of optic neuritis and transverse myelitis (Devic's syndrome). For example, transverse myelitis occurs in approximately 4% of patients with lupus erythematosis, probably caused by vasculopathy and cord ischemia. In a recent report of two patients with lupus and Devic's syndrome, MR (0.5T) showed abnormal high signal in a normal size cord corresponding to the level of transverse myelitis (optic nerve lesions were not successfully imaged).[29]

IMMUNE-MEDIATED MYELITIS

A group of childhood CNS syndromes have a pathologic picture and anatomic distribution similar to MS.[44a] They are known by a variety of names, including "acute disseminated encephalomyelitis" (ADEM), "immune-mediated encephalomyelitis" (IME), "immune-complex-mediated disseminated vasculomyelinopathy," "postinfectious encephalomyelitis," "postvaccinial encephalomyelitis," and "paraexanthematous allergic encephalomyelitis."[14,28,37,44,45] Symptoms in these postinfectious syndromes are seen within 3 days to 3 weeks after a variety of systemic viral illnesses, most commonly mumps, measles (rubeola), rubella, and varicella. Direct viral infection of the CNS is not present.[45] The incidence of postinfectious lesions is highest for measles at approximately 1 in 1 thousand cases.[37,45] Less frequently, vaccinations are the antecedent event (1 per 1 million measles vaccinations) and unusual inciting factors include bacterial and mycoplasma infections, as well as immunemediated diseases such as ulcerative colitis, acute rheumatic fever, thrombotic thrombocytopenic purpura, and drug reactions.[45] The common denominator of these lesions and MS is a perivenous inflammatory infiltrate in the acute phase of disease followed by local demyelination. Hemorrhagic necrosis may occur in rapidly progressive lesions.[45] The identification of immune-complex deposits in the walls of involved vessels and the similarity of these lesions to experimental acute encephalomyelitis (EAE) in animals (an experimental model for MS produced by an immune response to myelin basic protein) suggest an immune mechanism and imply a pathophysiology similar to MS.[24,28,44,45] These syndromes primarily affect the cerebral white matter. Lesions in the spinal cord may cause transverse myelitis and other cord symptoms, with the most severe cases resulting in cord necrosis.[25,37,44,45] Cord symptoms are usually associated with encephalitis but may be seen alone, as with post measles syndrome, which presents as acute transverse myelitis in 3% of cases.[45] Cord symptoms usually occur with a longer latency after infection than the encephalitis. They often begin with mid- or low back pain and urinary hesitancy that progress to paralysis, occasionally ascending to involve the brain stem. Most patients undergo moderate to complete recovery, but a higher mortality rate is seen with ascending involvement of upper cervical and brain stem levels.[45]

The major difference between immune-mediated lesions and MS is that the former are most common in younger patients (early to mid-childhood when most viral exanthems occur) and are almost always associated with a monophasic illness. Rare cases of relapsing ADEM have been reported that may mimic recurrent multifocal MS.[37] There appears no definitive way to differentiate acute encephalomyelitic lesions from initial MS plaques, except in cases with fever and meningismus, which are rare with MS.[41,45] CSF laboratory studies are not specific for the encephalomyelitis syndromes but are often suggestive of aseptic meningitis with lymphocytic pleocytosis (granulocytes and erythrocytes in hemorrhagic cases), which are also unusual findings in MS.[45] Mild elevation of CSF proteins may be present but there are few reports of electorphoresis characterization (e.g., presence or absence of oligoclonal bands) that might be compared to MS.[4,45] A dramatic clinical response to corticosteroid therapy may help to identify the immune-mediated lesions and discriminate them from MS, but both disease processes tend to resolve spontaneously and accurate assessment of therapy response may be difficult.[45]

MR images of immune-mediated myelitic lesions in the acute phase are likely to be very similar to acute MS plaques with high signal on T2W images and cord swelling, caused by the local edema accompanying the perivenous infiltrate. Few descriptions of spinal cord MR in these lesions are available but in one report of the childhood post-rubella syndrome, an MR abnormality was seen in the cord corresponding to transverse myelitis at T_{11}-T_{12}.[4] Enhancement of acute myelitic lesions with intravenous GdDTPA on MR has not been documented but is likely to occur, based on the pathologic similarity to MS, enhancement of EAE lesions on MR, and enhancement of cerebral IME lesions on CT scanning.[15,24] A dramatic response or resolution of MR lesions with corticosteroid therapy, which occurs with cerebral ADEM lesions (1.5T),[3] may help to discriminate myelitic lesions from MS plaques, which tend to respond more slowly. Chronic spinal cord myelitic lesions are likely to appear similar to chronic MS plaques on MR with high signal on T2W images as a result of persistent demyelination and, in severe cases, local gliosis and atrophy. Clinical history (e.g., typical antecedent infections) is especially important for differentiating chronic lesions from MS because helpful objective clinical findings in acute disease, such as fever and meningismus, are unlikely to be present in the chronic disease.

Spinal cord lesions may occasionally be seen with postinfectious immune-mediated peripheral nerve disease such as the Landry-Guillain-Barré syndrome. The ascending paralysis of Landry-Guillain-Barré syndrome is produced by a lymphocytic inflammation and demyelination in spinal nerves and dorsal root ganglia. Axonal destruction in some cases produces loss of anterior horn cells and Wallerian degeneration of fiber tracts in the posterior columns of the cord.[47]

NECROTIZING MYELOPATHY

Necrotizing myelopathies are another group of noninfectious nonneoplastic cord lesions that may be difficult to differentiate from MS on MR. The pathologic hallmark of these lesions is necrosis with little or no inflammation.[21] The age of occurrence is similar to that for acute MS, predominantly in the twenties to early forties, with a wide age range from 3 to 74 years.[21] Lesions are common after systemic infections that range from viral to protozoal (e.g., mumps, typhus, and malaria), but are also common after local infections (e.g., breast abscess, appendicitis, sinusitis, oral infection, and respiratory tract infections) and in association with carcinomas and heavy metal toxicity.[21] Progressive ascending sensory and motor deficits with loss of sphincter control develop rapidly, often ending with complete quadriplegia and intercostal paralysis.[21,22] Multiple spinal levels may be involved, but the initial and most severe lesions are usually at the thoracolumbar level. In most cases the pathophysiology of cellular death and necrosis is unexplained. Nutrient vessels are normal and, as mentioned, inflammatory infiltrates are absent. Acutely, the cord is swollen with liquifactive necrosis, usually nonhemorrhagic, affecting both grey and white matter. An area of demyelination is often seen at the edges of lesions. In patients who survive the acute episode, chronic lesions result in cord atrophy and cavitation (syrinx). Treatment (e.g., ACTH) is uniformly ineffective.[21]

One example of MR in necrotizing myelopathy is available in the literature: a case report of a patient with myelomonocytic leukemia and progressive ascending motor and sensory myelopathy.[22] MR (0.35T) showed high signal without swelling in the cervical cord from the foramen magnum to C_4, corresponding to neuropathologic findings of diffuse nonhemorrhagic necrosis affecting both grey and white matter. Leukemic infiltration, opportunistic infection, nutritional deficiency (B_{12}), radiation injury, chemotherapy toxicity, and vascular abnormality were excluded as causes, and the lesion was interpreted as a "paraneoplastic" necrotizing myelopathy.

SUMMARY

In clinically definite MS, spinal cord lesions showing high signal on MR, with or without cord swelling or contrast enhancement, can be best explained by the perivenous inflammatory, demyelinating, and gliotic pathology of MS plaques. However, when evidence for MS is equivocal or with single lesions and the initial onset of symptoms, clinical findings, clinical history, and behavior of the lesion over time may be needed to discriminate MS from CNS immune-mediated postinfectious/postvaccinial syndromes, noninflammatory necrotizing myelopathy, viral encephomyelitis, bacterial infection, neoplasia, and paraneoplastic syndromes.

REFERENCES

1. Allen IV. Demyelinating disease. In: Adams JH, Corsellis AN, Duchen LW, eds. Greenfield's neuropathology, Ed. 4. New York: John Wiley & Sons, 1984.
2. Asbury AK, Herndon RM, McFarland F, et al. National Multiple Sclerosis Society Working Group on neuroimaging for the Medical Advisory Board. Neuroradiology 1987;29:119.
3. Atlas SW, Grossman RI, Goldberg HI, et al. MR diagnosis of acute disseminated encephalomyelitis. J Comput Assist Tomogr 1986;10:798.
4. Bitzan M. Rubella myelitis and encephalitis in childhood: a report with magnetic resonance imaging. Neuropediatrics 1987;18:84.
5. Brian R, Wilkinson M. The association of cervical spondylosis and disseminated sclerosis. Brain 1957;80:456.
6. Carswell R. Pathologic anatomy: illustrations on the elementary forms of disease. London: Longman, Orme, Brown, Green and Longman, 1838.

7. Charcot JM. Histologie de la sclérose en plaque. Gaz Hôp (Paris) 1868;41:554.
8. Cobb SR, Mehringer CM. Wallerian degeneration in a patient with Schilder disease: MR imaging demonstration. Radiology 1987;162:521.
9. Coin CH, Hucks-Follis A. Cervical computed tomography in multiple sclerosis with spinal cord involvement. J Comp Assist Tomogr 1979;3:421.
10. Cruveilhier J. Anatomie pathologique du corps humain. Paris: J.B. Baillière, 1829-1842.
11. Cutler RWP. Multiple sclerosis. In: Scientific American Medicine, March, 1987.
12. Dejong RN. Multiple sclerosis: history, definition and general considerations. In: Vinken PJ, Bruyn GW, eds. Handbook of clinical neurology. Amsterdam: North-Holland Publishing Co., 1978.
13. DeLaPaz RL, Floris R, Enzmann D. High field MR imaging of spinal cord multiple sclerosis. (Submitted for publication).
14. Dunn V, Bale JF, Zimmerman RA, et al. MRI in children with postinfectious disseminated encephalomyelitis. Magn Reson Imaging 1986;4:25.
15. Enzmann DR. Imaging of infections and inflammations of the central nervous system: computed tomography, ultrasound, and nuclear magnetic resonance. New York: Raven Press, 1984.
16. Enzmann DR, Rubin JB. Cervical spine: MR imaging with a partial flip angle, gradient-refocused pulse sequence. Part II. Spinal cord disease. Radiology 1988;166:473.
17. Farlow MR, Edwards MK, Kolar OJ, et al. Magnetic resonance imaging in multiple sclerosis: analysis of correlations to peripheral blood spinal fluid abnormalities. Neurology 1987;37:1527.
18. Feasby TE, Paty DW, Ebers GC, et al. Spinal cord swelling in multiple sclerosis. Can J Neurol Sci 1981;8:151.
19. Floris R, Bianco F, Rossi F, et al. The role of spinal cord MRI in the diagnosis of multiple sclerosis. Riv Neurol 1987;57:170.
20. Fog T. The topography of plaques in multiple sclerosis. Acta Neurol Scand, Suppl. 41 1965;15:1.
21. Follis AGH, Netsky MG. Progressive necrotic myelopathy. In: Vinken PJ and Bruyn GW, eds. Handbook of clinical neurology, Amsterdam: North-Holland Publishing Co. 1978.
22. Gieron MA, Margraf LR, Korthals JK, et al. Progressive necrotizing myelopathy associated with leukemia: clinical, pathologic, and MRI correlation. J Child Neurol 1987;2:44.
23. Gonzalez-Scarano F, Grossman RI, Galetta S, et al. Multiple sclerosis disease activity correlates with gadolinium-enhanced magnetic resonance imaging. Ann Neurol 1987;21:300.
24. Grossman RI, Lisak RP, Macchi PJ, et al. MR of acute experimental allergic encephalomyelitis. AJNR 1987; 8:1045.
25. Hoffman HL, Norman RM. Acute necrotic myelopathy associated with perivenous encephalomyelitis. J Neurol Neurosurg Psychiatry 1964;27:116.
26. Honig LS, Sheremata A, Shapiro L, et al. Spinal cord abnormalities without cerebral lesions: magnetic resonance imaging study of demyelinating disease. Ann Neurol (abstract), 1986;20:152.
27. Hughes JT. Pathology of the spinal cord, ed. 2, Philadelphia: W.B. Saunders Co., 1978.
28. Johnson KP, Wolinsky JS, Ginsberg AH. Immune mediated syndrome of the nervous system related to virus infections. In: Vinken PJ, Bruyn GW, eds. Handbook of Clinical Neurology. Vol 34. Amsterdam: North Holland Publishing Co., 1978.
29. Kenik JG, Krohn K, Kelly RB, et al. Transverse myelitis and optic neuritis in systemic lupus erythematosus: a case report with magnetic resonance imaging findings, Arthritis Rheum 1987; 30:947.
30. Kurtzke JF. Clinical manifestations of multiple sclerosis. In: Vinken PJ and Bruyn GW, eds. Handbook of Clinical Neurology. Vol 9. Amsterdam: North-Holland Publishing Co., 1978.
31. Latack JT, Gabrielsen TO, Knake JE, et al. Computed tomography of spinal cord necrosis from multiple sclerosis. AJNR 1984;5:485.
32. Lumsden CE. Multiple Sclerosis - a reappraisal. In: McAlpine D, et al. ed. 2, Edinburgh: Churchill Livingston, 1972.
33. Lumsden CE. The neuropathology of multiple sclerosis. In: Vinken PH and Bruyn GW, eds. Handbook of clinical neurology, Vol 9. Amsterdam: North-Holland Publishing Co., 1978.
34. Maravilla KR, Weinreb JC, Suss R, et al. Magnetic resonance demonstration of multiple sclerosis plaqued in the cervical cord. AJNR 1984;5:685.
35. Mawad ME, Hilal SK, Fetell MR, et al. Patterns of spinal cord atrophy by metrizamide CT. AJNR 1983;4:611.
36. Miller DH, McDonald WI, Johnson G, et al. Detection of intrinsic inflammatory and demyelinating spinal cord lesions with MRI, p.9. Society of Magnetic Resonance in Medicine, Sixth annual meeting (abstract), August 1987.
37. Miller HG, Stanton JB, Gibbons JL. Acute disseminated encephalomyelitis and related syndromes. Br Med J 1957;1:668.
38. Miska RM, Pojunas KW, McQuillen MP. Cranial magnetic resonance imaging in the evaluation of myelopathy of undetermined etiology. Neurology 1987;37:840.
39. Nilsson O, Larsson E-M, Holtas S. Myelopathy patients studied with magnetic resonance for multiple sclerosis plaques. Acta Neurol Scand 1987;76:272.
40. Oppenheimer DR. The cervical cord in multiple sclerosis. Neuropathol Appl Neurobiol 1978;4:151.
41. Poser CM, Paty DW, Scheinberg L, et al. New diagnostic criteria for multiple sclerosis: guidelines for research protocols, Ann Neurol 1983;13:227.
42. Poser CM, Kleefield J, OReilly GV, et al. Neuroimaging and the lesion of multiple sclerosis. AJNR 1987a;8:549.
43. Poser CM. MRI, myelopathy, and MS. Neurology 1987b;31:1692 (letter).
44. Renkawek K, Majkowska-Wierzbicka J, Krajewski S. Necrotic changes of the spinal cord with immune-complex-mediated disseminated vasculitis in a case of atypical allergic encephalomyelitis. J Neurol 1985; 232:368.

44a. Reik L: Immune-mediated central nervous system disorders in childhood viral infections. Seminars Neurology 1982; 2:106.

45. Sriram S, Steinman L. Postinfectious and postvaccinial encephalomyelitis. Neurol Clin 1984;2:341.
46. Tashiro K, Ito K, Maruo Y, et al. MR imaging of spinal cord in Devic disease. J Comput Assist Tomogr 1987;11:516.
47. Thomas PK, Landon DN, King RHM: Diseases of the peripheral nerve. In: Adams JH, Corsellis AN, Duchen LW, eds. Greenfield's neuropathology, ed. 4. New York: John Wiley & Sons, 1984.
48. Waxman SG. Current concepts in neurology: membranes, myelin, and the pathophysiology of multiple sclerosis. N Engl J Med 1982;306:1529.

10

Degenerative Disc Disease

Dieter R. Enzmann

MR accomplished for the spine and spinal cord what CT accomplished for the brain. It opened up new, accurate methods of investigating spine and spinal cord diseases not accessible to previous imaging techniques. For this reason some previously long-held tenets and diagnostic criteria need to be modified for the new technology. The capabilities of a particular pulse sequence must be understood, especially when CSF flow characteristics can affect diagnostic capability. Understanding flow compensation and pulse sequences that circumvent CSF flow problems, i.e., variable flip angle/gradient echo pulse sequences, is important because CSF flow characteristics differ in the cervical spine compared with the thoracic and lumbar spine.[9,10] In the cervical region, the variable flip angle/gradient echo scans have major application in axial and sagittal imaging, whereas they are less applicable in the lumbar spine,[9,10,11] where conventional T1W or T2W spin echo (SE) axial or sagittal images (gated or ungated) are more appropriate. The thoracic region is a transition zone where T1W images or variable flip angle scans can be useful. The one constant in all spine imaging is that the initial scan should be a sagittal T1W scan.

Use of a local coil is required for the diagnosis of cervical disc disease and is recommended for lumbar disc disease. In the cervical spine either an anteriorly placed or posteriorly placed local (surface) coil can be used to diagnose disc herniation (Figure 10-1). A review of Chapter 2 is recommended for a discussion of MR scanning techniques.

MR has a greater sensitivity to disc abnormalities than CT or myelography. For this reason, it is important for the radiologist to be familiar with clinical syndromes indicative of disc disease because a higher level of interpretation skills are necessary for determining the clinical importance of a particular finding. An accurate clinical history is essential for proper interpretation of MR findings and their potential relevance to the patient's clinical symptoms. It should be apparent that the MR scan is obtained in a resting, static position and not in a weight-bearing or other position that could potentially accentuate nerve or cord impingement. Lesions need to be identified that could potentially involve clinically relevant nerve roots if stress were applied.[17] Fast variable flip angle scans offer the possibility of obtaining scans in flexion and extension positions. It is also apparent from MR scans that significant pathology, discs, and osteophytes, can be seen without associated clinical symptoms. The presence of an anatomic abnormality clearly does not automatically signify clinical expression.[27,36] Especially with MR the radiologist must relate the diagnostic imaging findings to the clinical symptoms.

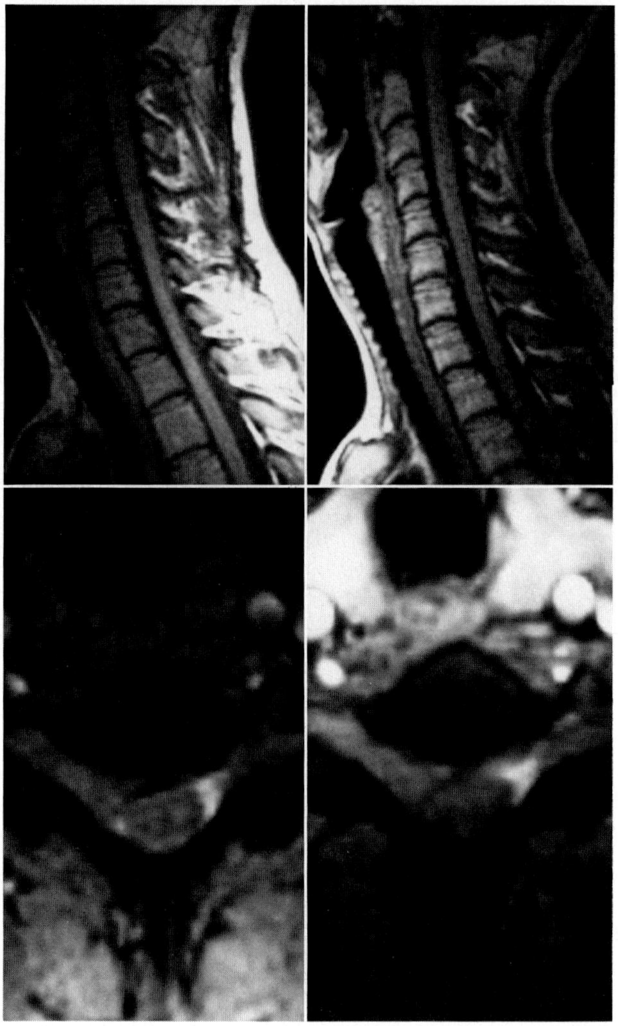

FIGURE 10-1. Surface coils. Comparison of anterior and posterior neck surface coil. Sagittal T1W scan (SE 800/20) obtained with anterior coil (**B**) shows midline herniated disc components at C_5-C_6 and C_6-C_7 better than image obtained with posterior surface coil (**A**). Axial variable flip angle scans (GRASS 25/13, 7°) are comparable for anterior (**D**) and posterior (**C**) surface coils in depiction of right C_5-C_6 lateral disc herniation.

CLINICAL FINDINGS

Cervical Spine

As a general rule, with clinical syndromes associated with cervical disc disease, motor findings are more accurate than sensory findings in localizing the disc level. For sensory findings pain distribution is helpful in localization whereas definite sensory loss is unusual and often not very specific (Figure 10-2). This occurs because of the significant overlap of nerve territories in the upper extremity. Sensory findings may range from tingling paresthesia to severe, localized pain. In addition, common reflex arcs can be attributed to specific nerve roots (Table 10-1). The C_5 root affects the biceps reflex, shoulder pain, and shoulder abduction. The C_6 root can affect pain in the biceps, lateral arm, and thumb and index finger; its motor effect is primarily elbow flexion. The C_7 root includes the triceps reflex and the following motor movements: shoulder abduction, elbow extension, and wrist extension and flexion. Pain with the

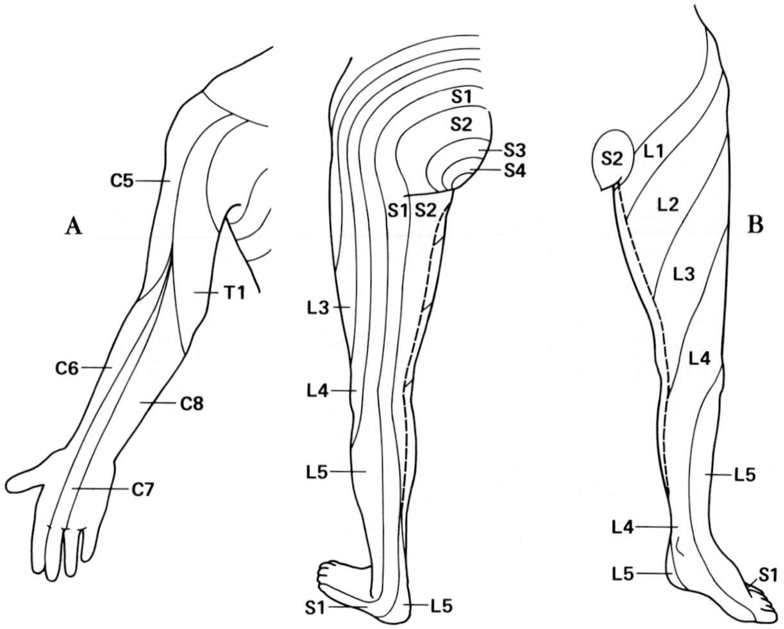

FIGURE 10-2. **A,** Cutaneous distribution of C_5-T_1 roots. **B,** Cutaneous distribution of L_1-S_4 roots.

TABLE 10-1

	Reflex	Pain	Motor
C_5	Biceps	Shoulder	Shoulder abduction (full 180°)
C_6		Biceps Lateral arm Thumb and index	Elbow flexion
C_7	Triceps	Diffuse: entire arm	Shoulder abduction Elbow extension Wrist extension Wrist flexion
C_8		Below elbow	Finger flexion Finger extension
T_1		Shoulder Medial arm	Intrinsic hand Muscles weakness and wasting

C_7 root is usually diffuse throughout the entire arm. The C_8 root may have pain below the elbow with its motor functions involving finger flexion and extension. The T_1 root may cause shoulder and medial arm pain; motor movement in the intrinsic hand muscles can be affected. Pain syndromes may be accentuated by cervical motion, as well as by activities that change CSF pressure such as coughing, straining, or sneezing.

Lumbar Spine

In contrast to the cervical spine, the lumbar spine sensory symptoms are more reliable than motor findings in localizing nerve root lesions because most muscles have their nerve supply derived from two roots. In addition, two other factors must be kept in mind: (1) the actual nerve roots arise from the spinal cord well above their exit point below their respective pedicle and thus have a long course in the spinal canal where they could be potentially affected, and (2) once the lumbar and sacral plexus has formed, individual nerves again course over long distances passing through the pelvis, adjacent to bone edges and foramina, which can impinge on these nerves. Lesions in these locations (i.e., the thoracolumbar region, the lumbar and sacral plexuses, and the pelvis) could be mistaken for disc disease (Figure 10-3). Table 10-2 lists the pertinent reflexes, pain distributions, and motor weaknesses associated with various lumbar and

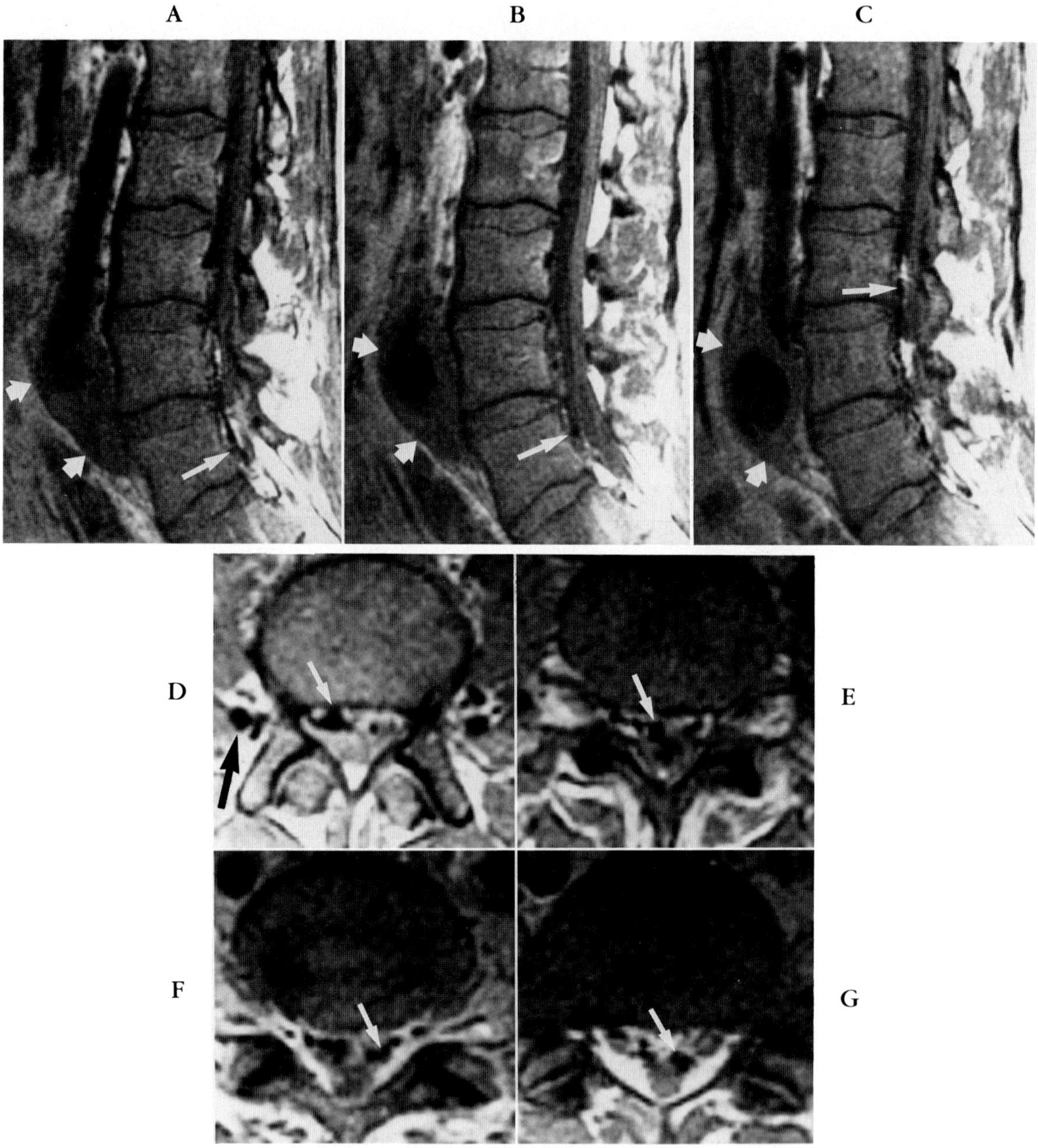

FIGURE 10-3. Mycotic aneurysm. Low back pain may not be result of lumbar degenerative disc disease; other salient findings can be seen on MR scans. **A-C,** Sagittal T1W scans (SE 800/20) show unusual prominence of epidural veins, round and linear areas of signal void, in anterior epidural space *(arrows)*. **D-G,** Axial first echo (TE 20) scans of T2W series (gated SE 2100/20) show prominent anterior inferior epidural veins as large round signal voids. Anterior inferior vertebral veins prominent at all levels *(white arrows)*. Longitudinal venous sinus outside spinal canal is also enlarged (*black arrow,* **D**). Enlarged veins are present because mycotic aneurysm (*arrows,* **A-C**) compresses iliac veins, resulting in collateral flow through vertebral venous plexus. **A-D.**

TABLE 10-2

	Reflex	Pain	Motor
L_2		Thigh	Hip flexion
L_3		Thigh	Knee extension
L_4	Knee	Medial leg	Foot inversion
L_5		Back thigh Lateral calf Dorsal calf Big toe	Foot dorsiflexion
S_1	Ankle	Back thigh Back calf Lateral calf	Foot plantar flexion
S_2		Inner thigh Inner buttocks Genitalia	

sacral roots. A diagram of the cutaneous distributions of the various nerve roots is helpful in localizing disc disease (see Figure 10-2). Most disc pathologic conditions affect the L_4, L_5, and S_1 roots. The L_4 root can decrease the knee jerk and cause pain medially in the lower leg. The L_5 root has no reflex but the pain distribution is in the back of the thigh, lateral calf, dorsal foot, and often the big toe. The S_1 root affects the ankle jerk and can cause pain in the back of the thigh, back of the calf, and lateral foot. The lower sacral roots supply the skin of the posterior inner thigh, inner buttocks, and genitalia.

OSTEOPHYTES

Cervical Spine

Clinically important osteophytes form on the posterior lip of the vertebral body on the superior and inferior end-plates; they may be confined to the midline but often extend laterally to involve the intervertebral foramina.[28] It is in this latter location where they have the most serious effect of compressing exiting nerve roots that occupy the lower half of the intervertebral foramen. It is not until these nerves have traversed this foramen and reached the region posterior to the vertebral artery that they form the dorsal root ganglion. The regions of greatest concern in cervical radiculopathy therefore are the posterolateral superior end-plates and the intervertebral foramina. These areas are best visualized on axial views, which are essential to the diagnosis of osteophytic spurs and osteophytic narrowing of foramina. Sometimes sagittal oblique views help, if the spurring is extensive.

Cortical bone and osteophytic bone produce little signal with conventional proton imaging and are thus seen as low signal on most of the currently used pulse sequences: T1W, T2W, and variable flip angles scans (T2*W). In some instances, osteophytes are large enough to produce signal where they are filled by marrow (see Figure 10-8). This usually occurs only with large osteophytes that are in a midline or paramidline location. They can be identified on T1W sequences by high signal fat within them. These types of osteophytes are common in spondylosis and may have a role in cervical myelopathy, but they tend not to be the more lateral osteophytes that cause radiculopathy. Osteophytes without marrow are difficult to detect on sagittal and axial T1W scans. Because adjacent ligamentous structures and CSF are nearly of the same low signal intensity, such osteophytes can be difficult to detect on any T1W image of the spinal canal (Figure 10-4). Some type of motion-compensated T2W or T2*W image is necessary (see Figure 10-4). Such osteophytes are somewhat easier to identify in the more lateral foramen where either epidural veins or epidural fat provides some contrast.

Uncompensated T2W images in a sagittal or axial projection have a handicap similar to T1W images because the low signal osteophyte cannot be differentiated from signal loss caused by CSF flow phenomenon in the subarachnoid space. When CSF gating or other flow compensation techniques are used with T2W imaging, the bright CSF signal provides excellent contrast for delineating osteophytes. Variable flip angle scans, by generating high signal CSF, also provide excellent contrast for detailing osteophytes (Figure 10-5).[9,10,11] Such scans provide sufficient contrast in the foramen because both epidural fat and epidural veins provide intermediate signal intensity that contrasts with low signal bone (Figures 10-5 and 10-6).[9,10,11] T2W images that have low signal intensity fat may not provide sufficient contrast. Variable flip angle/gradient echo scans appear to be the most efficacious scanning technique in the axial view for the diagnosis of cervical disc disease and the delineation of osteophytes.[9,10,11] False positive images are possible because of magnetic susceptibility

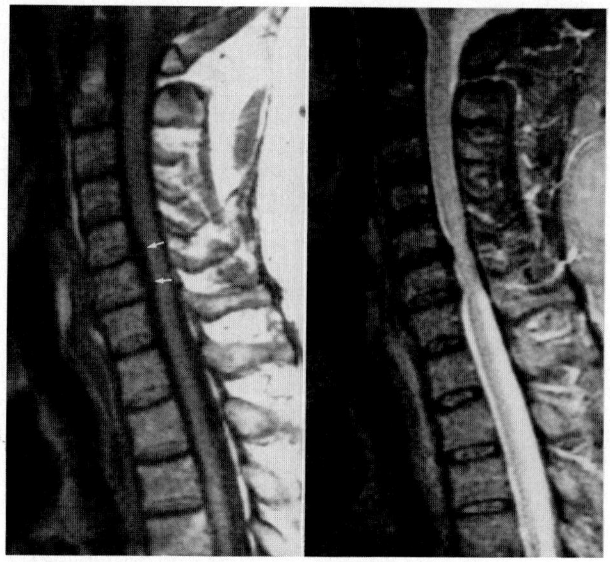

FIGURE 10-4. Osteophytes composed of dense sclerotic bone are very low signal intensity on all pulse sequences. On T1W (SE 800/20) images they can be particularly difficult to visualize because of lack of contrast with adjacent low signal structures such as posterior longitudinal ligament, dura, and CSF. **A,** Osteophytes at C_5-C_6 and C_6-C_7 are difficult to visualize on T1W image; their presence is suspected only because of slight deformity of anterior surface of cord at this level *(arrows)*. **B,** T2W image (SE gated, 2000/80) clearly shows osteophytes, which narrow spinal canal at C_5-C_7 level. Low signal osteophytes seen well because of high contrast afforded by high CSF signal.

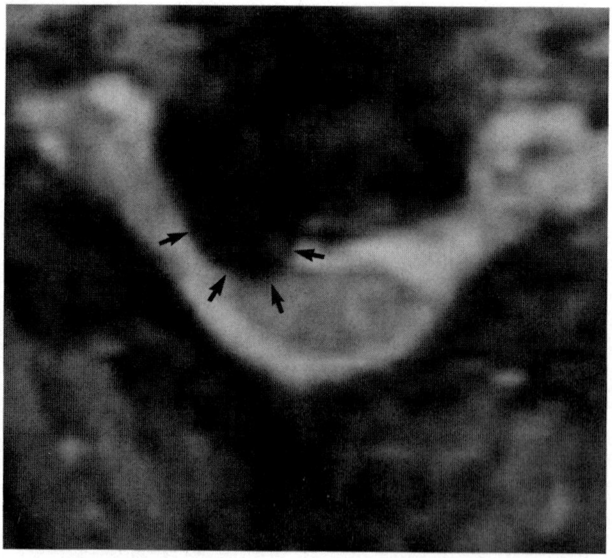

FIGURE 10-5. Osteophyte. Axial, variable flip angle/gradient echo scan (GRASS 30/13, 7°) shows osteophyte well depicted with this pulse sequence as an area of marked low signal intensity *(arrows)*. Osteophyte involving right uncinate process impinges on right neural foramen and right anterolateral recess of spinal canal. Osteophytes are well delineated because high contrast afforded by adjacent high signal CSF and intermediate signal from fat or venous structures in neural foramen.

A B C D

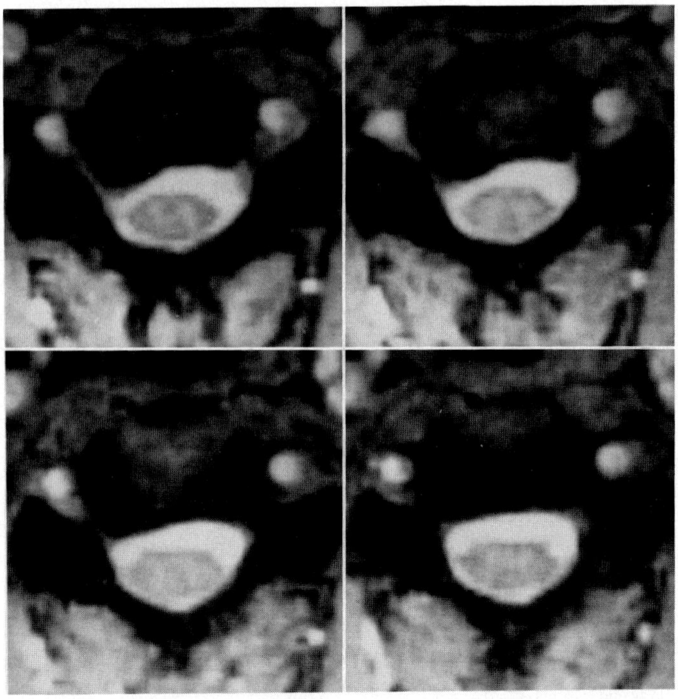

FIGURE 10-6. Osteophyte. Set of four axial variable flip angle/gradient echo scans (22/12, 7°) shows appearance of osteophyte involving right uncinate process, seen with 5 mm overlapping technique (see Chapter 2). Bone is of consistent low signal, impinging into right foramen on all slices through the foramen and allowing accurate differentiation from disc herniation.

effect caused by metallic shavings from surgery (Figure 10-7). In the sagittal view, although a T1W sagittal scan should be the initial scan, a sagittal variable flip angle scan or motion-compensated T2W scan should also be obtained for osteophyte delineation.

Thoracic Spine

Osteophytes of the thoracic vertebrae are uncommon but when present, they often appear with a myelopathic rather than a radiculopathy syndrome. The thoracic cord lies in close proximity to the posterior vertebral body border because of the thoracic kyphosis, thus osteophytes are somewhat easier to identify on T1W sagittal images because of the relative lack of an anterior subarachnoid space. Osteophytes of any significance cause cord indentation and a cord deformity is usually identifiable. Nevertheless, the same problem can occur with smaller osteophytes as in the cervical region because their low signal can be mistaken for the low signal seen in the anterior subarachnoid space caused by pulsating CSF. Symptomatic osteophytes in the thoracic region are normally midline or paramidline; lateral osteophytes are rare and usually of little clinical significance. Thoracic osteophytes can usually be detected by sagittal imaging, and axial imaging is used to confirm their presence and further delineate their effect on the cord. In the sagittal view, T1W sequences often suggest the diagnosis and a sagittal variable flip angle scan or a sagittal motion-compensated T2W scan definitively makes the diagnosis. In the axial view, either a T1W scan or a variable flip angle scan is sufficient to confirm the diagnosis and assess the effect on the cord.

Lumbar Spine

Osteophytes commonly occur in the lumbar region involving both end-plates of the vertebral body. They may be large enough to contain marrow or fat elements (Figure 10-8). It is often an osteophyte from the superior articulating facet

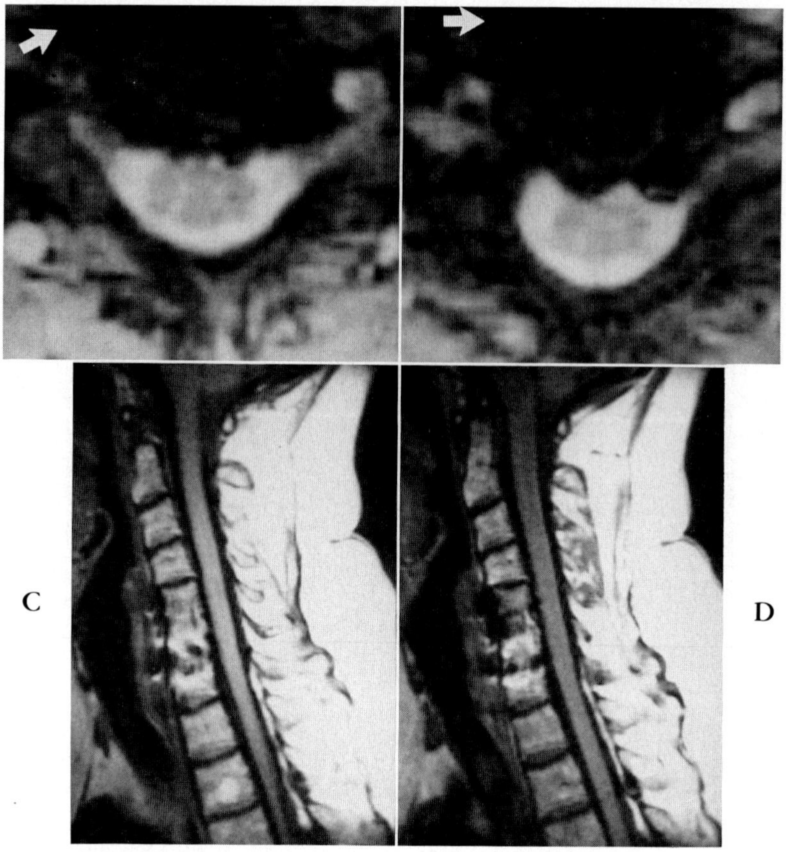

FIGURE 10-7. Magnetic susceptibility artifact. Axial, variable flip angle/gradient echo scans (22/12, 7°) show several anterior low signal areas extending into spinal canal and left neural foramen (**B**). Note large areas of low signal extending into prevertebral soft tissue beyond anterior margin of vertebral body *(arrows,* **A** and **B**). "Apparent impingement" into spinal canal is not caused by osteophytes but rather the result of magnetic susceptibility effect caused by residual metallic residue from previous fusion surgery. **C** and **D,** Sagittal T1W scans (SE 800/20) show postsurgical changes from C_6-C_7 anterior fusion. Multiple areas of very low signal immediately adjacent to areas of very high signal suggest metallic artifact. On gradient refocused scans (**A and B**) such artifacts are accentuated and when small can simulate osteophytes.

that impinges on the intervertebral foramen causing root impingement and a clinical radiculopathy syndrome.[5] To detect clinically relevant osteophytic changes therefore axial views are required to examine lateral recesses and sagittal views or oblique sagittal views perpendicular to the foramen to delineate nerve root impingement by an osteophyte. Such osteophytes are best seen on T1W scans because fat, which is of high signal, provides high contrast in the foramina. Impingement is seen on sagittal or oblique views as displacement of fat around the nerve by bone and distortion of the nerve. In severe cases, epidural fat is entirely replaced. The problem of poor contrast caused by adjacent low signal of moving CSF in the cervical and thoracic region is less relevant in the lumbar region. T2W scans show osteophytic impingement upon the dural sac or root sleeves because CSF is displayed as white and nerve roots are seen as low signal structures. Variable flip angle scans can also be used in the lumbar region, but results are generally inferior to SE scans.

Clinically significant osteophytes in the cervical, thoracic, and lumbar regions occur at different anatomic sites and because of this, different pulse sequences are needed to delineate them. In general, when osteophytes are adjacent

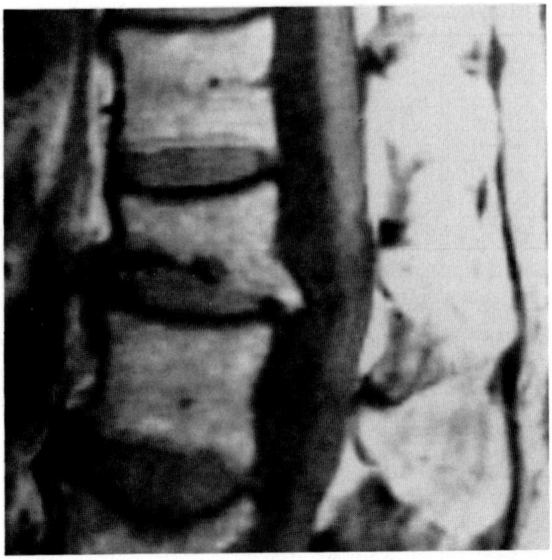

FIGURE 10-8. Osteophyte. Some osteophytes attain sufficient size so as to have marrow elements within them. Such elements usually contain fat giving the osteophyte a high signal appearance on T1W images (SE 800/20). In general, low siginal osteophytes are easier to see in lumbar region because adjacent CSF is higher signal intensity than in the cervical spine.

to moving CSF a variable flip angle scan or a motion-compensated T2W scan is necessary to delineate them. When osteophytes are adjacent to epidural fat, T1W scans are sufficient. These findings highlight a general principle in imaging the spine: in the cervical and upper thoracic region compensation for CSF pulsation is consistently required, whereas this is less important in the lumbar spine because of less CSF pulsation.

DISC DISEASE

Degenerative Disc Disease

Degeneration of the intervertebral disc is seen as loss of signal on T1W and T2W scans and can be easily diagnosed by MR. Disc degeneration is characterized by dehydration and fibrillation of cartilage, which results in narrowing of the disc space. Reduction of the disc's effectiveness as a "shock absorber" causes adjacent bony changes characterized by bone sclerosis, bone spur formation, and subchondral cyst formation. On T1W and T2W images a degenereated disc has lower signal than normal. This is particularly evident on a T2W image where the disc normally has an elliptical area of high signal intensity. The etiology of this high signal is thought to be related to the water content in the disc, although the shape of the high signal of a normal disc on the T2W image does not conform to any specific anatomic structure. Disc narrowing is readily identified by MR as a loss of height between the vertebral end-plates. Gas formation within a degenerated disc can be diagnosed by the complete loss of MR signal, although this can be difficult to detect because a degenerated disc is already of low signal. The presence of gas, however, does not signify any clinical importance other than the presence of a degenerated disc.

The contrast agent gadolinium diethylenetriamine penta-acetic acid (GdDTPA) is likely to receive considerable use in degenerative disc disease because its use can result in enhancement within the disc space diffusely or focally, such as along the end-plate (see Figure 10-49), representing enhancement of fibrous tissue within the disc. The normal avascular disc has vascular tissue encroaching on it and the fibrous tissue presumably represents a reparative attempt to the degenerative process.

Bone changes adjacent to degenerative discs have one of three major patterns. Lower than normal marrow signal is adjacent to the vertebral body end-plate on a T1W image in conjunction with increased signal intensity of the same region on a T2W image.[34] These findings are indicative of damage to the end-plates in the form of fissures and the development of subchondral fibrosis. This fibrous tissue is vascularized and high signal intensity on the T2W image represents an increase in extracellular water compared to normal marrow. In addition, this fibrous tissue exhibits contrast enhancement with GdDTPA (see Figures 10-47 and 10-49). Another pattern in this same subchondral region is low signal intensity on T1W and T2W scans, which correlates with bony sclerosis in the end-plate region. Low signal intensity on both types of pulse sequences reflects the relative paucity of mobile protons that can yield signal. Of these two manifestations of degenerative change, only the first could prove to be of some difficulty in differentiating degenerative change from an infectious spondylitis.[34] Nevertheless, in most instances the differentiation can be made by virtue of the lack of disc space changes usually seen in infection, lack of bone destruction, and the usual parallel orientation of the degenerative changes to the end-plate (see Figure 10-47). The third manifestation of degenerative change is the replacement of subchondral red marrow by yellow marrow or by adipose tissue (see Figure 10-36). In this instance the T1W scan shows increased signal intensity adjacent to the end-plate and low signal intensity (equivalent to normal marrow) on a T2W scan.

Disc Herniation

A variety of terms is used to describe the phenomenon of nucleus pulposus material escaping from the confines of the normal anulus fibrosus to cause nerve root or cord compression. The normal nucleus pulpolsus is confined to the intervertebral disc space by the anulus fibrosus, a concentric lamellar structure which is attached to cartilage of the adjacent vertebral end-plates. The outer fibers of the anulus, attached to bone of the adjacent vertebral apophyseal rings by Sharpey's fibers,[28] cannot be reliably distinguished from anulus although they are of very low signal at the periphery of the disc space.

The nucleus pulposus can migrate from its normal position in several directions. It can herniate through the end-plate into an adjacent vertebral body causing a Schmorl's node, which is probably of little clinical significance. For reasons that are not entirely clear, the posterior lamellar structure of the anulus fibrosus is more susceptible to degenerative weakening than other areas. The nucleus pulposus therefore is often displaced posteriorly. In this location, it may cause simple bulging of an intact anulus. The nucleus may also dissect through the entire anulus, escaping its confines to cause a herniated disc. This can occur posteromedially and posterolaterally. Furthermore, this herniated nucleus pulposus material may dissect either caudally or rostrally once it has penetrated the anulus, producing a "free" or sequestered disc fragment (Figure 10-9). In these latter instances the posterior longitudinal ligament may still confine the disc fragment to the immediate disc space or posterior vertebral body region (see Figure 10-9). Finally, disc material can rupture through the posterior longitudinal ligament, migrate further, and become lodged intradurally (see Figure 10-9).[14]

There is some confusion in nomenclature as to when a disc is bulging, protruding, herniated, extruded, "free", etc. Determining the status of anulus and the exact relationship of a herniated disc fragment to the anulus, posterior longitudinal ligament, and dura can be difficult by imaging tests alone; hence the somewhat nebulous and confusing terminology. Myelography and CT do not allow adequate definition of the nucleus pulposus and its relationship to these structures to allow more specific terminology. Although MR is an improvement, it also does not allow specific definition of what is disrupted by the disc fragment and cannot always differentiate a bulging disc (implying intact anulus) from a herniated disc (implying ruptured anulus). MR, however, is a valuable aid in assessing the integrity of the posterior anulus and posterior longitudinal ligament. A free fragment that has ruptured through the posterior longitudinal ligament has some characteristics that may distinguish it.[20] Disc fragments that have migrated away from the disc space are relatively easy to define. The status of the posterior longitudinal ligament in the presence of free fragments may be difficult to evaluate by MR. Despite these anatomic issues the most important finding is whether the disc, in whatever form, compresses a clinically relevant nerve root or cord and where. This is well delineated by MR.

This text uses the terms *bulging*, *herniated*, and *free* fragment, recognizing that the exact anatomic structural defects are not always known. A bulging disc is one where no focal expansion is noted, rather the anulus boundary extends beyond the vertebral body margin on a broad front. The outer anulus is intact (see Figure 10-9). Herniated disc refers to nucleus pulposus material that focally extends beyond the confines of the vertebral body margins; i.e., asymmetry is a prominent feature in the axial view. In addition, there will be some evidence of rupture (partial or complete) of the outer anulus (see Figure 10-9). Although some authors distinguish protrusion (partial rupture of the outer anulus) and herniation (complete rupture of the outer anulus) this is not practical because the distinction can rarely be made by imaging studies, including MR.[18] In our terminology they are both herniated discs.

Herniated discs are characterized by contiguity of the disc fragment with the native disc space (see Figure 10-9). The herniation may take place through a radial tear or through a transverse tear (see Figure 10-9).[41] The radial tear violates the lamellar structure from the nucleus to the anulus surface. The transverse tear refers to disc material dissecting between Sharpey's fibers and their attachment to the apophyseal ring (see Figure 10-9). These two tears are subtypes of disc herniation. The free disc fragment or sequestered disc refers to disc material that has migrated away from a contiguous position with the native disc space (see Figure 10-9). It ruptures through the anulus and comes to lie between it and the posterior longitudinal ligament, between this ligament and dura, or within the dural sac (see Figure 10-9). Identification of a free fragment is important because the surgical approach may be more extensive and percutaneous methods of disc removal will be contraindicated.

The above disc herniation classification was developed for the lumbar spine. These definitions are similar but less clear in the cervical spine in part because the ligamentous structures are more difficult to define. They may also be less important because in this confined anatomic area simple bulging can cause significant nerve compression. Nevertheless, cervical herniated discs have some distinguishing features especially when they are severe enough to penetrate the posterior longitudinal ligament.[11] When this occurs they cause a large anterior extradural defect on sagittal views and a large focal, sharply demarcated anterior defect on the dural sac in an axial view (Figure 10-10).[11] Free fragments are less common in the cervical spine.

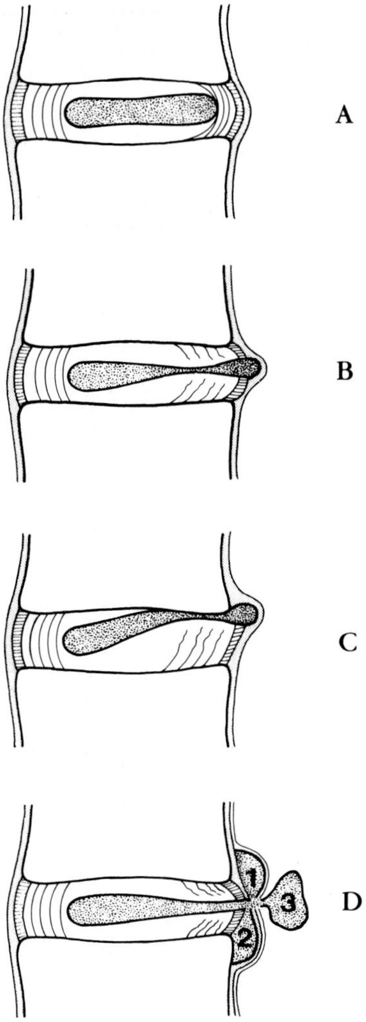

FIGURE 10-9. Diagrammatic representation of **A**, disc bulge **B** and **C**, disc herniation, and **D**, "free" disc fragment. Disc bulge refers to bulging but intact anulus (**A**). In herniated discs, nucleus pulposus material ruptures through a discontinuous anulus (**B** and **C**) but remains contiguous with native disc space. Tear in anulus may be radial (**B**) or transverse (**C**). The latter interrupts Sharpey's fibers. **D**, Free disc fragment or sequestered disc refers to nucleus pulposus material that migrated under posterior longitudinal ligament *(2)*, between ligament and dura *(1)*, or through dura *(3)*.

MR: cervical spine

Disc disease in the cervical spine can cause symptoms by two mechanisms: cord compression resulting in myelopathic conditions or root compression resulting in radiculopathic conditions. Disc herniations causing a myelopathy are usually extensive herniations with a large midline component (see Figure 10-10). To produce a myelopathy, disc herniations often have to be associated with a congenitally narrow canal or ligament hypertrophy, which compromises the spinal canal posteriorly. Central herniations are less severe, cause minimal or no cord compression (Figure 10-11), are quite common, and are easily diagnosed on T1W, T2W, and T2*W (variable flip angle) scans. Mild midline bulges or herniations are common enough that one needs to raise the diagnostic threshold in order to call only significant herniations (see Figure 10-11).[37]

The nucleus pulposus is of intermediate signal

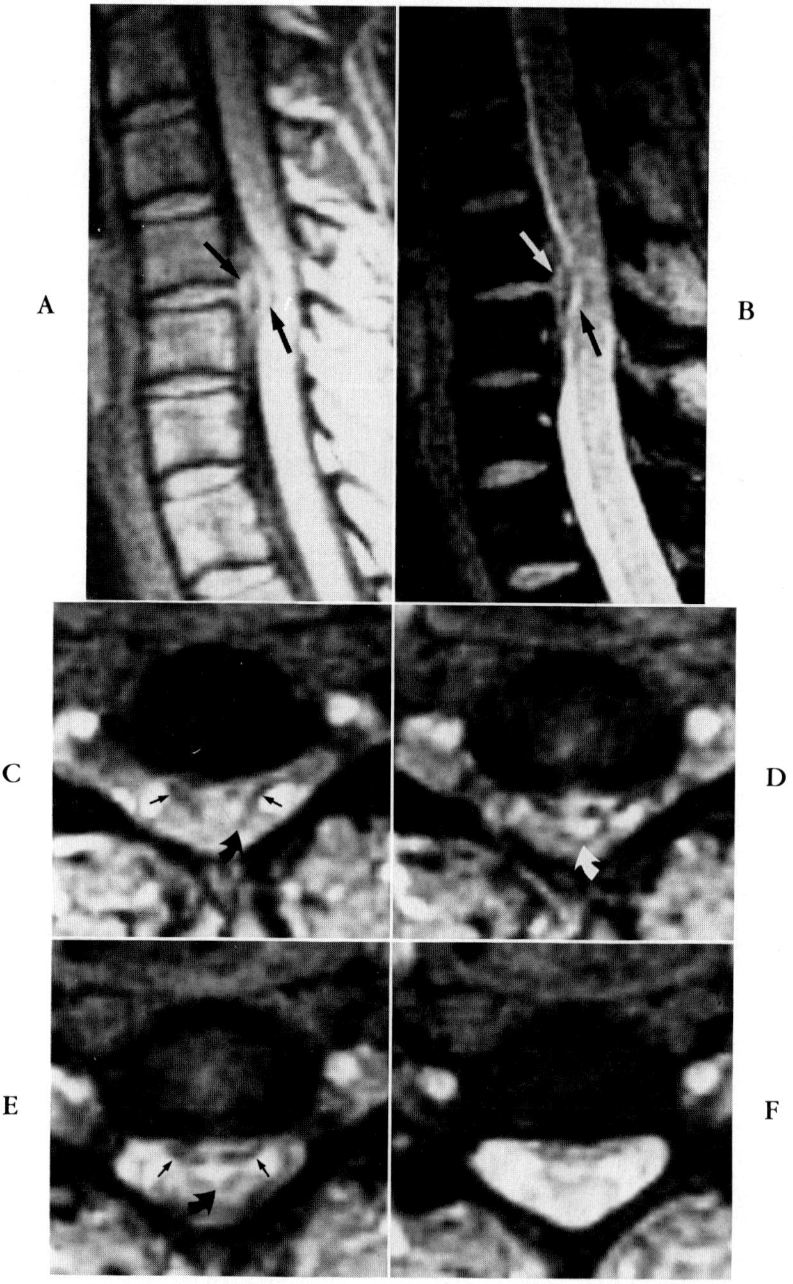

FIGURE 10-10. Cervical disc herniation. MR scan of severe cervical C_5-C_6 disc herniation with suggested rupture through anulus and posterior longitudinal ligament. **A,** Sagittal T1W scan (SE 800/20) shows large disc herniation compressing cord at C_5-C_6. Disc material appears to have two components *(arrows)* separated by thin, low signal intensity line. **B,** Sagittal variable flip angle/gradient echo scan (GRASS 40/20, 5°) confirms disc herniation and two components of fragment *(arrows)*. **C-F,** Axial, variable flip angle scans (GRASS 30/16, 7°) show large midline disc herniation and two compartments of disc material. Broad extradural defect outlined by thin line of low signal intensity probably represents anulus and posterior longitudinal ligament (*small arrows,* **C** and **E**). Second more focal rupture in midline with second thin line of low signal intensity separating disc material from compressed cord (*curved arrow,* **D** and **E**). Findings suggest posterior component of disc herniation represents fragment that has ruptured through posterior longitudinal ligament to lie between it and dura (**C-F**).

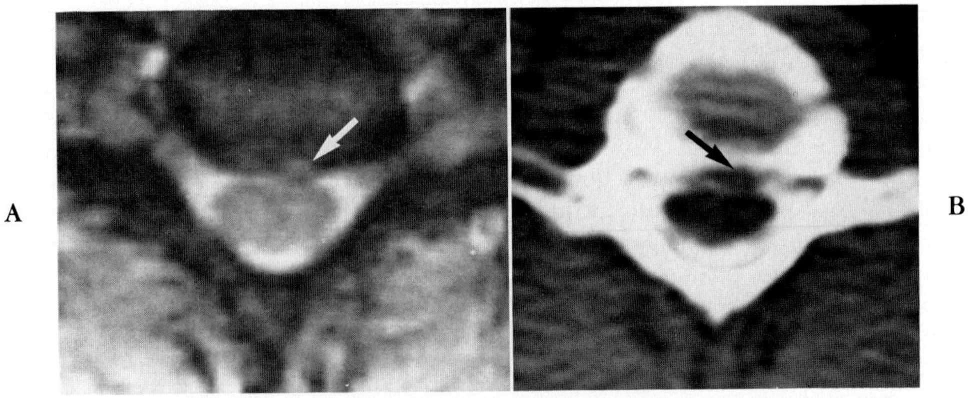

FIGURE 10-11. Small cervical disc herniation. Comparison of **A**, variable flip angle/gradient echo scan (GRASS 22/12, 7°) with **B**, metrizamide cervical CT scan at the C_6-C_7 disc level (CT, 3 mm) shows MR technique capable of detecting very small disc herniations *(arrows)*. Disc herniation is not important clinically but illustrates sensitivity of MR.

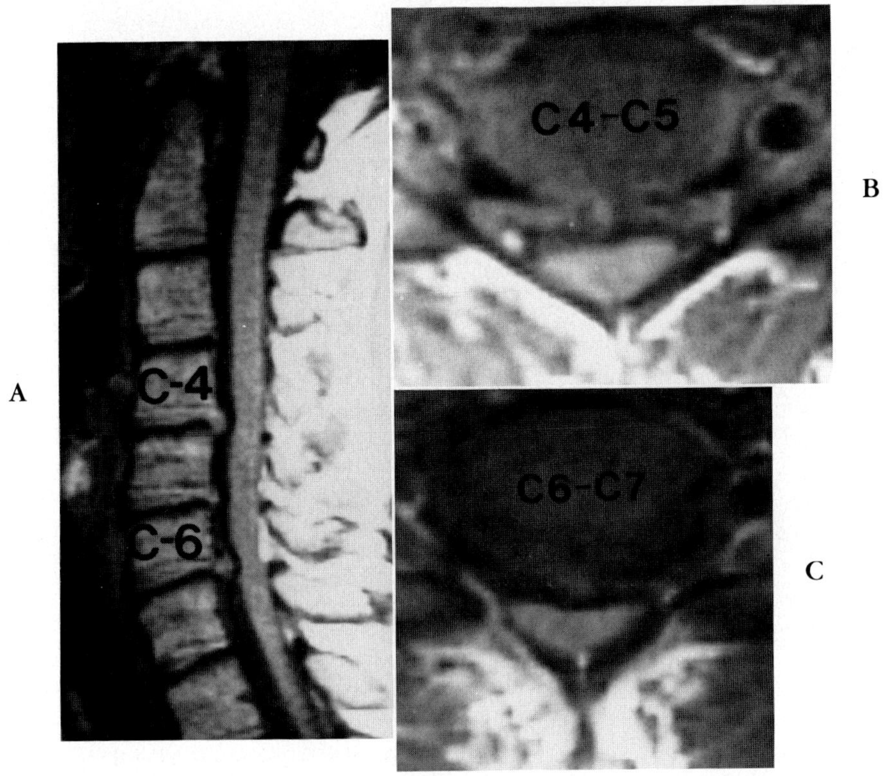

FIGURE 10-12. Cervical disc herniation. Use of only T1W sequences in diagnosis of cervical disc disease. **A,** T1W sagittal scan (SE 600/25) shows prominent disc herniations impinging on cord at C_4-C_5 and C_6-C_7. **B** and **C,** Axial T1W scans (SE 1000/25, 5 mm slice, NEX 4) show disc herniations. **B,** At C_4-C_5 level impingement on spinal canal seen as deformity of cord on right. Discrimination of borders of disc herniation is difficult especially in foramen because disc material is nearly same intensity as epidural fat and epidural venous sinus in this location. **C,** Midline herniation is evident at C_6-C_7 level by increased signal in midline and by cord deformity. (Courtesy of Dr. David Norman.)

on a T1W sagittal scan and extends beyond the confines of the vertebral body as demarcated by the vertebral marrow signal in both disc bulging and herniation. In many instances a bulging disc cannot be definitively distinguished from a small herniation. The thin line of low signal between the nucleus pulposus and the subarachnoid space or cord could represent remaining anulus and posterior longitudinal ligament and dura, or posterior longitudinal ligament and dura alone. The latter two structures cannot be distinguished.

A MR disc protocol can use only T1W scans (Figures 10-12 and 10-13) or probably better, a combination of T1W sagittal and T2*W axial scans (Figures 10-14 to 10-17). Impingement of disc material on the cord can best be seen on the sagittal view. Disc material impinges into what should be low signal subarachnoid space (see Figures 10-12 and 10-13). A T1W sequence shows indentation and sometimes subtle flattening of the cord contour whereas T2W or T2*W scans show low signal ligament abutting the cord, as well as flattening of the cord contour. The low signal line demarcating herniated disc from cord represents a combination of dura and posterior longitudinal ligament, if it is still intact (see Figures 10-12 and 10-13). In the axial view,

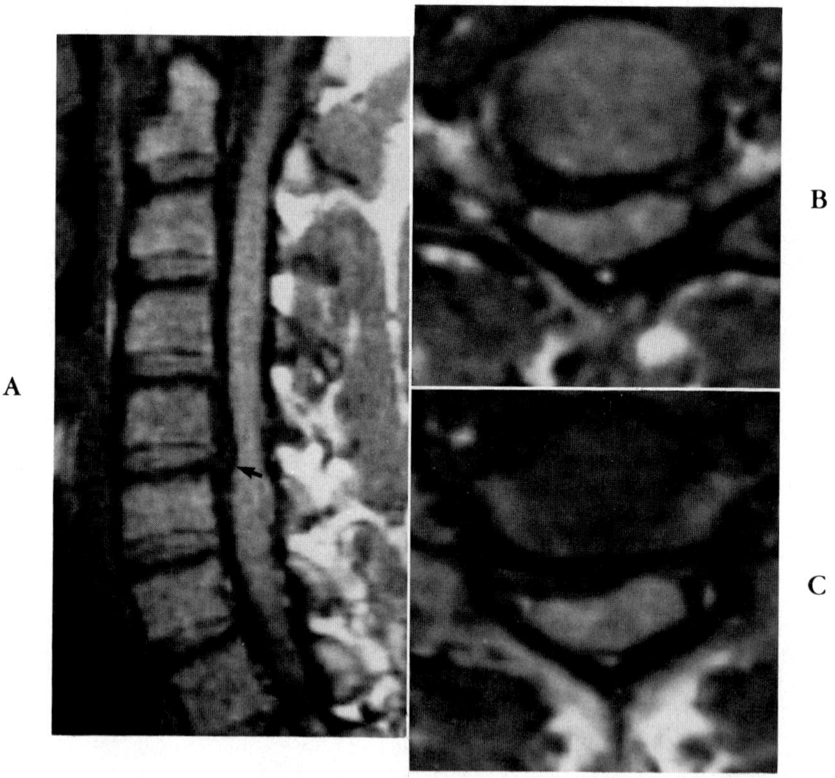

FIGURE 10-13. Cervical disc herniation. **A,** Sagittal T1W scan (SE 600/25) just right of midline shows extradural defect consistent with herniated disc at C_5-C_6 *(arrow)*. Slightly convex area of increased signal behind vertebral body represents disc material impinging on cord. **B** and **C,** Axial T1W scans (SE 1000/25) at C_5-C_6 level show disc herniation extending from midline toward right intervertebral foramen. On highest slice (**B**), herniated disc is well seen because it is outlined by black line representing some combination of anulus, posterior longitudinal ligament, and dura. On lower slice (**C**) lateral margin of herniated disc is more difficult to delineate in the foramen, because of similar signal intensity between disc material and epidural fat or venous sinus. Lesion is detectable by its extradural defect and cord deformity and black linear border. This shows difficulty with axial T1W images in diagnosis of disc herniation, i.e., similarity in signal intensity of herniated disc material and adjacent neural foramen tissue. (Courtesy of Dr. David Norman.)

disc bulging or herniation in the midline can be detected by visualizing the intermediate signal intensity of the nucleus pulposus posterior to the disc space in a convex contour (see Figures 10-12 and 10-13), which may have a broad base to the disc (bulging) or can be sharply localized (herniation). Most of the midline bulges or herniations are of little clinical significance. On T1W scans (sagittal or axial) the posterior anulus, posterior longitudinal ligament, dura, and pulsating CSF are essentially indistinguishable by signal intensity. On the axial view impingement on the cord is usually inferred by deformity of its normal elliptical shape even if the disc material itself is not well seen (see Figures 10-12 and 10-13).

Text continued on p. 459.

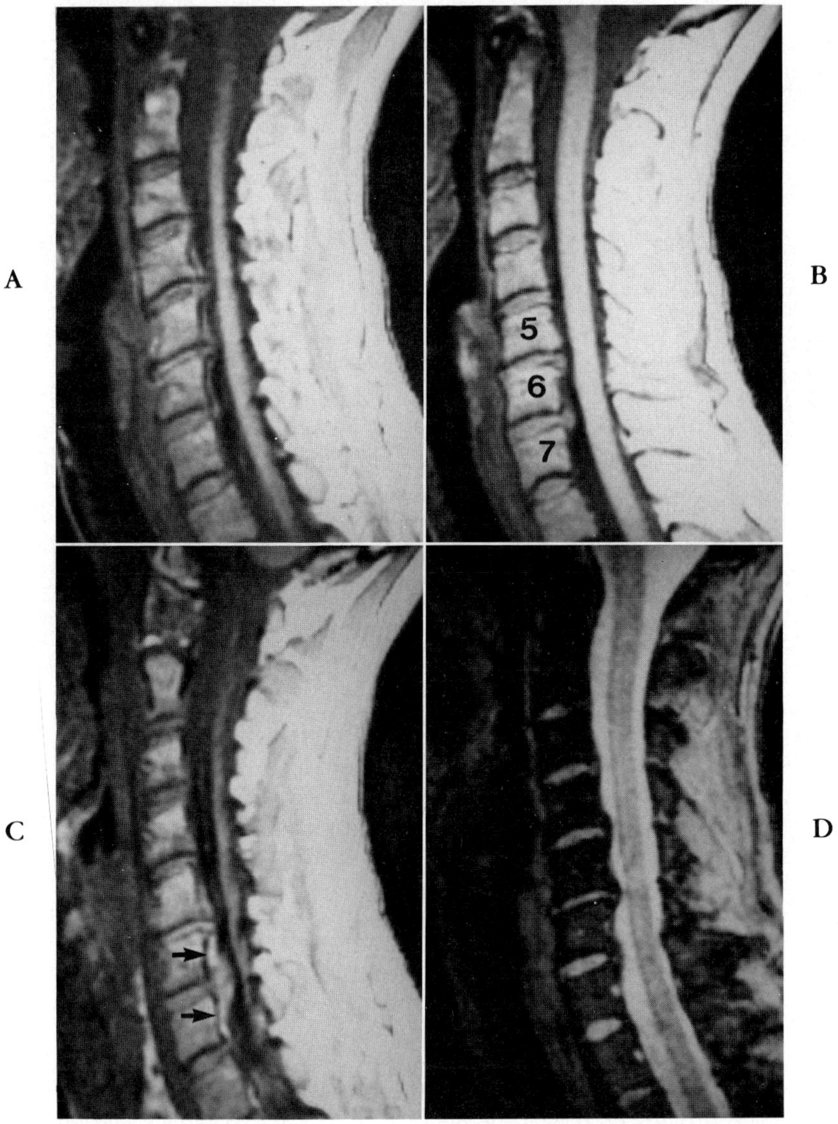

FIGURE 10-14. Cervical disc herniations. MR scans in patient with multiple disc herniations show value of sagittal scans and higher contrast afforded by axial variable flip angle/gradient echo scans compared to axial T1W scans. Sagittal T1W scans (SE 800/20) show, **A**, small disc herniations at C_4-C_5, C_5-C_6 to left of midline, **B**, in midline at C_5-C_6 and C_6-C_7 and, **C**, at C_6-C_7 to right of midline. Disc herniations off midline (**A** and **C**) are more evident because dura and ligament are lifted from vertebral body making epidural venous plexus more prominent (*arrows*, **C**). This is particularly evident with left C_6-C_7 herniation (**C**). **D**, Sagittal, variable flip angle scan (GRASS 25/13, 5°) confirms extradural defects. *Continued.*

E

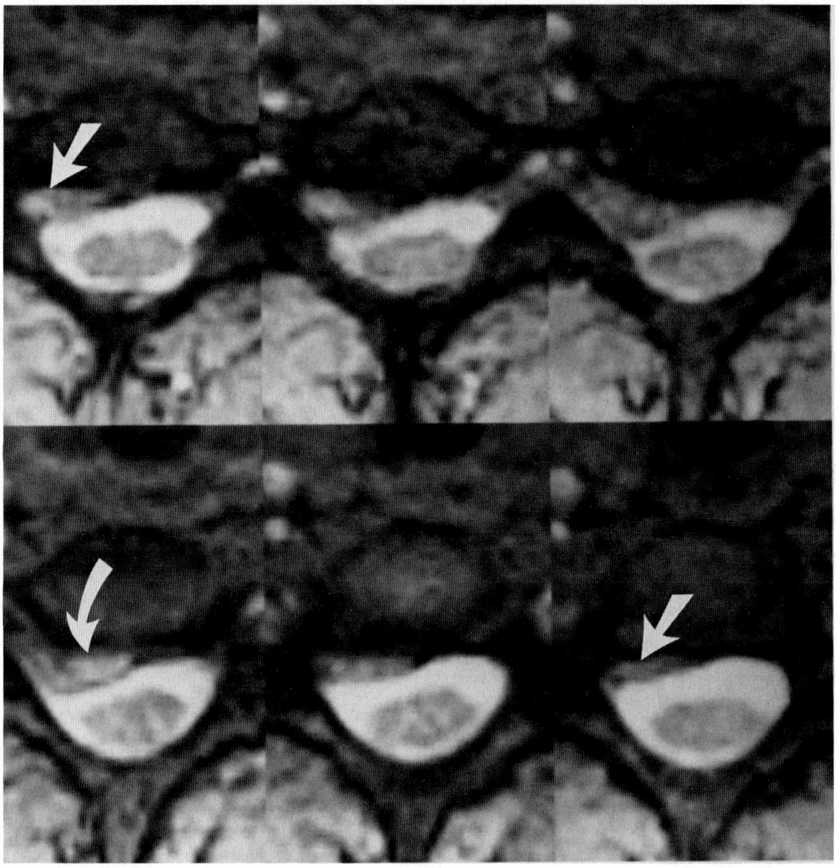

FIGURE 10-14, cont'd. **E,** Six axial, variable flip angle/gradient echo scans (GRASS 25/13, 7°) show large right disc herniation at C_6-C_7 that extends into neural foramen (**E**). Scans span distance between C_6 pedicle *(upper left)* to C_7 pedicle *(lower right)*. Large right extradural defect impinges on right anterolateral recess and into foramen *(curved arrow)*. Herniated disc material has intermediate signal intensity, which is typical; it is outlined by thin line of low signal intensity separating it from spinal canal. High signal at level of pedicles *(straight arrows)* is caused by dilated epidural venous plexus, not herniated disc. These views were obtained with 5 mm slice thickness and overlapping technique (FOV 24 cm, 256 × 256 matrix). **F,** Set of four axial T1W (SE 800/20) scans (3 mm slice) of same disc space using same in-plane resolution (FOV, 24 cm, matrix 256 × 256) shows right herniated disc. Disc material is intermediate signal intensity on T1W scans and easily seen because of large size. There is good contrast between low signal CSF and disc material in the spinal canal but contrast and delineation is less optimal in neural foramen. Cord deformity is evident and seemingly out of proportion to size of disc herniation. **G-J,** Comparison of large C_6-C_7 (**G** and **H**) and more subtle C_4-C_5 (**I** and **J**) disc herniation shows disc more evident on variable flip angle/gradient echo scans (GRASS 25/13, 7°) (**G** and **I**) than on T1W scans (SE 800/20) (**H** and **J**). Both show similar configuration to cord but actual disc herniation is more evident on variable flip angle scan.

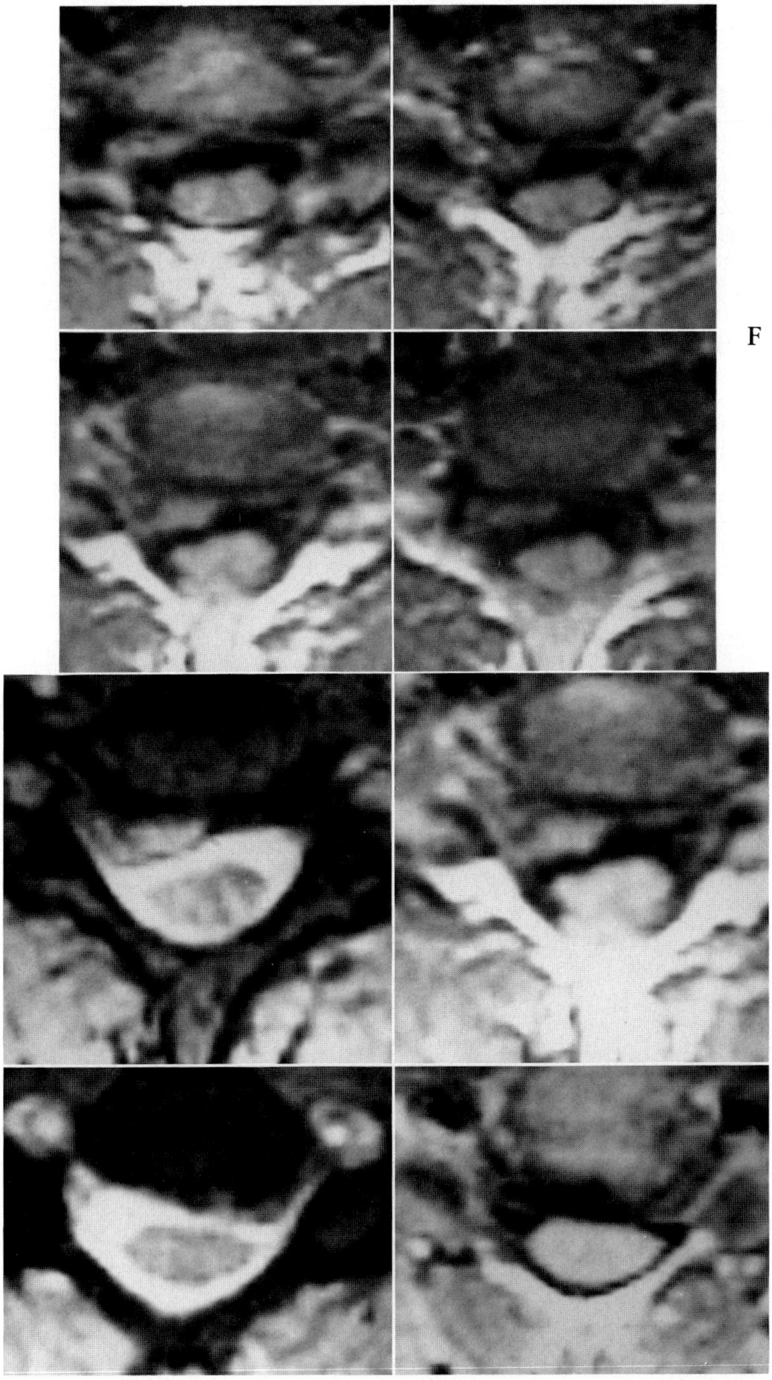

F

G

H

I

J

FIGURE 10-14, cont'd. For legend see previous page.

Continued.

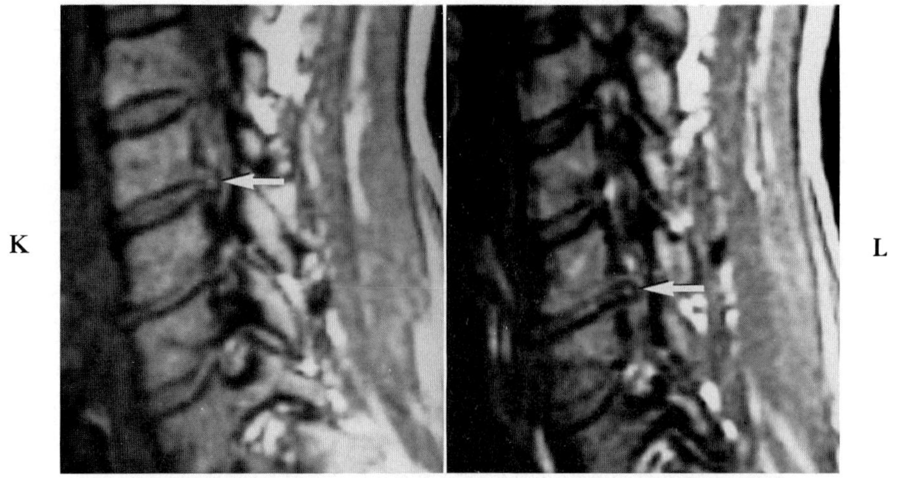

FIGURE 10-14, cont'd. **K** and **L,** Cervical, oblique T1W scans (SE 800/20) were also obtained on each side and angled perpendicular to axis of neural foramen. On right oblique, **K,** C_4-C_5 disc herniation is visualized *(arrow);* on left oblique **L,** C_6-C_7 herniation is also detected *(arrow)*. Oblique views are generally not necessary if axial variable flip angle scans are used.

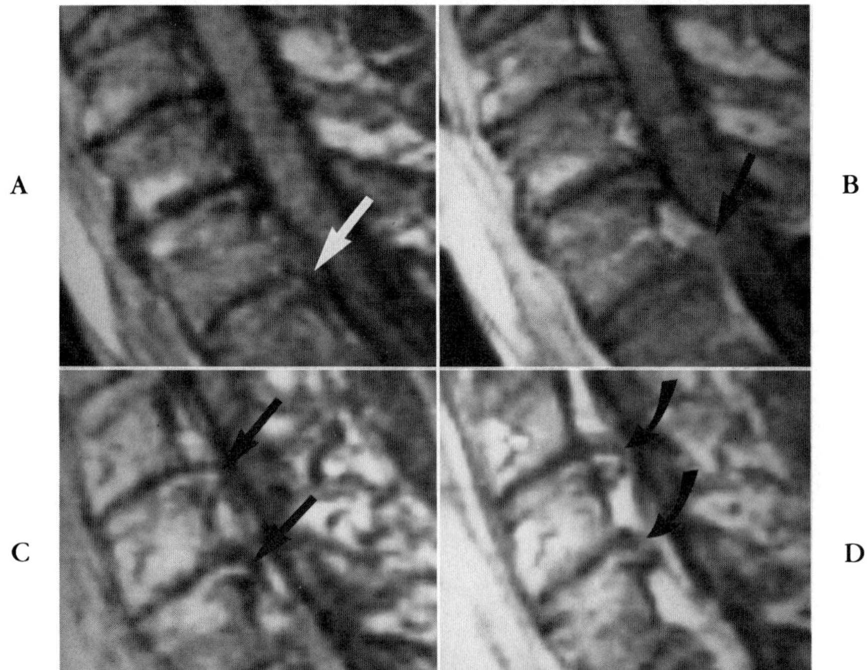

FIGURE 10-15. A-D, For legend see following page.

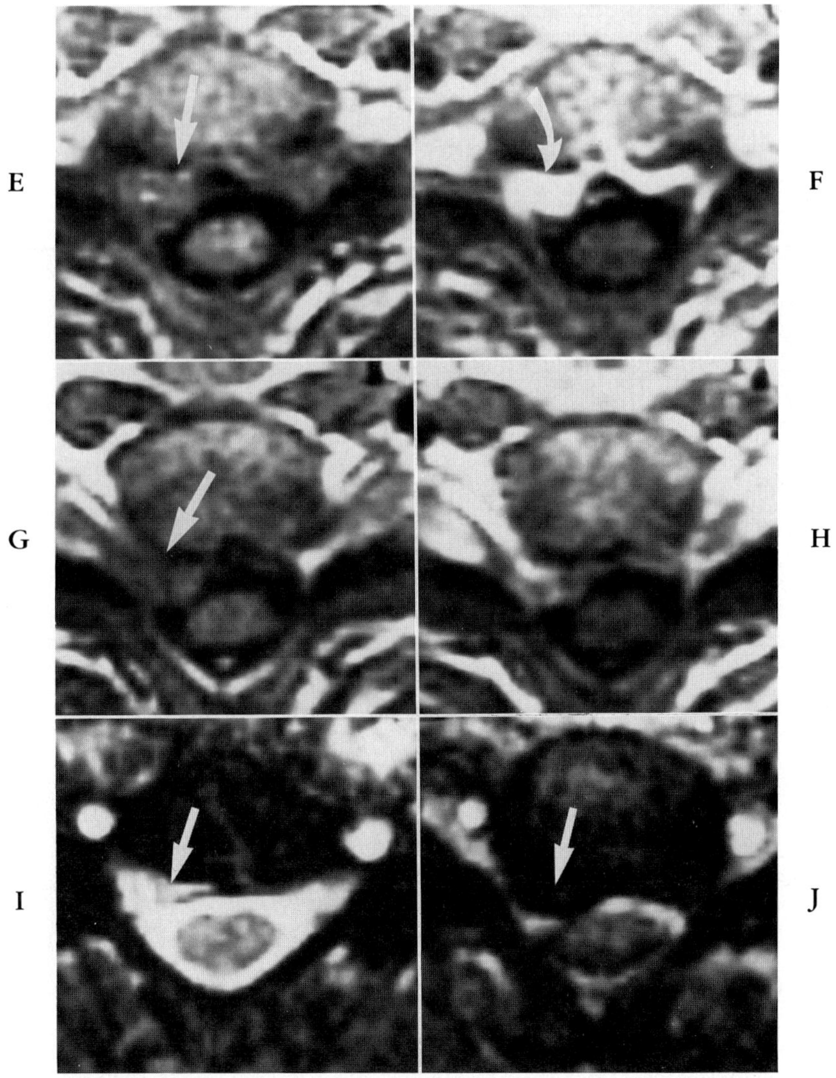

FIGURE 10-15, cont'd. Cervical disc with GdDTPA. Comparison of T1W images and variable flip angle scans. **A-D,** Sagittal precontrast (**A** and **C**) T1W scans (SE 800/20) show moderate cervical stenosis and lateral disc herniation on the right side (*arrows,* **C**). These disc herniations are visible by their continuity with native disc space and their contrast with the dilated epidural venous plexus. This disc-venous plexus contrast is increased after administration of GdDTPA on postcontrast scans (**B** and **D**) where disc herniations are more conspicuous (*arrows,* **D**). At C_7-T_1 level, disc herniation is somewhat subtle on the precontrast scan (**A,** *arrow*) and more evident on the postcontrast scan (*arrow,* **B**). **E-H,** Axial precontrast (**E** and **G**) T1W scan (SE 800/20) confirms presence of a disc herniation in the right anterolateral recess. Extent of herniation within the foramen, however, is difficult to determine (*arrow,* **G**). Postcontrast T1W scan shows two significant findings (**F** and **H**). At level slightly above disc space, precontrast scan (*arrow,* **E**) is seen to overestimate size of the disc herniation compared to the postcontrast scan (**F**) in that a large portion of soft tissue abnormality represents dilated venous plexus (*arrow,* **F**). Within the foramen the postcontrast scan (**H**) shows that there is enhancement indicative of venous plexus rather than disc herniation; the herniation is primarily medial to the foramen (**H**). **I** and **J,** Axial, variable flip angle scans (GRASS 33/17, 7°) not only show disc herniation (*arrow,* **J**), but also dilated venous plexus above the disc (**I,** *arrow*). Although administration of GdDTPA improves delineation of cervical disc disease on T1W images, the variable flip angle scan provides similar information without contrast.

A, B

C, D

E

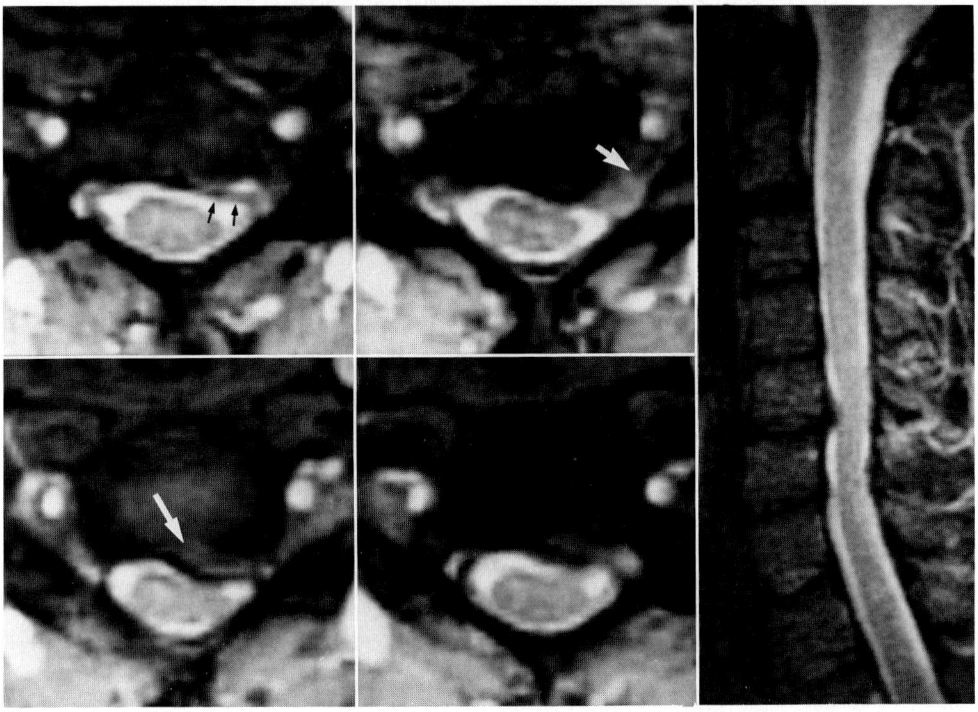

FIGURE 10-16. Cervical disc herniation. Cervical disc herniations have characteristic findings on variable flip angle/gradient echo images (GRASS 22/12, 7°). C_5-C_6 disc herniation depicted on four overlapped axial images spanning interval from C_4 pedicle (**A**) to C_5 pedicle (**D**). **A,** Asymmetric posterior displacement of dura on left *(arrows)* at level of C_4 pedicle. High signal between dura and bone is dilated venous plexus. **B,** On next level, left anterior extradural defect is larger and extends into neural foramen on left. Note disruption of normal dark line in foramen *(arrow)*. **C,** Next lower level shows intermediate signal intensity within extradural defect identical to and contiguous with signal intensity of disc space *(arrow)*. Black line separating herniated disc from deformed cord is combination of posterior longitudinal ligament, dura, and residual anulus. Disc extends into left neural foramen (**B** and **C**). **D,** At lowest level approaching C_5 pedicle the extradural defect, although smaller, is still seen. Two important features of diagnosis of cervical disc herniation are intermediate signal intensity of disc material in extradural space and thin black line demarcating disc material from subarachnoid space and cord. **E,** Sagittal T2W scan (gated SE 800/100) shows midline component of C_5-C_6 disc herniation but extent is only fully appreciated on axial views.

A

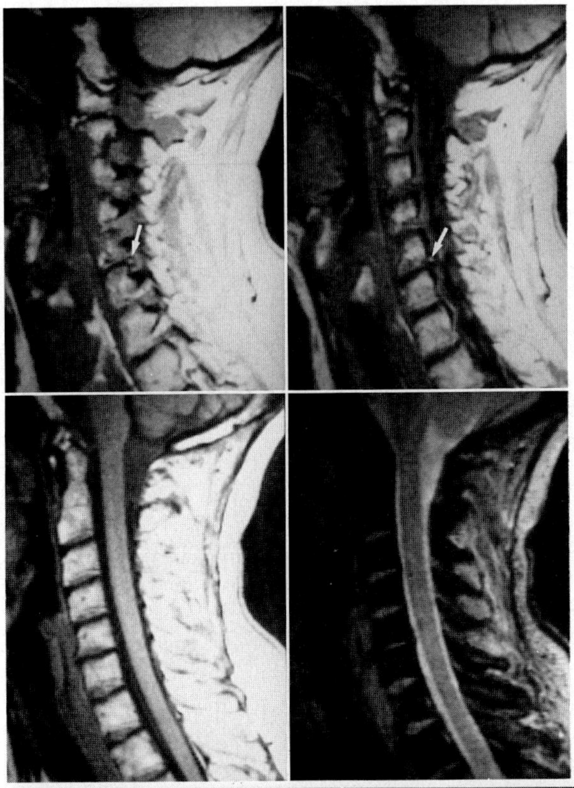

B

C, D

FIGURE 10-17. Subtle cervical disc herniation. Findings in cervical disc disease may be subtle and require close correlation between sagittal and axial images. **A** and **B,** Sagittal T1W scans (SE 800/20) to left of midline suggest small disc herniation at C_5-C_6 *(arrows)*. **C,** Midline T1W scan and **D,** midline variable flip angle scan (GRASS 22/12, 5°) show no evidence of disc herniation. **E-H,** Axial variable flip angle/gradient echo scans (GRASS 22/12, 7°) show subtle findings indicating lateral disc herniation on left within neural foramen. On axial variable flip angle scans, blunting of root sleeve seen on left side (**F** and **G**) when compared to normal root sleeve on right side *(arrows)*. Although no clear thin black outlines disc, signal intensity within left neural foramen is diffusely lower compared to right foramen. This in combination with root sleeve impingement is indicative of disc herniation limited to neural foramen.

E

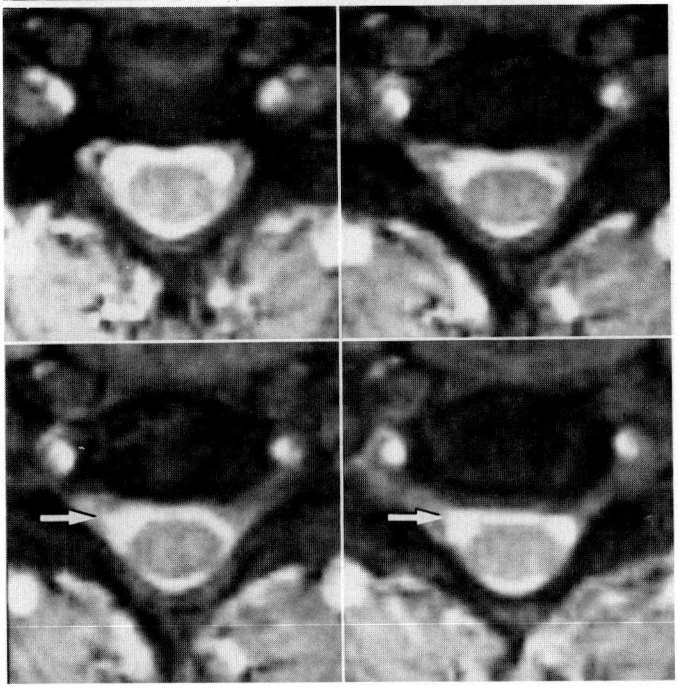

F

G

H

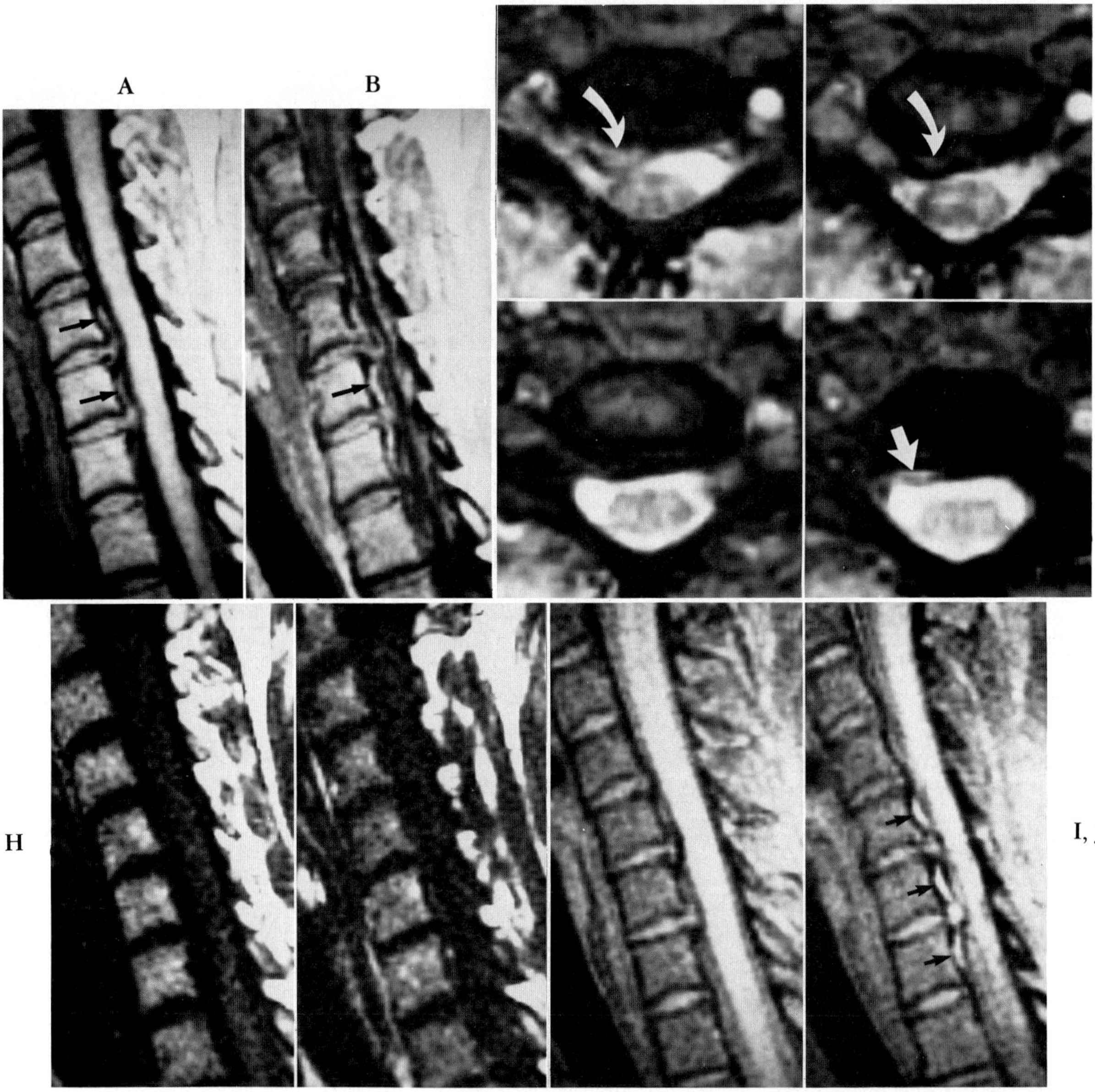

FIGURE 10-18. Epidural venous plexus. Disc herniations in cervical spine can cause prominent dilated epidural venous sinuses seen as areas of increased signal posterior to vertebral bodies. **A** and **B**, Sagittal T1W scans (SE 800/20) show two obvious disc herniations at C_5-C_6 and C_6-C_7. In addition to disc material posterior to vertebral body, increased signal is seen along posterior surface of C_5, C_6, and C_7 in midline, (*arrows*, **A**) and paramidline locations (*arrow*, **B**). Signal posterior to vertebral body should not be mistaken for migrated herniated disc material. **C-F**, Axial variable flip angles scans (GRASS 25/12, 7°) show herniated disc material (*arrow*, **C** and **D**) and **F**, increased signal caused by dilated epidural venous sinuses (*arrow*). **G** and **H**, "Fat" images (water signal suppressed) at same sagittal locations show signal posterior to vertebral body is not fat. **I** and **J**, "Water" images (fat signal suppressed) shows high signal in posterior location to be of water origin (*arrows*). Border between herniated disc material and dilated epidural veins, representing dura and posterior longitudinal ligament, is better delineated on water images (**I** and **J**).

Disc material is of intermediate signal intensity on T1W images and T2*W variable flip angle scans and thus almost always directly visualizable. Indirect findings on T1W images have to be carefully noted because of the similarity in signal intensity of anulus, ligament, bone, and CSF (see Figures 10-12 to 10-14). Also on T1W images displaced fat or epidural venous sinus in the intervertebral foramina may be difficult to distinguish from disc material because of similarity in signal intensity (see Figures 10-13 and 10-14). The "black line" border of the herniated disc helps in this localization (see Figure 10-13). The use of GdDTPA can help distinguish disc material from venous structures (see Figure 10-15).

Axial T2*W variable flip angle scans provide better delineation of herniated discs because the extradural defect can be readily appreciated as a result of high contrast afforded by high signal CSF (see Figures 10-14 and 10-15). Displacement of the dura and root sleeves is easily identified. In addition, venous structures in the intervertebral foramina, especially at the higher cervical levels, are of high signal intensity and displacement or compression is easily identified. In general the contrast available for diagnosing disc disease is higher with variable flip angle scans than with T1W scans (see Figures 10-14 and 10-15); thus they allow a thicker slice thickness if necessary. One must be aware of partial volume artifact, however; partial volume of an osteophyte can produce an intermediate signal suggestive of a herniated disc. Comparison of adjacent slices and an overlapping scanning technique (see Chapter 2) should eliminate this potential for a false positive diagnosis of disc herniation.

Major symptoms in the cervical spine occur when disc herniations are in a posterolateral location causing impingement on the nerve roots as they exit the dura through the root sleeve or slightly more distally in the intervertebral foramen.[19,27] Detecting posterolateral and lateral herniations is difficult on sagittal T1W or T2W scans alone; axial views are necessary. If there is a midline component to the herniated disc the sagittal views show it well. However, if the disc has only a lateral herniated component without a midline component, sagittal T1W scans may miss the diagnosis, although subtle findings can be present on the off-midline slices (see Figures 10-16 and 10-17). These usually consist of intermediate signal intensity behind the vertebral bodies rostral and caudal to the disc caused by a dilated epidural venous plexus that fills the space as a result of posterior displacement of the dura and posterior longitudinal ligament by the herniated disc (Figure 10-18). A disc entirely confined within the foramen can be missed on sagittal views (Figures 10-17 and 10-19).[15] Axial views are crucial and mandatory for the correct diagnosis of cervical disc disease—a T2*W image is more accurate than a T1W image. The diagnosis hinges on identifying the herniated disc material itself or on indirect findings such as dural and nerve root compression or displacement of fat or epidural veins in the intervertebral foramen (see Figures 10-14 to 10-19).

The thin dark line in the middle of the intervertebral foramina indicates where the nerve roots course toward the dorsal root ganglion and represents an important anatomic landmark (see Figure 10-16). Displacement or disruption of this dark line suggests nerve root displacement and compression. The dark line may represent perineurium and is consistently seen at the mid- and higher cervical levels, does not appear to be a chemical-shift artifact of variable flip angle pulse sequences (see Chapter 2) and is more difficult to visualize as a landmark at the lower cervical levels, C_6-C_7 and C_7-T_1. The landmark unfortunately can be obscured in patients with osteophytic narrowing of foramina. At times therefore it will be difficult to detect disc herniation when significant osteophytic disease is also present in the foramen. Even when both osteophyte and disc are present it is often possible to separate the two disease processes using axial variable flip angle scans (thin slices) and sagittal oblique T1W scans.[40]

Although anatomic specimens have been scanned in an oblique plane to show nerve roots and their configuration in the intervertebral foramen, this is not a widespread clinical scanning approach.[7,23,39] The oblique scanning technique works well with a T1W sequence because it relies on perineural fat for contrast. The oblique plane will probably not become a basic screening scan for detection of cervical spine disc disease but it can be useful in further delineating suspected lateral disc herniations or clarifying complicated cases where disc herniation may be difficult to separate from osteophyte (see Chapter 2).

A, B

C

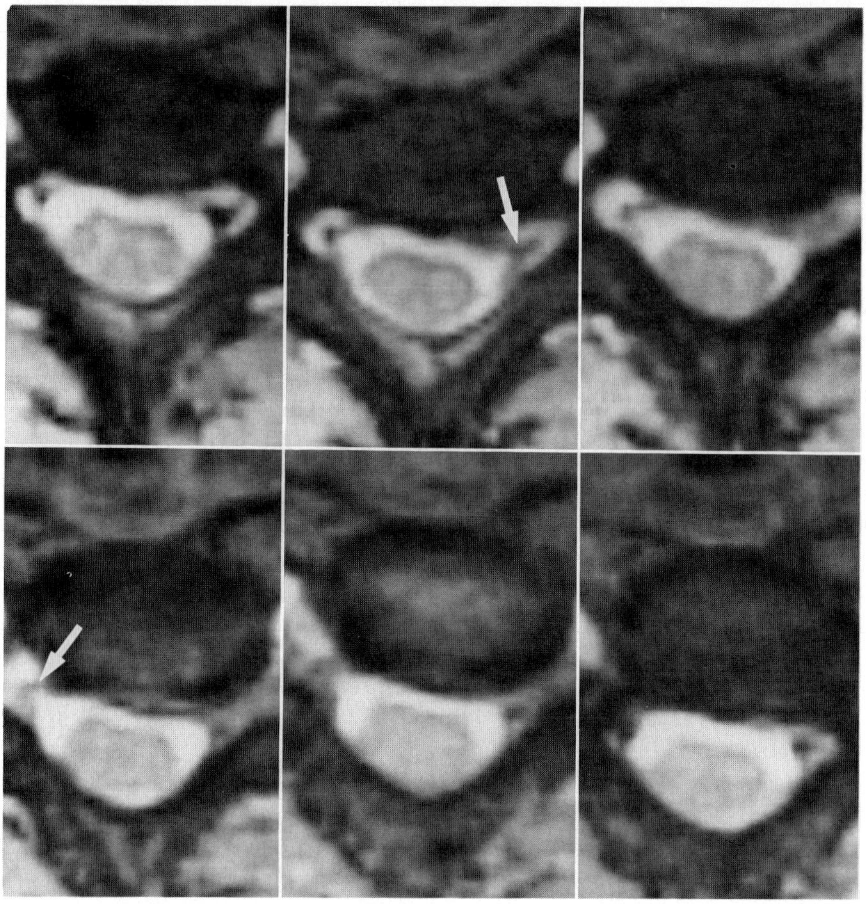

D, E

F

FIGURE 10-19. Subtle lateral cervical disc herniation. Findings in disc herniations can be limited to neural foramina and be more subtle compared to those that involve spinal canal. Subtle findings consist of asymmetry between right and left neural foramina on variable flip angle/gradient echo scans (GRASS 22/12, 7°). Scans are from pedicle to pedicle (**A-F**). Small anterolateral extension of subarachnoid space representing root sleeve is asymmetric with left C_6-C_7 root sleeve (*arrow,* **B**) appearing at higher level than right C_6-C_7 root sleeve (*arrow,* **D**). At every level signal intensity of left neural foramen (**C-E**) is consistently lower than signal intensity within right neural foramen (**D** and **E**). These findings indicate a lateral disc herniation on the left.

In comparing myelography, CT, and MR, MR detects a greater number of lesions in the cervical spine. This may result in a greater number of "positive" scans. The greater sensitivity of MR to disc disease needs to be put in clinical perspective. There has always been a discrepancy between imaging test findings in the cervical spine and clinical symptomatology for suspected disc disease.[27,36] It is not unusual to see disc disease by myelography at levels where there is no clinical radiculopathy accompanying pathologic conditions. This is also true with MR. There are no clear imaging criteria to distinguish herniated discs that are clinically symptomatic from those that are not. For MR interpretations to be clinically relevant, it is crucial to correlate imaging findings with clinical symptoms. Only in this way can MR scan interpretations be made relevant to the patient's clinical problems. It is also important to remember that in the cervical region, as well as in the thoracic and lumbar regions, that in the horizontal scanning position any existing pathologic conditions might be in a "decompressed" state. Anatomic derangements shift in a weight-bearing position and if this is visualized, nerve root compression might be

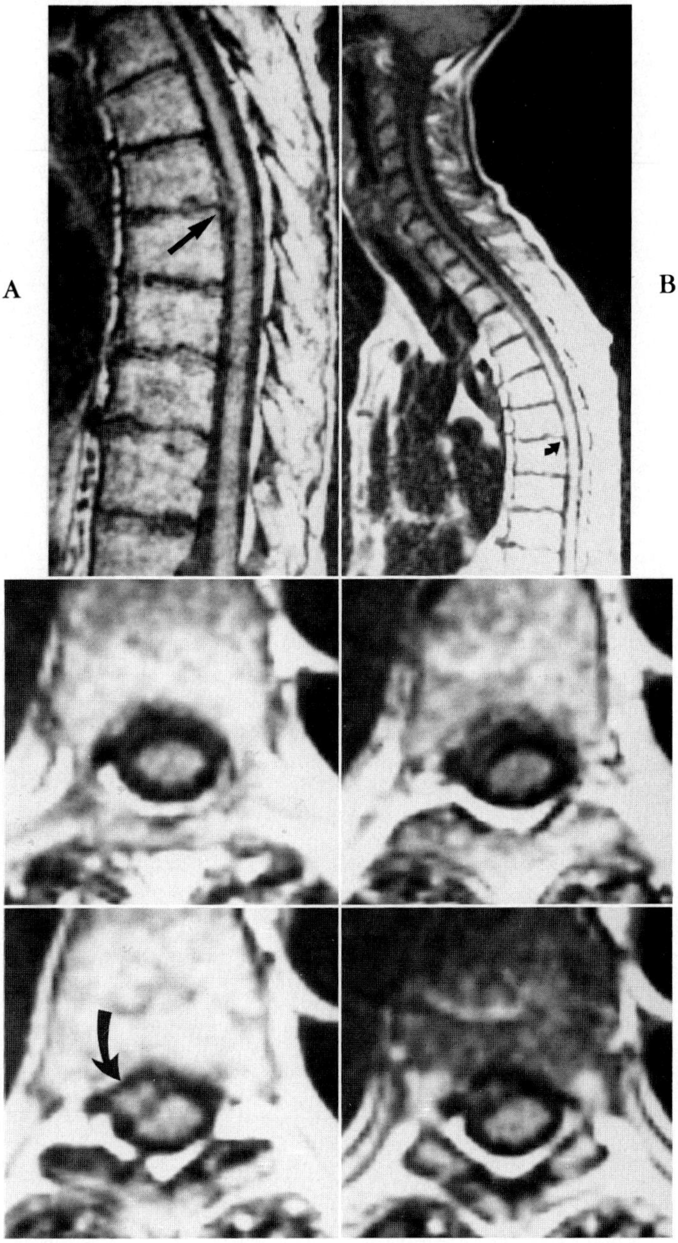

FIGURE 10-20. Thoracic disc herniation. **A,** The key to diagnosing thoracic disc disease is the sagittal T1W scan (SE 800/20) on which disc material extends beyond posterior margin of vertebral bodies, has similar signal intensity as bone marrow, and often indents cord *(arrow)*. **B,** With use of surface coil and thus limited field of view (FOV), specific thoracic level (T_7-T_8) cannot be ascertained without larger localizing view, which is useful for visualizing anatomic landmarks (SE 300/20, NEX 1, FOV 48 cm) but is not accurate in detecting disc herniation itself *(arrow)*. **C-F,** Axial T1W scans (SE 1000/20) are adequate for diagnosis of disc herniation in the thoracic spine. Herniated disc material is often isointense with spinal cord (*arrow,* **E**).

Continued.

G H

I J

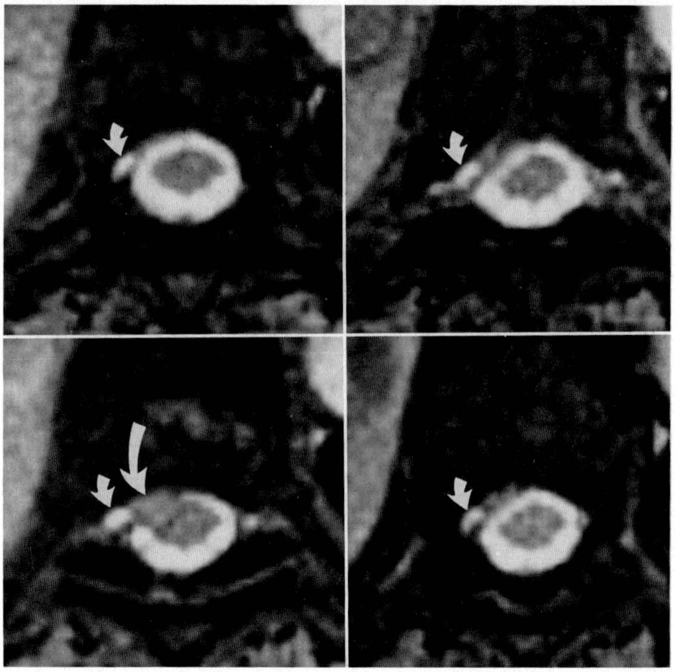

FIGURE 10-20, cont'd. **G-J,** Axial variable flip angle scans (GRASS 25/13, 7°) obtained at same levels as T1W scans show disc herniation equally well. **I,** Signal intensity of disc material is similar to that of spinal cord *(large curved arrow)*. In thoracic region as in cervical region when disc material strips dura away from bone resultant space is occupied by dilated venous structures *(small curved arrows)*.

A

B, C

D, E

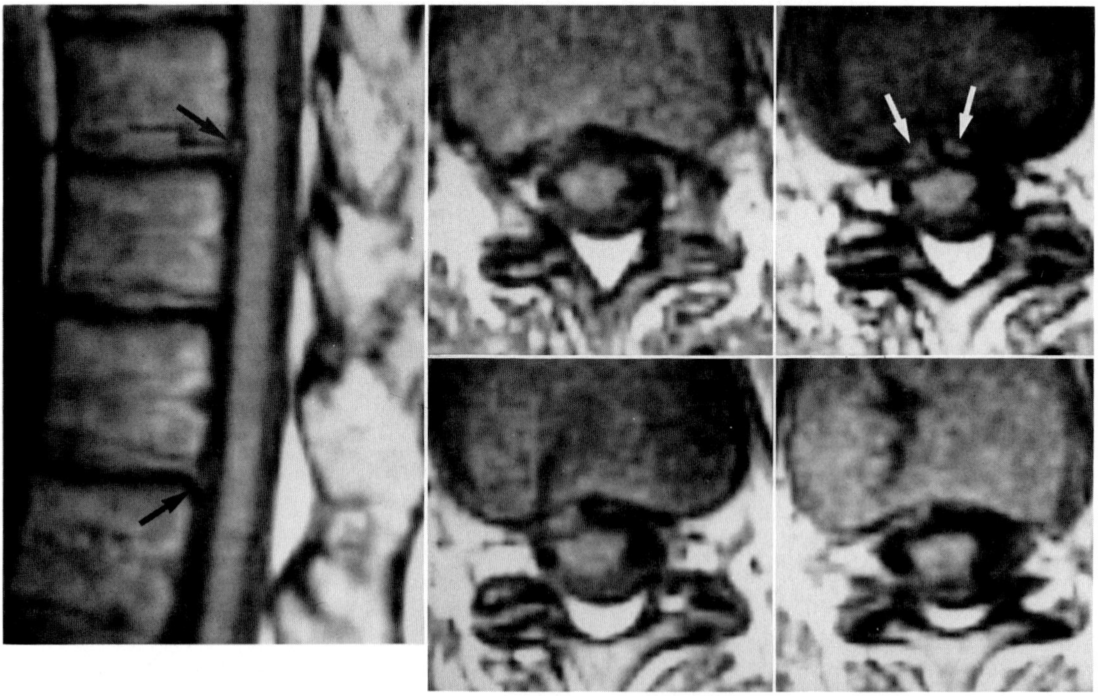

FIGURE 10-21. Thoracic disc herniation. **A,** Sagittal T1W scan (SE 600/25) of 37-year-old female with acute onset of lower extremity weakness and sensory changes referable to this level shows small disc herniations at T_9-T_{10} and T_{11}-T_{12} *(arrows)*. **B-E,** In most instances, axial T1W scans (SE 1000/25) show disc herniation well because of intermediate signal intensity. Note two apparent disc fragments at T_{11}-T_{12} disc space (*arrows,* **C**) that deform cord anteriorly.

more obvious (see Figure 10-59). Awareness of all potential nerve root compressions and their clinical correlates is useful in making MR scan interpretations.

MR: thoracic spine

Disc herniations in the thoracic spine are relatively uncommon, accounting for less than 5% of all disc herniations. This is in part a result of the difficulty in their diagnosis with the previous techniques of myelography and CT. Disc herniation does not correlate with calcification of thoracic discs.[32] Most thoracic disc herniations occur below T_8 with T_{10} to T_{11} and T_{11} to T_{12} the most common sites. Disc herniations at high thoracic levels are unusual.[1] The major clinical manifestation of herniation is pain and sometimes myelopathy. Radiculopathy is not a significant presentation for thoracic disc disease. Thoracic discs tend to be primarily midline in location and thus the sagittal T1W sequence is useful in their detection.[12] They can be off midline, however, and paramidline slices need to be examined thoroughly on the T1W sagittal sequence, the usual initial screening scan (see Figures 10-20 and 10-21). A localizing scan (see Chapter 2) is usually necessary to accurately determine the disc level (see Figure 10-20). A sagittal T2W or T2*W sequence more easily detects extradural defects caused by thoracic discs (see Figures 10-23 and 10-24). At times only a T2W or T2*W sagittal scan adequately delineates a thoracic disc (see Figures 10-23 and 10-24), especially when the herniated disc material is of low signal intensity, i.e., closer to CSF rather than marrow signal intensity (see Figure 10-24). Axial scans, either T1W or T2*W confirm the presence of a disc and better delineate its extent (Figures 10-20 to 10-25). Cord compression can usually be evaluated on the sagittal scan. Because the T1W scan plays an important role as a screening pulse sequence for detecting thoracic discs, it is important to understand the effect of changing the phase-encoding and frequency encoding axes (see Chapter 2) because having the frequency encoding axis perpendicular to the spine could result in a false negative examination (see Figure 10-25).[8]

In unusual circumstances a thoracic disc, if extensive, may cause a clinical syndrome of a slowly progressive myelopathy. In such instances, it is usually not a simple, acute, herniated disc but a more chronic one that causes marked impingement into the spinal canal (Figure 10-26).[29] The difficulty in diagnosis rests not with the imaging test but with the clinician thinking of the possibility and ordering the MR examination to pursue it.

MR: lumbar spine

Lumbar disc disease is common and a great deal is known about it by virtue of myelography and CT. Whereas MR improves the ability to diagnose cervical disc disease, the increment of improvement over CT in the lumbar spine is less, although more information is available because of better soft tissue discrimination (Figure 10-27). Anatomy is exquisitely shown.[6] There is also a wider latitude in MR techniques for studying lumbar disc disease compared to the cervical region. Generally axial scans are obtained in a plane parallel to the disc space (Figure 10-28). The entire examination can be carried out with T1W sequences in both sagittal and axial scans (Figures 10-29 and 10-30). Other combinations are possible: sagittal T1W scans and axial T2W scans, sagittal T1W and axial T2*W scans, sagittal T2W or T2*W and axial T1W scans, etc. Axial T2W scans often provide more detailed information about exiting nerve roots (Figures 10-31 to 10-34). Second echo images of a T2W sequence provide information comparable to intrathecally enhanced spine CT (Figures 10-31 to 10-33, 10-35, and 10-36). A variety of combinations of pulse sequences provide enough information for a confident diagnosis of disc disease. A T2W sequence can help considerably when some other disease entity such as tumor, inflammation, or arachnoiditis masquerades as disc disease.

Midline herniations are relatively easy to detect but usually are of little clinical significance unless they have a lateral component that impinges on exiting nerves. On T1W scans in sagittal and axial planes the nucleus pulposus is of intermediate signal intensity and its herniated portion extends beyond the confines of the vertebral body. The disc material may be lower, higher, or the same signal intensity as CSF in the dural sac (see Figures 10-29 to 10-31). The intermediate signal intensity of the disc is often outlined by a thin line of low signal, especially

Text continued on p. 477.

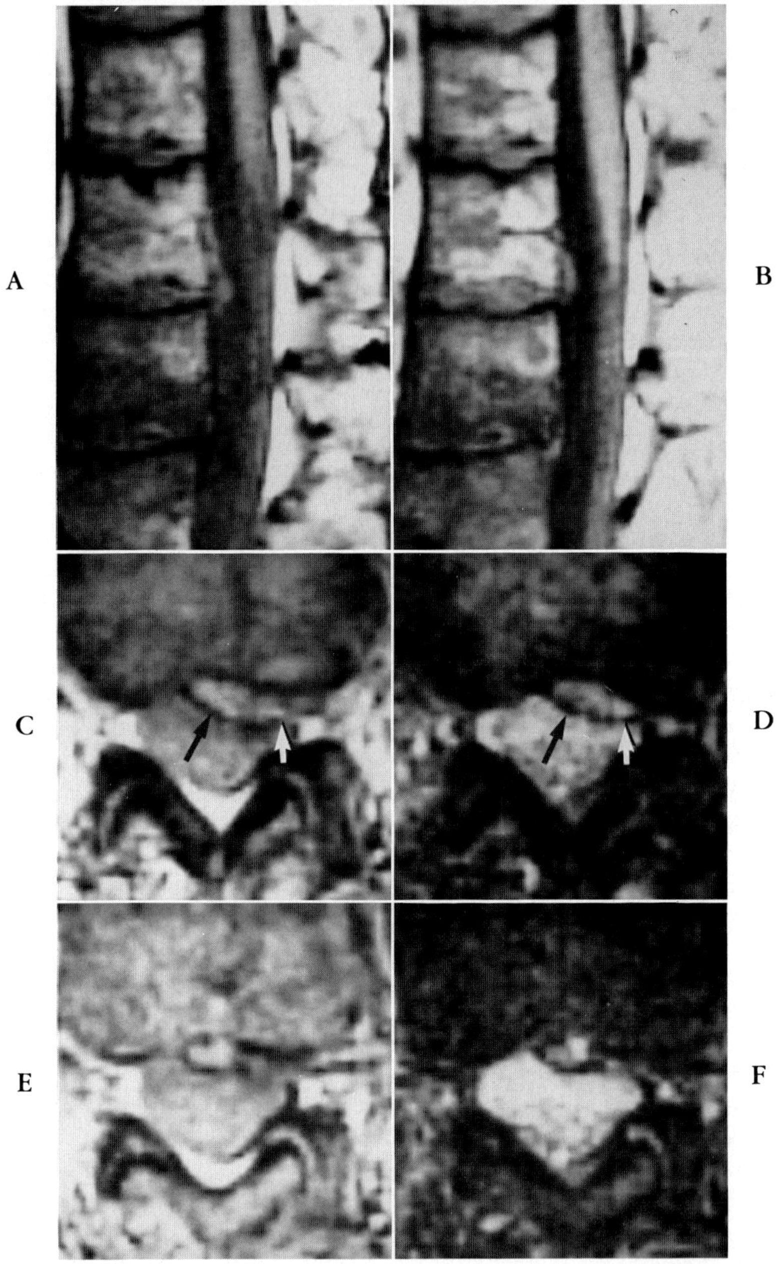

FIGURE 10-22. Thoracic disc herniation. Acute onset of T_{12} pain, on the left, of 46-year-old patient. **A** and **B,** Sagittal T1W scans (SE 800/20) show disc herniation on left side (**A**) and in midline (**B**). Scan suggests migration of disc material cephalad along lower posterior aspect of T_{12}. **C-F,** Axial T2W scans (SE gated 2100/20, 80) show large herniated disc in midline (*black arrows,* **C** and **D**) and extension toward left neural foramen (*white arrows,* **C** and **D**). Disc herniation shows high signal intensity on both first (**C** and **E**) and second (**D** and **F**) echos. Anterolateral extradural defect and compression of dural sac on left side is well shown on axial T2W scan. Roots of cauda equina are seen in the posterior dural sac (**D** and **F**) and are unaffected.

A B

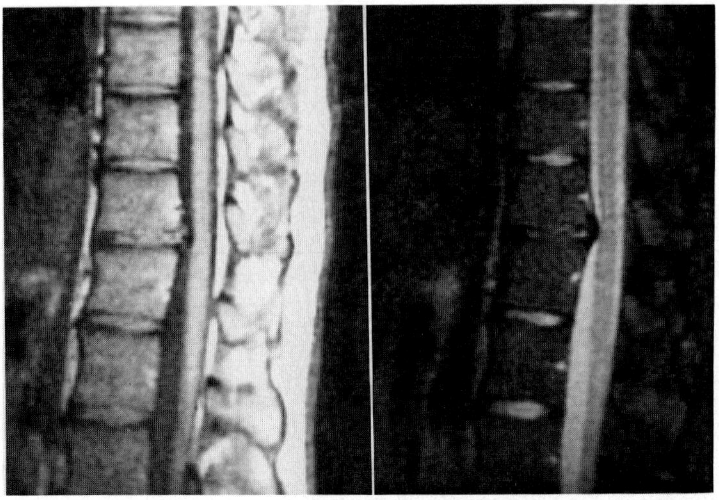

FIGURE 10-23. Thoracic disc herniation. Herniated thoracic disc at T_{11}-T_{12} detectable on **A,** T1W (SE 800/20) sagittal scan but findings were more prominent on **B,** sagittal T2W scan (SE gated, 2100/80), showing prominent extradural defect at T_{11}-T_{12}. Disc space is narrowed and lower than normal signal intensity (**B**); degree of impingement on spinal canal is better appreciated on T2W scan.

A B C D

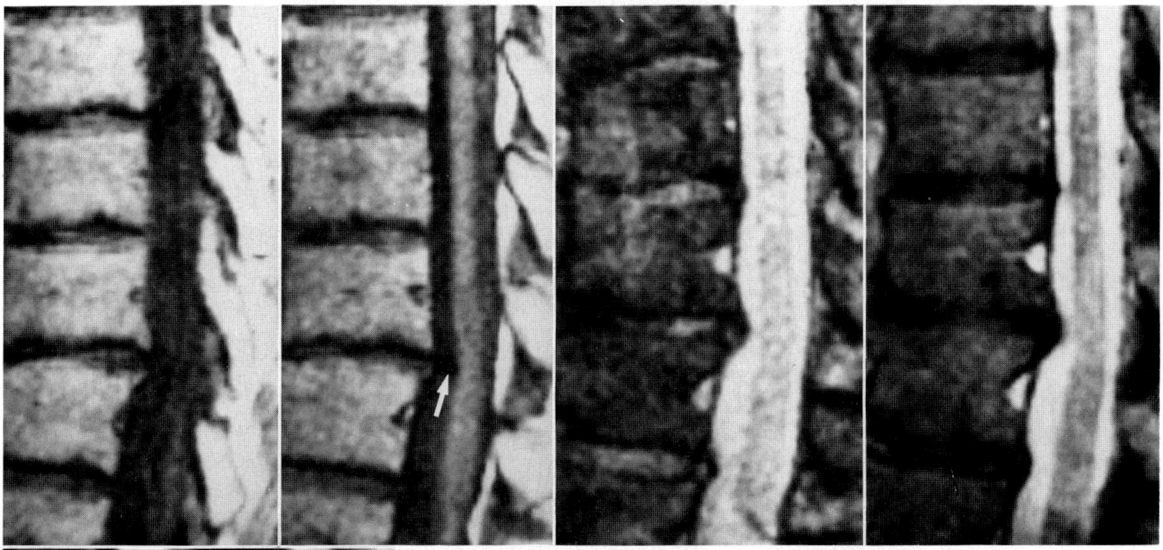

E

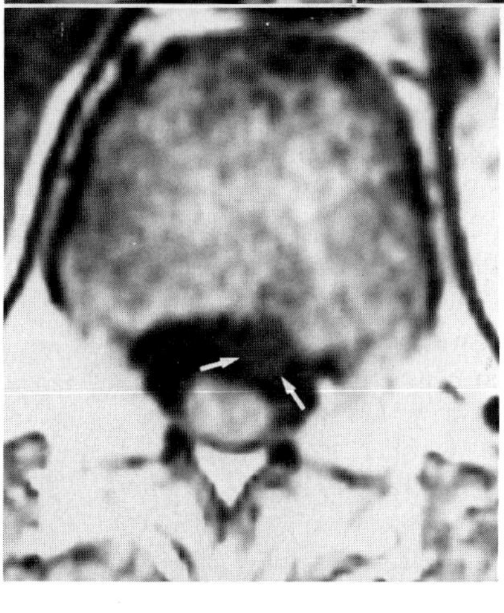

FIGURE 10-24. Subtle thoracic disc herniation. Thoracic disc herniation can be difficult to detect on sagittal T1W scans. **A** and **B,** Midline (**B**) and left paramidline (**A**) T1W scans (SE 800/20) of patient with prominent hyperreflexia shows slight deformity of cord at level of conus medullaris (**B**) although disc material causing this impression is difficult to visualize (**A**). Subtle area of low signal in anterior subarachnoid space suggests herniated disc material (*arrow*, **B**). **C,** Sagittal variable flip angle scan (GRASS 25/13, 5°) and **D,** sagittal T2W scan (gated and flow-compensated 2200/80) show anterior extradural defect at T_{11}-T_{12} accounting for posterior displacement of cord. **E,** Axial T1W scan (SE 800/20) shows paramidline disc herniation on left *(arrows)* displacing cord posteriorly and flattening its left anterolateral surface. Herniated disc material is low signal intensity *(arrows)*.

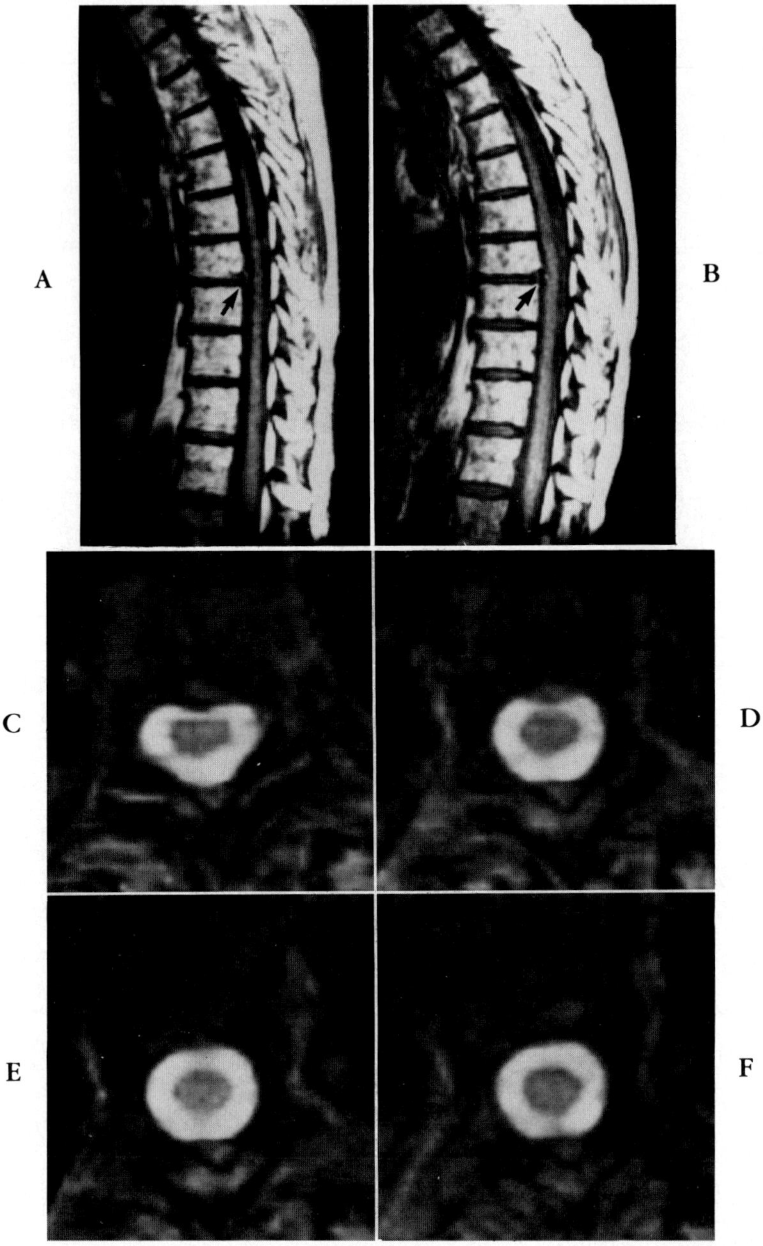

FIGURE 10-25. Thoracic disc—phase axis. Changing phase-encoding direction from **A**, perpendicular to **B**, parallel to spinal canal can obscure thoracic disc herniations on T1W scans (SE 800/20). With phase-encoding direction perpendicular to spine (frequency encoding direction parallel to spine) chemical-shift artifact occurs in superior-inferior direction. Subarachnoid space anterior to cord is well seen as is disc herniation, which impinges on subarachnoid space (*arrow*, **A**). With phase-encoding direction parallel to spine (frequency encoding axis perpendicular) chemical shift artifact is in anteroposterior direction resulting in falsely narrowed subarachnoid space, possibly obscuring a thoracic disc herniation. This technique of axes switching may be used to reduce ghost artifacts (arising from heart) from projecting over spinal canal. **C-F**, Axial variable flip angle/gradient echo scans (GRASS 22/12.5, 4°) confirm presence of midline disc herniation (**D**). This pulse sequence shows that sagittal image (**A**), rather than **B**, provides more accurate delineation of size of anterior subarachnoid space when compared to axial images. (From Enzmann DR, Griffin C, Rubin JB. Potential false-negative MR images of the thoracic spine in disc disease with switching of phase- and frequency-encoding gradients. Radiology 1987; 165:635. With permission.)

A

B

C, D

G

E, F

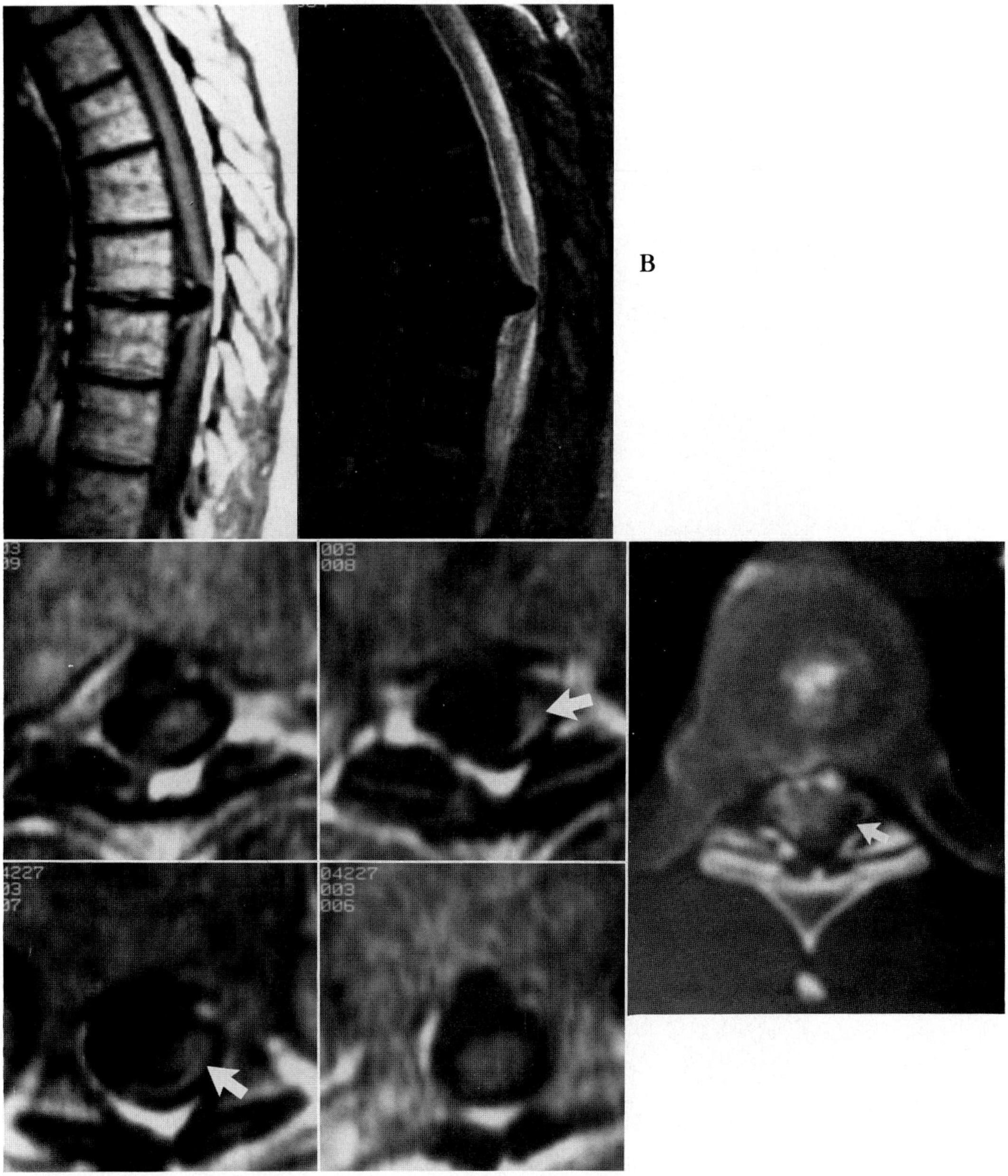

FIGURE 10-26. Calcified thoracic disc. Long history of numbness and lack of coordination in lower extremities of 66-year-old male. **A,** Sagittal T1W (SE 800/20) scan shows large, very low signal intensity, anteroextradural defect at T_7-T_8 level. Low signal intensity indicates heavy calcification or ossification. Cord is displaced posteriorly. **B,** Sagittal T2W scan (SE gated, 2000/80) shows marked posterior displacement and compression of spinal cord. **C-F,** Axial T1W scans (SE 1000/20) show area of low signal intensity occupying large portion of spinal canal at this level (**D** and **E**). Cord is compressed and displaced to left (*arrows,* **D** and **E**). **G,** Metrizamide CT scan at level of calcified herniated disc correlates closely to axial T1W image (**E**). The deformed and compressed cord is seen on images **E** and **G** *(arrow).*

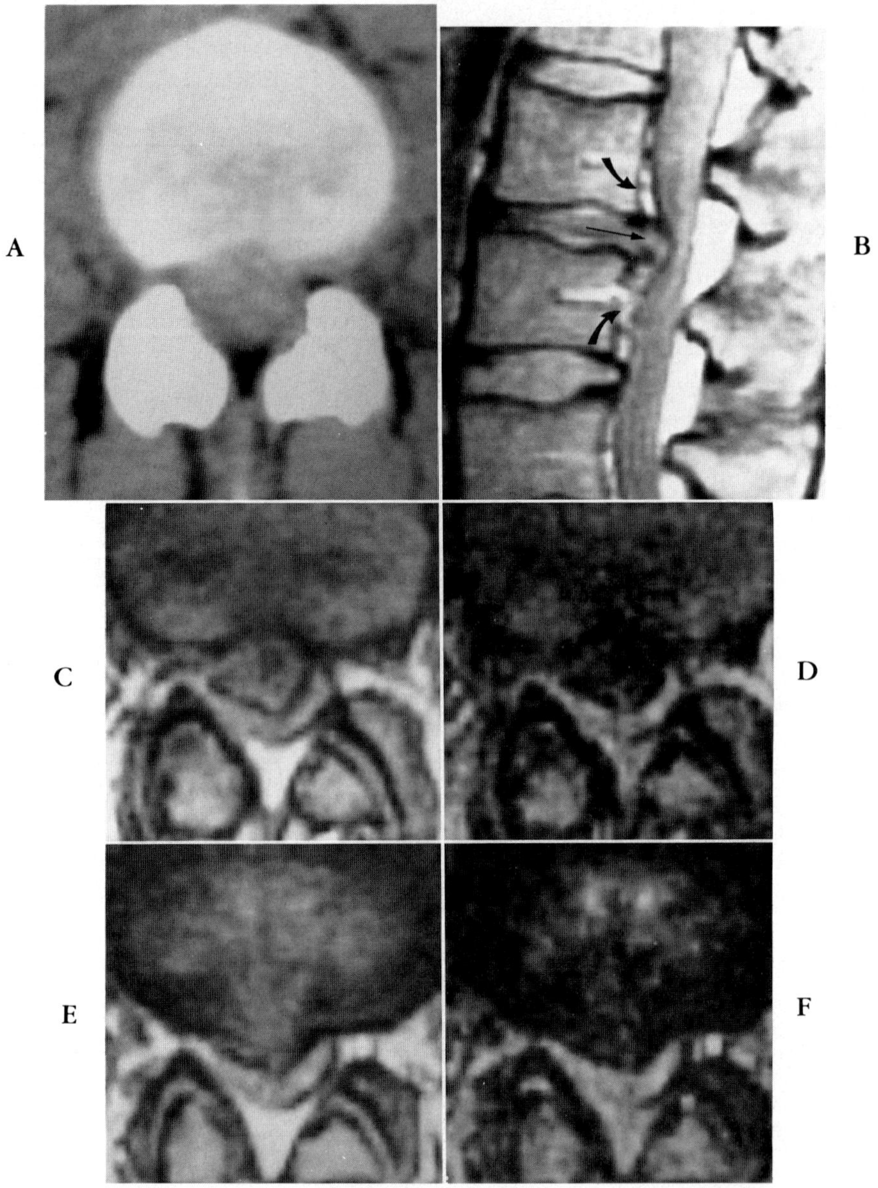

FIGURE 10-27. Lumbar disc herniation. Although CT is excellent for diagnosing lumbar herniated discs, at times the lack of disc–dural sac contrast makes diagnosis difficult. **A,** Large midline herniated disc occupying almost entire dural sac is difficult to detect on CT. **B,** Sagittal balanced image (SE 2500/20) shows obvious large midline disc herniation with gap in anulus *(straight arrow)* indicating radial tear. Dura and posterior longitudinal ligament are lifted off adjacent vertebrae causing dilatation of epidural venous plexus *(curved arrows)*. **C-F,** Axial T2W scan (gated 2400/20, 80) shows large herniated disc fragment on balanced images (**C** and **E,** TE 20) that has nearly same signal intensity as CSF, is contiguous with disc space, and is separated from CSF by thin black line representing dura and ligament. Second echo (**D** and **F**) shows disc material as low signal intensity compared to CSF.

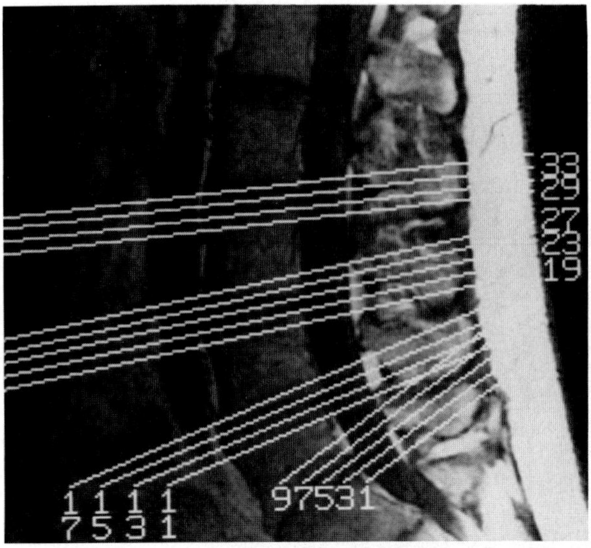

FIGURE 10-28. Localization. Sagittal T1W scan (SE 800/20) prescribes location of axial slices of T2W sequence at L_2-L_3, L_3-L_4, L_4-L_5, and L_5-S_1 disc spaces.

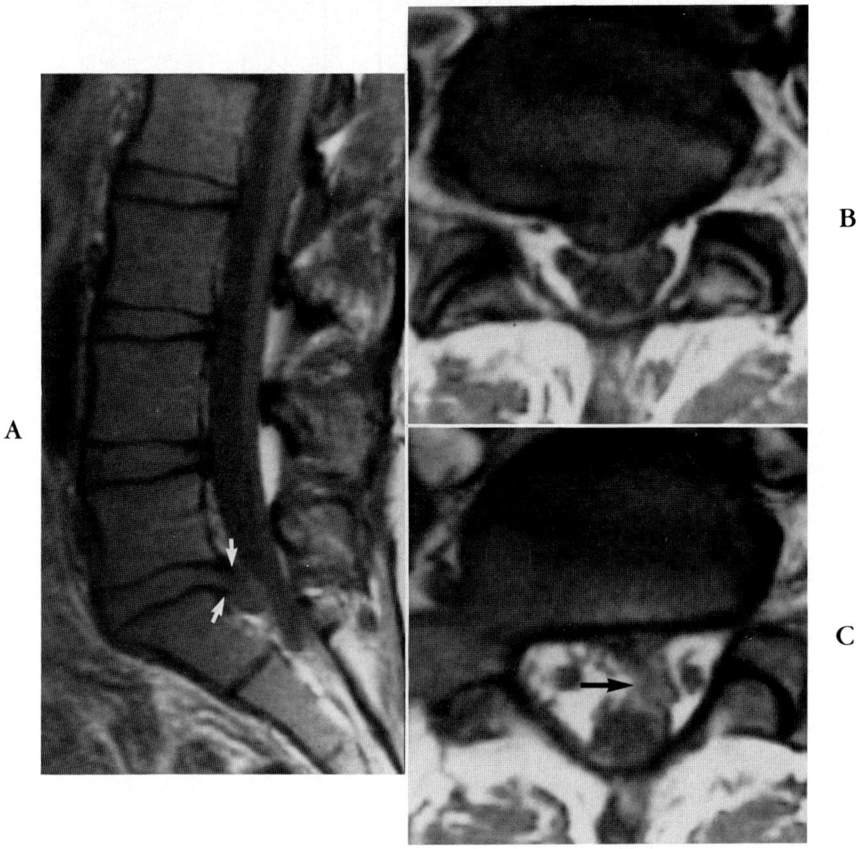

FIGURE 10-29. Lumbar disc herniation. Lumbar disc protocol using only T1W images. **A,** Sagittal and **B** and **C,** axial T1W scans (SE 1000/20) of patient with large L_5-S_1 herniated disc. Large fragment may be termed "extruded" because it extends from disc space. Rupture through anulus and posterior longitudinal ligament is seen as discontinuity in black line normally delimiting disc posteriorly (*arrows,* **A**). Disc material directly abuts dura. Axial views show central component of herniated disc (**B**) and more distal extruded fragment (*arrow,* **C**) situated between dural sac and left S_1 root. (Courtesy of Dr. D. Norman.)

A B

C D

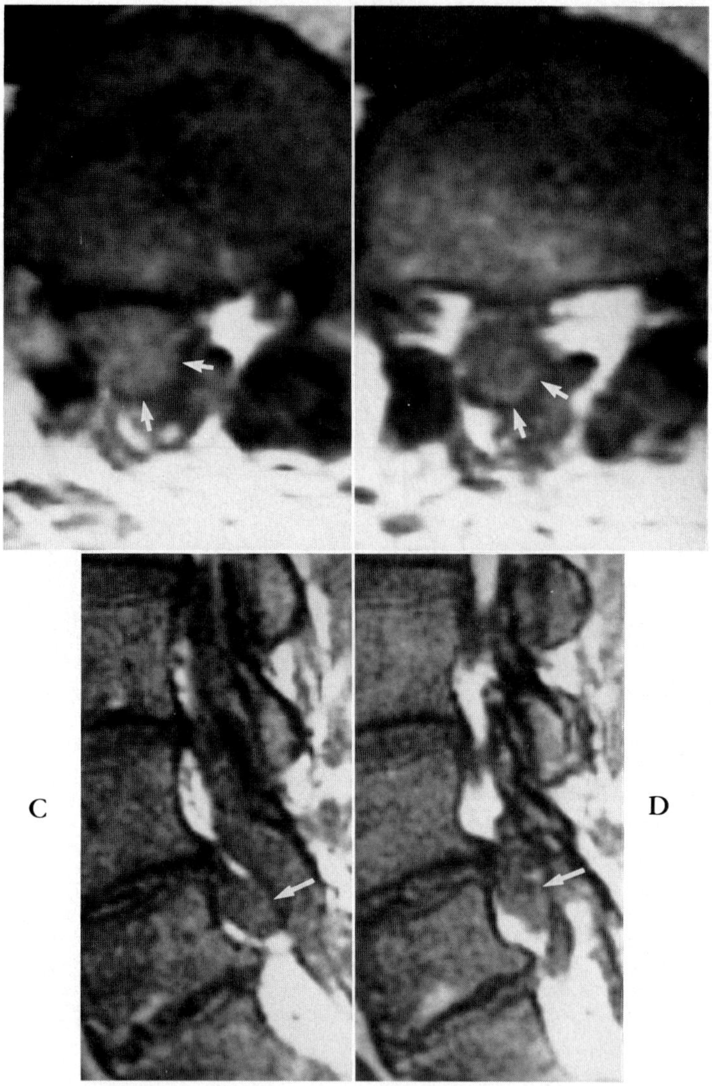

FIGURE 10-30. Lumbar disc herniation. **A** and **B**, Axial T1W scans (SE 800/20) show large herniated disc on right obliterating epidural fat and right L_5 nerve root sleeve. Disc material is easily identified by displacement of normal epidural fat. "Free fragment" is same signal intensity as disc material and slightly higher signal intensity than CSF. **C** and **D**, "Free" nature of disc fragment is better visualized on paramidline sagittal views (SE 1000/20) where large fragment *(arrows)* displaces normal epidural fat and deviates nerve root posteriorly.

A

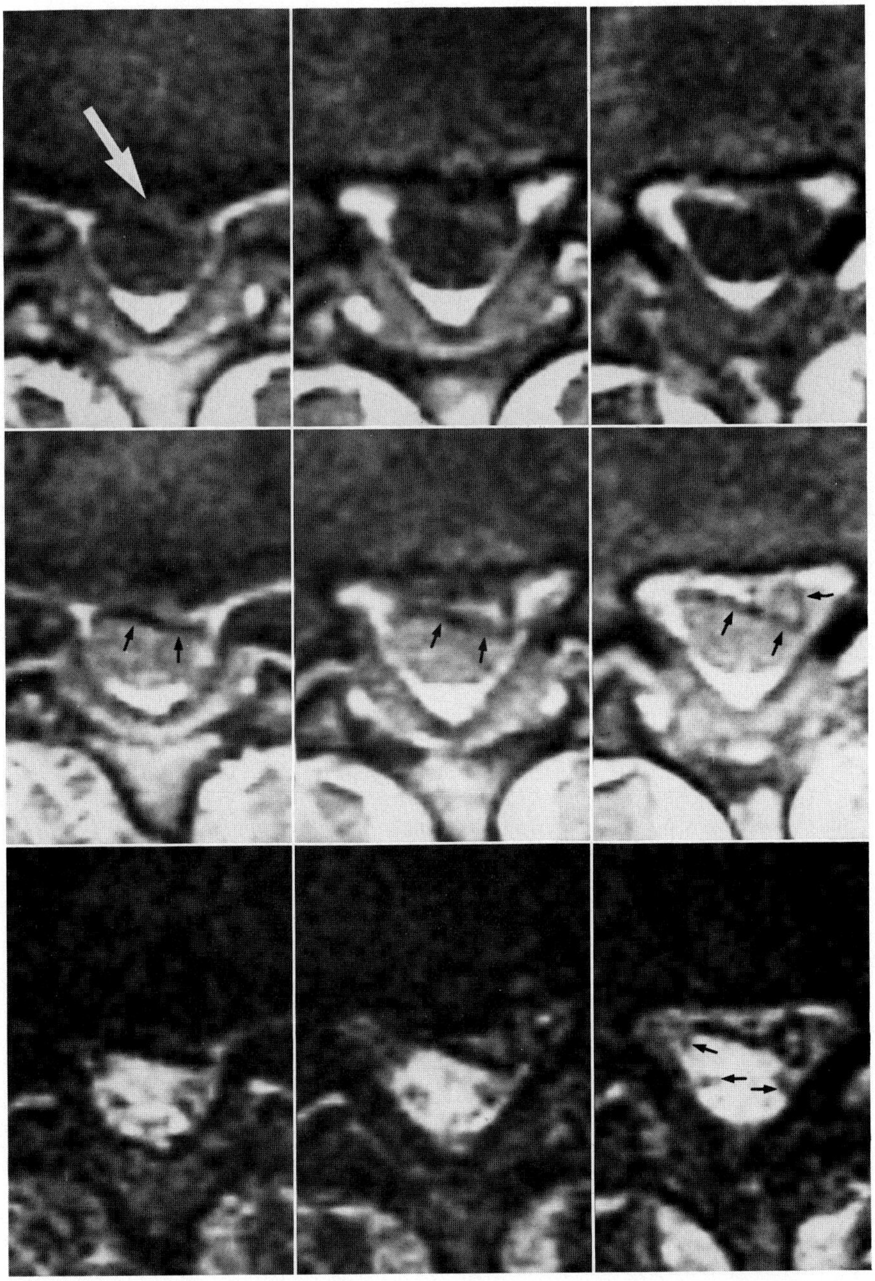

B, C

D

E, F

G

H, I

FIGURE 10-31. Lumbar disc herniation. Axial scans of patient with left herniated lumbar disc compare **A-C,** T1W technique (SE 800/20) with identical slices using T2W technique (gated 2300/20, 80; **D-F,** TE 20; **G-I,** TE 80). **A-C,** On T1W sequence, disc herniation, of slightly higher signal than CSF, is identified by anterior and anterolateral extradural defect. Herniated disc material is contiguous with disc space (*arrow,* **A**) and is higher signal than CSF at all levels (**A-C**). Similar findings are present on first echo of T2W sequence (**D-F**), although signal intensity of disc material is higher compared to CSF in dural sac (**E** and **F**). Demarcation between dura and herniated disc on balanced image is clearly outlined by thin low signal (*black*) line (*arrows* **D-F**). Configuration of extradural defect is better appreciated on second echo of T2W sequence (**G-I**). Signal intensity of herniated disc material is lower than that of CSF. More heavily T2W scans allow visualization of individual lumbar roots (*small arrows,* **I**) that helps define which root is compressed by herniated disc.

A

B, C

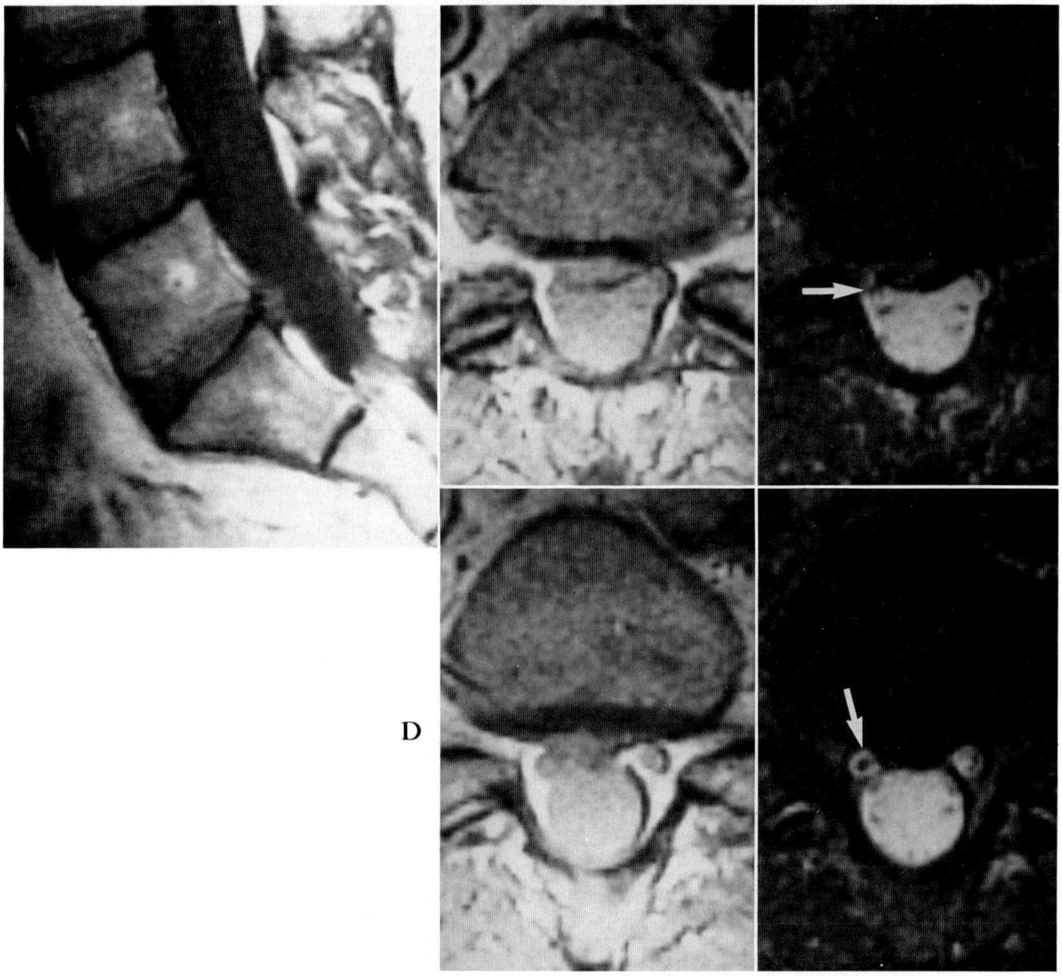

D

E

FIGURE 10-32. Lumbar disc herniation. **A,** Sagittal T1W scan (SE 800/20) shows midline disc herniation at L_5-S_1. In disc herniation, determination of nerve roots that can be affected by the herniated material is an important assessment. **B-E,** Axial T2W scans (SE gated, 1900/20, 80) demonstrate disc herniation and delineate individual nerve root(s) within dural sac or root sleeve that could be affected. Two adjacent axial T2W images **B** and **D,** first echo (TE, 20) and, **C** and **E,** second echo (TE, 80) show midline herniation, its displacement of epidural fat, and its impingement on dural sac. Although root sleeve and nerve within it (*arrow,* **E**) are spared, disc fragment displaces right L_5 root laterally and posteriorly just as it enters the root sleeve (*arrow,* **C**).

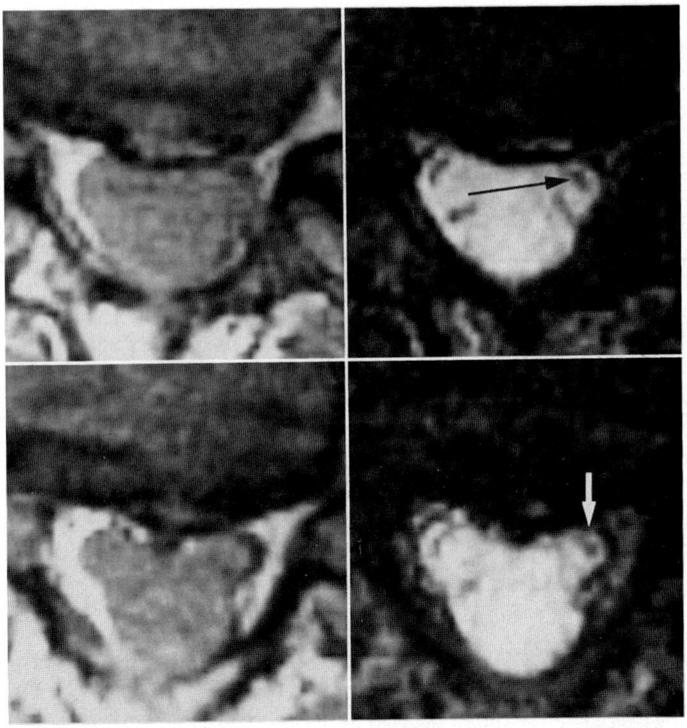

FIGURE 10-33. Subtle lumbar disc herniation. Axial T2W pulse sequence (SE gated, 2000/20, 80) is useful in determining status of nerve roots, even with subtle disc herniations. **A** and **C,** Balanced images show small disc herniation in midline and slightly off to left. **B** and **D,** More heavily weighted T2W second echo shows minimal impingement upon dural sac and slight posterior displacement of left L_5 root (*arrow,* **B**) with intact nerve root sleeve (*arrow,* **D**). This pulse sequence provides information comparable to intrathecally enhanced spine CT.

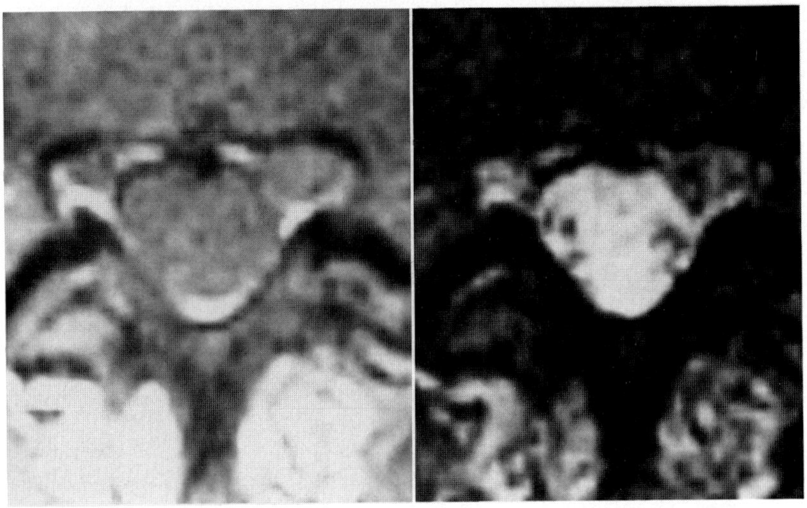

FIGURE 10-34. Subtle lumbar disc herniation. Some disc herniations are difficult to detect because of their coincidental simulation of normal anatomy. **A,** Axial T2W (SE gated, 2100/20, 80) scan shows mild asymmetry in nerve root sleeves on first echo, the balanced image. **B,** Second echo with more T2 weighting shows that structure on left is low signal intensity and does not represent nerve root sleeve; rather it is an extradural defect on left caused by disc fragment. Large root sleeve is expected to have higher signal intensity (**B**). Findings represent disc herniation on left.

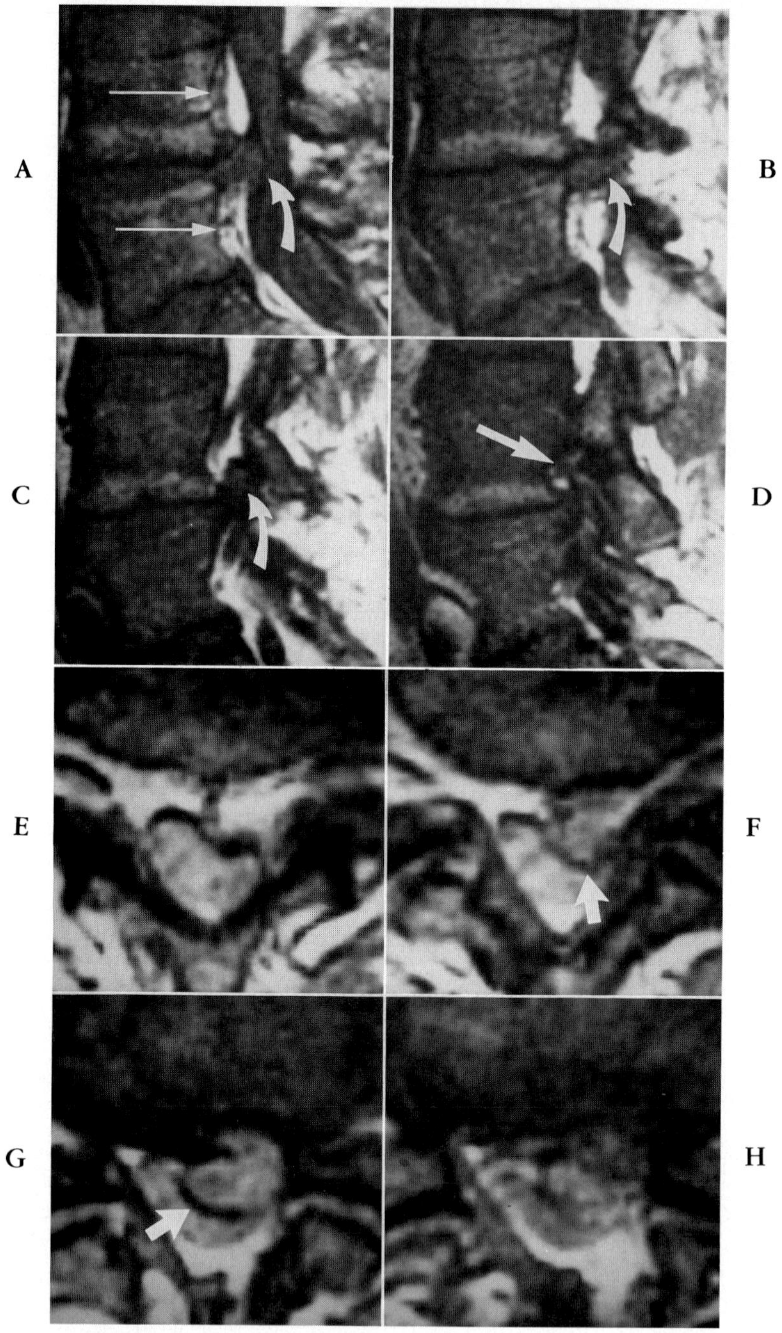

FIGURE 10-35. Lumbar disc herniation. Lumbar disc herniations can be accurately localized using axial and sagittal scan information. **A-D,** Sagittal T1W scans (SE 800/20) show large herniated disc fragment near midline extending to left (*curved arrows,* **A-C**). Herniated disc does not extend into bony neural foramina (**D**). L_4 nerve is seen surrounded by normal epidural fat (*arrow,* **D**) and is spared. **E** and **H,** Determination of lateral extent of disc herniation is more difficult in axial T2W scans (SE gated 2100/20/80). On first echo images (TE20) (**E-H**) despite having same signal intensity as CSF in dural sac, large herniated disc is evident because of dural and epidural fat displacement and low signal intensity line separating disc from dural sac (*arrows,* **F** and **G**).

I J K L

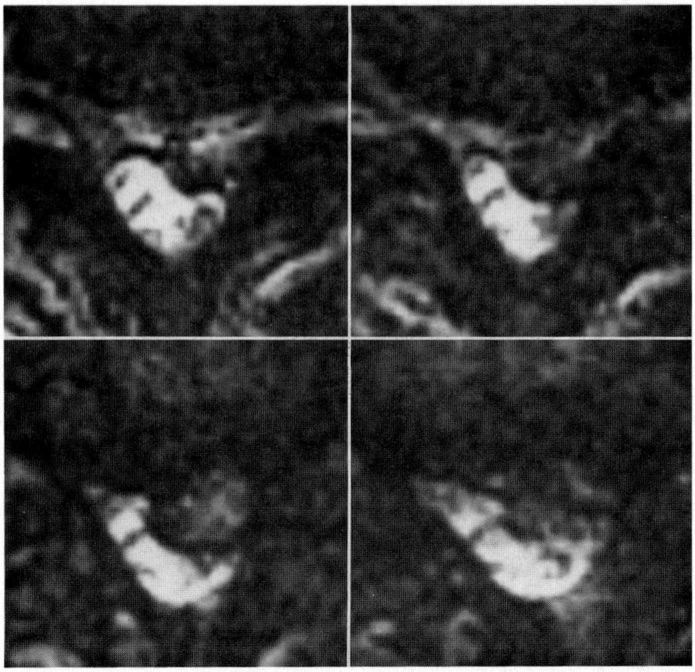

FIGURE 10-35, cont'd. **I-L**, Degree of extradural defect and impingement on lumbar roots is better demonstrated on second echo images (**I-L**). Large disc fragment markedly compresses exit point for L_5 root on left. Large disc herniation resulted in dilatation of **A**, epidural venous plexus *(long arrows)* between dura and ligament and vertebral body.

A B, C

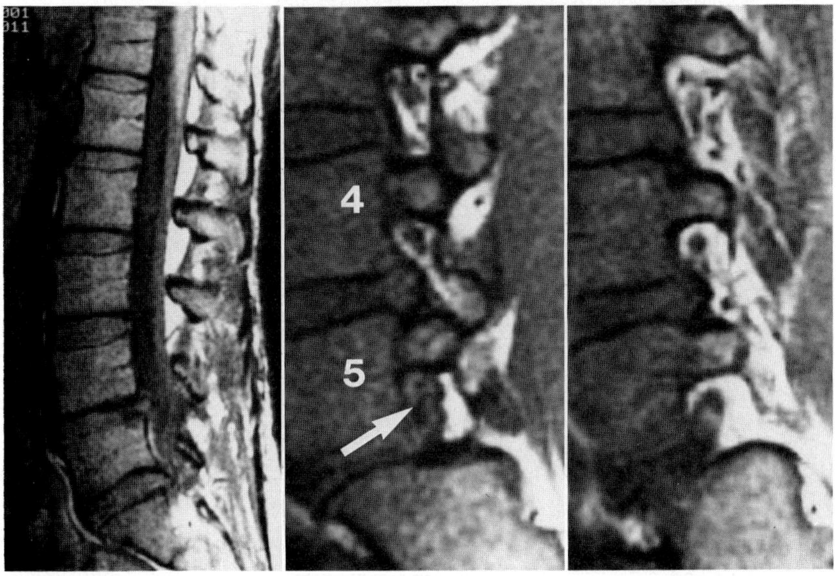

FIGURE 10-36. Lumbar disc herniation. **A**, Sagittal T1W scan (SE 800/20) provides sufficient contrast between disc and anulus-ligament to indicate intact thin black line representing posterior longitudinal ligament. Subligamentous disc herniations are present at L_4-L_5 and L_5-S_1. **B** and **C**, T1W sagittal oblique scans (SE 800/20) through foramina on left shows disc herniations in foramina (**B** and **C**). Only L_5-S_1 disc herniation impinges on root in intervertebral foramen (*arrow*, **B**).

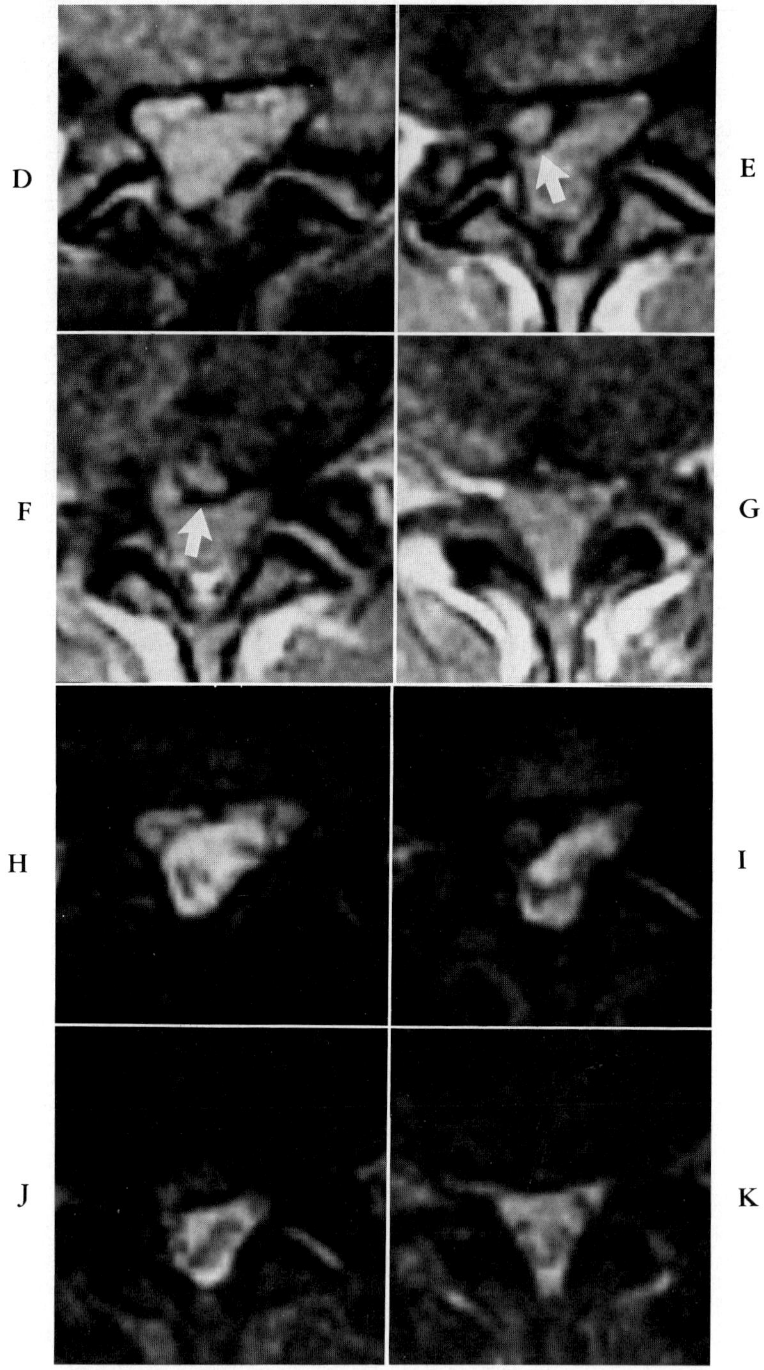

FIGURE 10-36, cont'd. **D-G,** Axial T2W scans (gated 2000/20, 80) show right sided herniated discs at L_4-L_5 (**D-K**) and L_5-S_1 (**L** and **M**). On balanced first echo images (**D-G**) L_4-L_5 herniated disc is same signal intensity as CSF in dural sac. Nevertheless, it is clearly outlined because of thin black line separating the two structures (*arrows* **E** and **F**). Black border is combination of dura, ligament, and sometimes, anulus. Disc herniation has complex nodular shape; oblique views (**B** and **C**) show that it does not extend significantly into foramen at L_4-L_5. **H-K,** Axial T2W second echo images show extradural defect on dural sac caused by low signal herniated disc.

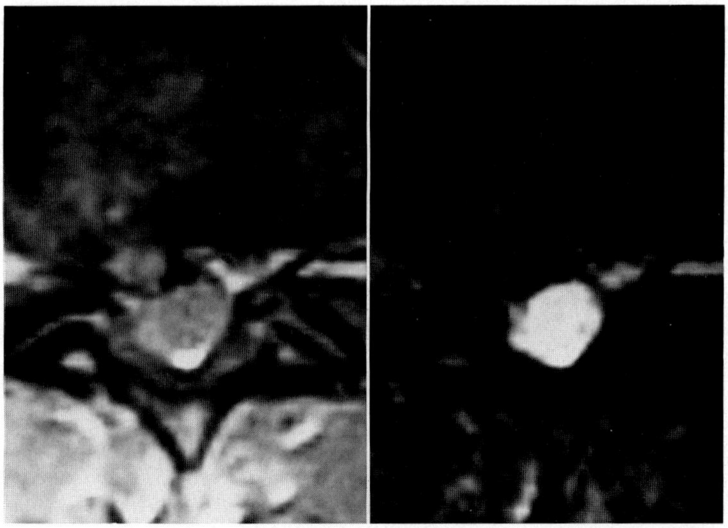

FIGURE 10-36, cont'd. **L** and **M**, At L_5-S_1 level, herniated disc has same signal characteristics as CSF on balanced image (**L**) but is lower in signal on more heavily T2W image (**M**). Extension into intervertebral foramina is better appreciated on oblique view (**B** and **C**) than on axial view (**L** and **M**).

on T2W images (see Figures 10-31 to 10-33, 10-35, and 10-36); depending on location this line represents residual anulus, posterior longitudinal ligament, dura, or a combination of these. Rupture of anulus and posterior ligament can be appreciated on T1W scans when this thin dark line is discontinuous or is not visualized (Figures 10-37 and 10-38; see Figures 10-29, 10-36, and 10-41). With large disc herniations the space between vertebral body and the "stripped away" dura and ligament becomes occupied by a dilated epidural venous plexus, epidural fat, or both (see Figures 10-35 and 10-37).

On sagittal, oblique, and axial T1W scans, displacement of normal epidural fat is an important finding in disc herniation, especially in lateral discs (Figures 10-39 and 10-40). On sagittal scans, the intervertebral foramina are well seen and show the exiting nerve root surrounded by epidural fat. Loss of this normal epidural configuration is usually evident on the sagittal scan, indicating a lateral herniation (see Figures 10-36 and 10-39). It can be seen on the axial view, but its effect on the nerve is somewhat more difficult to determine. Sagittal oblique T1W scans improve this visualization. In any event, disc herniation needs to be confirmed in two views to verify its presence and clinical significance. T2W axial scans are often helpful and superior to T1W scans in detecting subtle disc herniations and their effect on the dural sac and nerve root sleeves (see Figures 10-32 to 10-34). The second echo of a T2W pulse sequence provides axial images comparable to intrathecally enhanced CT spine studies where the CSF in the dural sac and root sleeves is high signal intensity highlighting nerve roots that are seen as low signal intensity structures. Such images clearly show extradural defects and nerve root compression that are helpful in evaluating the clinical significance of a particular finding.

Most lumbar disc herniations are easy to detect on T1W or T2W scans.[22] They are usually large enough to involve the midline and a paramidline location making them readily detectable on both sagittal and axial images. On T1W images they have a similar and sometimes higher signal intensity than CSF in the dural sac. On T1W images herniated discs are visualized not because of dural sac–disc contrast but because of displacement of epidural fat and deformity of the dural sac and rootsleeves. On T2W images findings are similar on the first echo, which is usually a "balanced" image, i.e., nearly equal T1 and T2 weighting and a strong proton density effect. On the second echo the diagnosis depends on abnormal signal in the disc fragment, as often occurs with sequestered fragments, or

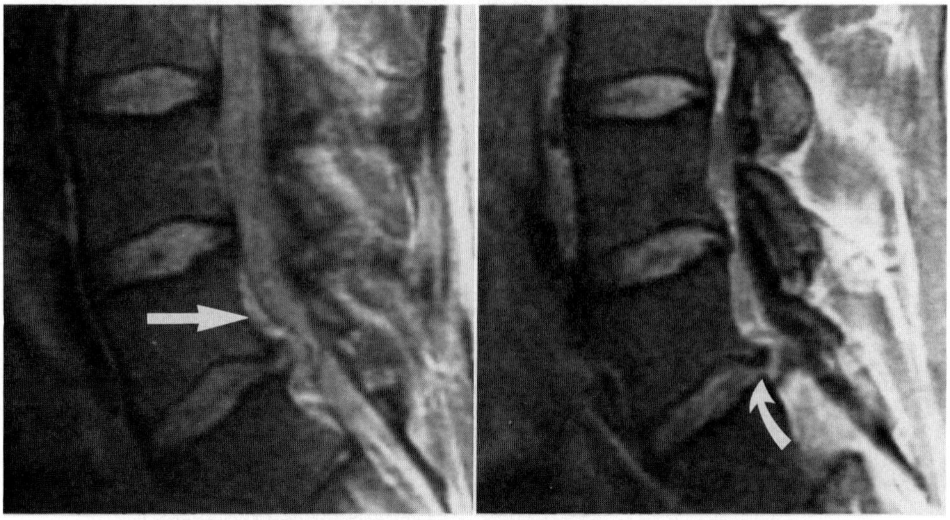

FIGURE 10-37. Lumbar disc herniation. Rupture through anulus is often well seen on T2W sagittal scan (SE 1500/40) because of increased contrast between anulus and ligament and CSF (**A** and **B**). Lack of continuous black line (*curved arrow,* **B**) connecting posterior margins of vertebral body is consistent with rupture of anulus and posterior longitudinal ligament. With larger disc herniations, dura and posterior longitudinal ligament are separated from posterior surface of vertebral body and is seen as thin black line (**A**) because it is highlighted by high signal CSF on one side and by dilate epidural veins between it and vertebral body (*arrow,* **A**) on other side.

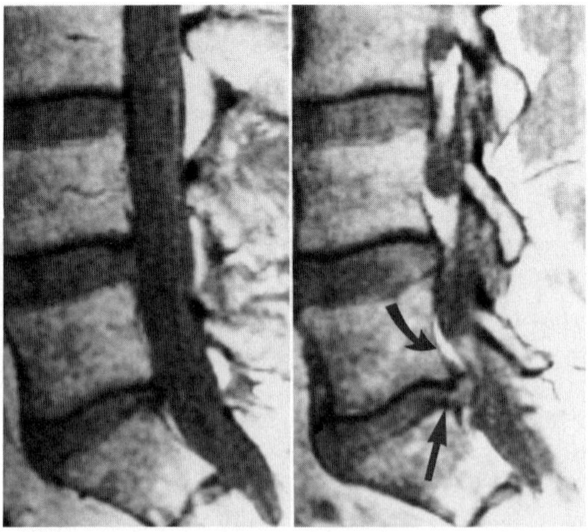

FIGURE 10-38. Lumbar disc herniation. MR scan of typical lumbar disc herniation at L_5-S_1 level using T1W sagittal scans and T2W axial scans. **A** and **B**, Sagittal T1W scans (SE 800/20) show nucleus pulposus herniating through disrupted anulus but intact posterior longitudinal ligament (*straight arrow,* **B**) on scan just to right of midline. Fat deposition is seen under elevated dura (*curved arrow,* **B**).

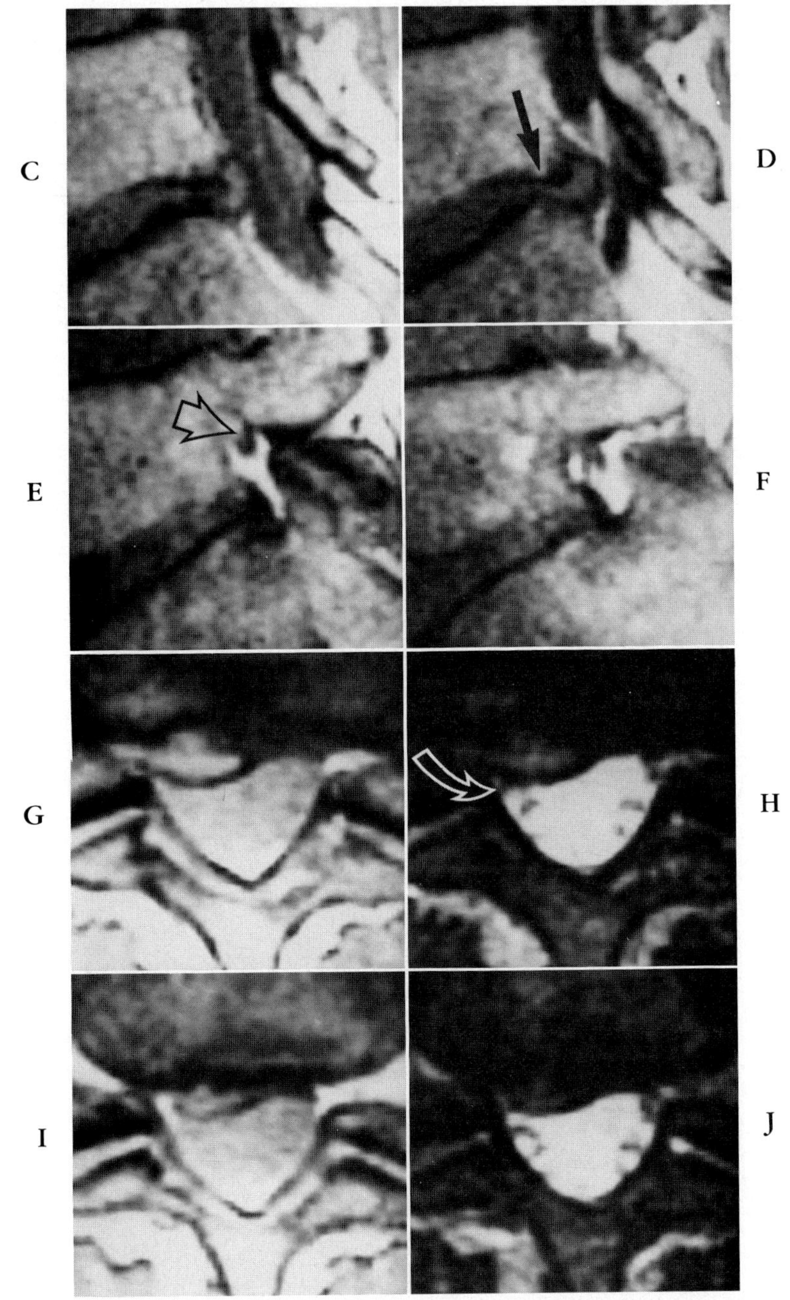

FIGURE 10-36, cont'd. C-F, Sagittal oblique, T1W scans (SE 800/20) of L_5-S_1 intervertebral foramina show disrupted anulus (*arrow*, **D**) and that subligamentous disc herniation (note residual black outline of disc) is limited to medial portion of foramen where it can affect S_1 root (**D**) rather than L_5 root (*arrow*, **E**). L_5 root appears unaffected. **G-J,** Axial T2W scans (SE 2400/20, 80) show herniated disc well on first echo (**G** and **I**) and second echo images (**H** and **J**). Extent of involvement of intervertebral foramen is difficult to assess accurately on axial images alone although right S_1 root involvement is discernable. Extradural defect and posterior displacement of right S_1 root (*arrow*, **H**) well seen on second echo image, which provides good contrast between CSF and nerve roots.

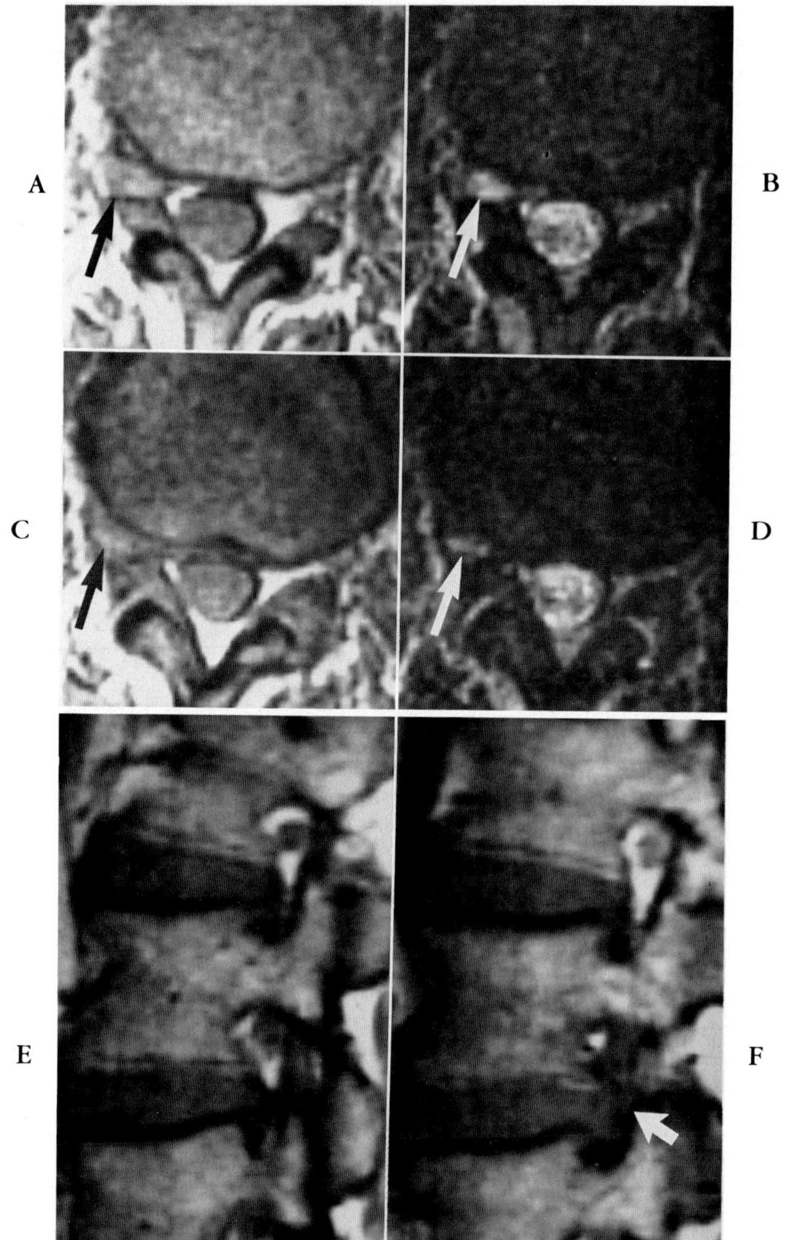

FIGURE 10-39. Lumbar disc herniation–lateral. Lateral lumbar disc herniations outside spinal canal can be difficult to diagnose. **A-D,** On axial T2W scans (SE gated 2000/20, 80) herniated disc material is seen to displace normal epidural fat within neural foramen on balanced images (*arrow,* **A** and **C**). On more T2W, second echo images disc material may have increased signal intensity compared to epidural fat normally in that location (*arrows,* **B** and **D**). **E** and **F,** Presence of lateral disc can be confirmed on routine sagittal views or on oblique sagittal views obtained with T1W scan (SE 800/20). Herniated disc material identified by displacement of normal epidural fat in foramen. Larger amount of disc material is seen on more lateral oblique view (*arrow,* **F**).

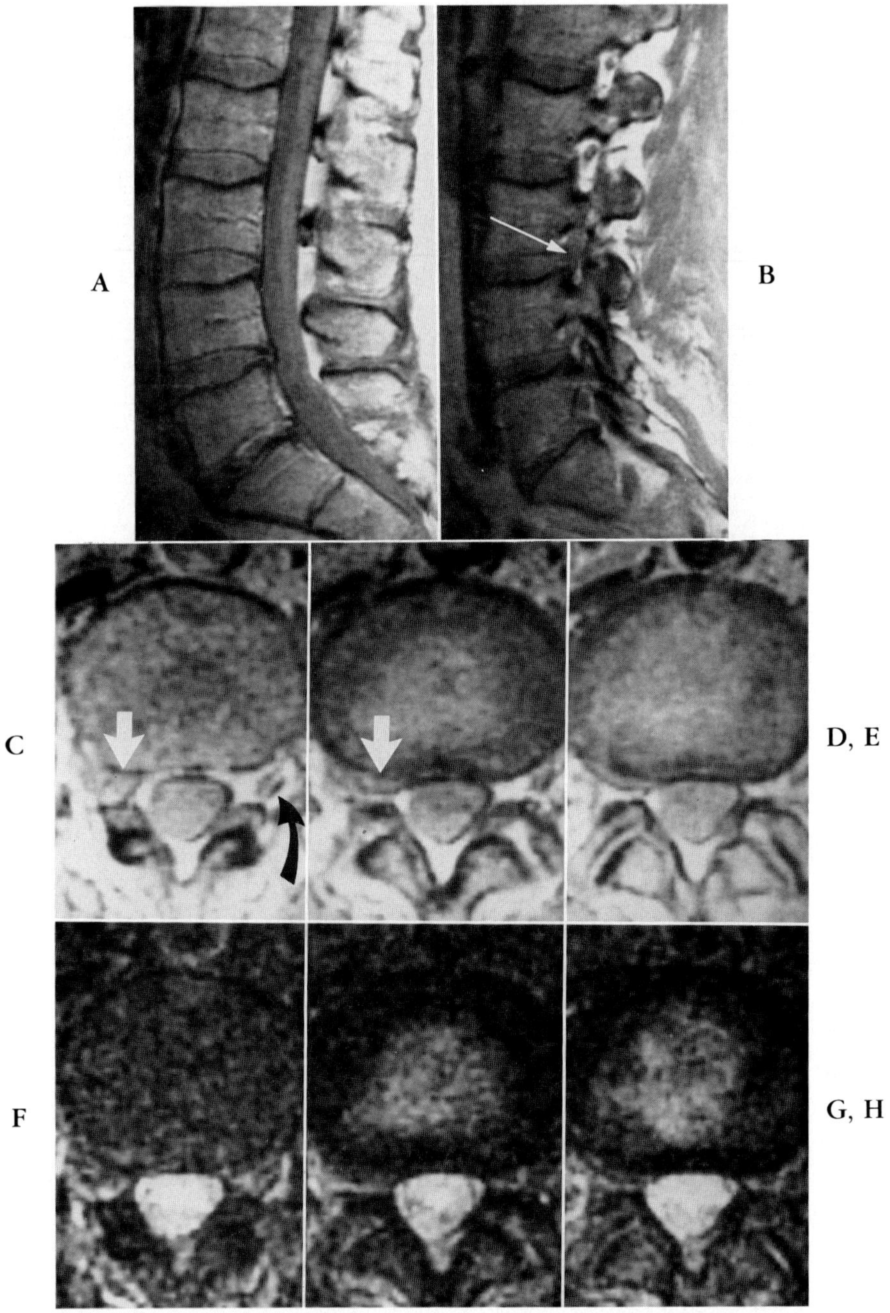

FIGURE 10-40. Lumbar disc herniation–lateral. Lateral disc herniations require careful scrutiny of all images because they may be subtle on sagittal and axial images. **A** and **B,** Sagittal T1W scan (SE 800/20) shows small midline herniation of L_4-L_5 and evidence for lateral disc herniation on right at L_3-L_4 (*arrow,* **B**). **C-H,** Lateral disc herniation is confirmed on axial T2W scan (SE gated 2000/20, 80). Focal disc herniation occupies neural foramen where ganglion normally resides (normal ganglion on left, *curved arrow,* **C**) but in this patient is displaced by herniated disc (*straight arrow,* **D**). Finding is confirmed on first echo image at next lower level (*arrow,* **E**). Note that second echo images (**F-H**) show no evidence of deformity of dural sac, and disc material is difficult to detect because it has nearly same signal intensity as adjacent fat. Side to side asymmetry is better visualized on first echo (**C-E**) than on second echo images (**F-H**). When using axial T2W technique, both first and second echo images must be scrutinized.

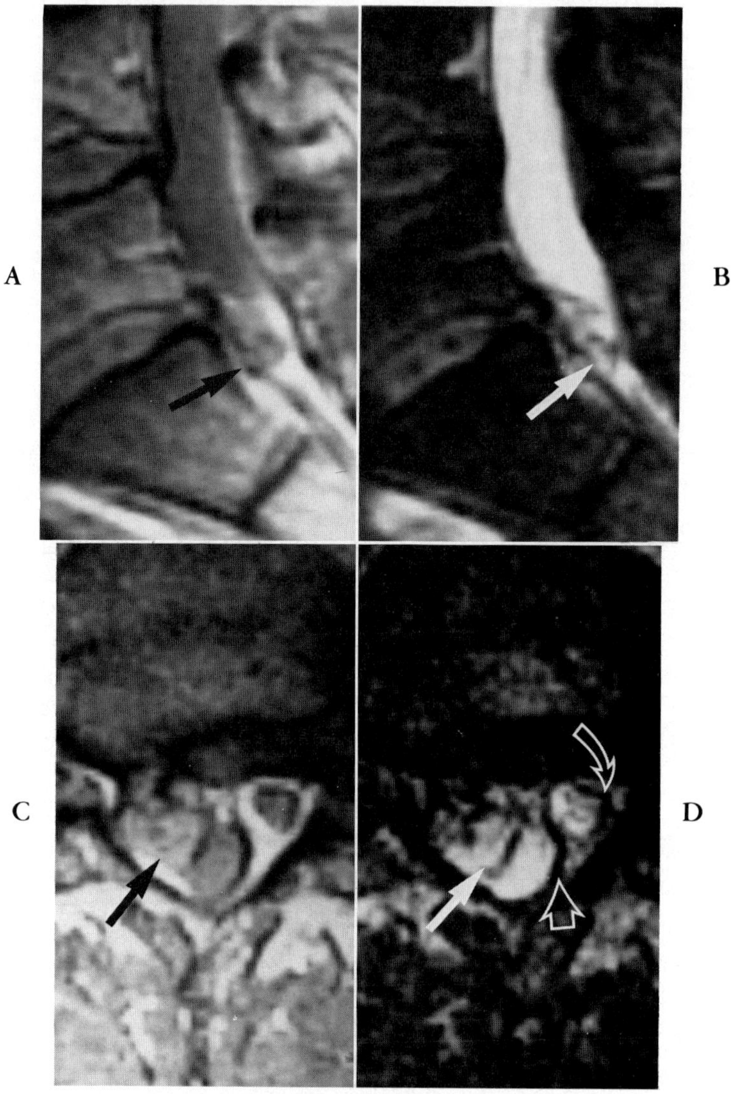

FIGURE 10-41. Lumbar disc–"free" fragment. Disc herniations resulting in "free" fragments show characteristics of other disc herniations but in addition the "free" fragment often has high signal intensity on second echo of T2W sequence; higher signal than disc fragments that are not "free". **A,** Sagittal T2W scan (SE 2000/20, 80) shows disruption of anulus and ligament on first echo indicating transverse tear (see Figure 10-9) with disc material extending inferiorly behind S_1 *(arrow)*. **B,** Second echo shows "free" disc material of high signal intensity *(arrow)*. **C,** Axial T2W first echo image shows large disc fragment occupying right half of spinal canal. Even on this image, signal intensity of disc material is higher than that of CSF in dural sac. **D,** On second echo T2W axial scan right root sleeve is obliterated *(curved arrow)* and extruded disc material *(closed straight arrow)* is same high signal intensity as CSF in dural sac. Thin black line, probably dura and ligament, separates these two structures. Black line on left side of dural sac *(straight open arrow)* and left root sleeve *(curved open arrow)* results from chemical shift artifact. Dural margin on right is obscured by this artifact.

deformity of the dural sac, which is well seen because of high contrast afforded by the relative high signal of CSF. Epidural fat has low signal on the second echo image and thus affords little contrast for disc herniaton detection.

The herniated disc may be far lateral, i.e., lateral to the intervertebral foramen at the pedicle (see Figures 10-39 and 10-40) making detection difficult, but both axial and sagittal T1W scans will show asymmetry and displacement of epidural fat near the spinal root ganglion. On T2W images, the first echo shows similar findings but the second echo could miss the disc material if it is of low signal intensity (see Figure 10-40). Both echo images need to be scrutinized. The disc material may be high signal on the second echo of a T2W sequence and thus easily identifiable (see Figure 10-39). Sagittal views help in assessing clinical significance of a lateral disc herniation.

Sequestered "free" fragments are best detected on sagittal scans showing migration from native disc space along the dorsal surface of the adjacent vertebral bodies (see Figure 10-9).[20] Such free fragments are seen on axial scans but their separation from the disc space is best appreciated on the sagittal scan, which readily differentiates between a free fragment and adjacent epidural fat (Figures 10-41 to 10-43). On a sagittal T2W sequence such extradural defects are well visualized (see Figure 10-41). The free fragment disc material often is still hydrated and thus shows relatively high signal intensity on a T2W image (see Figure 10-42). Disc herniations can stand out with this type of pulse sequence and this can be of help in lateral disc herniations (see Figure 10-39).

The use of GdDTPA in disc disease may show enhancement even in a non-operated disc, often on the periphery of the disc or extending into the disc space itself (see Figure 10-49). The sites of enhancement most likely represent vascular fibrous tissue, which is a response to tissue injury, i.e., anulus tear. This area of enhancement could change over time because it represents a tissue capable of remodelling. The reported decreased size of disc herniations may reflect a decrease in this granulation tissue over time. A large area of enhancement may suggest a significant component of granulation tissue; in such instances, a noncontrast scan could overestimate the herniation size (see Figure 10-50). The frequency of this is unknown, but it is probably uncommon.

Lumbar roots traverse a long distance from the spinal cord to their eventual destination and thus symptoms suggestive of disc disease can be mimicked by other disease entities. It is therefore important for a lumbar spine study to include examination of the cauda equina and the conus medullaris on the sagittal view. This is the analog to the conus view that was a standard part of lumbar myelography. It is also important to remember that pelvic disease (neoplastic or inflammatory) can mimic lumbar radiculopathy, as well as hip disease such as aseptic necrosis. Referred knee pain can enter the differential diagnosis. Reliance on the clinician's working diagnosis guides the MR examination. Nevertheless, in patients with known malignancies, it is important to scrutinize other areas. The examination should probably be carried through the sacrum, especially if the clinical picture suggests the potential involvement of sacral nerve roots that may be infiltrated by tumor far distal from their exit from the spinal canal. The short inversion time, inversion recovery sequences (STIR), may be valuable in visualizing the lumbar and sacral nerve plexus and any impingement thereon.

Recurrent Disc Herniation

A major clinical and imaging problem is that of detecting recurrent disc herniations once surgery has been performed. Surgical intervention disrupts normal anatomic landmarks and complicates the use of morphologic information in detection of residual or newly herniated disc material. In addition to bone defects after surgery, the epidural fat adjacent to the dural sac is replaced by fibrotic tissue. On T1W scans and T2W balanced images (first echo) this fibrotic tissue has similar signal intensity as CSF (Figures 10-44 and 10-45). A T2W scan, especially the axial view, can outline the margins of the dural sac, which may not be as easily seen on T1W scans, and therefore may be helpful to detect an extradural mass effect caused by a postoperative herniated disc (see Figures 10-44 and 10-45).

In some instances, residual or recurrent herniated disc is different signal intensity than the postsurgical scar tissue and thus can be

A

B, C

D, E

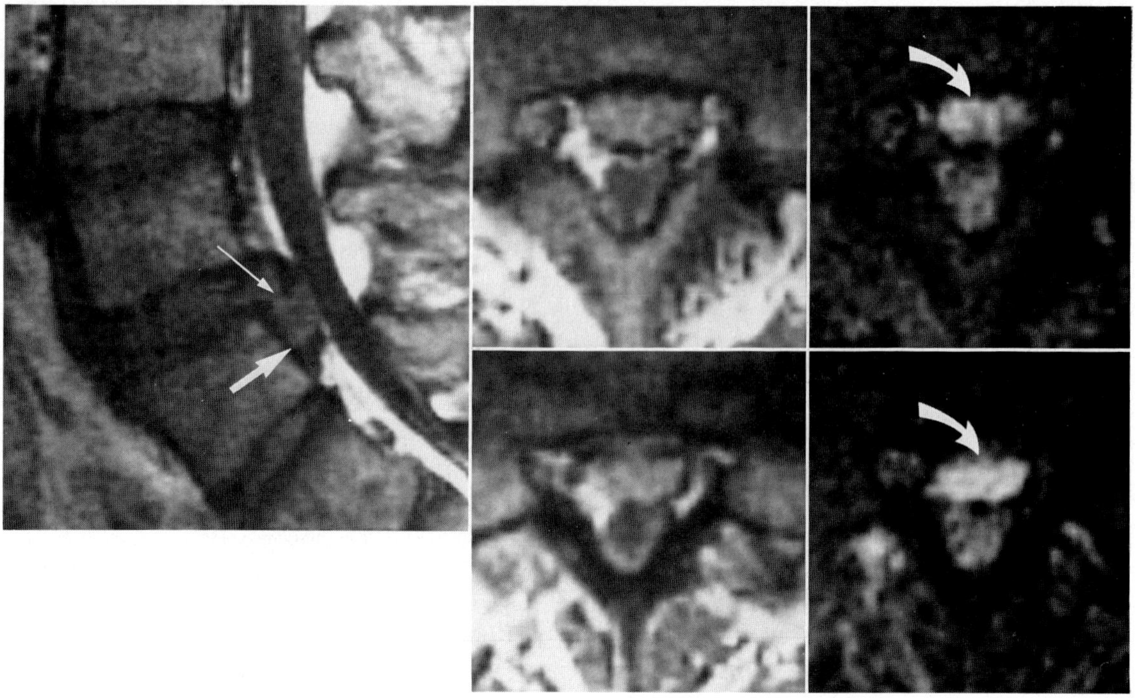

FIGURE 10-42. Lumbar disc–"free" fragment. It can be difficult to determine if a disc represents a "free" fragment. This should be suspected when a disc fragment is high signal on a T2W scan. **A,** T1W sagittal scan (SE 800/20) shows large disc herniation at L_4-L_5 with clear disruption of anulus-ligament complex *(small arrow)* and migration of disc fragment down posterior aspect of L_5 *(large arrow)*. **B-E,** Axial T2W scans (SE gated 1900/20, 80) show large midline disc herniation that on first echo (**B** and **D**) is slightly higher signal intensity than CSF in dural sac. On second echo images (**C** and **E**) disc material is relatively higher signal intensity than CSF in dural sac *(arrows)*. High signal intensity suggests disc fragment is similar to "free" fragment, although sagittal image suggests some persistent continuity between fragment and disc space. Classification of some disc herniations can be difficult, but considering disc signal intensity it would be reasonable to assume a "free" fragment.

A

B

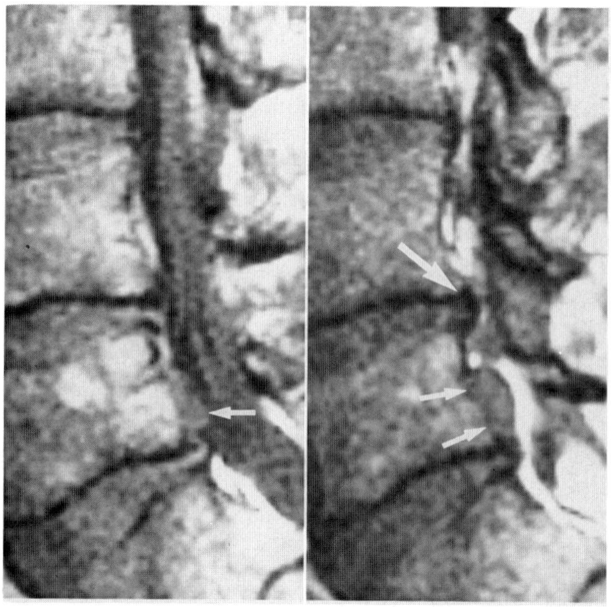

FIGURE 10-43. Lumbar disc–"free" fragment. A sequestered disc ("free" fragment) can present without myelographic findings. **A** and **B,** Sagittal T1W scan (SE 800/20) shows small disc herniation at L_4-L_5 *(large arrow)* and sequestered fragment arising from L_5-S_1 disc space that migrated rostrally behind L_5 in midline (**A**) and off to right (**B**) *(small arrows)*.

C D E F G H
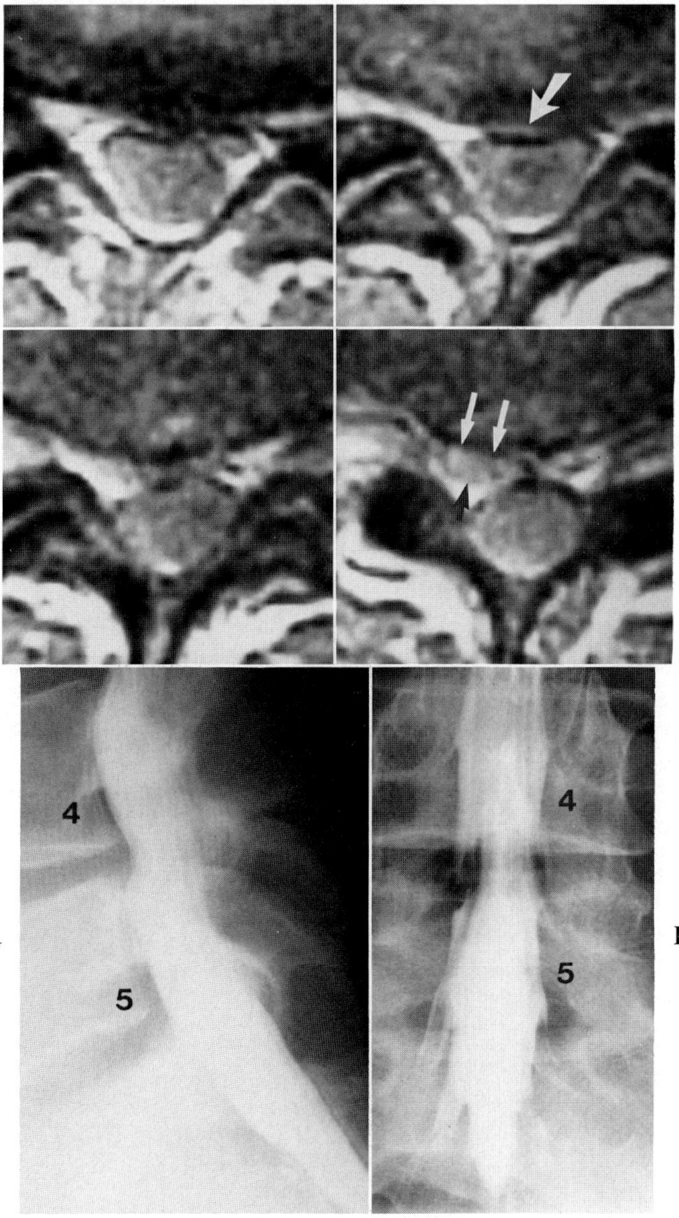

FIGURE 10-43, cont'd. C-F, On first echo, (TE 20) of axial T2W scan (SE gated 2200/20, 80) findings are also subtle. Only small extradural defect is present at level of L_5-S_1 disc space (*arrow*, **D**) whereas at higher level sequestered fragment is seen as abnormal soft tissue mass on right side of canal (*arrows*, **F**). Note asymmetry in right anterior epidural space compared to left side, which shows linear venous structures (**F**). Myelogram in AP (**G**) and lateral (**H**) show L_4-L_5 disc herniation well but there is no evidence of sequestered fragment arising from L_5-S_1 disc space.

A 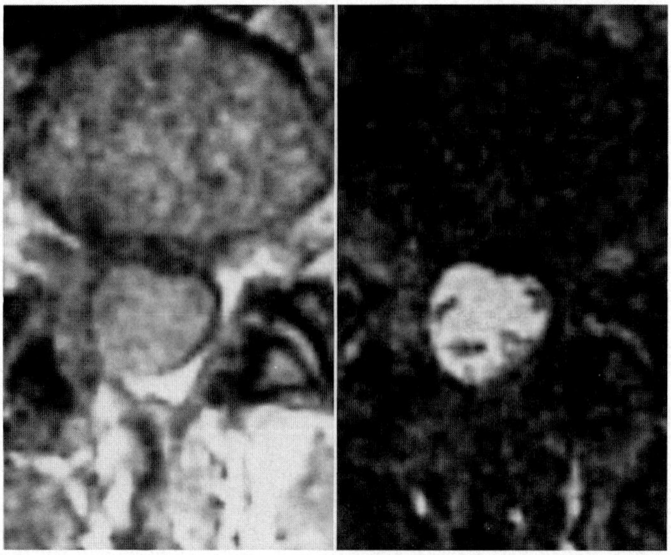 B

FIGURE 10-44. Postoperative lumbar spine. Abnormal signal intensity is noted on right side of spinal canal and in right neural foramen of postoperative patient. **A,** On first echo (TE 20) of axial T2W scan (SE gated 2000/20, 80) abnormal signal appears to be postoperative fibrosis because dural sac is not deformed. **B,** Second echo (TE 80) image shows normal margins of dural sac; fibrous tissue poorly seen because of low signal intensity. Individual lumbar nerve roots are seen, suggesting no significant arachnoiditis.

A, B, C, D 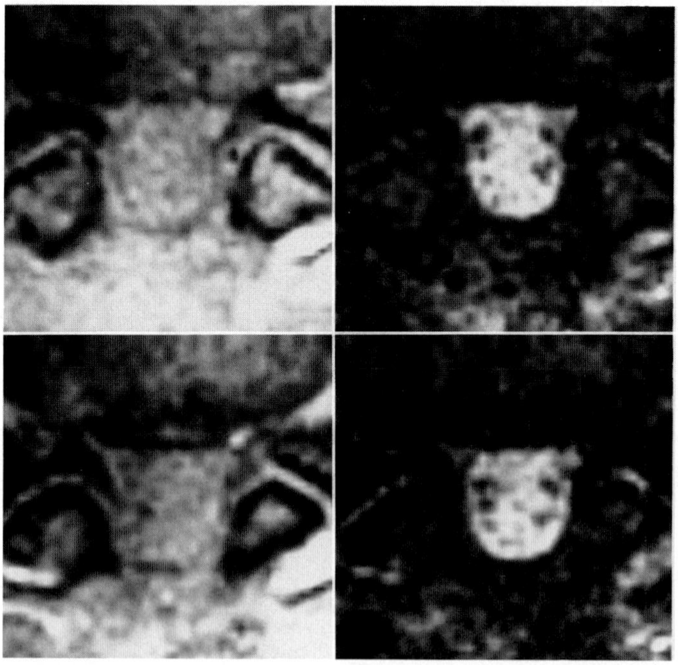

FIGURE 10-45. Postoperative lumbar spine. Postoperative spine can be difficult to evaluate for residual or recurrent disc herniation. Axial T2W scan (SE gated 2100/20, 80) is useful because it can accurately delineate dural sac and nerve roots within scar tissue. **A** and **C,** First echo (balanced) images show poor discrimination between dural sac and postoperative fibrosis around sac. **B** and **D,** Second echo images clearly demarcate high CSF signal within dural sac from surrounding low signal postoperative tissue. Because major criteria for detecting recurrent or residual disc is mass effect on dural sac, these images are important in detecting such extradural mass effects.

differentiated[4]; this is best seen on T2W images. In other instances, disc material may have the same signal intensity as scar tissue and thus differentiation is difficult or impossible; this occurs more frequently on T1W scans.[4] On T2W scans this may also be the case, but often disc material is higher signal intensity than scar tissue. Nevertheless, there will be instances when the disc is degenerated enough that its signal intensity cannot be differentiated from scar tissue. A major finding in differentiating herniated disc from scar tissue in such instances is that scar tissue usually does not cause a mass effect that results in focal indentation of the dural sac. There are exceptions, however. On a T2W sequence where the margin of the dural sac is well delineated, this mass effect should be readily apparent and, if present, suggests disc. Sagittal oblique T1W views perpendicular to the neural foramina may be of benefit in differentiating disc material from scar tissue by showing contiguity of the suspected disc herniation with the native disc space. This relationship is difficult to demonstrate on axial views alone.

GdDTPA

An effective technique for solving the dilemma of postsurgical change vs. recurrent or residual disc is the use of an MR contrast agent such as GdDTPA. Scar tissue enhances with this contrast agent whereas disc material does not. There may be some enhancement of disc material on delayed scans. Immediate scanning is therefore recommended. The enhancement probably represents vascular fibrous tissue that is closely associated with the disc material. Using a T1W sequence, without and with contrast, resolves the problem of separating postsurgical scar tissue from disc material (Figures 10-46 to 10-50), especially in the uncommon circumstance where fibrosis results in deformity of the dural sac suggesting a mass effect (Figures 10-48 and 10-50). Both sagittal and axial views are valuable in making this diagnosis. Sagittal oblique views are necessary on occasion, in which the disc material will stand out as lower signal intensity compared to the higher signal, enhanced granulation tissue (see Figures 10-46 and 10-50).

A

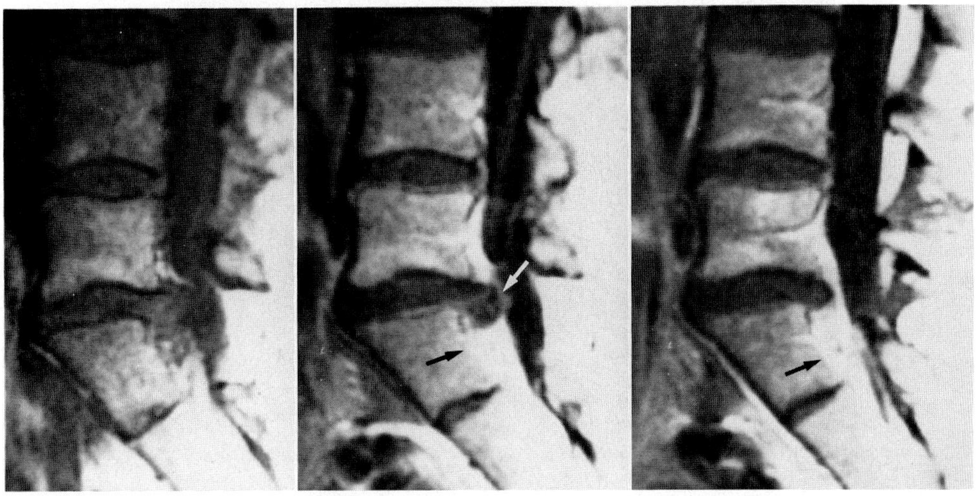

B, C

FIGURE 10-46. Postoperative lumbar spine–GdDTPA. Comparison of **A**, precontrast T1W scan (SE 600/20) and **B** and **C**, postcontrast T1W scans (SE 600/20) show value of GdDTPA as contrast agent in detecting recurrent disc herniation. Precontrast scan shows irregular soft tissue density posterior to disc space at L_5-S_1. Fibrotic tissue cannot be distinguished from possible disc herniation (**A**). PostGdDTPA scans show some enhancement of postoperative site posterior to L_5-S_1 (*black arrow*, **B**) but well-defined defect in epidural space does not exhibit contrast enhancement *(white arrow)*, which represents recurrent herniated disc. **C**, More lateral slice shows prominent enhancement of postsurgical scar *(arrow)*. (Courtesy of Dr. Allan Williams.)

A herniated disc may be "coated" by fibrous tissue after surgery. Differentiation of these two types of tissue is not possible on noncontrast T1W scans and thus the size of a disc herniation can be overestimated (Figure 10-50). Signal intensity of disc material and granulation tissue can be difficult to distinguish on T1W scans (Figure 10-50). Retraction of such granulation tissue may be responsible for "improvement" in disc herniations as seen on imaging tests. The use of GdDTPA allows such differentiation (Figure 10-50). Whether GdDTPA should be used for all disc disease to make such a distinction should be evaluated in the future. Such information may help in presurgical evaluation.

Contrast enhancement can be visualized in the disc space (Figures 10-49 and 10-50), presumably representing fibrotic tissue intermixed with disc material as a healing response to damage or surgery. The nerve and nerve root sleeve stand out as low signal compared to scar tissue (Figure 10-48). In this particular diagnostic problem, an MR contrast agent is of clear benefit and greatly facilitates image interpretation where conventional pulse sequences without contrast may fall short.

A

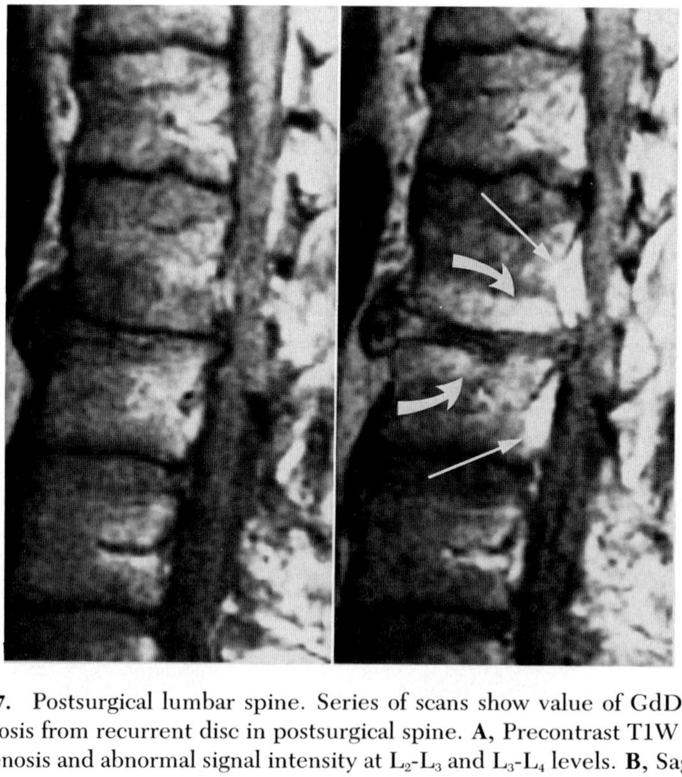

B

FIGURE 10-47. Postsurgical lumbar spine. Series of scans show value of GdDTPA in differentiating fibrosis from recurrent disc in postsurgical spine. **A,** Precontrast T1W scan (SE 800/20) shows stenosis and abnormal signal intensity at L_2-L_3 and L_3-L_4 levels. **B,** Sagittal postcontrast scan shows increased signal intensity along inferior end-plate of L_3 and superior end-plate of L_4 *(curved arrows)*. Marked enhancement is noted in anterior venous plexus of canal behind L_2 and L_3 vertebral bodies *(straight arrows)*. **C-J,** Precontrast axial T1W scans (SE 1000/20) (**C, E, G,** and **I**) obtained in rostal to caudal direction in area of previous surgery show poor definition of dural sac because of replacement of epidural fat by fibrotic tissue. PostGdDTPA axial T1W scans (**D, F, H,** and **J**) at same levels show prominent enhancement of fibrotic tissue *(arrows)* and lack of any recurrent disc herniation.

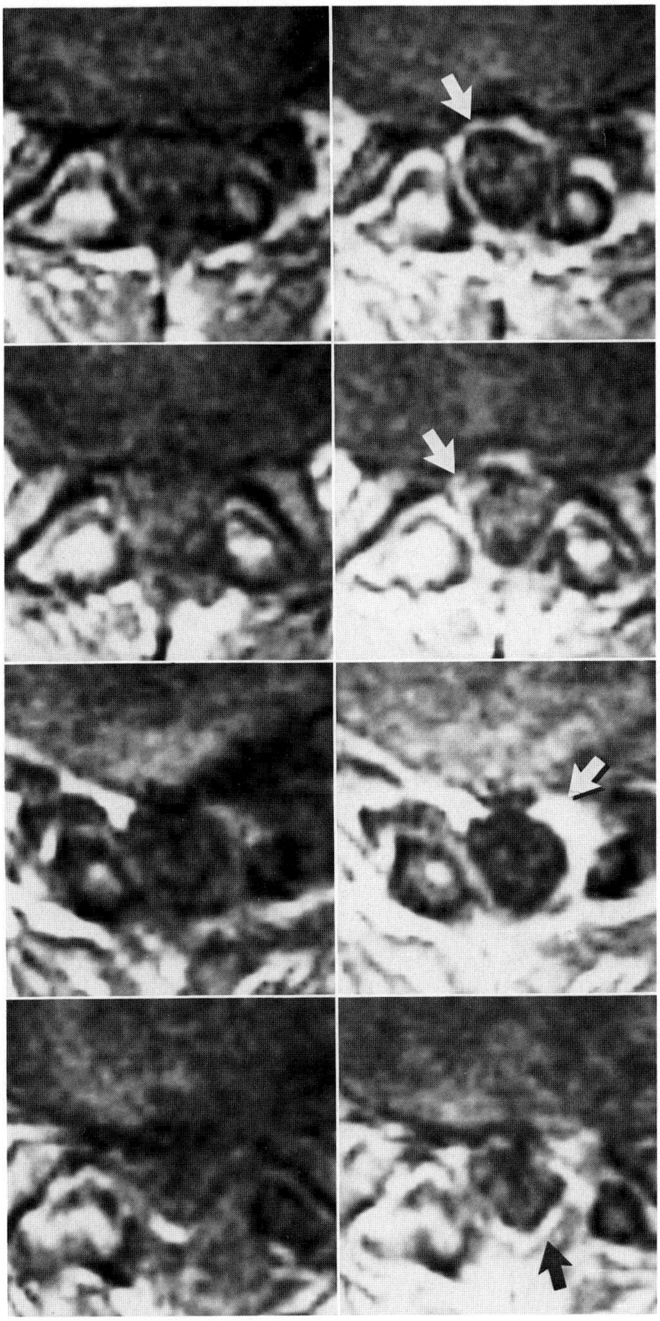

C D E F G H I J

FIGURE 10-47, cont'd. For legend see previous page.

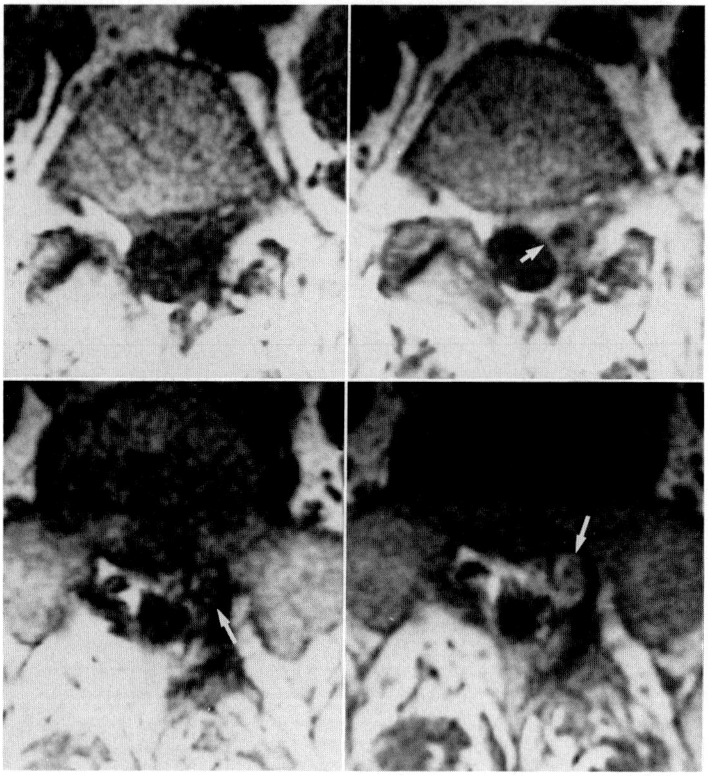

A B C D

FIGURE 10-48. Postoperative lumbar spine–GdDTPA. **A** and **C**, Precontrast T1W scans (SE 600/20) compared to **B** and **D**, postcontrast T1W scans show value of GdDTPA in differentiating postoperative scar from recurrent disc herniation at two lumbar levels: L_4-L_5 (**A** and **B**) and L_5-S_1 (**C** and **D**). On precontrast T1W scans (**A** and **C**) dural sac and postoperative sac cannot be adequately differentiated. At L_4-L_5 level scar tissure enhances and shows left root sleeve in relief. No disc herniation is identified, although dural sac is flattened on left (*arrow*, **B**). Preoperative scan was unavailable to determine if morphologic change occured after surgery. At L_5-S_1 level (**C**) precontrast T1W scan suggests possibility of free fragment *(arrow)*. **D**, PostGdDTPA scan shows enhancement indicating scar tissue and not disc *(arrow)*. (Courtesy of Dr. Allan Williams.)

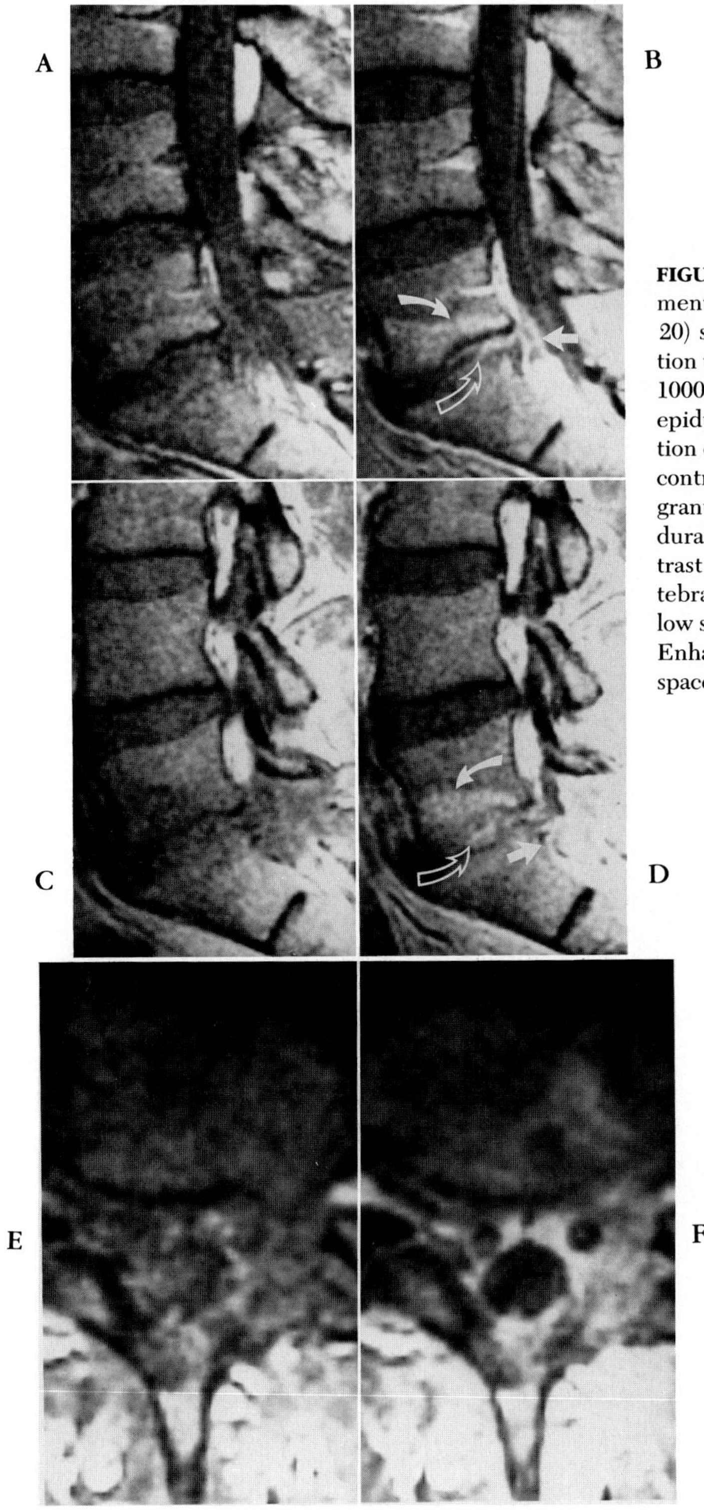

FIGURE 10-49. Postsurgical GdDTPA enhancement. **A** and **C**, Sagittal precontrast scans (SE 800/20) show replacement of epidural fat by granulation tissue at L_5-S_1 level. Precontrast axial scan (SE 1000/20) at L_5-S_1 disc level shows obscuration of epidural fat–dural sac interface (**E**). Disc herniation cannot be accurately assessed. **B** and **D**, Postcontrast (GdDTPA) scans show enhancement of granulation tissue *(straight arrows)*. On axial scan, dural sac and root sleeves are well seen on postcontrast scan (**F**). Note enhancement within L_5 vertebral body (*curved arrows*, **B** and **D**) changing low signal region into relatively high signal region. Enhancement is also identified within L_5-S_1 disc space (*open curved arrows*, **B** and **D**).

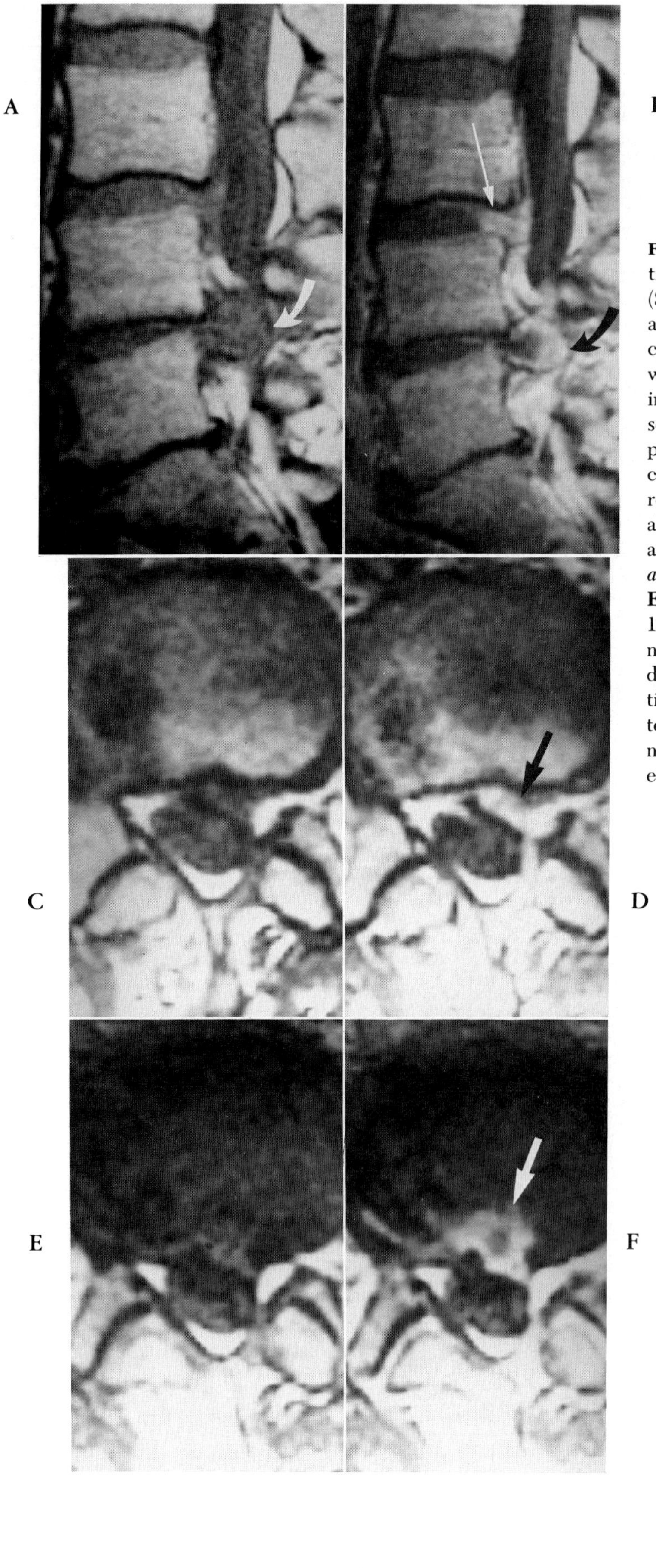

FIGURE 10-50. Postsurgical disc herniation and GdDTPA. Sagittal T1W scans (SE 800/20) preGdDTPA injection (**A**) and postGdDTPA injection (**B**). On noncontrast scan (**A**) large mass, isointense with native L_4-L_5 disc space impinging into spinal canal *(arrow)*. Postcontrast scan (**B**) shows contrast enhancement on periphery of mass *(curved arrow)* sparing central portion of mass, which represents recurrent disc herniation. Enhancement also in anterior epidural venous plexus and posterior disc space at C_3-C_4 *(straight arrow)*. **C** and **E,** PreGdDTPA and **D** and **E,** postGdDTPA axial T1W scans (SE 1000/20) at L_3-L_4 level show no disc herniation, but contrast enhancement of epidural granulation tissue allows differentiation (*arrows,* **D** and **F**) from disc material, a separation not possible on noncontrast scans. Note enhancement extends into disc space proper (**B** and **F**).

G H

I J

K L

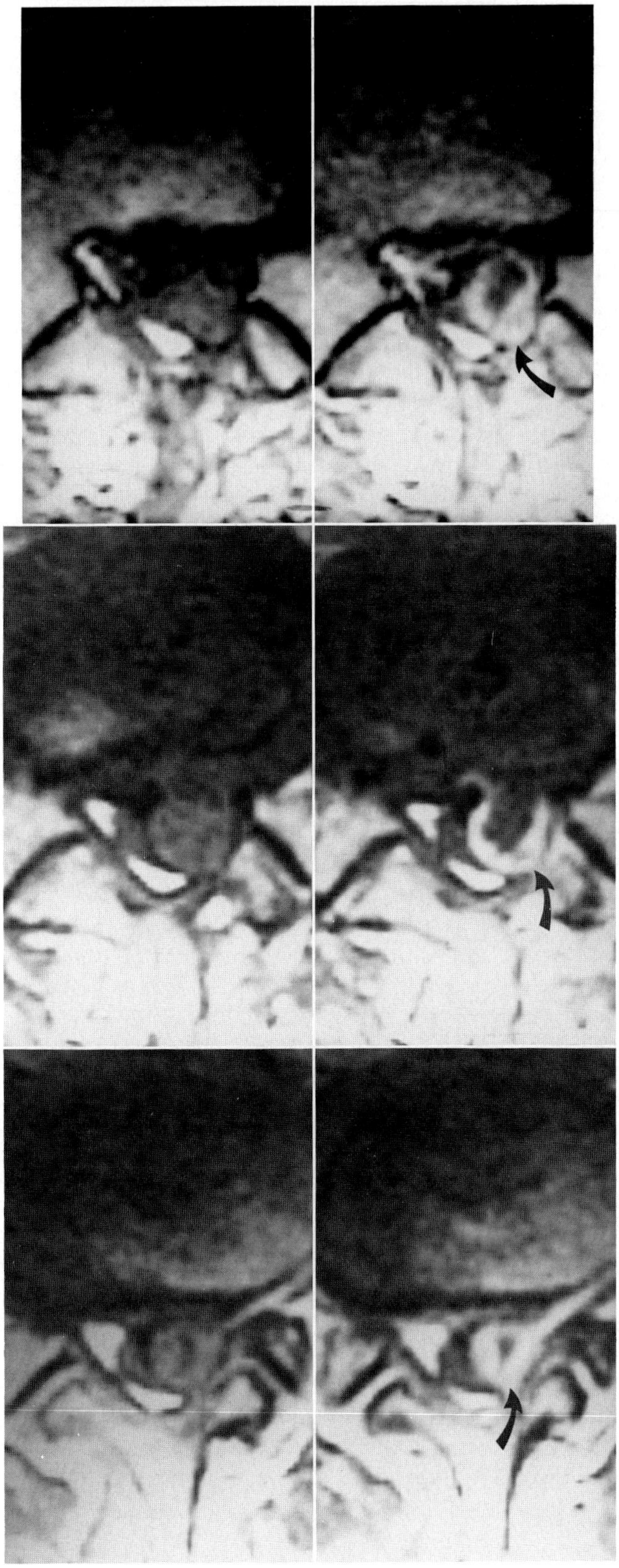

FIGURE 10-50, cont'd. PreGdDTPA (**G**, **I**, and **K**) and postGdDTPA (**H**, **J**, and **L**) axial T1W scans (SE 1000/20) at L_4-L_5 level show recurrent disc herniation evidenced by nonenhancing portion of extradural mass (**H**, **J**, and **L**). Contrast enhancement encircles recurrent disc herniation and probably represents "coating" of granulation tissue *(arrows)*, a differentiation not possible on noncontrast scans (**G** and **I**).

SPINAL STENOSIS

Patients with spinal stenosis usually present clinically in the fifth and sixth decade. Patients with congenitally narrow spinal canals are clearly at greater risk. In the cervical cord, the clinical picture is that of a slowly progressive myelopathy although radicular symptoms are possible. In rare instances it progresses rapidly.[27] The myelopathy is aggravated by hyperextension. It is characterized by mild to moderate paraparesis (upper extremity weakness is a later finding if it develops at all), normal sensory and bladder functions, and brisk reflexes. In general, these findings are associated with pain. In the thoracic region, although spinal stenosis is uncommon, it may present with either a radiculopathy or myelopathy. Both upper and lower motor neuron signs may be present. Symptoms include pain, sensory changes, paraparesis, claudication, urinary incontinence, and extensor plantar responses.[3,33,38] In the lumbar region, pain is also prominent but the typical presentation is a type of claudication that is exacerbated by hyperextension and relieved by flexion.

Pathogenesis

The major congenital factor is one of short, thick pedicles that narrow the spinal canal in an anteroposterior (AP) direction. The most important factors in spinal stenosis are the acquired factors, with congenital factors primarily lowering the threshold by setting the stage for stenosis. The acquired factors include ligamentum flavum hypertrophy, posterior longitudinal ligament hypertrophy or ossification,[24] osteophytes, disc bulging and herniation, and spondylolisthesis. Old trauma may play a role in causing or accelerating this process. All these factors may contribute in various proportions to narrowing of the spinal canal. Facet disease plays a larger role in the lumbar spine where it can cause narrowing of the lateral recesses. In general the most important factors are some type of disc protrusion in combination with hypertrophy of the ligamentum flavum.[35] Ligament hypertrophy may involve the posterior longitudinal ligament in addition to the ligamentum flavum. The former ligament may calcify, producing the well-known entity of ossification of the posterior longitudinal ligament (OPLL).

MR Findings

Cervical

Stenosis can simply compromise the size of the subarachnoid space in the cervical region, or it may cause cord deformity and cord compression. The diagnosis of cervical spine stenosis is often suspected on the T1W sagittal image when it shows a small or absent subarachnoid space around the cervical cord (Figure 10-51). In more severe degrees of stenosis actual deformity of the cervical cord is seen (see Figure 10-51). The deformities may be subtle but can be detected as either focal indentations or focal flattening of the cord, usually on its ventral surface. In some circumstances, cervical spine stenosis, is missed on a T1W sagittal scan because either the hypertrophied ligament or the osteophyte is of similar signal intensity as the anterior subarachnoid space, i.e., dark gray or black. In such instances, the T1W sagittal scan may be falsely negative (see Figure 10-4). This pitfall is avoided on the sagittal scan, if images with high signal CSF are obtained with a sagittal gated, flow-compensated, or variable flip angle scan. In each of these scans low signal intensity of either the osteophyte or hypertrophied ligament stands out in contrast to the high signal CSF. T2W or T2*W scans yield an appreciation of the degree and extent of cervical spinal stenosis (Figures 10-52 and 10-53; see Figure 10-51).

Axial scans are important to corroborate sagittal scan findings. On T1W axial scans, subarachnoid space can be difficult to delineate and spinal stenosis is usually seen as a deformity of the normal elliptical shape of the cervical cord. In its most subtle form, the cord shows slight flattening of its anterior surface. In its most severe form, the cord assumes a small, triangular appearance. On axial scans, in which CSF is seen as high signal, only a small amount if any CSF may be detected in severe stenosis (see Figure 10-52). The residual CSF is usually present in the anterolateral recesses and sometimes in the midline posteriorly. The relative lack of CSF is easy to detect, making the diagnosis straightforward. Increased signal intensity may be seen between dura and vertebral body that represents dilated epidural venous plexus (see Figure 10-52), often seen when multiple disc herniations contribute to cervical spinal stenosis (see Figure 10-52).

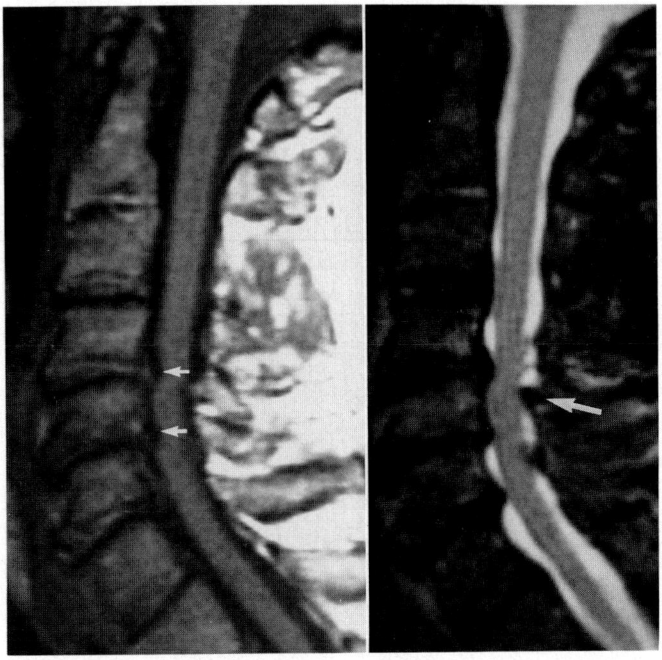

FIGURE 10-51. Cervical stenosis. Cervical spondylosis causing stenosis of canal usually suspected on **A,** T1W scan (SE 800/20) when extradural defects indent spinal cord *(arrows)*. Several impressions on spinal cord are seen from C_5-C_7 *(arrows)*. **B,** Sagittal T2W scan (SE gated, 2100/80) better demonstrates severity of impingement on subarachnoid space and cord. Cervical canal compromise is combination of anterior disc herniations and posterior ligament hypertrophy *(arrow)*. T2W scan can also indicate evidence of cord damage, which is not detected in this patient.

A number of patients with severe cervical stenosis on T2W sagittal scans and axial scans may show abnormal high signal within the cord (see Figures 10-52 and 10-53). The pathologic correlation of this abnormal signal is a combination of neuronal loss, demyelination, and infarction that is characterized by cavitation and necrosis[26]—findings often grouped under the term, *myelomalacia*.[2] Syrinx formation has also been reported.[2] These areas of cavitation (microcystic change) and syrinx formation have been detected before MR by virtue of their enhancement on delayed CT scans after the intrathecal instillation of metrizamide.[16,17] The MR abnormality is detected more frequently in patients who have a clinical myelopathy (see Figures 10-52 and 10-53). The prognostic significance of this finding has not been defined, although once such abnormal cord signal is present it is usually not reversed by subsequent decompressive surgery. The area of abnormal cord signal however localizes to the site of the most severe cervical stenosis, making it unlikely to be mistaken for other intrinsic cord lesions.

Thoracic

Spinal stenosis of the thoracic spine is less common than spinal stenosis in the cervical or lumbar spine. When it occurs, it is often related to hypertrophy of the lamina, apophyseal joints, ligamentum flavum, or combinations thereof.[33,39] A large osteophyte or a large herniated disc rarely causes stenosis (see Figure 10-26). The stenosis usually occurs at a single level, compared to cervical and lumbar regions where stenosis often occurs at multiple levels. Common levels are the T_{10} to T_{12} levels. Cord compression usually occurs posterolaterally[33]; cord deviation could be lateral and therefore subtle on the sagittal view. Axial views should be performed at any suspicious level on the sag-

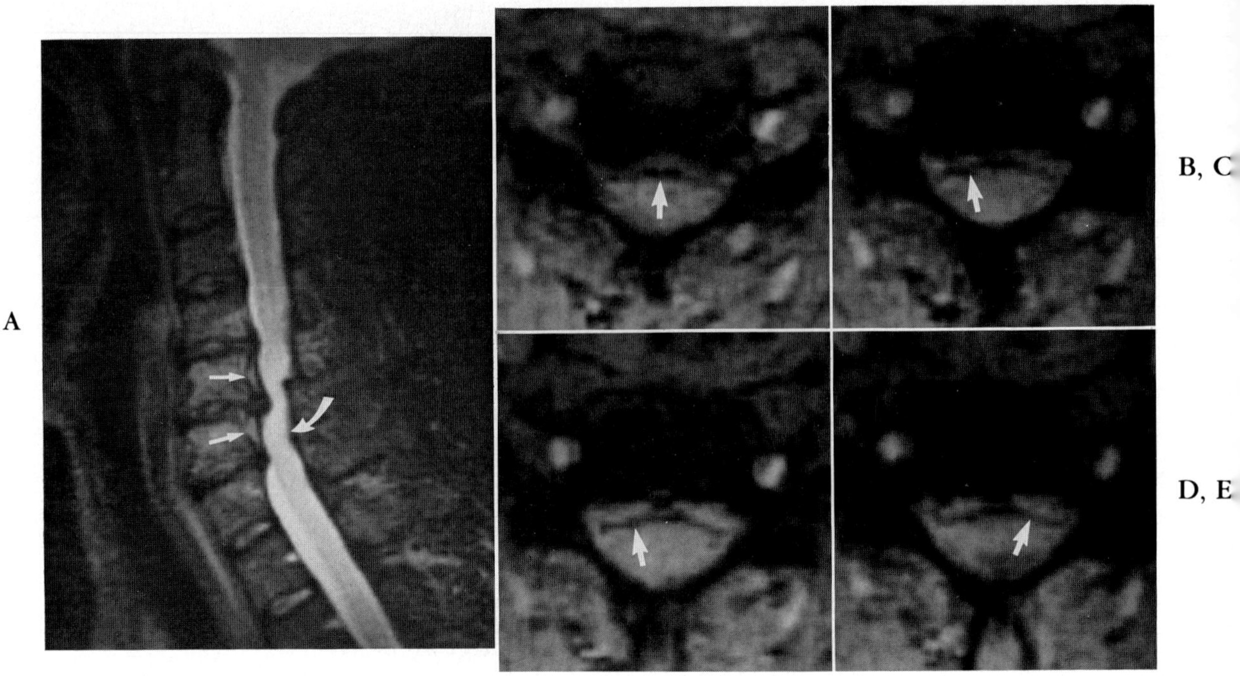

FIGURE 10-52. Cervical stenosis. **A,** Sagittal T2W scan (SE gated 2200/80) shows cervical stenosis at C_5 and C_6 that is combination of congenitally narrow canal and multiple disc herniations, which have separated dura from vertebral body resulting in thin layer of intermediate signal intensity between these two structures *(arrows)* and represent dilated epidural venous plexus *(arrows)*. In addition, abnormal high signal in cord at level of stenosis indicates cord damage, probably gliosis, at this level *(curved arrow)*. **B-E,** Axial variable flip angle/gradient echo scans (GRASS 25/13, 7°) show lack of high signal CSF at these levels. Thin black line in anterior third of spinal canal represents posteriorly displaced dura and posterior longitudinal ligament *(arrows)*. Axial variable flip angle scans and sagittal gated scan show absence of subarachnoid space at C_5 and C_6 levels.

ittal scan, or at any clinically relevant level. Lesions detectable on T1W sagittal and axial scans are often sufficient to make the diagnosis. T2W scans may add further information, especially with respect to cord damage but are usually not necessary for the diagnosis.

Lumbar

The development of stenosis in the lumbar spine, is again an interplay between the size of the spinal canal and the development of disc protrusions (bulge or herniation), osteophytes, and ligament hypertrophy (Figures 10-54 to 10-57). A congenitally narrow canal predisposes the patient for spinal stenosis with minimal to moderate degrees of soft tissue changes. Remember that lateral disc herniation may accompany lumbar stenosis and thus add to clinical symptomatology (see Figure 10-57). The diagnosis is often suspected on the T1W sagittal scan because it usually requires a combination of disc bulging or herniation plus ligament hypertrophy to cause true stenosis in the lumbar region (see Figures 10-54, 10-56, and 10-57). The disc bulging or herniation is usually identifiable in the midline on sagittal scans. It can, however, be difficult to detect if the disc material is low signal intensity (see Figure 10-56). Spondylolisthesis contributes to spinal stenosis in part because of the bony offset and also because disc bulging often accompanies displacement (Figure 10-58). Ligament hypertrophy can be appreciated as an area of intermediate signal in the posterior aspect of the canal at the disc space level (see Figures 10-54 and 10-57). Lumbar stenosis is suspected when

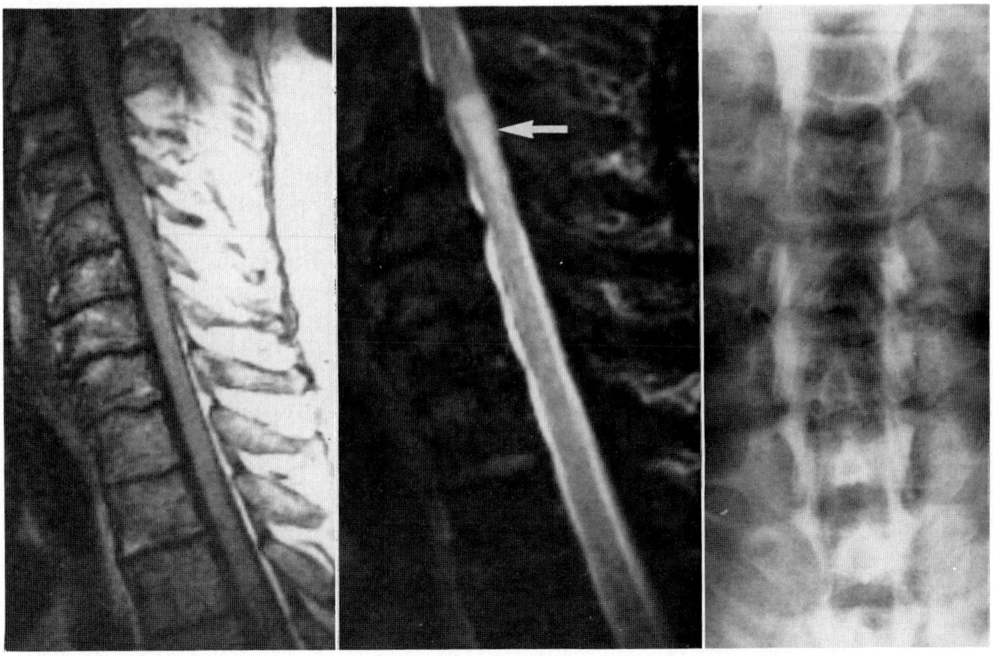

FIGURE 10-53. Cervical stenosis. Amount of cord damage in cervical stenosis can be extensive and could suggest possibility of cord tumor. **A,** Sagittal T1W scan (SE 800/20) suggests cervical stenosis, but cord damage is not detected. **B,** Sagittal T2W scan (SE gated, 1900/100) of patient who had myelopathy shows extensive area of high signal abnormality in upper cervical cord *(arrow),* representing myelomalacia related to cervical stensosis. Intraoperative ultrasound did not detect evidence of tumor or other type of intramedullary mass. **C,** Concurrent myelogram shows severe stenosis at C_4-C_5, same level as cord abnormality seen on MR (**B**).

the spinal canal is seen on only one midline slice and appears compromised on either side of midline when using a thin slice (3 mm) technique. As with other areas in the spine, a perpendicular confirmatory view is always advised. An axial T1W scan will show a bulging or herniated disc and hypertrophied ligamentum flavum. The low signal intensity dural sac will appear small and in severe cases will have a trefoil appearance. Even with this organized approach to scanning, spinal stenosis can be missed by MR when it is position dependent. In a supine position stenosis may not be detected whereas in an upright, weight-bearing position disc bulging, ligament bulging, or subluxation causes lumbar stenosis (Figure 10-59).

Sagittal T2W scans of the lumbar spine are less often used in the work-up of disc disease, but if obtained the area of stenosis is well seen as a result of high contrast between high signal CSF and all of the structures that can cause stenosis, because they are all of lower signal intensity (see Figure 10-57). There is a difference in signal intensity of CSF above and below the stenosis. Above the stenosis, CSF signal intensity is lower because of motion as compared to below the stenosis where CSF is relatively stationary (see Figure 10-57). This adheres to the basic principle that with conventional, nonmotion-compensated SE sequences, moving CSF has a lower signal intensity than stationary CSF.

Axial T2W sequences are commonly used in the work-up of disc disease and will show similar findings above and below the stenosis. On axial T2W scans, the dural sac is normally filled with high signal CSF and thus easily visualized. At the site of stenosis the dural sac will appear of low signal intensity because little CSF resides there (see Figures 10-54 to 10-57). Immediately above and below the area of stenosis, nerve roots may be "bunched" in the middle of the dural sac and can be seen as low signal in the high signal

A

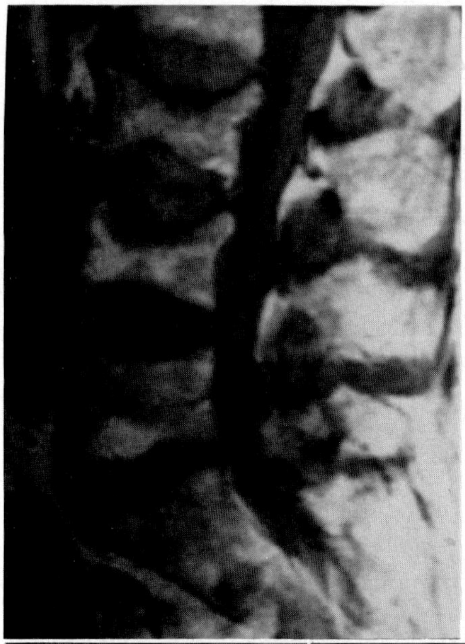

FIGURE 10-54. Lumbar stenosis. **A,** Sagittal T1W scan (SE 800/20) shows diffuse degenerative changes and compression fractures of L_3 and L_4, inhomogeneous pattern of fat replacement marrow, and suspected stenosis at L_4-L_5 that is difficult to determine with certainty. **B-G,** Set of six axial T2W scans (SE gated 2100/20, 80) more accurately shows severe degree of stenosis at L_4-L_5 level and **B-D,** (TE 20) demonstrate that stenosis is caused by combination of disc bulge and ligament hypertrophy (*arrow,* **D**). **E-G,** second echo images (TE 80) show virtually no visible CSF at level of disc space *(open arrow)*. High signal in facet joints indicates small effusions *(curved arrows)*.

B, C

D

E, F

G

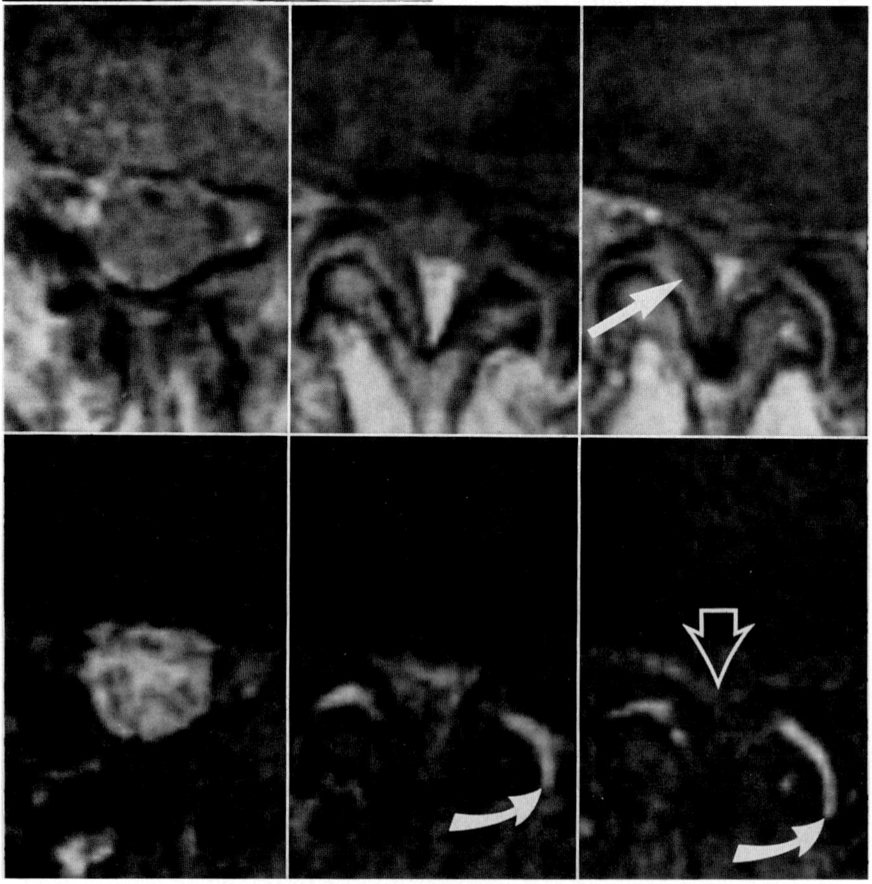

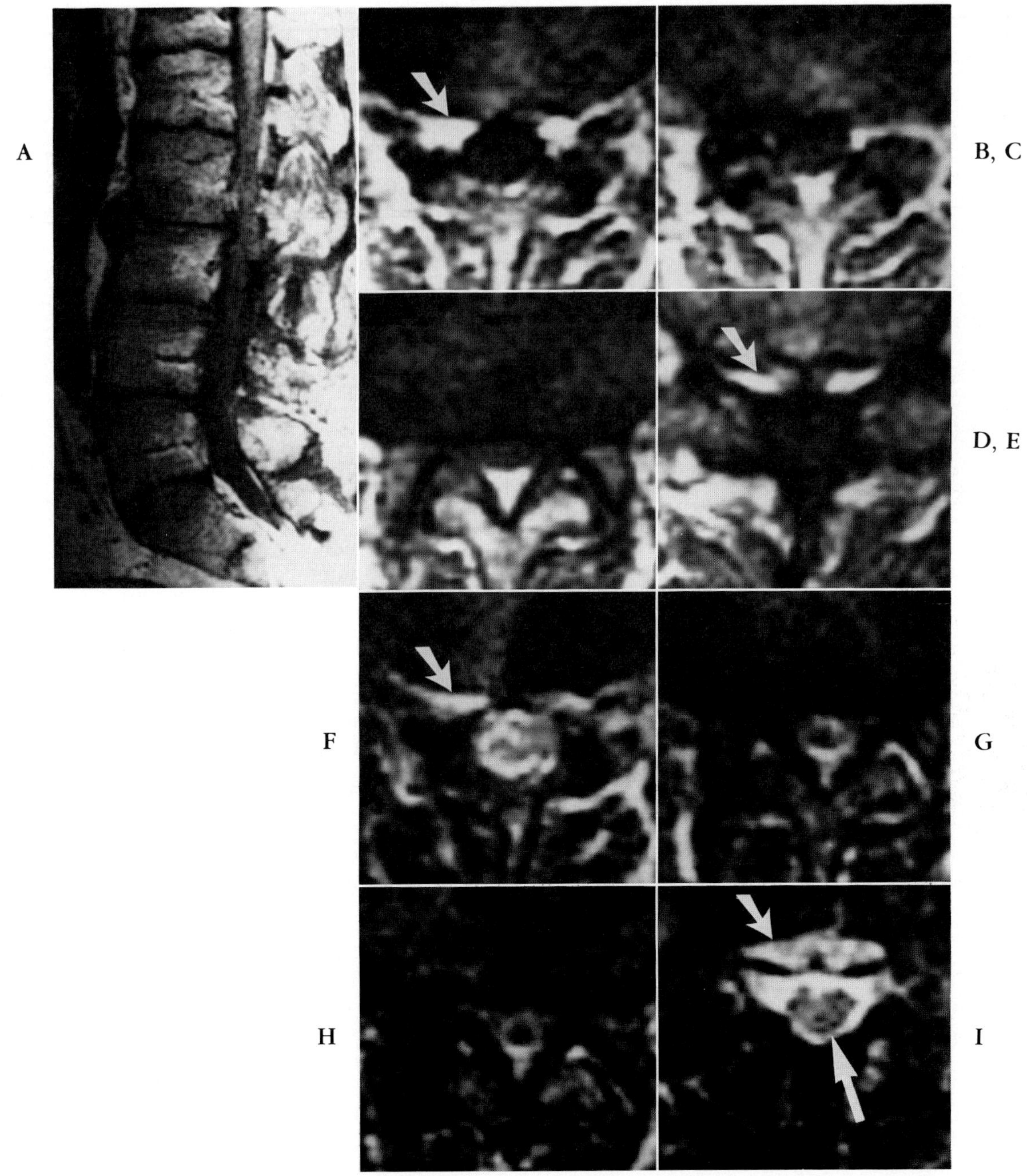

FIGURE 10-55. Lumbar stenosis. **A,** Sagittal T1W scan shows suspected area of lumbar stenosis at L_2-L_3 and L_3-L_4 levels (SE 800/20). **B-E,** Axial scans performed as series of stacked slices compare axial T1W scans (SE 1000/20) with axial T2W scans (SE, gated, flow-compensated 2700/80). Spinal stenosis diagnosed by very small dural sac (**D**). Areas of increased signal intensity in anterior spinal canal above and below area of stenosis represent dilated venous sinuses (*arrows,* **B** and **E**). **F-I,** Axial T2W images show marked narrowing of dural sac (**H**) at same level on T1W scan. Above and below area of stenosis, dural sac is relatively capacious but shows central congregation of nerve roots (*large arrow,* **I**). Note that dilated venous plexus is also high signal intensity on T2W scans above and below area of stenosis (*oblique arrows,* **F** and **I**).

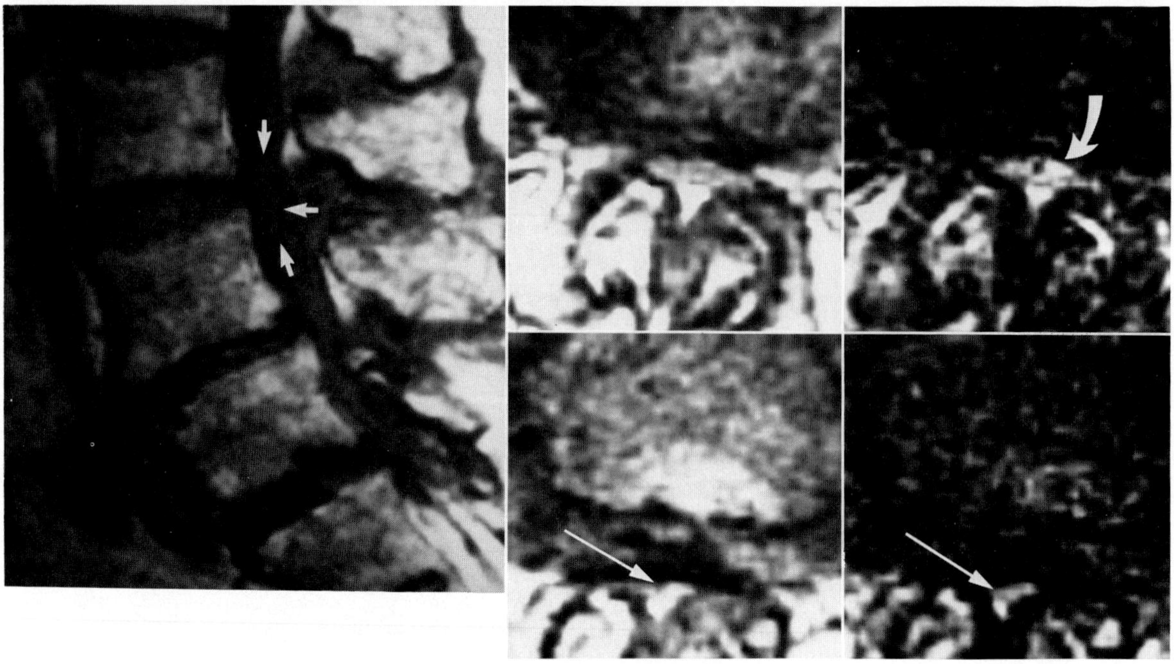

FIGURE 10-56. Lumbar stenosis. Degree of lumbar stenosis may be underestimated from sagittal T1W scans. **A,** Sagittal T1W scan (SE 800/20) shows diffuse degenerative changes in lumbar spine with disc space narrowing at L_4-L_5 and L_5-S_1. Spinal stenosis is suspected at these two levels, but L_3-L_4 level does not appear to be obviously stenotic. Close inspection of sagittal scan shows large disc herniation with disc material being nearly same signal intensity as adjacent CSF (*arrows,* **A**). **B-E,** Axial T2W scan (SE gated 2200/20, 80) shows severe degree of stenosis at L_4-L_5 level on first echo (**B**) and second echo (**C**) images. Only small amount of high signal representing CSF visualized at this level (*curved arrow,* **C**). At L_3-L_4 level, virtually no dural sac visualized except for tiny remnant *(arrows)* on either first echo (**D**) or second echo (**E**). At this level there is diffuse large disc herniation spanning entire spinal canal.

CSF (see Figures 10-54, 10-55 and 10-58) representing the MR equivalent of the "washboard" spine with bunched nerve roots seen on myelography in spinal stenosis. Because CSF is high signal on T2W sequences, they delineate the degree of spinal stenosis better than T1W sequences.

Ossification of the Posterior Longitudinal Ligament

Ossification of the posterior longitudinal ligament is a special subcategory of degenerative disease that can cause severe cervical spine and sometimes thoracic spine stenosis.[13,24,25] It is characterized by multilevel disease with marked hypertropy and prominent calcification of the posterior longitudinal ligament. This disease entity is more common in Japanese patients, but its etiology is unknown. The diagnosis can be made on sagittal T1W and T2W scans but an axial scan is required for accurate delineation of the prominent calcifications and ossifications that can be quite irregular and have bizarre shapes (Figure 10-60). The calcified–ossified ligament usually has its most severe involvement at the C_4 to C_6 levels and is seen as irregular low signal intensity on T1W and T2W images (see Figure 10-60). Delineation of the ossified ligament is better on T2W and T2*W images because of higher contrast. The distribution of ossification within the ligament is better seen on axial images. The large, often globular calcifications are usually in the midline but can be laterally situated (see Figure 10-60).[15,25] Midline calcific masses can markedly compress the cord and produce extensive parenchymal damage (see Figure 10-60).[13,24,25]

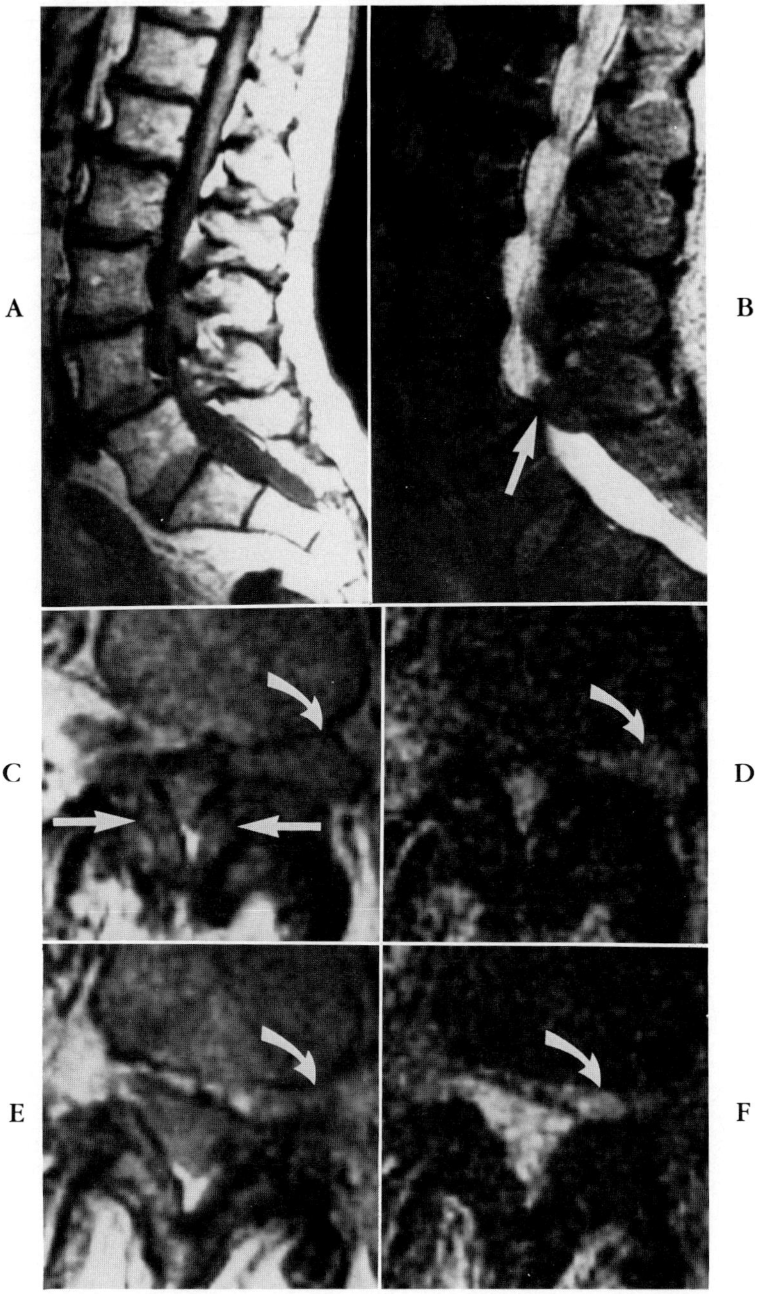

FIGURE 10-57. Lumbar stenosis. Combination spinal stenosis and lateral disc herniation. **A,** Sagittal T1W scan (SE 800/20) suggests spinal stenosis at L_4-L_5 level because spinal canal is poorly seen at this site. A grade I spondylolisthesis is present at L_4-L_5. **B,** Sagittal T2W scan (SE 2000/80) shows marked narrowing of spinal canal caused by combination of disc bulging anteriorly and marked ligament hypertrophy posteriorly *(arrow)*. **C-F,** Axial T2W scan (2000/20, 80) shows marked stenosis on first echo (**C**) and second echo images (**D**). Hypertophy of ligamentum flavum is better seen on balanced image *(straight arrows,* **C**). Lateral disc herniation at both levels is situated laterally in foramen *(curved arrows)*. On second echo images (**D** and **F**) herniated disc is of relative increased signal intensity. When different types of lesions are present, the MR scan is capable of detecting each of them.

A

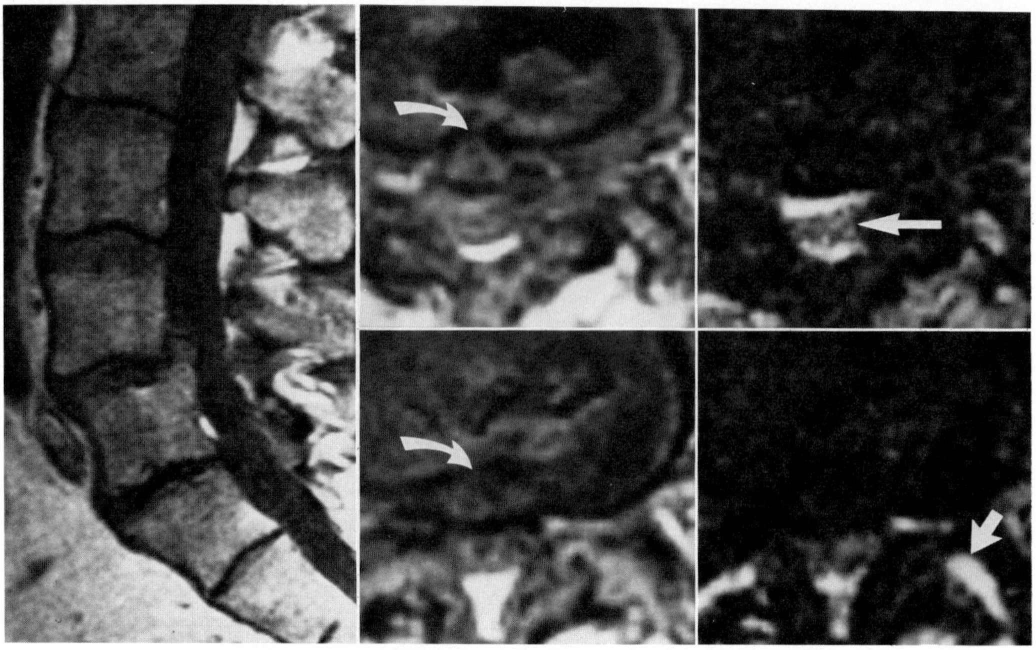

B, C

D, E

FIGURE 10-58. Lumbar stenosis. Spondylolisthesis is another cause of lumbar stenosis. **A,** Sagittal T1W scan (800/20) shows grade I spondylolisthesis of L_4-L_5. Forward displacement caused disc material to buckle and protrude posteriorly. Thin black line outlining disc material probably represents intact anulus, posterior longitudinal ligament, and dura. **B-E,** Axial T2W scans at this level show lumbar stenosis caused primarily by posterior bulging of disc (SE gated 2100/20, 80). First echo, balanced images, show canal compromise primarily caused by anterior disc (*arrow*, **B** and **D**); the ligamentum flavum is not hypertrophied. Axial second echo images show central "bunching" of nerve roots in canal (*arrow*, **C**) and marked narrowing of canal with minimal CSF still detectable at next lower level (**E**). Effusions in facet joints are evident on second echo images (*arrow*, **E**).

A

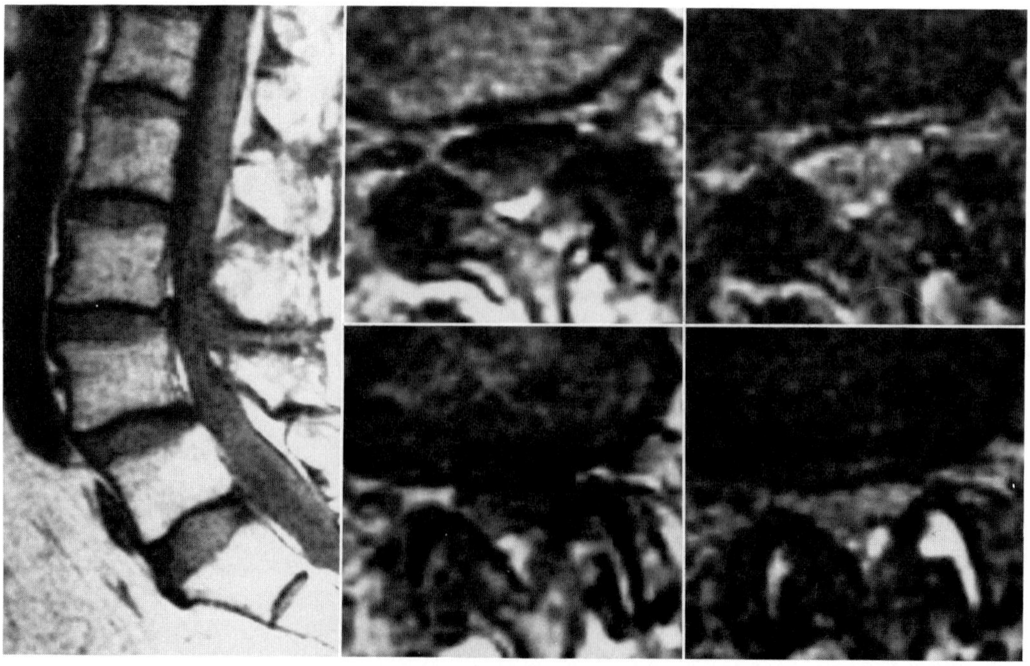

B, C

D, E

FIGURE 10-59. **A-E,** For legend see following page.

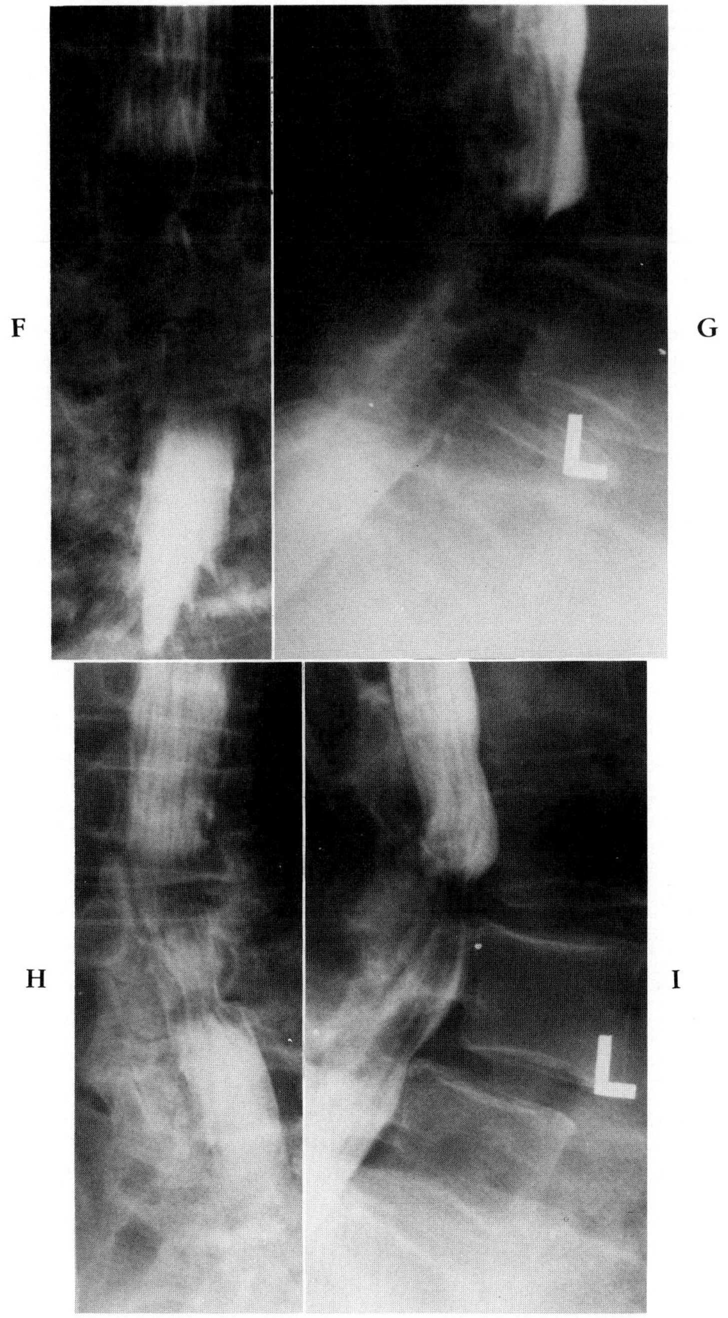

FIGURE 10-59. Lumbar stenosis–false negative MR. **A,** Sagittal T1W scan (SE 800/20) shows no significant stenosis on basis of disc protrusion or ligament hypertrophy. **B-E,** Axial T2W scans (SE gated 2600/20, 80) show only moderate stenosis at L_3-L_4 disc level. First echo images (**B** and **D**) show no significant disc bulge or ligament hypertrophy. Second echo images (**C** and **E**) show congregation of nerve roots in central canal but CSF is still identified, suggesting only moderate stenosis. **F-I,** Myelogram performed in upright position shows high-grade block at L_3-L_4 level on anteroposterior (AP) (**F**) and lateral (**G**) views. Note increased subluxation of L_4 on L_5 on lateral view (**G**) compared to sagittal MR scan (**A**). After flexion and more complete filling of lumbar canal, myelogram shows severe stenosis at L_3-L_4 on AP (**H**) and lateral (**I**) views. Increased disc bulging with weight bearing appears to be major cause of stenosis at this level. Subluxation at L_4-L_5 level does not cause stenosis.

A B C, D E, F G H

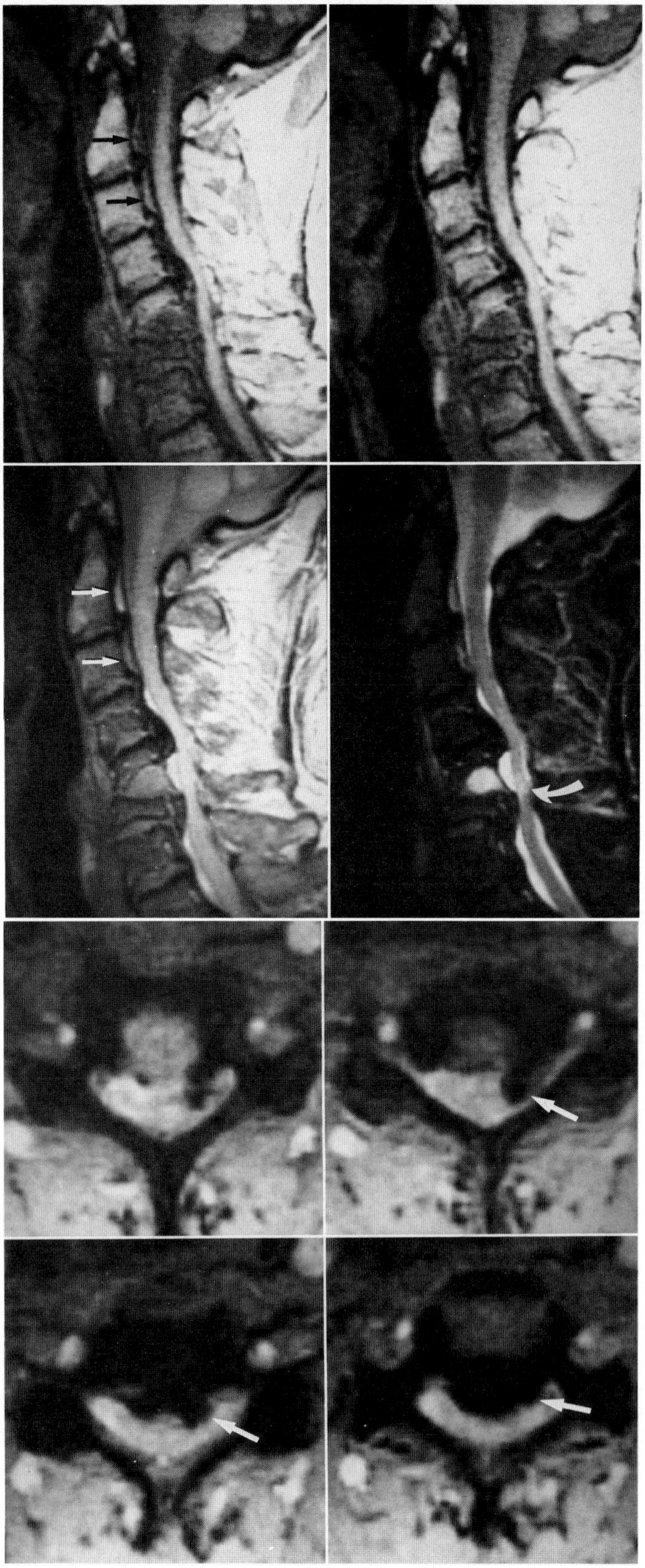

FIGURE 10-60. Ossification of posterior longitudinal ligament (OPLL). Patients with OPLL usually show dramatic findings indicative of cervical stenosis. **A** and **B,** Actual ossification of ligament may be difficult to detect on T1W images (SE 800/20) because low signal osteophytes may appear similar to low adjacent signal CSF. Cervical stenosis and compression and deformity of the cervical cord is obvious. **C** and **D,** Actual areas of ossification of the posterior longitudinal ligament are better appreciated on sagittal T2W images (SE gated, 2200/20, 80). Note that dura is stripped from back of vertebral bodies, particularly at C_2 and C_3 (**A-D**). This potential space is now filled by epidural venous plexus (*arrows,* **A** and **C**). Sagittal T2W scan (**D**) also shows abnormal cord signal at site of severe stenosis indicating cord damage (*curved arrow*). **E-H,** Set of four axial variable flip angle/gradient echo scans (GRASS 22/12, 7°) shows irregular calcification of posterior longitudinal ligament as areas of marked low signal intensity impinging into spinal canal (*arrows*). Cord is compressed and only small amount of subarachnoid space remains on right side.

MISCELLANEOUS

Facet Joints

MR does not yield the same degree of bone detail as CT but degenerative changes of the posterior articulating joints of the lumbar spine can be well seen. Subchondral cysts associated with degenerative arthritis can be focal areas of intermediate signal on T1W and high signal on T2W images within low signal bone. The normal facet joint of the lumbar spine shows minimal high signal within the synovial space. Increased fluid in these joints is easily visualized with T2W axial scans as increased high signal in an enlarged synovial joint space (see Figures 10-54 and 10-58).

Degenerative disease of the facet joint and its joint capsule can result in anterior displacement of the inferior articulating facet in relationship to the superior articulating facet. Because the ligamentum flavum extends into the neural foramen, such displacement can cause this ligament to buckle, resulting in nerve root compression as the nerve exits through the foramen. Sagittal (or sagittal oblique) T1W scans show such encroachment by virtue of displaced epidural fat and deformity of the nerve root (Figure 10-61). Hypertrophic bony changes of the inferior articulating facet can also cause impingement on the nerve as it exits through the foramen, termed lateral recess stenosis.[5]

Synovial cysts occur in the facet joints[18,21] and may reach considerable size and cause compressive symptoms. On T1W scans, synovial cysts may be seen as low signal intensity masses in the posterior spinal canal. They may be better delineated by axial T2W scans where their high signal fluid contents are similar to synovial fluid. The key to their diagnosis is location and the identification of a connection between the cyst and the synovial joint. Identification may be more easily accomplished on a T2W scan because of high signal fluid.

Postsurgical Spine (except disc)

Although bone is not seen as well on MR as on CT, its absence is certainly detectable. When laminectomies are performed, the usual areas of expected low signal in the posterior spinal canal (cervical or lumbar) are replaced by areas of immediate or high signal intensity. The normal well-delineated muscle and fat planes dorsal to the spinal canal are disrupted and obscured. Soft tissue signal intensity replaces epidural fat signal intensity in the spinal canal (see Figures 10-44 and 10-45). The lumbar dural sac may be difficult to delineate on T1W images when epidural fat is replaced by fibrosis. A T2W scan is useful in identifying the dural sac. In the case of bony fusion, the large bone mass is usually seen as an inhomogeneous mixture of high and low signal. Bone detail, because of this inhomogeneous signal intensity, is inferior to that seen with CT. In the lumbar region, a pseudomeningocele after surgery can be visualized on T2W sagittal and axial scans. Not uncommonly the MR shows multiple round areas of signal void in and around a surgical site. On the border of the signal void there may be a thin rim of very high signal, which is caused by strong, local ferromagnetic effects produced by miniscule metal shavings from the instruments used at surgery.[30] These MR findings usually pose no diagnostic difficulty although they can obscure areas of interest especially on variable flip angle/gradient echo scans in the cervical region (see Figure 10-7).

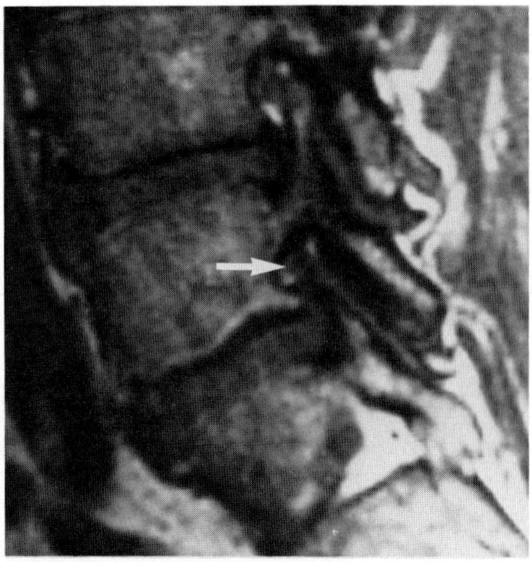

FIGURE 10-61. Root compression. Nerve root impingement can occur in neural foramen without disc disease, occurring secondary to buckling of ligamentum flavum because of forward subluxation of inferior facet on superior articulating facet. The nerve, instead of being round, is flattened *(arrow)* by a buckled ligamentum flavum.

Arachnoiditis

Arachnoidits results from several etiologies: myelography, surgery, infection, traumatic injury, etc. No matter what the etiology, arachnoiditis has the same appearance on MR as it does on myelography and intrathecally enhanced spine CT. The diagnosis by imaging tests is made consistently and reliably only in the lumbar region. When severe characteristic findings are detected in the cervical and thoracic regions (see Figures 7-20, 7-21, and 12-12), the diagnosis can be made on T1W images although it is more difficult than on T2W images.

On T1W sagittal scans of lumbar arachnoiditis seen after surgery, the normal differentiation between the conus and the cauda equina may be obscured. Normally the conus is well defined and of slightly higher signal intensity than the cauda equina, which is of slightly lower signal intensity but may be of similar AP dimension as the cord (see Figure 10-36). With arachnoiditis, this difference in signal intensity is obscured with the cauda having a similar intensity to the cord. In severe cases, because of this similarity in signal intensity it may be difficult to determine where the cord ends, and the cauda may appear as a wavy ribbon of tissue in the lumbar sac.

On the axial T1W scan, there is an area of increased intermediate signal where normally punctate, posteriorly located nerves would be seen. Because the nerves are not as well seen on T1W axial scans, it usually requires a more severe degree of arachnoiditis to produce enough abnormal signal intensity to detect them. On T2W scans, the diagnosis is facilitated because of the high contrast between high signal CSF and low signal intensity nerves. On an axial T2W scan, arachnoiditis can be seen as clumped nerves below the cord causing a low signal intensity defect in the subarachnoid space (see Figure 7-21). In the normal axial view, lumbar and sacral roots are seen as small, individual, low signal intensity dots within the high CSF space (see Figures 10-31 and 10-32; see Figure 10-22). The roots are normally located symmetrically along the posterolateral walls of the dural sac (see Figures 10-31 to 10-33). An axial T2W image is the most sensitive MR sequence for detecting arachnoiditis because adhesion of even a few nerves can be detected by the displacement and enlargement of normally small punctate dots (Figure 10-62).[31] With severe arachnoiditis, large clumps of roots may be visualized in the high signal CSF as multiple clumps or as one large single clump in the middle of the dural sac (see Figure 7-21). A T2W scan, especially the axial view, is essential for detecting minor degrees of arachnoiditis and is usually helpful in confirming the more severe forms (see Figure 10-62), if no contrast agent is used.

GdDTPA is increasingly used in postoperative MR disc examinations because it enhances epidural postoperative granulation tissue, as well as arachnoiditis within the dural sac. Enhancement can be seen even in subtle forms of arachnoiditis where individual nerve roots of the cauda equina exhibit contrast enhancement (Figure 10-63). This finding is not unlike that seen with leptomeningeal tumor (see Chapter 10). One may be able to detect subtle arachnoiditis that is the result of previous myelography rather than previous surgery (Figure 10-64).

Pantopaque

Although Pantopaque is now rarely used as a contrast agent for myelography, many patients have residual Pantopaque in their spinal canal from previous myelograms and it is important to be aware of its appearance on MR scans. Not surprisingly, Pantopaque, which is a lipid solution, exhibits high signal intensity on T1W images. (see Figure 12-13). It is usually seen as small globular areas of increased signal intensity situated in various locations in the dural sac. It may be posterior in the thoracic regions and commonly is in root sleeves in the lumbar regions (see Figure 12-13). It may be widely scattered throughout the spine. On T2W images, again as expected, the lipid component has lower signal intensity and Pantopaque is usually seen as a negative defect in high signal CSF spaces (see Figure 2-17). If both T1W and T2W sequences are obtained, there should be little confusion as to the diagnosis when such findings are seen.

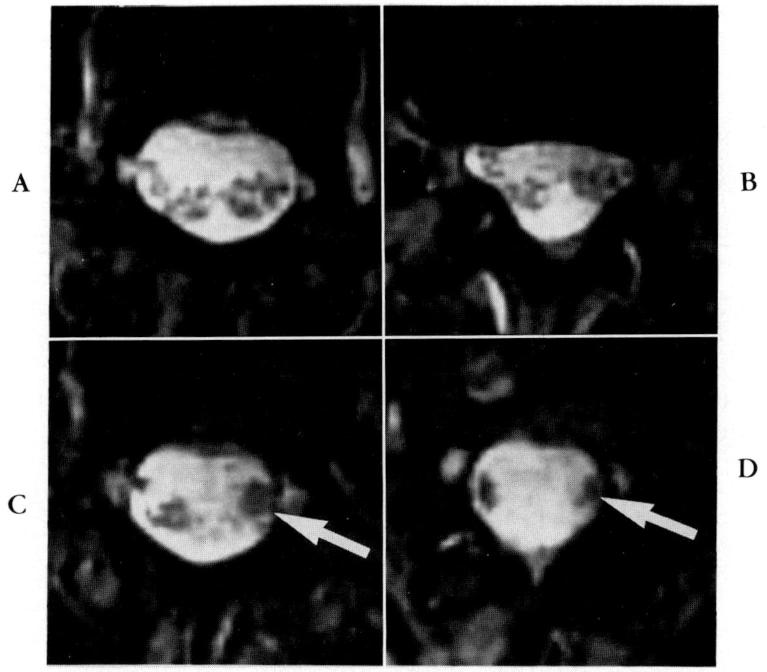

FIGURE 10-62. Mild arachnoiditis. Subtle postoperative changes such as mild arachnoiditis can be detected with T2W technique. **A,** Second echo of axial T2W scan (SE gated, 2200/80) shows capacious dural sac with individual nerve roots identifiable rostrally. Further caudally nerve roots begin to adhere and form two clumps of roots (*arrows*, **C** and **D**). Individual lumbar roots are normally visible at periphery of sac (**D**), but in this patient they are clumped (**B, C,** and **D**). These changes represent relatively mild postoperative arachnoiditis.

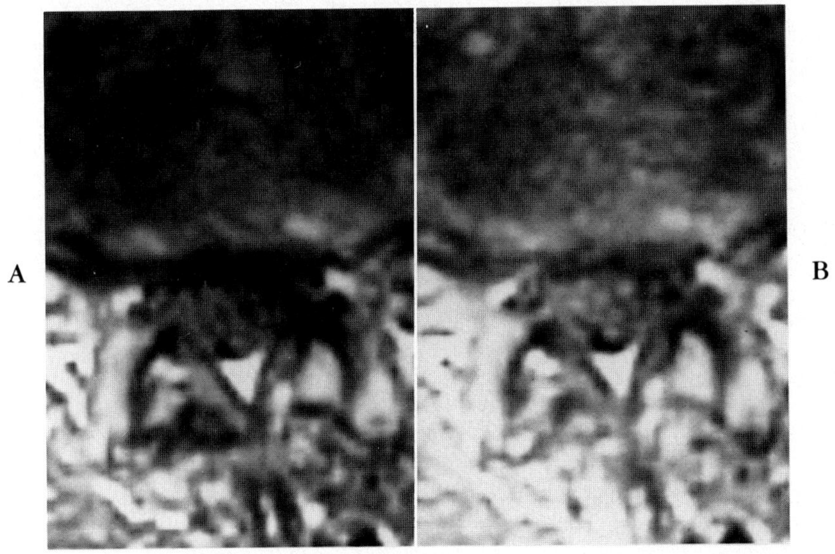

FIGURE 10-63. Postoperative arachnoiditis. **A,** Precontrast axial T1W scan (SE 1000/20) of cauda equina shows mild adhesion of roots. **B,** PostGdDTPA scan demonstrates multiple areas of punctate enhancement in cauda equina representing mild postoperative arachnoiditis. Appearance similar to what might be seen in leptomeningeal carcinomatosis.

A, B

C

D, E

F, G

H

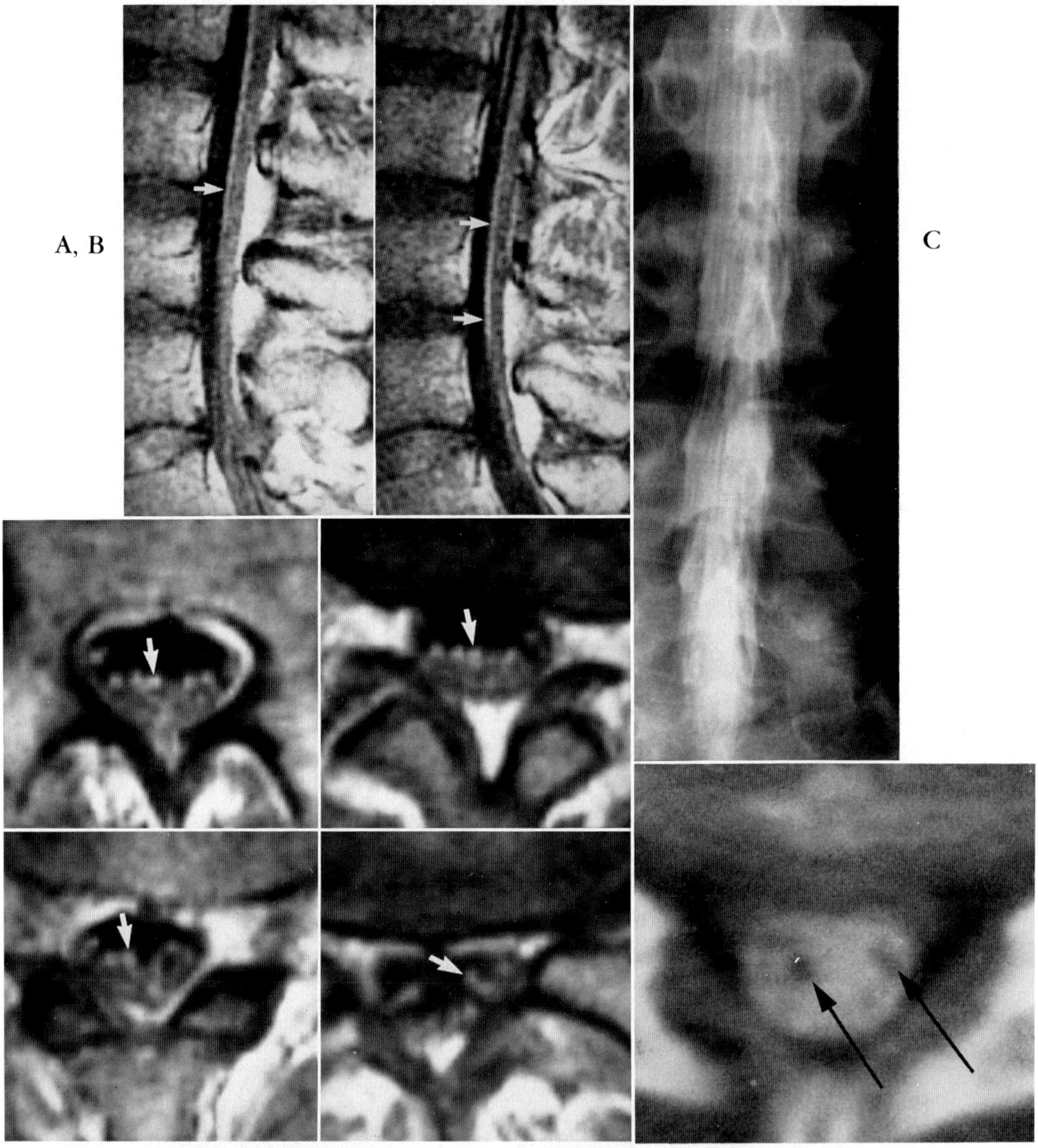

FIGURE 10-64. Mild postmyelographic arachnoiditis. Mild lumbar arachnoiditis secondary to multiple previous myleograms in 25-year-old male. There is no history of surgery, tumor, or infection. **A** and **B,** PostGdDTPA T1W scans (SE 800/20) show thin line of enhancement along anterior border of cauda equina *(arrows)*. No nodules are identified. **C,** Anteroposterior (AP) view of lumbar myelogram shows adhesion of nerve roots and irregularity and tortuosity of other individual roots. **D-G,** Axial postGdDTPA T1W scans (SE 1000/20) show enhancement of individual nerve roots located on anterior border of cauda equina *(arrows)*. There is mild adhesion of roots within cauda equina. **H,** Intrathecal contrast, spine CT performed after myelogram shows adhesion of nerve roots indicative of mild arachnoiditis *(arrows)*.

REFERENCES

1. Alberico AM, Sahni KS, Hall JA, et al. High thoracic disc herniation. Neurosurgery 1986; 19:3.
2. Al-Mefty O, Harkey LH, Middleton TH, et al. Myelopathic cervical spondylotic lesions demonstrated by magnetic resonance imaging. J Neurosurg 1988; 68:217.
3. Barnett GH, Hardy RW, Little JR, et al. Thoracic spinal canal stenosis. J Neurosurg 1987; 66:338.
4. Bundschuh CV, Modic MT, Ross JS, et al. Epidural fibrosis and recurrent disk herniation in the lumbar spine: MR imaging assessment. AJNR 1988; 9:169.
5. Ciric I, Mikhael MA, Tarkington JA, et al. The lateral recess syndrome. J Neurosurg 1980; 53:433.
6. Clarke LP, Schnitzlein HN, Murtagh FR, et al. High resolution MRI: imaging anatomy of the lumbosacral spine. Magn Reson Imaging 1986; 4:515.
7. Daniels DL, Hyde JS, Kneeland JB, et al. The cervical nerves and foramina: local-coil MR imaging. AJNR 1986; 7:129.
8. Enzmann DR, Griffin C, Rubin JB. Potential false-negative MR images of the thoracic spine in disk disease with switching of phase- and frequency-encoding gradients. Radiology 1987; 165:635.
9. Enzmann DR, Rubin JB. Cervical spine: MR imaging with a partial flip angle, gradient-refocused pulse sequence. Part I. General considerations and disk disease. Radiology 1988; 166:467.
10. Enzmann DR, Rubin JB. Cervical spine: MR imaging with a partial flip angle, gradient-refocused pulse sequence. Part II. Spinal cord disease. Radiology 1988; 166:473.
11. Enzmann DR, Rubin JB, Wright A. Cervical spine MR imaging: generating high-signal CSF in sagittal and axial images. Radiology 1987; 163:233.
12. Francavilla TL, Powers A, Dina T, et al. MR imaging of thoracic disk herniations. J Comput Assist Tomogr 1987; 11:1062.
13. Harsh GR, Sypert GW, Weinstein PR, et al. Cervical spine stenosis secondary to ossification of the posterior longitudinal ligament. J Neurosurg 1987; 67:349.
14. Holtas S, Nordstrom C-H, Larsson Em, et al. Case report: MR imaging of intradural disk herniation. J Comput Assist Tomogr 1987; 11:353.
15. Isu T, Iwasaki Y, Miyasaka K, et al. A reappraisal of the diagnosis in cervical disc disease: the posterior longitudinal ligament perforated or not. Neuroradiology 1986; 28:215.
16. Iwasaki Y, Abe H, Isu T, et al. CT myelography with intramedullary enhancement in cervical spondylosis. J Neurosurg 1985; 63:363.
17. Iwasaki Y, Tashiro K, Kikuchi S, et al. Cervical flexion myelopathy: a "tight dural canal mechanism." J Neurosurg 1987; 66:935.
18. Kjerulf TD, Terry DW, Boubelik RJ. Lumbar synovial or ganglion cysts. Neurosurgery 1986; 19:415.
19. Lesoin F, Biondi A, Jomin M. Foraminal cervical herniated disc treated by anterior discoforaminotomy. Neurosurgery 1987; 21:334.
20. Masaryk TJ, Ross JS, Modic MT, et al. High-resolution MR imaging of sequestered lumbar intervetebral disks. AJNR 1988; 9:351.
21. Mercader J, Gomez JM, Cardenal C. Intraspinal synovial cyst: diagnosis by CT. Neuroradiology 1985; 27:346.
22. Modic MT, Masaryk T, Boumphrey F, et al. Lumbar herniated disc disease and canal stenosis: prospective evaluation by surface coil MR, CT and myelography. AJNR 1986; 7:709.
23. Modic MT, Masaryk TJ, Ross JS, et al. Cervical radiculopathy: value of oblique MR imaging. Radiology 1987; 163:227.
24. Murakami N, Muroga T, Sobue I. Cervical myelopathy due to ossification of the posterior longitudinal ligament. Arch Neurol 1978; 35:33.
25. Murakami J, Russell WJ, Hayabuchi N, et al. Computed tomography of posterior longitudinal ligament ossification: its appearance and diagnostic value with special reference to thoracic lesions. J Comput Assist Tomogr 1982; 61:41.
26. Ono K, Ota H, Tada K, et al. Cervical myelopathy secondary to multiple spondylotic protrusions. A clinicopathologic study. Spine 1977; 2:109.
27. Penning L, Wilmink JT, van Woerden HH, et al. CT myelographic findings in degenerative disorders of the cervical spine: clinical significance. AJNR 1986; 7:119.
28. Resnick D, Niwayama G. Degenerative disease of the spine. In: Diagnosis of bone and joint disorders. Philadelphia: W.B. Saunders Co., 1981.
29. Roosen N, Dietrich U, Nicola N, et al. Case Report: MR imaging of calcified herniated thoracic disk. J Comput Assist Tomogr 1987; 11:733.
30. Ross JS, Masaryk TJ, Modic MT. Postoperative cervical spine: MR assessment. J Comput Assist Tomogr 1985; 11:955.
31. Ross JS, Masaryk TJ, Modic MT, et al. MR imaging of lumbar arachnoiditis. AJNR 1987; 8:885.
32. Ryan RW, Lally JF, Kozic Z. Asymptomatic calcified herniated thoracic disks: CT recognition. AJNR 1988; 9:363.
33. Smith DE, Godersky JC. Thoracic spondylosis: an unusual cause of myelopathy. Neurosurgery 1987; 20:589.
34. Sobel DF, Zyroff J, Thorne RP. Diskogenic vertebral sclerosis: MR imaging. J Comput Assist Tomogr 1987; 11:855.
35. Stollman A, Pinto R, Benjamin V, et al. Radiologic imaging of symptomatic ligamentum flavum thickening with and without ossification. AJNR 1987; 8:991.
36. Tamaki N, Kojima N, Tanimoto M, et al. Myelopathy due to diffuse thickening of the cervical dura mater in maroteaux-lamy syndrome: report of a case. Neurosurgery 1987; 21:416.
37. Teresi LM, Lufkin RB, Reicher MA, et al. Asymptomatic degenerative disk disease and spondylosis of the cervical spine: MR imaging. Radiology 1987; 164:83.
38. Wilberger JE, Chedid MK. Acute cervical spondylytic myelopathy. Neurosurgery 1988; 22:145.
39. Yamamoto I, Matsumae M, Ikeda A, et al. Thoracic spinal stenosis: experience with seven cases. J Neurosurg 1988; 68:37.
40. Yenerich DO, Haughton VM. Oblique plane MR imaging of the cervical spine. J Comput Assist Tomogr 1986; 10:823.
41. Yu S, Sether LA, Ho PSP, et al. Tears of the annulus fibrosus: correlation between MR and pathologic findings in cadavers. AJNR 1988; 9:367.

11
Vascular Diseases

Dieter R. Enzmann

There has been some misunderstanding about the true nature of spinal cord atrioventricular malformations (AVMs) in radiologic literature.[2,11,15] In general, there are two main categories of spinal cord AVMs: intradural and dural (Figure 11-1). Intradural AVMs can be further subcategorized into juvenile AVMs, glomus AVMs, and direct arteriovenous (AV) fistulas.[11,14,15] In juvenile AVMs the vascular nidus lies within the cord, but cord tissue can be found in the interstices of the vascular mass.[15] The glomus type of AVM is also intramedullary but no cord tissue exists within the tangle of abnormal vessels. Both of these intradural, intramedullary AVMs are characteristically fed by a medullary artery, i.e., an Adamkiewicz-type artery that also normally feeds the anterior spinal artery.[11] (see Figure 11-1). Feeders may be multiple in the juvenile AVM type. Venous drainage can be extensive, involving veins on the ventral and dorsal surfaces of the cord that may travel for long distances rostrally and caudally before they drain into epidural veins. Flow in medullary veins is away from the cord in intradural AVMs whereas in dural AVMs flow is toward the cord (see Figure 11-1). The intradural direct AV fistula does not have a vascular mass but consists of a direct arteriovenous connection within the cord or on its surface.[15]

Over the last few years, the more common dural type of AVM has been mistaken for the intradural type. The dural type of spinal cord AVM is fed by the dural branch of the radiculomedullary-dural artery, which arises from the intercostal artery. The dural artery feeds the AVM nidus, which is located only in the dura (see Figure 11-1) and these AVM feeders rarely give rise to vessels that feed the anterior spinal artery. The AVM nidus is drained by a medullary vein that drains into the dorsal coronal venous plexus on the cord (see Figure 11-1). In this type of AVM only the venous drainage is intradural, and it lies on the dorsal surface of the cord. The medullary vein characteristically penetrates the dura 1 or 2 mm cephalad or caudal to the exit of the nerve root.[9] The venous drainage is slow. Because there are no valves between the dorsal coronal plexus and radial veins within the cord, the resultant elevated venous pressure is transmitted to the cord. The key to treatment of dural AVMs is clipping of the arterial feeder(s), the draining vein(s), and removal of the dural AVM nidus. Surgery need involve only the dura; it does not require any intervention on the spinal cord. Specifically, the enlarged coronal veins do not need to be removed.

CLINICAL

Intradural AVM

Intradural AVMs have characteristics that dictate their clinical presentation. They are more often associated with arterial and venous aneurysms (50% of the intradural AVMs) and therefore subarachnoid hemorrhage may be an acute presentation. This is especially true of the glomus type of AVM. Unfortunately the cause of spinal subarachnoid hemorrhage is not always evident because no AVM or aneurysm is identified by angiography (see Figure 11-17). Intradural AVMs become symptomatic early in life, usually before age 30. Because they typically appear in cervical or thoracic locations, clinically they can involve both arms and legs. Spastic paraparesis, pain, temperature, and sensory deficits are common.[15]

Dural AVM

Clinical presentations of dural AVMs differ from intradural AVMs in that patients are usually older (>40 yrs) and have a history of gradual but steady deterioration. These AVMs are thought to be an acquired rather than a congenital lesion. Because dural AVMs always appear in the lower spine, the symptoms involve the lower extremities but not the upper extremities[15] and also involve pain and temperature deficits. Acute subarachnoid hemorrhage is not part of the clinical presentation. Symptoms may exacerbate with exertion.[15] Occasionally patients with dural AVMs develop sudden neurologic deterioration, with cause unknown, but possibly secondary to venous thrombosis. MR investigations may clarify this suspected pathogenesis.

MR FINDINGS

Intradural AVM

MR findings in intramedullary spinal cord AVMs are usually quite obvious (Figure 11-2), whereas in the dural type of AVM they can be much more subtle and may be mistaken for tumor or other lesions. Glomus and juvenile types of intradural AVMs represent those in which a nidus is in the parenchyma of the spinal cord and the findings are similar to those seen in brain AVMs. The cord is usually enlarged at the level of the nidus. On both T1W and T2W sequences multiple, serpigenous "signal void" areas can be seen in the mass where there is rapid blood flow through abnormal vasculature (Figures 11-2 and 11-3). Multiple, round, discrete signal voids are seen in all projections on T1W and T2W images, some becoming quite large, if there are large draining veins. Depending on the size of the veins, signal voids may extend for significant distances in both cranial and caudal directions, usu-

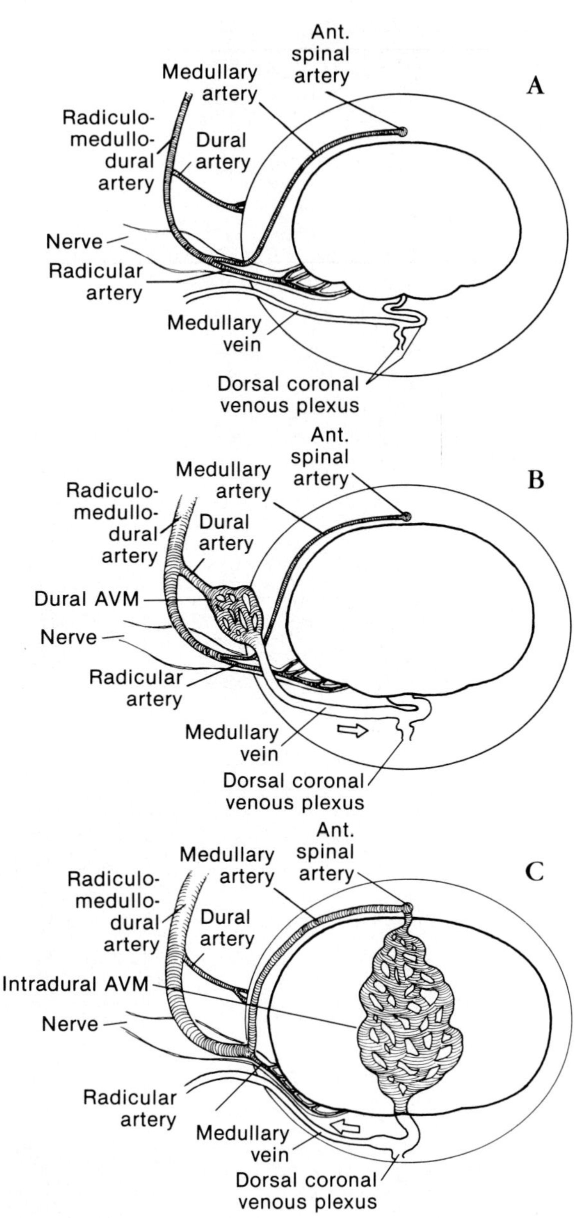

FIGURE 11-1. Diagrammatic representation of arterial supply and venous drainage of spinal cord. **A,** Normal cord. Normal radiculo-medullary-dural artery branching into dural branch, medullary branch, and radiculary artery. Small medullary vein penetrates dura near root exit. **B,** Dural AVM. Enlarged radiculo-medullary-dural artery and large dural branch. AVM nidus resides in dura. Venous drainage is toward cord by way of medullary vein. Cord is enlarged. **C,** Intradural AVM. Enlarged radiculo-medullary-dural artery and large medullary branch. AVM nidus is within cord parenchyma fed by anterior spinal artery. Venous drainage is by way of dorsal coronal plexus. Flow in medullary vein is away from cord.

A

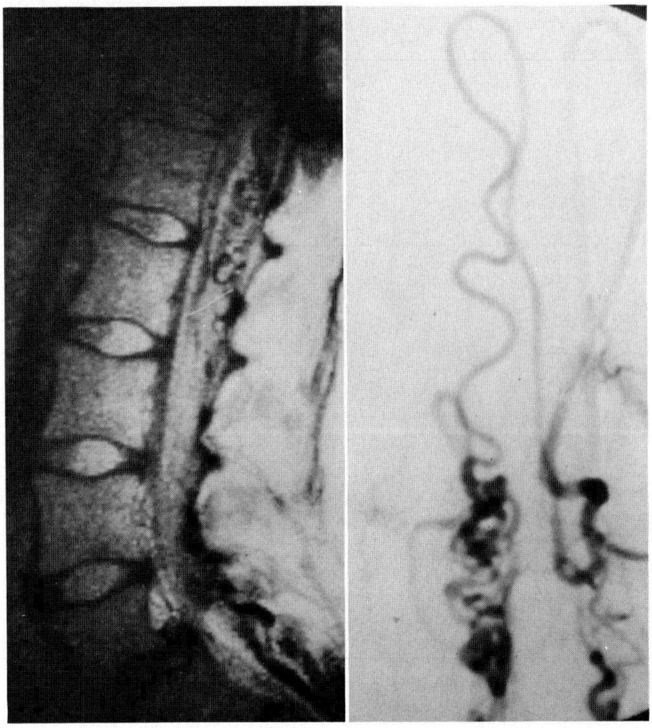

B

FIGURE 11-2. **A,** Sagittal balanced image (SE 1500/40) (midfield machine, .35T) shows obvious linear, serpigenous signal voids around conus. Findings are typical of intradural AVM, confirmed by spinal angiography, **B.**

A, B

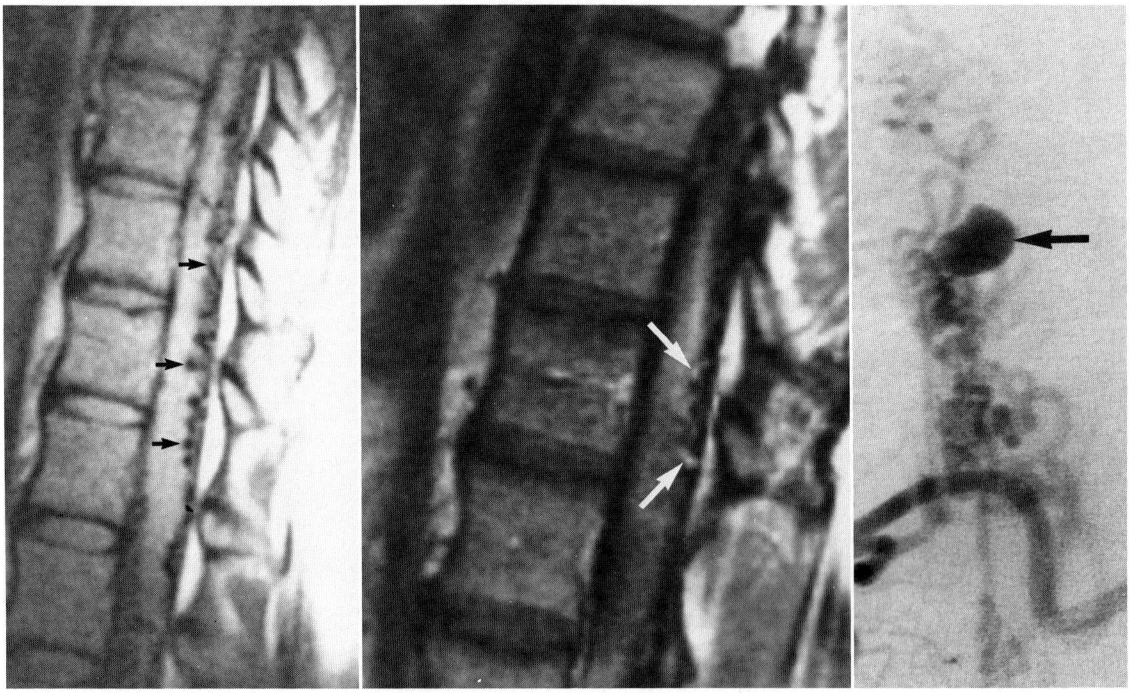

C

FIGURE 11-3. **A,** Sagittal T1W (SE 740/40) MR scan on midfield machine (.35T) shows markedly enlarged draining vein on dorsal surface of cord *(arrows)* indicative of spinal cord AVM. **B,** GdDTPA may prove useful in detecting small spinal cord AVMs (see Figure 11-5) for identifying nidus and for delineating draining veins, which are usually on dorsal surface. Some small draining veins are seen at level of conus as high signal *(arrows)* after administration of GdDTPA but other veins with rapid blood flow still show signal void. Slow venous blood flow may show enhancement with GdDTPA because of large blood pool of contrast, especially if scan is performed immediately after injection when blood levels are high. Intramedullary AVM as demonstrated by spinal angiography is fed by medullary artery; it also has associated aneurysm (**C,** *arrow*). (Courtesy of William Dillon, M.D.)

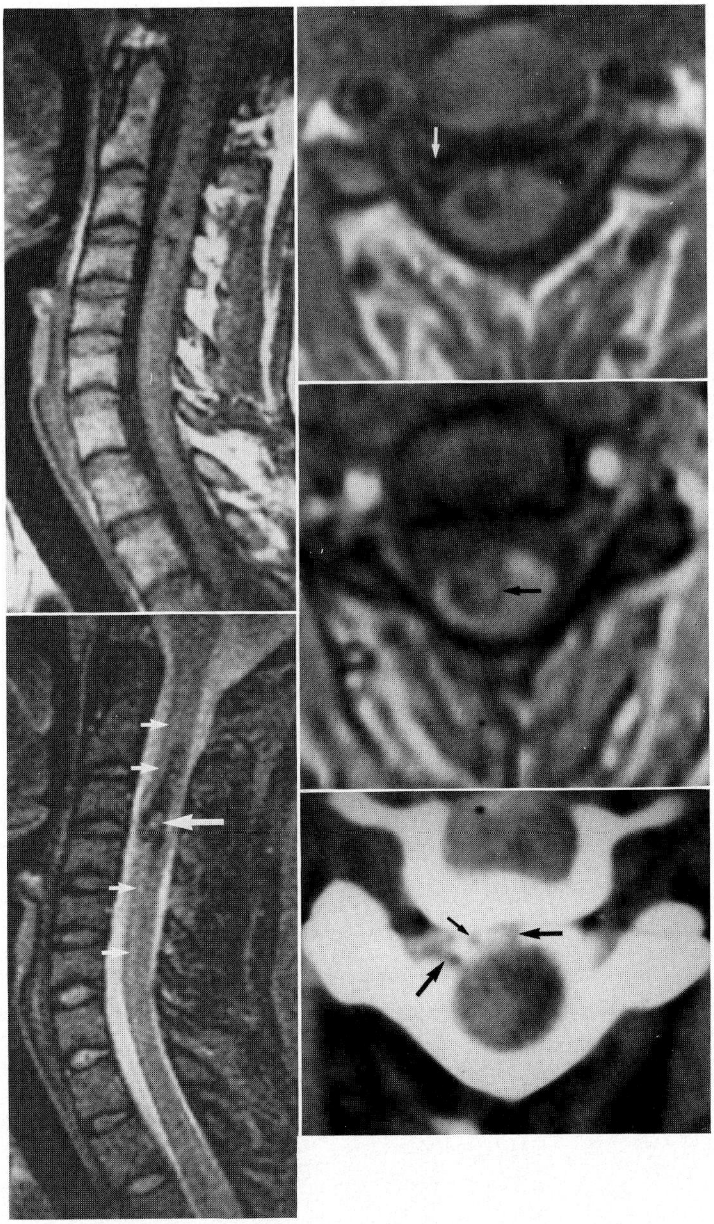

FIGURE 11-4. **A,** Sagittal T1W (SE 600/20) scan shows focal cord enlargement at level of C_3 in intradural AVM. Signal intensity is inhomogeneous at this site and several small areas of low signal intensity are visualized. **B,** T2W scan (SE, gated and flow compensated, 2300/70) shows larger area of low signal intensity extending further in cord tissue than suspected on T1W scan, suggesting hemosiderin magnetic susceptibility effect. In center of mass, an area of slightly high signal is visualized *(large arrow)*. Lesion disrupts normal thin line of minimally higher signal intensity stripe normally seen in anterior third of cord, representing grey matter *(small arrows)*. No definite signal voids representing vessels are visualized. **C,** Axial T1W scan (SE 1000/20) shows asymmetrically located region of low signal intensity on right of minimally enlarged cord. Focal area of low signal intensity in right anterolateral recess displaces ventral root *(arrow)*. Finding suggests presence of enlarged feeding vessel. Ventral root is displaced posteriorly as demonstrated by its anterior concavity *(arrow)*. An axial variable flip angle/gradient echo scan (GRASS 380/10) with large flip angle appropriate for detecting blood flow shows high signal in vertebral arteries and increased signal intensity in area of low signal on T1W scan (**C**). Increased signal suggests inflow of blood into lesion (**D,** *arrow*). **E,** Positive contrast CT scan confirms presence of abnormal vasculature in right anterolateral recess *(arrows)*.

Continued.

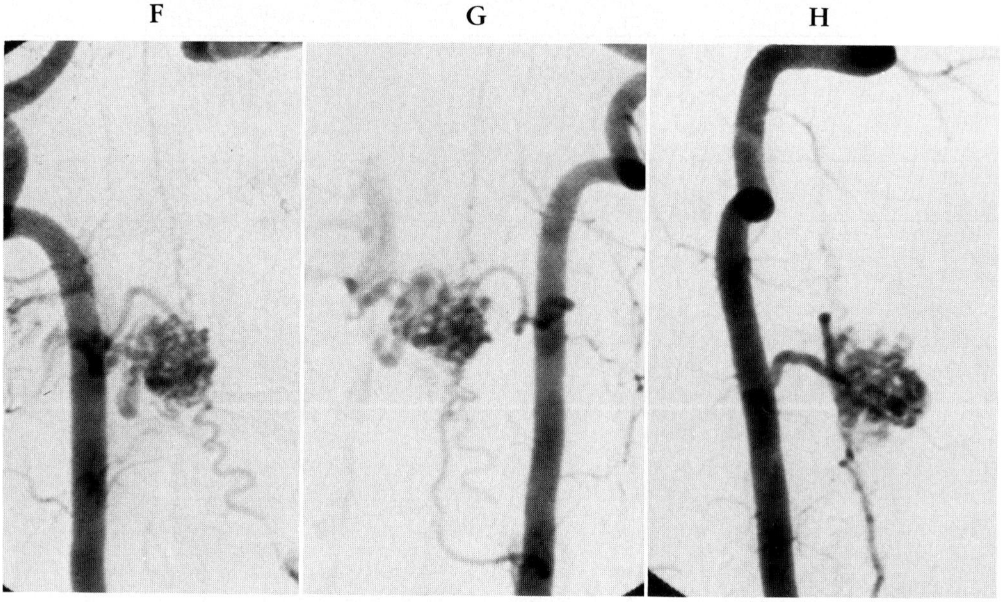

FIGURE 11-4, cont'd. Three arteriographic views (**F**, right vertebral AP view; **G**, left vertebral AP view; and **H**, left vertebral lateral view) show intramedullary vascular malformation fed by medullary arteries from vertebral arteries and venous drainage in both rostral and caudal directions. In addition, large draining vein exits spinal canal on right and drains into epidural venous plexus (**G**). (Courtesy of Dr. Grant Hieshima.)

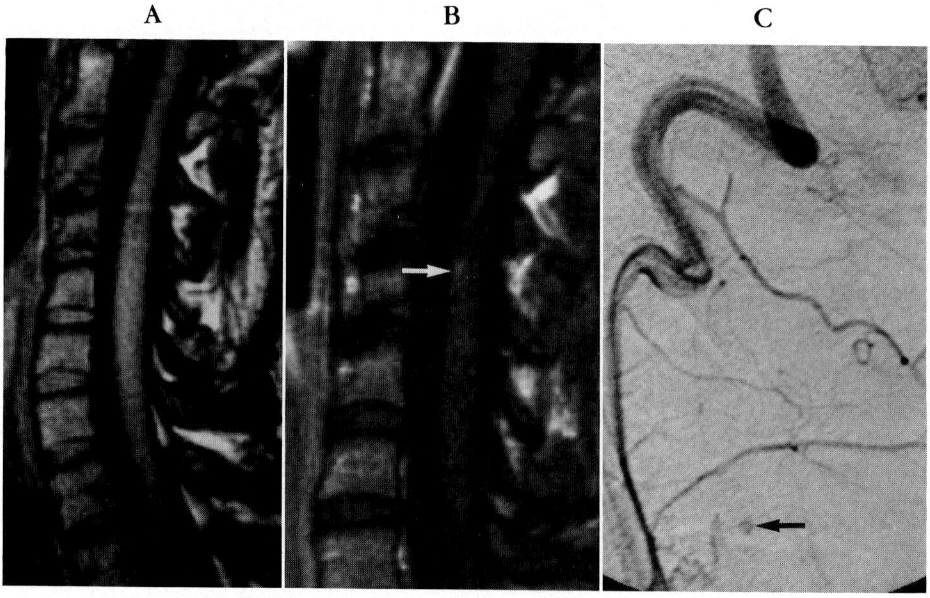

FIGURE 11-5. Small spinal cord AVM may require contrast-enhanced MR scans for detection. **A**, Sagittal T1W (SE 600/20) precontrast view shows no abnormality. **B**, PostGdDTPA T1W scan (SE 600/20) reveals small nodule of enhancement *(arrow)*. **C**, Vertebral arteriogram in late arterial phase demonstrates small AVM *(arrow)*. (Courtesy of William Dillon, M.D.)

ally on the dorsal surface but occasionally also on the ventral side. It is possible for only a previous hemorrhage to be the major detectable abnormality of the AVM nidus without obvious, identifiable signal voids representing feeding or draining vessels (Figure 11-4). On T2W images areas of high signal may be interspersed between areas of low signal indicating the presence of abnormal, gliotic cord tissue or old hemorrhage (see Figure 11-4). This may be more prominent in the juvenile AVM type. If there has been previous hemorrhage, evidence for a chronic hematoma may be present as delineated by an area of high signal intensity surrounded by a low signal intensity rim indicative of the hemosiderin effect (see Figure 11-4 and Figure 11-7).[6] This rim may be difficult to differentiate from other low signal structures in the nidus, but it usually has more indistinct margins compared to vessels; it also "blooms" (i.e., enlarges) on later echoes and on variable flip angle/gradient echo scans; vessels do not (see Figure 11-7). Depending on the presence of methemoglobin, high signal density may be present on a T1W sequence indicative of previous hemorrhage (see Figure 11-7).[6]

Intradural AVMs involving the spinal cord parenchyma are usually of substantial size and should pose no difficulty in detection or diagnosis. They may, however, be small and without obvious vascular signal voids, making them difficult to detect (Figures 11-5 to 11-7) or difficult to differentiate from other lesions such as low flow (cryptic) AVMs (see Figure 11-4). In such instances the use of a contrast agent such as Gadolinium diethylenetriamine penta-acetic acid (GdDTPA) may be valuable in detecting the nidus or the feeding or draining vessels (see Figures 11-5 to 11-7). The most difficult lesion to detect is the direct AV fistula, which does not have an abnormal collection of vessels (nidus); it may not cause a significant mass effect (see Figure 11-6) or a disruption of the blood-cord barrier. GdDTPA may be necessary to define its presence by MR, and even then it could be missed because detection will depend on enhancement of a small venous blood pool. It may be similar to the dural AVM lesion in that only indirect evidence of its presence can be detected. Clinical expertise and persistence will be necessary to pursue the imaging workup of patients who have these small, subtle spinal cord AVMs. GdDTPA helps detect small spinal AVMs and aids in differentiating hemorrhagic neoplasm from cryptic AVMs, which generally show no enhancement.[17] If tumor were associated with a chronic hematoma, the tumor mass would enhance and differ from enhancement seen with AVMs. Contrast enhancement by GdDTPA may be secondary to a permeability defect in the blood-cord barrier or because of enhancement of a blood pool, i.e., blood in the draining veins. In spinal AVMs the latter is most common. As long as the venous blood velocity is not too high (signal loss caused by high velocity) blood enhancement can be visualized (see Figure 11-7). CNS venous blood flow in small veins is constant velocity and thus does not lose signal because of pulsatility. Enhancement is therefore usually well marginated and serpigenous and seen on the surface of the cord, usually the dorsal surface where the coronal venous plexus is located. Enlarged veins within the cord may be detected.

Myelography is valuable in detecting abnormal veins in the subarachnoid space that are difficult to detect by MR, even with intravenous contrast media. Using MR as a screening examination with large fields of view (FOVs) (i.e., low spatial resolution) increases the likelihood of missing small AVMs. Small surface coils and high spatial resolution techniques are necessary for the diagnosis and characterization of spinal AVMs. Spinal angiography is, of course, the gold standard, but the extent to which it is pursued or repeated depends on clinical assessment and the results of MR and myelography.

Dural AVM

The AVM nidus with a dural lesion is usually small and subtle, even on high quality, magnified spinal angiography. The nidus is characteristically located near a nerve root sleeve and is situated in the dura itself (Figure 11-8; see Figure 11-1). It is so small that it can usually not be detected directly by any MR pulse sequence. Thus no areas of signal void are expected at the nidus site. What can be seen with dural AVMs are the secondary effects: i.e., the enlarged draining veins on the dorsal surface of the cord and the cord enlargement thought to be caused by congestive myelopathy secondary to elevated venous pressure.[5,10] Enlargement of the conus appears characteristic of this type of AVM and may be the only finding.[5] If MR images have sufficient spatial resolution, small, subtle, ser-

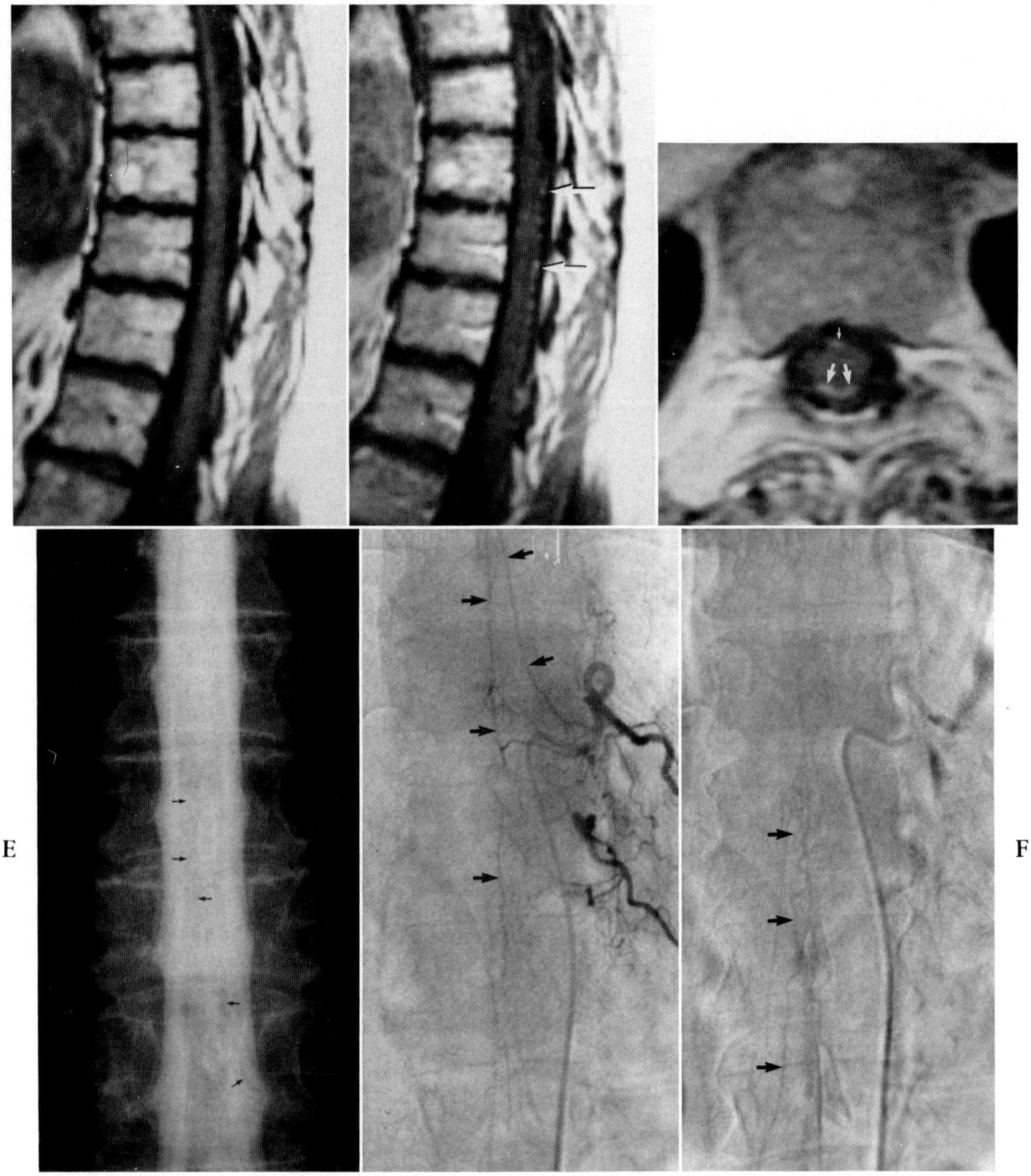

A, B C D, E F

FIGURE 11-6. Use and value of GdDTPA demonstrated in detection of small spinal cord AV fistula. **A,** Precontrast T1W (SE 600/20) image of low thoracic cord shows no evidence of AVM. **B,** Postcontrast GdDTPA scan shows thin line of enhancement along dorsal surface of cord representing draining vein *(arrows)*. **C,** Axial T1W (SE 600/20) postcontrast GdDTPA scan shows faint area of enhancement on dorsal surface of cord *(large arrow)* representing draining coronal venous plexus. Additional draining vein on ventral surface also enhances *(small arrow)*. Findings are subtle but lesion is very small AV fistula. **D,** Water soluble myelogram demonstrates subtle serpigenous vessels projected over cord *(arrows)*. **E,** Spinal arteriogram in early arterial phase shows t_{11}, radiculomedullary artery *(arrows)* leading to small fistula at its caudal end; fistula then drains in caudal direction by way of a small vein (**F,** *arrows*). Fistula itself is difficult to visualize. Subtle lesions such as this one show value of GdDTPA in detecting small vascular malformations of spinal cord. Additional draining vein on ventral surface also enhances *(small arrows)*. Blood flow must be slow, accounting for lack of signal void. Increased signal from blood vessels with use of GdDTPA depends on velocity of blood flow in the vessel. (**A-C,** From Dillon WP, et al.: Radiology 1989, 170:229.)

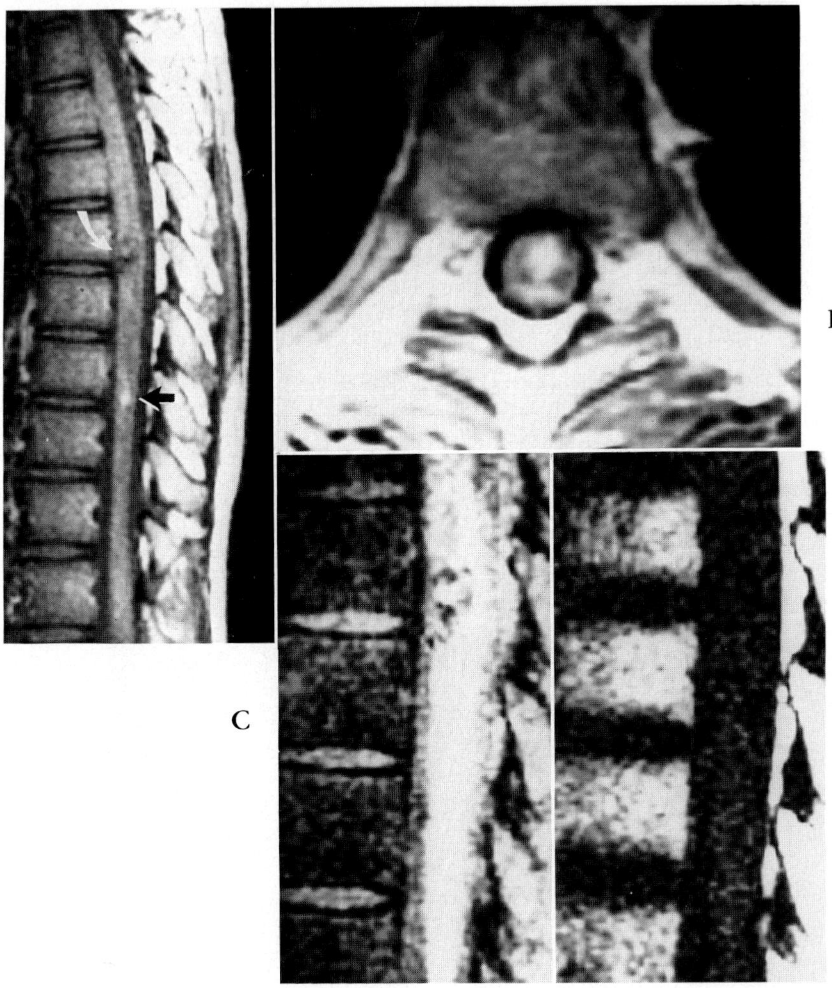

FIGURE 11-7. Spinal cord AVM. MR scans of 18-year-old male with 4 day history of decreased pain and temperature sensation in T_4-L_2 distribution and history of "transverse myelitis" with paraplegia that resolved completely 4 years ago. **A,** Sagittal T1W scan (SE 800/20) with large FOV (32 mm) shows cord enlargement in midthoracic region, focal abnormal high signal within cord *(straight arrow)* and focal area of mixed high and low signal more cephalad *(curved arrow)*. **B,** Axial T1W scan (SE 1000/20) through area of high signal shows intraaxial location. Minimal adjacent low signal is also seen. **C,** "Water" and **D,** "fat" images (SE 800/20 using suppression techniques) show no evidence of fat tissue (**D**) indicating high signal lesion (**A** and **B**) is hemorrhage. "Water" image accentuates circular low signal lesion suggesting hemosiderin effect in upper lesion (*curved arrow,* **A**). *Continued.*

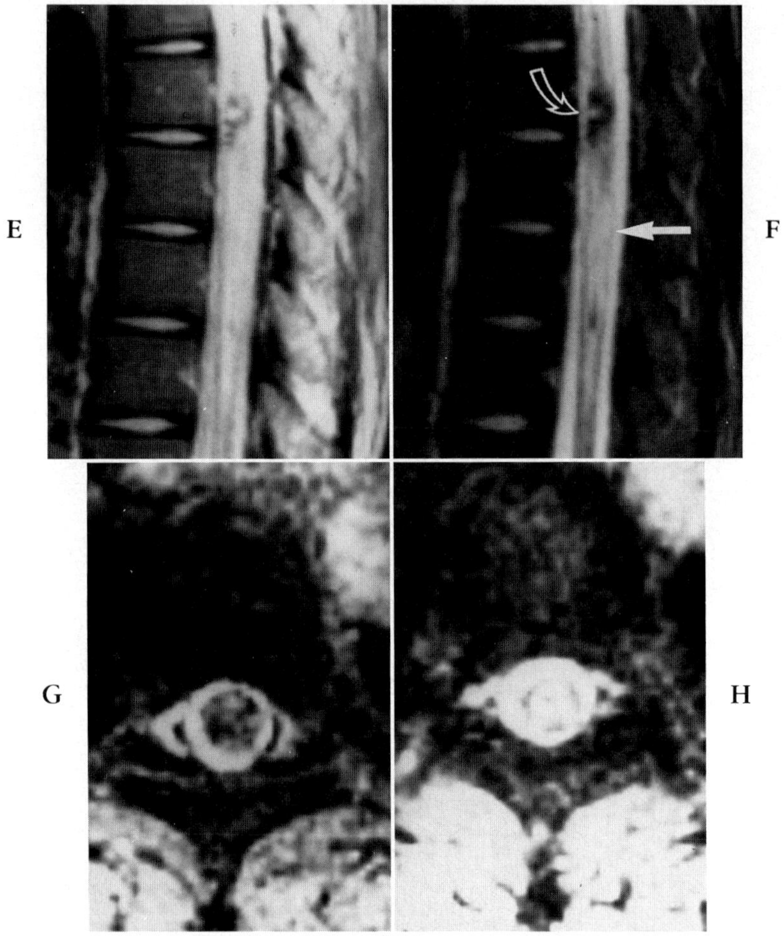

FIGURE 11-7, cont'd. **E**, (First Echo) and **F**, second echo of sagittal T2W scans (SE, gated 2700 20/80) show abnormal signal intensity in cord above, between, and below both lesions (*straight arrow*, **F**). Note "blossomed" circular low signal intensity around upper lesion (*curved arrow*, **F**) indicative of hemosiderin effect. **G** and **H**, Axial variable flip angle/gradient echo scans (SE 40/16, 5°) through (**G**) and below (**H**) upper lesion show marked loss of signal at site of hemosiderin deposition (**G**) and abnormal high signal within cord (**H**).

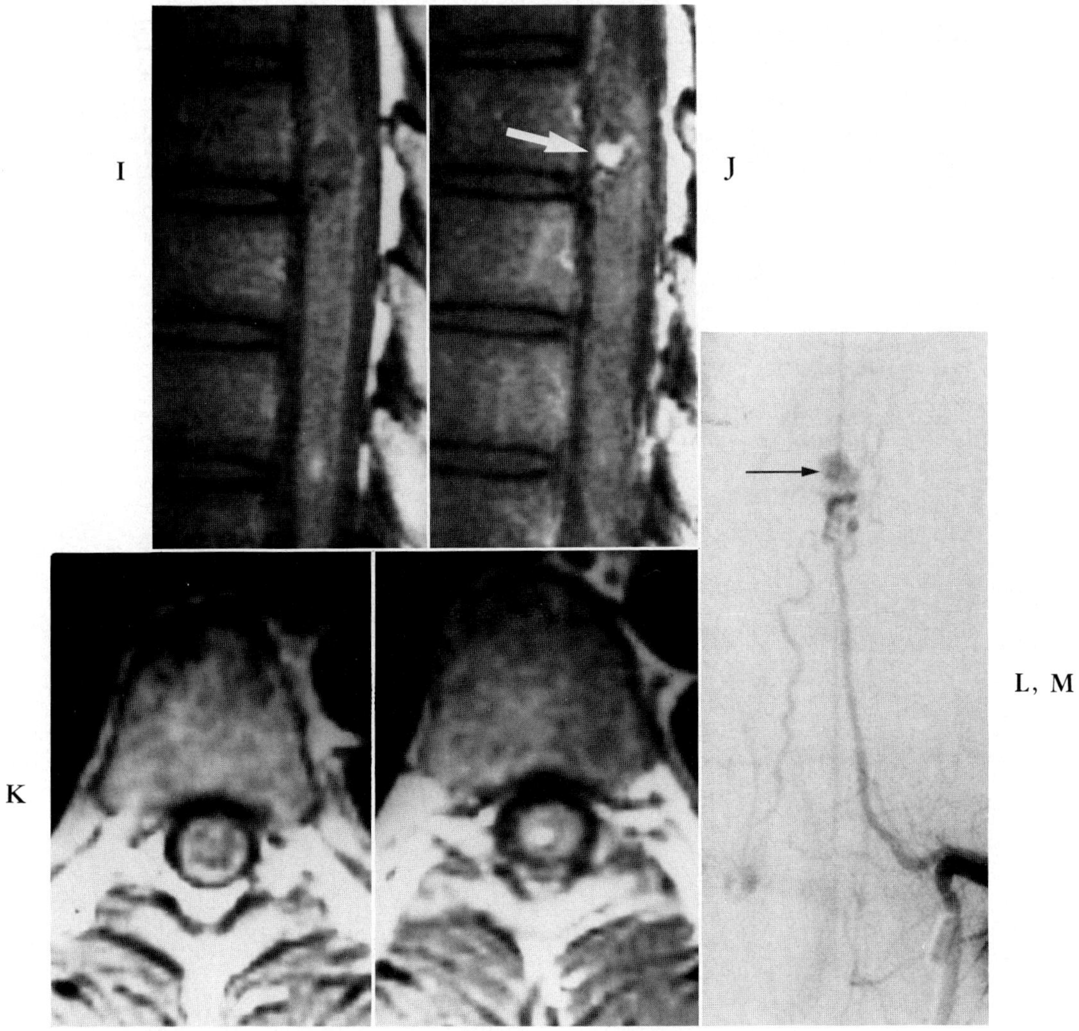

FIGURE 11-7, cont'd. Sagittal T1W scans (SE 800/20) pre- (**I**) and post- (**J**) GdDTPA injection. Abnormal cord enhancement is in upper lesion within circular area of low signal intensity (*arrow*, **J**), representing enhancement of blood pool in varix identified on arteriogram (*arrow*, **M**). Axial T1W scans (SE 1000/20) pre- (**K**) and post- (**L**) GdDTPA injection show location within cord of abnormal contrast enhancement (**L**). **M**, Spinal arteriogram shows enlarged feeding radiculomedullary artery, small AVM nidus, and small varix. The latter represents area of contrast enhancement seen on MR (**J** and **L**).

A, B

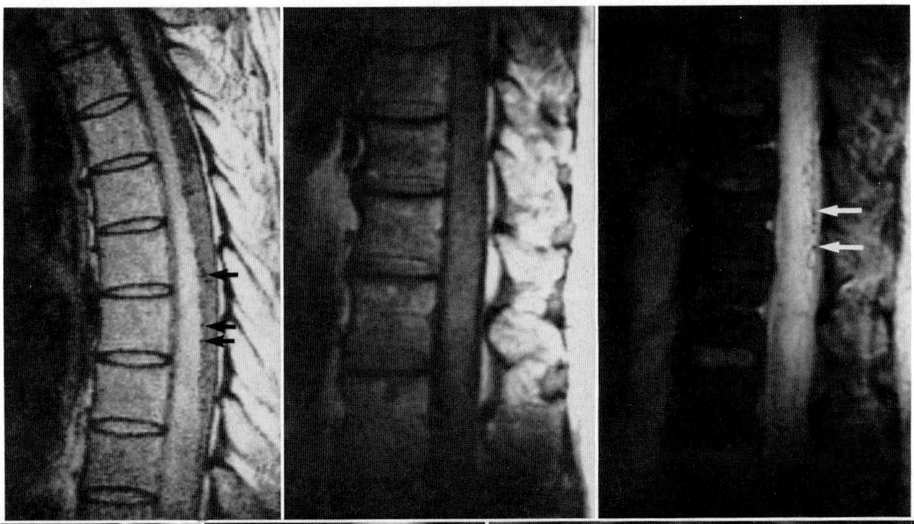

C

D, E

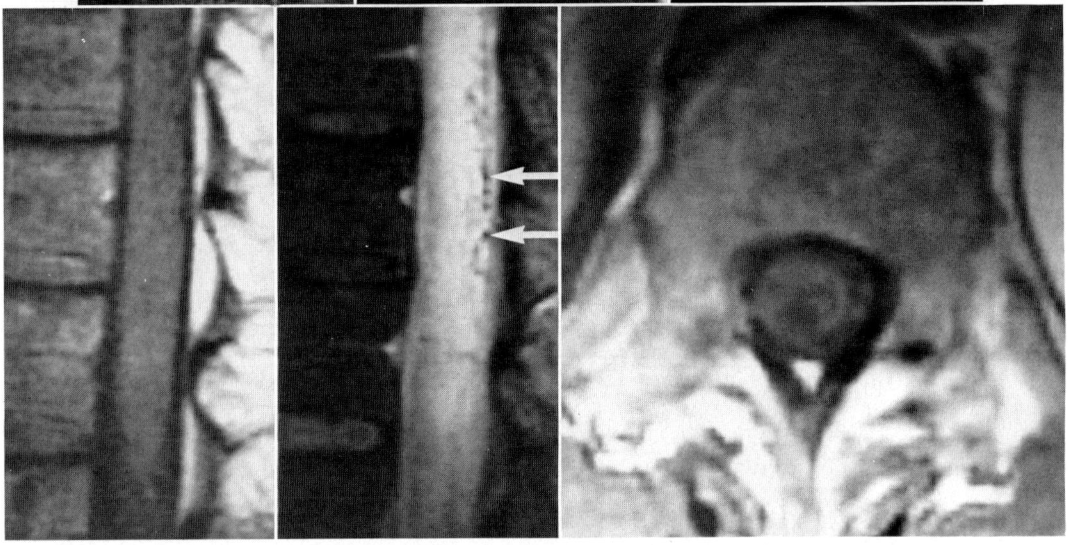

F

FIGURE 11-8. MR scans, myelogram, and spinal arteriogram of patient with spinal dural AVM fed by right T_9 intercostal artery. An outside sagittal T1W scan (.35T) of thoracic cord shows cord enlargement that led to provisional diagnosis of cord tumor. **A,** Small punctate areas of signal void on dorsal cord (*arrows*) were not appreciated but are crucial to correct diagnosis. Because lesion was already localized, a subsequent sagittal T1W scan (SE 800/20) and sagittal T2W scan (SE, gated 2200/80) was performed with small surface coil, improving SNR and permitting greater spatial resolution. **B,** Sagittal T1W scan shows diffuse enlargement of distal thoracic cord because it is same size as conus. Small dorsal veins are difficult to appreciate on this scan. **C,** T2W scan shows prominent abnormal vasculature dorsal to cord (*arrows*) and also demonstrates abnormal high signal intensity in distal thoracic cord and conus. Images **D** and **E** are magnifications of images **B** and **C** to better show abnormal signal intensity within cord and abnormal veins of dorsal coronal plexus (*arrows,* **E**). **F,** Axial T1W scan (SE 1000/20) confirms cord enlargement with abnormal low signal intensity within it. Confirmatory water-soluble contrast myelogram shows subtle but definite abnormal veins (*arrows,* **G**).

G 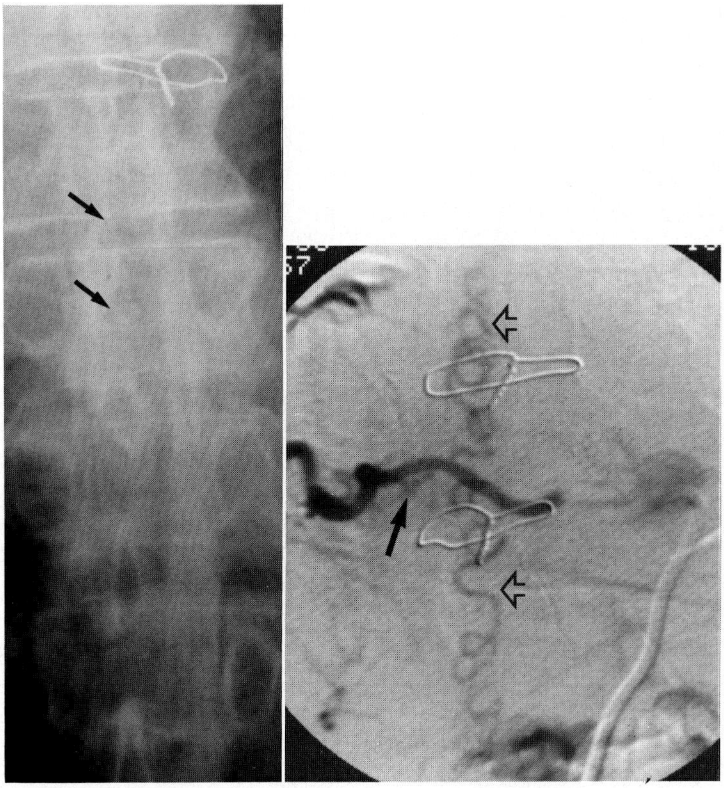 H

FIGURE 11-8, cont'd. **H,** AP view of spinal arteriogram shows small dural blush fed by right T_9 radiculo-medullo-dural artery. Veins can be seen draining in caudal and rostral direction *(open arrows)*. Nidus is indicated by solid arrow.

piginous areas of signal void representing the coronal venous plexus may be identified on the dorsal surface of the cord in sagittal and axial views on T1W and T2W images (see Figure 11-8). Pulse sequences sensitive to high velocity blood flow such as variable flip angle/gradient echo scans may help identify suspected signal voids dorsal to the cord as vessels. Contrast media, such as GdDTPA, may increase the conspicuity of such vessels.[4] Most often, the abnormality that will call attention to this lesion is enlargement of the cord. On T1W sequences, cord enlargement is apparent on both sagittal and axial scans and moderate low signal intensity may be identified within the cord (see Figure 11-8). On T2W scans the enlargement will again be noted, as well as abnormal, moderate high signal intensity within the cord extending for several vertebral body levels. The size and signal changes within the cord may be indistinguishable from a small localized, cord neoplasm. One distinguishing feature is that the abnormal signal intensity on T1W and T2W scans is relatively homogeneous with dural AVMs, more so than is typical for neoplasm. A careful search should be made for abnormal dorsal venous structures using a small surface coil to maximize the signal to noise ratio (SNR) and spatial resolution.

The correct diagnosis of the dural AVM rests with the detection of what may be subtle, abnormal dorsal venous structures. High resolution MR scan therefore is necessary. Definitive diagnosis may not always be possible with MR and a myelogram may be indicated for those patients with a suggestive history or with suggestive but inconclusive MR findings. The ultimate diagnosis rests with a spinal arteriogram.

SLOW FLOW VASCULAR MALFORMATIONS—"CRYPTIC"

The term *cryptic AVM* is used to describe vascular malformations in the brain that are difficult or impossible to detect with conventional angiography. They may be completely thrombosed or have such slow flow that vasculature is not demonstrated by angiography. They are, however, not cryptic by CT or MR. Pathologically, this "cryptic" type of lesion includes thrombosed AVMs, cavernous hemangiomas (cavernomas), capillary telangiectasias, and venous angiomas. In most instances, venous angiomas have a characteristic large draining vein allowing their diagnosis by angiography, CT, and MR. The other three entities are difficult to differentiate by imaging studies, although some investigators believe cavernous hemangiomas and capillary telangiectasias are the same lesion. In any event, vascular malformations that are angiographically occult occur in the spinal cord, as well as in the brain.[3,18,19,20]

The MR appearance of these spinal cord AVMs is similar to those seen in the brain. It has been suggested that the cavernous hemangioma has characteristic MR features differentiating them from the other types, i.e., a multiloculated appearance of numerous hemorrhagic cystic cavities. When present this feature may be helpful. What aids the diagnosis of slow flow AVMs in the spinal cord is the fact that in up to 25% of patients, such AVMs are multiple.[7] If detected in the spinal cord, a scan of the brain may detect other lesions of similar nature, securing the diagnosis (Figure 11-9). Variable flip angle/gradient echo scans, because of their magnetic susceptibility sensitivity, are recommended for brain screening. Depending on size, lesions may or may not enlarge the cord. Characteristic MR findings are those of a chronic hematoma. T1W scans may show a central area of isointensity or hyperintensity surrounded by a ring of low signal intensity (Figure 11-10; see Figure 11-9) that is caused by the magnetic susceptibility effect of hemosiderin in macrophages.[6] These features of the AVM require high resolution images because some of the characteristic findings are less evident on low resolution images (see Figure 11-10).

On T2W scans the central portion of the lesion is high or intermediate signal intensity surrounded by a low signal intensity rim that is more prominent than on T1W images (Figure 11-11). If pulse sequences using gradient refo-

A

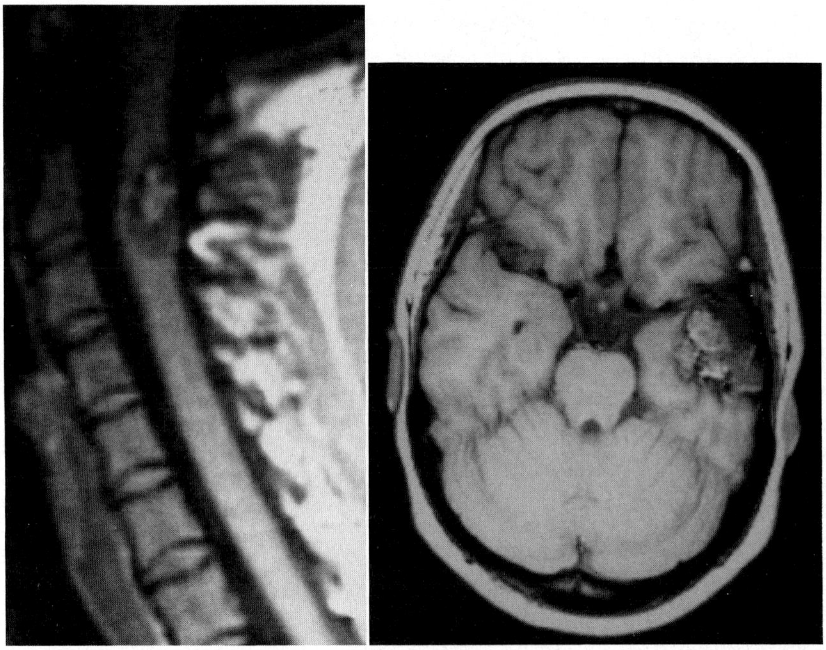

B

FIGURE 11-9. MR scans of patient with multiple cavernous hemangiomas in cervical cord and brain. Sagittal T1W (SE 600/20) scan shows typical findings of low signal intensity rim around center of higher signal intensity. Low signal intensity rim is caused by magnetic susceptibility effect of hemosiderin (**A**). AVM causes focal cord enlargement. **B**, Axial T1W (SE 600/25) scan shows larger but similar lesion in left temporal lobe.

cused echoes are used, the magnetic susceptibility effect is accentuated, and the low signal intensity rim around the lesion is further exaggerated and thickened (see Figures 11-10 and 11-11). The same pulse sequences accentuate the hemosiderin effect and may show this effect throughout the lesion (see Figure 11-11). This type of pulse sequence is useful in the spine and head to identify small, additional lesions that might otherwise be missed with conventional spin echo (SE) images. The magnetic susceptibility effect when enhanced by gradient echo pulse sequences may reveal small lesions that are nothing more than small punctate areas of signal loss.[7] A central area of isointensity or hyperintensity may not be identifiable in these small lesions. Nevertheless, their presence is strong confirmatory evidence of a slow flow AVM.

Confirmatory evidence is important because neoplasms involving the spinal cord may hemorrhage and thus simulate an AVM (Figure 11-12). The presence of multiple small hemorrhagic lesions, especially with brain involvement, suggests AVM over tumor. Vascular malformations are usually more localized than cord tumors although ependymomas can be well circumscribed lesions. In addition, spinal cord tumor will often show abnormal high signal on T2W images outside of the low signal intensity rim, indicating edema or tumor outside the borders of the hemorrhagic component of lesion. Cord enlargement beyond the areas of hematoma is indicative of neoplasm. If cord enlargement is limited to only the immediate area of the hematoma a vascular malformation is more likely. Abnormal high signal around the outside of a slow flow AVM is unusual, but can occur if there has been a recent hemorrhage within the AVM or previous surgery (see Figure 11-10). Signal outside the hemorrhagic component of a lesion, however, should suggest the diagnosis of tumor and lead to close interval follow up if no immediate action is taken.

A, B

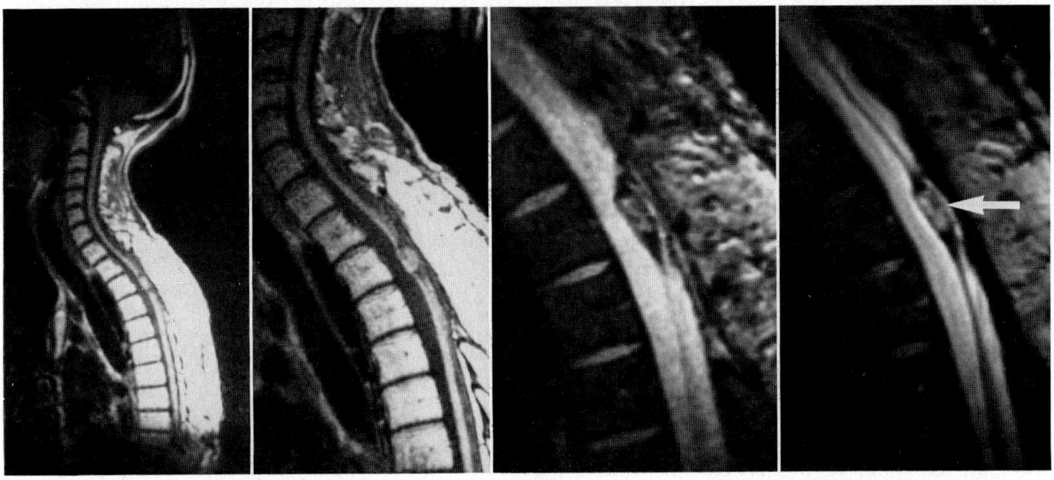

C, D

FIGURE 11-10. Series of MR scans in 41-year-old patient with cavernous hemangioma of spinal cord show value of increasing spatial resolution in identifying characteristic features. **A,** T1W scan (SE 400/20) with large field of view (FOV 48 cm) to localize lesion shows lesion but does not characterize it well. Image was obtained with large surface coil. **B,** Lesion at T_3 level is better seen on sagittal T1W scan (SE 800/20) obtained with smaller FOV (24 cm) but same surface coil. **C,** Sagittal, variable flip angle scan (40/13, 5°) shows prominent magnetic susceptibility effect in hemangioma. **D,** Sagittal T2W scan (SE, gated, flow-compensated 2400/80) shows lesion in detail with surrounding low signal area caused by hemosiderin deposition around higher signal intensity center (*arrow*). Cord appears narrower than on T1W scans because abnormal signal in cord makes it indistinguishable from adjacent CSF. This abnormal cord signal is not typical and is probably related to previous surgery in this patient. Appropriate use of surface coils to increase SNR and pulse sequences to highlight magnetic susceptibility effects is important in diagnosis of this disease.

A B C D, E

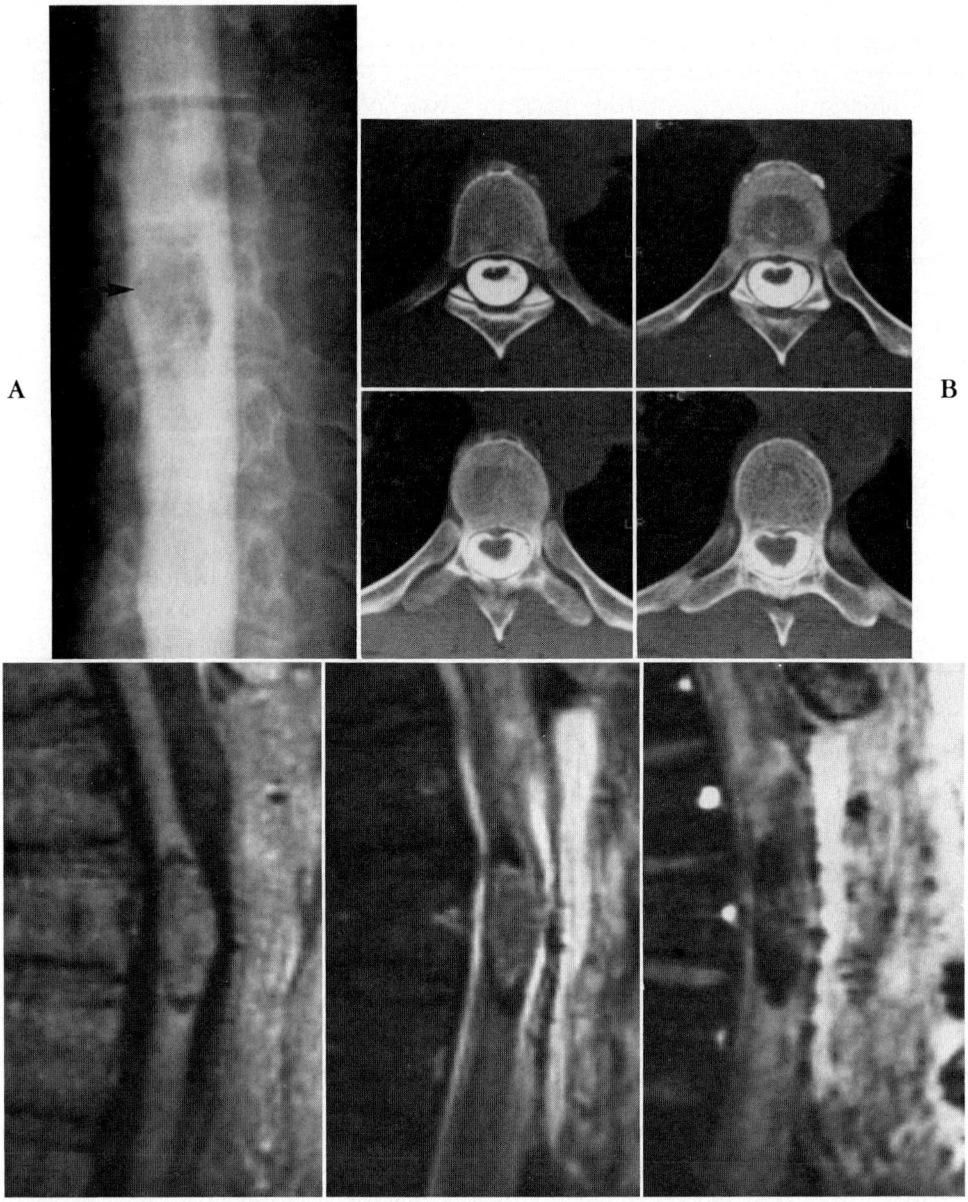

FIGURE 11-11. CT and MR scans of 38-year-old female with slowly progressive paraparesis caused by cavernous hemangioma. **A,** Water soluble contrast myelogram shows focal, irregular cord enlargement at level of T_7 (*arrow*). (The round lucency is an air bubble.) **B,** Axial CT scan obtained with intrathecal water soluble contrast shows somewhat atrophic cord above lesion (*upper left*) and irregular cord enlargement at level of lesion at T_7 (*lower right*). Sagittal MR scans were performed using three different pulse sequences: (1) **C,** T1W scan (SE 800/20) shows focal enlargement of cord at T_7 with decreased diameter of cord above lesion. Border between lesion and adjacent cord shows marked decreased signal in thin band configuration. (2) **D,** Sagittal T2W scan (SE, gated, 2000/80) shows main body of mass remains similar intensity as adjacent cord. There is no evidence of abnormal signal outside of mass within cord. Areas of low signal intensity at border between mass and cord appear wider and of lower signal intensity. Areas of low signal represent magnetic susceptibility effect expected from hemosiderin deposition. (3) **E,** Sagittal variable partial flip angle/gradient echo scan (GRASS 25/15, 33°) shows no evidence of blood flow within lesion. Note increased signal from penetrating veins in middorsal vertebrae. Mass lesion has prominent low signal intensity suggesting prominent magnetic susceptibility effect throughout entire lesion. Scan shows postsurgical changes dorsal to spinal canal from previous exploration where lesion was only visualized but not surgically manipulated.

F

G

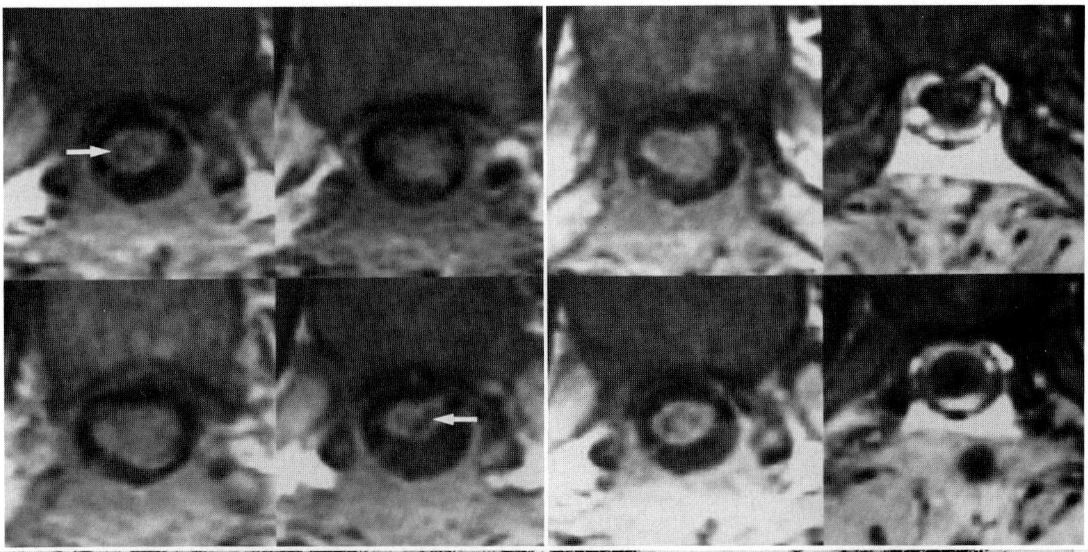

H

I

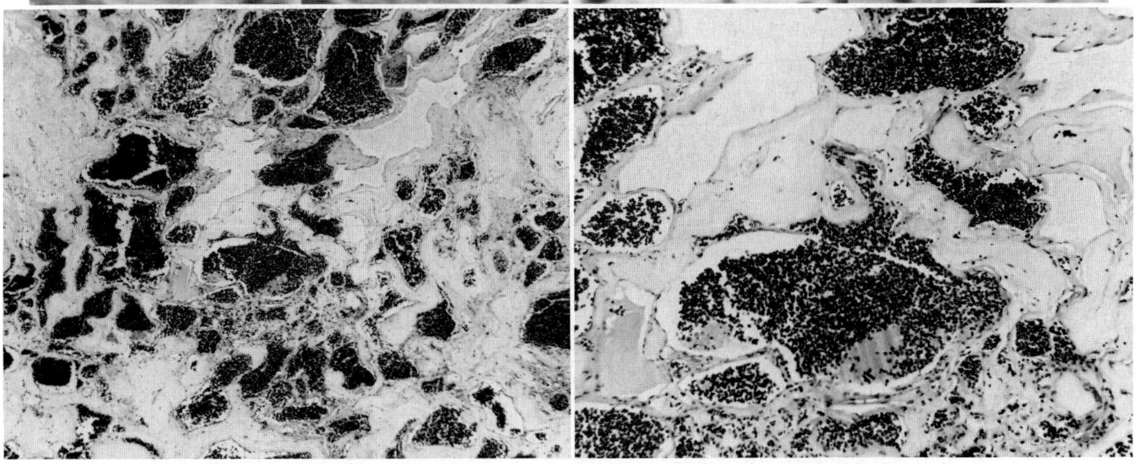

FIGURE 11-11, cont'd. Set of four axial T1W scans (SE 800/20) confirms irregular cord enlargement, as well as inhomogeneous signal intensity within mass (**F**). Areas of low signal intensity are seen above and below major region of enlargement (*arrows* in upper left and lower right images). There is no evidence of high signal on T1W images to suggest presence of paramagnetic effect caused by methemoglobin. Magnetic susceptibility effect caused by hemosiderin is prominent and seen on sagittal (**E**) and in axial (**G**) variable flip angle/gradient echo scans (GRASS 25/13, 33°). **G,** Four images compare equivalent levels using T1W pulse sequence (left column) with variable flip angle sequence (right column). Note that entire cord is low signal intensity on variable flip angle scan (right two images). There was no evidence of blood flow in this sequence. Size of cord, judged by area of low signal intensity, is artifactually large compared to T1W image (lower two images). Findings that suggest "cryptic" vascular malformation are localized nature of mass magnetic susceptibility effect at periphery of lesion and within lesion, and lack of abnormal signal intensity in cord adjacent to mass. The only atypical finding is lack of high signal intensity on T1W images, which would suggest presence of methemoglobin. Photomicrographs (H and E; **H,** 40× and **I,** 100×) of cavernous hemangioma shows typical microscopic features: network of various sized vessels, with walls composed of collagen, lined by single layer of endothelium. Some collagen exhibits hyalinization. **I,** Magnified view of central region shows that no vascular channels have features of arteries or veins. And also shows lack of neural tissue between vessels distinguishing this lesion from other AVMs. (Photomicrographs courtesy of Dr. Dikran Horoupian.)

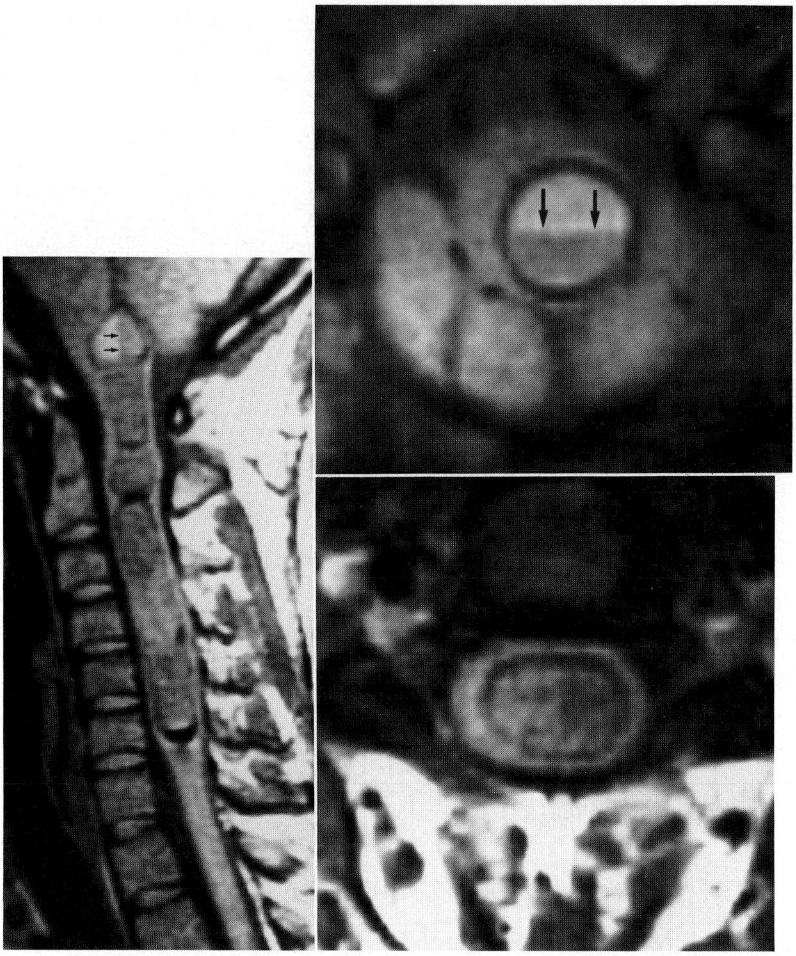
A B C

FIGURE 11-12. Astrocytoma. Sagittal T1W (SE 800/20) scan shows long lesion extending from medulla to C_6 level. **A,** Lesion is well circumscribed, has low signal rim around most of lesion (most prominent around inferior component), and appears to have four different compartments with cephalad compartment showing fluid level (*arrows*). Dependent fluid is lower signal intensity than upper fluid layer (**A** and **B**) (patient is horizontal). This pattern of fluid intensity is consistent with hemorrhagic cyst. Thin rim of signal intensity appearing to circumscribe entire lesion is consistent with magnetic susceptibility effect of hemosiderin deposition. Balanced (1500/25) axial views show same layering of fluid within hemorrhagic cyst (**B**) and confirms thin rim of signal intensity around cyst (**B** and **C**), a combination pathognemonic of hemorrhagic cyst (**B**, *arrows*). **C,** Axial view at level of C_2-C_3 confirms cord enlargement with abnormal high signal intensity enveloped by thin rim of low signal intensity indicative of hemosiderin effect. Except for extent of lesion and presence of a hemorrhagic cyst, findings are suggestive of slow flow vascular malformation. Lesion, however, represents hemorrhagic astrocytoma. (Courtesy of Dr. David Norman.)

EPIDURAL HEMORRHAGE

Epidural hemorrhage in the spinal canal is an uncommon disease process, although with the availability of MR imaging this diagnosis will be made more often. It is an important diagnosis because rapid neurosurgical intervention may be necessary to obtain a satisfactory outcome. A delay in diagnosis can result in significant morbidity and mortality. In most instances, the epidural hemorrhage is considered "spontaneous" in that no direct cause can be established. In a number of patients minor trauma may precede epidural hemorrhage but it is not clear that the trauma has had a cause and effect relationship. It is thought that at times even coughing or sneezing may be an initiating event; this is plausible because epidural veins that are thought to be one source of hemorrhage communicate directly with abdominal and retroperitoneal veins. Because there are no valves in this venous system, intraabdominal pressure is transmitted directly to the epidural venous plexus. Although venous bleeding is thought to be the primary source of epidural hemorrhage, arterial bleeding has also been identified.[1]

Associated considerations or events that have been temporally related to epidural hemorrhage fall into two categories: procedures and predisposing conditions. The procedures most often implicated are a lumbar puncture and spinal anesthesia.[13] Predisposing conditions are a bleeding diathesis, with anticoagulation therapy the most common condition.[13] Others include pregnancy and hypertension. Two spine lesions implicated as a source of hemorrhage are vertebral body hemangioma and spinal cord vascular malformations.[21] These aspects of the clinical history are important in considering the diagnosis.

The common site for epidural hemorrhage is the thoracic spine.[9,12,13] The hemorrhage may extend into the cervicothoracic region or caudally into the thoracolumbar region and can be localized or extend for several segments.[8] Because the epidural space in the thoracic region is larger posteriorly, this is the usual site for the hemorrhage, which may be localized unilaterally

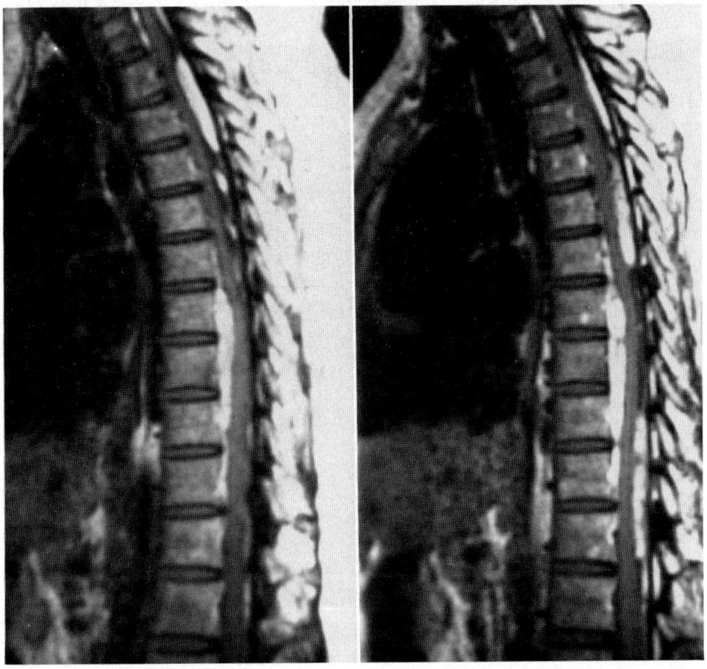

FIGURE 11-13. Epidural hemorrhage. Sagittal T1W (SE 600/20) scans show several discontinuous areas of high signal intensity anterior and posterior to cord representing spontaneous epidural hemorrhage. Although scattered, hemorrhages are sufficient size to cause cord deviation and compression. With this distribution there is little concern about confusion with fat. (Courtesy of Dr. Michael Brant-Zawadzki.)

on one side of the spinal canal or it may involve it circumferentially.[12]

The clinical presentation of spinal epidural hemorrhage is usually that of a sudden, acute onset of back or neck pain that may have a radicular distribution.[9,21] Shortly after the onset of pain, from minutes to hours and sometimes days, the signs and symptoms of cord or cauda equina compression develop. Patients develop long track signs and a sensory level. Depending upon the location, tetra or paraplegia may progress rapidly to total paralysis. Less commonly, the progression of disease may be less acute and even have an undulating pattern. Spinal epidural hemorrhages are a disease of old age although they can appear in the child age group.

A B C D

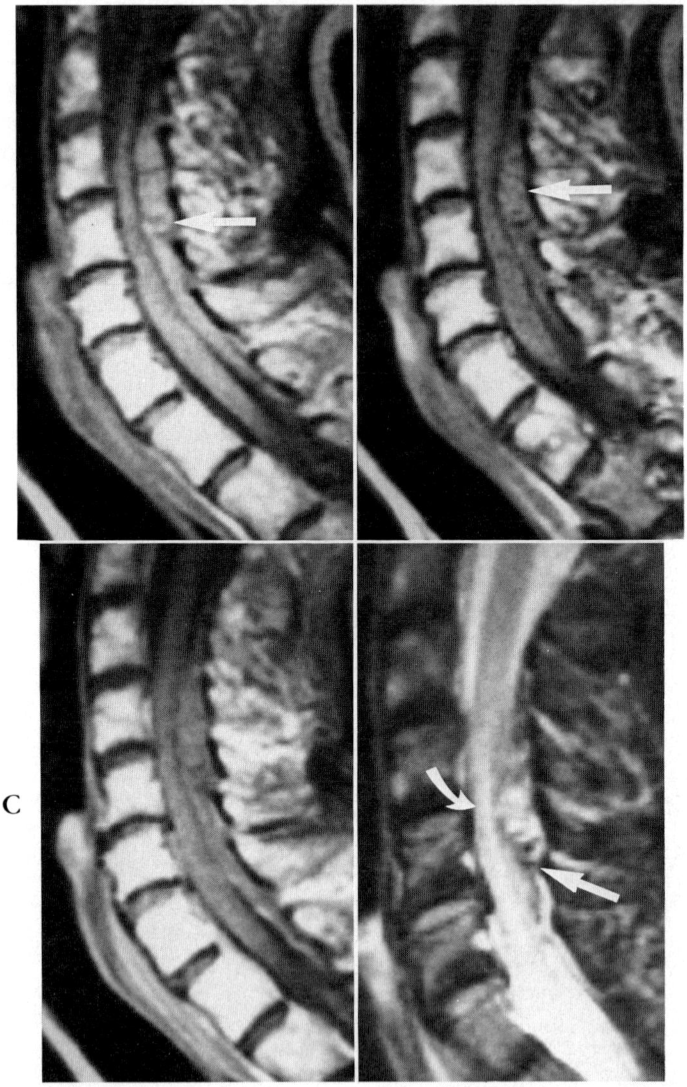

FIGURE 11-14. Epidural hematoma. MR scans of 46-year-old female with sudden onset of neck pain and lower extremity weakness. **A** and **B**, T1W sagittal (SE 800/20) images show extensive posterior mass (*arrows*) compressing cervical cord. Mass has intermediate signal intensity that does not show contrast enhancement on postGdDTPA scan (**C**). **D**, Sagittal T2W scan (SE gated 2200/80) reveals inhomogeneous signal intensity in posterior mass including areas of marked low signal intensity that suggest hemorrhagic component (*straight arrow*). Abnormal high signal intensity within cord at site of compression (*curved arrow*) indicates edema.

MR Findings

The key to diagnosis by MR is to choose pulse sequences that delineate the hemorrhagic nature of the lesion. The appearance of acute hemorrhage can vary in the first few days and between different field strengths.[6] In some instances, on a T1W image the extradural lesion will have high signal intensity, but often it has intermediate signal intensity (Figures 11-13 and 11-14; see Figure 11-18). It does not have a segmental distribution similar to normal epidural fat and it will show distortion or compression of the underlying spinal cord (see Figures 11-14 and 11-18).[16] On axial scans it may be unilateral and asymmetric (see Figures 11-14 and 11-18). A component of the hemorrhage may extend into the neural foramen. On a T2W scan the appearance will depend on the age of the hemorrhage. In an acute state it may demonstrate a variety of signal intensities ranging from marked low signal intensity caused by the magnetic susceptibility effect of deoxyhemoglobin to high signal intensity indicative of high proton density or high water content (see Figure 11-14).[6] The key to the diagnosis is the clinical history, the lesion site, and the extent of the lesion. In an acute situation, the major differential diagnosis is epidural abscess because it can have a similar clinical presentation and also exhibit hemorrhagic characteristics. Subdural hemorrhages have similar characteristics as an epidural hemorrhage (Figure 11-15).

Subarachnoid hemorrhage is easily differentiated from subdural or epidural hemorrhage in that it usually outlines and abuts the cord continuously for several segments (Figures 11-16 and 11-17). There is a clear line of demarcation between hemorrhage and epidural fat (see Figure 11-16). Because subarachnoid hemorrhage is more often associated with AVMs an intrinsic cord abnormality may be detected (see Figure 11-17). Additional features are seen on axial scans. Evidence for hemorrhage is seen as high signal in T1W images in areas where one normally sees signal voids caused by CSF pulsation (see Figure 11-16; see also Figures 1-8 and 1-9). Finally spinal ganglia may become enlarged and exhibit abnormal signal intensity (see Figure 11-16). This is an indirect sign of leptomeningeal disease and can be seen with leptomeningeal carcinomatosis.

The availability of MR scans will no doubt demonstrate the existence of less severe forms of epidural hemorrhage that do not have im-

E F G H

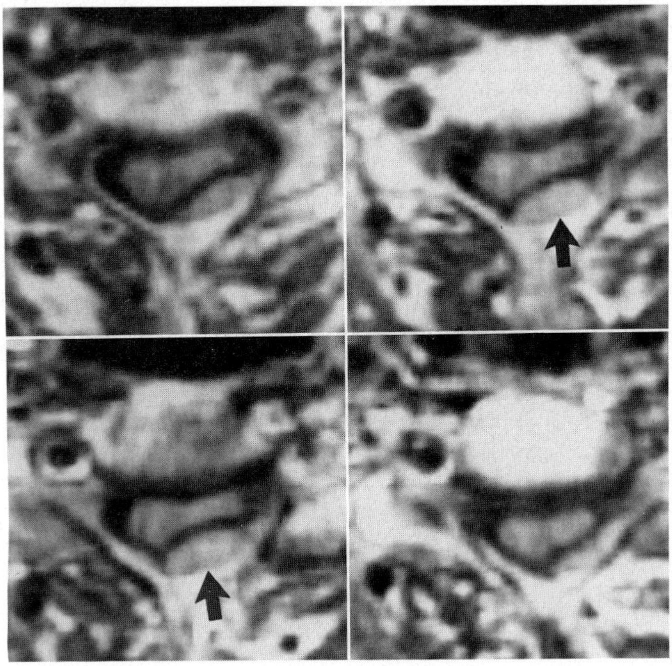

FIGURE 11-14, cont'd. E-H, Axial T1W scans (SE 1000/20) show asymmetric dorsal location of epidural hemorrhage confirmed by surgery (*arrows*).

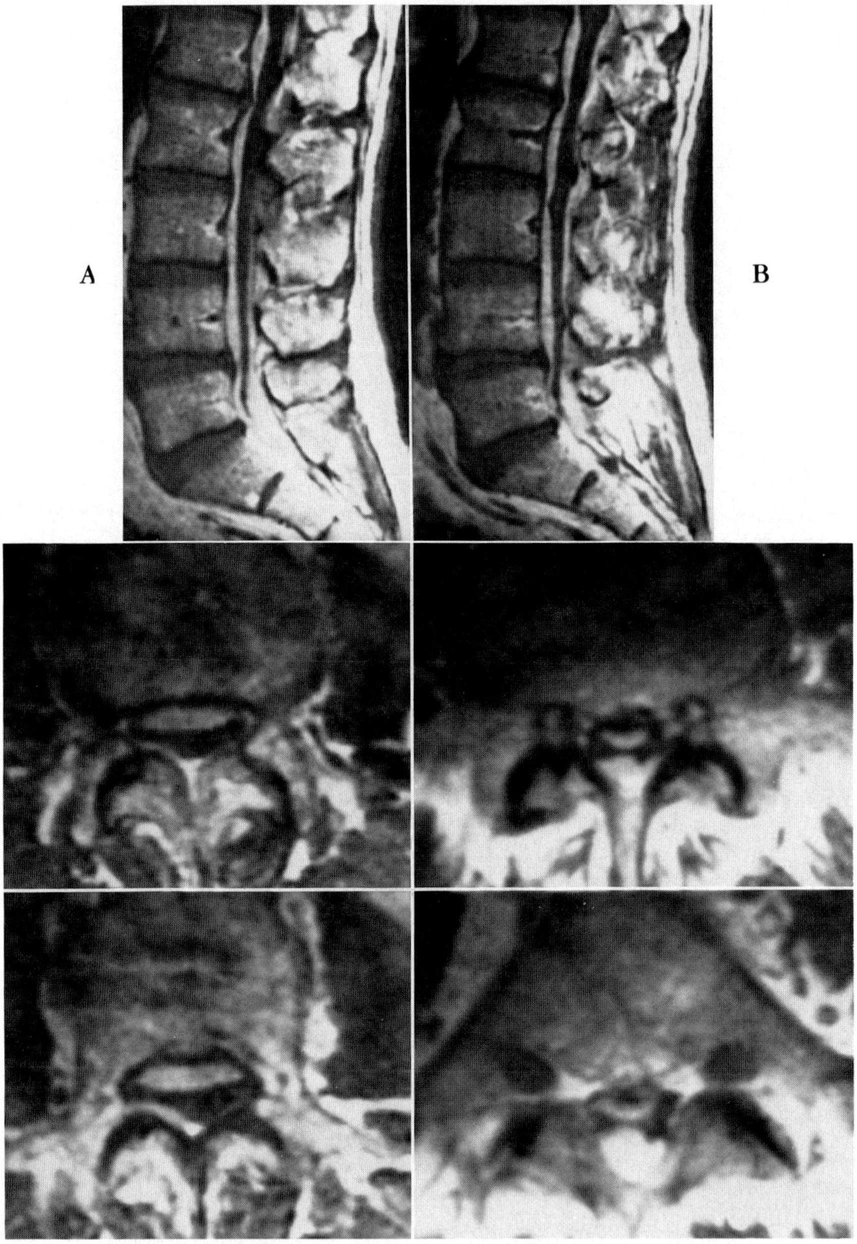

FIGURE 11-15. MR scan of patient with spontaneous subdural hematoma in lumbar spinal canal after minimal trauma. Patient had variant of von Willebrand's disease indicating a bleeding diathesis. **A** and **B**, Sagittal T1W (SE 600/20) scans show extensive area of high signal intensity lining lumbar spinal canal anteriorly and posteriorly, narrowing residual subarachnoid space. **C-F**, Axial T1W (SE 600/20) scans show localized increased signal intensity in anterior and posterior spinal canal. In midlumbar region (**C** and **D**) hemorrhage is more prominent anteriorly whereas in distal region (**E** and **F**) hemorrhage is more prominent in dorsal location. Subdural location is suggested because hemorrhage configuration conforms to dural margins and thin line of demarcation between hemorrhage and dorsal epidural fat (**A**). An axial T2W scan can help define displaced dura. (Courtesy of Dr. Michael Brant-Zawadzki.)

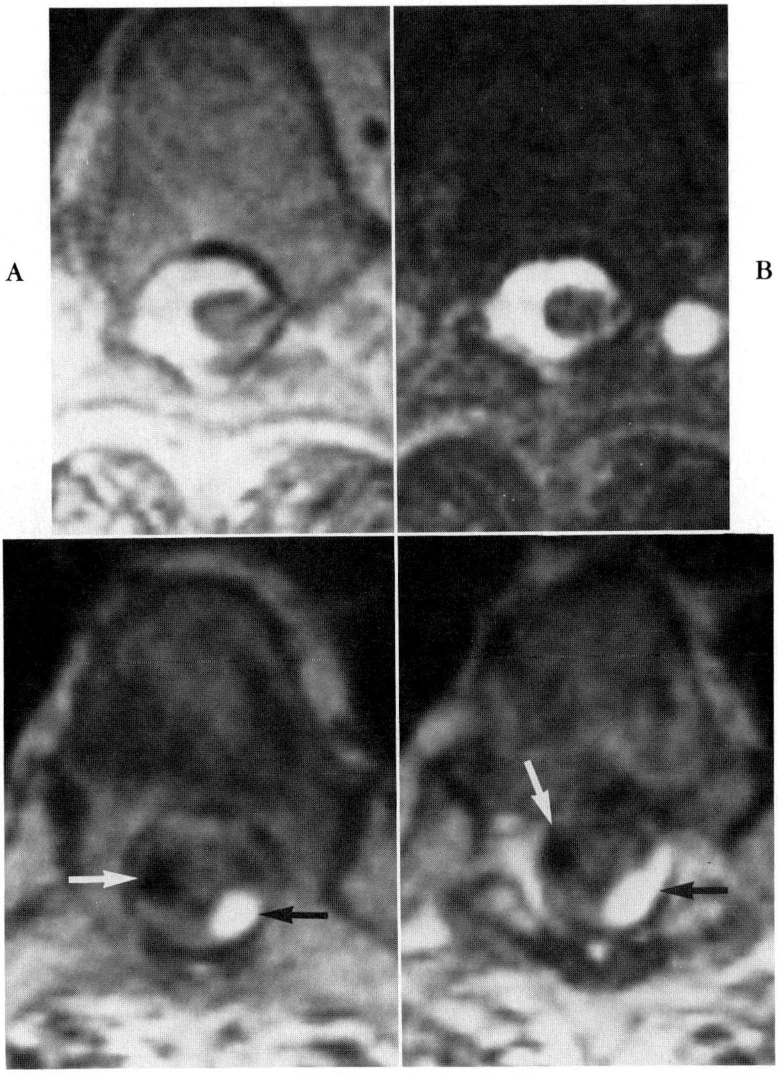

FIGURE 11-16. Subarachnoid hemorrhage of spinal (not intracranial) origin but without specific etiology. Spinal arteriogram was negative. T2W scan (gated, 2100/20, 80) shows marked increased signal intensity in subarachnoid space surrounding cord and displacing cord to left. This is evident on both first (**A**) and second (**B**) echo. Note abnormal signal and increased size of left ganglion on second echo. At upper margin of subarachnoid hemorrhage T1W (SE 800/20) scans **C** and **D**, show high signal in area that typically shows signal void caused by CSF pulsation (*black arrows*). Note on right side, area of CSF pulsation continues to show expected signal void (*white arrows*). Distribution of high signal confirms subarachnoid location of blood.

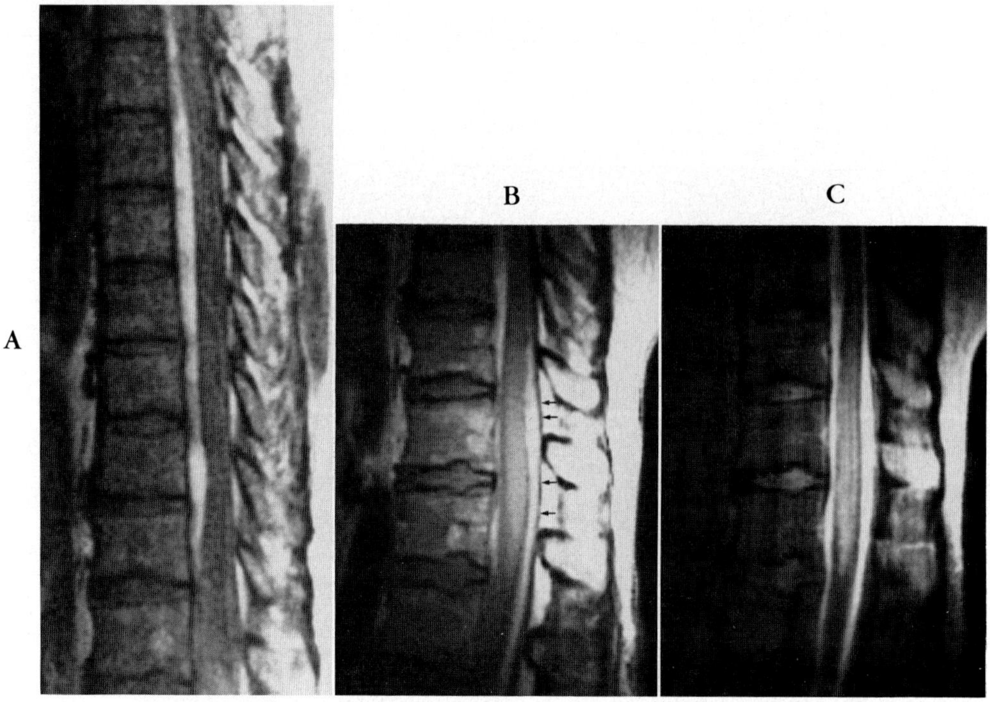

FIGURE 11-17. MR scans of patient with spinal subarachnoid hemorrhage probably arising near conus. Specific etiology was not clear because spinal arteriogram showed only somewhat dilated anterior spinal artery but no AVM or aneurysm. **A**, T1W image (SE 800/20) shows long segment of increased signal intensity anterior to cord, displacing it posteriorly. **B**, Close up view of conus using small surface coil shows subarachnoid hemorrhage anterior and posterior to conus on T1W (SE 800/20) image. In addition to slight anterior displacement abnormal high signal intensity is seen within conus. High signal on T1W image suggests component of parenchymal hemorrhage within cord. **C**, T2W scan (SE gated 1800/80) of conus also shows abnormal high signal within conus, as well as diffuse increased signal in subarachnoid space.

mediate and dire consequences. They may resolve spontaneously and are probably more common than expected. MR findings may be more nonspecific with the more chronic form because the obvious hemorrhagic characteristics may not be present (Figure 11-18) or may be more localized. In such patients, the differential diagnosis includes extraaxial lesions such as neuromas and synovial cysts. The diagnosis may become evident only when spontaneous resolution of the epidural masses is documented.

INFARCTION

Little is known about spinal cord infarction because it is difficult to diagnose and verify. The diagnosis is usually made on clinical grounds. In abdominal aortic aneurysm surgery spinal cord infarction is thought to be caused by interruption of vessels feeding the anterior spinal artery. A variety of vasculitides can cause cord infarction. In other situations the pathogenesis is not clear.

MR findings are similar to infarctions elsewhere in the central nervous system (CNS). T1W images can be relatively insensitive to infarctions in the cord unless they are large or show mass effect in the acute stage (see Figure 11-20), but they can detect cord swelling in the subacute stage (1 to 3 weeks). T2W images detect abnormal water accumulation (cytotoxic and vasogenic edema) and are especially important in diagnosis to detect abnormal increased signal in the cord even when cord size is normal (Figures 11-19 and 11-20). The extent of infarction depends on the anatomic distribution of the spinal arteries of the individual patient. Infarcts can be limited to a few segments or be quite exten-

D E F G

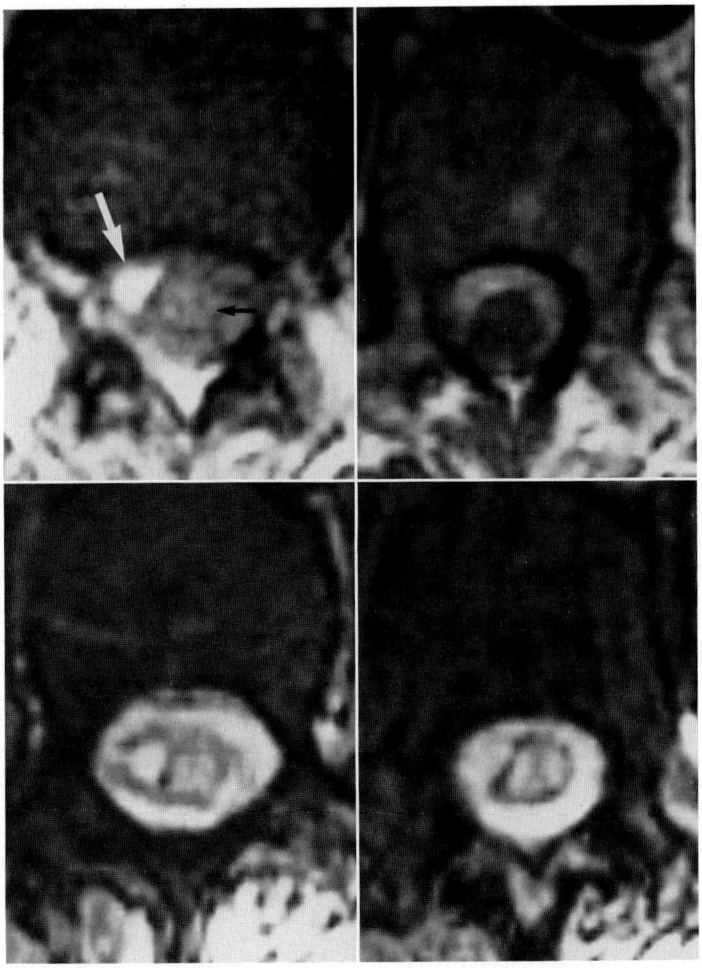

FIGURE 11-17, cont'd. **D** and **E**, Axial T1W (SE 800/20) scans show focal area of high signal adjacent to cord on left (*arrow*, **D**) and moderately increased signal throughout subarachnoid space at same level. Abnormal increased signal is seen within cord (*black arrow*, **D**). At higher level, cord signal returned to normal but increased signal still seen in subarachnoid space indicative of hemorrhage (**E**). **F** and **G**, Variable flip angle/gradient echo scans at same levels as **D** and **E** confirm local hematoma to right of cord that appears to be trapped in right part of cauda equina. Increased signal within conus is confirmed at both levels. Etiology of abnormal cord signal was not determined.

sive. Abnormal signal persists even in late stages when tissue loss results in cord atrophy. This narrowing of cord diameter is detectable on T1W and T2W images for variable lengths.

FOIX-ALAJOUANINE SYNDROME (SUBACUTE NECROTIC MYELITIS)

The Foix-Aljouanine syndrome refers to an uncommon and poorly understood disease process involving the spinal cord and conus.[5a,9a,20a] The term *subacute necrotic myelitis* is more descriptive and refers to the same disease process. A number of cases described in the literature reveal a consistent clinical pathologic pattern. Although the syndrome has been attributed to spontaneous thrombosis of spinal cord AVMs, this is not the essence of the disease process because it characteristically occurs without the presence of a spinal AVM.[20a]

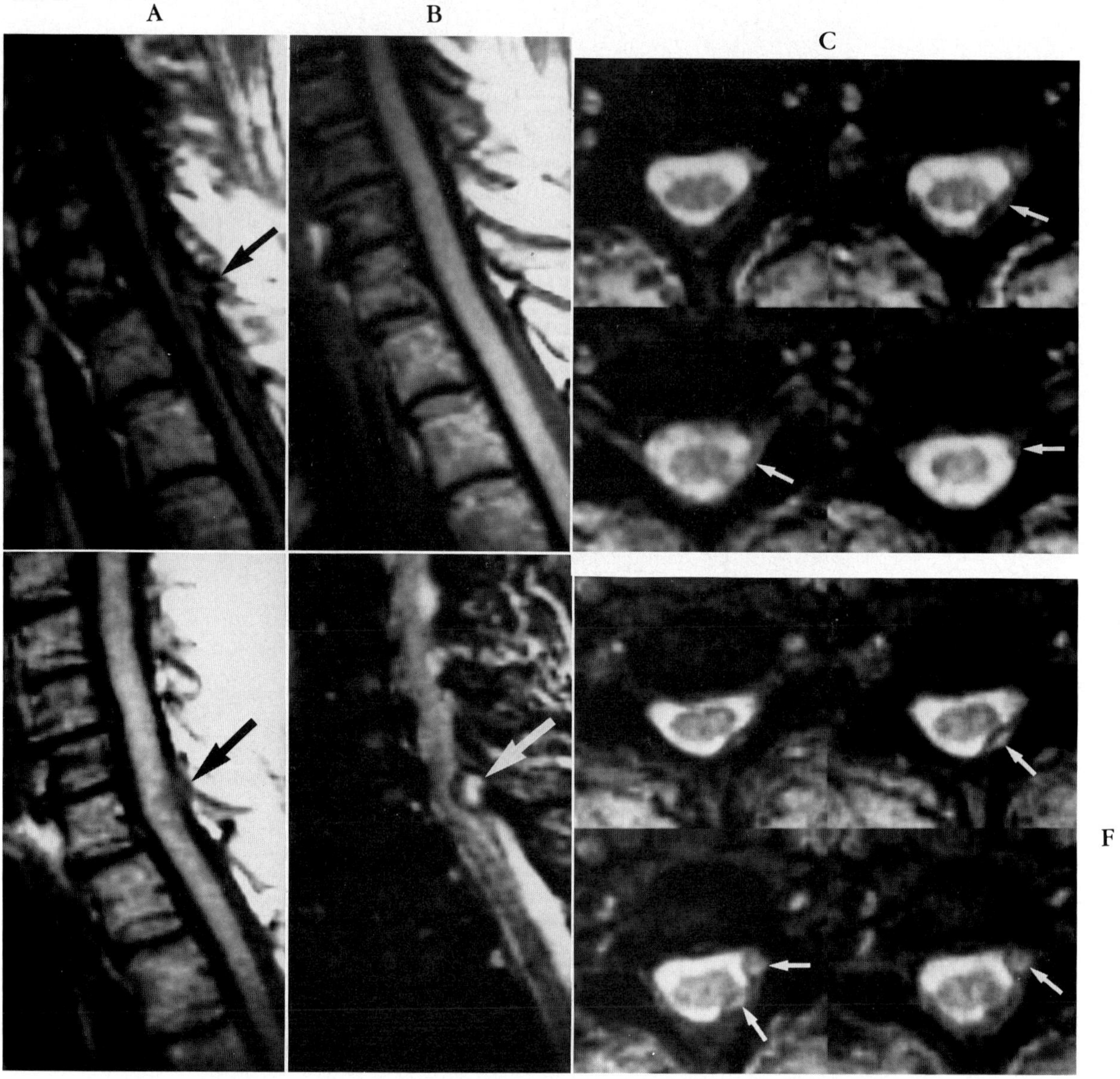

FIGURE 11-18. Serial scans of 59-year-old woman with focal cervical epidural hematoma that resolved spontaneously. At initial presentation patient complained of neck pain and left arm pain. **A,** T1W (SE 800/20) scan shows low signal intensity mass lesion at C_6-C_7 indenting cord posteriorly (*arrow*). **B,** Sagittal T2W (SE 2000/80) scan shows focal, circumscribed lesion in same location consisting of high signal intensity center and low signal intensity rim (*arrow*). **C,** Set of four axial variable flip angle/gradient echo scans (22/12, 7°) shows lesions unilateral involving epidural space adjacent to lamina and extending into left neural foramen (*arrows*). All lesions have similar features, i.e., medium to high signal intensity demarcated from subarachnoid space by thin rim of low signal (**C**). Patient had several intervening scans that showed progressive decrease in size of epidural masses without any therapy. Follow-up scan performed one year later shows almost complete resolution of epidural masses with sagittal T1W (SE 800/20) scans showing only minimal residua of dorsal epidural mass (*arrow,* **D**). Cord is no longer displaced (**E**). Set of four variable flip angle scans (25/13, 7°) shows almost complete resolution of epidural masses although minimal masses remain adjacent to left lamina and left neural foramen at C_6-C_7 (*arrow,* **F**).

A

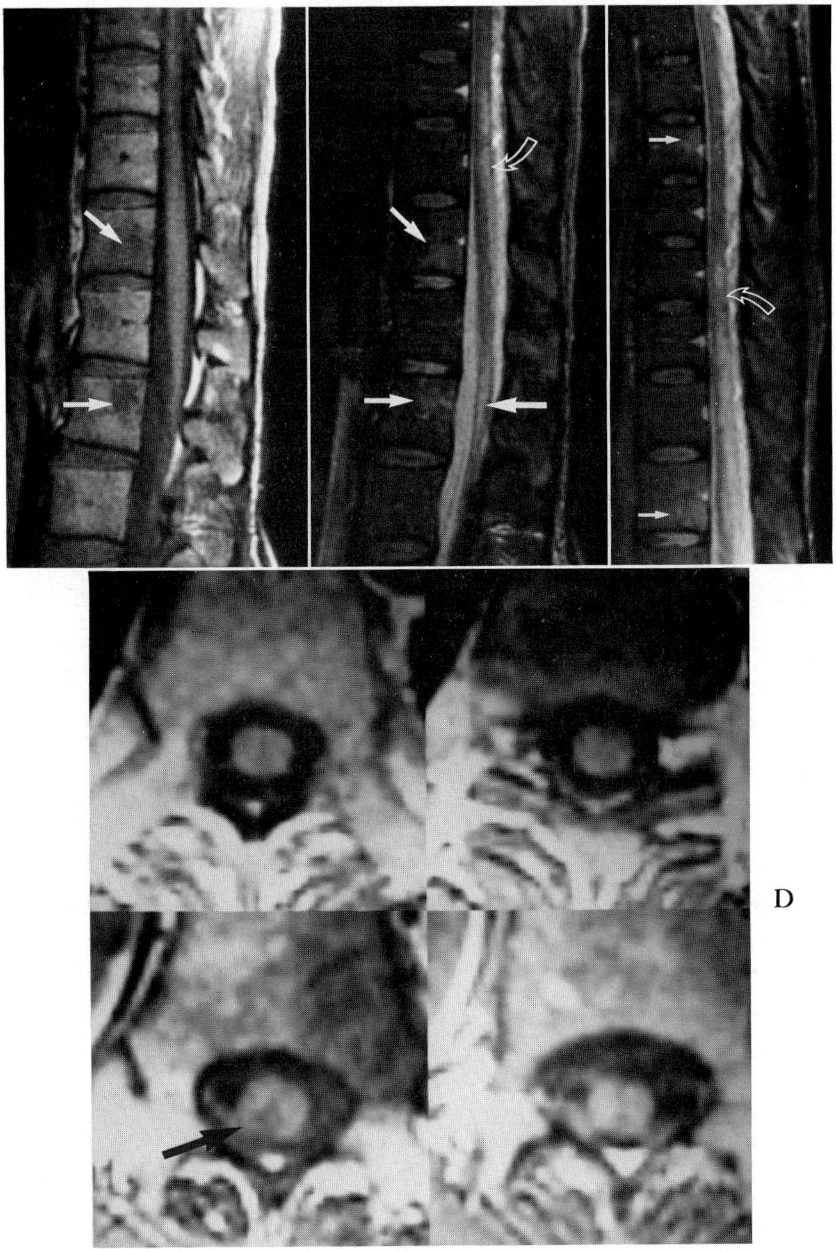

B, C

D

FIGURE 11-19. MR scan of suspected cord infarction in 46-year-old female with breast carcinoma, seen metastatic to L_1 and T_{11} (*arrows*, **A** and **B**), and T_6 (*top arrow*, **C**). Metastatic lesions are of increased signal compared to marrow on T2W scans (*arrows*, **B** and **C**). **A,** T1W scan (SE 800/20) shows normal conus size whereas T2W scan (SE gated 2200/80) shows abnormal high signal within cord from midthoracic level to conus (*curved arrows* **B** and **C**). Cord is not enlarged at sites of abnormal signal, which extends from T_8-T_{12}. Note increased signal within cauda equina that represents CSF (*large arrow*, **B**). Set of four T1W images (SE 1000/20) at conus suggests minimal enlargement on right side and some inhomogeneous low signal intensity in posterior cord (*arrow* **D**). Patient experienced sudden, acute loss of motor and sensory function below T_{12} highly suggestive of cord infarction and did not have CSF evidence of leptomeningeal carcinomatosis. Clinical history and lack of mass effect do not suggest cord metastases or paraneoplastic syndrome.

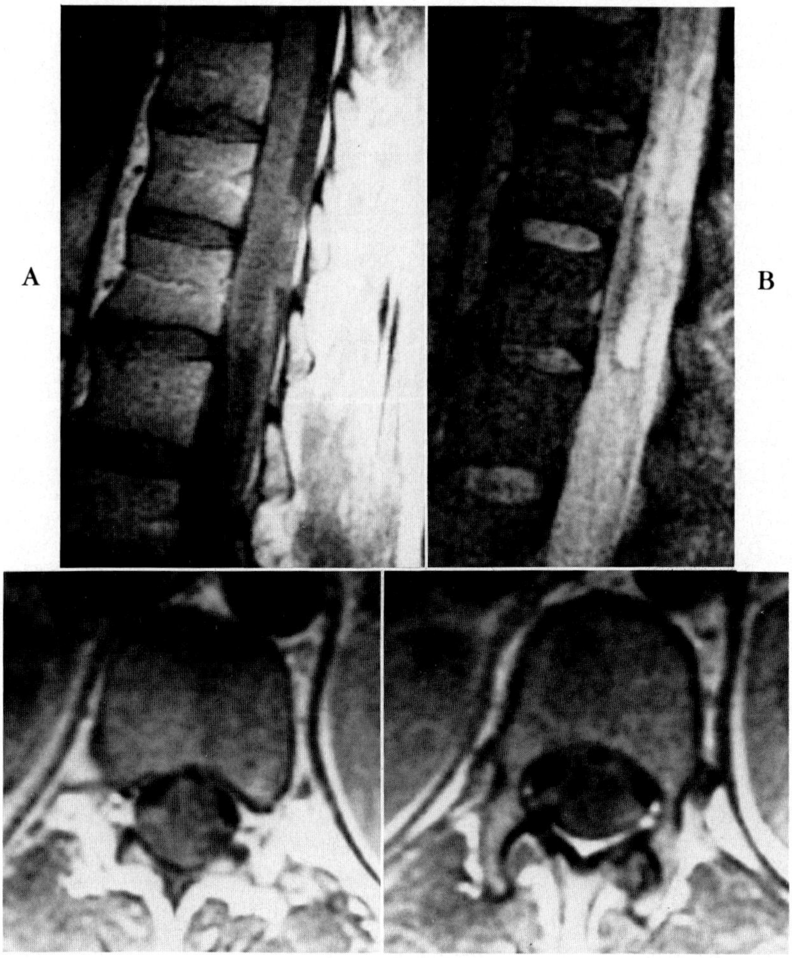

FIGURE 11-20. Cord Infarction. MR scans of female with systemic lupus erythematosis (SLE) and abrupt onset of conus symptoms indicative of acute infarction. T1W sagittal scan (SE 600/20) shows abnormal low signal in conus and unusual, posterior, asymmetric cord enlargement (**A, C,** and **D**). Signal abnormality and enlargement are better appreciated on axial T1W scans (SE 800/20) (**C** and **D**). **B,** Sagittal T2W scan (SE 2400/100) shows abnormal high signal within distal cord delineating extent of infarction.

Clinical

Subacute necrotic myelitis affects males more than females and the old more than the young. It has been associated with cor pulmonale. Typically, cauda equina and the distal cord symptoms have a gradual onset, progressing slowly over a period of 6 months to 4 years.[5a,20a] Weakness of the lower extremities shows a slowly ascending pattern. Early in the course of the disease, spasticity is prominent, and later flaccidity is characteristic.[5a,20a] Therefore, upper and lower motor neuron signs and symptoms can be present. Dorsal column and other sensory findings appear, usually after the onset of lower extremity motor changes. Clinically the differential diagnosis may include amyotrophic lateral sclerosis, various tumors, and spinal cord vascular malformations.

Pathology

Subacute necrotic myelitis shows characteristic histologic features that involve the spinal cord parenchyma and leptomeninges, in particular the veins in the cord parenchyma and on the surface.[9a,20a] The cord shows extensive areas of coagulative necrosis involving both gray and white matter. The leptomeninges are thickened

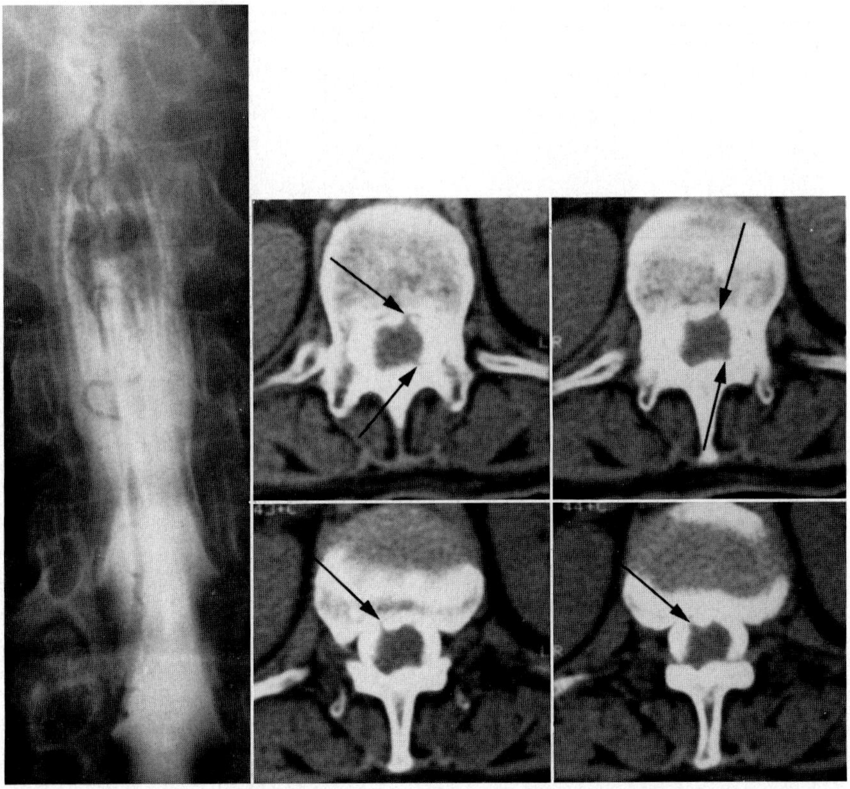

FIGURE 11-21. Foix-Alajouanine syndrome. Myelogram, CT scan, MR scan, and intraoperative ultrasound scan of a 73-year-old female who had a 2-year history of progressive lower extremity paraparesis and more recent sensory loss in both feet. Surgical exploration showed the presence of dilated tortuous superficial veins on both the ventral and dorsal surfaces of the conus but no AVM. Some veins were thrombosed, and others were patent. Necrotic material was found within the cord parenchyma. There was no evidence of an AVM either by spinal angiography or surgical exploration. **A,** AP myelogram shows an enlarged conus with prominent tortuous vessels overlying the conus and extending in both a cephalad and caudad direction. Findings appear typical for a spinal cord AVM. **B-E:** Axial CT scans performed after the myelogram shows an enlarged irregular conus with focal filling defects on the surface of the cord consistent with dilated vessels *(arrows)*. *Continued.*

and show evidence of focal arachnoiditis with associated inflammatory cellular infiltrates. The most characteristic pathologic finding involves the veins within, as well as on the anterior and posterior surfaces of the cord parenchyma. The veins are thick-walled, with the thickening caused by connective tissue deposition and infiltration by macrophages and lymphocytes.[9a,20a] The vein walls also may show extensive calcification. The veins themselves are large, tortuous, and in some segments, thrombosed. Some of these thrombosed veins show evidence of recanalization. Despite these extensive venous changes the arteries, even within the thickened leptomeninges, are typically normal.[20a] This combination of findings suggests a subacute thrombophlebitis.[9a,20a] Cord damage is presumed secondary to a venous type of infarction.

MR Findings

Findings on MR, CT, and conventional myelography are suggestive of a spinal cord vascular malformation (Figure 11-21). The distal thoracic cord and conus may be enlarged. All studies show evidence of abnormal prominent vasculature, which may be most evident on conventional myelography that shows the serpiginous filling defects. The intrathecally enhanced CT scan shows similar findings where the surface of

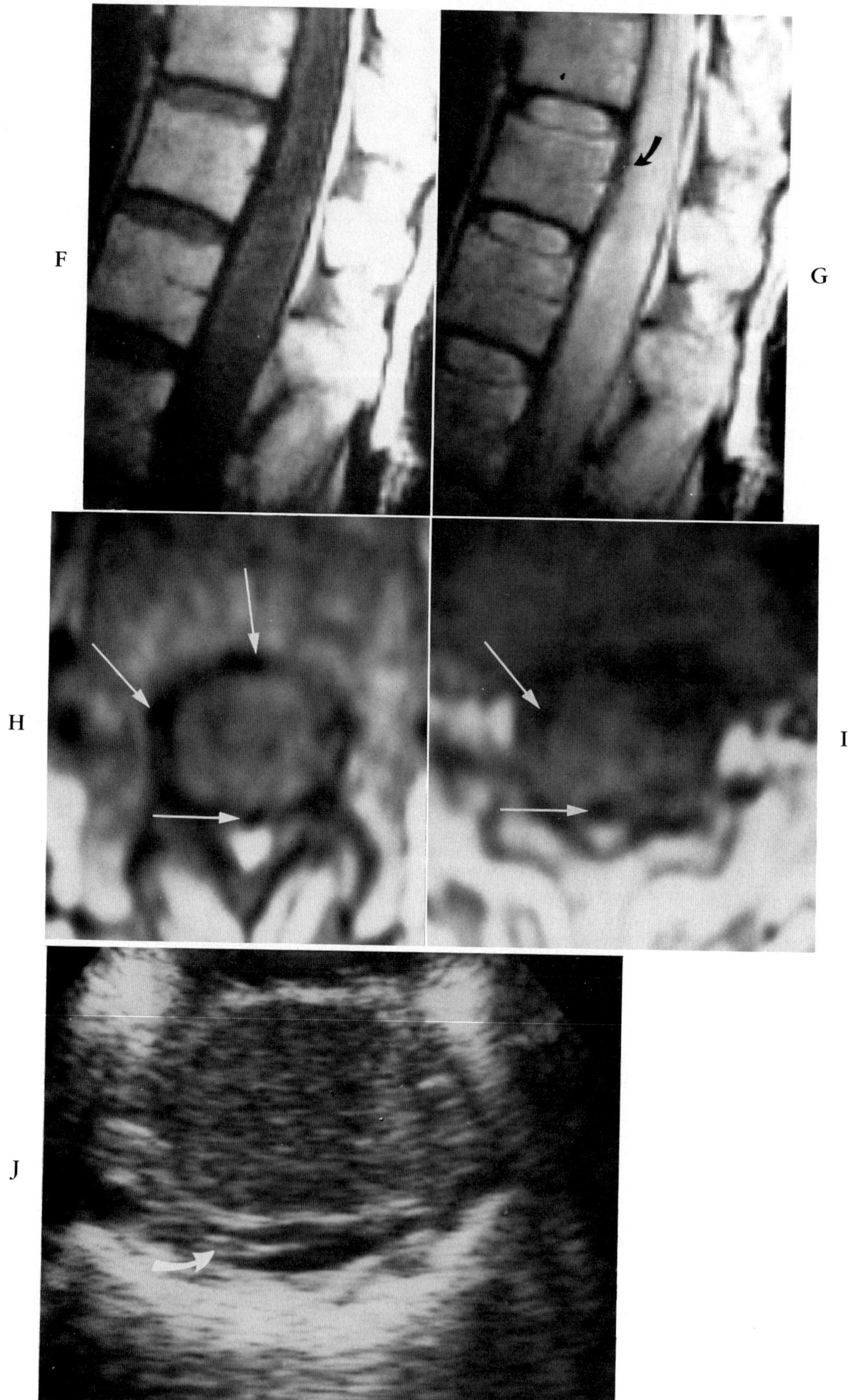
F
G
H
I
J

FIGURE 11-21, cont'd. F, Sagittal T1W scan (SE 500/17) obtained with a small surface coil shows diffuse enlargement of the distal thoracic cord and conus. Cord parenchyma is abnormal low signal intensity, which is relatively homogenous and central in the cord. Obvious regions of signal loss resulting from dilated vessels are not easily identified on this view. **G,** Sagittal T2W scan (SE 2100/30) (balanced image) confirms enlarged cord and conus. Cord parenchyma shows only mild inhomogenity. One area suggests small signal voids indicative of dilated vessels *(curved arrow)*. Axial T1W scans (SE 1000/25) show inhomogeneous signal intensity within enlarged conus (**H**). Numerous small focal areas of signal loss, adjacent to surface of the cord, could present channels of CSF flow and pulsation or dilated vessels. Dilated vessels proved to be superficial veins on surgical exploration (*arrows,* **H** and **I**). Ascending lumbar veins are somewhat prominent (**H**). **J,** Axial view of the conus by intraoperative ultrasound. Conus is diffusely enlarged and relatively hypoechoic, but the echo pattern is homogeneous. Increased echogenicity seen on the ventral surface of the cord represents enlarged superficial veins *(arrow)*. (**H,** Courtesy of Dr. Solomon Batnitzky).

the cord has an irregular appearance. The MR scan visualizes this same irregular cord surface. If the veins are patent, they appear as tortuous serpiginous signal voids on the surface of the cord (see Figure 11-21). The cord parenchyma may exhibit some inhomogenous signal intensity on both T1W and T2W MR scans at the site of enlargement and beyond. These cord parenchymal changes and the associated surface vascularity can be quite similar to the MR findings seen in the dural type of spinal AVM (see Dural AVM). In dural AVMs the dilated vessels are not likely to be as large and are usually limited to the dorsal surface of the cord, rather than dorsal and ventral, in this disease process. A characteristic of all these patients with subacute necrotic myelitis, despite this prominent vasculature on the imaging studies, is an invariably negative spinal arteriogram. The MR scan and a negative spinal arteriogram decreases confusion between this entity and the other spinal vascular malformation and the cryptic AVMs (see Slow Flow Vascular Malformations—"Cryptic").

REFERENCES

1. Beatty RM, Winston KR. Spontaneous cervical epidural hematoma. J Neurosurg 1984;61:143.
2. Cahan LD, Higashida RT, Halbach VV, et al. Variants of radiculomeningeal vascular malformations of the spine. J Neurosurg 1987;66:333.
3. Cosgrove GR, Bertrand G, Fontaine S, et al. Cavernous angiomas of the spinal cord. J Neurosurg 1988;68:31.
4. Dillon WP, Bolla K, Mark A, et al. Gadolinium DTPA MR of intradural spinal cord diseases. Radiology 1989; 170:229.
5. Dormont D, Gelbert F, Assouline E, et al. MR imaging of spinal cord arteriovenous malformations at 0.5 T: study of 34 cases. AJNR 1988;Z9:833.

5a. Foix C, Alajouanine T. Rev Neurol 1926;2:1.

6. Gomori JM, Grossman RI, Hackney DB, et al. Variable appearances of subacute intracranial hematomas on high-field spin-echo MR. AJNR 1987;8:1019.
7. Griffin C, DeLaPaz R, Enzmann DR. Magnetic resonance appearance of slow flow vascular malformations of the brainstem. Neuroradiology 1987;29:512.
8. Haykal HA, Wang A-M, Zamani AA, et al. Computed tomography of spontaneous acute cervical epidural hematoma. J Comput Assist Tomogr 1984;3:229.
9. Lanzieri CF, Sacher M, Solodnik P, et al. CT myelography of spontaneous spinal epidural hematoma. J Comput Assist Tomogr 1985;9:393.

9a. Mair WGP, Folkers JF. Necrosis of the spinal cord due to thrombophlebitis (subacute necrotic myelitis). Brain, 1953;76:563.

10. Masaryk TJ, Ross JS, Modic MT, et al. Radioculomeningeal vascular malformations of the spine: MR imaging. Radiology 1987;164:845.
11. Oldfield EH, DeChiro G, Quindlen EA, et al. Successful treatment of a group of spinal cord arteriovenous malformations by interruption of dural fistula. J Neurosurg 1983;59:1019.
12. Pear BL. Spinal epidural hematoma. AJR 1972;115:155.
13. Post MJD, Seminer DS, Quencer RM. CT diagnosis of spinal epidural hematoma. AJNR 1982;3:190.
14. Riche MC, Modenesi-Freitas J, Djindjian M, et al. Arteriovenous malformations (AVM) of the spinal cord in children. Neuroradiology 1982;22:171.
15. Rosenblum B, Oldfield EH, Doppman JL, et al. Spinal arteriovenous malformations: a comparison of dural arteriovenous fistulas and intradural AVMs in 81 patients. J Neurosurg 1987;67:795.
16. Rothfus WE, Chedid MK, Deeb ZL, et al. MR imaging in the diagnosis of spontaneous spinal epidural hematomas. J Comput Assist Tomogr 1987;11:851.
17. Sze G, Krol G, Zimmerman RD, et al. Intramedullary disease of the spine: diagnosis using gadolinium-DTPA-enhanced MR imaging. AJNR 1988;9:847.
18. Ueda S, Saito A, Inomori S, et al. Cavernous angioma of the cauda equina producing subarachnoid hemorrhage. J Neurosurg 1987;66:134.
19. Vaquero J, Martinez R, Martinez P. Cavernomas of the spinal cord: report of two cases. Neurosurgery 1988; 22:143.
20. Veerapen RJ, Sbeih IA, O'Laoire SA. Surgical treatment of cryptic AVMs and associated hematoma in the brain stem and spinal cord. J Neurosurg 1986;65:188.

20a. Wirth FP, Post KD, DiChiro G, et al. Foix-Alajouanine disease: spontaneous thrombosis of a spinal cord arteriovenous malformation: a case report. Neurology 1970; 20:1114.

21. Zilkha A, Irwin GAL, Fagelman D. Computed tomography of spinal epidural hematoma. AJNR 1983;4:1073.

12
Syringomyelia

Dieter R. Enzmann

ETIOLOGY

The term *syringomyelia* is confusing when it is used indiscriminately to refer to any type of cyst in the spinal cord. In this chapter, *syrinx* will refer only to a non-neoplastic cystic cavity of the spinal cord. The cystic cavity is not associated with an intraaxial tumor and does not have neoplastic tissue in its walls. A syrinx cavity, however, may be associated with an extraaxial tumor such as meningioma.[16,17,20]

Neither the etiology nor pathogenesis of syringomyelia is well understood. Contrast media and CT have not clarified the pathogenesis because enhancement of the cyst even on delayed scans is not specific for syrinx.[2,6,8,10,19] MR may be more informative. Syrinx occurs in specific clinical settings, suggesting some associated and predisposing factors that may have a causative role in its formation. Syringomyelia is associated with a number of congenital lesions.[23,24] One of the most common is the Chiari malformation, both I and II (Figure 12-1). With Chiari II malformation and its associated myelomeningocele, syrinx cavities may be seen anywhere in the cord but are often seen in the lower thoracic cord or in the distal portion of a tethered cord (Figures 12-2 to 12-4). Syrinx cavities are also seen in very complex congenital malformations such as diastematomyelia or even double spinal cords (see Chapter 5, Figure 5-9). MR demonstrates cavities that were undetectable with previous imaging methods.

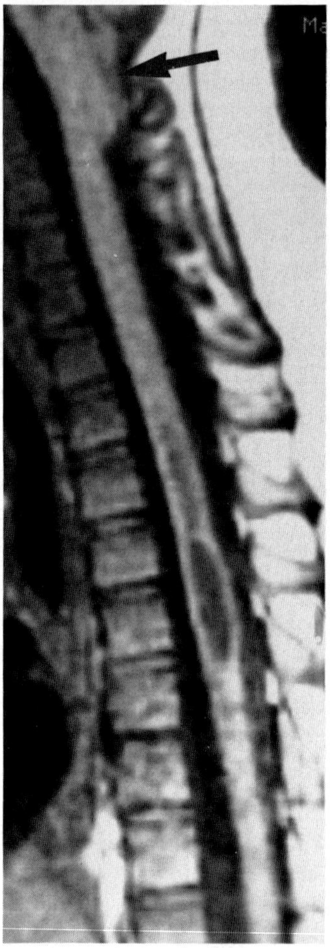

FIGURE 12-1. Sagittal T1W (SE 800/20) scan shows syrinx in upper thoracic cord associated with Chiari II malformation. Note tonsillar ectopia extending down to C_3 *(arrow)*. Fluid in syrinx did not exhibit motion.

A 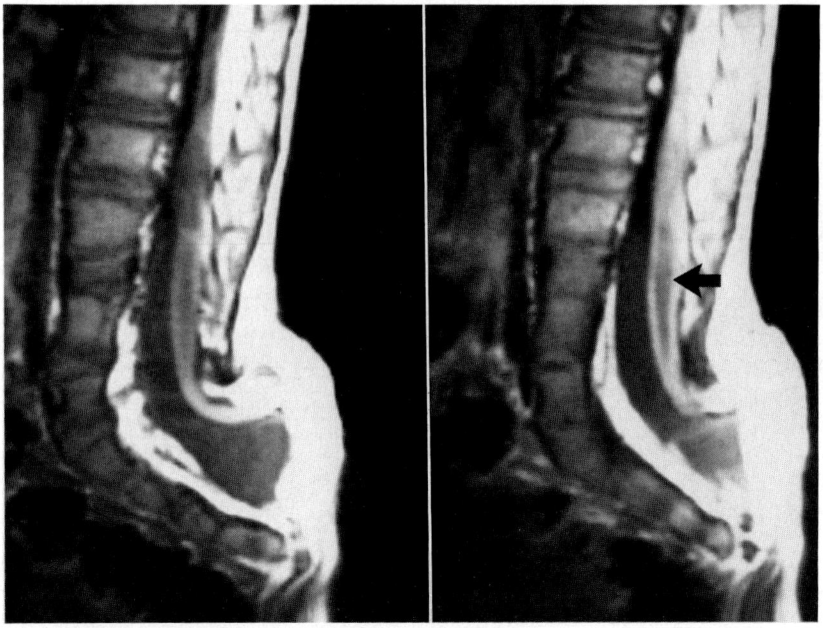 B

FIGURE 12-2. Syringomyelia associated with meningomyelocele in four-year-old male. **A** and **B**, Sagittal T1W scans (800/20) show vertebral body anomalies: widened lumbar canal with tethered cord ending in small lipoma within meningomyelocele. A small syrinx is seen in tethered cord *(arrow)*. *Continued.*

Syrinx cavities are probably more common than suspected in patients with Chiari I malformation (Figures 12-5 and 12-6). The syrinx cavity is detected early in most congenital lesions but in Chiari I malformation the syrinx usually presents later in life. The fact that patients with Paget's disease with narrowing of the foramen magnum also develop syrinx suggests that abnormal CSF flow around the foramen magnum contributes to the development of syringomyelia in patients with Chiari I and its propensity for a cervical location (see Figures 12-5 and 12-6).

Another relatively common cause for the development of syrinx is the posttraumatic spinal cord (see Figures 12-9 and 12-16).* Syrinx may present clinically within a few months to many years after trauma; the trauma is usually severe enough to have resulted in partial or complete paraplegia or tetraplegia.[5] The syrinx often initially develops at the specific site of injury where the cord has been damaged and usually extends rostrally, but caudal extension is also seen. The time course of syrinx development has not been elucidated (Figures 12-7 to 12-9). Rostral extension is more common with the syrinx often extending all the way to the cranial-cervical junction (see Figure 12-9). MR scans reveal a much higher incidence of syrinx in posttraumatic patients, primarily because the diagnosis of syrinx with other imaging techniques is difficult in that atrophic cords, even with a syrinx cavity present, often do not show enlargement. CT with metrizamide can show contrast accumulation in areas that are microcystic without a true syrinx.[9] Although syrinx is an important cause for neurologic deterioration in posttraumatic spinal cord injury, it is not the only cause and other disease entities, such as subarachnoid cysts that can cause cord compression (Figure 12-10; see Figure 12-13)[1,13] and abnormal hypertrophy of the posterior longitudinal ligament, resulting in severe spinal stenosis and cord compression, must be considered. Subarachnoid cyst must be differentiated from a dilated subarachnoid space (Figure 12-11).

The pathogenesis of syrinx formation in posttraumatic patients is not well understood, although abnormal CSF flow and pulsation pat-

*References 5, 7, 9, 17, 18, 21, 22, 25, 26.

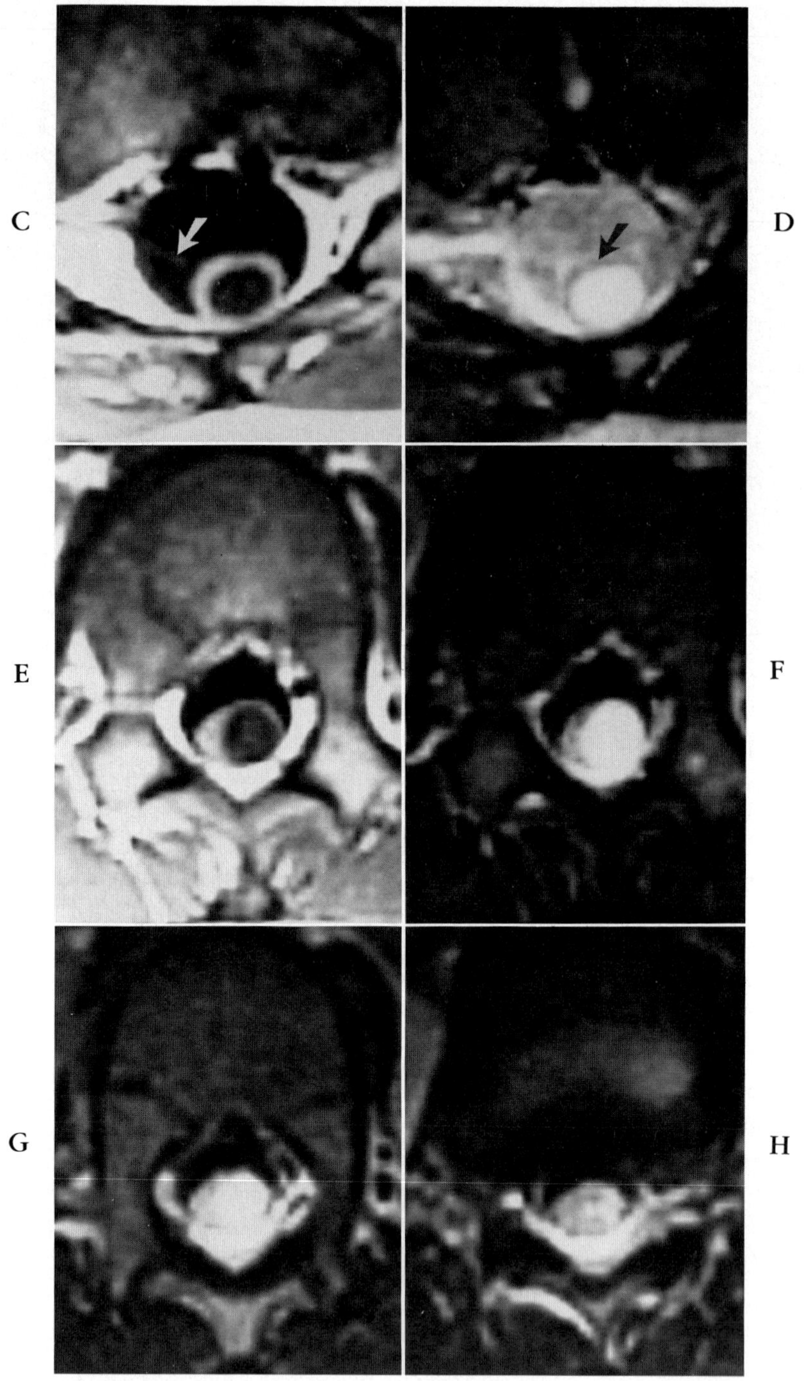

FIGURE 12-2, cont'd. **C** and **E**, Axial T1W scans (SE 800/20) show well-defined cyst within cord. **D** and **F**, Axial T2W images (2000/80) at same levels as T1W scans show high signal in cyst fluid indicating lack of fluid motion. Note cord signal intensity is normal on T2W images (*arrow*, **D**). At lower level, nerve root exits cord on right (*arrow*, **C**). Note difference in fluid pulsation within subarachnoid space in lower lumbar sac (**D**) compared to higher levels (**F**) where motion is greater; thus signal loss is greater. This difference in signal intensity can be appreciated on T1W sagittal scan (**B**) where approximately three different zones are seen: (1) very low signal at level L_1 and L_2, (2) intermediate signal at L_3-L_5, and (3) higher signal in meningomyelocele. Signal intensity differences reflect degree of CSF motion. T2W images at rostal end of syrinx show abnormal high signal within cord immediately above cyst (**G**) and normal cord above this level (**H**).

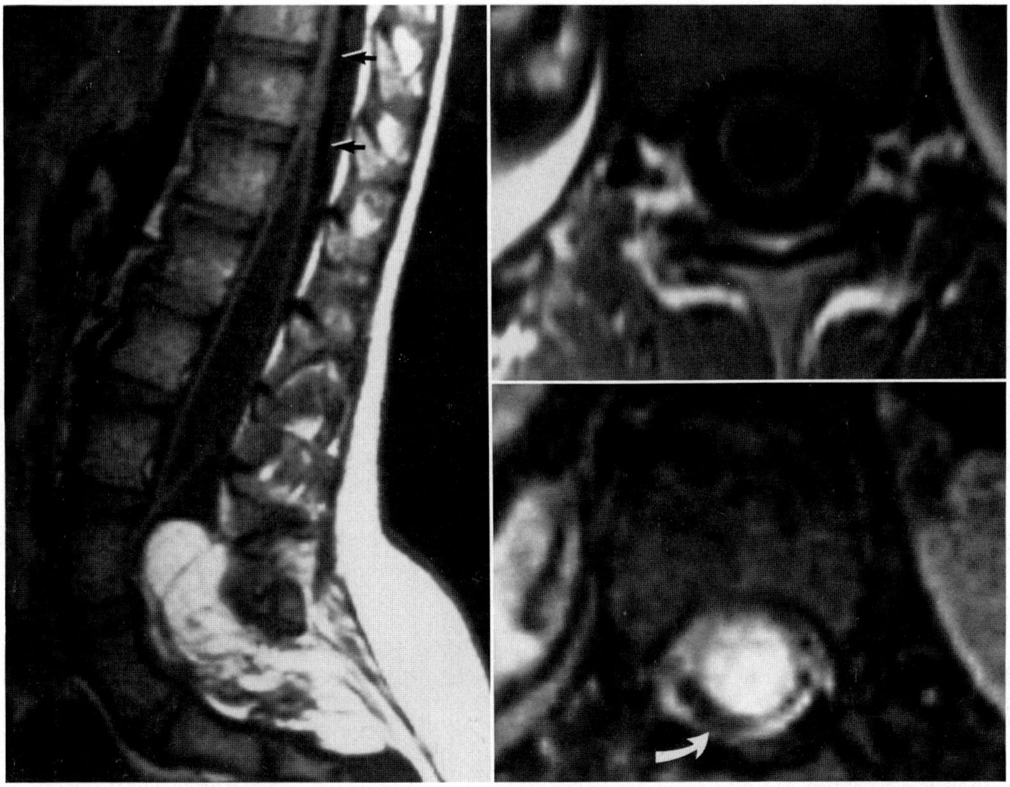

FIGURE 12-3. **A**, Sagittal T1W scan (SE 800/20) shows large syrinx in distal tethered cord that ends in large intradural and extradural lipomeningocele. The thin channel of **CSF** motion can also be seen as a thin strip of low signal intensity dorsal to the cord (*arrows*, **A**). **B**, Axial T1W scan (SE 1000/20) through midsyrinx shows well-defined centrally located cyst surrounded by thin rim of cord tissue. **C**, Axial ungated T2W scan (SE 2000/80) at same level shows high signal intensity in cyst fluid indicating no significant motion of fluid. Cord tissue signal intensity is normal, an intermediate shade of gray. Outside the cord the posterior, irregular, curvilinear area of low signal (*arrow*) indicates motion of subarachnoid CSF. The channel of CSF motion is seen as thin strip of low signal intensity dorsal to cord (*arrows*, **A**).

terns caused by the injury are thought to play a role. Actual rents in the cord leading to cysts have been identified but their development is not clear.[14] Posttrauma patients also develop local but significant arachnoiditis at the injury site that can alter CSF flow but the role of such changes is not known. Similarly, diffuse arachnoiditis has been associated with syrinx. The arachnoiditis can be caused by infectious chronic meningitis, arachnoiditis associated with Pantopaque, surgery, and other inflammatory diseases such as ankylosing spondylitis (Figures 12-12 and 12-13). These patients are also susceptible to subarachnoid cyst formation (see Figures 12-10 and 12-13). Syrinx has even been reported with severe spondylosis.[32]

Spinal subarachnoid cysts have been reported in conjunction with posttraumatic syrinx.[1] Their association suggests a common pathogenesis secondary to arachnoiditis and abnormal CSF dynamics but this remains to be proven. Arachnoid cysts cause symptoms by compressing the cord or nerve roots. Clinical manifestations, as well as the symptoms attributable to syrinx, are delayed after trauma. Their identification is important because syrinx treatment failure may be the result of enlargement of such arachnoid cysts rather than failure to decompress the syrinx.[1,13] These cysts and a syrinx may be in a type of dynamic equilibrium in that a decrease in syrinx size may result in an increase in subarachnoid cyst size and a lack of clinical relief of symp-

Text continued on p. 552.

A

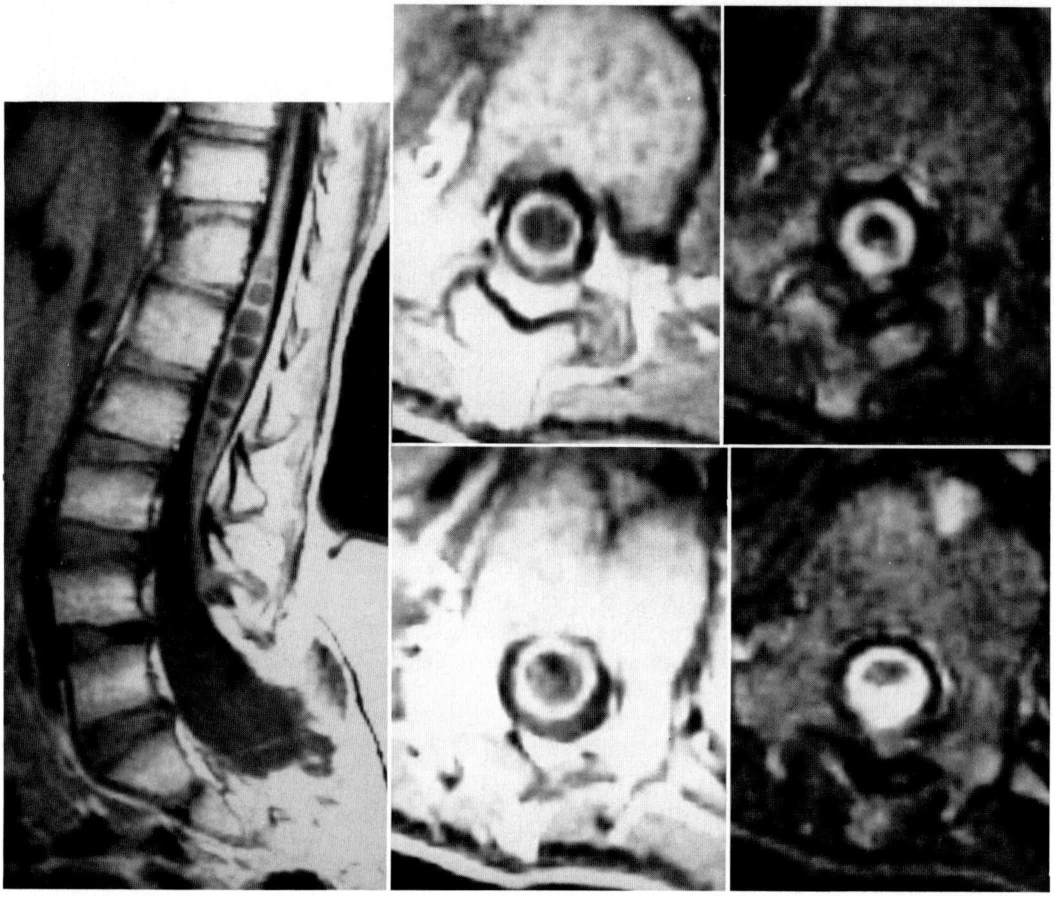

B, C

D, E

FIGURE 12-4. Syrinx of distal cord, in addition to tethered cord and myelomeningocele, in nine-year-old male. **A,** Sagittal T1W scan (SE 800/20) shows multiloculated appearance of syrinx. Note lower signal intensity of CSF anterior to syrinx compared to higher signal CSF lower in myelomeningocele indicating greater pulsation around syrinx compared to distal sac. **B** and **D,** Axial T1W (SE 1000/20) and **C** and **E,** axial T2W ungated (SE 2000/80) scans show morphology of syrinx cavity and signal loss in central cavity indicating fluid motion. This motion is complex. At one level fluid motion is in central region of the cyst (**B** and **C**). At higher level (**D** and **E**) only anterior portion of cavity shows signal loss; posterior portion retains signal indicating static fluid. Patient underwent surgery with release of tethered cord and a myelotomy for treatment of syrinx.

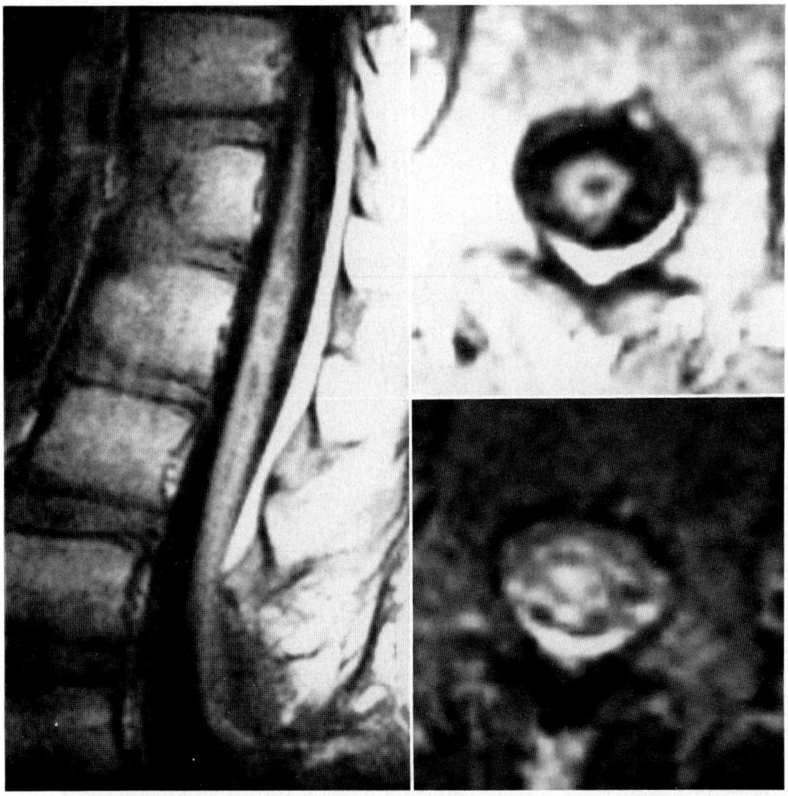

F G H

FIGURE 12-4, cont'd. **F,** Postoperative sagittal T1W scan (SE 800/20) shows collapse of syrinx with only small central cystic space remaining. **G,** Postoperative axial T1W (SE 1000/20) scan shows small, residual central low signal cyst, which on **H,** ungated T2W scan (SE 2000/80) exhibited high signal, indicating lack of fluid motion.

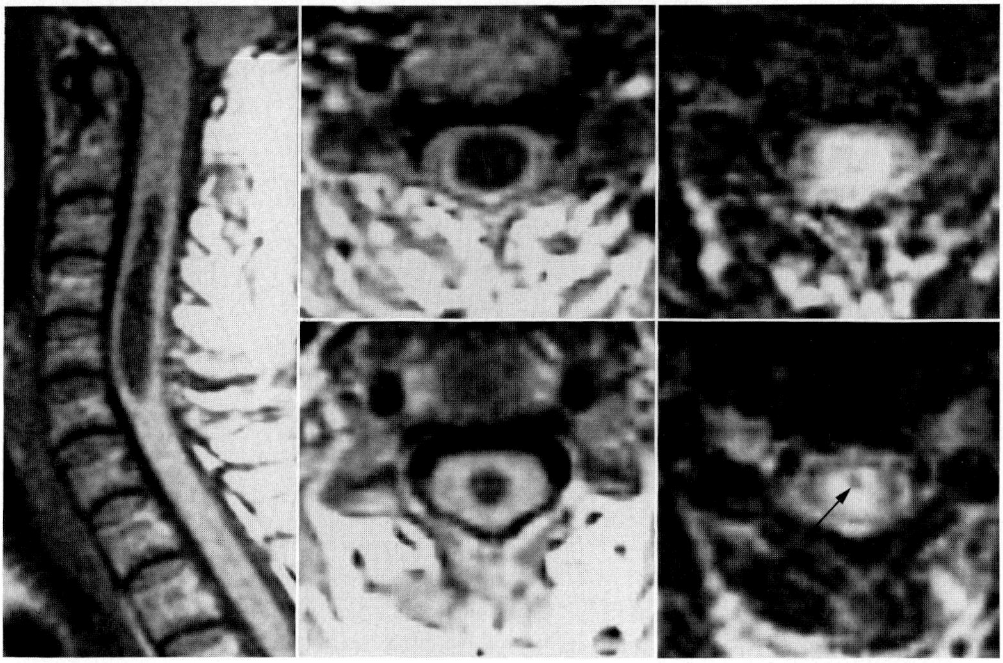

A B, C D, E

FIGURE 12-5. **A,** T1W sagittal scan (SE 800/20) shows focal cystic cavity extending from C_3-C_6. **B** and **D,** Axial T1W scans (SE 1000/20) show well-circumscribed cystic cavity in enlarged cord. Axial ungated T2W scans (2000/80) show prominent high signal within cyst indicating lack of fluid motion (**C**) except for one small area in lower portion of cyst (*arrow,* **E**). Comparing cyst size and area of abnormal signal at upper level (**D** and **E**), high signal intensity area is larger than cyst size, indicating adjacent area of abnormal cord tissue suggestive of myelomalacia. Syrinx shows essentially static fluid by SE technique with only one punctate area of minimal motion (see Figure 12-15).

A, B 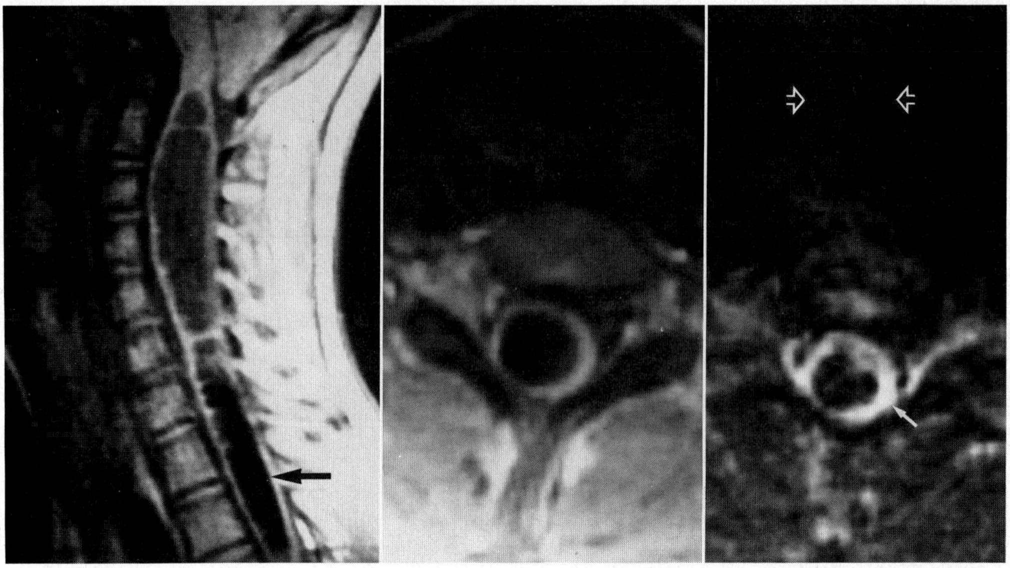 C

FIGURE 12-6. MR scan of 11-year-old female with symptoms of pain in upper back and right shoulder shows extensive syrinx extending from foramen magnum to conus medullaris in Chiari I malformation. **A**, T1W scan (SE 800/20) shows syrinx was a long-standing process indicated by enlargement of upper cervical spinal canal. Note greater signal loss in lower cervical cord *(arrow)* compared to upper cord indicating greater motion. **B**, Axial T1W scan (SE 1000/20) shows syrinx to be large single cystic cavity. **C**, Ungated axial T2W scan (SE 2000/80) at same level shows marked signal loss within cavity indicating fluid motion, and mismapping in phase-encoding direction of signal derived from this moving fluid *(paired open arrows)*. Note also diffuse abnormal high signal intensity of cord *(single arrow)*. Low signal is seen in subarachnoid space where CSF is pulsating. Maximal amount of CSF motion did not occur at rostral end of syrinx where it is largest diameter but rather in middle of syrinx in cervical and thoracic regions. Distribution of CSF motion does not suggest rostral (obex) to caudal transmission.

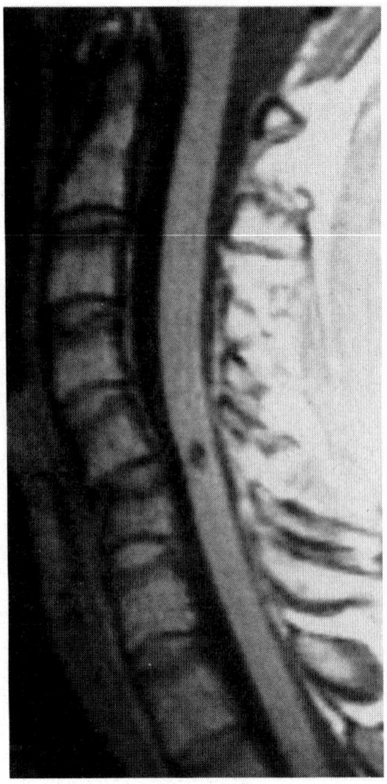

FIGURE 12-7. Sagittal T1W scan (SE 800/20) shows sequellae of posttraumatic injury to midcervical cord resulting in formation of small cyst, representing a very small syrinx. This stage does not show fluid motion. Whether this stage of cord damage progresses to a larger cyst and if so, at what rate, has not been determined.

A B

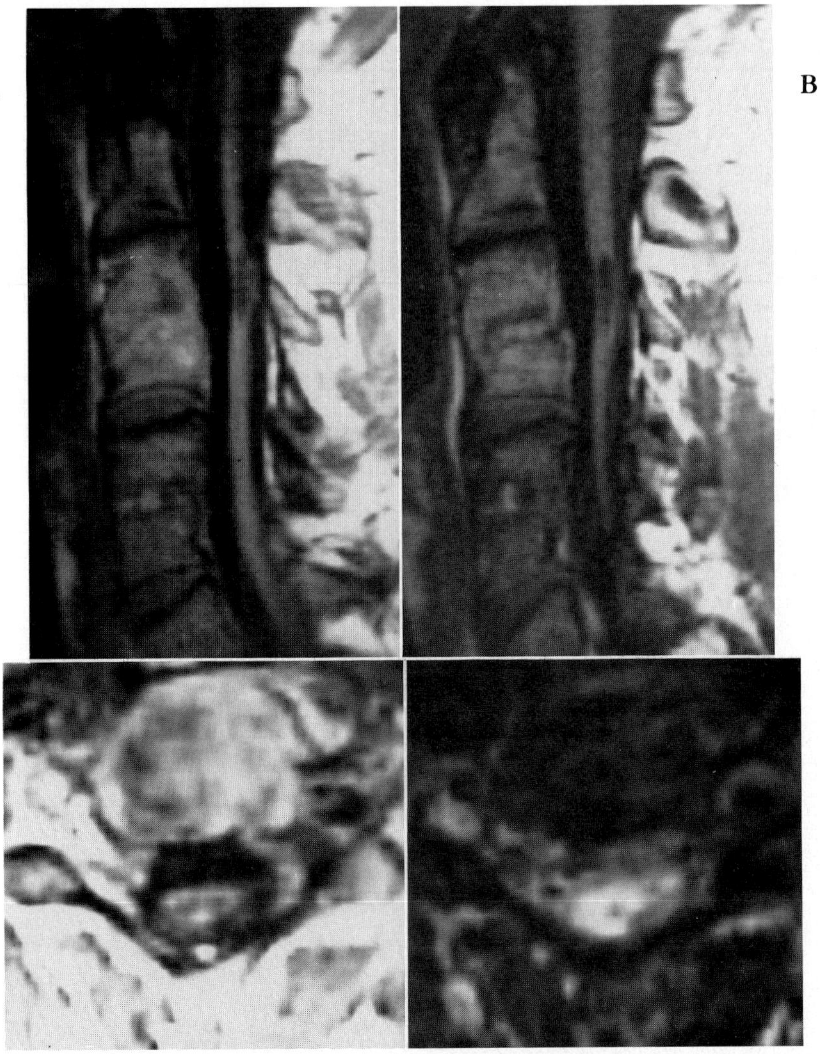

C D

FIGURE 12-8. **A** and **B,** Posttraumatic spine shows partial fusion of C_3 and C_4 at site of trauma. Sagittal T1W scans (SE 800/20) show cord atrophy and focal area of low signal intensity at site of trauma. Axial views through this low signal area suggest part that is cystic and part that represents myelomalacia. **C,** Axial T1W scan (SE 1000/20) shows atrophic cord and horizontal area of low signal intensity within cord. **D,** Second echo of T2W scan (SE 2000/80) shows abnormal signal within cord parenchyma and in the small cystic region, indicating abnormal cord tissue (myelomalacia) and static cyst fluid. Relatively high signal in CSF around cord in dilated subarachnoid space indicates decreased CSF pulsation even in anterolateral recesses where normally prominent CSF pulsation is seen.

A B

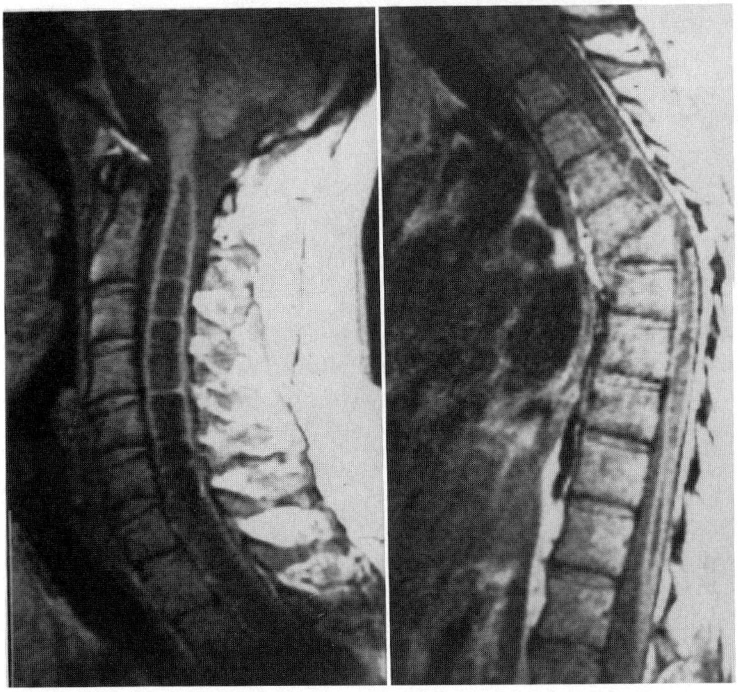

FIGURE 12-9. **A** and **B,** Posttraumatic syrinx in 26-year-old male. Cyst propagated in both caudal and rostral directions. Site of trauma resulted in wedged vertebra and spinal canal narrowing. T1W scan (SE 800/20) shows syrinx septated and largest in cervical region.

Continued.

C
D
E
F
G
H

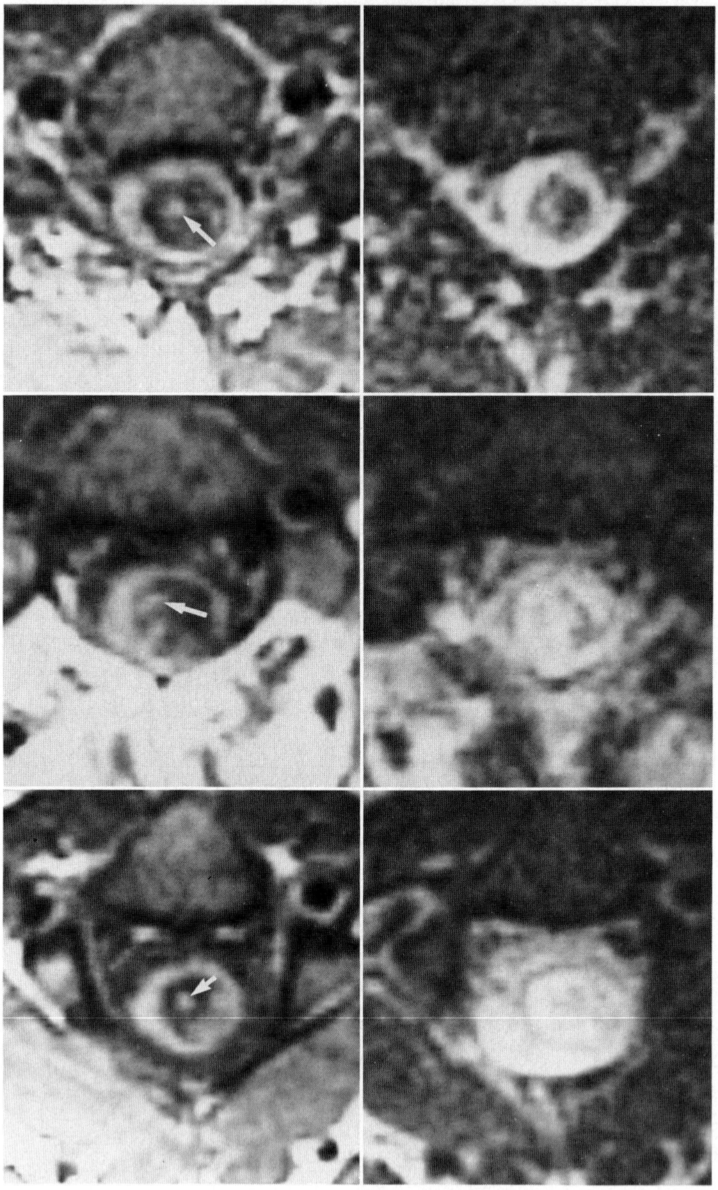

FIGURE 12-9, cont'd. **C**, **E**, and **G**, Axial T1W scans (SE 1000/20) show slightly asymmetrically placed cyst with complex internal septations *(arrows)*. **D**, Axial ungated T2W scans (2000/80) show signal loss in midcervical level but high signal within cyst at rostral end (**F** and **H**), indicating fluid motion in midportion of syrinx but little at its rostral limit (see Figure 12-16).

A

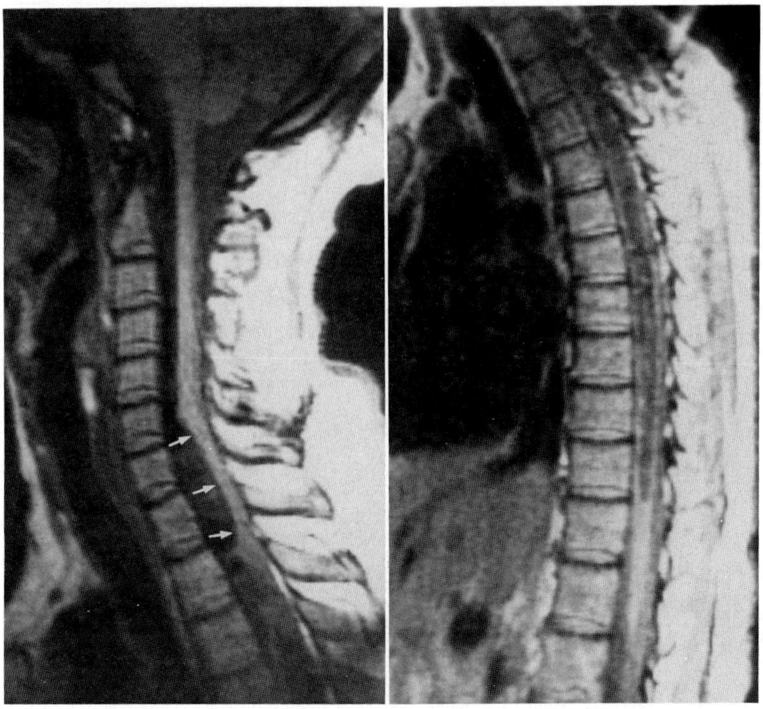

B

FIGURE 12-10. Sagittal T1W scans in patient with syringomyelia and subarachnoid cysts secondary to previous Tb meningitis. **A,** Sagittal view of cervical spine shows large low signal extramedullary area extending from C_6-T_2 causing convex indentation of cord anteriorly *(arrows)*. **B,** Sagittal view of thoracic cord shows long syrinx. No other subarachnoid cysts are identified. Diffuse increased signal intensity in subarachnoid space is secondary to arachnoiditis. In patients with syringomyelia associated with arachnoiditis, subarachnoid cysts as potential cause of clinical deterioration should be considered. (Courtesy of Dr. Alexander Marks.)

A, B

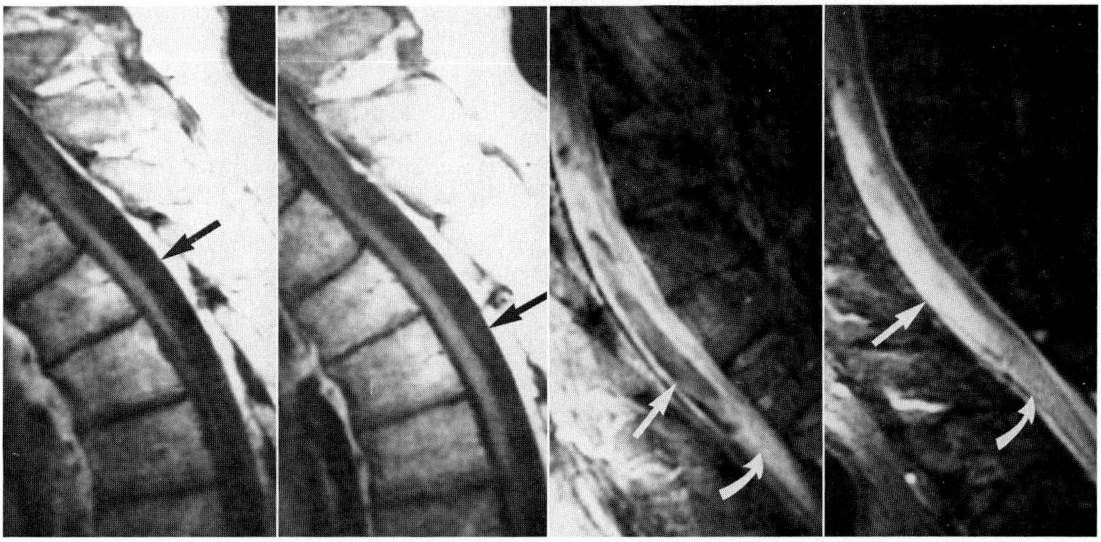

C, D

FIGURE 12-11. MR scan in posttraumatic patient in which findings could be mistaken for subarachnoid cyst. **A** and **B,** Sagittal T1W scans (SE 800/20) at cervical thoracic junction show prominent low signal intensity subarachnoid space behind thin spinal cord *(arrows)*, which could be mistaken for an asymmetrical dorsal syrinx. **C,** Sagittal T2W scan (gated and flow-compensated SE 1800/80) shows abnormal high signal intensity in distal cervical cord *(curved arrow)* and region of prominent high signal intensity CSF dorsal to thin cord *(straight arrow)*. T2W image and T1W images suggest possibility of dorsal posttraumatic subarachnoid cyst compressing spinal cord. **D,** Nonmotion-compensated T2W scan (SE 2000/80) shows signal loss in region dorsal to cord indicating CSF motion *(straight arrow)*. Area of high signal intensity in distal cervical cord is again noted *(curved arrow)*.

Continued.

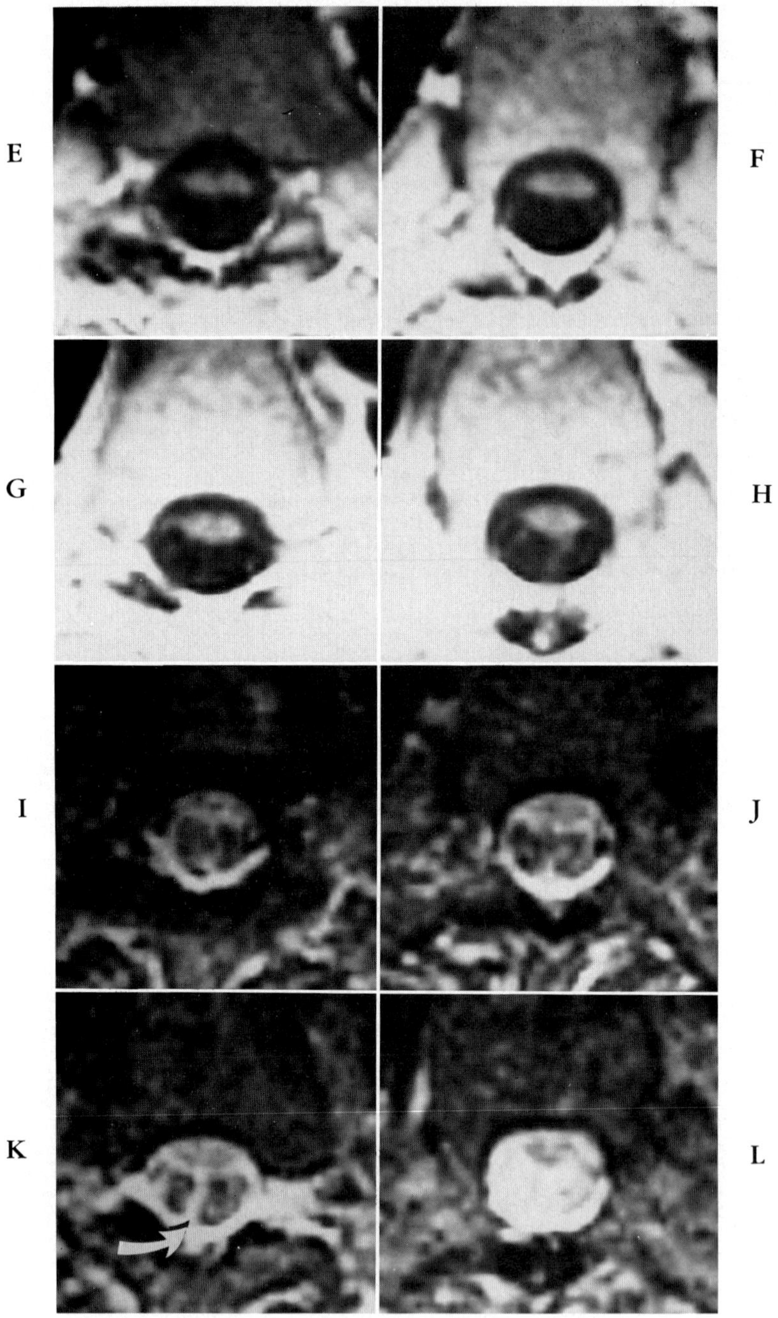

FIGURE 12-11, cont'd. **E-H,** Close inspection of axial T1W scans (SE 1000/20) shows prominent subarachnoid space dorsal to cord has fine arachnoid septations within it. No single cyst could be identified. **I-L,** Axial ungated and uncompensated T2W scans (SE 2000/80) at same levels as axial T1W scans show prominent areas of signal loss in dorsal subarachnoid space. Multiple compartments and arachnoid septations are confirmed on these scans. Septations are well visualized because they are accentuated by adjacent static fluid (*arrow,* **K**).

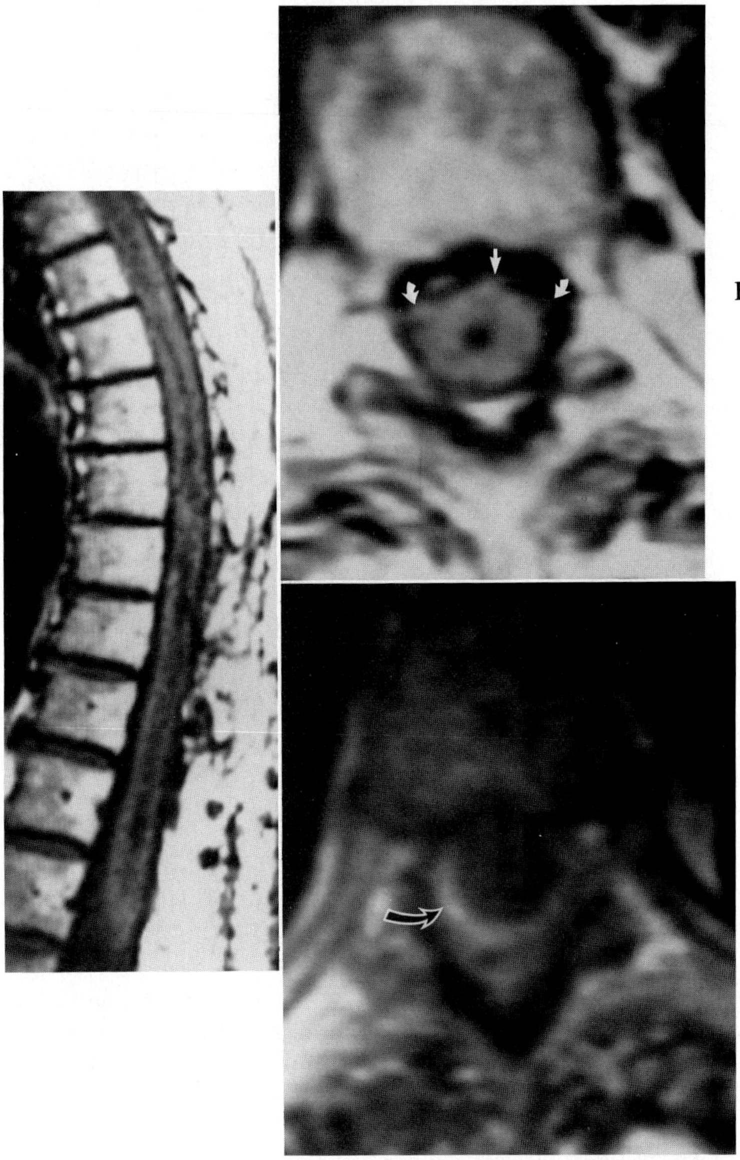

FIGURE 12-12. **A,** Sagittal T1W scan (SE 600/20) of patient with biopsy proven chronic arachnoiditis and syringomyelia. Cord appears enlarged and has "shaggy," poorly defined margin. In addition, it has central area of low signal intensity indicative of syrinx (**A** and **B**). **B,** Axial T1W scan (SE 1000/20) confirms cord enlargement, irregular margin secondary to leptomeningeal arachnoiditis *(arrows)*, and small, central cyst representing syrinx. **C,** PostGdDTPA scan (SE 600/20) shows prominent enhancement of arachnoiditis surrounding cord *(arrow)*. This finding unfortunately is similar to appearance of leptomeningeal carcinomatosis although clinical history usually allows differentiation. (Courtesy of William Dillon, M.D.)

A, B 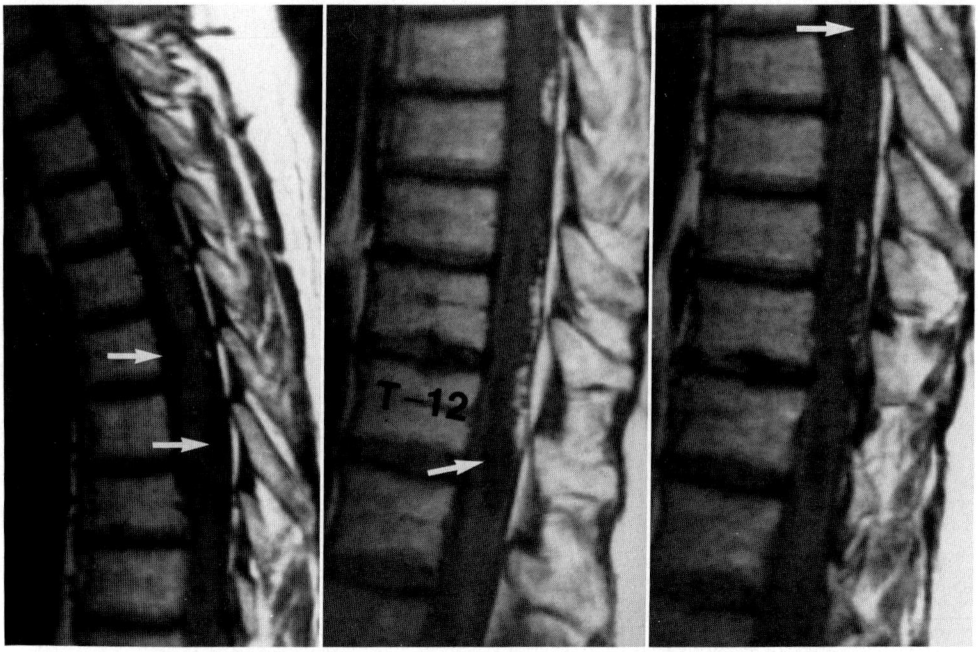 C

FIGURE 12-13. **A,** Sagittal T1W scan (SE 600/25) of upper thoracic cord and **B** and **C,** scans of lower (**C** is lateral to **B**) thoracic cord showing syrinx in conus (**B,** *arrow*) and multiple extradural defects (**A,** *arrows;* **C,** *arrow*) representing multiple subarachnoid cysts impinging on cord and deforming it. Subarachnoid cysts secondary to diffuse arachnoiditis. High signal intensity, small globules dorsal to cord but separate from dorsal epidural fat, are residual Pantopaque droplets in spinal canal. (Courtesy of Dr. David Norman.)

toms.[1,13] MR is the most accurate diagnostic tool available to identify the concurrent presence of such lesions and their response (or lack of response) to treatment.[1,13]

CLINICAL PRESENTATION

Clinically the diagnosis of syringomyelia can be suspected when one of the clinical entities mentioned previously is present. The syrinx cavity in congenital lesions associated with spinal dysraphism often does not have specific symptoms referable to it, in part, because the other abnormalities may simply overshadow its presence. Most of the other disease entities associated with syringomyelia occur over time and appear in the second to fourth decade. Clinically patients seem not to show symptoms until the syrinx has extended into the cervical cord. The classic presentation is that of a patient with decreased pain and temperature sense in the upper extremities that is disassociated from the sense of touch, which is usually preserved. The deficits have a segmental distribution. Associated with sensory findings is muscle wasting of the intrinsic muscles of the hand, sometimes involving the shoulder. These muscle changes are associated with fibrillation and involve one or both of the upper extremities. In some patients, the initial presentation and often the most severe clinical problem is that of increasing pain. The syrinx may be extensive enough to affect long tracks in the spinal cord and thus result in spasticity and ataxia involving the lower extremities and a loss of bladder control. Patients may also experience hyperhidrosis and autonomic dysfunction.

In general, there is no direct correlation between the size of the syrinx as visualized by MR and the severity of clinical symptoms across the different disease entities. In fact, one is struck by how large the syrinx can be in the face of minimal clinical symptoms in patients with Chiari I malformation. In other patients, often posttrauma patients, clinical symptoms may appear with relatively small cysts.

A B, C D E, F

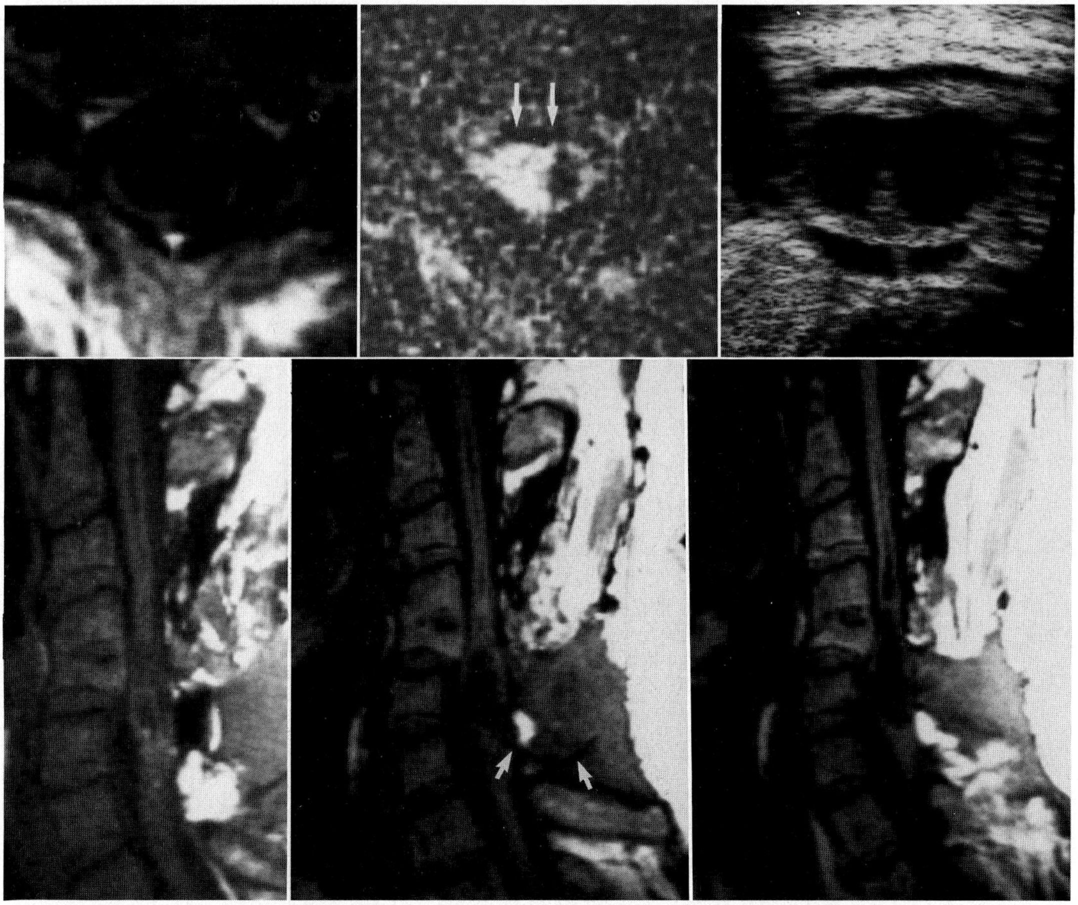

FIGURE 12-14. Posttraumatic (note fusion of C_4-C_5) syrinx patient with **A,** two separate cysts seen on axial T1W scan (SE 1000/20). **B,** Axial T2W scan (SE ungated 2000/80) shows high signal from right cyst and signal loss in left cyst indicating static fluid on right and fluid motion on left. Signal loss in anterior subarachnoid space indicates normal CSF pulsation *(arrows)*. **C,** Intraoperative ultrasound confirmed presence of two cysts. Syringosubarachnoid shunt placed and communication established between cysts. **D,** After surgery, sagittal T1W scan (SE 600/20) shows some residual cyst at C_2-C_3 and C_5-C_6 levels. Scan was obtained shortly after surgery and shows extent of decompression; low signal behind C_6 level represents postoperative air. Note size of residual cyst at C_5-C_6 level. **E** and **F,** One year later with patient experiencing recurrent symptoms, cyst at C_5-C_6 level increased in size while thin syrinx at C_2-C_3 remained unchanged (SE 800/20). Position of shunt tube ends just short of inferior border of lower cyst (*arrows*, **E**). ***Continued.***

MR FINDINGS

Syringomyelia is characterized by two major features: a cyst within the cord parenchyma and associated abnormal cord signal.* The cysts fall into two general categories: (1) a cyst with stationary fluid (see Figures 12-1 to 12-4 and 12-15) and (2) a cyst with fluid in motion (see Figures 12-4, 12-6, 12-9, 12-16 to 12-18, and 12-20).[7,28] The major cord abnormality, myelomalacia, is a nonspecific characterization because of the lack of detailed knowledge of the neuropathologic changes in such spinal cords (Figure 12-14; see Figures 12-5, 12-9, and 12-18). However, cord tissue associated with syrinx undergoes extensive gliosis, presumably on the basis of reaction to the stress of CSF and

*References 11, 12, 15, 27, 30, 31.

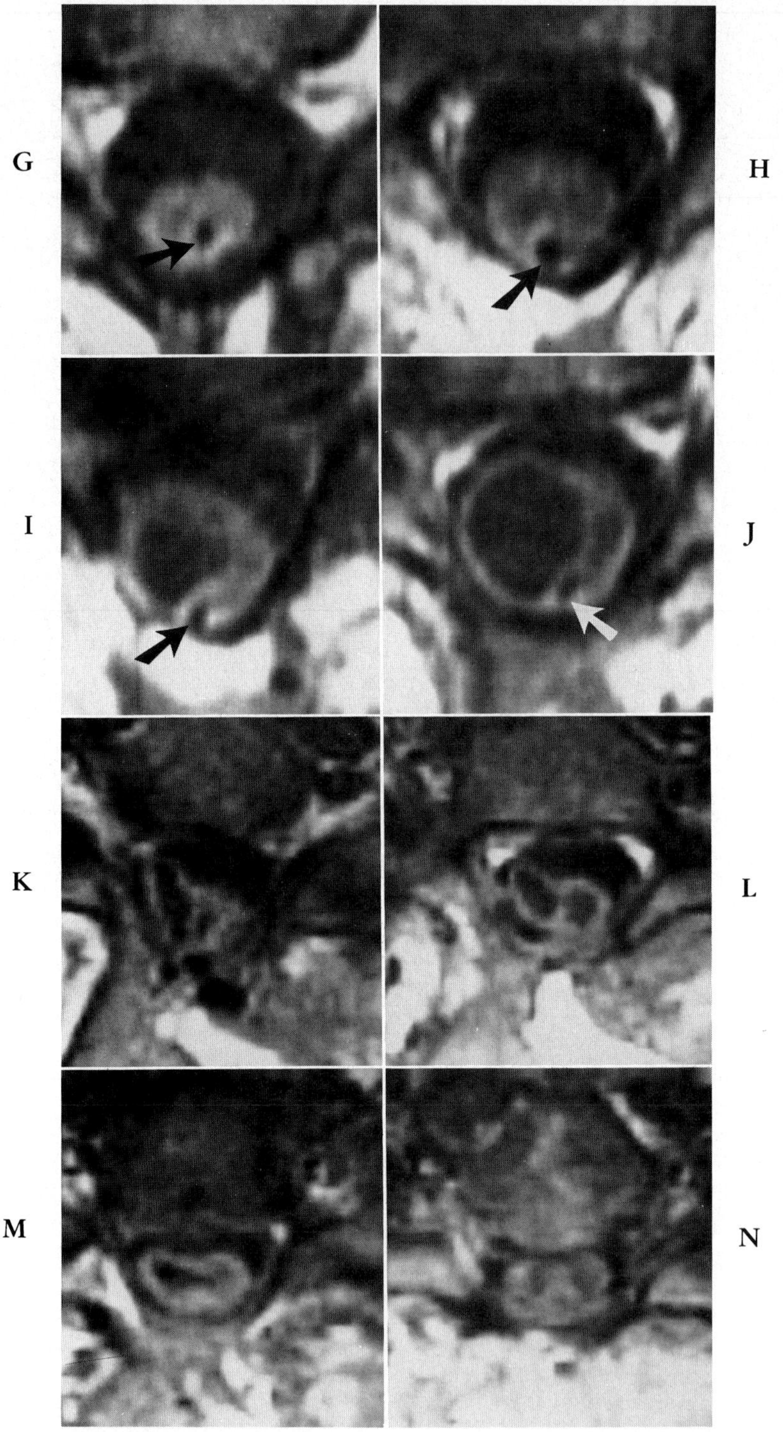

FIGURE 12-14, cont'd. G-J, Set of four axial T1W (SE 1000/20) scans show round area of low signal within posterior cord representing shunt tube *(arrows)*. It is evident that shunt tube does not communicate with enlarging cyst. There was no fluid motion within cyst. Revision of shunt produced subsequent partial collapse of cyst (**K-N**) as seen on set of four T1W images (SE 1000/20) obtained after shunt revision. (From Enzmann DR, O'Donohue J, Rubin JB, et al. With permission. AJNR 1987; 8:517.)

cyst fluid pulsation. T1W and T2W images are required to fully delineate the extent of cord damage, the syrinx size, and CSF-cyst fluid dynamics.

T1 Weighted Images

T1 weighted (T1W) scans are optimal for delineating cord size and cyst size. The extent of the syrinx can be determined on sagittal images, and axial images can confirm the presence of the cyst and also delineate the size of the cyst in relationship to the cord. The cyst may be asymmetrically dorsal in the cord. The axial scan is also useful for delineating multiple cysts, which can occur but usually cannot be differentiated on sagittal scans (see Figures 12-14 and 12-20). These multiple cysts have been documented with intraoperative ultrasound (see Figure 12-14).[30] The T1W image may show the cyst in an enlarged cord or it may demonstrate the cyst in an atrophic cord such as is often seen in the posttraumatic type of syrinx. The cyst and cord also appear atrophic after successful shunting (see Figures 12-18, 12-20, and 12-21).[3,4] With large syrinx cavities the cyst may have a "haustral" pattern representing fibroglial tracks within the cyst (see Figures 12-4 and 12-20). These septa may be within a single cyst or in separate, multiple cysts. It is important to recognize that some areas of low signal intensity on T1W images may not represent cystic fluid but myelomalacia, which can be the end stage of a previous cord infarction such as might occur in posttrauma patients. The first echo, the balanced image, (TE 20 to 30 msec) of a T2W sequence will help differentiate cyst from myelomalacia: cysts are of lower signal intensity than cord; myelomalacia is of higher signal intensity than cord.

T2 Weighted Images

T2 weighted (T2W) scans confirm morphologic features seen on the T1W scan but also provide further information about the cord and fluid dynamics. To maximize this type of information, the T2W image should be nonmotion-compensated and ungated in the axial view and performed with a thin slice technique to maximize the spin echo (SE) technique's sensitivity to CSF motion. The first echo (TE 20 to 30 sec) of a long TR, long TE sequence, can often help differentiate cyst from myelomalacia. This image is a balanced image because of the combined T1 and T2 weighting. On this image, cysts are low signal intensity because of their long T1, whereas myelomalacia is high signal intensity because of the relatively shorter T1 and breakthrough of the long T2 effect, which is similar to that seen with periventricular multiple sclerosis (MS) plaques and their detectability on the first and second echo images of a long TR, long TE sequence. On the axial T2W scan the cord around the cyst often shows abnormal high signal (myelomalacia) (see Figures 12-6, 12-9, 12-14, 12-17). Part of this signal may represent local edema (i.e., increased interstitial fluid), which is reversible with treatment. If it represents gliosis, it is not reversible with treatment. In cysts with fluid motion, the cord usually exhibits this abnormal signal at the level of the cyst and for short distances above and below the syrinx itself. The area of myelomalacia, however, may extend for some distance above and below the actual cyst. The cord may be of normal signal intensity at the level of the cyst (i.e., its walls) but this is usually only seen in cysts without significant fluid motion (see Figures 12-2 and 12-5).

If fluid within the cyst is relatively stationary, it will exhibit high signal intensity on the second echo (TE 80 msec) of a T2W sequence. The cyst will show a transition from low signal to high signal from the first to second echos of a long TR, long TE sequence for stationary fluid (Figure 12-15; see Figures 12-2, 12-3, and 12-5). If fluid within the cyst is in motion, it will show low signal intensity on the first and second echos of a long TR, long TE sequence (see Figures 12-4, 12-6, 12-9, 12-14, and 12-20).[7] Signal intensity will decrease from the first to the second echo. Signal loss is profound and caused by a combination of mismapping of the signal from moving CSF and intravoxel dephasing caused by turbulence[7] (see Chapter 1). The amount of motion that will cause this signal loss depends on the scanning technique used. The important parameters determining sensitivity to motion on axial imaging are: gradient strength (related to machine and field strength), slice thickness (gradient strength), and TE. The images presented in this chapter were obtained at 1.5T with 3 mm slices and a TE of 80 msec and show signal loss at pulsation amplitudes of as little as .5 mm.

A, B 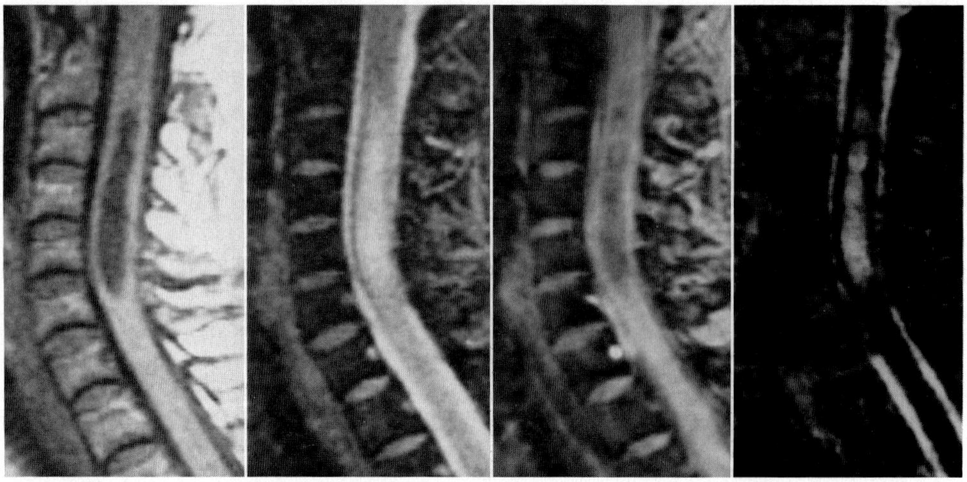 C, D

FIGURE 12-15. Sagittal and axial differential flip angle (DFA) imaging of Chiari I-associated syrinx in 51-year-old man—same patient as in Figure 12-5. **A,** T1W (SE 800/20) scan. Variable flip angle scans (GRASS) with **B,** flip angle of 6° and **C,** flip angle of 80°. **D,** Sagittal-DFA image. Morphology of cord cavity is well delineated on T1W image (**A**). Sagittal-DFA image (**D**), calculated from low and high flip angle GRASS images (**B** and **C**), qualitatively shows CSF motion within syrinx cavity and spinal subarachnoid space. Moving CSF depicted as high signal (i.e., white). CSF motion present in subarachnoid space ventral and dorsal to cord and within cyst (**D**). Syrinx fluid shows no significant motion with axial scans. Sagittal (**E**) and axial T1W scans (**F**) (SE 800/20) show morphology of cyst. Arrow denotes level of axial scan (**E**). Axial ungated T2W scan (SE 2000/20, 80) shows low signal on first echo (**G**) and high signal on second echo (**H**) in cyst. High signal on second echo means no significant motion (**H**). Quantitation of CSF motion accomplished using axial-DFA technique. Variable flip angle scans (GRASS) were obtained with flip angles of 10°, 20°, and 30° respectively (**I, J,** and **K**). Axial-DFA image calculated from images **I-K** reveals no significant through-plane motion within syrinx cavity (**K**), seen as low signal within cyst. In contrast, CSF within subarachnoid space has pulsation amplitude of 15 to 18 mm (*arrow*, **L**). Sagittal DFA technique extremely sensitive to CSF motion because it detects some motion whereas axial DFA technique shows this to be very low amplitude <.5 mm. DFA techniques are fully described in Chapter 1.

The areas of signal loss can be quite complex. In some portions of the cyst, CSF motion may exactly match the cyst size seen on the T1W axial image. In other areas the extent of signal loss on the nonmotion-compensated T2W scan may be smaller than the T1W image of the cyst because in some regions of the cyst, fluid adjacent to its walls may be relatively stationary and thus of higher signal (see Figures 12-4 and 12-9). This relative stationary fluid may be difficult to differentiate from adjacent myelomalacia cord on a second echo T2W image. In a large cyst the area of the signal loss caused by turbulence can be quite irregular and often does not match exactly the size of the cyst as seen on T1W images, especially at its rostral and caudal ends.

The term *relative stationary* is used because the SE pulse sequence with a 3 mm slice is sensitive to a certain magnitude of CSF pulsation. Quantitative studies show that signal loss can be seen with through-plane flow of as little as .5 mm,[23] suggesting a component of turbulence. With thicker slices, however, sensitivity to CSF motion is reduced. Therefore the technique used to study CSF motion is important in assessing a particular sequence's sensitivity to CSF motion. Some pulse sequences are extremely sensitive to CSF motion and could show CSF motion in all syrinxs. The previous discussion of relatively stationary fluid compared to mobile fluid refers to the categorization of signal loss as seen with an axial ungated scan, with TR 2000; TE 20 and 80, and a 3 mm slice thickness.

E, F G, H

I, J K, L

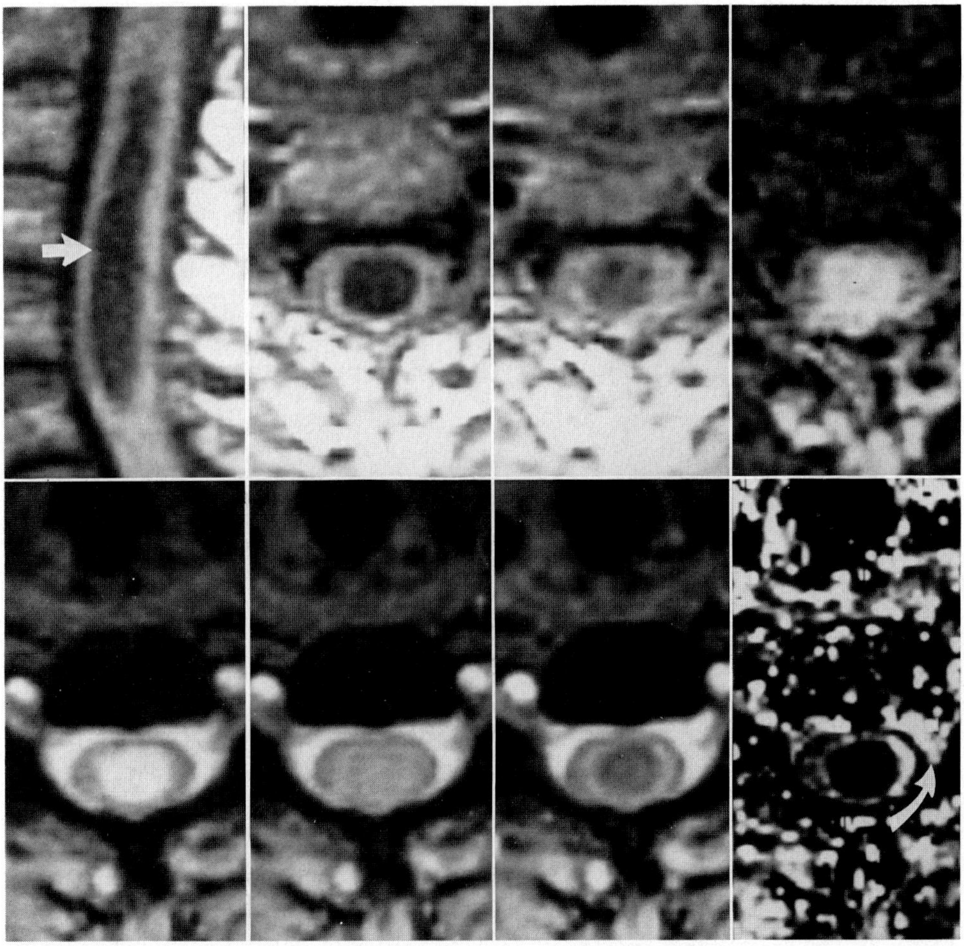

FIGURE 12-15, cont'd. For legend see previous page.

A, B C, D

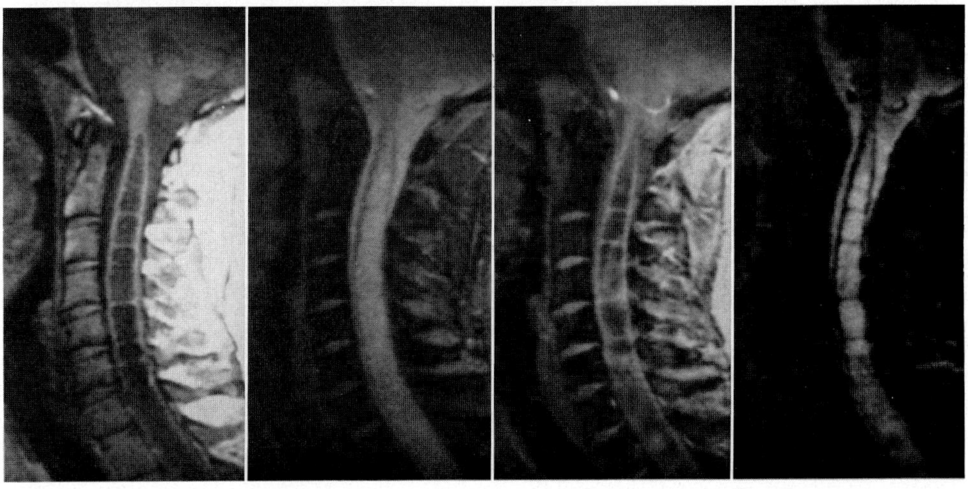

FIGURE 12-16. A-D, For legend see following page.

E

F, G

H, I

J, K

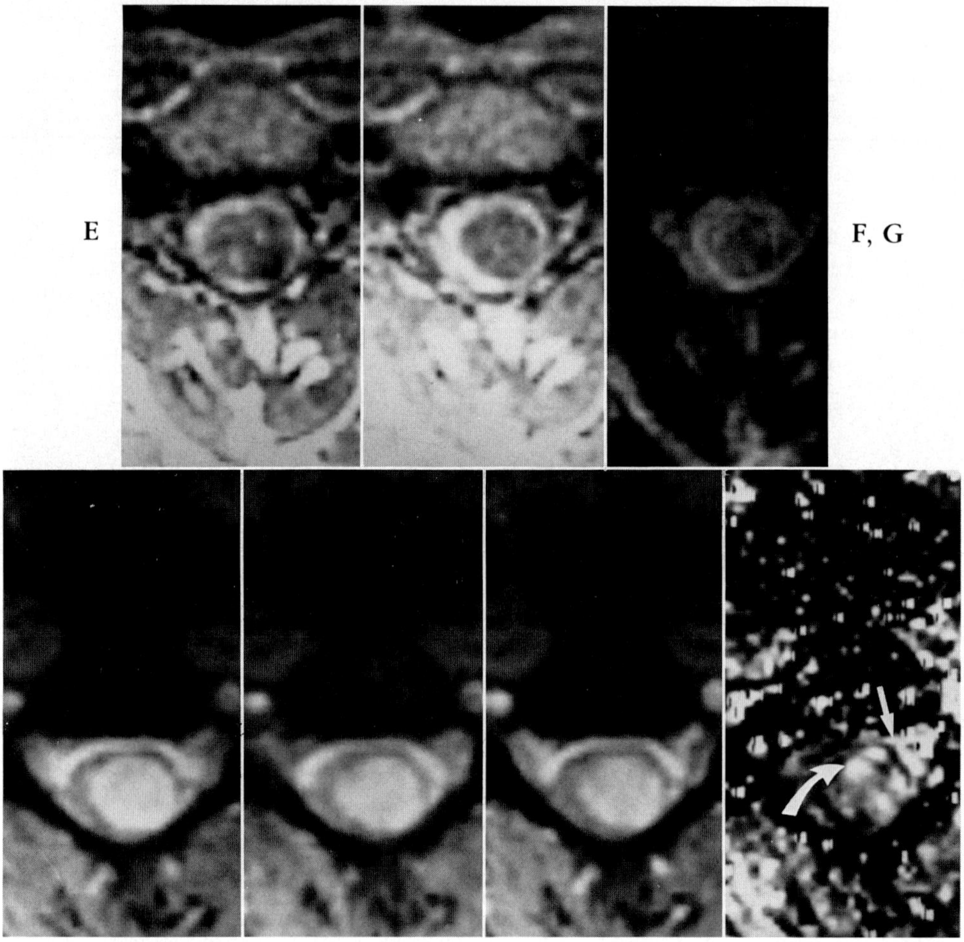

FIGURE 12-16. Qualitative and quantitative assessment of posttraumatic syrinx in 26-year old man. **A,** Sagittal T1W scan (SE 800/20); variable flip angle scans (GRASS) with **B,** flip angle of 6° and **C,** flip angle of 80°. Images **B** and **C** were used to calculate **D,** sagittal-DFA image. T1W scan shows large syrinx cavity with multiple internal septations in cervical spinal cord of same patient as in Figure 12-9. Sagittal-DFA image, calculated from low and high flip angle GRASS images, qualitatively shows CSF motion within entire syrinx cavity and within spinal subarachnoid space. Axial T1W scan (SE 800/20) shows cyst and septations (**E**). Axial ungated T2W scans (SE 2000/20, 80) show low signal intensity on both echoes (**F** and **G**) indicating fluid motion. Complex patterns of low signal intensity are present on T2W image (**G**) within syrinx cavity secondary to fluid motion. Low CSF signal intensity secondary to CSF motion also in subarachnoid space. Note high signal intensity of abnormal cord tissue. Quantitation of CSF motion was achieved using axial-DFA technique. Variable flip angle scans (GRASS) were obtained with flip angles of 10°, 20°, and 30° respectively (**H, I,** and **J**). Axial-DFA image (**K**) calculated from images (**H-J**). Axial-DFA image quantitated CSF motion within syrinx cavity and spinal subarachnoid space (**K**). Complex pattern of CSF motion within syrinx cavity is result of septations. CSF in central regions of cyst within subarachnoid space had pulsation amplitude ranging from 16 to 22 mm (*straight arrow,* **K**). Axial-DFA technique is fully described in Chapter 1.

Variable flip angle/gradient echo scans

Variable flip angle/gradient echo scans are a generic type of pulse sequence having complex interactions with pulsatile motion and flip angle (see Chapter 1) that can be used to advantage to detect fluid motion. Very low flip angles are insensitive to in-plane or through-plane flow whereas higher flip angles cause a change in signal intensity with changing fluid velocity.[23] When these images are processed and subtracted, a map of moving CSF can be generated (Figure 12-16; see Figure 12-15). In the sagittal plane (in-plane flow) this method is only qualitative but very sensitive to even minimal flow (<.5 mm) (see Figure 12-15). Moving CSF is displayed as high signal intensity. In the axial plane (through-plane flow) this dual flip angle (DFA) technique can be quantitative with signal intensity of CSF representing actual pulsation amplitude.[23] Higher amplitudes are seen as higher signal intensity (see Figure 12-16). Thus the fluid dynamics of a syrinx can be characterized accurately both qualitatively and quantitatively.

CYST FLUID MOTION

Only a limited amount of data is available to characterize fluid motion within a syrinx. Some syrinxes display unusual characteristics in their development. Cyst fluid may actually migrate within the cord without the fluid exhibiting detectable pulsation (Figure 12-17). Fluid motion clearly takes place in some cysts. The motion, however, appears complex in that it seems to have a more turbulent character than expected. Craniocaudad pulsation is the dominant pattern although it may not be uniform within the syrinx, especially those with septations. In Chiari I malformations there is no consistent evidence of transmitted pulsation through the obex through the central canal into the cyst (see Figure 12-21). The fluid at the rostral and caudal ends of a syrinx moves less than fluid in the middle of the cyst. The pulsation amplitude of syrinx fluid can vary greatly; from less than .5 mm to over 2 cm. CSF in the subarachnoid space seems to pulsate less than expected in some syrinx patients. This is especially true after the cyst is decompressed and the subarachnoid space is widened. How these fluid dynamics relate to the pathogenesis of syrinx remains unclear. Fluid motion seems to correlate best not with etiology of the syrinx but simply its size.[7] The larger the syrinx, the more likely it has fluid motion. Cause and effect have not been determined; it is simply a correlation.

SYRINX TREATMENT

A common, currently practiced method of treating syrinx is by means of a shunting procedure in which one end of the shunt is placed in the syrinx cavity and the other end is placed in the subarachnoid space or peritoneal cavity (Figures 12-18 and 12-19). The rationale for this type of treatment is empirical because such treatment usually halts progression of neurologic deterioration. Motor and sensory deficits usually remain stable, rarely the neurologic deficits are partially reversed. Pain, however, may be reduced. Despite the lack of knowledge about the pathophysiology of syrinx formation and its treatment, MR scans have confirmed the efficacy of this type of shunting procedure by demonstrating decreased cyst size.[4,7] The shunt itself is often detectable in the cord and in the syrinx cavity (see Figures 12-14 and 12-19). Recent results suggest other methods than direct cyst shunting may be beneficial. In patients with Chiari I malformation, for example, posterior fossa decompression with release of the cerebellar tonsils is enough to decompress the syrinx cyst and decrease its size (Figure 12-20). The mechanism of this cyst decompression is not understood.

T1W Images

T1W images show cyst and cord morphologic conditions to best advantage, and after successful shunting a decrease in cyst size and consequently also cord size. The shunt itself is often seen as a thin line of low signal intensity well demarcated from the cord and cyst (see Figures 12-14 and 12-19). If the shunt is placed within the cyst, the cyst will show a decrease in size. If the shunt is not within a cyst or adjacent to a multiloculated cyst, the cyst will remain enlarged (see Figures 12-14 and 12-19). The T1W image yields good information with regard to morphologic changes of the syrinx.

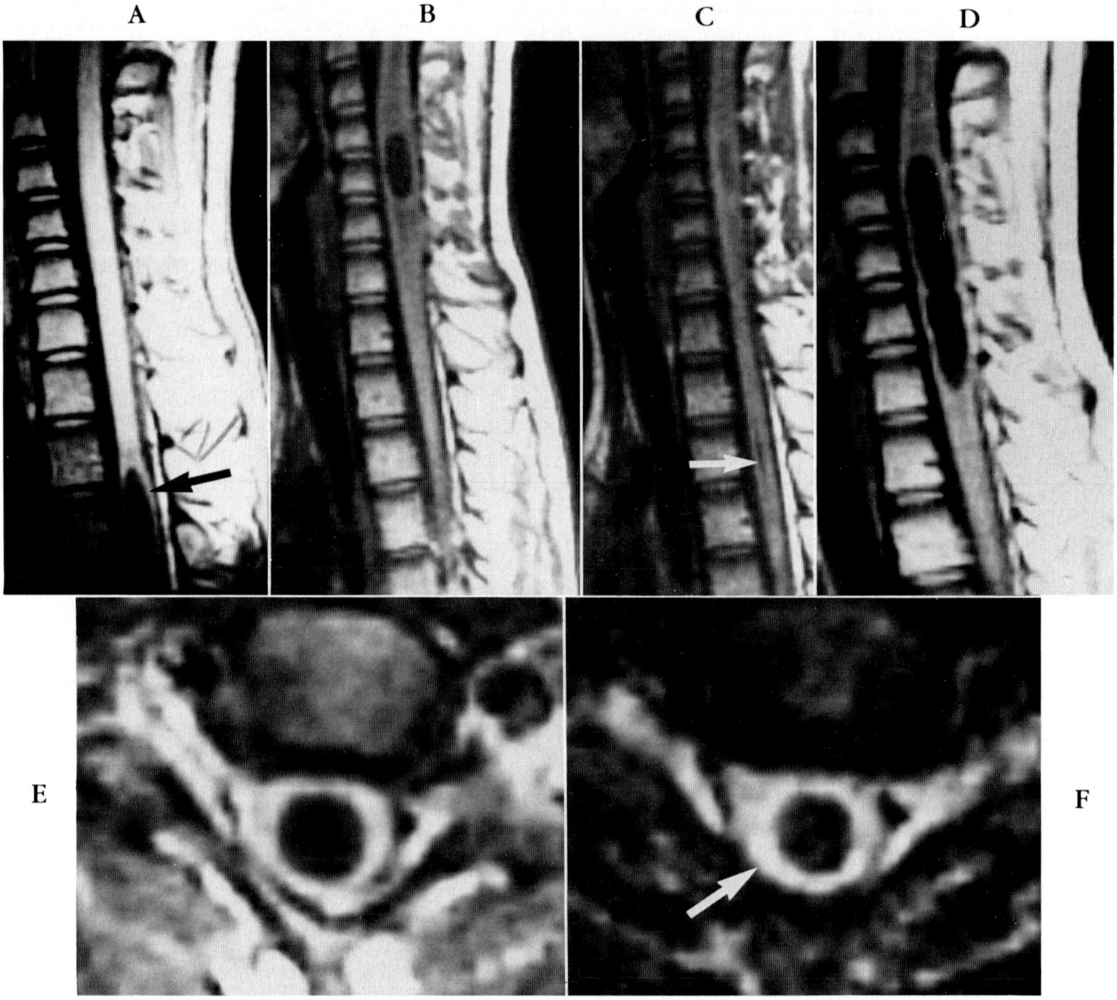

FIGURE 12-17. Series of sagittal T1W scans show unusual behavior of syrinx formation in 13-year-old female with etiology unidentified. **A,** Initial T1W scan (SE 1000/25) shows localized syrinx at T_2-T_4 level *(arrow)*. Fluid showed no evidence of motion at this time. **B,** Ten months later, sagittal T1W scans (SE 800/20) showed migration of cyst to C_4-C_5 level with collapse of cyst at T_2-T_4 level (*arrow,* **C**). At this time cyst fluid, although migrated, still did not show evidence of motion on ungated T2W scans. Sagittal T1W scan (SE 800/20) four months later shows **D,** increase in cyst size and **E,** development of fluid motion within it. Motion was documented on axial, ungated T2W scans (SE 2000/80) where signal void (**F**) was identified within cyst cavity conforming to cyst size seen on axial T1W scan (SE 1000/20) (**E**). Cord tissue around syrinx was also of abnormal high signal (*arrow,* **F**).

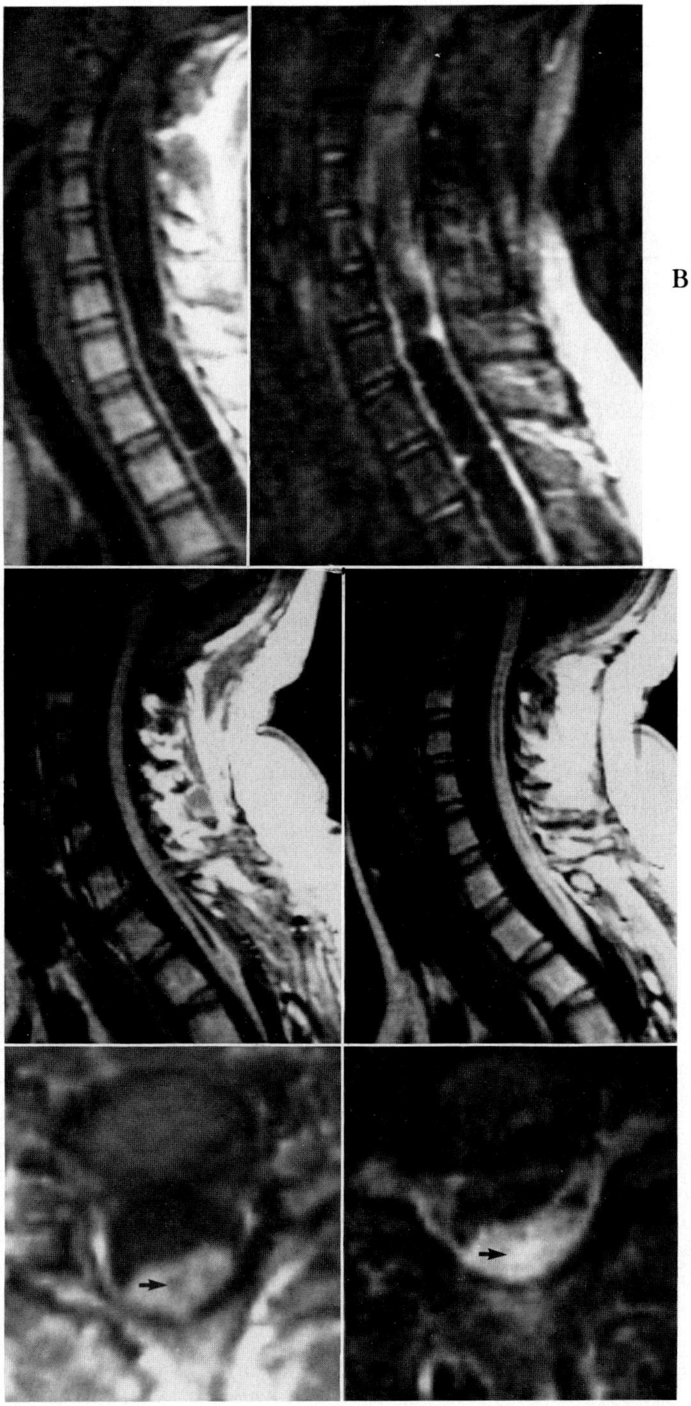

A B C D E F

FIGURE 12-18. **A,** 12-year-old patient with Chiari I malformation and syrinx involving cervical cord had minimal symptoms despite chronic nature of large syrinx in cervical canal (SE 400/20). **B,** Fluid in syrinx demonstrated significant motion seen by signal void within syrinx and phase shift artifact on ungated sagittal T2W scan (SE 2000/80). Ghost artifacts indicative of fluid motion are in anteroposterior phase-encoding direction. Patient underwent posterior fossa decompression and cyst shunting, which resulted in marked decrease of cyst size (**C** and **D**) as seen on T1W sagittal scan (SE 800/20). Axial T1W scan (SE 1000/20) in midcervical region shows small, residual center area of low signal representing collapsed cyst (*arrow*, **E**). Ungated axial T2W scan (SE 2000/80) shows prominent signal loss in anterior subarachnoid space indicating CSF motion, but high signal in central cyst indicates lack of fluid motion within collapsed syrinx (*arrow*, **F**).

A, B

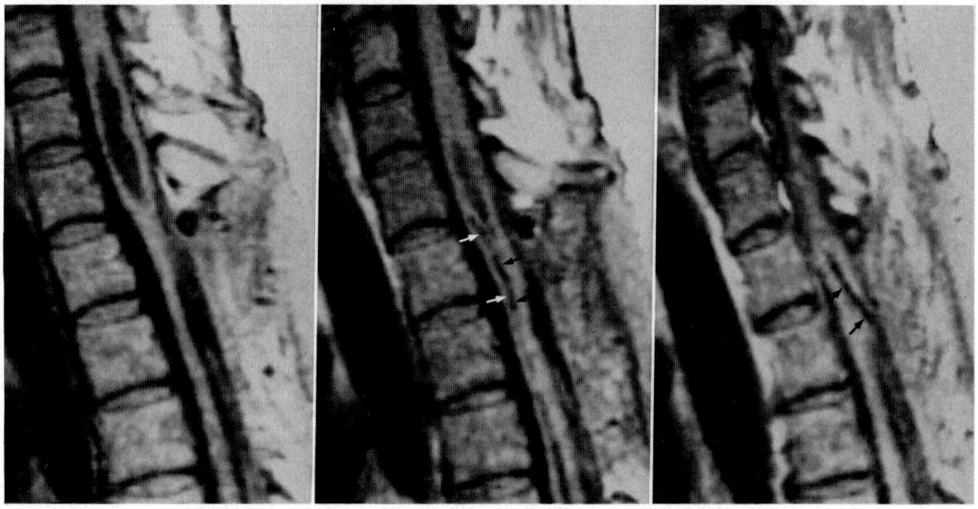

C

FIGURE 12-19. **A-C,** Sagittal T1W scans (SE 800/20) show failure of shunt tubing (*arrows,* **B** and **C**) to reach and decompress upper portion of syrinx. Syringosubarachnoid shunt is seen as linear low signal intensity (*arrows,* **B** and **C**).

A

B

C

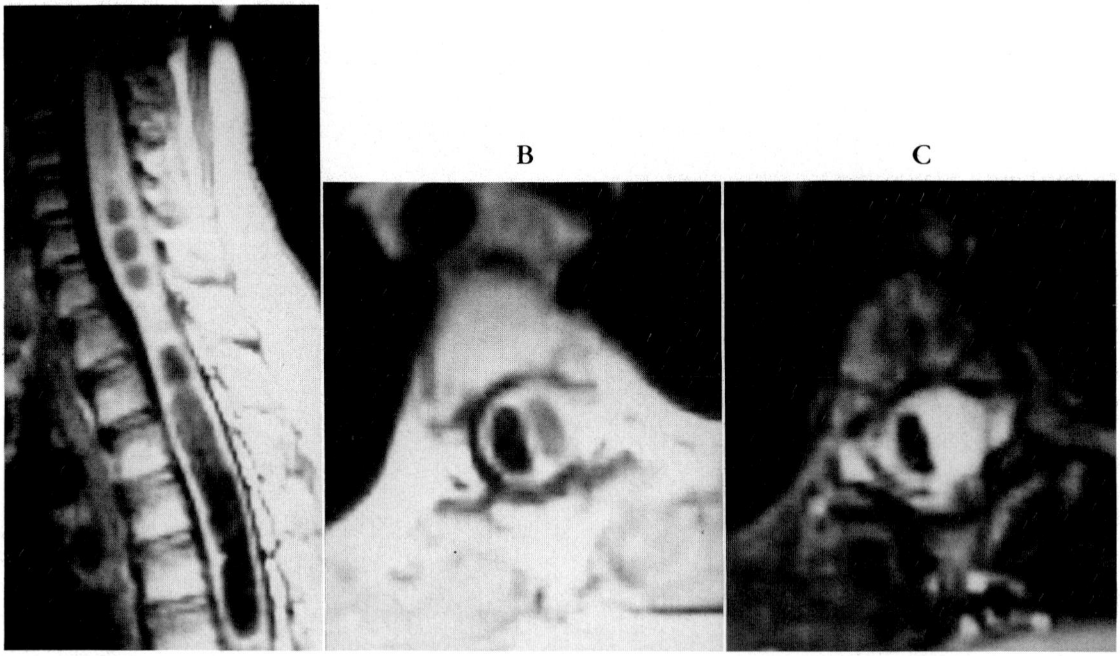

FIGURE 12-20. Two-year-old female with cervical and thoracic syrinx secondary to Chiari I malformation. **A,** Preoperative T1W scan (SE 800/20) shows large syrinx involving lower cervical and upper thoracic spinal cord. **B,** Axial T1W scan (SE 1000/20) demonstrates two cysts of different signal intensity: right cyst of lower signal intensity has fluid motion; left cyst with relatively higher signal intensity does not. **C,** Axial T2W scan (SE ungated 2000/80) shows pair of cystic cavities with left cyst exhibiting bright signal indicating stationary fluid and right cyst showing signal void indicating moving fluid. Patient did not undergo direct shunting of cyst; rather only posterior fossa decompression was performed.

D

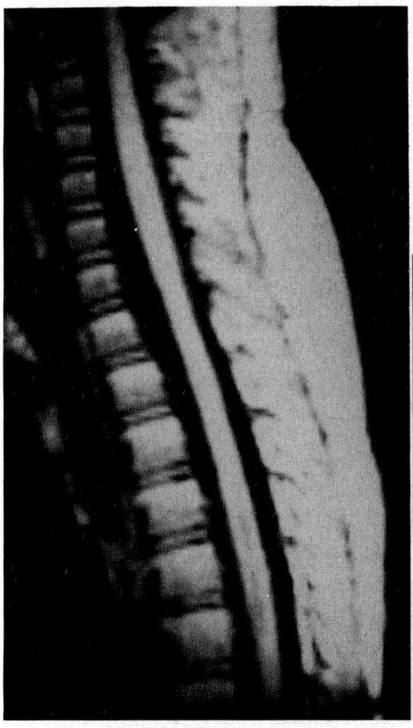

E F

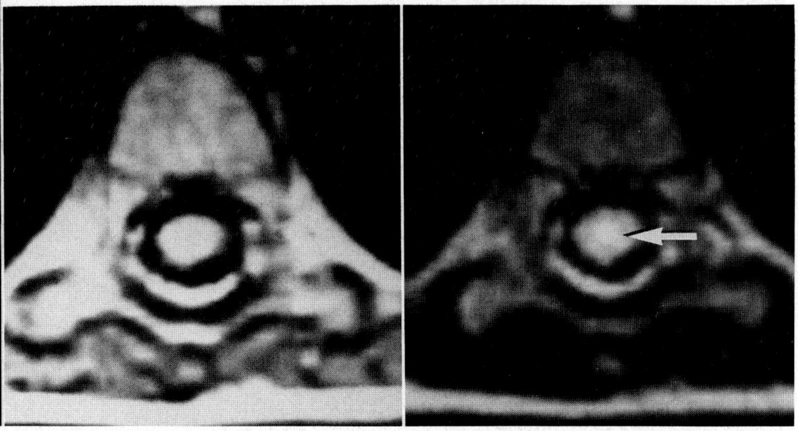

FIGURE 12-20, cont'd. **D,** Postsurgical T1W sagittal scan (SE 800/20) shows complete collapse of syrinx. Postoperative axial T2W scans (SE ungated 2000/20, 80) show no residual low signal cyst on **E,** first echo and only small central area of high signal indicative of residual myelomalacia on second echo (**F,** *arrow*). Peripheral portion of cord shows normal signal intensity. Cyst decompression was achieved with posterior fossa decompressive operation and no direct intervention of cyst itself.

T2W Images

The T2W scan provides more information with regard to pathophysiology than the T1W scan. It confirms the decrease in size of the cyst. On axial imaging, the presence or absence of a signal void within the cyst cavity indicates presence or absence of fluid motion. In a successfully shunted syrinx, not only does cyst size decrease but CSF motion decreases or ceases (see Figures 12-18 and 12-20). The signal voids compared to pretreatment scans become smaller or disappear entirely.[7] The axial T2W scan also provides the best information with regard to abnormal cord signal representing myelomalacia, which is usually unchanged after shunting although it may decrease somewhat at the extreme caudal or rostral end of a syrinx. Specialized techniques such as DFA can be used to quantitatively measure changes in fluid motion (see previous discussion on cyst fluid motion.)

Syrinx Recurrence

Clinical symptoms of a syrinx can recur when either one of the major MR findings, increased size or increased fluid motion, reappears. As expected when a syrinx recurs, its size increases (Figure 12-21). This is well seen on a T1W sagittal scan where the size of the syrinx increases compared to the immediate posttreatment scan. Axial scans may show that the shunt catheter in the cord, well seen on high resolution axial T1W images (see Figure 12-14), does not extend into the cyst that has increased in size (see Figures 12-14 and 12-21). The T2W scan confirms the increase in cyst size and often shows recurrence of fluid pulsation as well. A more subtle form of recurrence, however, is seen in which only fluid motion in the cyst recurs without a significant change in cyst size. Only T2W images or other motion sensitive sequences can detect this form of syrinx recurrence. This may represent the

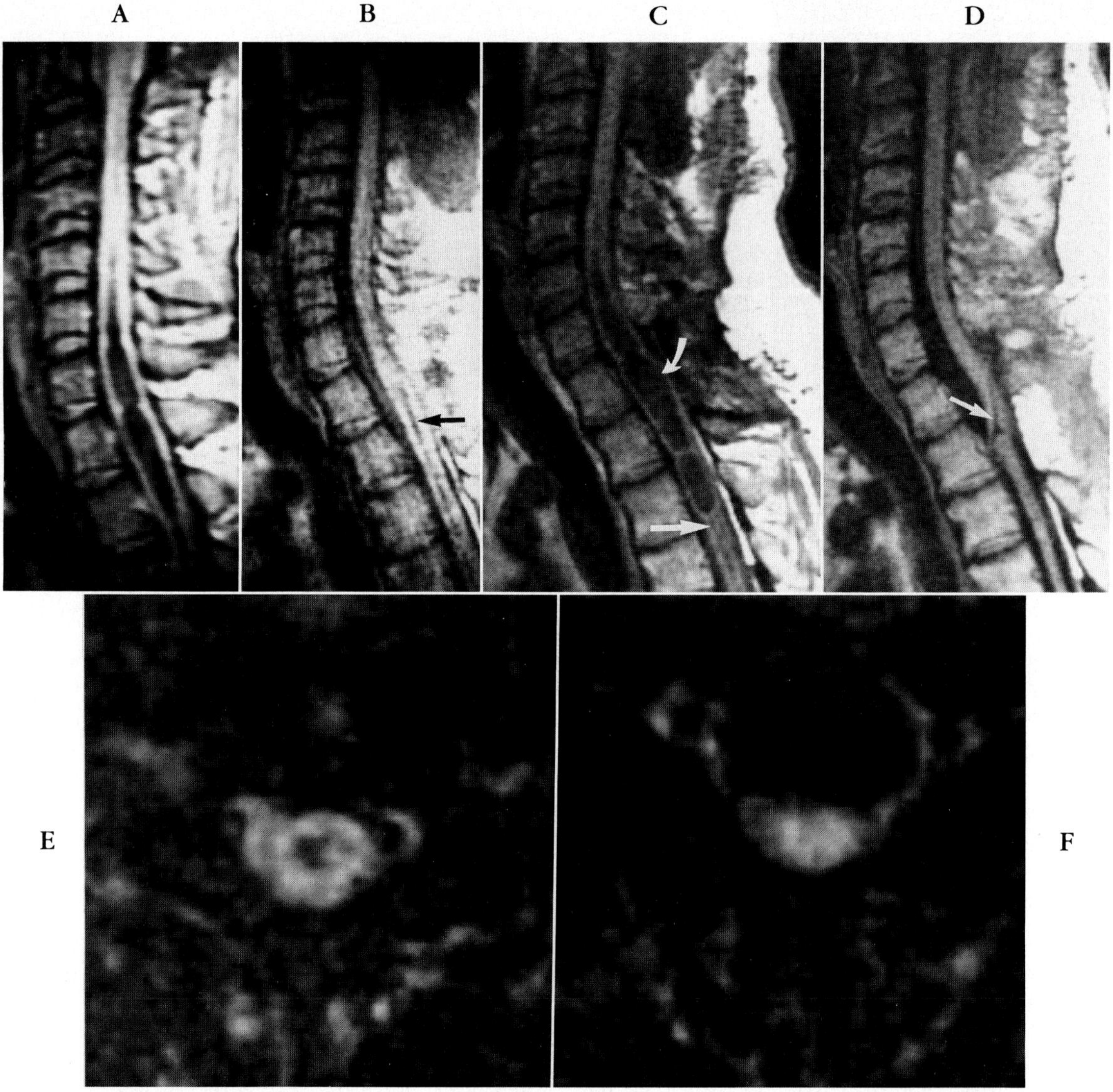

FIGURE 12-21. Series of sagittal scans show **A**, initial syrinx responding to **B**, shunting by decreasing in size with subsequent recurrence of syrinx shown as **C**, increased cyst size and **D**, repeated successful shunting. Initial scan (SE 2000/35) shows syrinx at cervical thoracic junction with pulsatile fluid (i.e., low signal). T1W scan (SE 800/20) shortly after surgery shows collapse of syrinx by placement of syringosubarachnoid shunt (*arrow*, **B**). Six months later patient had recurrent symptoms, and T1W scan (SE 800/20) showed recurrent cyst (*curved arrow*, **C**) rostral to shunt tube (*straight arrow*, **C**). Shunt (*arrow*, **D**) was revised causing complete collapse of cyst. Axial T2W scans (SE 2000/80) at time of second recurrence (**C**) showed fluid motion (i.e., signal loss) in middle of syrinx (**E**) but not at rostral end (**F**).

earliest stage of recurrence, with cyst enlargement to follow shortly thereafter. The signal character of the cord itself usually does not change with the recurrence of the cystic cavity.

As previously mentioned, in post traumatic patients or patients with severe arachnoiditis the presence of subarachnoid cyst could explain the lack of response to syrinx decompression.[1] These cysts can enlarge as the syrinx decreases in size.[1] The diagnosis of subarachnoid cyst has pitfalls (see Figure 12-11). For a subarachnoid cyst to be symptomatic it must be unequivocally a cyst that causes a mass effect on the adjacent cord (see Figures 12-10 and 12-13).

SYRINX VS. TUMOR

An isolated, non-neoplastic cyst must be distinguished from an extramedullary tumor with a cyst and from an intramedullary tumor with a cyst. The first is a true syrinx, the second is also, the last is not. The latter may be a cyst within a tumor or a cyst associated with hemangioblastoma. Syrinx formation may take place when an intradural-extramedullary tumor is present or it may appear after its removal. After it has been removed, syrinx formation is presumably related to abnormal CSF dynamics caused by adhesions formed after surgery.

Cysts associated with cord tumors, gliomas, ependymomas, and hemangioblastomas have some differentiating features from non-neoplastic syrinx. The diagnosis of tumor cyst is usually not difficult because with cord tumors an area of cord enlargement that is not caused by the cyst can be identified, confirming the presence of tumor (Figure 12-22). Noncystic cord enlargement is a key to the correct diagnosis. Tumor cysts, however, can become quite large. Despite their possible large size, tumor cysts do not show fluid motion as would a comparably sized syrinx (see Figure 12-22). Therefore on T1W and T2W images, signal intensity of the cystic fluid is higher compared to what it would be in a cyst

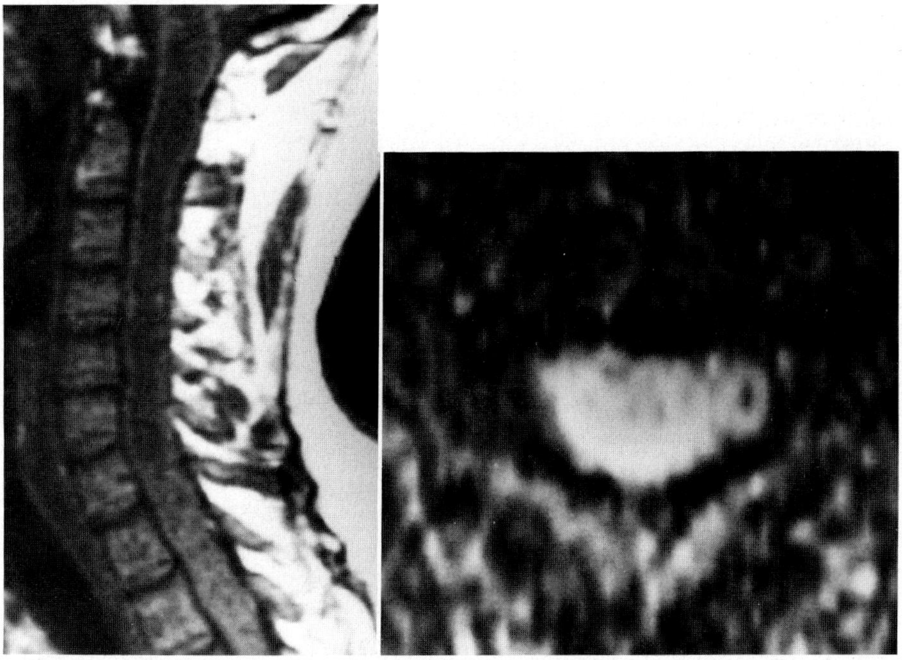

FIGURE 12-22. Sagittal T1W scan (SE 600/25) of cervical cord ependymoma shows large cyst in upper cervical cord extending into medulla. Note cord enlargement below cyst at levels C_1-T_2 indicating cyst is associated with intramedullary tumor. Axial ungated T2W scan (3 mm slice) (SE 2000/80) shows high signal intensity of cyst fluid indicating lack of fluid motion, a characteristic of cyst associated with intramedullary neoplasm. (From Enzmann DR, O'Donohue J, Rubin JB, et al. AJNR 1987;8:517.)

with fluid motion. Fluid motion is easily determined with ungated axial T2W scans. Tumor cysts characteristically show a homogeneous high signal within the cyst (see Figure 12-22). No signal voids are noted. Although there may be a small amount of motion caused by transmission of CSF pulsations through the cyst wall, it is minimal and not detected by this conventional SE technique.

There is more subtle differentiation at the level of the cyst on an axial T2W image. In a tumor cyst, cord tissue around the cyst is often near normal, intermediate signal intensity and can be differentiated from high signal of the cyst within it and from high signal CSF around it. The CSF around the cord is often high signal because cord enlargement has sufficiently damped CSF pulsation, virtually eliminating normal CSF pulsation (i.e., flow voids) in the subarachnoid space. As previously mentioned, in syrinxes the cord around the cyst is usually high signal intensity because of myelomalacia, making it difficult to differentiate from surrounding static CSF. Therefore the inability to differentiate cord tissue from adjacent CSF or cyst fluid indicates the possibility of a syrinx. Remember that small syrinxes may not show fluid motion. Therefore, the absence of fluid motion is not as diagnostic as the presence of fluid pulsation, which is virtually pathognemonic of nonneoplastic syrinx.[7]

Finally, probably the easiest method to make the tumor-syrinx differentiation is the use of a contrast agent such as GdDTPA. No contrast accumulates in the cord in syrinx and no areas of T1 shortening are detected.[29] Tumors such as astrocytomas, ependymomas, and hemangioblastomas (especially the latter two) are likely to show prominent contrast enhancement; hence bright signal on T1W images (see Chapter 8). With some astrocytomas, contrast enhancement may be more subtle. Although not yet reported, there will no doubt be astrocytomas that will have an intact blood-brain barrier and not show contrast enhancement with GdDTPA. This would be unusual and when it happens the above enumerated criteria for noncontrast scans can be invoked.

REFERENCES

1. Andrews BT, Weinstein PH, Rosenblum ML, et al. Intradural arachnoid cysts of the spinal canal associated with intramedullary cysts. J Neurosurg 1988;68:544.
2. Aubin ML, Vignaud J, Jardin C, et al. Computed tomography in 75 clinical cases of syringomyelia. AJNR 1981;2:199.
3. Barbaro NM, Wilson CB, Gutin PH, et al. Surgical treatment of syringomyelia, favorable results with syringoperitoneal shunting. J Neurosurg 1984;61:531.
4. Barkovich AJ, Sherman JL, Citrin CM, et al. MR of postoperative syringomyelia. AJNR 1987;8:319.
5. Barnett HJM, Jousse AT. Nature, prognosis and management of post-traumatic syringo-myelia. In: Barnett HJM, Foster JB, Hudgson P, eds. Major problems in neurology, syringomyelia. I. London: W. B. Saunders Co. 1973.
6. Bonafe A, Manelfe C, Espagno J, et al. Evaluation of syringomyelia with metrizamide computed tomographic myelography. 1980;4:797.
7. Enzmann DR, O'Donohue J, Rubin JB, et al. CSF pulsations within nonneoplastic spinal cord cysts. AJNR 1987;8:517.
8. Foster NL, Wing SD, Bray PF. Metrizamide ventriculography in syringomyelia. Neurology 1980;30:1323.
9. Gebarski SS, Maynard FW, Gabrielsen TO, et al. Posttraumatic progressive myelopathy. Clinical and radiologic correlation employing MR imaging, delayed CT metrizamide myelography, and intraoperative sonography. Radiology 1985;157:379.
10. Kan S, Fox AJ, Vinuela F. Delayed metrizamide CT enhancement of syringomyelia: postoperative observations. AJNR 1985;6:613.
11. Kokmen E, Marsh WR, Baker HL. Magnetic resonance imaging in syringomyelia. Neurosurgery 1985;17:267.
12. Lee BCP, Zimmerman RD, Manning JJ, et al. MR imaging of syringomyelia and hydromyelia. AJNR 1985; 6:221.
13. Mark AS, Andrews BT, Hodes J, et al. MRI of syringomyelia secondary to arachnoid adhesions. (Submitted for publication.)
14. Post MJD, Quencer RM, Green BA, et al. Radiologic evaluation of spinal cord fissures. AJNR 1986;7:329.
15. Pojunas K, Williams AL, Daniels DL, et al. Syringomyelia and hydromyelia: magnetic resonance evaluation. Radiology 1984;153:679.
16. Quencer RM, El Gammal T, Cohen G. Syringomyelia associated with intradural extramedullary masses of the spinal canal. AJNR 1986;7:143.
17. Quencer RM, Green BA, Eismont FJ. Posttraumatic spinal cord cysts: clinical features and characterization with metrizamide computed tomography. Radiology 1983;146:415.
18. Quencer RM, Sheldon JJ, Post MJD, et al. Magnetic resonance imaging of the chronically injured cervical spinal cord. AJNR 1986;7:457.
19. Resjo IM, Harwood-Nash DC, Fitz CR, et al. Computed tomographic metrizamide myelography in syringohydromyelia. Radiology 1979;131:405.
20. Rhyner PA, Hudgins RJ, Edwards MSB, et al. Magnetic resonance imaging of syringomyelia associated with an extramedullary spinal cord tumor: case report. Neurosurgery 1987;21:233.

21. Rossier AB, Foo D, Naheedy MH, et al. Radiography of posttraumatic syringomyelia. AJNR 1983;4:637.
22. Rossier AB, Foo D, Shillito J, et al. Progressive late post-traumatic syringomyelia. Paraplegia 1981;19:96.
23. Rubin JB. Differential flip angle CSF flow imaging. Part I, Theoretical basis and clinical implementation. (Submitted for publication.)
24. Samuelsson L, Bergstrom K, Thomas K-A, et al. MR imaging of syringohydromyelia and Chiari malformations in myelomeningocele patients with scoliosis. AJNR 1987;8:539.
25. Scher AT. Syringomyelia secondary to paraplegia due to fractures of the thoracic spine. S Afr Med J 1976; 21:1406.
26. Seibert CE, Dreisbach JN, Swanson WB, et al. Progressive posttraumatic cystic myelopathy: neuroradiologic evaluation. AJNR 1981;2:115.
27. Sherman JL, Barkovich AJ, Citrin CM. The MR appearance of syringomyelia: new observations. AJNR 1986;7:985.
28. Sherman JL, Citrin CM, Gangarosa RE, et al. MR appearance of CSF pulsations in the spinal canal. AJNR 1986;7:879.
29. Slasky BS, Bydder GM, Niendorf HP, et al. MR imaging with Gadolinium-DTPA in the differentiation of tumor, syrinx, and cyst of the spinal cord. J Comput Assis Tomogr 1987;11:845.
30. Wilberger JE, Maroon JC, Prostko ER, et al. Magnetic resonance imaging and intraoperative neurosonography in syringomyelia. Neurosurgery 1987;20:599.
31. Yeates A, Brant-Zawadzki M, Norman D, et al. Nuclear magnetic resonance imaging of syringomyelia. AJNR 1983;4:234.
32. Yu YL, Moseley IF. Syringomyelia and cervical spondylosis: a clinicoradiological investigation. Neuroradiology 1987;29:143.

Index

A

D

E

P